Atlas of General Surgery

Third Edition

Atlas of General Surgery

Third Edition

Selected from
Operative Surgery
Fifth Edition

Compiled by

Sir David Carter MD, FRCS(Ed), FRCS(Glas)
Regius Professor of Clinical Surgery, Royal Infirmary,
Edinburgh, UK

R. C. G. Russell MS, FRCS
Consultant Surgeon, The Middlesex Hospital, London, UK

Henry A. Pitt MD
Professor and Vice Chairman, Department of Surgery,
The Johns Hopkins Hospital, Baltimore, Maryland, USA

Consulting Editor

Hugh Dudley ChM, FRCS(Ed), FRACS, FRCS
Formerly Professor of Surgery, St Mary's Hospital, London, UK

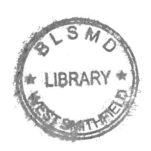

 CHAPMAN & HALL MEDICAL
London · Weinheim · New York · Tokyo · Melbourne · Madras

A. Cuschieri MD, MCh, FRCS, FRCS(Ed)
Department of Surgery, University of Dundee, Ninewells Hospital and Medical School, Dundee DD1 9SY, UK

J. A. DeWeese MD
Professor of Surgery and Chief Emeritus of Cardiothoracic and Vascular Surgery, University of Rochester Medical Center, 601 Elmwood Avenue, Rochester, New York 14642-8410, USA

H. T. Debas MD
M. Galante Distinguished Professor of Surgery and Dean of the School of Medicine, University of California, 513 Parnassus Avenue, S-320 San Francisco, California 94143-0104, USA

E. Deslandres MD
Assistant Professor, Department of Medicine, University of Montréal, Division of Gastroenterology, Hôtel-Dieu de Montréal, 3840 Rue St Urban, Montréal, Québec, Canada H2W 1T8

P. G. Devitt MS, FRCS, FRACS
Senior Lecturer, Department of Surgery, Royal Adelaide Hospital, Adelaide, South Australia 5000, Australia

H. B. Devlin MA, MD, MCh, FRCS, FRCSI
Consultant Surgeon, North Tees General Hospital, Stockton-on-Tees, Cleveland TS19 8PE and Lecturer in Clinical Surgery, University of Newcastle upon Tyne, UK

A. Duranceau MD
Professor of Surgery, University of Montréal, Division of Thoracic Surgery, Hôtel-Dieu de Montréal, 3840 Rue St Urban, Montréal, Québec, Canada H2W 1T8

G. R. Ekelund MD, PhD
Associate Professor and Chairman, Department of Surgery, Malmö General Hospital, University of Lund, S-21401 Malmö, Sweden

V. W. Fazio FRACS, FACS
Chiarman, Department of Colorectal Surgery, Cleveland Clinic Foundation, 9500 Euclid Avenue, Cleveland, Ohio 44106, USA

L. P Fielding MB, FRCS, FACS
Chief of Surgery, St Mary's Hospital, Waterbury, Connecticut 06706, USA

P. Frileux MD
Professor of Surgery, Hôpital Laennec, 42 rue de Sevres, F-75007 Paris, France

O. J. Garden BSc, MD, FRCS(Ed), FRCS(Glas)
Senior Lecturer and Honorary Consultant Hepatobiliary Surgeon, University Department of Surgery and Scottish Liver Transplantation Unit, Royal Infirmary, Edinburgh EH3 9YW, UK

H. S. Goh BSc, FRCS
Goh Hak-Su Colon and Rectal Centre, Suite 04-08 Gleneagles Medical Centre, 6 Napier Road, Singapore 258499

D. Gough FRCS, FRCS(Ed), FRACS, DCH
Consultant Paediatric Surgeon, Department of Surgery, Royal Manchester Children's Hospital, Pendlebury, Salford, UK

R. H. Grace FRCS
Consultant Surgeon, The Royal Hospital, Cleveland Road, Wolverhampton, West Midlands WV2 1BT, UK

J. L. Grosfeld MD
Surgeon-in-Chief, James Whitcomb Riley Hospital for Children, 702 Barnhill Drive, Indianapolis, Indiana 46202-5200, USA

J. D. Hardcastle MA, MChir, FRCS, FRCP
Professor of Surgery, University Hospital, Nottingham NG7 2U, UK

P. L. Harris MD, FRCS
Consultant Vascular Surgeon, Royal Liverpool University Hospital, Liverpool L7 8XP, UK

P. R. Hawley MS, FRCS
Senior Consultant Surgeon, St Mark's Hospital for Diseases of the Rectum and Colon and Consultant Surgeon, King Edward VII Hospital, London, UK

R. J. Heald MA, MChir, FRCS, FRCS(Ed)
Consultant Surgeon, Colorectal Research Unit, Basingstoke District Hospital, Basingstoke, Hampshire RE24 9NA, UK

G. Hellers MD, PhD
Chairman, Department of Surgery, Huddinge University Hospital, S-14186 Huddinge, Sweden

J. T. Hobbs MD, FRCS
Honorary Senior Lecturer in Surgery, University of London, London, UK

P. Hornick FRCS
Department of Cardiothoracic Surgery, Harefield Hospital, Middlesex, UK

T. T. Irvin PhD, ChM, FRCS(Ed)
Consultant Surgeon, Department of Surgery, Royal Devon and Exeter Hospital, Exeter, Devon EX2 5DW, UK

M. H. Irving MD, ChM, FRCS
Professor of Surgery, University Department of Surgery, Hope Hospital, Salford M6 8HD, Lancashire, UK

C. W. Jamieson MS, FRCS
Consultant Surgeon, St Thomas' Hospital, London SE1 7UT, UK

G. G. Jamieson MS, FRACS, FACS
Dorothy Mortlock Professor of Surgery, Department of Surgery, The University of Adelaide, Royal Adelaide Hospital, Adelaide, South Australia 5000

H. Jiborn MD, PhD
Associate Professor, Department of Surgery, Malmö General Hospital, University of Lund, S-214 01 Malmö, Sweden

G. W. Johnston MCh, FRCS
Honorary Professor, Queen's University Belfast and Consultant Surgeon, Royal Victoria Hospital, Belfast, UK

M. Killingback FRCS, FRCS(Ed), FRACS
Sydney Adventist Hospital, Sydney, NSW, Australia

J. E. J. Krige FRCS, FCS(SA)
Associate Professor, Department of Surgery, University of Cape Town, Observatory 7925, Cape Town, South Africa

Z. H. Krukowski PhD, FRCS(Ed)
Consultant Surgeon, Aberdeen Royal Infirmary, Foresterhill, Aberdeen AB9 2ZB, UK

B. Launois MD, FACS
Professor, Digestive and Transplantation Surgery, Hôpital de Pontchaillou, Rue Henri Le Guilloux, 3500 Rennes, France

H. W. C. Loose FRCR
Consultant Radiologist, Freeman Hospital, Newcastle-upon-Tyne NE7 7DN, UK

P. H. Lord OBE, MChir, FRCS
Formerly Consultant Surgeon, Wycombe General Hospital, High Wycombe, Buckinghamshire HP11 2TT, UK

J. S. P. Lumley MS, FRCS
Professor in Vascular Surgery, St Bartholomew's Hospital, London EC1A 7BE, UK

N. Madden MA, FRCS
Consultant Paediatric Surgeon, Westminster Children's Hospital, London SW1, UK

G. Maddern PhD, MS, FRACS
Jepson Professor of Surgery, Department of Surgery, University of Adelaide, The Queen Elizabeth Hospital, Woodville, South Australia 5011

M. A. Malias MD
Resident Surgeon, Department of Surgery, University of Louisville School of Medicine, Louisville, Kentucky 40292, USA

C. V. Mann MA, MCh, FRCS
Consulting Surgeon, The Royal London Hospital and St Mark's Hospital for Diseases of the Rectum and Colon, London, UK

A. Mannell FRACS, FRCS, MS
Specialist Surgeon, The Rosebank Clinic, and Consultant Surgeon, Baragwanath Hospital, University of the Witwatersrand, Johannesburg, South Africa

A. O. Mansfield ChM, FRCS
Consultant Vascular Surgeon, St Mary's Hospital, London W2 1NY, UK

M. Marberger MD
Professor and Chairman, Department of Urology, University of Vienna, Alser Strasse 4, A-1090 Vienna, Austria

C. J. Martin FRACS
Professor of Surgery, University of Sydney and Head of Surgical Division, Nepean Hospital, PO Box 63, Penrith, NSW 2751, Australia

R. B. Mateo MD
Assistant Instructor in Medicine, Brown University School of Medicine, Providence, Rhode Island 02907, USA

N. A. Matheson ChM, FRCS, FRCS(Ed)
Consultant Surgeon, Aberdeen Royal Infirmary, Foresterhill, Aberdeen AB9 2ZB, UK

T. Mätzsch MD, PhD
Associate Professor, Department of Surgery, Lund University, Malmö General Hospital, S-214 01 Malmö, Sweden

J. E. Meilahn MD
Assistant Professor of Surgery, Department of Surgery, Temple University School of Medicine, Philadelphia, Pennsylvania 19140, USA

W. S. Moore MD
Professor of Surgery and Chief, Section of Vascular Surgery, UCLA School of Medicine, Los Angeles, California 90024, USA

M. W. Mulholland MD
Associate Professor of Surgery, University of Michigan, 2920 Taubman Health Center, 1500 E Medical Center Drive, Ann Arbor, Michigan 48109-0331, USA

S. J. Mulvihill MD
Associate Professor of Surgery, Department of Surgery, University of California, 533 Parnassus Avenue, California 94143-0788, USA

J. J. Murray MD
Staff Surgeon, Department of Colon and Rectal Surgery, Lahey Clinic Medical Center, Burlington, Massachusetts 01805, USA

A. Nakeeb MD
Surgical Resident, Department of Surgery, The Johns Hopkins Medical Institutions, Blalock 688, 600 N Wolfe Street, Baltimore, Maryland 21287-4688, USA

G. L. Newstead FRACS, FRCS, FACS
Associate Director, Division of Surgery, Prince of Wales and Prince Henry Hospitals, Randwick, NSW 2301, Australia

M. J. Notaras FRCS, FRCS(Ed), FACS
Consultant Surgeon, 11 Harmont House, 20 Harley Street, London W1N 1AA, UK

S. O'Dwyer MD, FRCS
Consultant Surgeon, The General and Queen Elizabeth Hospitals, Birmingham B4 6NH, UK

J. R. Oakley MD, FRACS
Staff Surgeon and Head, Section of Enterostomal Therapy, Department of Colorectal Surgery, Cleveland Clinic Foundation, 9500 Euclid Avenue, Cleveland, Ohio 44106, USA

K. R. Palmer MD, FRCP(Ed)
Consultant Physician, Western General Hospital, Edinburgh EH4, UK

S. Paterson-Brown MS, MPhil, FRCS(Ed), FRCS
Consultant Surgeon, University Department of Surgery, Royal Infirmary, Edinburgh EH3 9YW, UK

R. K. S. Phillips MS, FRCS
Consultant Surgeon, St Mark's Hospital for Diseases of the Rectum and Colon, London EC1V 2PS, UK

H. A. Pitt MD
Professor and Vice Chairman, Department of Surgery, The Johns Hopkins Medical Institutions, Blalock 688, 600 N Wolfe Street, Baltimore, Maryland 21287-4688, USA

H. C. Polk MD
Senior Professor and Chairman, Department of Surgery, University of Louisville School of Medicine, Louisville, Kentucky 40292, USA

J. P. Pryor MS, FRCS
Consultant Uroandrologist, King's College and St Peter's Hospital at the Middlesex Hospital, London, UK

S. C. Rakić MD, PhD, FACS
Department of Surgery, Leyenburg Hospital, Postbus 40551, The Hague 2504 LN, The Netherlands

J. J. Ricotta MD
Professor of Surgery and Director, Division of Vascular Surgery, State University of New York at Buffalo, 3 Gates Circle, Buffalo, New York 14209, USA

W. P. Ritchie Jr MD, PhD
Professor and Chairman, Department of Surgery, Temple University School of Medicine, Philadelphia, Pennsylvania 19140, USA

A. W. Robbins MD
Surgical Director, The Hernia Center, 222 Schanck Road, Suite 100, Freehold, New Jersey 07728-2974, USA

D. A. Rothenberger MD
Clinical Professor of Surgery and Chief, Division of Colon and Rectal Surgery, University of Minnesota Medical School, St Paul, Minnesota 55102, USA

C. V. Ruckley MB, ChM, FRCS(Ed), FRCPE
Consultant Surgeon, Vascular Surgery Unit, Royal Infirmary, Edinburgh EH3 9YW, UK

R. C. G. Russell MS, FRCS
Consultant Surgeon, The Middlesex Hospital, London W1N 8AA, UK

I. M. Rutkow MD, MPH, DrPH
Surgical Director, The Hernia Center, 222 Schanck Road, Suite 100, Freehold, New Jersey 07728-2974, USA

J. M. Sackier FRCS
Associate Professor of Surgery, University of California, San Diego, California 92103, USA

J. H. Scurr BSc, FRCS
Consultant Surgeon, Department of Surgical Studies, The Middlesex Hospital, London W1N 8AA, UK

A. E. Siperstein MD
Department of Surgery, Mount Zion Medical Center of University of California, San Francisco, California 94143-1610, USA

J. Terblanche ChM, FRCS, FCS(SA)
Professor and Head, Department of Surgery and Co-Director, ILRC Liver Research Unit, University of Cape Town, Observatory 7925, Cape Town, South Africa

J. P. S. Thomson DM, MS, FRCS
Consultant Surgeon and Clinical Director, St Mark's Hospital for Intestinal and Colorectal Disorders, Northwick Park, Harrow, Middlesex HA1 3UJ, UK

R. Udelsman MD, FACS
Associate Professor and Director of Endocrine and Oncologic Surgery, The Johns Hopkins Hospital, Blalock 688, 600 N Wolfe Street, Baltimore, Maryland 21287-5674, USA

M. C. Veidenheimer MD
Vice-Chairman, Department of Surgery, HCI International Medical Centre, Clydebank G81 4HX, UK

A. Watson MD, FRCS, FRCS(Ed), FRACS
Consultant Surgeon, The Wellington Hospital, London NW8 9LE, UK

S. D. Wexner MD, FACS, FASCRS, FACG
Director of Anorectal Physiology Laboratory, Cleveland Clinic, Fort Lauderdale, Florida 33309, USA

H. N. Whitfield MA, MChir, FRCS
Consultant Urologist, St Bartholomew's Hospital and St Mark's Hospital for Diseases of the Colon and Rectum, London, UK

C. B. Williams FRCP
London Clinic Endoscopy, The Clinic, 20 Devonshire Place, London W1N 2DH, UK

K. A. Zucker MD, FACS
Professor of Surgery, University of New Mexico School of Medicine, Albuquerque, New Mexico 87131, USA

Contributing Medical Artists

Antoine Barnaud
11 Rue Jacques Dulud,
92200 Neuilly Sur Seine, France

Andrew Bezear
6 Queen Street, Godalming,
Surrey GU7 1BD, UK

Diane Bruyninckx MMAA, AIMI
20 Van Halmaelelei,
B-2930 Brasschaat, Belgium

Joanna Cameron BA(Hons), MMAA
11 Pine Trees, Portsmouth Road,
Esher, Surrey KT10 9JF, UK

Angela Christie MMAA
14 West End Avenue, Pinner,
Middlesex HA5 1BJ , UK

Peter Cox RDD, MMAA, AIMI
Canon Frome Court,
Canon Frome, Ledbury,
Herefordshire HR8 2TD, UK

Susan Darrington
P.O. Box 581, Subiaco,
Western Australia 6008

Marc Donon
45 Avenue Felix, Faure,
75015 Paris, France

Patrick Elliott BA(Hons), ATC, MMAA, AIMI
46 Stone Delf,
Sheffield S10 3QX, UK

Raymond Evans BA(Hons), MMAA
Unit of Art in Medicine,
Department of Cell and Structural Biology,
University of Manchester, Manchester M13 9PT, UK

Jenny Halstead MMAA
The Red House, 85 Christchurch Road,
Reading, Berkshire RG2 7BD, UK

Mark Iley BA(Hons)
12 High Street, Great Missenden,
Buckinghamshire HP16 9AB, UK

Diane Kinton BA(Hons)
Gillian Lee Illustrations,
15 Little Plucketts Way, Buckhurst Hill,
Essex IG9 5QU, UK

The late Robert Lane MMAA
Studio 19A, Edith Grove,
London SW10, UK

Gillian Lee FMAA, HonFIMI, AMI, RMIP
Gillian Lee Illustrations,
15 Little Plucketts Way, Buckhurst Hill,
Essex IG9 5QU, UK

Marks Creative Consultants
4 Harrison's Rise, Croydon,
Surrey CR0 4LA, UK

Richard Neave FMAA, AIMI
Unit of Art in Medicine,
Department of Cell and Structural Biology,
University of Manchester, Manchester M13 9PT, UK

Gillian Oliver MMAA, AIMI
15 Bramble Road, Hatfield,
Hertfordshire AL10 9RZ, UK

Paul Richardson BA(Hons)
54 Wellington Road,
Orpington, Kent BR5 4AQ, UK

Denise Smith BA(Hons), MMAA
Unit of Art in Medicine,
Department of Cell and Structural Biology,
University of Manchester, Manchester M13 9PT, UK

Philip Wilson FMAA, AIMI
23 Normanshurst Road, St Paul's Cray,
Orpington, Kent BR5 3AL, UK

Contents

Preface

Rob and Smith's *Operative Surgery* has been a landmark in the presentation of surgical technique, combining succinct description with appropriate illustrations. The multi volume work was conceived in the 1940s by Professor Charles Rob (then of St Mary's Hospital, London) and Mr Rodney Smith (now Lord Smith of Marlow). That it was a timely and appropriate venture is clear from the fact that a second edition was required by 1968 and a third in 1977–80. A fourth edition was prepared during the 1980s and now, in the mid 1990s, the present editors are half way through a revision of the whole series.

The very wide span of the work has entailed a volume for every subspeciality of surgery, with the result that what is considered by the trainee to be general surgery may be found scattered amongst many volumes. In order to help the trainee to encompass common surgical procedures easily, a selection from the fourth edition was made and published as the *Atlas of General Surgery*.

This new edition of the *Atlas of General Surgery* is a selection from the fifth edition. Material has been completely revised and a new selection of chapters made. In order to compress the operations from multiple volumes into one volume difficult choices have had to be made. The choice has been guided by the requirement of the surgical trainee during his general professional training and will be of value to the general surgeon during his early years of specialist training. The editors hope that this edition will whet the appetite of the reader to look at alternative procedures described in the main volumes and to use those volumes when he or she is a specialist trainee.

D. C. Carter
R. C. G. Russell
H. A. Pitt

Minor operations: excision and skin closure, small flaps, small grafts

Bernard W. Chang MD
Assistant Professor, Division of Plastic and Reconstructive Surgery, Johns Hopkins University School of Medicine, Baltimore, Maryland, USA

History

The origins of wound closure date back to ancient history. Some of the earliest recorded attempts at wound closure are alluded to in the Edwin Smith Surgical Papyrus from Egypt in the 17th century BC[1]. In this treatise, suturing technique was described such that 'Thou shouldst draw together for him his gash with stitching'. The concept of flaps of tissue was first described in ancient India (600BC) for nasal reconstruction after nasal amputation which was used as a form of punishment[2]. Celcus (25BC) later described the use of advancement flaps for reconstructing defects. Skin grafting was not described until the early 1800s by Baronio of Italy in his publication *Degli Innesti Animali* (On Grafting in Animals), and the first recorded successful human skin graft was performed by Sir Astley Cooper in 1817[2].

Principles

Surgical excision and proper skin closure are fundamental skills necessary for any operation. Wounds that are created by trauma or by surgical intervention require meticulous attention to achieve a good result, and closure of these wounds has many basic principles in common. Clean wound margins must be obtained with removal of all devitalized tissue. This goal can be accomplished by gentle handling of tissue and by the use of sharp instruments for excision or debridement. Infection must be minimized by using sterile technique and appropriate timing of wound closure. Ischaemic conditions must be avoided at the wound edges to avoid poor wound healing. In addition, avoidance of dead space and adequate haemostasis are necessary to prevent late infectious complications. Finally, to ensure fine wound healing, tension should be minimized and careful tissue approximation must be obtained by layered closure and fine suture for the cutaneous closure.

When a large defect is present and primary closure is not feasible, tissue may be used from an adjacent area to reduce tension on the wound closure (local flap) or a skin graft may be used from a distant location. Advantages of local flap coverage include better colour match, texture and contour. Local flaps are designed so that the donor site may be closed primarily.

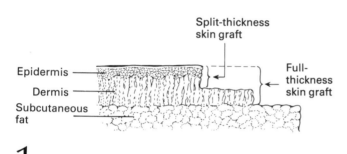

1

1 A skin graft may also be used, but involves harvesting skin from a distant site as a full-thickness (epidermis and dermis) or split-thickness (epidermis and partial dermis) graft. Full-thickness skin graft donor sites must be closed primarily and, thus, are limited in size. Split-thickness skin graft donor sites will re-epithelialize spontaneously and are therefore not limited in size. Full-thickness skin grafts and thick split-thickness skin grafts have less tendency to contract over time and have better contour and consistency than thinner grafts. The colour match and skin consistency with skin grafts are generally not as good as with a local flap. Skin grafts are used more commonly for large non-weight-bearing defects with well vascularized wound beds and no exposed vital structures.

Delayed primary closure is indicated in wounds that are highly contaminated, wounds with extensive injury or an uncertain zone of injury, and after tumour excision with unclear margins. Many of these wounds require serial debridement before closure. In some cases wounds may be left to heal by secondary intention.

Preoperative

Open wounds must be assessed for the level of contamination, severity of surrounding tissue injury and involvement of deeper anatomical structures. Contaminated wounds must be debrided thoroughly.

2 Minor degrees of contamination may be treated by irrigation with normal saline using a syringe with a 14 gauge needle. Moderate to heavy levels of contamination may be debrided sharply.

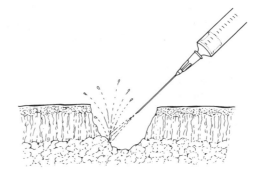

2

Injury to the surrounding tissue must be assessed with regard to mechanism of injury. High energy injuries such as gunshot wounds or motor vehicle injuries may involve a large surrounding zone of injury and may require serial debridements. Low energy injuries often may be closed primarily.

Wounds may also be created surgically by the excision of skin tumours or scar revision. It is important to plan the excision so that adequate margins are obtained. Primary closure may then be obtained if skin tension is not excessive. Skin tension is determined by the width of the wound and by the degree of laxity of the surrounding skin. Areas that require wider excision will require a skin graft or local flap. Preoperative assessment of colour match, durability and sensibility must be considered in choosing the type of coverage. In general, skin graft donor sites closer to the area of excision provide skin with a better colour match (that is, preauricular or postauricular skin grafts for facial lesions). Local flaps are often used as well and will provide coverage with better colour match and texture.

Preparation of the skin involves proper cleansing followed by application of an antiseptic solution such as a povidine-iodine solution. Sterile drapes are then placed around the operative site. It is important that the drapes are wide enough to include donor sites and to avoid the creation of an oxygen tent beneath the drapes. Preoperative intravenous antibiotics may also be given at this time.

Anaesthesia

In most cases local anaesthesia with 1% lignocaine (Xylocaine) and 1/100 000 adrenaline is sufficient for small wounds, although adrenaline is contraindicated for use in the digits as it may cause irreversible ischaemia. For prolonged anaesthesia, 0.25% or 0.50% bupivacaine (Marcain) may be used as well. A 27-gauge or 25-gauge needle may be used for infiltration.

3 Regional anaesthetic blocks are useful in many regions of the body. Digital blocks (using 1% plain lignocaine) are useful for surgery on the digits. Infiltration is performed in the web space on both sides of the affected digit at the level of the common digital nerve which is located just beneath the palmar fascia. Approximately 2–3 ml of the local anaesthetic are necessary to block each common digital nerve.

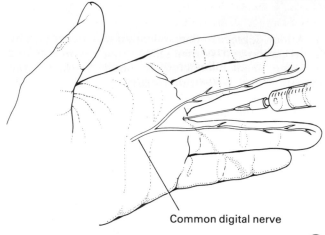

Common digital nerve

3

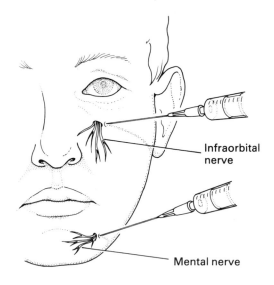

Infiltration nerve

Mental nerve

4

4 Regional nerve blocks may also be performed in the facial region. The three divisions of the trigeminal nerve may be blocked effectively to anaesthetize the upper, middle and lower thirds of the face (i.e. the supraorbital, infraorbital and mental nerves). These nerves may be blocked as they exit the facial skeleton at their respective foramina.

If larger areas require anaesthesia, general anaesthesia is preferable.

Operations

PRIMARY SKIN CLOSURE

5a–d For deeper wounds a layered skin closure is necessary. Deeper subcutaneous tissue (Scarpa's fascia) may be closed with a braided or monofilament absorbable suture. Cuticular closure may be accomplished in several ways. Buried intradermal sutures with inverted knots using an absorbable suture material may be followed by the application of sterile adhesive tapes (*Illustration 5b*), simple interrupted sutures using a non-absorbable monofilament (*Illustra-*tion 5c) or a simple running suture (*Illustration 5d*). It is important to include more tissue in the deeper portion of the suture so that the wound edges may be everted. The sutures should be spaced apart by approximately the same distance as the transverse suture length. Finer suture material is used in the facial region (5/0 or 6/0) than on the trunk or extremities (4/0 or 5/0).

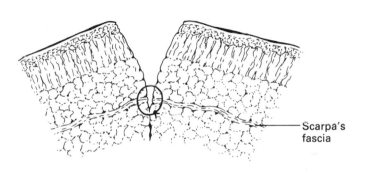

Scarpa's fascia

5a

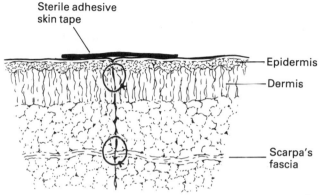

Sterile adhesive skin tape

Epidermis

Dermis

Scarpa's fascia

5b

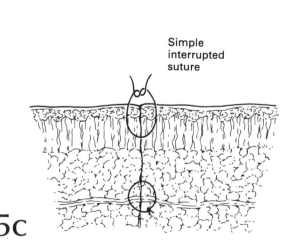

Simple interrupted suture

5c

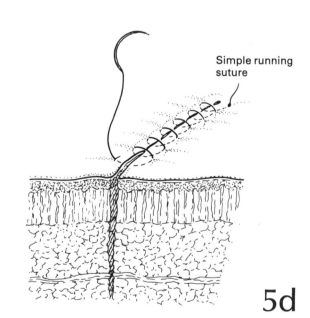

Simple running suture

5d

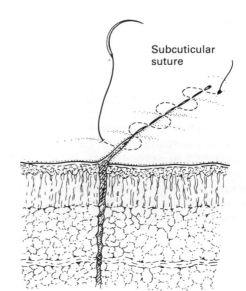

6a

6a–c Another method of cutaneous closure involves the use of a running subcuticular suture. Absorbable or non-absorbable suture material may be used. If a non-absorbable material is used the suture must be brought out through the skin every few centimetres to facilitate removal. The suture may be brought out through the skin surface at the ends of the incision or a buried knot may be placed. Other methods of skin closure include the horizontal mattress suture (*Illustration 6b*) and the vertical mattress suture (*Illustration 6c*).

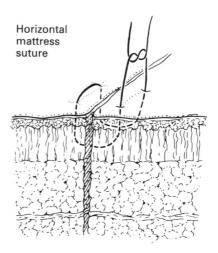

6b

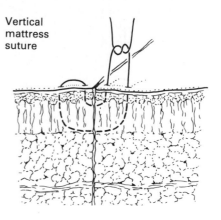

6c

SMALL GRAFTS

Split-thickness skin grafts

Split-thickness skin grafts are useful for covering defects that are too large to close primarily. The recipient site must be clean and well vascularized. The most common donor sites include the lower extremities and the gluteal region. The donor and recipient sites are prepared and drapes are placed so that both sites may be accessed. The donor site is cleansed with saline and mineral oil is applied lightly.

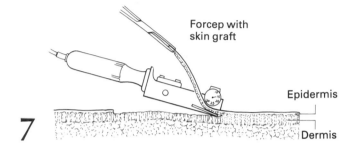

Forcep with
skin graft

Epidermis

Dermis

7

7 A powered dermatome is used for harvesting skin and is typically set to between 13/1000 and 18/1000 inch in thickness, depending on the thickness of skin graft desired.

The donor site is covered with either a fine mesh gauze or an occlusive non-permeable drape. The skin graft may be placed as a sheet graft with small holes cut for drainage ('pie crusted') or may be meshed with a meshing device that can adjust the amount of expansion of the skin graft (1.5 to 1, 3 to 1, etc.). The graft is fixed to the recipient bed with staples or a running suture.

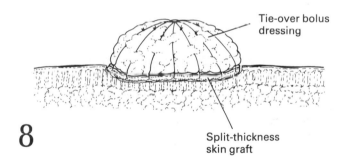

Tie-over bolus
dressing

Split-thickness
skin graft

8

8 In recipient areas where there is much motion, a tie-over bolus dressing may be applied to minimize shearing. A tie-over bolus dressing is created by placing circumferential 3/0 silk sutures and tying the sutures over a bolus of cotton balls soaked in mineral oil surrounded by fine mesh gauze. The tie-over bolus dressing is left intact for 3–5 days and then removed.

Full-thickness skin grafts

Full-thickness skin grafts include the epidermis and the entire dermis. Since no dermal elements are left, re-epithelialization occurs from the periphery of the defect if the wound is left open. The donor site is therefore usually closed primarily. The most common donor sites for full-thickness skin grafts include the groin and the preauricular and postauricular regions. The donor area is prepared as usual and marked in an elliptical pattern to encompass a portion of skin sufficient to cover the recipient site.

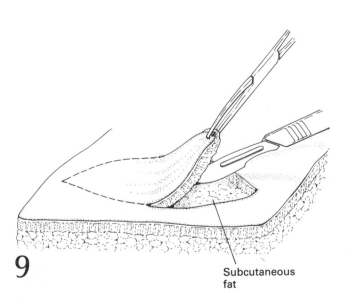

Subcutaneous
fat

9

9 The graft is harvested with a scalpel down to the level of the subcutaneous fat and the deep layer of the graft is trimmed with scissors to remove adherent fat.

The graft is then fixed to the recipient bed with a running suture and a tie-over bolus dressing is placed as previously described. The donor site is closed primarily.

SMALL FLAPS[3,4]

Various types of small local flaps may be used for closure of small cutaneous defects. These flaps all use adjacent tissue for closure of the wound with primary closure of the donor site. By using local flaps, tension may be distributed away from the primary defect facilitating closure of the wound.

Rotation flap

10 A hemi-ellipse is designed adjacent to the defect. The length of the ellipse should be at least twice the length of the base The flap is elevated in the subcutaneous plane and rotated to cover the defect. The distal tip of the flap is trimmed to fit the defect, and the donor site is closed primarily. Deep dermal absorbable sutures are used followed by fine non-absorbable sutures for the skin.

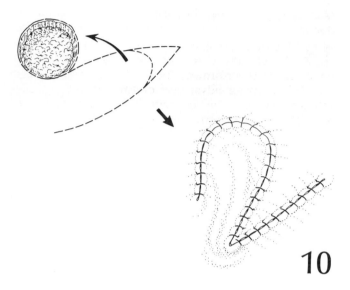

10

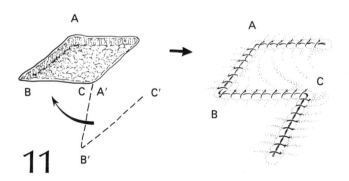

11

Rhomboid flap

11 The rhomboid flap is a variation of a rotation flap which enables the entire flap to be used for coverage with primary closure of the donor site. Irregular shaped defects may be converted to a rhomboid shaped defect. A straight line is drawn from the obtuse corner of the rhomboid and then angled to parallel the side of the rhomboid defect. The flap is elevated in the subcutaneous plane and rotated into the defect. The donor site is able to be closed primarily as the flap rotates into place.

Bilobed flap

12 A double rotation flap is utilized in this technique. Two lobes with a common base are designed adjacent to the defect. The first lobed flap is elevated in the subcutaneous plane and rotated into the primary defect. The second lobed flap is designed slightly smaller than the first lobe and rotated into the defect created by the first lobe. The defect from the second lobe is closed primarily.

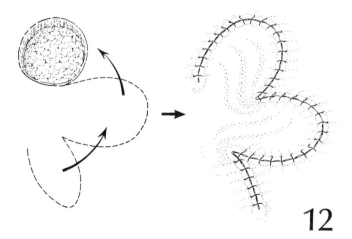

12

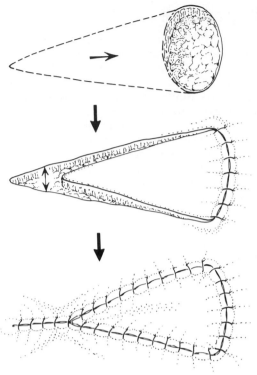

V–Y advancement flap

13 Incisions are made in a V pattern adjacent to the defect down to the subcutaneous fat. No undermining is performed. The flap is advanced towards the defect taking advantage of the mobility of the subcutaneous fat. The resultant donor deficit is closed primarily in a Y pattern.

13

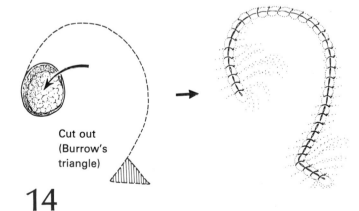

Cut out
(Burrow's
triangle)

14

Rotation advancement flap

14 A large semicircular incision is made adjacent to the defect and the flap is undermined in the subcutaneous layer. The flap is advanced and rotated, closing the defect Due to the elasticity of the skin, the tension of the closure is distributed along the entire length of the incision. A small triangle of tissue is often excised at the base of the flap to avoid redundancy (Burrow's triangle). The incisions are all closed primarily.

Postoperative care

A sterile gauze dressing is applied to the wound postoperatively. The patient may be allowed to get the suture line wet in 24–48 h. When external cutaneous sutures are present, they are removed as soon as possible to avoid suture marks in the skin. The amount of time the sutures are left in place varies with the region of the body due to differential healing. In the facial region, sutures are typically removed in 3–5 days. Elsewhere in the body, sutures are usually left in place for 7–10 days. Sterile tapes may be applied to the closure after suture removal.

Outcome

If proper surgical principles are adhered to, a closed healed wound will be the ultimate result. The incidence of wound infection or wound dehiscence should be minimal. Long-term sequelae including hypertrophic scarring or keloid formation are often dictated by the amount of tension, the location of the wound and the patient's wound healing physiology. Attempts to control the degree of scarring may be improved by further research in wound healing.

References

1. Jurkiewicz MJ, Krizek TJ, Mathes SJ, Ariyan S. *Plastic Surgery; Principles and Practice.* St Louis: CV Mosby, 1990.

2. Davis JS. *Plastic Surgery: Its Principle and Practices.* Philadelphia: Blakiston's Son and Co, 1919.

3. Smith JW, Aston SJ, eds. *Grabb and Smith's Plastic Surgery.* 4th edn. Boston: Little, Brown, 1991.

4. Georgiade NG, Georgiade GS, Riefkohl R, Barwick WJ. *Essentials of Plastic, Maxillofacial, and Reconstructive Surgery.* Baltimore: Williams and Wilkins, 1987.

Excision of skin cancers

Bernard W. Chang MD
Assistant Professor, Division of Plastic and Reconstructive Surgery, Johns Hopkins University School of Medicine, Baltimore, Maryland, USA

Skin cancers (non-melanoma) are one of the most common types of cancers in the world. Basal and squamous cell cancers comprise most of these skin cancers. In addition, many premalignant skin lesions exist, and other lesions can mimic skin cancers. In many cases visual inspection alone is not sufficient to make a diagnosis, and excisional biopsy of suspicious lesions is indicated. Early skin cancers, if left untreated, may continue to enlarge and become difficult to excise and close the defect primarily. Predisposing lesions for basal and squamous cell cancers include sebaceous naevus, actinic keratosis and porokeratosis. Malignant skin lesions include basal cell cancers, squamous cell cancers, Merkel cell cancers and dermatofibrosarcoma protuberans. Lesions that may mimic malignant lesions include trichoepitheliomas, desmoplastic trichoepitheliomas, eccrine epitheliomas and keratoacanthomas[1].

History

Skin tumours have been treated throughout the ages with various forms of ablative treatment including cautery, freezing, chemical application, radiation and surgical excision. Of these forms of treatment, surgical excision has been the mainstay of therapy. Historical observations of cutaneous malignancy date back to Hippocrates and his description of what appeared to be a cutaneous melanoma. In the early 1800s Marjolin noted the appearance of cancers in ulcerated wounds or in wounds that failed to heal. Shortly after the discovery of X-rays, many reports of radiation-induced neoplasia of the skin were reported[2].

Principles

For any suspicious skin lesion a biopsy is performed initially. Specimens of larger lesions may be taken by punch biopsy or incisional biopsy, while excisional biopsy may be performed for smaller lesions. Once the histopathology of the lesion is determined, the necessary margins for excision may be determined. In some cases, Moh's micrographic surgery (surgical excision performed with serial microscopic examination of margins) may be indicated (i.e. recurrent basal or squamous cell cancers, tumours with poorly defined borders and tumours adjacent to critical structures such as the eyelid, nose, etc.).

For small nodular basal cell carcinomas a 5-mm margin of excision is adequate. For larger basal cell carcinomas with infiltrative or morpheaform characteristics, a 10-mm or greater margin is necessary. Moh's micrographic surgery may be useful for these larger lesions[3].

For squamous cell cancers of the skin a 10-mm margin is adequate for tumours less than 10 mm in diameter, a 15-mm margin for tumours of 10–20 mm diameter and a 45-mm margin for tumours larger than 20 mm (95% cure rates)[3].

Preoperative assessment

Preoperative assessment consists of a careful history and physical examination. Important historical information includes duration of presence of the lesion, change in characteristics of the lesion (i.e. size, colour, shape, etc.) and prior history of skin cancers. Some syndromes may be associated with basal and squamous cell cancers such as the basal cell naevus syndrome, Basex syndrome and xeroderma pigmentosum.

Careful physical examination should include close examination of the margins of the lesion and proximity to local anatomical structures. Local lymph node drainage should also be examined. The lesion should be examined closely for irregularities in pigmentation, peripheral borders and contour.

Anaesthesia

For smaller lesions local anaesthesia alone or in conjunction with intravenous sedation may be used. Larger lesions, which may require a skin graft or local flap, may require general anaesthesia.

Operation[4]

Depending on the type of lesion present, the surgical margins of excision are carefully marked prior to infiltration of local anaesthesia. The margins are drawn uniformly around the periphery of the lesion and the incision is made through the entire thickness of the skin. The specimen is orientated and labelled with sutures before being sent for pathological examination. In some cases a frozen section may be obtained to check selected margins. If primary closure is deemed feasible, several considerations must be made in planning the skin closure including direction of least skin tension, natural skin lines and adjacent anatomical landmarks. Simple elliptical excision is used most commonly. Variations of elliptical excision may be used to hide scars in natural anatomical transition zones. Skin cancers that cannot be excised and closed primarily may be closed with the use of a split-thickness skin graft or a local flap.

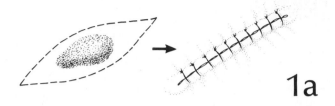

1a

Simple elliptical excision

1a,b An ellipse is drawn around the defect so that the length of the ellipse is approximately four times the width. The axis of the ellipse should be in parallel with natural skin lines. The incision is made down to the subcutaneous tissue. Slight undermining of the skin edges may be performed to facilitate closure which is performed in layers using fine suture technique.

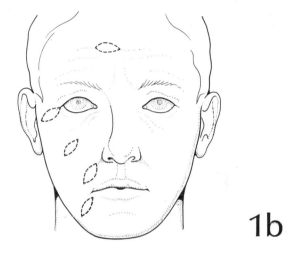

1b

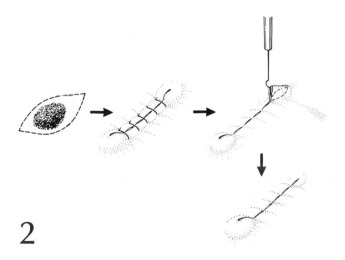

Removal of 'dog ears'

2 If an elliptical excision is performed with a shorter length to width ratio, excess skin may protude at the ends of the closure forming a 'dog ear'. This excess tissue may be excised by elevating the skin at the corner with a single hook and trimming the excess.

2

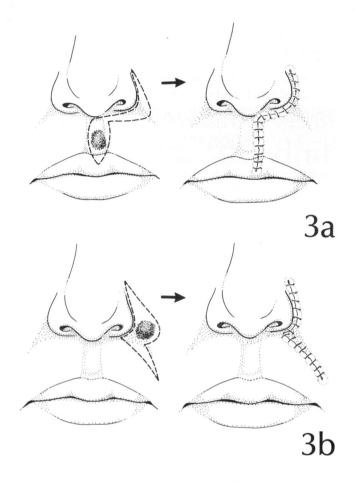

3a

3b

Discontinuous ellipse

3a,b If there are natural anatomical transition areas in the region of a planned excision for skin cancer, the ellipse may be made as a discontinuous ellipse to hide the scars. This technique is especially useful for lesions in the perioral and nasal regions.

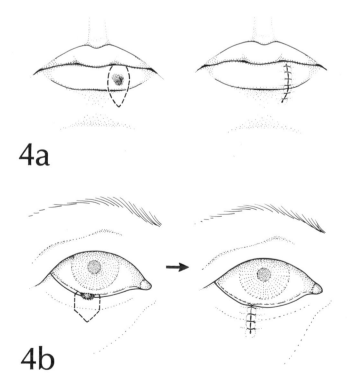

4a

4b

Hemi-elliptical excision

4a,b For lesions near the margin of the lip or eyelid a hemi-elliptical excision may be performed with primary closure. In the lips, careful anatomical alignment of the vermilion and white roll are of utmost importance. An absorbable fine suture material is used to approximate the muscle and a fine nylon suture is used to align the white roll and to close the skin. The mucosa is closed with gut suture.

In the eyelid the hemi-ellipse is modified into a pentagonal shape to prevent notching in the lid margin. A fine absorbable suture material is used to approximate the orbicularis muscle and the grey line and tarsus, as well as the skin.

Nasolabial flap

5   A nasolabial rotation flap may be based superiorly or inferiorly and may be used to close defects of the lateral portion of the nose and the upper and lower lips. The donor site is closed primarily in the natural skin lines of the nasolabial fold.

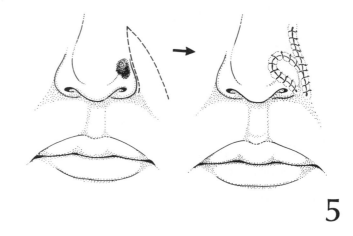

5

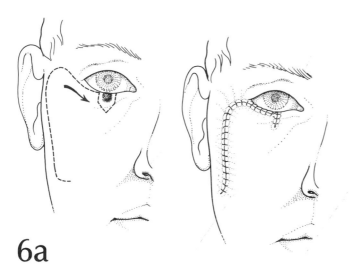

6a

Cheek advancement flap

6a,b   For lesions of the mid face and lower eyelid a cheek rotation advancement flap may be used for closure. The flap is undermined and raised in the subcutaneous plane, rotated towards the defect and the incisions are all closed primarily.

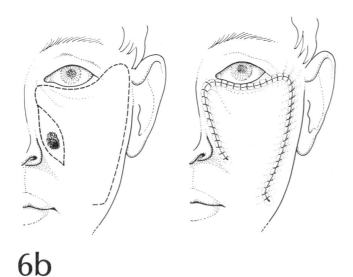

6b

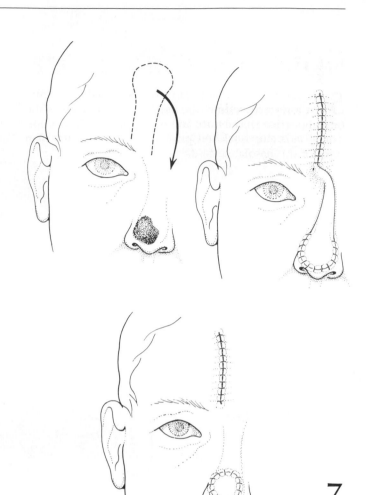

Forehead flap

7 The forehead flap is most commonly used for nasal reconstruction. It is designed on the paramedian forehead and is rotated most commonly to cover defects in the distal nose. The donor site is closed primarily and the base of the flap is divided approximately 3 weeks later.

7

Postoperative care

A sterile gauze dressing is applied to the wound after surgery. Sutures are removed in 3–5 days for facial incisions and in 7–10 days elsewhere in the body, depending on the degree of tension of the wound. Re-excision of the tumour site is sometimes necessary if a positive margin is found on microscopic examination.

Outcome

Patients should be followed on a regular basis after excision of skin tumours to determine if there are any signs of local recurrence or other primary lesions. For basal cell carcinomas the recurrence rate for well differentiated tumours may be less than 10% and 25% for less well differentiated lesions. For squamous cell cancers, well differentiated lesions have a cure rate of 95% whereas poorly differentiated lesions have a recurrence rate of up to 30%. Metastases for either basal or squamous cell cancers are uncommon[2].

References

1. Moschella SL, Hurley HJ. *Dermatology*. 2nd edn. Philadelphia: WB Saunders, 1985.

2. Jurkiewicz MJ, Krizek TJ, Mathes SJ, Ariyan S. *Plastic Surgery: Principles and Practice*. St Louis: CV Mosby, 1990.

3. Cottel WI. Skin Tumors I. Basal and squamous cell carcinoma. *Selected Readings in Plastic Surgery*. 1988; 5:1.

4. Smith JW, Aston SJ, eds. *Grabb and Smith's Plastic Surgery*, 4th edn. Boston: Little, Brown, 1991.

Epigastric hernia

H. Brendan Devlin   MA, MD, MCh, FRCS, FRCS(I)
Consultant Surgeon, North Tees General Hospital, Stockton on Tees, Cleveland;
Associate Lecturer in Clinical Surgery, University of Newcastle upon Tyne

Introduction

An epigastric hernia is a protrusion of extraperitoneal fat between the decussating fibres of the linea alba. These hernias usually occur in the midline of the epigastrium between the xiphisternum and the umbilicus; but small hernia can occur away from the midline and may protrude into the rectus muscle sheath. If these hernias enlarge considerably they may develop a peritoneal sac, which may be subcutaneous in the midline hernia or interstitial, within the rectus sheath in more lateral hernias.

Preoperative

Indications

Epigastric hernias may cause symptoms quite out of proportion to their size as the very narrow opening in the linea alba predisposes to attacks of strangulation of the peritoneal fat in which the patient may suffer severe abdominal pain when the swelling becomes tense and tender. The occurrence of such attacks is an adequate indication for operative treatment. It is, however, important to investigate the patient fully, as a small innocent epigastric hernia is sometimes blamed for symptoms which are in fact due to some intra-abdominal condition, such as a peptic ulcer. At the same time it is true to say that an epigastric hernia may sometimes produce symptoms which closely resemble those due to a peptic ulcer.

Anaesthesia

A general anaesthetic is usually employed but repair can be quite satisfactorily performed under local infiltration with lignocaine or bupivacaine.

The operation

Position of patient

The patient is placed supine on the operating table.

Suture materials

For repair metric 3 polypropylene sutures are used.

Drapes

Drapes are arranged so that the whole of the epigastric area from the costal margin to just below the umbilicus is exposed for surgery. Not infrequently the hernia is found to be larger than anticipated and placing the drapes widely has the advantage of facilitating an extended incision.

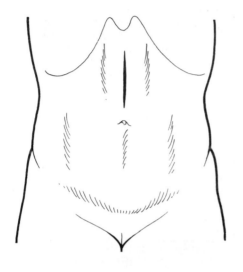

1

The incision

A vertical incision has the advantage that the abdomen can easily be opened if this is deemed necessary.

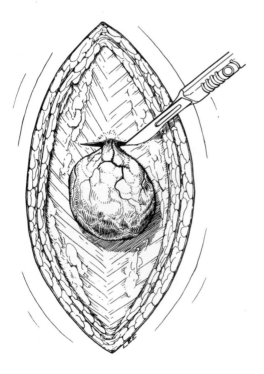

2

The fatty hernia which is enclosed within a fine capsule is dissected out from the surrounding abdominal fat. The opening in the linea alba which is usually tiny should be enlarged by incisions from opposite sides running laterally into the linea alba.

3 & 4

The hernia is incised at its neck to determine whether there is a peritoneal sac and to reduce its contents if present into the abdomen.

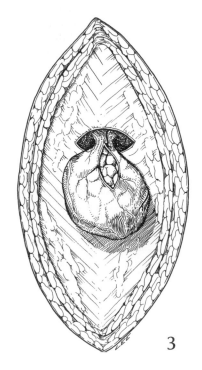

3

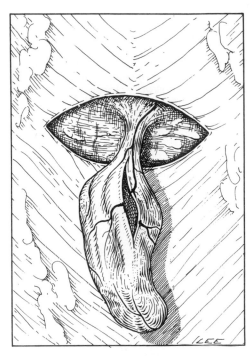

4

5 & 6

The neck of the hernia is then ligated with a transfixion suture of metric 3 chromic catgut and the hernia excised.

The opening in the linea alba is then closed by overlapping its edge as shown with two rows of interrupted polypropylene or nylon sutures, the first row inserted as mattress sutures and the second as simple sutures.

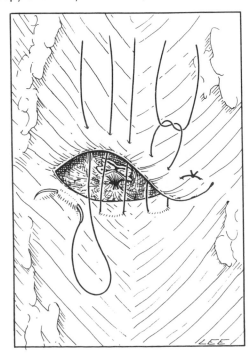

5

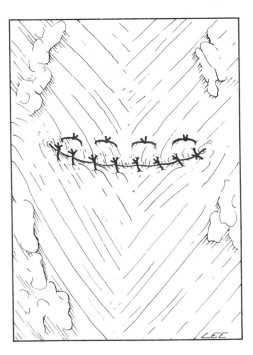

6

7

The subcutaneous fat is closed with interrupted catgut sutures. No 'dead space' should be left and the fat should be closed so that the skin is closely approximated.

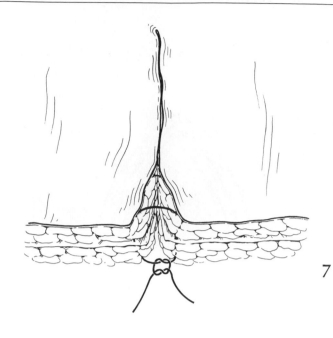

7

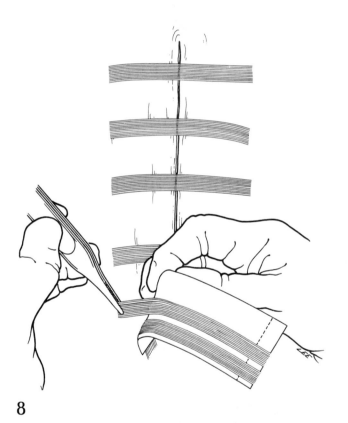

8

8

The skin is closed with microporous adhesive tape or a strip of gauze impregnated with collodion or similar adhesive. Non-penetrating skin clips give an equally good closure but require skilled attention when they are removed. Sutures should not be used.

Postoperative care

No special postoperative care is needed.

Illustrations by Peter Cox and Gillian Oliver

Umbilical hernia in children

J. L. Grosfeld MD
Professor and Chairman, Department of Surgery, Indiana University School of Medicine, and Surgeon-in-Chief, James Whitcomb Riley Hospital for Children, Indianapolis, Indiana, USA

Principles and justification

An umbilical hernia is a common occurrence in infants and young children. The hernia sac protrudes through a defect in the umbilical ring due to a failure of complete obliteration at the site where the fetal umbilical vessels (umbilical vein and the two umbilical arteries) are joined to the placenta during gestation.

Approximately 20% of full-term neonates may have an incomplete closure of the umbilical ring at birth. However, 75–80% of premature infants weighing between 1.0 kg and 1.5 kg may show evidence of an umbilical hernia at birth. Umbilical hernia is more common in girls than boys. Black children have a higher incidence than white children.

The umbilical bulge becomes more apparent during episodes of crying, straining, or even during defecation, and may result in considerable protrusion of the sac and, at times, visceral content through the ring. The hernial protrusion is composed of peritoneum adherent to the undersurface of the umbilical skin. The hernia often causes considerable parental anxiety and frequent requests for operative repair in early infancy.

Although rupture or incarceration of an umbilical hernia occurs, this is an exceptionally rare event in the author's experience (three cases during the past 22 years). The hernia is rarely a cause of pain or other symptoms. Almost 80% of umbilical hernias will decrease in size and close spontaneously by 5–6 years of age. Careful counseling will usually allay unnecessary parental anxiety and fear.

Indications

As the majority of these very low-risk hernias will close spontaneously, it is safe to wait until the child is 5 years of age (particularly if the umbilical ring is less than 1.5 cm in diameter) before attempting repair. In contrast, defects of more than 2.0 cm diameter rarely close spontaneously. Since there is a significant risk of complications including incarceration and strangulation in adults with umbilical hernia, those hernia defects that do not close by 5 years of age should be electively repaired. The umbilical defect can also be repaired in children under 5 years of age with a ring of more than 2.0 cm in whom a general anesthetic is anticipated for another condition (including repair of an inguinal hernia).

Preoperative

The child is kept without oral intake for 6 h before the anticipated time of the procedure. The operation can safely be carried out on an outpatient basis.

Careful preparation of the skin is essential as the umbilicus is often a repository of surface debris, lint, etc. and is not always kept immaculate. Preoperative cleansing with cotton applicator sticks may be useful.

Anesthesia

After administration of mild preoperative sedation, the procedure is carried out under general endotracheal anesthesia.

Operation

1 After appropriate skin preparation and application of sterile linen drapes, a curved ('smile') incision is made in a natural skin crease immediately below the umbilicus. A supraumbilical incision is also acceptable, especially if a supraumbilical defect is encountered. Placement of four quadrant traction by the assistant on the abdominal wall and slight upward traction of the defect allows selection of the site of the incision. The curved incision should not extend beyond 180°.

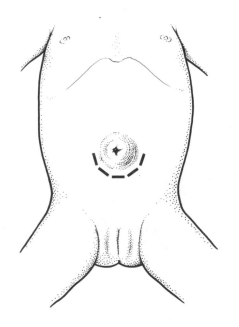

1

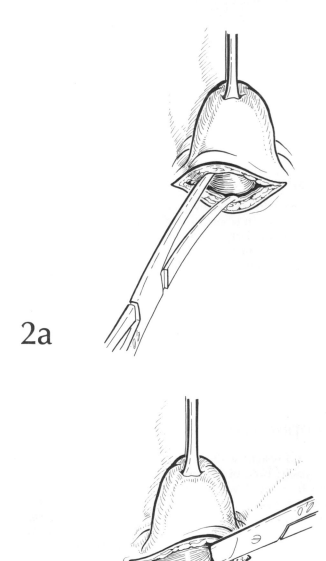

2a

2b

2a, b The subcutaneous tissue is incised and bleeding points controlled with a fine tip electrocoagulator. With upward traction on the inner margin of the upper lip of the incision, dissection is carried out down along the sac to the level of the anterior abdominal wall fascia. By blunt dissection with a mosquito clamp a plane is developed on either side of the sac, extending superiorly to gain control of the entire circumference of the sac. Any contents in the sac should be reduced into the peritoneal cavity. If the sac is large, the surgeon or assistant places an index finger in the skin defect to evert the sac where it is attached to the skin. The sac is dissected free from its skin attachments, preserving the umbilical skin for an umbilicoplasty. Bleeding points are controlled with an electrocoagulator. Separation of the sac may require its transection near the skin to preserve the umbilicus for cosmetic purposes.

3a, b The entire sac is elevated by mosquito clamps to maintain control of the edge of the defect and to have direct visualization during placement of sutures to avoid visceral injury. The sac is opened and any contents reduced. The rim of the defect is identified and the sac incised to allow placement of sutures starting at the corner farthest from the surgeon. Interrupted 3/0 (infants and young children) or 2/0 (older children and teenagers) non-absorbable sutures are placed but not initially tied. The sutures are elevated to maintain upward traction on the abdominal wall. The sac is partially excised at the level of the abdominal wall as more sutures are placed. A traction suture is also placed at the corner of the transverse wound closest to the operating surgeon, and the remaining sac is excised. All of the sutures are then tied. If a lot of redundant tissue is present or the initial tissue layer seems sparse, a layer of fascia can be imbricated over the initial line of repair with interrupted non-absorbable sutures.

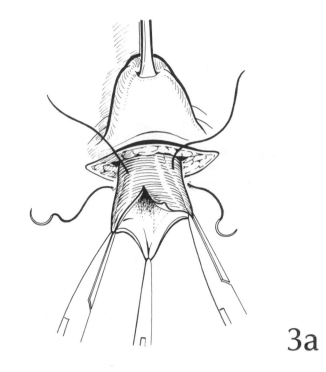

3a

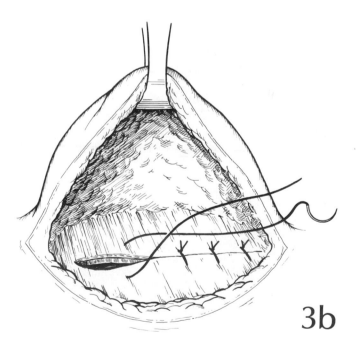

3b

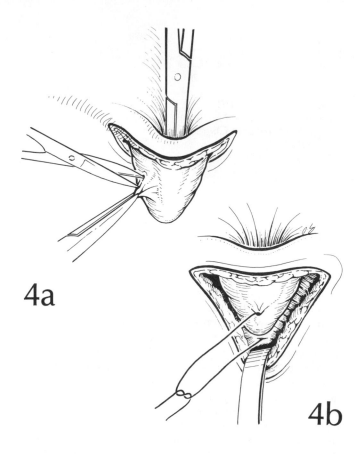

4a

4b

4a, b An umbilicoplasty is performed for cosmetic purposes by inverting the undersurface of the redundant umbilical skin to the anterior abdominal wall fascia with one or two interrupted 4/0 absorbable sutures. Any remnant of the peritoneum on the umbilical sac that is adherent to the skin may be safely left behind.

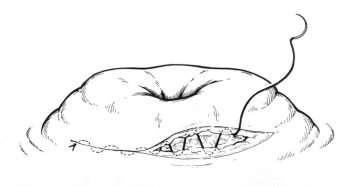

5

5 The wound is closed by a few interrupted inverted 4/0 polyglactin sutures in the subcutaneous fascia. The skin edges are opposed with a collodion dressing. No skin sutures are placed. When the collodion dries, a pressure dressing is applied to obliterate any dead space and prevent hematoma formation.

Postoperative care

Oral fluids can be offered when the infant is alert. Acetaminophen with codeine may be used for pain control for 24–48 h. Postoperative activity restrictions are the same as for inguinal hernia repair.

Complications

Complications are unusual and are limited to a wound infection (1%) or an occasional wound hematoma. Recurrence is rare, the only recurrence observed by the author being in a child with renal failure on long-term continuous ambulatory peritoneal dialysis.

Illustrations by Gillian Lee

Umbilical hernia in adults

H. Brendan Devlin   MA, MD, MCh, FRCS, FRCS(I)
Consultant Surgeon, North Tees General Hospital, Stockton on Tees, Cleveland;
Associate Lecturer in Clinical Surgery, University of Newcastle upon Tyne

Introduction

Umbilical hernias in adults can be a cause of considerable morbidity and if complications supervene they can lead to death. Umbilical hernias are much less frequent in the adult population than inguinal hernias (in the last 9 years the author has operated on 19 cases – 10 male and 9 female – compared with 603 primary inguinal hernias).

Preoperative

Indications for operation

Most patients with umbilical hernias complain of a painful protrusion at the umbilicus and this discomfort may be indication enough for operation. Absolute indications for surgery include obstruction and strangulation. Irreducibility is not an absolute indication for surgery: many long-standing umbilical hernias have many adhesions in a loculated hernia and are thus irreducible. In larger hernias the overlying skin may become damaged and ulcerated. Such hernias are best treated by operation after the skin sepsis has been controlled. In general the author's policy is to advise surgery for all umbilical hernias unless there are strong contraindications which would include obesity, chronic cardiovascular or respiratory disease, or ascites (umbilical hernias can be manifestations of cirrhotic or malignant peritoneal effusions).

Suture materials

For repair of the aponeurosis, metric 4 polypropylene or metric 3.5 nylon is used. The subcutaneous fat is closed with metric 3.5 chromic catgut. The skin is best closed with metal clips.

Anaesthesia

General anaesthesia with full muscle relaxation should be employed.

Patients who require an extensive intraperitoneal dissection often have considerable adynamic ileus after surgery and may require a postoperative regimen of nasogastric suction and fluid and nutritional support.

Position of patient

The patient is laid on his back on the operative table.

Drapes are applied to allow good access to the umbilical area and the abdomen if extended access is required.

Preoperative preparation

Sepsis is the great hazard to herniorrhaphy using non-absorbable suture material. Scrupulous surgical technique is vital if infection is to be avoided. The skin is routinely covered at the site of operation with sterile adherent film which is not removed until the subcutaneous fat is closed. Sutures are never used to close the skin for, by their very nature, sutures have the potential of introducing dermal and epidermal bacteria into the subcutaneous tissue along their tracks. Each suture is a linear abscess lined with granulation tissue and, if the 'infection' in these abscesses spreads and involves the buried sutures, sinuses may result.

For haemostasis both ligation with catgut and diathermy are used. Careful haemostasis is most important if haematoma and consequent sepsis are to be avoided.

The operation

1

The incision

Two semilunar incisions joined at their extremities are used. The ellipse of stretched skin and the enclosed umbilical cicatrix are excised. Care must be taken when deciding the dimensions of the incisions. Though the umbilical cicatrix is best excised, removal of too much skin will place the final wound under tension and jeopardize its healing. It is better to aim on the side of caution and take little skin away at the commencement of the operation; more skin can always be excised later.

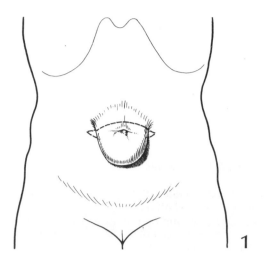

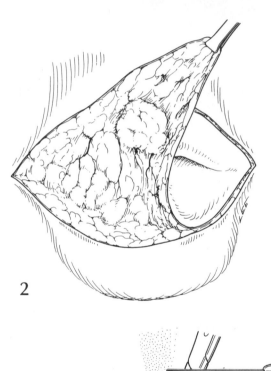

2 & 3

Removal of redundant skin and fat

The area of skin and subcutaneous fat enclosed by the semilunar incisions is removed. The incisions are deepened down to the muscular aponeuroses, care being taken to ensure that the incisions are vertical and at right angles to the fascia and that the skin is not undermined and its blood supply hazarded. This part of the dissection can be very bloody, and a cautious aproach and careful sequential haemostasis are recommended. The avoidance of blood loss at this stage is very important if blood transfusion and its considerable hazards in an obese and elderly patient is to be avoided.

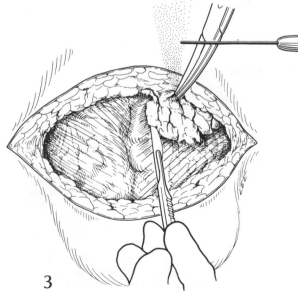

Identification of neck of the sac

When the incisions have been deepened to the aponeurosis the margins of the aponeurosis about the peritoneal neck of the sac can be sought and dissected.

4, 5 & 6

Management of the Sac I

Having isolated the neck of the sac all the overlying fat and skin can be dissected off leaving the peritoneum of the sac protruding bare through the defect in the abdominal wall. The sac can now be opened and its contents inspected. Often the contents are densely adherent to the lining of the sac particularly at the fundus. Adhesions must be divided and ligated where necessary to control bleeding. Again the admonition about the avoidance of blood loss should be remembered. Densely adherent omentum, particularly if it is partly ischaemic, is best excised. After the contents have been freed from the sac they are ready to be returned to the main peritoneal cavity.

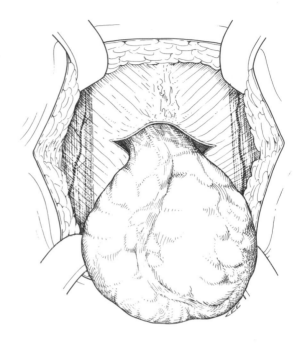

4

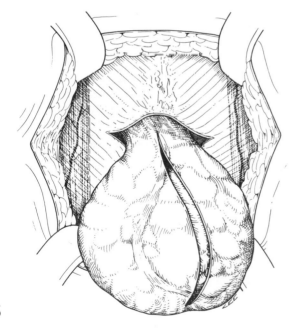

5

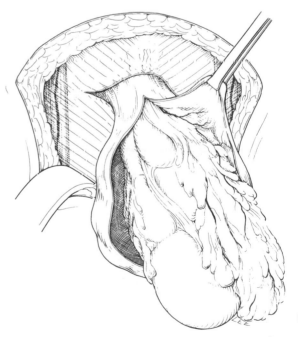

6

Management of the sac II

If the sac is vast and multiloculated an alternative strategy can often usefully be employed.

7

Once the peritoneum of the neck at any one point has been identified it should be opened and a finger inserted.

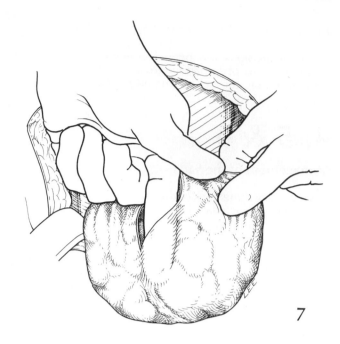

7

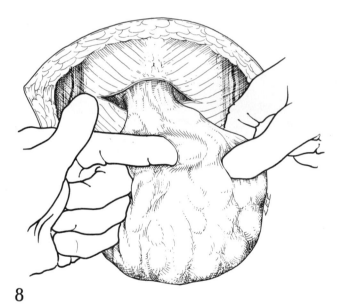

8

8

The whole mass of sac, contents and overlying fat and skin is then held up by assistants while the neck is dissected around using the finger in the sac as a direction finder. This dissection can be tedious if the sac is multiloculated and the contents very adherent. It is well for the operator to change from side to side of the operating table to facilitate this manoeuvre. Once the neck has been divided attention can be turned to the contents of the sac. Adhesions are divided and doubtfully viable omentum excised.

Enlargement of the aponeurotic aperture

9

The opening in the abdominal wall is next enlarged laterally for 3 or 4 cm on either side, the rectus muscle being retracted as the posterior rectus sheath is divided, taking care not to injure the epigastric vessels.

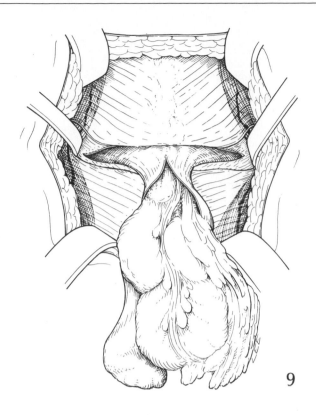

9

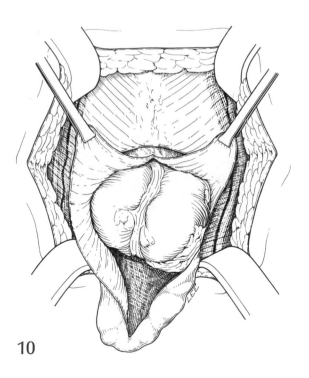

10

10

Once the fibrous ring of the neck has been divided the contents of the sac can be reduced back into the abdomen.

The repair of the defect – Mayo technique[1]

11

The margins of the opening – aponeurosis, posterior rectus sheath and peritoneum – are now grasped in large haemostats and held up by assistants.

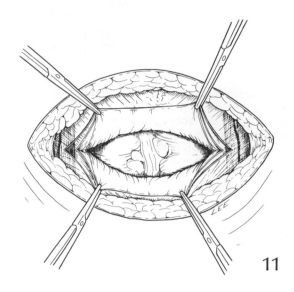

11

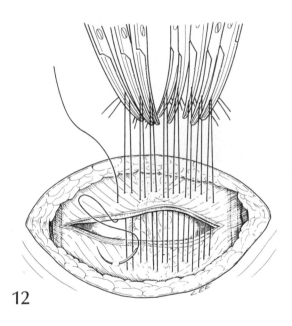

12

12

The deep sutures are next placed. Strong non-absorbable material (metric 4 polypropylene or metric 3.5 nylon) is used on a round-bodied needle.

The suture enters the upper (cephalad) flap from without, between 2 cm and 3 cm from its margin. The needle is then grasped on the deep surface of the upper flap, passed across the defect and then from the outside through the lower flap. Then the needle is pulled back through the lower flap, across the defect and through the deep surface of the upper flap. The suture thus placed is held in a clip. Many more such sutures are now inserted and held untied until all are in place.

There are four useful technical points.

1. In the upper flap the sutures must all be placed further than 2 cm from the margin – up to 4 cm is permissible.
2. In the lower flap the sutures must all be at a distance greater than 1 cm from the margin.
3. It adds to the stability of the suture lines if the sutures are staggered, not all at the same interval from the margins of the defect.
4. The more sutures that are put in the easier they are to close and tie, and the strain is more evenly distributed.

13

After the sutures have all been placed the flaps are brought together, the upper being 'railroaded' down the sutures until it lies overlapping the lower flap.

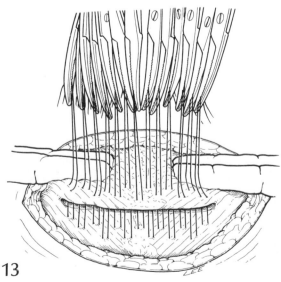

13

14

The sutures are now tied, fixing the tissues firmly (but not too tightly) together. A triple-layer, double-throw knot is used. When all the knots are complete the ends are cut short.

A fine suction drain is now placed in between the two flaps of the aponeurosis.

The edge of the upper flap is now sutured to the anterior surface of the lower flap using the same non-absorbable suture material as previously. Suture bites of over 1 cm into both upper and lower flaps are used.

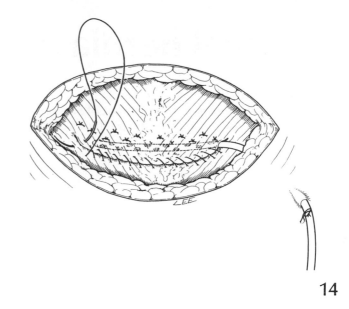

14

Closure

Meticulous haemostasis, suction drainage and obliteration of any dead space are the essential components of this part of the operation.

The subcutaneous fat is closed in terraces using fine (metric 3) chromic catgut. Suction drainage is employed.

15

The skin is closed using skin clips. Suturing of the skin is not recommended: it is often poor and infected in the vicinity of a longstanding umbilical hernia and sutures may carry skin bacteria along their tracks to the deeper parts of the wound or introduce sepsis adjacent to the non-absorbable hernia repair.

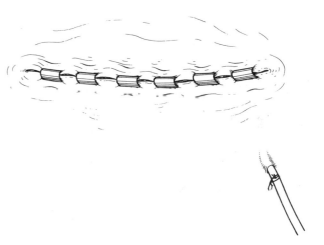

15

Postoperative care

If there has been extensive handling and dissection of the small gut and omentum during the operation, postoperative nasogastric suction and parenteral metabolic support will be needed until normal peristalsis is re-established.

Early ambulation and breathing excercises are essential. The postoperative problem which most frequently arises is respiratory embarrassment caused by the wound pain and the newly raised intra-abdominal pressure.

Reference

1. Mayo, W. J. Further experience with the vertical overlapping operation for the radical cure of umbilical hernia. Journal of the American Medical Association 1903; 41: 225–228

Illustrations by Peter Cox and Gillian Oliver

Inguinal hernia in children

J. L. Grosfeld MD

Professor and Chairman, Department of Surgery, Indiana University School of Medicine, and Surgeon-in-Chief, James Whitcomb Riley Hospital for Children, Indianapolis, Indiana, USA

History

The first reference to hernia repair in children is credited to Celsus who in AD25 recommended removal of the hernia sac and testes through a scrotal incision. Paré recommended treatment of childhood hernia; however, the first accurate description was made by Pott in 1756. Czerny performed high ligation of the hernia sac through the external ring in 1877. Ferguson recommended that the spermatic cord should remain undisturbed during inguinal hernia repair in 1899. In 1912, Turner documented that high ligation of the sac was the only procedure necessary in most children. Herzfield was the first advocate of outpatient surgical repair of inguinal hernia in children in 1938. Early repair in infancy was recommended by Ladd and Gross in 1941. The concept of bilateral inguinal exploration was promoted by Duckett, Rothenberg and Barnett, among others. Advances in neonatal intensive care have resulted in improved survival of premature infants who have a high incidence of hernia and an increased risk of complications. These cases have stimulated great interest into considerations regarding the timing of operation and choice of anesthesia. Recently, Puri and others have challenged the necessity of routine bilateral inguinal exploration.

Principles and justification

The occurrence of congenital inguinal hernia is related to descent of the testis which follows the gubernaculum testis as it descends from an intra-abdominal retroperitoneal position to the scrotum. Those factors affecting descent (androgenic hormonal influences for the abdominal descent phase and local hormonal influences, such as GFRH release from the genitofemoral nerve for the scrotal descent phase) are beyond the scope of this chapter. However, as the testis passes through the internal ring it drags with it a diverticulum of peritoneum on its anteromedial surface referred to as the 'processus vaginalis'. In girls the persistence of the processus vaginalis that extends into the labia majora is known as the canal of Nuck. The layers of the processus vaginalis normally fuse in >90% of full-term infants, obliterating the entrance to the inguinal canal from the peritoneal cavity. Failure of obliteration may result in a variety of inguinal–scrotal anomalies including complete persistence resulting in a scrotal hernia, distal processus obliteration and proximal hernial patency, complete patency with a narrow opening at the internal ring referred to as a communicating hydrocele, hydrocele of the canal of Nuck in girls or inguinal canal in boys, and a hydrocele of the tunica vaginalis.

Clinical presentation

The majority of inguinal hernias in infants and children are indirect hernias. Boys are more commonly affected than girls in a ratio of 9:1; 60% present on the right side due to later testicular descent and obliteration of the processus vaginalis on the right, 25% occur on the left side, and 15% are bilateral. The diagnosis is often apparent as a bulge and can be observed in the groin with crying or straining. Scrotal enlargement and frequent change in scrotal size resulting from transfer of fluid between the peritoneal cavity and the sac may be noted. Physical examination will often confirm these observations: however, diagnosis may depend on visualization of these events by the referring pediatrician or parent.

Inguinal hernia is a high-risk hernia as it is frequently complicated by incarceration, occasionally leading to strangulation and obstruction. In young infants with undescended testes and associated hernia the testis is sometimes at risk of torsion or atrophy caused by compression of the vascular supply by a hernia sac filled with bowel compressing the testicular vessels at the level of the internal inguinal ring. The incidence of incarceration is highest in the youngest patients, particularly premature infants and infants under the age of 1 year where an incarceration rate of 31% has been reported. The incarceration rate in children up to 18 years of age is 12–15%.

Indications

Because of the high rate of complications associated with inguinal hernia there is no place for conservative management except in instances of an isolated hydrocele of the tunica vaginalis. The natural history of this particular abnormality is often associated with spontaneous involution at 6–12 months of age. As long as the hydrocele does not change in size, this can be watched. All other inguinal scrotal anomalies require surgical intervention. In addition to instances of incarceration seen in boys, girls can present with a mass in the labia majora due to a sliding hernia of the ovary and fallopian tube. This may be associated with a risk of torsion of the ovary in the hernia sac.

The operation is usually performed shortly after the diagnosis is made. Attempts to reduce an incarcerated hernia using sedation and manual reduction are successful in more than 80% of cases. An elective operation is then carried out within 24 h of the reduction. In the case of hernias in small premature infants already hospitalized in the neonatal intensive care unit because of other illnesses, elective repair is carried out just before discharge. For infants diagnosed after discharge from the hospital who require ventilatory support or experience episodes of apnea and/or bradycardia in the neonatal period, elective repair is usually delayed until 44–60 weeks of corrected conceptional age. Although most infants and children can be managed in an ambulatory setting, infants with bronchopulmonary dysplasia or those who required ventilator support at the time of birth should be observed after surgery in an extended observation (23-h) center and monitored for episodes of apnea and bradycardia.

Preoperative

The operation is usually performed under general anesthesia, although some surgeons prefer spinal anesthesia in very premature infants.

The lower abdomen, inguinal scrotal area, perineum and thighs are prepared with iodophor solution and draped appropriately for herniorrhaphy.

Operation

1 A transverse incision is made in the lowest right inguinal crease above the external inguinal ring. Scarpa's fascia is incised and the external oblique fascia identified. The inguinal ligament is located and traced down to expose the external inguinal ring.

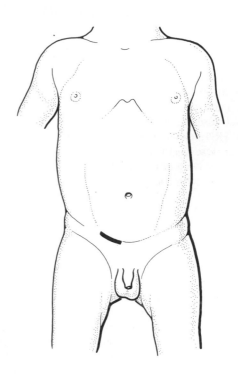

1

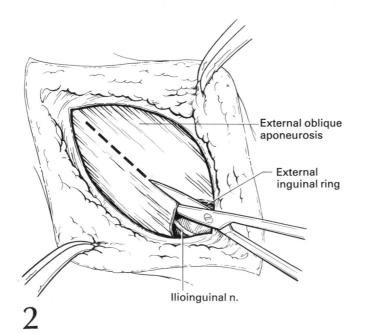

2 The external oblique fascia is opened along the axis of its fibers, perpendicular to the external inguinal ring, for 1–2 cm.

External oblique aponeurosis

External inguinal ring

Ilioinguinal n.

2

3   The spermatic fascia covers the cord structures. The ilioinguinal nerve can be seen on the outer vestment of the fascia. The cremasteric muscle is teased open by blunt dissection on the anteromedial surface of the cord, exposing the glistening hernia sac.

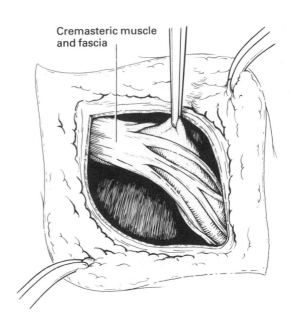

4   The sac is elevated anteromedially and the vas deferens and spermatic vessels are carefully dissected free from the diverticular structure of the inguinal hernia sac. The vas deferens should never be grasped with a forceps or a clamp as this can result in an injury.

The hernia sac often extends to the testicular area. Once the vital structures are identified and mobilized laterally, the sac can be divided between clamps and the upper end dissected superiorly to the level of the internal inguinal ring. The extent of the superior dissection is identified by the presence of retroperitoneal fat at the neck of the sac.

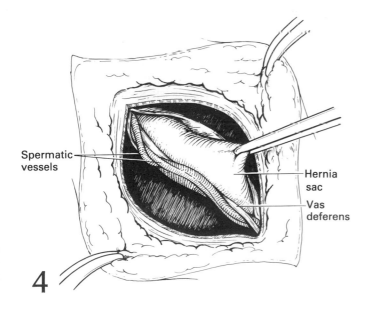

5 The contents of the sac should be reduced and a clamp placed on the sac which is twisted in a clockwise manner to ensure that all of the contents are reduced. A pair of DeBakey forceps is placed at the base of the sac to protect the cord structures. The neck of the sac is transfixed with a 4/0 (in small infants) or 3/0 non-absorbable suture ligature. A free tie should never be used as distension of the abdomen may push the tie off the peritoneum.

The distal end of the hernia sac is opened on its anterior surface. If a separate hydrocele is present, this should be excised at the same time. If the internal ring is excessively large, this can be snugged (made smaller) inferior to the cord vessels with an interrupted 3/0 silk suture. The floor of the canal usually requires no specific therapy and, during the dissection, the surgeon should avoid any injury to the transversalis fascia. High ligation of an infant hernia is usually all that is required. In rare cases where there is an associated direct hernia, this can be repaired by inserting two or three sutures between the conjoined tendon and Poupart's or Cooper's ligament. The testis should be returned to a normal intrascrotal location at the end of the procedure. Administration of a local anesthetic (e.g. bupivacaine) along the ilioinguinal and hypogastric nerves will reduce postoperative pain.

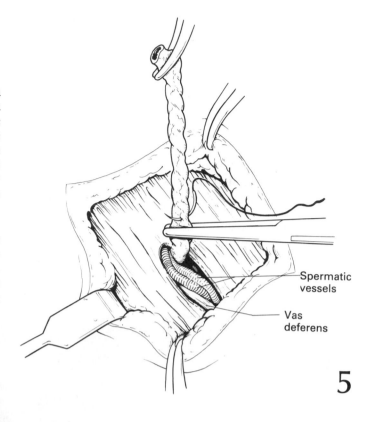

Spermatic vessels

Vas deferens

5

6 Wound closure is accomplished with interrupted 4/0 silk or polyglactin (Vicryl) sutures on the external oblique fascia.

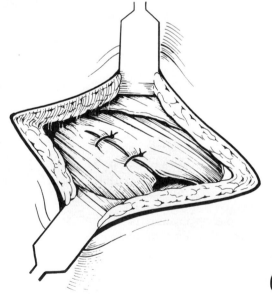

6

7 Scarpa's fascia is closed with one or two interrupted 4/0 polyglactin sutures, burying the knot. The skin edges are opposed with interrupted 4/0 or 5/0 plain gut or polyglactin subcuticular sutures. The skin edges are opposed with a collodion dressing in infants before they are toilet-trained or with sterile skin closure strips (e.g. Steristrips) and a semipermeable adhesive film dressing (e.g. Opsite) in older children.

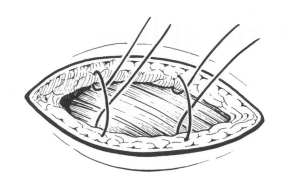

7

The author routinely explores the contralateral side in some cases, particularly those infants younger than 1 year, girls less than 5 years, and in selected patients with a clinically apparent left inguinal hernia. Contralateral exploration is reasonable if the operator is experienced and skilled in performing inguinal hernial repairs in infants, if the anesthetist has considerable expertise in administering anesthesia to young infants, and if the patient has no serious underlying condition that increases the risk of an operation. An operation is always performed first on the side with the clinically obvious hernia.

Postoperative care

With the exception of infants who require extended observation, most patients are discharged from the day surgery room within 2 h after operative repair. Oral intake may be resumed when the child awakens. Tylenol with codeine is used for analgesia for 48 h following the procedure. Baths can be resumed on the third postoperative day. There are no activity restrictions for infants but older children should refrain from bicycle riding or other vigorous physical activity for one month.

Complications

Injury to the spermatic vessels or vas deferens is unusual. If the vas deferens is divided it should be repaired with interrupted 7/0 or 8/0 monofilament sutures. The use of magnifying loupes or an operating microscope will make the repair more precise.

Intraoperative bleeding is also an unusual complication unless the floor of the canal is weakened and requires repair. Needle-hole injury to the epigastric vessels or the femoral vein can usually be controlled by withdrawal of the suture and direct pressure.

Postoperative complications include wound infection, scrotal hematoma, postoperative hydrocele and recurrent inguinal hernia. The wound infection rate at most major pediatric centers is quite low (1–2%). An increased incidence of infection might be expected in incarcerated hernias.

Recurrent inguinal hernia is a relatively uncommon complication in children with recurrence rates of less than 1% having been reported by experienced pediatric surgeons. Of these, 80% are noted within the first postoperative year. The major causes of recurrent inguinal hernia in children include: (1) a missed hernial sac or unrecognized peritoneal tear; (2) a broken suture ligature at the neck of the sac; (3) failure to repair (snug) a large internal inguinal ring; (4) injury to the floor of the inguinal canal, resulting in a direct inguinal hernia; (5) severe infection; (6) increased intra-abdominal pressure; and (7) connective tissue disorders.

Postoperative hydrocele may rarely occur after high ligation of the proximal hernial sac and incomplete excision of the distal portion. To avoid this complication the anterior surface of the distal hernial sac can be split and the anterior and lateral aspects of the sac partially resected. The postoperative hydrocele often resolves spontaneously. Rarely, long-term persistence of the hydrocele may require a formal hydrocelectomy.

Testicular atrophy has been observed after incarcerated hernias and acute tense hydroceles in young infants.

Inguinal hernia in adults

H. Brendan Devlin   MA, MD, MCh, FRCS, FRCS(I)
Consultant Surgeon, North Tees General Hospital, Stockton on Tees, Cleveland;
Associate Lecturer in Clinical Surgery, University of Newcastle upon Tyne

Historical note

The surgical literature abounds with descriptions of operations for inguinal hernia. However, few of these essays describe new or original principles. The foundations underlying the modern approach to inguinal hernia were laid by Marcy[1] who observed the anatomy and physiology of the deep inguinal ring and correctly inferred the import[2] of the obliquity of the canal. Bassini[3], who built on Marcy's observations, had heard Marcy lecture in 1881, and grasped the significance of the anatomical arrangement, and in particular the role of the transversalis fascia and transversus abdominis tendon. Bassini originally stressed the importance of dividing the transversalis fascia and reconstructing the posterior wall of the canal by suturing the transversalis fascia and transversus muscle to the upturned, deep edge of the inguinal ligament. In his repair, Bassini included the lower arching fibres of the internal oblique muscle where they form the conjoint tendon with the transversus muscle. He called the upper leaf of his repair the 'triple layer', that is, transversalis fascia, transversus abdominis and internal oblique. Bassini's original observations about the fascia transversalis and 'triple layer' have somehow been lost from the later literature. Many of the failures of 'Bassini's operation' occur in cases where the fleshy conjoint tendon only has been sutured to the inguinal ligament.

The three main principles in the operative management of inguinal hernia are as follows.

1. The normal anatomy should be reconstituted as far as possible. The first layer to be defective, in either indirect or direct hernias, is the transversalis fascia; this should therefore be repaired first.
2. Only tendinous/aponeurotic/fascial structures should be sutured together. Suturing red fleshy muscle to tendon or fascia will not contribute to permanent fibrous union of these structures; nor will it result in anything resembling the normal anatomy.
3. The suture material must retain its strength for long enough to maintain tissue apposition and allow sound union of tissues to occur. A non-absorbable or very slowly absorbable suture material must therefore be employed.

Non-absorbable suture materials do have their own inherently disadvantageous properties: proneness to sepsis, adverse tissue reaction and sinus formation. These have led surgeons to seek compromise suture materials which have often not proved effective when used for inguinal hernia repair.

These three principles of repair of the inguinal hernia have been admirably combined in the repair operation outlined by Dr Earl Shouldice of Toronto about 1951[4]. This is the operation described in this chapter.

Dr Shouldice's own results, and the combined results from his clinic, are most impressive. More than 78 000 hernias have been repaired since 1951 with a recurrence rate of 0.8 per cent at 5 years[4]. Myers and Shearburn[5], using the same technique, reported a recurrence rate of 0.1 per cent in 953 consecutive operations for primary inguinal hernia.

Preoperative

Suture materials

The suture material of choice for the repair is metric 3 polypropylene. In the original Shouldice series from Toronto monofilament stainless steel wire was used[4]. Myers and Shearburn[5] and Devlin et al.[6] originally used stainless steel wire but have subsequently used polypropylene. Stainless steel wire is a most effective suture material but it is difficult to use; prolypropylene is as effective and is much easier to handle.

Indications and contraindications to surgery

Successful surgical repair is the treatment of choice for inguinal hernias in males. The Shouldice operation is therefore recommended for all male hernia patients from pubescence to retirement. With the elderly male aged over 70 years a less definite policy must be adopted; if the hernia is direct and spontaneously reducible the patient often has few if any symptoms attributable to it and surgery is not advisable. Indeed, the risk of anaesthesia and surgery in this age group are greater than the chances of developing complications necessitating urgent surgery[7].

Administrative and management arrangements for inguinal hernia surgery

A careful administrative policy is necessary if the greatest benefits (for the patients and the community) are to be obtained using the Shouldice technique. At North Tees General Hospital patients are treated on a 'planned early discharge' basis; that is, an assessment of the patient's clinical and social status is made preoperatively and a decision taken about the duration of his hospital stay prior to his admission. In general three regimens are used.

1. Day case – 8 hour stay – applicable to all healthy males who have good home circumstances.
2. Two night – 48 hour stay – applicable to healthy males with less appropriate social status.
3. Five-day stay – most suitable for older patients, patients with contemporaneous medical conditions or patients who are socially disadvantaged.

About one-third of patients fall into each of these categories.

The advantages of this 'planned early discharge' system – apart from the discipline it imposes on the surgical team – are that it keeps the patient mobile and not institutionalized, that there is a challenge to keep complications to a minimum, and finally that it is socially and economically advantageous to the patient and to the community[8,9].

Anaesthesia

Local or general anaesthesia may be employed. General anaesthesia seems more acceptable to British patients, but the clinical and economic advantages of local anaesthesia should not be overlooked. The Shouldice Clinic uses local anaesthesia routinely.

Local anaesthesia

The iliohypogastric and ilioinguinal nerves should be blocked lateral to the inguinal canal, and the skin and subcutaneous tissues in the line of the incision should be infiltrated. The region of the peritoneal neck of the sac will need infiltration during the operation. Traction on the peritoneum is uncomfortable for the patient and the site where the cord comes through the transversalis fascia is infiltrated as soon as the cord is exposed. The anaesthetic agent of choice is 0.5 per cent lignocaine with 1:200 000 adrenaline. About 50–100 ml of this solution are all that is needed for adequate anaesthesia. The maximum dose that can be given to a 70 kg healthy male is 100 ml of the 0.5 per cent lignocaine with adrenaline solution. The infiltration is made easier if a continuously rechargeable syringe is used.

An alternative local anaesthetic is bupivacaine hydrochloride (Marcaine) 0.25 per cent with adrenaline 1:400 000 up to a maximum dosage of 2 mg/kg body weight.

General anaesthesia

General anaesthesia is quicker than local anaesthesia and more comfortable for the patient. No preoperative narcotic drugs are given. Atropine is injected immediately preoperatively and then a short-acting barbiturate and halothane are used, accompanied by muscle relaxants and endotracheal intubation. Light general anaesthesia without any preoperative narcotic agents is safe and allows early discharge after surgery.

The operation

Position of patient

The patient is placed on his back on the operating table. Access is improved if the head of the table is tilted downward by about 15°.

For haemostasis, the larger vessels are ligated, especially the veins in the subcutaneous tissue, using metric 3.5 chromic catgut. Otherwise, diathermy is used for haemostasis. Careful haemostasis is most important if haematoma and consequent sepsis are to be avoided.

Sepsis is the great hazard to herniorrhaphy, particularly when non-absorbable suture material is used. Scrupulous surgical technique is vital if infection is to be avoided. The skin is routinely covered at the site of operation with sterile adherent film which is not removed until the subcutaneous fat is closed. Sutures are never used to close the skin. By their very nature sutures have the potential for introducing dermal and epidermal bacteria into the subcutaneous tissue along their tracks. Each suture is a linear abscess lined with granulation tissue, and if the 'infection' in these abscesses spreads and involves the buried sutures sinuses may result.

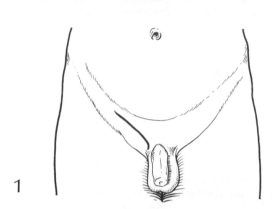

1

The incision

The incision is placed 1 cm above and parallel to the inguinal ligament. Laterally the incision begins over the deep inguinal ring, runs to the pubic tubercle, then curves caudally (vertically) and runs down over the pubic tubercle. It is important to keep the knife at right angles to the patient's skin on this corner in the incision in order to avoid undercutting the flap on its lower outer side. More importantly, the extension provides good access to the cord as it emerges from the superficial inguinal ring.

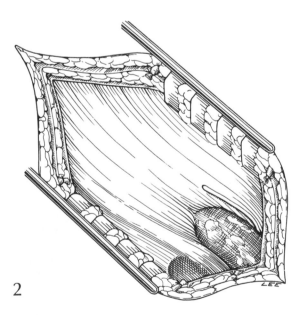

2

Exposure

After the skin has been divided the subcutaneous fat is opened in the length of the incision down to the external oblique aponeurosis. Carefully, haemostasis is now attained. The superficial pudendal and superficial epigastric vessels are tied with catgut and the smaller vessels dealt with using diathermy. A self-retaining retractor is now introduced and opened. This retractor serves two purposes: it opens the wound to facilitate access and the slight traction it exerts on the skin ensures haemostasis in the small vessels in the immediate subdermal tissues.

After the subcutaneous fat has been opened down to the external oblique aponeurosis, the deep fascia of the thigh is opened to allow access to the femoral canal. The femoral canal is exposed below the inguinal ligament and checked to make sure it is intact. It is important not to overlook a concomitant femoral hernia which may present in the postoperative period.

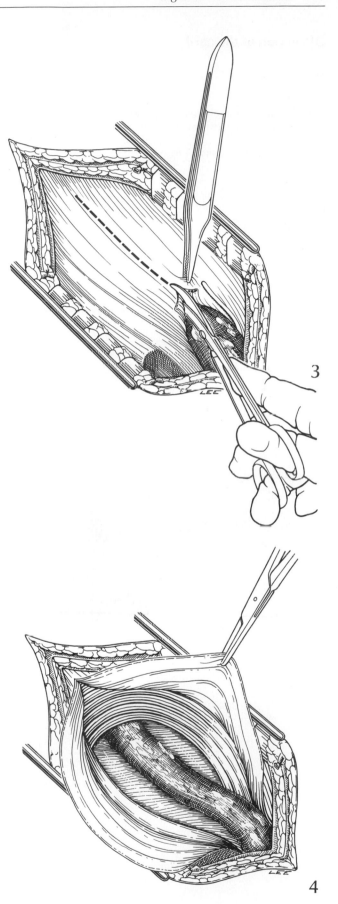

3

4

3 & 4

Dissection of the canal

The external oblique aponeurosis is next opened in the long axis of the inguinal canal. This incision extends down to the external inguinal ring, the margin of which is divided. With the ring opened, the upper medial flap of the external oblique is grasped in a haemostat and lifted up off the underlying cremaster fascia. The aponeurosis is gently freed from underlying structures by gauze dissection up to its fusion into the lateral rectus sheath.

Similarly, the lower lateral leaf of the external oblique is mobilized and freed of the underlying cord coverings down to the upturned deep edge of the inguinal ligament, which is exposed.

Thus the whole of the cord is exposed.

Dissection of the cord

5

The cremaster muscle/fascia is now divided in its long axis from its proximal origin down to the level of the pubic tubercle.

The cremaster is made into two flaps, an upper medial and a lower lateral flap. These flaps are raised off the pampiniform plexus of veins, the other contents of the cord and the vas deferens. The flaps of the cremaster are each traced proximally to their origin from the conjoint tendon and distally to the pubic tubercle. The cremaster is clamped, divided and ligated with catgut at its origin from the conjoint tendon and similarly dealt with distally at the level of the pubic tubercle.

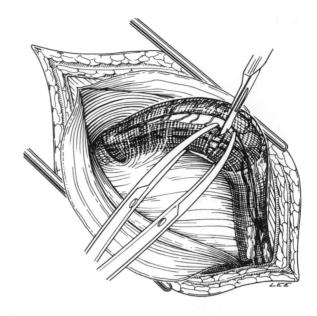

5

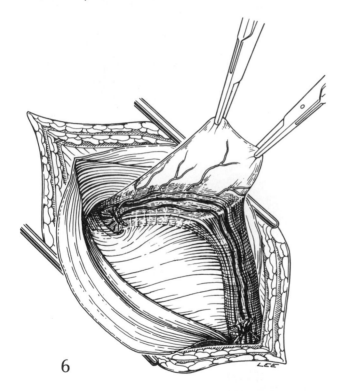

6

6

After the cremaster has been removed the contents of the cord and any hernia contained therein should be visualized. If there is a lipoma in the cord it is excised at this stage, but removal of a lipoma must not be used as an excuse to strip out all the fat and areolar tissue in the cord. If this is done the patient will suffer considerable post-operative testicular oedema and may even develop a hydrocele.

Identification of the transversalis fascia

After the contents of the cord have been adequately visualized they are lifted up and the continuation of the transversalis fascia on to the cord at the deep ring is identified. The condensation of the transversalis fascia about the emerging cord is the deep ring and it must be identified accurately. The correct identification and dissection of the deep ring is crucial to the subsequent repair operation.

Hernial sacs

Indirect

If an indirect hernial sac is present it should be easily found now. It lies on the anterosuperior aspect of the cord structures. Further management depends on the presence and nature of the contents of the indirect hernial sac.

7

No contents   If the sac is empty, it is lifted and freed from the adjacent structures by gauze dissection. It is traced back to its junction with the parietal peritoneum, transfixed with a catgut suture which is tied around it securely and the redundant sac excised.

Small bowel and/or omentum, with or without adhesions   Unless the hernia is strangulated and the small bowel non-viable, any adhesions are divided and the small bowel is returned to the abdominal cavity. Strangulated omentum or small bowel can be resected at this stage. The diagnostic decision as to what should be done about very adherent and frequently partially ischaemic omentum is a difficult one. If there is any doubt about omentum it is best excised, because to return omentum of doubtful viability to the peritoneal cavity invites the formation of adhesions.

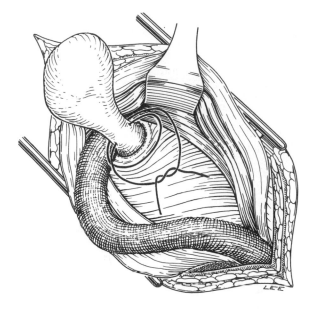

7

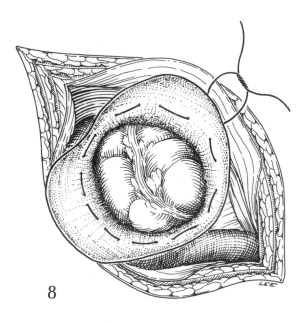

8

8

The sliding hernia   Such a hernia may contain the caecum and appendix (on the right side) in its wall, the sigmoid colon (on the left side) or the bladder (in the medial wall on either side). The following guidelines apply in these circumstances.

1. No attempt should be made to separate caecum or sigmoid colon from the sac wall. This may compromise their blood supply and lead to further unnecessary problems.
2. The appendix must not be removed, as this could introduce sepsis.
3. Appendices epiploicae must never be removed from the sigmoid colon – they may harbour small colonic diverticula excision of which will precipitate sepsis.
4. On the medial side of a sac there should be no attempt to dissect the bladder clean. If the bladder is inadvertently opened, a two-layer closure and urethral drainage are required. Recovery will obviously be delayed.

A sliding hernia is dealt with by clearing as much peritoneal hernia sac as possible and then closing it using an 'inside-out' purse-string suture. When it is closed it is pushed back behind the transversalis fascia.

9a & b

Direct

The direct sac may be either a broad-based bulge behind and through the transversalis fascia (*a*) or, less commonly, have a narrow neck (*b*). In the first type interference with the peritoneum is not needed – the sac should be pushed back behind the transversalis fascia, which will be subsequently repaired. In the second, which is usually at the medial end of the canal, extraperitoneal fat is removed, the sac carefully cleared, redundant peritoneum excised and the defect closed with a catgut transfixion suture. Care must be taken to avoid the bladder which is often in the wall of such a sac.

Combined direct and indirect

Lastly a combined direct and indirect 'pantaloon' sac straddling the deep epigastric vessels may be found. In such a case the sac should be delivered to the lateral side of the deep epigastric vessels and dealt with as described for an indirect hernia.

10

Dissection of transversalis fascia

The most essential part of the Shouldice operation is the repair of the transversalis fascia. This structure should already have been identified at its condensation around the cord forming the deep inguinal ring. The condensed deep inguinal ring is freed from the emerging cord by sharp dissection. When this is completed the medial margin of the ring is grasped in a dissecting forceps or a haemostat and lifted up off the underlying extraperitoneal fat. Dissecting scissors are now passed through the ring between the fascia and the underlying fat. By this manoeuvre the fascia is separated from the underlying structures, particularly the deep epigastric vessels. The transversalis fascia is now divided along the length of the canal, beginning at the deep inguinal ring and continuing down to the pubic tubercle. The upper medial flap is lifted up away from the underlying fat.

Attention is now turned to the lower flap. It is penetrated by the cremasteric vessels arising from the deep epigastric vessels; these should now be ligated and divided close to their origin using catgut. If care is not taken with the cremasteric vessels they may be torn off the deep epigastric vessels and troublesome haemorrhage will follow. If a direct hernia is present it will bulge forward at this time and must be pushed back in order to free the lower lateral flap of the transversalis fascia. This flap must be freed down to its fusion to the deep part of the inguinal ligament.

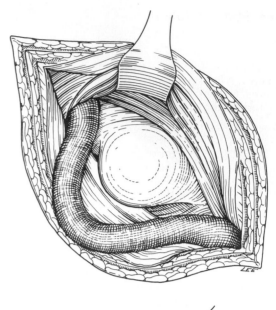

9a

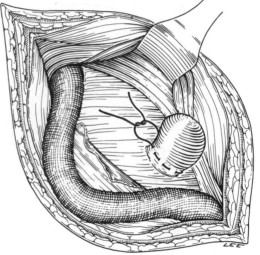

9b

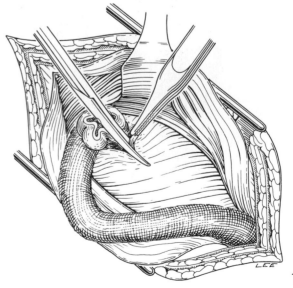

10

Repair of transversalis fascia

11

If the previous dissection has been carried out carefully, and if haemostasis is now complete, the remainder of the operation should be easy. First the transversalis fascia is repaired and the deep ring is carefully reconstituted using a 'double-breasting' technique. The posterior wall of the canal must be reconstituted so that *all* of the peritoneum and the stump of a hernial sac are retained behind it. To do this the lower lateral flap of the transversalis fascia is sutured to the deep surface of the upper medial flap. The repair is begun at the medial end of the canal, the first suture being placed in the transversalis fascia where that structure becomes condensed into the aponeurosis and periosteum on the pubic tubercle. The lower lateral flap of the transversalis fascia is then sutured to the undersurface of the upper flap at the point where the upper flap is just deep to the tendon of the transversus abdominus (conjoint tendon). At this point there is a thickening or condensation of the transversalis fascia which holds sutures easily. The fascia is sutured laterally until the stump of an indirect hernia lies behind it and it has been snugly fitted around the spermatic cord.

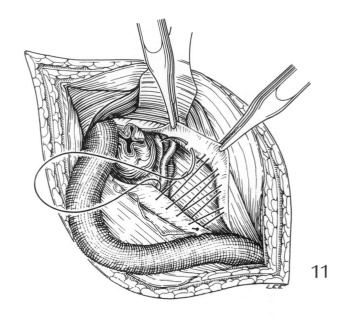

11

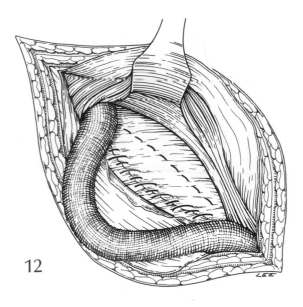

12

12

The direction of suturing is then reversed. The free margin of the upper medial flap is brought down over the lower lateral flap and sutured to the transversalis fascia at its condensation into the upturned deep edge of the inguinal ligament in the floor of the canal. Suturing is continued back to the pubic tubercle, where the suture is tied. By this manoeuvre the transversalis fascia is 'double-breasted' on itself, the 'direct area' of the canal is reinforced and the internal ring carefully reconstituted and tightened.

It is important not to split the fascial fibres. Sutures should be placed about 2–4 mm apart and bites of different depth taken with each so that an irregular 'broken saw-tooth' effect is produced.

The repair of the fascia transversalis is the crucial part of the operation. The fascia must be dissected and handled with care if its structure is to be maintained.

13 & 14

Reinforcement with the conjoint tendon

The conjoint tendon is now used to reinforce the repair of the transversalis fascia. A suture is started laterally through the upturned deep edge of the inguinal ligament at the medial margin of the reconstituted deep inguinal ring and continued to the deep tendinous surface of the conjoint tendon which is directly to the medial side of the deep ring. Sometimes, particularly if the cord is bulky, it is easier to proceed in reverse by passing the needle first through the undersurface of the conjoint tendon and then under the cord and through the upturned edge of the inguinal ligament.

At the point where this suture is inserted, the deep surface of the conjoint tendon is just beginning to become aponeurotic (the tendon of the transversus muscle) and it should hold sutures easily. The suture is continued in a medial direction, picking up the upturned edge of the inguinal ligament and the undersurface – the aponeurotic part – of the conjoint tendon down to the pubic tubercle. The direction is then reversed, suturing the aponeurotic part of the conjoint tendon loosely to the external oblique aponeurosis about 0.5 cm above the inguinal ligament. The 'broken saw-tooth' technique previously mentioned is again used, and as it is done the suture is gently pulled snug, not tight, so that the conjoint tendon and rectus sheath are rolled down on to the deep surface of the external oblique aponeurosis. Suturing is continued laterally until the conjoint tendon is brought up flush with the medial edge of the emergent spermatic cord. The suture is then tied.

The reconstruction of the posterior wall and the floor of the inguinal canal is now complete. The cord is now to be placed back in the canal.

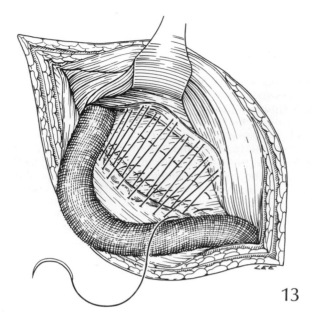

13

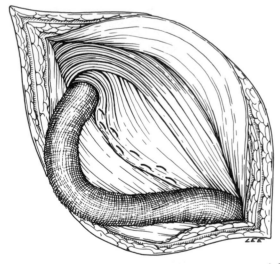

14

Closure

15

The external oblique aponeurosis

Now that the cord has been replaced the external oblique aponeurosis can be closed over it. Again a 'double-breasting' technique is used. The suturing is commenced medially, the lower lateral flap being sutured to the undersurface of the upper medial flap. Suturing is from medial to lateral and back again so that the upper flap is brought down over the lower flap and a new external inguinal ring is constructed at the medial end of the canal.

The repair is now complete and if all the layers have been sutured exactly as described the loads on the suture lines should be well distributed; there should be no undue tension and no splitting of fibre bundles. Indeed the structures should have just 'rolled together'.

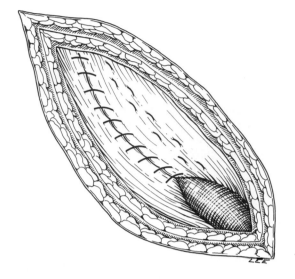
15

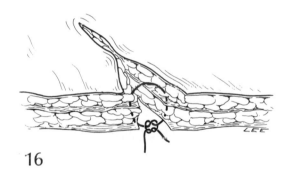
16

16

The subcutaneous tissue

The subcutaneous tissue is carefully closed with interrupted catgut sutures. No 'dead spaces' should be left and the fat should be closed so that the skin is closely approximated.

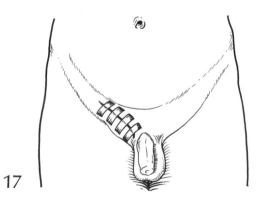
17

17

The skin

The skin is closed with microporous adhesive tape or a strip of gauze impregnated with collodion or similar adhesive. Non-penetrating skin clips give an equally good closure but require skilled attention when they are removed. Sutures should not be used.

18

Suture technique if monofilament stainless steel wire is used.

As an alternative to polypropylene, 34-gauge stainless steel wire can be used. This is the original material used by Dr Shouldice. Stainless steel is an excellent suture material which is strong and causes little tissue reaction. However, special attention must be given to technique if it is not to be broken or kinked in use. It is best to carry the wire as a loop on a long hook between each suture. The assistant must wield the hook carefully while at the same time keeping out of the operating surgeon's way and simultaneously maintaining the tension in the loop constant.

BILATERAL HERNIA

Bilateral hernia must never be repaired simultaneously for three reasons.

1. If sepsis occurs it may be bilateral if introduced at the same operation.
2. After simultaneous bilateral herniorrhaphy there is often much oedema and swelling of the penis and scrotum, which can make voiding tiresome and will delay convalescence.
3. There is evidence that simultaneous bilateral herniorrhaphy using the Shouldice technique may stretch the transversalis fascia unduly and predispose the patient to subsequent femoral hernia[4].

It is usual to allow an interval of 3–5 weeks between operations in bilateral hernias.

RECURRENT INGUINAL HERNIA

Recurrent inguinal hernias are always difficult and operation should only be undertaken by an experienced surgeon who is interested in this problem. If there is sepsis or sinus formation, operation should not be undertaken until it has settled. It may be necessary to remove all foreign suture material from the wound at a first operation and then wait some months before attempting the repair.

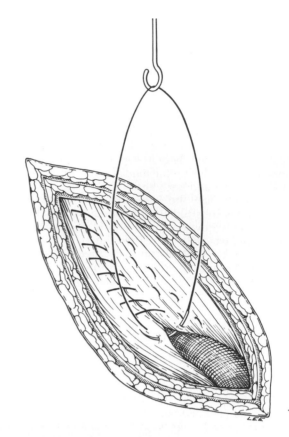

18

it is always wise to use wire on a recurrent hernia because this material is least likely to cause the sepsis to flare up. The technique is identical to that described above. Generally, tissue planes can be identified if a slow and gentle dissection is made. To date the author has never had to divide the cord in order to repair a recurrent hernia.

THE STRANGULATED HERNIA

The same operative technique can be used to treat a strangulated inguinal hernia. If additional access is required to deal with gangrenous gut the deep ring can be enlarged medially by dividing the deep epigastric vessels between ligatures, taking care to avoid the bladder. It is preferable to perform a standard paramedian incision for access to the main peritoneal cavity rather than to have to do an awkward resection of gangrenous tissue through the groin incision.

Postoperative care

Immediate active mobilization is the key to rapid convalescence. The 'client with a hernia' must not be allowed to become institutionalized into the 'postoperative patient'.

If the operation has been performed under local anaesthesia the patient should be helped to *walk* from the operating table. If general anaesthesia has been used the patient must be made to get up and walk as soon as he is conscious. There may be slight pain after surgery and a suitable mild analgesic should be prescribed. Analgesics with narcotic properties are never needed.

The wound dressing is removed *by the patient* on the fifth postoperative day. After the dressing is removed the patient can shower or bath normally.

Light office or professional work can be resumed after about 7 days and most other heavier jobs after about 8 weeks. Patients are told that they may undertake any work which does not cause pain to their wounds.

Some personal results

Over a period of 9 years 603 primary hernia repairs have been performed using this technique. So far, there have been only 5 recurrences. In 4 of these, multistrand polyester suture material had been used and the wound became septic and formed sinuses. In the remaining recurrence, steel wire had been used; in this case the wound became slightly inflamed some 4 days after the patient had gone home, and the wound was immediately reopened by another surgeon and the wire removed. All 5 primary recurrences were reoperated on and to date these second repairs have been sound[10].

Of 81 patients operated on for recurrent hernia, only one has developed a recurrence.

Conclusion

The Shouldice operation can be recommended for three reasons.

1. It has given uniformly excellent results in Toronto, Philadelphia and Stockton on Tees[4,5,6] and the results are significantly better than those of other techniques reported in the British literature[11,12].

2. It conforms to the principles of good repair surgery, namely, careful and accurate restoration of anatomical planes and their approximation by non-irritative suture material until firm biological union is accomplished.

3. It is, when combined with good management policies, cost effective.

References

1. Marcy, H. O. The cure of hernia. Journal of the American Medical Association 1887; 8: 589–592

2. Zimmerman, L. M., Anson, B. J. Anatomy and surgery of hernia. 2nd ed. Baltimore: Williams and Wilkins, 1967

3. Bassini, E. Ueber die Behandlung des Leistenbruches. Archiv für Klinische Chirurgie 1890; 40; 429–476

4. Glassow, F. The shouldice repair of inguinal hernia. In: Varco, R. I., Delaney, J. P., eds. Controversy in surgery. Philadelphia: W. B. Saunders, 1976

5. Myers, R. N., Shearburn, E. W. The problem of recurrent inguinal hernia. Surgical Clinics of North America 1973; 53: 555–558

6. Devlin, H. B., Russell, I. T., Muller, D., Sahay, A. K., Tiwari, P. N. Short stay surgery for inguinal hernia. Lancet 1977; 1: 847–849

7. Neuhauser, D. Elective inguinal herniorrhaphy versus truss in the elderly. In: Bunker, J. P., Barnes, B. A., Mosteller, F., eds. Costs, risks and benefits of surgery. New York: Oxford University Press, 1977

8. Russell, I. T., Devlin, H. B., Fell, M., Glass, N. J., Newell, J. J. Day-case surgery for hernias and haemorrhoids. Lancet 1977; 1: 844–846

9. Department of Health and Social Security. Administrative arrangements: planned early discharge of patients undergoing surgery. London: HMSO, 1978 (Notes on good practices No. 12)

10. Datta, D., Zaidi, A., Devlin, M. B. Short stay surgery for inguinal hernia. Lancet 1980; 2: 99–100

11. Marsden, A. J. Inguinal hernia: a three year review of one thousand cases. British Journal of Surgery 1958; 46: 234–243

12. Shuttleworth, K. E. D., Davies, W. H. Treatment of inguinal hernia. Lancet 1960; 1: 126–127

Femoral hernia

H. Brendan Devlin MA, MD, MCh, FRCS, FRCS(I)
Consultant Surgeon, North Tees General Hospital, Stockton on Tees, Cleveland;
Associate Lecturer in Clinical Surgery, University of Newcastle upon Tyne

Introduction

A femoral hernia is a protrusion of a peritoneal sac covered with extraperitoneal fat through the femoral canal medial to the femoral vessels as they proceed from the abdomen into the thigh. A femoral hernia sac may contain all or part of an abdominal viscus.

Femoral hernias occur much less frequently than inguinal and, in contradistinction to the latter, are more frequent in females than males. In the author's experience, the ratio of femoral to inguinal hernias is 18:1, and in femoral hernia the ratio of female to male is 3.9:1.

The aetiology of femoral hernia is ill understood. In contrast to inguinal hernia, there is no easy embryological explanation. The fact that femoral hernias are most frequently found in middle-aged and elderly females and the disparity in incidence between parous and nulliparous women suggests that intra-abdominal pressure and the stretching of aponeurotic tissue consequent on pregnancy are important factors. Chronic cough, intestinal obstruction, constipation and excessive physical labour may also contribute to raised intra-abdominal pressure. Weight loss in the elderly female is also associated with femoral hernia.

Operation should always be advised, for two reasons.

1. It is impossible to make and fit an adequate truss to control such a hernia.
2. The incidence of strangulation in these hernias is high – and strangulated hernia in the elderly carries considerable morbidity.

When a patient presents with intestinal obstruction and a femoral hernia, and the hernia is not tender and therefore not strangulated, reduction by taxis may be employed in the short term, but if there is any suggestion that strangulation has occurred taxis should not be employed. Urgent operation is obligatory for all cases of strangulated femoral hernia.

1

Anatomy

Femoral hernia has a sinister reputation because of the unyielding anatomy of the femoral canal. The whole canal (that is, the space between the pubis and the iliopsoas muscle) is bounded anteriorly by the inguinal ligament, posteriorly by the pectineal ligament at its attachment to the pubic bone, medially by the sharp lateral margin of the lacunar ligament and laterally by the iliopsoas muscle with its overlying fascia. The canal is divided into two compartments, the lateral being occupied by the femoral artery and femoral vein, and the smaller medial by areolar tissue, some lymphatics and a lymph node. It is through this small medial compartment that a femoral hernia penetrates into the thigh. In its advancement into the thigh the hernial sac carries with it some extraperitoneal fat about its fundus and it may draw the extraperitoneal anterolateral wall of the bladder down with it on its medial aspect. Once the sac is entrenched in the thigh its medial wall is pressed up against the sharp unyielding margin of the lacunar ligament medially, the unyielding pectineal fascia and pubic bone posteriorly, the inguinal ligament anteriorly and the femoral vein laterally. Compression of the femoral vein and the saphenous vein by a femoral hernia may occur; indeed, visible distension of these veins has been described as a diagnostic sign in the differential diagnosis of a femoral hernia from other groin swellings.

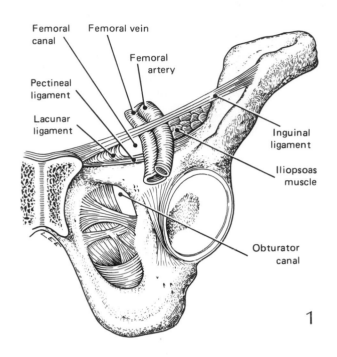

1

Types of operation

Because of its complex anatomical relationships there is no simple access to the femoral canal. Three approaches to femoral herniorrhaphy are described here because no one operation is ideal or uniformly suited to each case.

1. The abdominal, suprapubic or extraperitoneal operation developed by Henry[1]. This is often known as the McEvedy, though Henry used a midline incision and McEvedy a pararectus approach[2].
2. The inguinal or 'high' operation[3, 4].
3. The crural or 'low' operation[5].

The extraperitoneal approach gives excellent access to the femoral canal and to the general peritoneal cavity, should that be necessary to deal with a strangulated viscus. However, this approach to the pelvis is unfamiliar to most surgeons and therefore not to be recommended to the inexperienced surgeon operating on his first strangulated femoral hernia at dead of night.

The inguinal approach is familiar but has the twin drawbacks of disrupting the inguinal canal mechanism and not providing adequate access to a strangulated viscus.

The crural approach to the femoral sac is good and bloodless and repair of the hernia is easy by this method. Its very significant disadvantage is that access to a strangulated viscus is often very inadequate.

The crural approach is recommended to the occasional or novice surgeon. If a visceral strangulation is present it is best to perform a standard lower paramedian incision and deal with the crisis through an incision which is familiar to most abdominal operators. With an emergency situation, or for the inexperienced surgeon, there is no place for an anatomical extravaganza. The 'low' operation will be described in detail.

CRURAL OPERATION

Preoperative

Preoperative management

In the uncomplicated case no special preoperative management is required. The lower abdominal and upper thigh area should be shaved and it is best to have the patient catheterized before surgery (the bladder is often involved in the medial wall of the hernial sac and preoperative catheterization will lessen the likelihood of bladder injury).

If the hernia is obstructed or strangulated, preoperative nasogastric aspiration and appropriate fluid replacement will be required.

Anaesthesia

General anaesthesia is preferred, but local anaesthesia can be employed. If it is, the operating surgeon must remember that the parietal peritoneum is very sensitive and manipulation of it can cause the patient much discomfort unless the anaesthesia is adequate. Wide local infiltration with 0.5 per cent lignocaine with adrenaline 1:200 000 is adequate. Up to 500 mg of lignocaine (100 ml of 0.5 per cent solution) can be administered safely to a healthy 70 kg adult but this quantity will need to be reduced in the elderly or in debilitated patients. As an alternative to lignocaine there is bupivacaine hydrochloride 0.25 per cent with adrenaline 1:400 000 which could be used. The dosage should not exceed 2 mg per kg of body weight. Bupivacaine has the advantage that anaesthesia lasts longer than with lignocaine.

Suture materials

The suture material for the repair of the fascia of the femoral canal is metric 3 polypropylene. For haemostasis metric 2 chromic catgut and diathermy are used. The hernial sac and parietal peritoneum are closed with metric 3.5 chromic catgut. The subcutaneous tissue is sutured with metric 3.5 and the skin closed with hypoallergenic microporous adhesive tape.

For the repair of the fascia of the femoral canal a J-shaped 30 mm tapercut needle is best, as it facilitates the deep suturing to the pectineal fascia.

The operation

Position of patient

The patient is placed flat supine on the operating table.

Draping

If the hernia is not strangulated, towels are placed to allow access to the affected groin area only. If strangulation is present or suspected the sterile towels should be placed so that there is easy access to the lower abdomen.

2

The incision

A skin incision is made directly over the hernia and about 2.0 cm below the inguinal ligament. The incision should be about 6.0 cm long and oblique so that it is parallel to the inguinal ligament.

After the skin has been divided it is easy to separate the subcutaneous fat down to the coverings of the hernial sac. Secure haemostasis should be attained before the sac is mobilized.

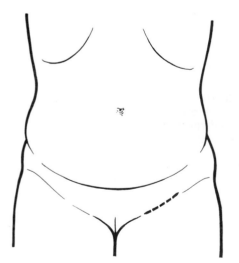

2

3

Mobilization of the sac

The sac, having emerged from the femoral canal, carries before it transversalis fascia and extraperitoneal fascia in front of which is the attenuated cribriform fascia and femoral vessel fascial layer in the thigh. Because of these fascial layers the sac usually makes a forward and upward turn in its path and its fundus can be found lying over the inguinal ligament. It is important to appreciate this before mobilization is attempted. Once the sac is identified the fascial layers are cleaned from it by blunt dissection, which is best achieved by wiping the fascia off with a gauze swab. These extraperitoneal coverings of the sac are frequently quite thick.

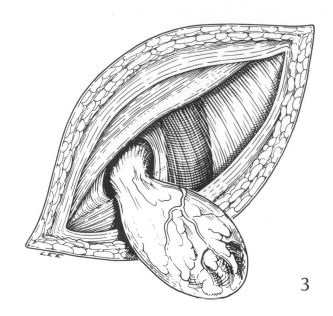

3

Identification of femoral opening

The neck of the sac is now cleared of fat and fascia so that the boundaries of the femoral canal can be identified. It is best to identify the medial and anterior margins of the canal first. The medial margin is the lacunar ligament and is easily seen as it sweeps around from the inguinal ligament to the subjacent pubic bone. Anteriorly, the rolled-over edge of the inguinal ligament can readily be separated from the sac underneath it and the sac should next be lifted up. The fascia on the pectineus muscle is easily recognizable and if this is traced back to the ramus of the pubis, the posterior margin of the canal – the pectineal ligament – can be recognized.

Attention is now turned to the lateral boundary of the canal – the femoral vein. This is the most vulnerable structure in this area and is difficult to identify because it is covered with a quite opaque fascial sheath. One manoeuvre is to identify the femoral artery by touch; the artery lies immediately lateral to the vein so the vein *must* be in any space between the sac and the palpable artery. A careful dissection is made on the lateral side of the sac, preferably using 'curved on the flat' dissecting scissors

and keeping close to the sac. The dissection of the sac is only complete when the entire circumference of its neck has been clearly defined.

Inspection of contents of sac

The lateral side of the fundus of the sac should now be opened. The medial side should be avoided, as it may be partly formed by the bladder. There is always much adherent extraperitoneal fat on the fundus which generally contains many distended veins. If these bleed they can confuse the anatomy, so the fat should be gently broken through with a haemostat point and the bleeding carefully controlled.

Inside the extraperitoneal fat the true peritoneal hernial sac will be found. It is grasped in a haemostat and then opened.

Any contents of the sac can now be gently freed, adhesions divided and the contents reduced back into the general peritoneal cavity. If strangulation is present an alternative approach to the remainder of the operation may be necessary (*see* p. 57 in this chapter).

4 & 5

Closure and excision of sac

When it is certain that the neck of the sac is isolated and that the sac is empty it can be closed and excised. Traction is applied to the open sac and, using metric 3.5 catgut on a 40 mm round needle, a transfixion suture should be securely tied around the neck. The redundant sac is cut off, leaving a generous cuff beyond the transfixion suture, and the stump of the sac will now recede through the femoral canal and out of sight.

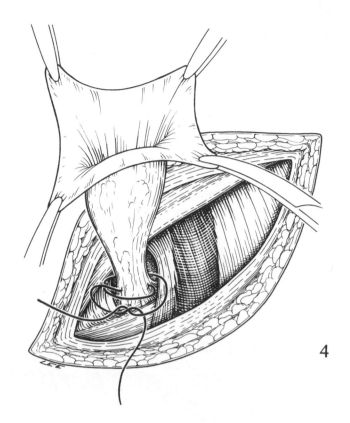

4

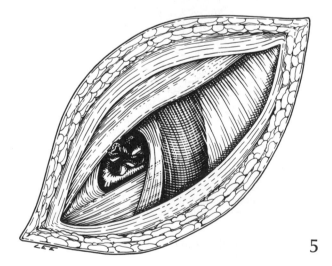

5

Repair of canal

First stage

The canal is repaired using a single figure-of-eight suture of metric 3 polypropylene on a J-shaped needle.

6

The femoral vein is retracted laterally and the pectineal ligament clearly identified on the superior ramus of the pubic bone. The first suture is placed through this ligament from its deep aspect at the point where the medial margin of the femoral vein would lie if it were not retracted. It is necessary to experiment with the retractor and identify this point correctly. If the suture is placed too far laterally the vein will be compromised, and if placed too far medially the repair will be unsound.

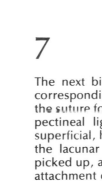

6

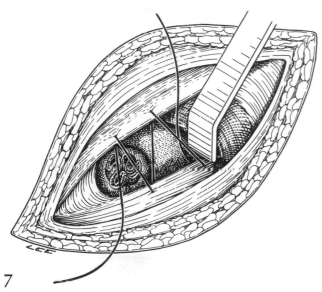

7

7

The next bite must pick up the inguinal ligament at a corresponding distance from its pubic attachment so that the suture forms the base of an isosceles triangle. Next the pectineal ligament is picked up, again from deep to superficial, halfway between the first pectineal suture and the lacunar ligament, and last the inguinal ligament is picked up, again halfway between the first suture and the attachment of the ligament to the pubis.

8

Now the free end of the suture is passed deep to the two loops and the two ends are tied securely. When the suture is pulled tight, the medial 0.75 cm or so of the inguinal ligament will be approximated to the pectineal line and the femoral canal closed. Futhermore, if the knot is placed at the medial side it will be away from the femoral vein which will not be damaged by it.

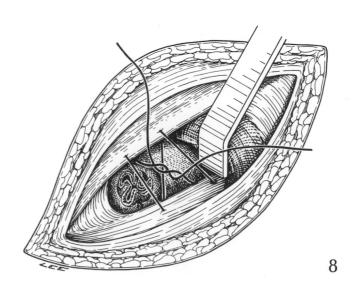

8

9 & 10

Second stage

So far the canal has been closed by the apposition of two tendinous structures under some degree of tension. According to the rules of biological repair tendinous structures drawn together under tension and subject to varying stresses such as respiration and movement do not heal readily. Therefore it is advisable to reinforce the union with a further aponeurotic patch which is not under tension. This is easily achieved by raising a flap of fascia off the surface of the pectineus muscle and suturing it to the external oblique aponeurosis in such a way that it covers the initial repair of the femoral canal. A continuous polypropylene suture is used for this double-breasting manoeuvre.

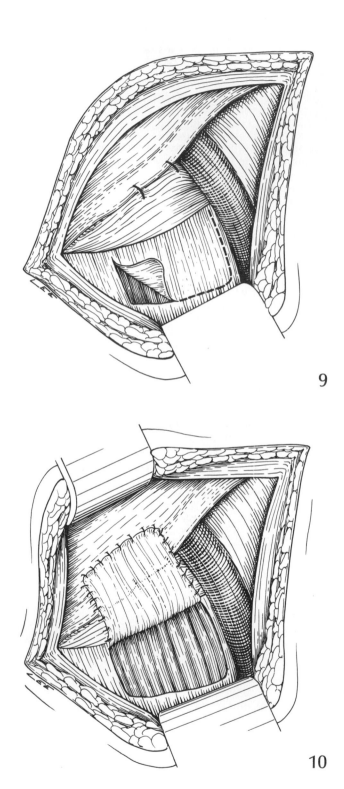

9

10

Closure

11

The subcutaneous fat is closed meticulously with interrupted metric 3.5 chromic catgut sutures. Haemostasis must be secure and any dead space must be avoided.

The skin is closed with microporous adhesive tape or gauze impregnated with Collodion.

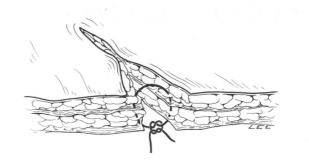

11

Postoperative care

No special postoperative care is required. There should be no postoperative restriction of activity save that imposed in the first few days by postoperative pain which in any case should be minimal.

Strangulation

If strangulation is suspected the sac is approached as described. Once the sac is identified it will be seen to contain blood-stained fluid if strangulation has occurred. The sac should be opened on the lateral aspect of its fundus and the contents inspected. A variety of intra-abdominal viscera may be found in the femoral hernia sac. No viscus should be returned to the peritoneal cavity unless it is definitely viable. Viability of any viscus can only be assessed after its blood supply has been normalized by removing the constriction at the neck of the sac.

Any blood-stained fluid in the sac is sucked out (and some sent for microbiological culture) and the contents of the sac are gently manipulated so that the neck of the sac is revealed clearly. It is very important to be careful with a strangulated loop of gut, as operative perforation can seriously weaken the patient's condition. Quite frequently, careful dissection of the neck of the sac and removal of oedematous extraperitoneal fat about it are all that is required to release the strangulation. The constricting agent is usually the thickened peritoneal neck of the sac and the oedematous extraperitoneal fat about it rather than the ligamentous structures which form the anterior, posterior and medial margins of the sac. The femoral vein is very rarely involved in the strangulation process, which confirms that the neck of the sac itself is most usually the constricting agent.

When the sac has been opened the inguinal ligament can generally be retracted upwards and the femoral vein laterally so that the neck of the sac can be divided.

After the strangulation has been released any contained viscera are wrapped in warm saline packs and left alone for a full 5 min before being inspected. Omentum of doubtful viability is best excised. Small intestine must only be returned to the peritoneal cavity if it has all been inspected and shown to be vital. Often there is a linear necrosis of the bowel where it has been compressed by the neck of the sac and this should be oversewn.

If a considerable segment of gangrenous small bowel needs resection more gut is prolapsed into the wound. Alternatively, if there is technical difficulty, an ipsilateral lower paramedian incision can be made and bowel resected through the groin wound (to avoid contamination of the peritoneal cavity). Anastomosis is then carried out through the main peritoneal cavity. It is worth stressing the importance of not contaminating the main peritoneal cavity and not returning non-viable bowel into it. The use of an ipsilateral lower paramedian incision for all cases of difficulty is strongly recommended.

INGUINAL OPERATION[3,4]

This operation achieves the same objective of fastening the medial portion of the inguinal ligament to the pectineal ligament in order to reduce the size of the femoral canal as has been described above using the crural approach. However, in the inguinal approach the femoral canal is exposed by opening the posterior wall – the transversalis fascia – of the inguinal canal.

The incision and dissection for this operation are exactly the same as those employed in the Shouldice operation for inguinal hernia (see pp. 40–43 in this volume). After the transversalis fascia in the posterior wall of the inguinal canal has been opened the extraperitoneal fat on the neck of the femoral hernia can be identified and removed by blunt dissection. The sac can now either be delivered above the inguinal ligament or opened below the ligament and its contents reduced. The neck of the sac is then transfixed and ligated.

The medial extremity of the inguinal ligament is now sutured to the pectineal. Again a figure-of-eight polypropylene suture is used but in this operation it is inserted from above, that is, through the incision in the posterior wall of the inguinal canal. The inguinal canal is then repaired using the Shouldice technique (see pp. 45–48 in this volume), care being taken to reinforce the femoral repair with the overlapped transversalis fascia at the medial part of the canal.

The inguinal approach for the repair of femoral hernia is not recommended as the operation of choice because it is technically more difficult and more time-consuming than the crural operation and because it disrupts an otherwise normal inguinal canal.

EXTRAPERITONEAL OPERATION[1]

This operation illustrates the genius of an expert surgical anatomist exploiting fascial plane dissection at its most elegant. Henry's extraperitoneal approach to the anterior pelvis gives an excellent exposure of both femoral canals simultaneously, but it is not an operation for the tyro. In the hands of an expert it is a fine operation enabling bilateral femoral hernia to be dealt with simultaneously through one incision.

The patient is placed on the operating table and the bladder emptied by catheterization. A vertical midline suprapubic incision is made, the aponeurotic layer is opened and the peritoneum exposed. The recti are retracted to either side and the space between the peritoneum and the abdominal wall muscles is opened by gentle blunt dissection in order to approach the femoral canal on either side. Femoral sacs are dealt with by reduction of their contents, transfixion of their necks and resection of redundant sac. If strangulation is present the subjacent peritoneum can easily be opened, the contents of the sac inspected, and so forth. The femoral canal is repaired using a non-absorbable suture as described in the inguinal operation (see p. 45 in this volume). The anterior abdominal wall is closed layer by layer.

References

1. Henry, A. K. Extensile exposure. 2nd ed. Edinburgh and London: Livingstone, 1957

2. McEvedy, P. G. Femoral hernia. Annals of the Royal College of Surgeons of England 1950; 7: 484–496

3. Annandale, T. Case in which a reducible oblique and direct inguinal and femoral hernia existed on the same side, and were successfully treated by operation. Edinburgh Medical Journal 1875; 21: 1087–1091

4. Lotheissen, G. Zur Radikaloperation der Schenkelhernien. Zentralblatt für Chirurgie 1898; 21: 548–550

5. Lockwood, C. B. The radical cure of femoral and inguinal hernia. Lancet 1893; 2: 1297–1302

Hernia repair: the mesh plug hernia repair

Ira M. Rutkow MD, MPH, DrPH
Surgical Director, The Hernia Center, Freehold, New Jersey, USA

Alan W. Robbins MD
Surgical Director, The Hernia Center, Freehold, New Jersey, USA

Principles and justification

Since the early 1980s, the surgical techniques used in repairing groin hernias have undergone a profound transformation. These changes are highlighted by the fact that, in 1996, over 50% of all groin hernia repairs incorporated a mesh prosthesis as part of the repair[1,2]. American surgeons are increasingly enamoured with the concept of a 'tension-free' hernia repair in which the mesh prosthesis is not utilized to buttress or support a primary sutured herniorrhaphy but *is* the actual repair.

It is estimated that, in 1996, almost 750 000 groin herniorrhaphies were completed in the USA. Of this total, approximately 620 000 were unilateral repairs, 100 000 were repaired bilaterally, and 30 000 were femoral hernias. In addition, there were some 90 000 umbilical herniorrhaphies, 75 000 epigastric, Spigelian and other abdominal wall hernia repairs, and 80 000 incisional herniorrhaphies. Since one million hernia operations are completed annually, it is self-evident that enormous socioeconomic forces relate to the practice of hernia surgery. Among the most evident of these socioeconomic influences is the fact that over 80% of inguinal hernia repairs are now conducted on an ambulatory basis. In the USA it would be considered out of the ordinary to be hospitalized overnight for any type of elective groin herniorrhaphy.

Unfortunately, no recent reliable studies have been published concerning the incidence or the prevalence of abdominal wall hernias in the general population. Such important, yet basic, questions as the percentage chance of an individual being in need of a herniorrhaphy over the course of his or her lifetime or the absolute number of hernias that exist in the USA on any given day are therefore statistically undefined. What is available are data regarding age and sex characteristics of individuals who undergo herniorrhaphy. For instance, 92% of all persons undergoing an inguinal hernia repair are men, while for femoral hernia only 26% are men. Regarding age at the time of hernia repair for inguinal herniorrhaphy, 18% are under the age of 15 years, 26% are aged 15–44 years, 30% are 45–64 years old, and 26% are over the age of 65, while for femoral hernia, 27% are aged 15–44 years, 31% are 45–64 years old, and 42% are above 65 years of age. All other abdominal wall hernias, including umbilical, epigastric, and incisional, are in a ratio of 65% women to 35% men. As a group, abdominal wall hernias are performed most frequently in the 45–64 year age group[3].

One of the newer methods of prosthetic based hernioplasties is that of laparoscopic hernia repair. Over the last 5 years the laparoscopic companies and the surgeons who represent them have tried to persuade surgeons and the lay public of the perceived benefits of laparoscopic hernia repair. Laparoscopic instrument makers had hoped that, by 1995, 25–35% of all herniorrhaphies performed in the USA would be done laparoscopically. This goal has not been achieved, and the reality is that currently less than 5% of all hernioplasties are completed using a laparoscope.

Unlike laparoscopic cholecystectomy, laparoscopic hernia repair has not been accepted by the American surgical profession[4]. There are four likely explanations for this: (1) technical (laparoscopic hernia surgery is difficult to perform), (2) clinical (scarcity of long-term studies examining recurrence and complication rates), (3) experience and learning curve (for many surgeons the learning curve exceeds the number of hernia operations they perform in a given year), and (4) cost reimbursement (laparoscopic hernia surgery is expensive and insurance carriers are increasingly reluctant to pay for the unnecessary use of advanced technologies).

The surgical literature on hernia repair suggests a better short-term and long-term result when the repair is performed by a specialized hernia surgeon or service than that obtained by general surgeons not dedicated to the field of hernia repair. At present a dozen or so surgeons in private practice in the USA have developed a special interest in hernias and operate on them to the exclusion of other surgical procedures. The collective experience of these surgeons, not just relative to the actual operative repair but with regard to a more complete understanding of hernias as part of the human condition, deserves closer attention. By dealing only with a single surgical condition 'hernia specialists', who perform hundreds of hernia repairs annually, gain insight into the disease process which a general surgeon cannot achieve.

What has become increasingly evident is that time honoured methods of evaluating hernia surgery are, in fact, outmoded and, perhaps, even deleterious to the practice of surgery. For instance, recurrence rates have long been considered the 'gold standard' upon which herniorrhaphies are measured. However, it has been reliably demonstrated that low recurrence rates can be achieved regardless of which of a number of hernia repair techniques is utilized. Regardless of whether it is a tissue-to-tissue or sutured hernia repair, a tension-free or mesh-based technique, or even a laparoscopic repair, there is a relative agreement of recurrence rates in the hands of hernia specialists. Accordingly, the outcome measures must include (1) recurrence rates, (2) technical difficulty, (3) overall complication rates and seriousness of the complications, (4) overall rehabilitation including short-term and long-term postoperative discomfort and return to daily and work activities, and (5) socioeconomic factors, notably cost.

By incorporating these five outcome measures into the evaluation process, the once straightforward task of determining clinical efficacy becomes a more complicated process. Which relevant end point, if any, should take precedence over the others? For example, in the difficult economic times of the 1990s, are socioeconomic factors and recurrence rates equally important? Some might suggest that the former are significantly more critical than the latter[5,6]!

The use of mesh prosthetics in hernia surgery has caused many time-honoured surgical precepts to be reconsidered. For instance, the concept of having to repair each layer of the defect in a discrete manner is no longer applicable. There should be no attempt to approximate weakened tendinous-aponeurotic-fascial structures with sutures. Instead, the mesh prosthesis itself becomes the repair. Tissue dissection should always be kept to a minimum, especially in recurrent hernia repairs. Misguided manoeuvres to identify anatomical structures, including fused abdominal wall layers, only leads to unacceptable postoperative complications.

Of the newer mesh-based hernioplasties, the mesh plug or 'PerFix' repair has garnered the support of a growing number of American surgeons[7]. Through its simplicity of performance and reliance on a low cost hernia plug, it has been found applicable for all inguinal and femoral hernias. The 20 minute mesh plug repair is conducted on an ambulatory basis with most patients being discharged less than 2 h after completion of the operation.

Preoperative

For patients under the age of 40 years with no signs or symptoms of medical problems, no preoperative investigation is required. Individuals over 40 years of age undergo an electrocardiogram and a fingerstick haemoglobin assay. When it is deemed appropriate (e.g. cardiac or pulmonary difficulties, etc.), the patient is advised to consult an internal medicine or family practice specialist to receive medical clearance specifically for ambulatory surgery.

The operative site is shaved just before the start of the procedure and involves only the section of skin where the incision is to be made. Skin is prepared with povidone-iodine and alcohol. Even though a mesh prosthesis is the mainstay of the hernia repair, antibiotics are not routinely administered as part of the surgical routine. Marlex mesh, of which the PerFix plug is composed, is particularly resistant to infection, and in over 3000 plug repairs dating back to 1989 there has not been a single case in which the mesh plug has had to be removed because of a wound infection.

Anaesthesia

Oral intake, except for cardiac or antihypertensive medication, is stopped after midnight of the night before surgery. Epidural anaesthesia is routinely used. This method allows the patient to cough or strain on command during the operation, and aids in testing the integrity of the plug repair. The epidural regimen, using 3% chloroprocaine (2 ml of fentanyl is added to the 30 ml vial of chloroprocaine) in addition to 1 mg of intravenous midazolam, preserves most motor function which permits patients to move their lower extremities while under a profound sensory block with little peritoneal sensation. Since chloroprocaine has rapid onset and ultrashort duration, patients are able to walk within 60 min of the end of the procedure.

Operation

PRIMARY INGUINAL HERNIA REPAIR

Skin incision

1 With the patient supine, the operating room table is placed in a head down or Trendelenburg position. This provides easier access to the inguinal canal, especially in obese individuals. A 6-cm skin incision is used starting at the pubic tubercle and extending towards the anterior iliac crest. The orientation of such an incision directly overlies the inguinal canal, in particular the external and internal inguinal rings. A scalpel is used only to provide an incision in the epidermis. The remainder of the incision and all subsequent tissue dissection, including that of the hernia sac off the spermatic cord, is accomplished with electrocautery. This instrument provides excellent haemostasis and markedly decreases postoperative haematoma and seroma formation. Average blood loss during a PerFix herniorrhaphy should be less than 5 ml.

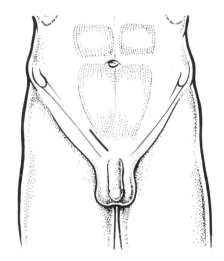

1

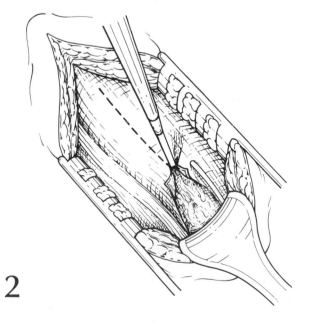

2

Exposure

2 The subcutaneous tissues are opened down to the external oblique aponeurosis. The aponeurosis is split from the external ring to just above its location over the internal ring. A self-retaining blunt Beckman retractor and a hand-held Goelet retractor provide excellent exposure.

Exposure of the spermatic cord

3 With the sweeping motion of a finger, the external oblique fascia is separated medially from the underlying tissues to provide a simple form of abdominal wall relaxation. The lateral leaf of the external oblique fascia is similarly freed from the underlying structures in order to expose the entire inguinal canal and spermatic cord. A rubber drain is placed around the cord at the level of the pubic tubercle.

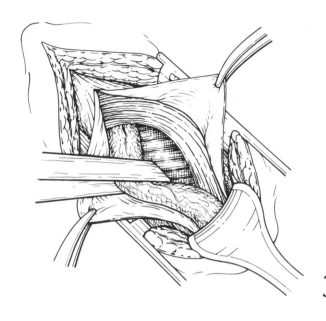

3

Dissection

The essential feature of the PerFix hernia repair is minimal dissection. For too long, surgeons have laboured under the misconception that every anatomical structure in the inguinal canal has to be dissected and identified. This unnecessary trauma leads to increased 'pain and suffering', the phrase which has given groin hernia surgery such an ugly epithet.

Indirect hernias

4 For the indirect hernia, the sac is approached by separating the cremasteric fibres longitudinally along the spermatic cord, so as not to destroy the cremasteric reflex. The cremasteric muscles should never be removed.

The indirect sac is dissected free to the level of the internal ring, along with any lipomata of the cord. The sac is rarely opened, except in cases of acutely incarcerated or strangulated hernia. Sacs do not therefore need to be ligated, nor should they be sent for routine but unnecessary pathological evaluation. The key element in completing a mesh plug indirect hernia repair is a high dissection, not a high ligation. The high dissection, characterized by visualizing the preperitoneal fat pad at the level of the internal ring, is essential in creating a pocket for positioning the PerFix hernia plug. The high dissection is greatly aided by pulling on the sac much like a taut rubber band and breaking up all adhesions between the sac and surrounding soft tissues.

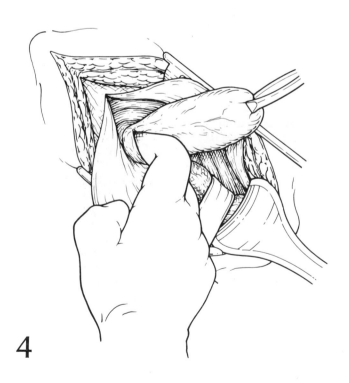

4

Direct hernias

5 In direct hernias the attenuated fusiform or sacular transversalis fascia is elevated with an Allis clamp. The base (e.g. neck) of the sac is completely circumscribed with electrocautery to allow the preperitoneal fat to 'pout' through. This is an essential step which creates an opening into the preperitoneal plane where the PerFix plug must ultimately be situated. It is important in completing the circumscription that this manoeuvre is not carried too far wide into areas of intact transversalis fascia. The posterior inguinal wall is rarely a heavy aponeurotic fascial structure. It is usually thin and may even be translucent. It is important for the surgeon to realize that the transversalis fascia is frequently intact in areas where it seems attenuated. To carry the dissection too wide creates a larger opening into the retroperitoneum than is needed.

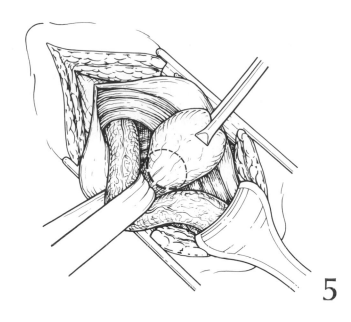

5

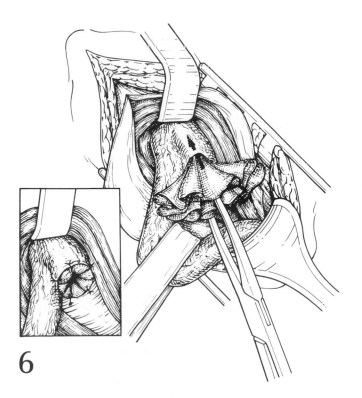

6

Placement of PerFix plug

Indirect hernia

6 The freely dissected indirect sac and any adjacent lipomata are placed back through the internal ring into the abdominal cavity. A PerFix plug is inserted, tapered end first through the internal ring and placed into position just beneath the crura. The fluted outside layer of the plug, combined with its inside configuration of eight mesh 'petals', maintains the overall contour of the device while allowing it to conform tension-free to the configuration of the internal ring. If the overall bulk of the PerFix plug is deemed excessive, then some of the inside 'petals' can be removed.

Regardless of the size of the internal ring, all PerFix plugs must be secured to the crura with a minimum of one or two interrupted sutures. This prevents any possible migration of the plug. With internal rings that are grossly attenuated, the plug should be secured to the crura with multiple interrupted sutures. The patient is requested to cough or strain to verify correct positioning of the plug and to ensure that the hernia sac remains securely reduced behind the prosthesis.

Direct hernia

7 The freed sac and overlying attenuated transversalis fascia and transversus abdominis aponeurosis layer are invaginated. As with the indirect repair, a plug is inserted narrow end first through the newly created floor defect and secured to surrounding intact tissue using multiple interrupted sutures. Because Marlex mesh has a well documented 'Velcro-like' reaction to tissue, any surface, regardless of how flimsy it may appear, usually suffices to hold the plug in position. The patient is requested to cough or strain to verify correct positioning of the plug.

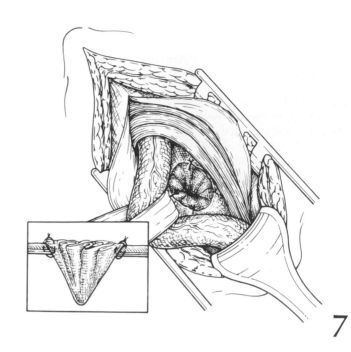

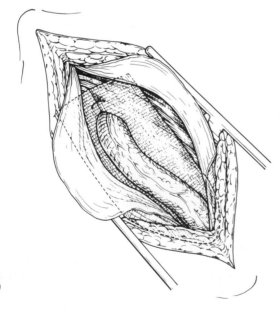

Placement of onlay patch

8 All indirect and direct primary hernias are reinforced with a second piece of flat Marlex mesh. This onlay patch is placed on the anterior surface of the posterior wall of the inguinal canal from the pubic tubercle to above the internal ring. The lateral portion of the onlay patch includes an aperture for the spermatic cord. This split section is sutured back together to itself, thereby providing an opening for the cord while functioning as a pseudo-internal ring. It is important to understand that the onlay patch is intended solely to strengthen the direct space in an indirect repair and the area of the internal ring in a direct repair. The onlay patch is not an integral part of the current repair, but acts merely as a future prophylaxis.

Any successful PerFix plug repair is strictly related to the presence of a preperitoneally positioned plug placed through a small (6 cm) anterior surgical incision using minimal tissue dissection. For this reason, the onlay patch need not be secured with sutures but is laid in position, taking advantage of the 'Velcro-like' effect of Marlex. Despite the presence of an onlay patch, the PerFix plug procedure should not be confused with another well known tension-free mesh-based technique, the Lichtenstein repair, which consists solely of a circumferentially 'sutured' onlay patch.

Closure

9 Cord structures are placed on the anterior surface of the onlay patch. The external oblique aponeurosis is reapproximated over the cord structures with a continuous suture. Scarpa's fascia and subcutaneous tissues are brought together with interrupted sutures, and the skin edges are coapted with a running subcuticular stitch. A transparent, self-adhesive dressing is secured over the incision.

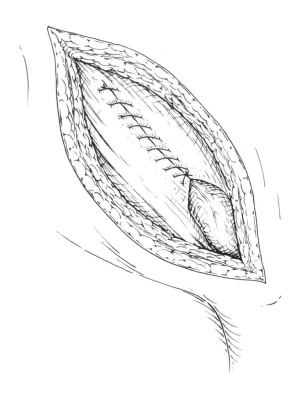

9

RECURRENT INGUINAL HERNIA REPAIR

The PerFix plug hernioplasty is also applicable to recurrent inguinal hernias. In operating on such defects, the generic surgical principle is to perform as little overall dissection as possible. Accordingly, routine attempts to identify fused anatomical layers are never made. Unlike primary repairs, the spermatic cord is not routinely mobilized with a recurrent hernia since attempts at such mobilization cause further damage to an already compromised cord.

The key to the mesh plug repair of a recurrent hernia is to locate an edge of the 'pearly-white' hernia sac using minimal tissue dissection. The recurrent direct sac, be it fusiform or saccular, is simply dissected down to its base on the inguinal floor. The base is circumscribed to allow preperitoneal fat to 'pout' through. This step helps release the sac completely from adjacent scarred areas and also permits full access to the preperitoneal space. The recurrent indirect sac is similarly freed, albeit with a high dissection beyond the internal ring. A finger is inserted through the direct defect or the internal ring to evaluate the integrity of the rest of the previous repair as well as the femoral area. The recurrent sac is then reduced without ligation or excision.

Using a similar technique as with primary hernia repair, the PerFix plug is inserted into the internal ring or placed into the direct defect. It is mandatory with all recurrent hernias that the mesh plug be secured with multiple anchoring sutures between it and the scarred margins of the rigid inguinal floor defect or the scarred internal ring. An onlay patch may be used, depending on whether the spermatic cord was mobilized and whether there is sufficient space to lay down such a flat piece of Marlex mesh.

SLIDING INGUINAL HERNIA REPAIR

A sliding inguinal hernia is treated with the same principle of minimal dissection. The sac is separated off the spermatic cord structures, a high dissection is completed, and the entire structure is placed back into the abdominal cavity. Attempts to reconstruct the sac wall are unnecessary.

FEMORAL HERNIA REPAIR

Operative approach

10 Using an infrainguinal approach, the mushroom like appearance of a femoral hernia is noted emanating from the femoral canal. Adhesions between the hernial sac and surrounding tissues are freed. If the femoral opening is too small and the sac too bulky to be adequately reduced, the sac is divided and ligated. It should then be possible to reduce the remaining proximal portion of the sac.

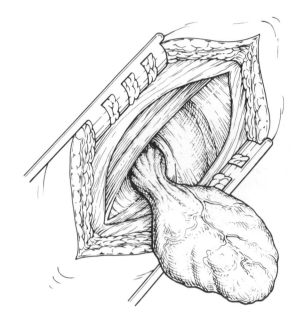

10

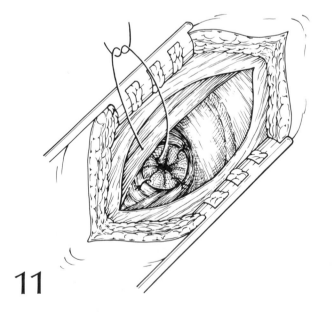

11

Placement of PerFix plug

11 The sac is reduced from outside in through the femoral canal. Using a PerFix hernia plug, all the inside 'petals' are removed and only the outside fluted layer of mesh is placed through the opening of the femoral canal. After proper positioning, the plug is secured by interrupted sutures to the surrounding fascia or other tissues which compromise the opening of the femoral canal. The patient is asked to cough or strain to verify positioning and complete reduction of the femoral hernia sac. An onlay patch is not required.

Closure is similar to that of an inguinal hernia repair.

Postoperative care

Neither oral nor hypodermic narcotic pain medicines are used postoperatively. Instead, a 60 mg intramuscular injection of ketorolac tromethamine is given in the recovery room. At discharge patients are provided with a prescription for 15 propoxyphene napsylate and paracetamol (acetaminophen) tablets. However, they are routinely instructed not to take these tablets unless discomfort becomes difficult to tolerate. Patients treated with a PerFix plug remain amazingly pain-free, and over 85% of them required nothing more than non-prescription pain medicine in the immediate postoperative period.

Every patient is permitted to begin lifting up to 9–10 kg whenever desired. Assuming that the individual will feel well, they may resume normal day-to-day activities (dinner engagements, light exercise, walking, etc.) including return to work at their own discretion. Heavy manual labour can be started in 2 weeks and other less intensive activities (aerobic workouts, bicycling, jogging, tennis, etc.) in a proportionally shorter amount of time.

Outcome

Since 1989, 3000 patients have had this hernia repair; the clinical effectiveness and universal application of the PerFix plug hernioplasty has been well demonstrated[7,8]. It is a technically simple surgical operation, which in a standardized form can be utilized to repair virtually any groin hernia. Most impressively, the mesh plug hernioplasty helps to reduce operative morbidity and short-term and long-term postoperative discomfort. From an anatomical and physiological standpoint, the plug repair is a preperitoneal procedure via an anterior surgical incision.

The PerFix plug is preferable to a mesh patch. It is easier to work with and far simpler to secure to surrounding tissues than a sutured onlay patch, especially those that lie in a preperitoneal plane. The cone-shaped configuration of the PerFix plug handles easily and forms a total occlusion of the defect. The interstices of the mesh become completely infiltrated with fibroblasts and the plug remains permanently strong. The mesh is not subject to deterioration or rejection and is not felt postoperatively by patients.

References

1. Goussous HG. Effectiveness of the mesh plug technique (letter). *Surgery* 1995; 117: 600.

2. Robbins AW, Rutkow IM. The mesh-plug hernioplasty. *Surg Clin North Am* 1993; 73: 501–12.

3. Rutkow IM, Robbins AW. Demographic, classificatory and socioeconomic aspects of hernia repair in the United States. *Surg Clin North Am* 1993; 73: 413–26.

4. Brooks DC. A prospective comparison of laparoscopic and tension-free open herniorrhaphy. *Arch Surg* 1994; 129: 361–6.

5. Rutkow IM. Laparoscopic hernia repair. The socioeconomic tyranny of surgical technology. *Arch Surg* 1992; 127: 1271.

6. Rutkow IM. The recurrence rate in hernia surgery: how important is it? *Arch Surg* 1995; 130: 575–6.

7. Rutkow IM, Robbins AW. 'Tension-free' inguinal herniorrhaphy: a preliminary report on the 'mesh plug' technique. *Surgery* 1993; 114: 3–8.

8. Rutkow IM, Robbins AW. Mesh plug hernia repair: a follow-up report. *Surgery* 1995; 117: 597–8.

Illustrations by Gillian Lee Illustrations

Hernia repair with mesh using local anaesthetic techniques

M. J. Notaras FRCS, FRCS(Ed), FACS
Honorary Consultant Surgeon, Barnet and Edgeware Hospitals, London and Consultant Surgeon, London Hernia Centre, London, UK

Principles and justification

The open mesh repair performed under sedation and local anaesthesia is ideal for ambulatory surgery. Avoiding general anaesthesia and using infiltration local anaesthesia has a significant impact in minimizing morbidity, especially for the elderly and patients with high ASA gradings. Obesity is not a contraindication. Bilateral hernias are repaired at one session. The technique is safe, simple, effective, economical, and is without post-anaesthesia side effects.

Modern pre-emptive and postoperative pain management, combined with local anaesthesia infiltration before incision, increases the duration of postoperative analgesia and is important in the overall management of hernia repair. This multimodal approach complements the surgical technique in reducing pain and stress in response to surgery. It results in an early return to normal activity within 1–2 weeks. Patients are able to walk and to urinate within hours of surgery.

Many patients are apprehensive about local anaesthetic techniques. It is important that they are well informed before admission with explanatory sheets on what is to be expected before, during and after the procedure. At admission, further reassurance helps to overcome any anxieties. Premedication before entering the theatre is not required.

Mesh

A monofilament polypropylene mesh such as Marlex or Prolene is preferred. These have a larger porosity than other monofilament meshes. It is essential that only monofilament synthetic sutures (000) are used for fixation. If infection occurs it should resolve with time. Multifilament suture materials such as silk, linen, cotton or braided synthetics should not be used as they predispose to persistent sinuses if the wound should become infected. A broad-spectrum antibiotic is given peroperatively in a single dose for prophylaxis against infection. When operating in a dedicated 'clean' theatre it has been shown that prophylactic antibiotics do not affect outcome.

Preoperative

Patients are starved of food for 4 h in case of the need to convert to general anaesthesia. Clear fluids may be taken up to 2 h before operation. The author prefers patients to be shaved with an electric razor on admission and then to walk to the theatre. Patients are monitored with pulse oximeter, continuous electrocardiographic and intermittent blood pressure recording. An intravenous cannula is inserted into the dorsum of the hand for drug administration.

Pre-emptive analgesia and local anaesthesia

Providing there are no contraindications, a diclofenac suppository (100 mg) is inserted before operation. Sedation is achieved and maintained by giving intravenous diazepam (5–25 mg) and intravenous pethidine (25–50 mg) titrated according to response. The elderly usually require less than 5 mg diazepam, while young adults or those with a history of a high alcohol intake may require high doses of diazepam (20–30 mg).

A surgeon-administered local anaesthetic 'infiltration as you proceed' technique is used in preference to a field block of the ilio-inguinal and ilio-hypogastric nerves. The latter technique is a blind and unreliable method. When inefffective, there is a tendency to inject large volumes of local anaesthetic in the area, which may result in excessive diffusion causing unwanted femoral nerve paresis. The technique is unsuitable for ambulatory surgery.

A mixture of 0.5% lignocaine and adrenaline 1/200 000 (40 ml) and 0.5% bupivacaine with adrenaline 1/200 000 (20 ml) is used. The lignocaine provides a rapid onset of anaesthesia and the bupivacaine provides pain relief of a longer duration. Plain local anaesthetic is required for patients receiving monoamine oxidase inhibitors or tricyclic antidepressants as the adrenaline may produce prolonged hypertension. About 30 ml of the local anaesthetic mixture is used for a single hernia. For simultaneous bilateral repair, the mixture is diluted with an equal volume of normal saline to a concentration of 0.25%.

Operations

Position of the patient

The supine patient is placed in a slight Trendelenburg position which assists venous return. Heparinization is unnecessary. A strap is placed just above the knee to prevent knee bending. The arms are crossed in front of the chest and gently secured to prevent their inadvertent downward movement. The hernia contents are reduced after the patient has been sedated. The patient's head should not be screened with drapes which are placed up to neck level. Conversation and music help to relax the atmosphere. The patient should be able to test the repair by coughing or attempting to raise the shoulders or legs.

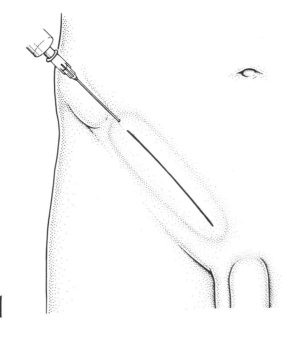

INGUINAL HERNIA REPAIR

1   The line of incision is marked with a 'Pentel' pen so that it does not rub off with the skin preparation which should be aqueous rather than alcohol-based. The latter may be painful if applied to the unanaesthetized scrotal area.

The local anaesthetic is infiltrated subcutaneously as the needle (23 gauge) is advanced along the line of the proposed incision. The tip of the needle is not in place long enough to cause an intravascular infusion of the drug. After incision, further anaesthetic is introduced deep to Scarpa's fascia and then the external oblique aponeurosis is exposed.

2 Approximately 10 ml of local anaesthetic is injected just underneath the aponeurosis at the lateral part of the incision. This will flood and distend the inguinal canal. The nerves of the inguinal canal are thus anaesthetized and the fluid dissection separates them from the external oblique aponeurosis. With this technique the nerves are more easily identifiable and less likely to be damaged on entering the inguinal canal. Occasionally, the ilio-inguinal nerve does not exit through the external ring and has to be freed so that it may be mobilized with the cord (inset).

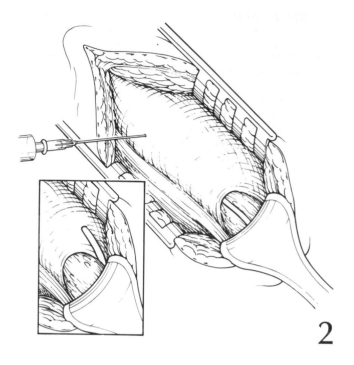

2

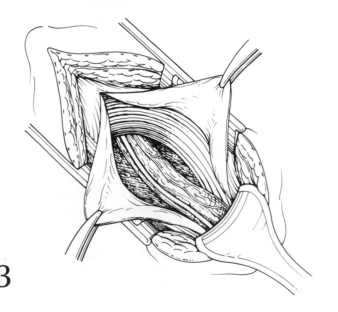

3

3 If there was difficulty in reducing the contents of a large sac before operation then, once the inguinal canal and external ring are opened, reduction may be achieved after further infiltration of local anaesthetic around the internal ring, into the cord and into other selected points. If reduction is difficult, then the hernia may be a sliding type or have adherent omentum or bowel in its sac. With sharp and finger dissection, the upper and lower leaves of the external oblique muscle are separated from the spermatic cord and the posterior wall of the inguinal canal. If the indirect sac is small or there is a direct hernia, then the cord is fully mobilized before dealing with the hernia. With a large indirect hernia it is sometimes better to open up the cord by incising the cremasteric muscle, identifying the sac and dissecting it free from the vas deferens and vessels. Local anaesthetic is injected between the sac and other structures to assist in the dissection. Once the indirect sac is dealt with or a sliding hernia has been returned to the abdominal cavity, the bulk and diameter of the spermatic cord is reduced, making it easier to complete its mobilization and free it from its attachments.

4 The spermatic cord is elevated with its cremaster muscle covering. Its medial attachments to the conjoint area are divided. The cremasteric (external spermatic) vessels with the adjacent genital branch of the genitofemoral nerve are identified in the spermatic fascia just inferior to the bulk of the cord. Local anaesthetic is injected between these structures and the inguinal ligament to increase the space separating them. This space is opened with the scissors to create a window which is entered with the finger to free the cord from its attachments to the floor of the inguinal canal. The cord is freed to at least 2 cm beyond the pubic tubercle. Just lateral to the pubic tubercle there are often small vessels supplying the external spermatic fascia and these may need coagulating before division.

For retraction, a soft rubber Paul's tube is placed around the mobilized cord to include the cremasteric (external spermatic) vessels, the ilio-inguinal nerve and the genital (cremasteric) nerve. The cremasteric muscle and fibres are preserved except for some fibres which may be cut medial to the cord at the internal ring for improved exposure of the posterior wall. Skeletonization or stripping and excision of the cremasteric muscle fibres is unnecessary, especially when using a mesh repair. It may injure the nerves and small blood vessels of the cord. The cuff of cremasteric muscle at the internal ring cushions the cord contents against the surrounding mesh. Lipomas of the cord at the internal ring are excised.

A small indirect sac is mobilized from its attachments to the cord and internal ring to just proximal to its neck. It is either excised or invaginated into the abdominal extraperitoneal space. The posterior wall of the inguinal canal and the femoral ring may be tested by digital

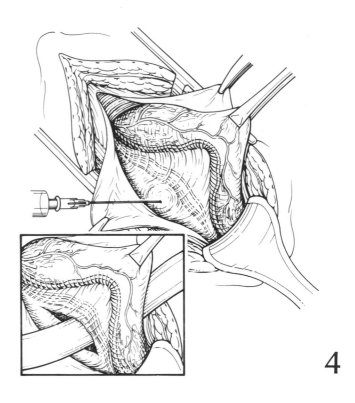

4

examination through the sac opening. With a Gilbert type I hernia, which only has a small internal ring and an intact canal floor, a simple onlay mesh repair is performed (*see Illustration 7*).

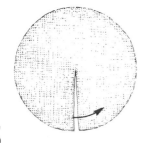
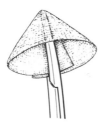

5

5 A sliding hernia is returned to the abdominal cavity after freeing it from the cord and internal ring. If there is a moderately enlarged internal ring admitting 1–2 fingers (Gilbert type II hernia) and there is attenuated transversalis fascia which cannot be used to repair the ring, a piece of mesh approximately 4–5 cm in diameter, shaped like an umbrella with a radial slit for overlap, may be inserted through the internal ring along the path of the former hernial protrusion to lie and spread in the extraperitoneal area adjacent to the internal ring. This helps to block the opening from within the extraperitoneal space. An onlay mesh repair is then performed (*see Illustration 7*).

6 A large indirect sac extending into the scrotum is transected just below the internal ring and the distal part left in the cord after reducing its contents. Adherent omentum or small bowel are easily dissected free and reduced as the diazepam provides considerable muscle relaxation. The anterior wall is incised and left open to prevent hydrocoele formation. Avoiding full sac dissection reduces bleeding, haematoma formation and testicular vessel damage which may result in testicular ischaemia.

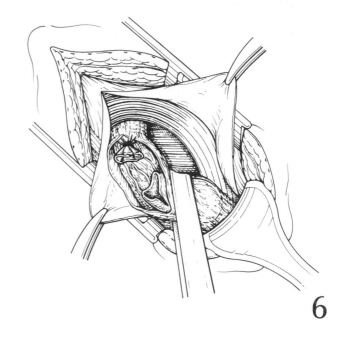

6

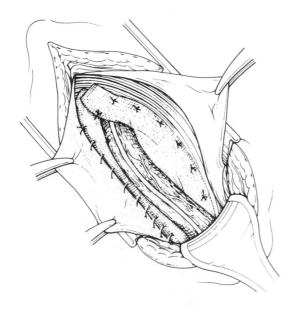

7

7 A large scrotal or sliding hernia with a large internal ring of two finger breadths or more (Gilbert type III hernia) might need some form of intenal ring and posterior wall reconstruction. Usually one can appose or imbricate the transversalis fascia to 'normalize' the posterior wall in preparation for an onlay mesh. Rarely, it may be necessary for an inlay mesh graft to be placed in the preperitoneal space and sutured behind the conjoint area and to the inguinal ligament (*see Illustration 13*).

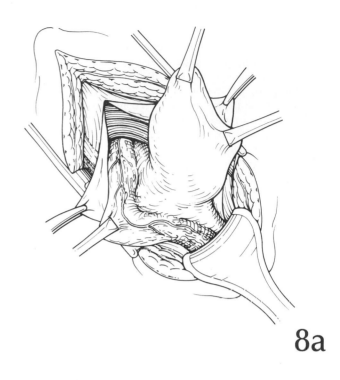

8a

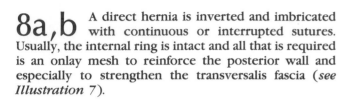 A direct hernia is inverted and imbricated with continuous or interrupted sutures. Usually, the internal ring is intact and all that is required is an onlay mesh to reinforce the posterior wall and especially to strengthen the transversalis fascia (*see Illustration* 7).

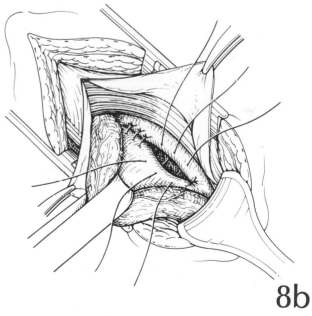

8b

9 Before inserting the mesh, the most medial border of the inguinal canal is displayed by separating the external oblique from the underlying internal oblique muscle. The dissection extends beyond, above and medial to the pubic tubercle. To improve exposure, an oblique cut upwards and medially onto the external oblique aponeurosis is sometimes necessary to release the most medial part of its upper leaf where it forms the external ring and becomes attached to the rectus aponeurosis. This creates a triangular flap of external oblique aponeurosis just above the pubic tubercle which can be used for both attachment and covering of the most medial part of the mesh.

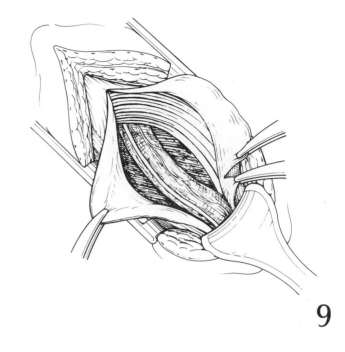

9

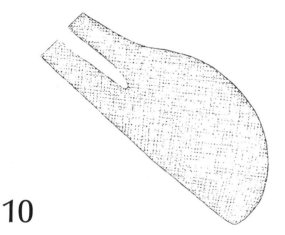

10

10 The mesh is prepared by cutting it into a shape to fit the posterior wall of the inguinal canal. The lateral end of the mesh is slit and trousered with two tails, the upper tail is about 3 cm in width and the lower tail approximately 2 cm in width. The tails are positioned to surround the cord at the internal ring and lie lateral in a pocket between the external and internal oblique muscles.

11 With the cord retracted upwards, a continuous 000 monofilament non-absorbable synthetic suture (e.g. Prolene) is used to suture the most medial lower edge of mesh to the aponeurotic tissue above and medial to the pubic tubercle, then proceding laterally to the insertion of the inguinal ligament, along the external aponeurosis just above the shelving border of the inguinal ligament, and finally lateral to the internal ring. Rather than suturing the inferior mesh edge directly to the inguinal ligament, the author prefers a side-to-side suture apposition of the mesh to the inguinal aponeurosis just above the shelving margin of the inguinal ligament (*see* inset). This technique ensures that the femoral vessels are not accidentally punctured or sutured and leaves an overlap of the inferior part of the mesh extending over the reflected part of the inguinal ligament onto the transversalis fascia. It is a danger area if staples are used.

The superior edge of the mesh is then sutured to the rectus sheath and to either the internal oblique aponeurosis or muscle (as described by Lichtenstein) or the reflected part of the external oblique muscle just where it meets the internal oblique muscle. The ilio-hypogastric nerve must be in a position not to be entrapped by the suturing of the mesh. The author uses an extremely loose continuous monofilament suture to position the mesh, leaving tension-free anchoring points. Lichtenstein prefers interrupted absorbable sutures. Lateral to the internal ring and cord, the upper trouser of the mesh is overlapped over the lower one and sutured to it or the external oblique aponeurosis. The preserved ilio-inguinal and genital nerves, the cremasteric vessels and cord are thus surrounded by the new 'internal ring'. The opening should be at least 1.5 cm in diameter. The external oblique muscle is closed over the cord with a continuous suture.

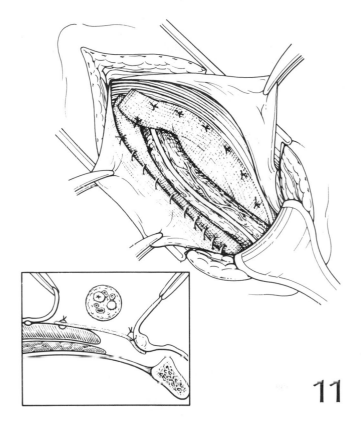

11

TUMESCENT TECHNIQUE FOR RECURRENT INGUINAL HERNIA REPAIR

It is important in the preoperative assessment of the patient to record the size and state of the testes. If the testis on the side of the recurrence is already atrophied, then is should be explained to the patient, and the possibility of excision of the testis to close the inguinal canal totally in the repair should be discussed. The elderly may accept orchidectomy if they have had repeated recurrences. A tension-free mesh repair should still be performed. If possible, information on the previous repair should be obtained.

In planning the incision one may find that the previous scar is too horizontal and this would reduce exposure of the inguinal canal. It is better for the new incision to follow the line of the inguinal canal and hernia, especially if the recurrence is large and extending into the scrotum. The same local anaesthetic approach is used as for primary hernia repair except that one has to be extremely cautious with the subcutaneous dissection in case the cord might have been previously exteriorized with the external oblique muscle repaired behind it. Fortunately, this is extremely rare. It is best to dissect just superior to the scarred subcutaneous tissue, keeping in 'virgin' territory until the external oblique aponeurosis is exposed. The most lateral part of the aponeurosis free of scar tissue is selected as the intitial site for infiltration of local anaesthetic. A large volume of local anaesthetic is injected to cause overdistension of the inguinal canal as it helps to separate the spermatic cord from the external oblique muscle and the posterior wall of the canal. Other points for injection may also be selected. Further dissection superficial to the aponeurosis is made down to the scar of the previously closed aponeurosis. After opening the external oblique muscle further fluid dissection is employed by continually introducing the local anaesthetic to separate and assist sharp dissection of the vital structures of the cord. With first-time repair of a recurrent hernia, the dissection is usually not difficult.

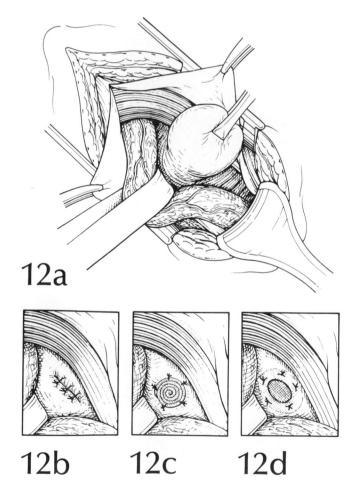

12a

12b　　12c　　12d

12a–d
An indirect sac recurrence is excised or inverted. Umbrella mesh plugging may be necessary. Small direct hernias are invaginated and the wall defect closed, plugged or inlaid with mesh before the final onlay mesh repair.

13 If the posterior wall is thinned out by a large direct defect, then the weakened transversalis fascia is opened, preserving as much tissue as possible while dissecting the hernia. The sac is returned to the abdominal cavity and either an underlay or onlay mesh technique is used for the repair, depending on what is left of the inguinal anatomy of the posterior wall. Closure of the posterior wall without tension for an onlay mesh may not be possible, and therefore an inlay of mesh sutured behind the internal oblique and transversalis muscles may be necessary. If the inguinal ligament is weak and regarded as insecure for stitching of the inferior edge of the medial part of the mesh, it is attached to the pectineal ligament and then laterally to the inguinal ligament. If excessive dissection is required, a vacuum drain may be necessary.

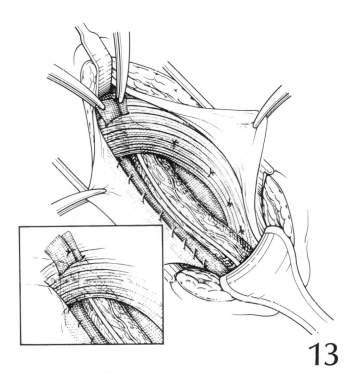

13

14a–c If the anterior approach should prove difficult, it is best to convert to the extraperitoneal one. This takes the dissection above and outside the inguinal canal into virgin extraperitoneal tissue behind Hesselbach's triangle. When repairing multirecurrent or prevascular hernias, the extraperitoneal approach is usually required. Either a vertical or transverse incision is used. The preperitoneal approach allows the surgeon to repair a recurrent hernia without the need to dissect out the cord.

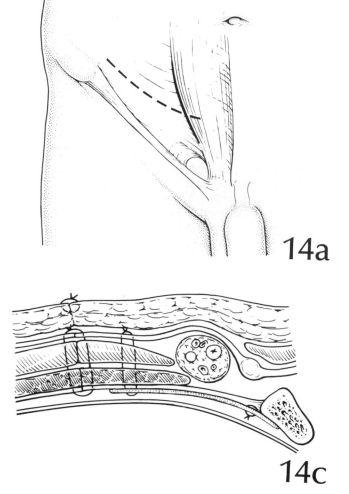

14a

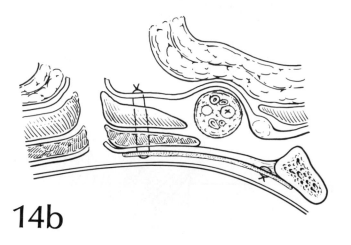

14b

14c

15 The mesh prosthesis lies in the extraperitoneal space and covers Hesselbach's triangle. The inferior edge of the most medial part of the mesh is sutured to the pectineal ligament, arches over the iliac vessels and is then sutured to the iliopubic tract. The internal ring is reconstructed as shown. The upper edge of the mesh is sutured to the anterior abdominal wall muscles with sutures that loosely pass through all layers.

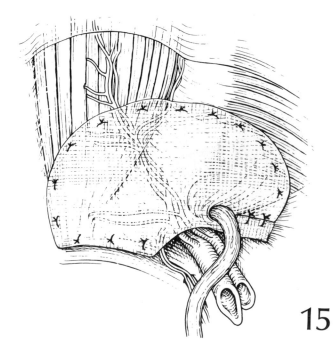

15

FEMORAL HERNIA REPAIR

The mesh technique is ideal for repair of a femoral hernia. An uncomplicated small femoral hernia may be repaired with the local anaesthetic infiltration technique.

16 The local anaesthetic is introduced by the 'infiltrate as you go' technique. The author prefers a slightly indirect approach to the hernia. The incision is made just slightly below that which would be used for an inguinal incision, rather than directly over the femoral hernia. The lower external oblique aponeurosis is exposed at its most medial point near the pubic tubercle and is followed down to where the inguinal ligament fuses with Scarpa's fascia which is then opened where it lies over the femoral canal area. Frequently, the sac is surrounded by extraperitoneal fat which may need to be removed to reduce its bulk in order to permit its excision or reduction into the abdominal cavity. The margins of the femoral canal are defined and prepared for the repair. A prosthetic plug of rolled mesh may be inserted and sutured to block the femoral canal opening as described by Lichtenstein.

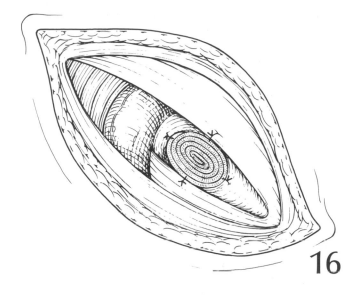

16

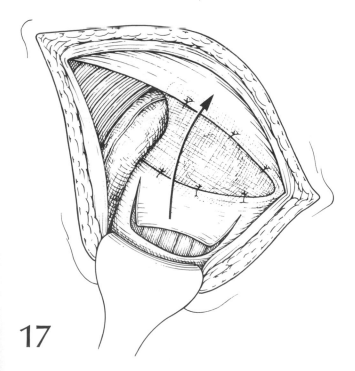

17

17 The author prefers to patch the femoral canal with a small piece of mesh to cover the femoral canal from within and overlap its edges. It is sutured to the inguinal and pectineal ligaments. The mesh is then covered with a flap of pectineal fascia.

In the extremely rare event of any difficulty with a femoral hernia when using the infrainguinal approach, one simply converts to an inguinal approach by opening up the inguinal canal and approaching the femoral canal through the transversalis fascia. Both the inguinal and femoral canals are then patched with mesh.

MESH REPAIR OF EPIGASTRIC AND SMALL UMBILICAL HERNIAS

Small aponeurotic epigastric and umbilical hernias may be repaired with local anaesthesia using mesh techniques, especially on thin patients. The defects should not be larger than 5 cm in diameter. They are often herniations of extraperitoneal fat with a small sac and, when dissected free, are simply invaginated back into the extraperitoneal space of the umbilical area. It is essential that the defect is repaired without tension so it may need to be fortified with mesh. The traditional overlap Mayo repair for umbilical hernia is a poor technique which requires a tension closure and should be avoided as it is more prone to recurrence. The author prefers an apposition closure if it can be performed without tension. The local anaesthetic technique is especially suited for men who often have a small defect as there is minimal divarication of the recti. Most women with an umbilical hernia have divarication of the recti with an attenuated linea alba as a result of multiparity and mesh reinforcement is required to prevent recurrence. General anaesthesia is required for large hernias, but infiltration of local anaesthetic during the operation should still be used as part of the multimodal management to reduce postoperative pain.

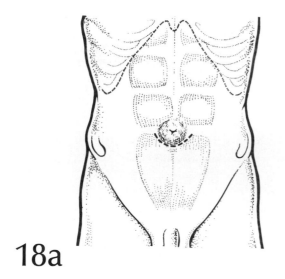

18a

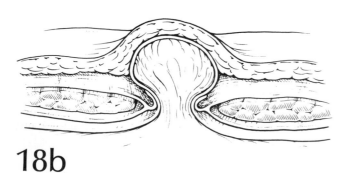

18b

18a,b After subcutaneous infiltration of local anaesthetic around the hernia, a curved incision is made around its inferior aspect. The upper umbilical skin flap is adherent to the sac and needs to be separated from it by further infiltration of local anaesthetic and sharp dissection. Once the sac is isolated and the fascial edges of the rectus are well exposed (*Illustration 18b*), further local anaesthetic is infiltrated into the extraperitoneal space and deep into the rectus sheath and muscle bordering the defect. The extraperitoneal tissue attachments to the posterior rectus sheath at the margins of the hernia defect are separated, making a space which extends 1–2 cm beyond its edges. Small sacs with extraperitoneal fat are invaginated rather than excised. Slightly larger sacs with adherent omentum are left unopened and replaced back into the extraperitoneal space of the abdominal cavity. The omentum will protect the small bowel from further adhesions to the operative area. Any obvious small bowel adhesion to the sac wall is freed and the peritoneum closed. It is important that the mesh is sandwiched between the peritoneum and muscle and that there is no direct contact with bowel.

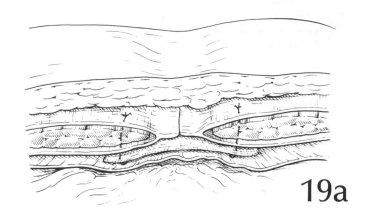

19a

19a,b A mesh patch with a diameter at least 2 cm larger than the defect is inserted into the preperitoneal space and sutured into position with minimal tension. Any redundant attenuated aponeurosis present is used to cover the mesh and sutured over it.

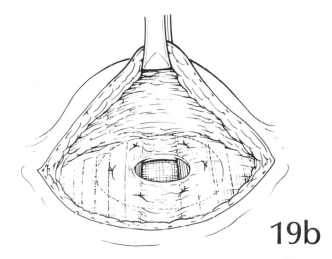

19b

Skin closure

Following each of the above procedures, the skin is closed with a subdermal continuous absorbable suture as it simplifies wound care. Steristrips may be used to tidy up the closure to ensure good dermal apposition. If there has been excessive dissection, as with a giant scrotal or recurrent hernia, a small vacuum drain may be required. Dressings are removed on the first postoperative morning and, as the wound is sealed, patients may take a shower or bath.

Postoperative care

Patients may be discharged within a few hours after the operation. Non-steroidal anti-inflammatory drugs and a mild analgesic are given for pain. Unrestricted activity is encouraged as soon as possible within the limitations of postoperative discomfort. Most patients return to normal activities within a week depending upon their motivation and type of work. Driving is left to the patient's discretion but they are advised to first test their reaction to pressure on the brake pedal in a stationary vehicle. Most are driving within a week. Patients are forewarned that ecchymoses and swelling may extend onto the shaft of the penis and the scrotum, and that there may be a rope-like induration under the scar. Patients who have repairs of a large scrotal hernia or simultaneous bilateral hernia repair are advised to wear a scrotal support as the scrotum may become swollen.

Further reading

Gilbert AI. Prosthetic adjuncts to groin hernia repair: a classification of inguinal hernias. *Contemp Surg* 1988; 32: 128–35.

Lichtenstein IL, Shulman AG, Amid PK, Montllor MM. The tension-free hernioplasty. *Am J Surg* 1989; 157: 188–93.

Lichtenstein IL, Shulman AG, Amid PK. The cause, prevention, and treatment of recurrent groin hernia. *Surg Clin North Am* 1993; 73: 529–44.

Notaras MJ. Experience with mersilene mesh in abdominal wall repair. *Proc R Soc Med* 1974; 67: 1187–90.

Notaras MJ. Repair of difficult and recurrent inguino-femoral hernias with synthetic mesh. In: Maingot R, ed. *Abdominal Operations*. 7th edn. New York: Appleton-Century Crofts, 1980: 1643–9.

Wheatley RG, Samaan AK. Postoperative pain relief. *Br J Surg* 1995; 82: 292–4.

Breast surgery

Kirby I. Bland MD
Chairman, Department of Surgery, Rhode Island Hospital, Providence, Rhode Island, USA

Romeo B. Mateo MD
Assistant Instructor in Surgery, Brown University School of Medicine, Providence, Rhode Island, USA

Until the last decade, breast carcinoma was the leading cause of cancer-related mortality in women. Suspicious mammographic or palpable lesions of the breast need both complete diagnostic evaluation and a multidisciplinary approach to treatment. Surgical diagnostic modalities include needle aspiration of cystic lesions, fine needle aspiration biopsy and open biopsy of solid breast masses. Segmental mastectomy and modified radical mastectomy are currently the most common approaches to the surgical management of breast carcinoma. A precise knowledge of the anatomy of the breast, as well as the details of these procedures and their variations, will ensure optimal therapeutic results and cosmesis.

Needle aspiration of a breast cyst

Breast cysts with no evidence of ductal atypia comprise a large number of breast lumps in women between the ages of 35 and 50 years. Fluid from these cysts is readily aspirated with a 22 gauge needle and a syringe.

1 After the breast and chest wall are prepared, the cyst can be supported and controlled between two fingers. Local anaesthesia, although usually unnecessary, should be administered only in small volumes to avoid compromising adequate palpation. Aspiration of greenish-brown fluid virtually confirms the diagnosis of benign (non-proliferative) cystic disease and should not be submitted for cytological examination. A bloody aspirate is more likely to be indicative of malignancy and should always be submitted for cytological review. A report of an equivocal or suspicious cytological examination necessitates excision of residual tissue to confirm the presence or absence of malignancy.

After aspiration the cyst should not be palpable. If a residual mass is evident following aspiration, then repeat fine needle aspiration biopsy, core needle biopsy or open biopsy is indicated. Follow-up examination and mammography is indicated if the mass recurs within 6 weeks of aspiration.

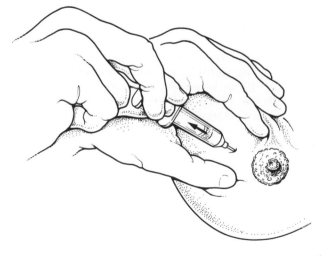

1

FINE NEEDLE ASPIRATION BIOPSY

Fine needle aspiration biopsy of breast masses is a safe and reliable diagnostic technique that can be performed in the clinic using local anaesthesia. Although relatively easy to perform it is essential that the proper equipment is available, adequate samples are obtained, and smears are prepared in a manner suitable for an experienced pathologist to interpret.

Equipment

If 20 or 22 gauge needles are used to procure tissue, a local anaesthetic is unnecessary. When larger needles are selected, a local anaesthetic should be administered with a 27 gauge needle and only a small volume should be infiltrated to avoid disturbance of the lesion. Two commonly used syringe holders can accommodate 10 or 20 ml syringes.

Materials essential for cytopathological examination of fine needle aspiration biopsy samples are listed in *Table 1*.

Table 1   Inventory list for cytopathology trolley

Microscope and power cord
Block (10 × 10 × 7 inches) to raise microscope for ease of viewing
All frosted slides (one box at least three-quarters full)
Clear glass slides with frosted labels (one box at least three-quarters full)
Sterile rubber gloves (two pairs)
20-, 22-, and 19-gauge needles, especially 20-gauge
Centrifuge tubes (1–3 ml, 1–6 ml)
Sterile syringes (20 ml)
Needle holder (autoclaved) (2)
Three tubes of normal saline and 50% ethanol; fill tubes one-quarter full with saline and one-quarter with alcohol so that tube is half full
Two tubes (6 ml) of tissue culture medium
Requisition forms
Paper towels
Black pen, pencil
Two Coplan jars of 95% ethanol
One Coplan jar of water to rinse slides after staining
DiffQuik solutions I and II
Tweezers

A cytology trolley is prepared for fine needle aspiration cytology. The services of a cytotechnologist can be very helpful in preparing the slides following aspiration.

Technique

The skin preparation solution should be allowed to dry thoroughly so that no residual liquid iodine or alcohol remains on the surface. Before percutaneous introduction of the needle tip, 5 ml of air is aspirated into the syringe to allow the maximal volume of procured epithelial cells to remain in the barrel of the needle, rather than being displaced into the lumen of the syringe. After locating and stabilizing the mass with one hand, the surgeon introduces the needle tip through the skin and into the mass at a slightly oblique angle to minimize inadvertent penetration of the chest wall. Once the needle has penetrated the tumour, maximum suction (-40 cm H_2O) is applied to the syringe. As the surgeon manoeuvres the needle into the mass at variable angles over an area of no more than 1 cm^2, clumps of cells are dislodged from the tumour and enter the hub of the needle.

The goal of fine needle aspiration biopsy is to fill the needle (not the syringe) with cellular contents. Therefore, before removal of the needle from the mass the plunger and the suction are released and the plunger assumes its original position in the syringe cylinder (5 ml).

The needle is withdrawn and the contents are meticulously expressed onto glass slides. This volume should not exceed a drop with a diameter of no more than 5 mm. Additional slides for extra aspirate volume are used as needed. A second empty slide is laid on top of the specimen slide, causing the cellular sample to diffuse slowly between the two glass surfaces. The slides are then turned apart, just as one opens the pages of a book, without pulling the slides apart or producing smear artifact. One slide is used for air-dried stains, e.g. DiffQuik, while the other slide is fixed in 95% ethanol to be later stained with DiffQuik or Papanicolaou stain, or used for detection of cellular antigens using immuno-peroxidase techniques.

After expressing the cellular material onto slides, the practitioner may obtain any residual cells within the syringe and needle by aspirating culture medium (e.g. Eagle's MEM or RPMI 1640) into the syringe and harvesting the cells by filtration or cytocentrifugation. If the removed needle contains small tissue fragments, these can be prepared for cell block and paraffin embedding. If a cyst associated with a solid mass is entered, the aspirated fluid is forwarded for cytological examination; fine needle aspiration biopsy should be repeated when a residual mass is palpable following cyst fluid drainage.

Complications

Complications of fine needle aspiration biopsy include pneumothorax, haematoma formation, acute mastitis and, rarely, tumour growth within the needle track. The likelihood of causing a pneumothorax is diminished when the needle is placed at an acute angle to avoid entry into the chest wall. Haematomas are common and may elicit false positive readings on mammograms obtained after aspiration. Mammography should therefore be performed before fine needle aspiration biopsy; if it is done afterwards a delay of 2 weeks will usually allow resolution of the haematoma. Acute mastitis is rare and needle track involvement with tumour is also less likely to occur because of the small gauge of needles used and because the track is included in subsequent resection specimens.

Diagnostic reliability of fine needle aspiration biopsy

The sensitivity of fine needle aspiration biopsy of breast masses ranges from 80% to 98%, the principal cause of false negative results being sampling and slide preparation error. The specificity and positive predictive value approaches 100% because false positive results are exceedingly rare. Diagnostic accuracy ranges from 84% to 99.5% because reported false negative rates range from 0.7% to 22%.

False negative findings may be reduced by (1) increasing the number of aspirates (minimum of three), (2) paying proper attention to technical preparation of the procured tissues by avoidance of air drying and loss of cellular material, and (3) using an experienced clinician to perform the aspiration. Nevertheless, in cases where samples of suspicious breast lesions fail to yield a definitive diagnosis of malignancy, an incisional or excisional biopsy must be performed.

CUTTING NEEDLE BIOPSY

The standard Tru-Cut needle is the most commonly used cutting needle for breast biopsy. Although a core of tissue is incised from the breast mass, as with fine needle aspiration biopsy decisions for therapeutic management following cutting needle biopsy are useful only when results are positive for malignancy. Incomplete or suspicious masses which undergo an inadequate biopsy for technical reasons should be excised.

Technique

Because cutting needles are 12 gauge or larger, local anaesthesia is necessary. A No. 11 scalpel blade is used to make a very small skin incision, just large enough to allow entry of the tip of the biopsy needle into the breast parenchyma in the closed position. The central needle is then advanced into the mass. The outer cutting sheath is closed over the central needle while the breast and the central needle are both stabilized. The entire apparatus is then removed with the procured tissues while still in the closed position. A tubular core of tissue can be found after opening the sheath and removing the specimen from the central needle

Because a larger core of tissue is obtained with the cutting needle biopsy, the risk of haemorrhage and tissue disturbance is greater than in fine needle aspiration biopsy. The central needle should not be advanced beyond the suspect mass, since this action may implant the contiguous normal breast or chest wall with tumour cells.

Open biopsy of breast lesions

Indications

The surgeon's decision to perform a breast biopsy depends on a full evaluation of the patient's personal and family history, other risk factors, the physical examination, and the mammographic ultrasonography findings.

Certain clinical presentations warrant a breast biopsy without reservation, e.g. a newly recognized, discrete, non-cystic mass necessitates tissue diagnosis with various techniques including fine needle aspiration cytology, core needle biopsy, or incisional/excisional biopsy. As already mentioned, indeterminate, suspicious or negative findings on fine needle aspiration biopsy of the mass also mandate open biopsy. Skin dimpling, peau d'orange, or bloody nipple discharge requires biopsy of any underlying suspicious mass detected on physical examination or by mammography. Moreover, failure of an apparent infection to resolve despite appropriate antibiotics and therapy should lead the physician to take a biopsy specimen, not only of the underlying breast tissue, but also of the overlying skin to evaluate subdermal lymphatic extension of a neoplastic process. Factors associated with an increased risk of malignancy in nipple discharge include: (1) yellow, pink, bloody, or watery discharge; (2) discharge accompanied by a mass or a lump; (3) unilateral discharge from a single duct; (4) discharge associated with excoriation of the epithelium as in Paget's disease; and (5) age greater than 50 years. Finally, women presenting with an axillary mass should undergo complete physical examination and mammography before biopsy of the axillary mass to detect any suspicious breast lesions.

Mammographic indications for breast biopsy include: (1) a suspicious soft tissue mass identifiable within the breast parenchyma; (2) architectural distortion, including contracture of trabeculae leading to stellate changes, with severe asymmetrical periductal and lobular thickening; and (3) mammographically suspicious microcalcifications, either clustered, branching or linear.

Finally, the patient who presents with a lesion which appears clinically and radiographically to be benign and with associated risk factors requires biopsy of the lesion to determine its pathology and to evaluate the patient's subsequent risk for breast malignancy. Approximately 70% of patients who undergo breast biopsy have histologically benign disease and therefore are not at increased risk for developing cancer; the remaining 30% of patients whose biopsies show proliferative or atypical changes (i.e. moderate hyperplasia, including sclerosing adenosis, papillomas and atypical hyperplasia) have a two-fold increased risk for breast cancer. It is only in this latter group (atypia) that the risk of cancer is further increased by family history, reproductive history, calcification and age.

General principles

All breast biopsies should be performed with the assumption that the suspicious mass is malignant. In planning an open biopsy the following should therefore be considered: (1) adequate anaesthesia; (2) an incision designed for cosmesis with consideration of the need for potential subsequent procedures; (3) standardized specimen handling with laboratory processing; and (4) meticulous haemostasis and closure.

Operation

Position of the patient

The patient is placed in a supine position on the operating table and the ipsilateral thorax on the side of the lesion is slightly elevated with folded drapes. The patient's arm is placed in a relaxed position on an arm board.

Anaesthesia

Most palpable and non-palpable breast lesions can be excised with local anaesthesia (1% plain lignocaine) and sedation. Plain lignocaine may be preferable to avoid epidermolysis of the skin, which occurs when adrenaline is included. Extensive infiltration of the subcutaneous tissue with a local anaesthetic is not recommended as this makes palpation of the suspicious mass more difficult, especially if the mass is less than 1 cm. Furthermore, injection of the tumour is contra-indicated as this adds little to patient comfort and creates the potential for regional dissemination of tumour cells.

Contraindications to local anaesthesia include: (1) a palpable or non-palpable lesion located deep within the breast parenchyma which may require significant manipulation of tissue near the fascia; (2) an anxious or apprehensive patient or one who prefers general anaesthesia; and (3) a patient who agrees to have a biopsy, frozen section and definitive operative therapy during a single procedure (one-stage or single-stage).

Whether local or general anaesthesia is used, the surgeon may infiltrate the skin and subcutaneous tissues with a longer acting agent such as 0.5% bupivacaine after the procedure to provide extended analgesia until adequate levels of oral analgesic agents are administered.

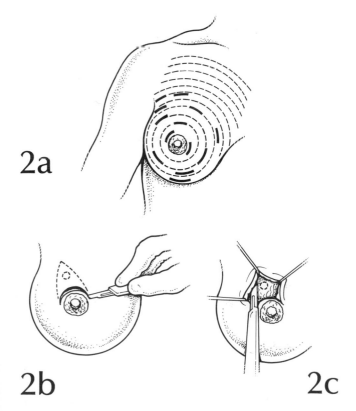

2a

2b

2c

PALPABLE LESIONS

Incision

2a–c The lines of tension (Langer's lines) in the skin of the breast are generally concentric and parallel with the nipple-areolar complex. Incisions that parallel these lines of tension result in thin and cosmetically acceptable scars. Periareolar incisions are especially useful in this regard, but thin skin flaps must be assiduously avoided to ensure cosmetically contoured and viable tissues around the areola. The biopsy incision should also be planned and completed within the boundaries of the subsequent mastectomy or tylectomy specimen, should such a more radical procedure be necessary.

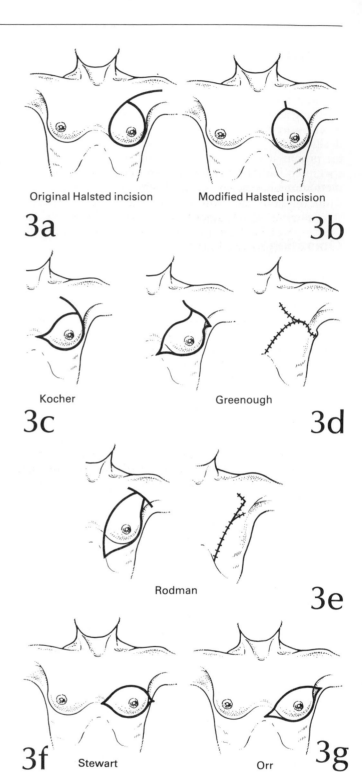

3a–h Variants of the radical mastectomy incision which may be used subsequently are illustrated. The subsequent modifications of the original Halsted incision preserve the cephalic vein.

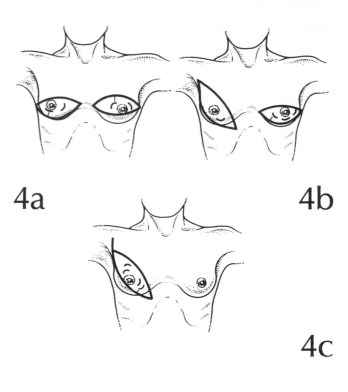

4a–c The mastectomy incision shown allows a margin of normal tissue between the tumour and the skin edges. Radial scars are not recommended, but inner lower quadrant lesions may be best approached by a radial incision as long as it lies within the proposed mastectomy scar.

Dissection

Excision of breast masses should be done sharply, preferably with the cold scalpel or electrocautery. Because hormone receptors are heat labile, the use of electrocautery on the tumour surface can theoretically decrease hormone receptor levels. Judicious use of electrocautery is recommended, but preferably on normal tissue already separated from the specimen. Assays for oestrogen and progesterone receptors should be requested on all neoplastic tissues removed at biopsy, instead of at mastectomy, because the more prolonged warm ischaemia time of mastectomy may alter (diminish) the oestrogen and progesterone receptor content.

Excision of the mass should include a surrounding 0.5–1.0 cm margin of normal breast parenchyma. If the mass is contiguous with the chest wall, it is essential to avoid incision of the pectoralis fascia at biopsy as re-excision by segmental or total mastectomy should encompass this barrier *en bloc*. It is preferable not to apply crushing clamps or extensive torque on the lesion to avoid disruption and exfoliation of cells within the wound. A 'figure-of-eight' traction suture may be placed to provide purchase around the lesion and to allow non-traumatic manipulation of the mass. Careful retraction with skin hooks will minimize trauma to the skin edges and improve cosmetic results.

Incisional biopsies are indicated in patients with large (≥ 4 cm) primary breast lesions. The actual biopsy of the tumour is best performed with the cold scalpel; electrocautery is avoided entirely to obviate tissue necrosis and tumour artifact. Careful attention to haemostasis is mandatory to prevent dissemination of potentially malignant cells.

Closure

After removal of the biopsy specimen, meticulous haemostasis is imperative. The wound is copiously irrigated with saline and re-inspected for any other bleeding points. Obliteration of the dead space is not mandatory, although the authors routinely use 2/0 or 3/0 interrupted absorbable suture (polyglycolic acid or chromic catgut) in multiple layers to facilitate closure of the breast tissue defect. As an option, a small (0.25 in) Penrose drain may be placed and secured at the deepest portion of the wound and removed within 48 h.

The surrounding skin and subcutaneous tissue is infiltrated with 0.5% bupivacaine for extended analgesia. The subcutaneous tissue is approximated with 3/0 or 4/0 interrupted absorbable sutures. The skin may be closed with subcuticular absorbable 4/0 or 5/0 sutures followed by Steri-strips to approximate the skin edges. A light occlusive dressing is applied.

NON-PALPABLE LESIONS

Arrangements should be made for the patient to have needle localization of the suspicious lesion confirmed by mammography. Precise placement by the radiologist of a self-retaining wire contiguous with the suspicious lesion allows guidance to the suspicious lesion. It is imperative to have available both the initial diagnostic mammographic films and those after placement of the wire for confirmation of accurate localization. Care must be exercised with positioning of the patient after placement of the wire and in antiseptic preparation of the skin and the exposed length of the wire.

Two methods can be used to perform the biopsy.

5a–c Circumferential tissue planes parallel to the localization wire can be developed to excise a core of tissue which can then be grasped with Allis clamps. Dissection can then be continued more deeply to incorporate the lesion and the wire circumferentially.

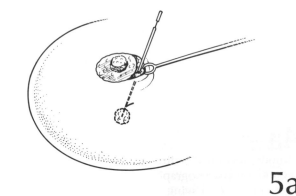

5a

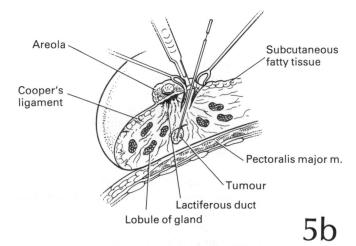

Areola

Cooper's ligament

Subcutaneous fatty tissue

Pectoralis major m.

Tumour

Lactiferous duct

Lobule of gland

5b

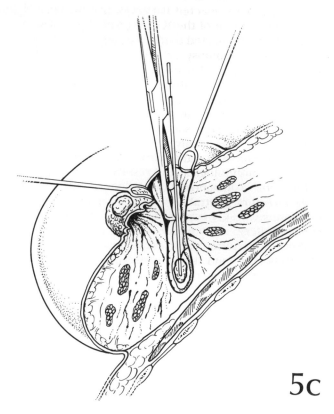

5c

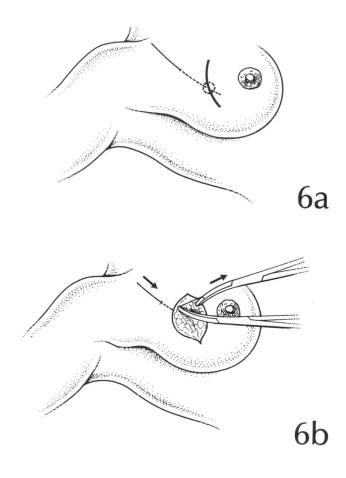

6a,b Alternatively, an incision can be made directly over the site of the suspicious lesion based on the direction and final location of the wire tip at mammography. Palpation of the wire can be facilitated by leaving the needle sheath in place. Thereafter, with exposure the wire is grasped and its external portion manipulated into the wound. The wire can then be used to direct circumferential dissection around the suspected lesion.

After removal of the specimen it should be orientated three-dimensionally with markers, paint or sutures. The entire specimen with the localization wire in place should be examined radiographically to confirm complete removal of the suspected lesion.

SPECIAL SITUATIONS

Patients who present with a nipple discharge without a definable mass on clinical or radiographic examination may undergo breast biopsy in two ways. The involved duct can be cannulated with a thin probe and the surrounding tissue can be excised circumferentially, or the duct can be injected with a vital dye followed by complete excision of the stained tissues.

In patients suspected of harbouring Paget's disease of the nipple, the biopsy specimen should include the subareolar mass and a portion of skin of the nipple-areola complex. In the absence of a palpable breast mass in patients with suspected Paget's disease, a segment of the areolar complex and subareolar tissue should be excised. Alternatively, should the areolar and surrounding skin present as a scaly and encrusted lesion, a sterile glass slide may be used to scrape this area to obtain a specimen for cytological examination. The treatment of choice for a diagnosis of Paget's disease is total mastectomy or central segmental mastectomy.

Patients who present with the peau d'orange appearance of inflammatory breast carcinoma are best treated with preoperative multi-drug, cyclic, neoadjuvant chemotherapy and should therefore only undergo incisional biopsy as the initial diagnostic approach. In addition, a wedge biopsy of skin adjacent to the underlying mass should be examined for dermal and subdermal lymphatic invasion to confirm diagnosis of the clinical presentation.

Complications and follow-up

Major complications following breast biopsies are rare, and complications of any nature occur in less than 5–10% of cases. Large haematomas and infections should be treated aggressively with evacuation, drainage and antibiotics.

After open biopsy the timing of the definitive surgical procedure is critical. No deleterious effects on the rates of recurrence or survival have been found if definitive surgery is completed within 2 weeks of biopsy.

Segmental mastectomy (lumpectomy/tylectomy)

Indications

Prospective randomized trials show that breast conservation surgery has long-term results equivalent to those for radical mastectomy with regard to locoregional control, disease-free survival rates and overall survival rates. As both procedures have similar outcomes, surgeons are increasingly advising the breast-conserving option when technically feasible.

Criteria for eligibility for conservation surgery include: (1) tumours 4 cm or less in transverse diameter; (2) absence of tumour multicentricity; (3) a breast of adequate size and volume to allow both a margin-free resection and a cosmetic result without gross deformity; (4) negative tumour margins at the time of resection; (5) completion of axillary nodal sampling of levels I and II to obtain 10 or more nodes; and (6) comprehensive postoperative irradiation to the intact breast administered by an experienced and competent radiotherapist.

Operation

Patient positioning and anaesthesia are similar to those for open biopsy.

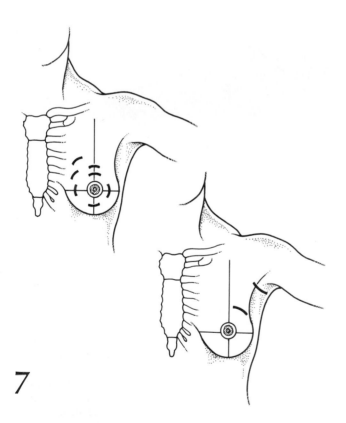

7

7 The various sites for curvilinear (non-radial) incisions in the breast that are preferable for cosmetic appearance and enhanced wound repair are shown.

8 Radial incisions are not recommended. Incisions for axillary dissection should be separate (discontinuous) from the breast incision to improve cosmesis.

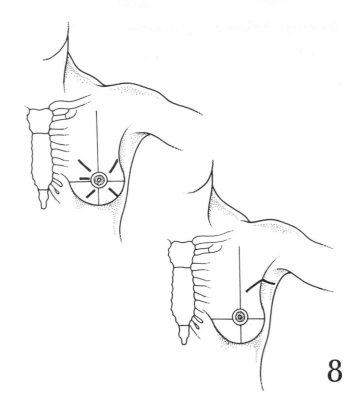

8

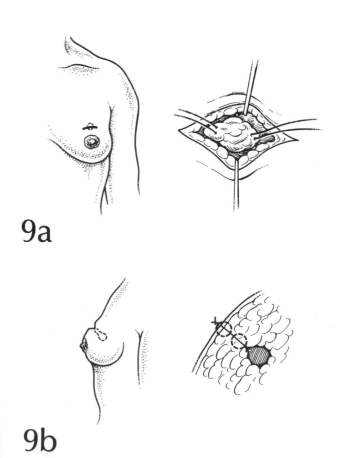

9a

9b

9a,b Ideally, incisions should be placed directly over the tumour and parallel to Langer's lines. Distant 'tunnelling' through remote breast tissue and the creation of skin flaps are to be avoided to ensure maximal cosmesis. The breast incision should be made with the consideration that a subsequent conventional mastectomy may be necessary if tumour-free margins cannot be obtained. Finally, in those patients who have had previous incisions over the tumour (i.e. incisional or excisional biopsies), *en bloc* excision of the involved skin of the previous biopsy site should be completed. When the diagnosis was established by fine needle aspiration or cutting needle biopsy, skin excision is not required unless there is concern about tumour implantation of a superficially invasive lesion.

Dissection and specimen preparation

The goal of the segmental mastectomy is the removal of residual tissue and a volume of normal tissue in all dimensions around the tumour to achieve tumour-free margins. This breast conservation approach can be achieved by avoiding undermining the skin margins, tunnelling into remote tissues and flap elevation. Deeper dissection should avoid removal of the pectoralis fascia unless the lesion invades the fascia or is closely adherent. As in open biopsy, the technique involving judicious use of the electrocautery is advised with segmental mastectomy.

10 Following removal of the specimen, its margins should be identified and orientated three-dimensionally for the pathologist. Markers or indelible, multicoloured paints should be placed on all margins to identify the superior, inferior, lateral, medial, superficial (anterior) and deep (posterior) aspects of the specimen.

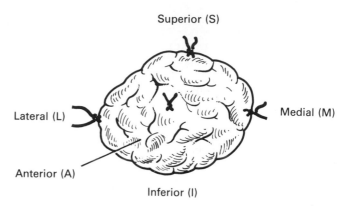

Superior (S)

Lateral (L)

Medial (M)

Anterior (A)

Inferior (I)

10

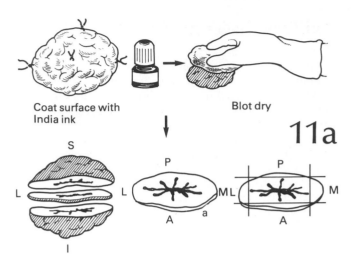

Coat surface with India ink

Blot dry

11a

11b

- Palpate for tumour
- Bisect tumour and specimen transversely (horizontally)

- Obtain A–P, L–M diameters of tumour and partial SI measurement (a)
- Take aliquots for receptors, frozen if required

- Take blocks of L, M, A, P, margins and blocks of tumour

11a–d The entire specimen should be coated with India ink or coloured with indelible tissue dyes which would concurrently mark and orientate the specimen. Before cutting and fixation of the specimen, the pathologist should measure the three dimensions of the excised specimen and inspect it for gross tumour involvement of the margins. This is essential to achieve clear surgical margins.

After cutting the specimen, any grossly 'close' margins should undergo frozen section examination. If the margin is close but free of involvement on frozen section, routine re-section at the site of involved tissue and submission of this tissue as a new section is recommended.

The specimen is then divided for steroid-receptor, cellular, biochemical and molecular marker studies and for permanent blocks.

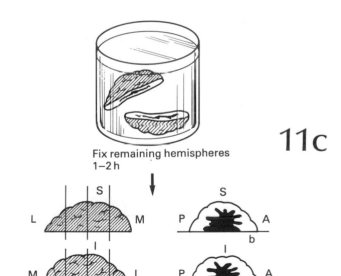

Fix remaining hemispheres 1–2 h

11c

11d

- Place cut surface down
- Take sagittal blocks through superior and inferior portions

- Blocks viewed from side. Each may be transected to give SA, SP, IA, IP margins
- Measure SI diameter of tumour a + b + c

Closure

Meticulous haemostasis and precise approximation of skin edges are essential for cosmetically acceptable closures. Large breasts with adequate volumes of residual tissue may be left with 'dead space'. This 'dead space' should not be closed, if such closure leaves a concave deformity as occurs in large superficial tumour excisions of moderate-sized breasts; in this case the subcutaneous fat alone may be approximated. Preferably, drains should not be placed within lumpectomy wounds. The surrounding skin and subcutaneous tissue is infiltrated with 0.5% bupivacaine for extended local analgesia and the skin is closed with subcuticular 4/0 or 5/0 sutures followed by Steri-strips to ensure precise skin approximation.

Axillary dissection (sampling)

Axillary dissection, for which a better term is axillary sampling, is performed to determine histological evidence of regional nodal involvement as an *indicator* of metastic disease. This procedure represents a staging technique without therapeutic benefit to the patient. Preferably, a minimum of 10 nodes from levels I and II are obtained to stage infiltrating breast neoplasms. *In situ* carcinomas of the breast, whether of lobular or ductal origin, do not require nodal sampling because the incidence of regional metastasis in such carcinomas is less than 2%.

12 Preferred (P) and optional (O) incisions used in axillary dissections are shown. After the incisions are made, thick axillary flaps are elevated superiorly and inferiorly. Level I and II nodes are identified and removed *en bloc* with regional loose areolar tissue of the axillary fat, as described for modified radical mastectomy (*see* below). Thus, axillary sampling is inclusive of the external mammary, subscapular and lateral axillary nodal groups of level I and the central nodal group of level II. Removal of the pectoralis muscle, however, is not necessary because careful elevation of the muscle will allow adequate access and resection to the highest level of planned sampling (level II). Improved cosmesis and motor function is achieved if the medial pectoral nerve, lying lateral to the pectoralis minor muscle, is identified and preserved.

Following removal of the nodal tissues, a closed Silastic drain (e.g. Jackson–Pratt, 10-mm) is placed via an inferior stab wound and connected to vacuum suction. The skin and subcutaneous tissues are infiltrated with 0.5% bupivacaine for prolonged analgesia. Subcutaneous tissues are optionally approximated with absorbable sutures and the skin is closed in a subcuticular fashion.

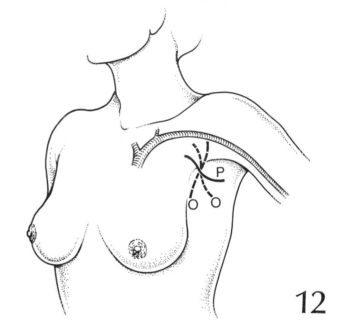

12

Modified radical mastectomy

13 The patient is positioned with the ipsilateral arm and shoulder in a relaxed extended position on an armboard. The ipsilateral shoulder and hemithorax are slightly elevated with a sheet roll. Draping should include the supraclavicular fossa and the entire shoulder up to and including the elbow. This allows full range of motion of both the shoulder and the elbow joints.

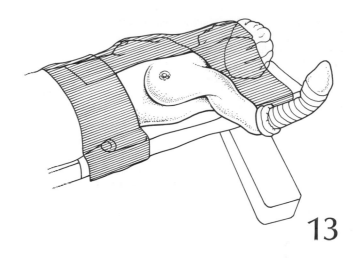

13

First assistant

Surgeon

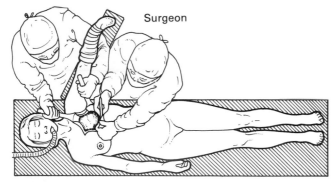

14 An occlusive stockinette dressing is secured distal to the elbow with a Kling or Kerlix cotton roll to isolate the hand and the forearm. The first assistant is positioned cephalad to the armboard and shoulder and can provide traction, control rotation and protection of the arm, shoulder and axillary contents.

14

Incisions

15a,b The classic Stewart elliptical incision may be used for central and subareolar primary lesions of the breast. The incision extends medially to the margin of the sternum and laterally to the anterior margin of the latissimus dorsi. A margin at least 2–3 cm from the edges of the tumour should be obtained with the skin incision. If immediate reconstruction is anticipated when adequate tumour-free margins can be achieved, the 'skin-sparing' mastectomy is advisable. Frozen section margin control, to assure histologically clear margins, is mandatory with this technique.

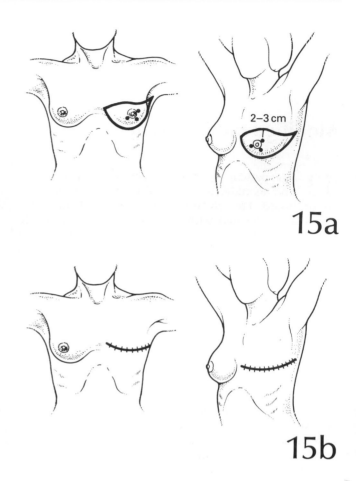

15a

15b

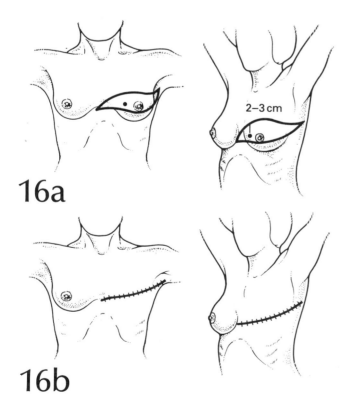

16a

16b

16a,b Inner quadrant lesions may be approached with the more obliquely placed modified Stewart incision where the medial extent of the incision extends to the reconstruction with myocutaneous flaps.

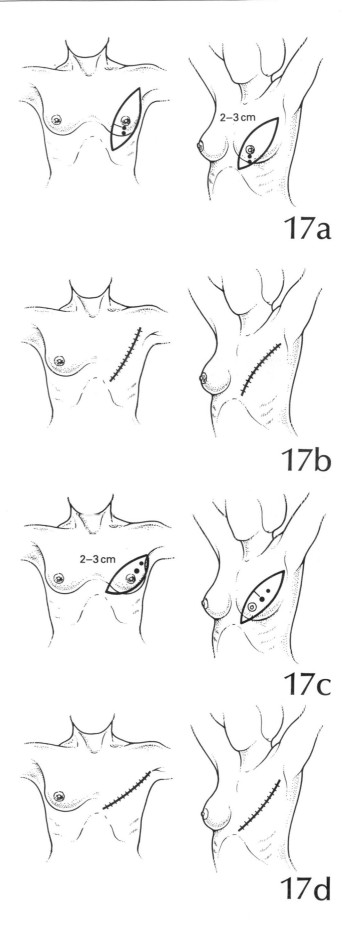

17a–d The classic oblique (Orr) incision is used for upper outer quadrant lesions (*Illustrations 17a,b*), while a slight variation can be used for lower inner and vertically placed lesions of the breast (*Illustrations 17c,d*). This incision is especially advantageous to consider with skin-sparing mastectomy, as all incisions are oblique, lateral and placed in the upper outer quadrant.

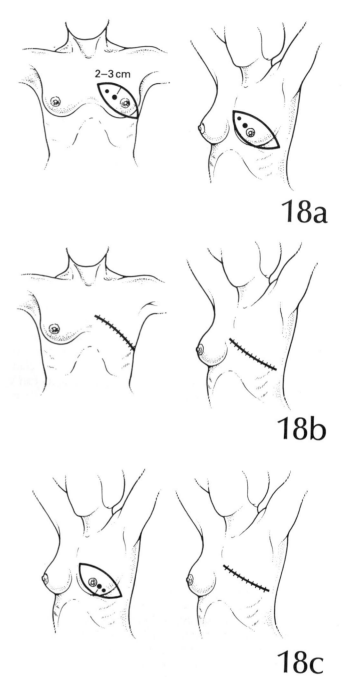

18a–c Upper inner lesions are often difficult to manage because of their location and their subsequent effect on cosmesis. The superior flap must allow access for axillary dissection and still provide flap margins 2–3 cm from the tumour (*Illustrations 18a,b*). Similar incisions can be used for lower outer quadrant lesions (*Illustration 18c*).

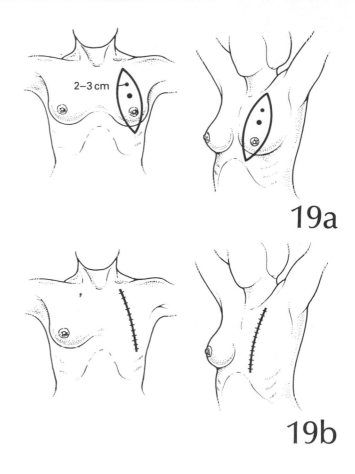

19a

19b

19a,b Large lesions (T2, T3 and T4) that are high lying, infraclavicular or fixed to the pectoralis major often need Halstedian incisions or their modifications (*see Illustrations 3a–h*) and subsequent skin grafting. T1 lesions in these locations can be approached with a vertically placed elliptical incision.

Dissection

The following describes the Patey technique for the modified radical mastectomy whereby removal of the pectoralis minor muscle allows easy access to level III (apical) nodes to facilitate removal of nodes from all three levels. The techniques of modified radical mastectomy described by Auchincloss and Madden preserve both the pectoralis major and minor muscles and therefore allow only incomplete dissection (levels I and II) with preservation of level III nodes.

20 Regardless of the skin incision selected, the limits of modified radical mastectomy are delineated laterally by the anterior margin of the latissimus dorsi muscles, medially by the midline of the sternum, superiorly by the subclavius muscle, and inferiorly approximately 1–2 cm inferior to the infra-mammary fold. For any incision used, the skin edge should have a 2–3-cm margin from the tumour. Attention is first directed towards developing inferior and superior flaps. Flap thickness varies with the build of the patient, but ideally should be 7–8 mm thick. The level of dissection extends just cephalad to the cutaneous vasculature and is accentuated by flap traction. The skin flaps are retracted and exposed by an assistant with skin hooks or towel clips while the operator provides caudal traction on the breast tissue. A skin flap of constant thickness must be developed in order to avoid creating devascularized subcutaneous tissues that contribute to wound seroma, skin necrosis or flap retraction.

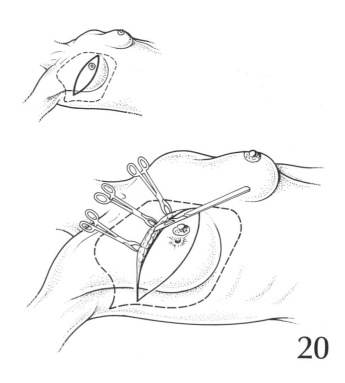

20

21 The superior skin flap is elevated to the level of the subclavius muscle and the pectoralis major fascia is dissected from the pectoralis musculature by placing countertraction on the breast and fascia in a caudal direction. Multiple perforating vessels may be encountered and should be carefully clamped and ligated. Fascial excision, which allows minimal haemostasis, is achieved by traction at the fascial margin by the operator's fingers while an incision is made parallel to the pectoralis major muscle fibres. The inferior flap is then elevated in a similar fashion medially to the midline, inferiorly to the aponeurosis of the rectus abdominus tendon, and laterally to the anterior margin of the latissimus dorsi. The superolateral margin of the pectoralis major is cleared, leaving the most inferior portion of the breast in continuity with the axillary contents.

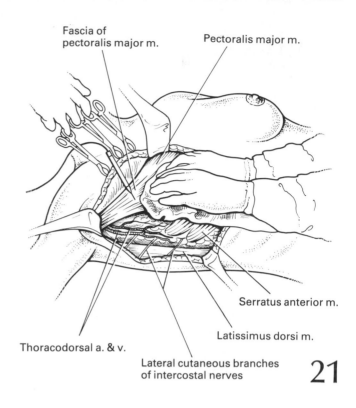

Fascia of pectoralis major m.

Pectoralis major m.

Serratus anterior m.

Latissimus dorsi m.

Lateral cutaneous branches of intercostal nerves

Thoracodorsal a. & v.

21

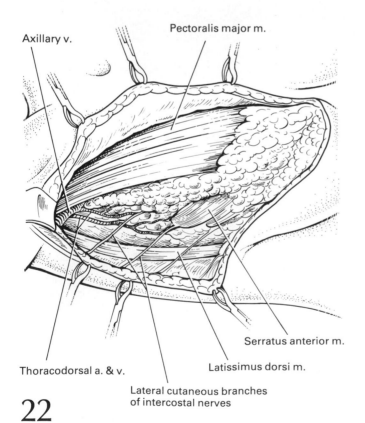

Axillary v.

Pectoralis major m.

Serratus anterior m.

Latissimus dorsi m.

Thoracodorsal a. & v.

Lateral cutaneous branches of intercostal nerves

22

22 Areolar and nodal tissues surrounding the latissimus dorsi muscle are dissected; this muscle delineates the lateral boundary of the axillary dissection. Intercostobrachial sensory nerves providing cutaneous innervation to the lateral chest, axilla and medial upper arm are commonly divided in the course of dissection of the axilla and lateral skin flaps. Selective preservation of these sensory nerves is possible without compromise of the *en bloc* dissection principles, as long as these fibres are freely dissected from the axillary contents. Sacrifice of this nerve is appropriate when involvement with fixation is evident.

23a,b Elevation of the loose areolar tissue of the lateral axillary space may aid in the identification of the most lateral extent of the axillary vein, otherwise the superficial investing fascia of the axillary space must be incised (*Illustration 23b*) to further expose the axillary vein. Finger dissection of the lateral and inferior margin of the pectoralis major will allow identification of the insertion of the tendinous portion of the pectoralis minor muscle.

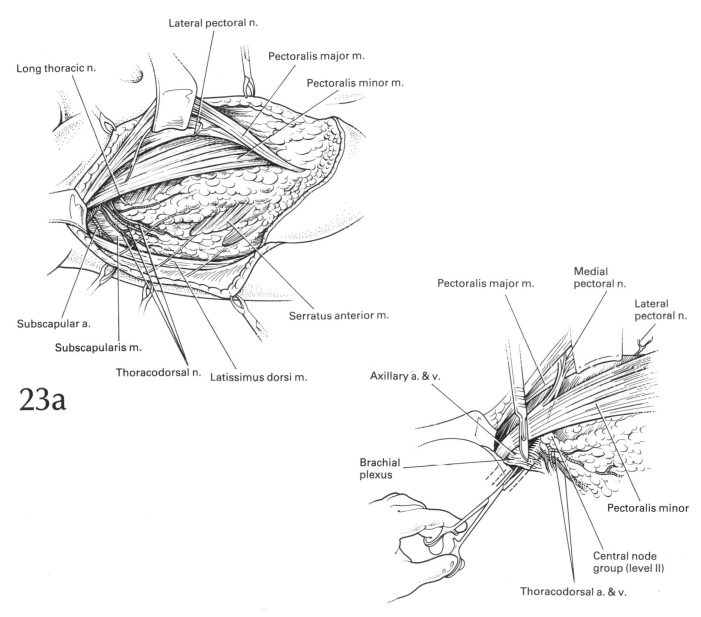

23a

23b

24a,b In the Patey technique the tendinous portion of the pectoralis minor muscle is divided near its insertion on the coracoid process while protecting the medial and lateral pectoral nerves. With this division, levels II and III nodes are thoroughly exposed. Interpectoral nodes (Rotter's nodes) are readily included *en bloc* with the operative specimen. Caudal to the axillary vein, nodal dissection commences from lateral to medial after identification of the long thoracic and thoracodorsal nerves.

The long thoracic nerve is constant in its location anterior to the subscapularis muscle and is closely applied to the investing fascial compartment of chest wall musculature (serratus anterior). Its entire course must be carefully isolated and dissected from the axillary contents. Its identification can be verified by a gentle pinch initiating a 'twitch' in the serratus anterior muscle. The inadvertent division of this neural structure will result in a 'winged scapula'. The thoracodorsal

nerve lies lateral to the long thoracic nerve and has a variable inferolateral course en route to its innervation of the latissimus dorsi muscle. Isolation and dissection throughout its courses is recommended to avoid denervation and motor loss to this muscle.

The lateral axillary nodal group, the subscapular and the external mammary nodal groups (all level I) are then carefully dissected *en bloc*. The nodal contents are swept together for extirpation with the central nodal group (level II) and the apical (subclavicular) level III group. The most superior and medial extent of the dissection is the clavipectoral fascia (Halsted's ligament); this nodal group should be marked with a clip or a suture for specimen orientation at the time of pathological processing and study. During dissection constant and repeated reorientation with respect to the location of the two nerves noted above must be achieved to avoid injury or inadvertent ligation.

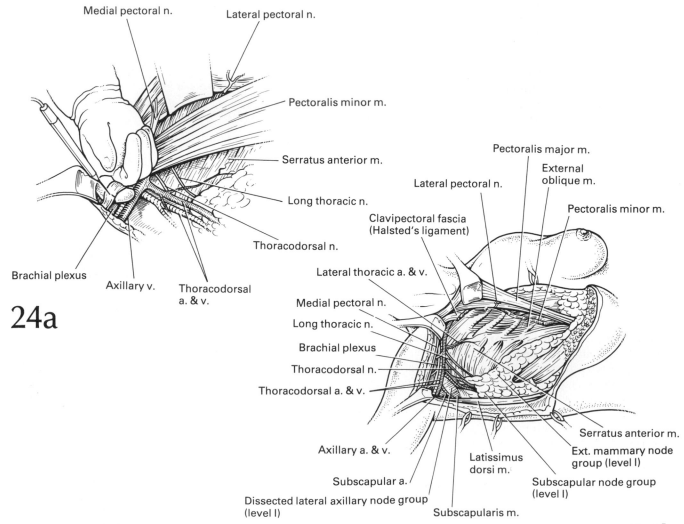

24a

24b

25 After the axillary nodes are dissected free, the origins of the pectoralis minor from ribs 2–5 are transected. The remaining attached breast and fascia are cleared medially and inferiorly from the aponeurosis of the rectus abdominus muscle.

The specimen should immediately be sent to the pathology department to obtain samples for measurement of steroid hormone receptors if this procedure was not completed at the initial biopsy.

Meticulous haemostasis is achieved. It is advisable at this point for the surgeon and all assistants and nurses to reglove and, optionally, regown. Moreover, a separate small instrument tray is requested for wound closure to avoid the potential for implantation of exfoliated tumour cells in the wound. The wound is copiously irrigated and re-examined for bleeding points. Two closed suction Silastic drains are placed, one in the axillary space inferior to the vein and a second in the superomedial aspect of the defect, anterior to the pectoralis major. These drains are brought out through inferior incisions and secured to the skin with monofilament nylon sutures. They are then attached to portable suction bulbs or vacuum bottles.

Subcutaneous tissue is approximated with 2/0 or 3/0 absorbable sutures and the skin is closed with staples or subcuticular 4/0 absorbable sutures and Steri-strips. A light bulky dressing is applied and secured with tape. Optionally, the surgeon may immobilize the ipsilateral arm in an arm sling. Drains are removed when their outputs diminish to less than 20–30 ml in a 24 h interval.

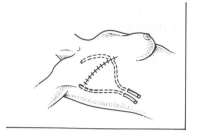

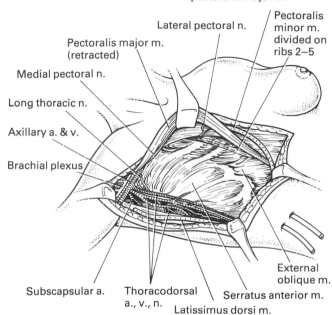

Drain anterior to pectoralis major m.

Lateral pectoral n.

Pectoralis minor m. divided on ribs 2–5

Pectoralis major m. (retracted)

Medial pectoral n.

Long thoracic n.

Axillary a. & v.

Brachial plexus

External oblique m.

Subscapsular a.   Thoracodorsal a., v., n.   Serratus anterior m.

Latissimus dorsi m.

25

Postoperative care

Closed suction catheter drainage is generally necessary for 4–7 days after the operation. Most patients can be discharged with their closed suction catheter drainage system (eg. Hemovac, Davol or Jackson-Pratt) and followed up by a visiting nurse. The drains may be removed when measured serosanguineous output is 20–30 ml within a 24-h period.

Patients are encouraged to resume activity on the evening of their operation. A normal or light meal is usually well tolerated that night as well as some early ambulation. Based on results from randomized prospective clinical trials, it is advisable for patients to continue immobilization of the ipsilateral shoulder and upper arm in an arm sling, while mobility is permitted below the elbow in the forearm and hand. During the first postoperative week patients are encouraged to begin graded, active range-of-motion exercises of the ipsilateral arm and shoulder. Physical and psychological rehabilitation of the post-mastectomy patient has been greatly facilitated by support agencies which are often provided by post-mastectomy patients.

Although rare, the immediate postoperative complications of pneumothorax and haemorrhage should be identified and corrected quickly. Postoperative assessment should include evaluation of all wounds for infection or tissue necrosis. The patient must be counselled for any complaints of hypaesthesias and paraesthesias, or findings consistent with peripheral nerve injury. Moreover, any signs of lymphoedema or seroma formation must be addressed with long-term interventions which will prevent recurrence or progression.

Flexible endoscopy of the upper digestive tract

André Duranceau MD
Professor of Surgery, Department of Surgery, University of Montréal, Division of Thoracic Surgery, Hôtel-Dieu de Montréal, Montréal, Québec, Canada

Eric Deslandres MD
Assistant Professor, Department of Medicine, University of Montréal, Division of Gastroenterology, Hôtel-Dieu de Montréal, Montréal, Québec, Canada

Principles and justification

Upper digestive flexible endoscopy has evolved considerably over the last 25 years. It presently plays a dominant role in the evaluation of the upper gastrointestinal tract. Specifically, it provides both direct and complete visualization of the area and direct access for tissue sampling and/or therapeutic intervention. The technique should be mastered by any clinician with a special interest in diseases of the oesophagus, stomach, or duodenum.

Preoperative

Patient preparation

Preparation for upper gastrointestinal endoscopy begins with the initial consultation. Following radiological assessment of the oesophagus and stomach, the indications and advantages of the technique are discussed with the patient. The procedure is explained in simple terms. During the clinic evaluation, allergies, current medication and previous medical history are reviewed. The need for antibiotic prophylaxis is assessed.

The patient should fast overnight before the procedure. Outpatients should be accompanied, particularly if intravenous sedation is to be used.

In the endoscopy suite, the procedure is explained again to minimize the patient's anxiety. Having a calm and relaxed patient avoids to some extent the need for sedation. A tense patient should not be submitted to upper digestive endoscopy under simple topical anaesthesia. Proper sedation dictates the use of pulse oximetry and electrocardiography. Aggressive or uncooperative patients should not be submitted to endoscopy under local anaesthesia.

A lignocaine gargle or spray is used for topical anaesthesia of the pharynx and hypopharynx. The patient is instructed to undertake a Valsalva's manoeuvre in order to protect the larynx from the spray.

It is difficult to be dogmatic about which patients will require intravenous sedation. The advantages of topical anaesthesia are a rapid recuperation after the procedure and a rapid return to normal activities. When this is explained to the patient, it encourages some to undergo the procedure with topical anaesthesia. This is so particularly if the atmosphere and the behaviour of the staff are calm and confident. When needed, adequate sedation may be obtained with benzodiazepines (diazepam, midazolam). Pethidine hydrochloride may be added for relaxation and analgesia. This medication should be administered slowly in small doses until the desired level of sedation is obtained.

Technique

Introduction of the endoscope

Blind insertion

1 The patient sits facing the surgeon or lies in the left lateral decubitus position. The endoscope lies on the right shoulder of the endoscopist. Following appropriate topical anaesthesia, the index and third finger of the left hand are placed on the back of the patient's tongue. Forward traction by the two fingers permits the introduction of the slightly flexed end of the endoscope over the back of the tongue into the buccopharynx.

The endoscopist removes the fingers from the patient's mouth and holds the head of the patient slightly bent forward. The endoscope is gently advanced until resistance is felt. Voluntary swallowing at this point allows the instrument to pass into the cervical oesophagus. The mouthpiece, previously positioned around the shaft of the endoscope, is installed between the patient's teeth and the examination is started.

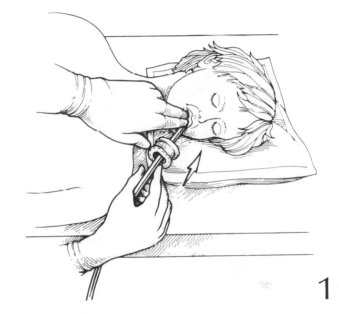

1

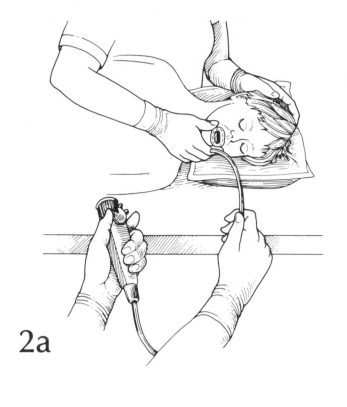

2a

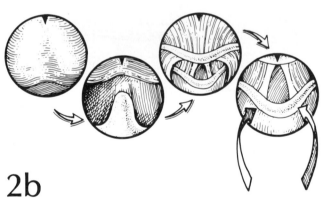

2b

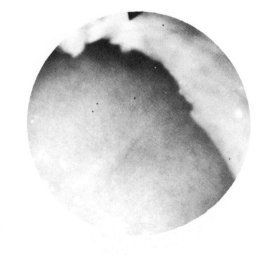

2c

Visual insertion

2a–e The patient lies in the left lateral position after buccopharyngeal and hypopharyngeal topical anaesthesia has been applied. A mouthpiece is installed between the teeth or gums and the flexible tip of the endoscope is advanced, taking care to stay in the midline and at the interface between the tongue and hypopharyngeal mucosa. Tongue, uvula, epiglottis and cricoarytenoid cartilages are seen. Passing beside the midline, the cricoarytenoid cartilages are passed and the tip of the endoscope stops on the cricopharyngeus which closes the entry to the oesophagus. Gentle local pressure while asking the patient to swallow allows the tip of the endoscope to pass into the cervical oesophagus.

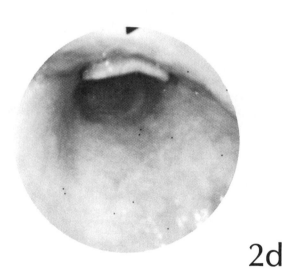

2d

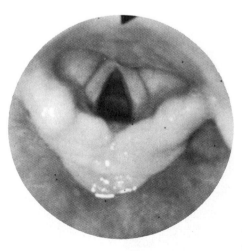

2e

Examination of the oesophagus

The instrument is advanced under direct vision, with the tip of the endoscope always central in the lumen, using optimal insufflation to keep the lumen of the oesophagus well distended. Systematic routine examination of the oesophagus is completed first in order to document as meticulously as possible any mucosal abnormality. This 'first-hand' inspection is important, because no trauma has been caused by manipulation or passage of the instrument. Two rules must always be observed: (1) the endoscope must be advanced with clear vision of the central lumen; (2) if direct vision is obscured or there are any doubts, the endoscope should be withdrawn.

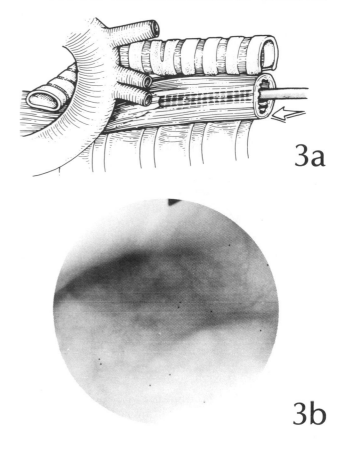

3a

3a, b Distal to the cricopharyngeal sphincter, the first landmark in the oesophagus is the extraluminal compression by the left main bronchus and the aortic arch. Pulsations of the left heart over the distal half are identified. A large oesophagus may be 'moulded' on the descending thoracic aorta.

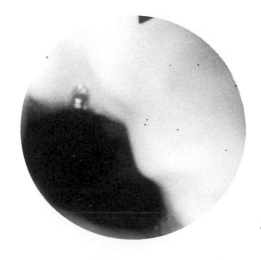

3b

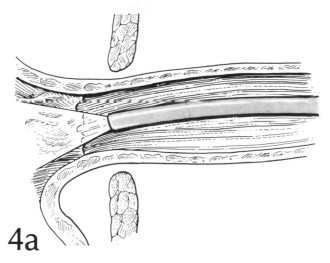

4a

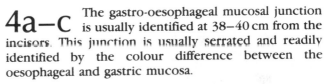

4a–c The gastro-oesophageal mucosal junction is usually identified at 38–40 cm from the incisors. This junction is usually serrated and readily identified by the colour difference between the oesophageal and gastric mucosa.

The position of the oesophageal hiatus in the diaphragm is identified by asking the patient to inhale deeply; the diaphragmatic hiatus during inspiration creates an imprint on the oesophageal or gastric wall. The positions of both the hiatus and the mucosal junction are recorded in order to document the possibility of a hernia or of a columnar-lined oesophagus.

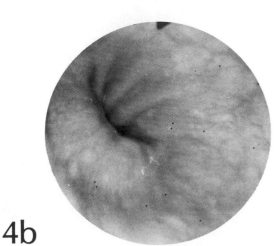

4b

4c

Passage into the stomach

Passage of the endoscope into the stomach requires appropriate observations to be made at the gastro-oesophageal junction. This junction may be closed or widely patulous. Passage into the gastric lumen is usually a simple manoeuvre that occurs without resistance. Occasionally however, mucosal, submucosal, or extrinsic lesions can distort the normal junction and cause difficulty in progression into the stomach. Absence of any mucosal lesion, but a progressive 'giving' of the lower oesophageal sphincter area under pressure, raises the possibility of a motor disorder.

Examination of the stomach

5a, b On entering the stomach, it becomes distended with air and this often causes discomfort to the patient. By tipping the end of the endoscope slightly down and towards the left, a view of the greater curvature and of the posterior gastric wall is obtained. Aspiration of all retained liquid is carried out to decrease the risk of aspiration and also to allow proper examination of the stomach.

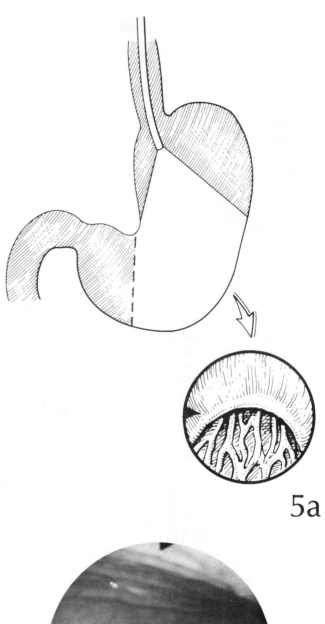

5a

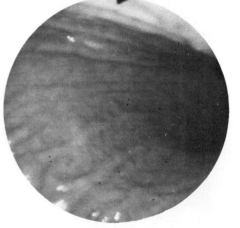

5b

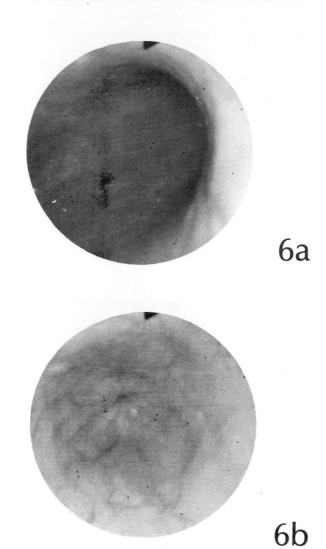

6a

6b

6a–c A rotation movement of the tip of the instrument allows examination of the anterior and posterior walls of the body of the stomach. The lesser curvature down to the angulus and the greater curvature are viewed by the same motion. The most proximal part of both curvatures are better examined when using the J manoeuvre (see below).

The endoscope is advanced along the greater curvature and the endoscopist rotates the instrument toward the right while angulating its tip. Progression toward the antrum and pylorus is accomplished with the same rotating movement of the tip, allowing complete circumferential assessment of the antrum.

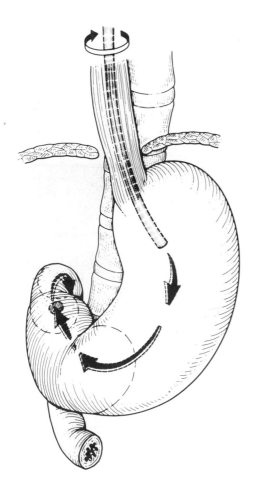

6c

The prepyloric area and the pyloric ring are always approached directly, with passage through the pylorus being done under direct vision. The tip of the endoscope must always visualize the pyloric lumen while pressure is put on the advancing instrument. When the pylorus 'yields', complete assessment of the first part of the duodenum is undertaken as far as the superior duodenal angle. When pathology is thought to be confined to the oesophagus or stomach, the examination is not carried further and the endoscope is pulled back into the distal stomach.

7a–h While the tip of the endoscope lies along the distal lesser curvature and while the stomach is distended, rotation of the instrument is accomplished toward the greater curvature. Complete 180° upwards angulation of the endoscope tip completes the J manoeuvre. The endoscope is pulled back gently while the stomach is distended. Swinging of the retroflexed tip allows proper visualization of the subcardial area and of the fundus of the stomach. Simultaneous rotation of the endoscope gives an excellent view of the lesser curvature from the cardia to the angulus.

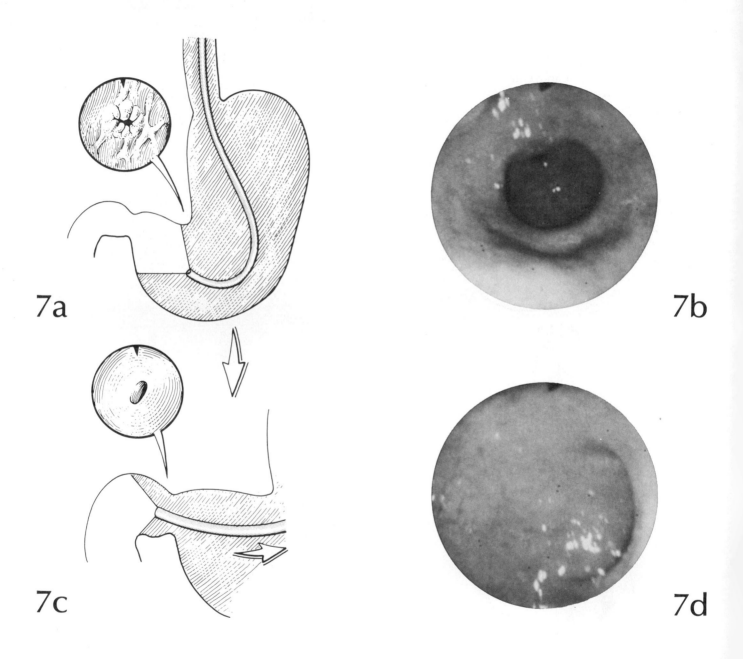

7a

7b

7c

7d

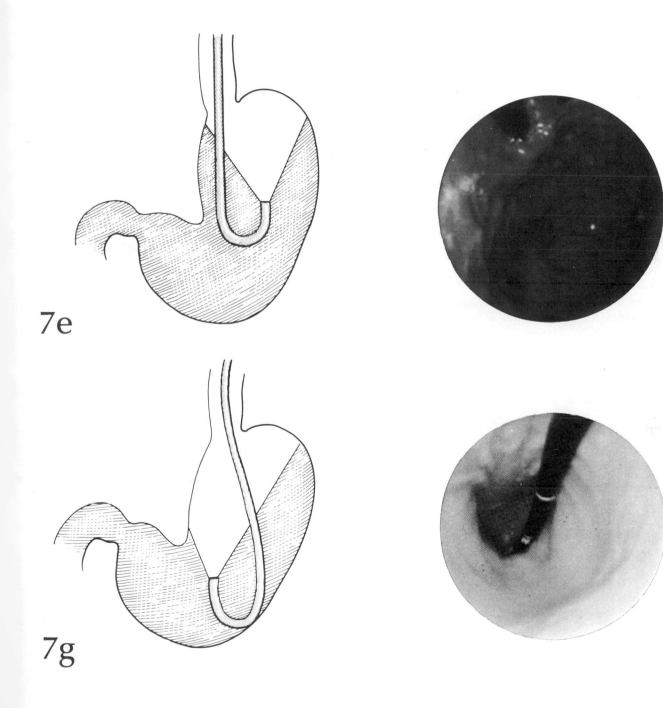

7e

7f

7g

7h

Taking tissue specimens

8a–c Biopsies are taken from any lesion seen in the oesophagus or stomach using cup forceps. The presence of a dependable cytopathology division encourages the use of brush cytology for diagnosis of all mucosal abnormalities. The diagnostic yield of cytology is higher than that of biopsies in the authors' hands, particularly for obstructive oesophageal lesions.

Recovery

Patients are encouraged to avoid drinking or eating for approximately 30 min after termination of the procedure.

The results of the endoscopy should be discussed with the patient immediately if no sedation has been given. If the patient has received sedation, explanations are delayed until the patient has recovered. This information should be given in the presence of the person accompanying the patient, as the effects of sedation on a patient's memory may persist for some time.

Patients are advised not to drive or engage in regular working activities for a few hours if they have been given sedation.

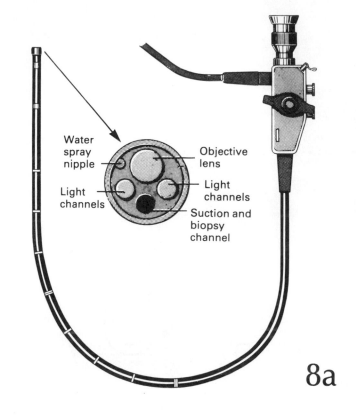

Water spray nipple

Objective lens

Light channels

Light channels

Suction and biopsy channel

8a

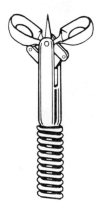

8b

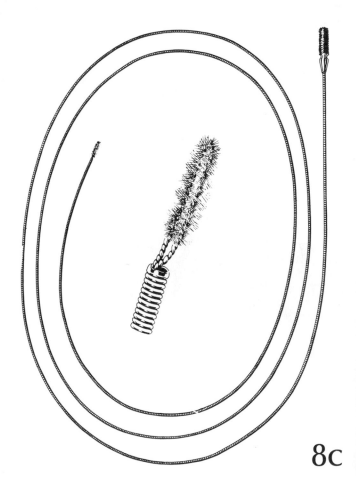

8c

Injection sclerotherapy of oesophageal varices

J. E. J. Krige FRCS, FCS(SA)
Associate Professor, Department of Surgery, University of Cape Town, South Africa

John Terblanche ChM, FRCS, FCS(SA)
Professor and Head, Department of Surgery and Co-Director, MRC Liver Research Centre, University of Cape Town, South Africa

Techniques

The three techniques of injection sclerotherapy are intravariceal, paravariceal and the combination of both intravariceal and paravariceal methods.

Intravariceal technique

Injection of sclerosant directly into the varix to induce variceal thrombosis is the most widely used technique. The injections are localized to the lower 5 cm of the oesophagus. The authors use 5% ethanolamine oleate.

Paravariceal technique

Sclerosant is injected into the submucosa adjacent to a varix, as described by Wodak[1] and Paquet[2]. The most widely used sclerosant is polidocanol (0.5% or 1% concentration). The sclerosant is administered as 30–40 separate injections (0.5–1 ml each) in a helical fashion, commencing at the gastro-oesophageal junction and extending approximately one-third of the way up the oesophagus. The aim is to produce oedema to compress the varix during acute bleeding and subsequently to provoke tissue reaction, fibrosis and thickening of the mucosa over the varices to prevent bleeding. This technique will not be described further.

Combined technique

The combination of intravariceal and paravariceal injections is used in Cape Town for the emergency management of actively bleeding varices, and in the elective management of large varices to prevent needle-puncture bleeding[3]. The authors use 5% ethanolamine oleate although other agents have been used successfully by other groups. A small volume (1 ml) of sclerosant is injected paravariceally to partially compress the varix, followed by an intravariceal injection of a larger volume (up to 5 ml) to thrombose the varix. As with the intravariceal injection technique, the injections are restricted to the lower 5 cm of the oesophagus.

Equipment

Endoscopes

1 Either single- or twin-channel endoscopes are suitable for injection sclerotherapy. The single-channel endoscope should have a large channel so that suction is not reduced after the injector has been inserted. The twin-channel endoscope is useful for acute bleeding because one channel allows unimpeded suction during injection. Either end- or oblique-viewing endoscopes are effective for injection sclerotherapy. For general purposes an end-viewing instrument is more versatile, enabling both diagnostic and therapeutic functions to be performed. The advantages of an oblique-viewing endoscope are better visualization of the greater and lesser curves of the stomach and the built-in forceps elevator which is helpful in aiming the injector, particularly when small varices are being injected electively.

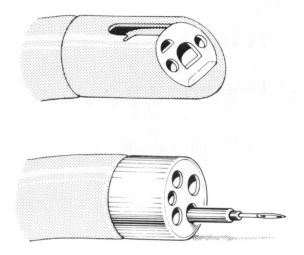

1

Injectors

Several types of sclerotherapy injectors with retractable needles are commercially available (*Illustration 1*). The flexible metal injectors are robust and reusable, but the narrower internal calibre and greater resistance during injection restricts the volume of sclerosant administered per unit time compared with the disposable injectors. Injectors are equipped with either 23 or 25 gauge needles. The larger needle is preferred as it facilitates injection of viscous sclerosant solutions and is not associated with any greater risk of bleeding after withdrawal of the needle.

Sclerosants

Several different sclerosant agents have been successfully used. The Cape Town group uses 5% ethanolamine oleate for both the intravariceal and the combined injection technique[3]. The most widely used alternative solutions are sodium tetradecyl sulphate (1%) and sodium morrhuate (2%) while polidocanol (0.5% or 1%) is used almost exclusively by proponents of paravariceal sclerotherapy[4].

Procedures

ELECTIVE SCLEROTHERAPY

Preparation of patient

The procedure is explained to the patient and signed consent obtained. Two assistants, including a qualified nurse trained in endoscopy techniques, should be present throughout the procedure. One assistant provides suction of the patient's mouth to avoid aspiration, ensures that the bite guard is not dislodged and comforts the patient. The other assistant advances and retracts the injector needle and administers the sclerosant under the direction of the endoscopist. The posterior tongue and pharynx are sprayed with a local anaesthetic (10% xylocaine). A small butterfly needle is inserted into a superficial hand vein and remains in place for the duration of the procedure. The appropriate analgesia and sedation are administered intravenously according to the medical status of the patient. The desired sedation is achieved by injecting small incremental doses, being cautious to avoid oversedation in the aged and in those with liver compromise. The authors' preference is 2.5 mg midazolam and 25 mg pethidine.

Before passing the endoscope the fully connected instrument should be checked for satisfactory function of the light source and lens, focus and tip deflection controls, air, suction and water channels. The assistants should be familiar with the technique and equipment. Commands such as 'advance needle' and 'retract needle' should be rehearsed before injection. The endoscopist indicates the volume to be injected and the assistant acknowledges that the desired volume has been injected. It is important that the assistant should comment when more resistance than expected is encountered during injection, because the varix may be thrombosed or the needle incorrectly positioned.

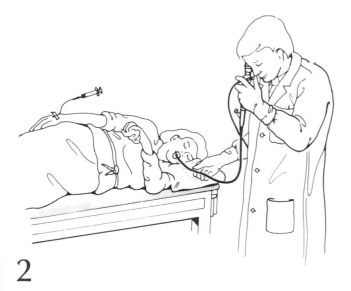

Position of patient

2 The patient is placed in the left lateral decubitus position at the top of the bed with the head on a pillow and the neck slightly flexed. The distal endoscope tube is lubricated with a water-soluble medical-grade lubricant, dentures are removed and a comfortable mouthpiece (bite guard) is used in patients with teeth to protect the endoscope.

2

Endoscopy

3 Passage of the fibreoptic endoscope is initiated by guiding the gently flexed tip over the tongue and then extending the tip in the upper pharynx. The opening of the cricopharynx is identified and negotiated with gentle pressure coinciding with a swallow. The instrument is passed under direct vision, keeping the oesophageal lumen in full view by controlling the tip. Intermittent insufflation of air is used to maintain sufficient distension of the lumen for visibility. Constant or excessive air insufflation should be avoided. Mucus and fluid are removed through the suction channel and the lens cleared with a jet of water when necessary. After passing the cricopharynx, the entire oesophagus is examined for oesophageal varices. The extent, number and size are noted for documentation. Unless varices are bleeding, panendoscopy is first performed to exclude other lesions before commencing injection of varices.

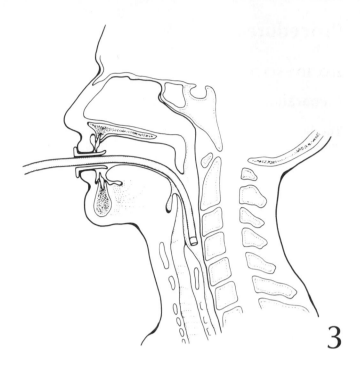

3

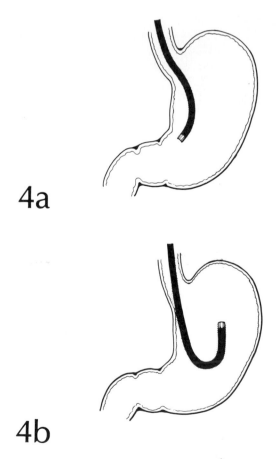

4a

4b

4a, b When the stomach is reached, the tip is passed distally under vision, insufflating only enough air to display the channel ahead. The pylorus is centred in the field of view and air is insufflated to distend the distal stomach and relax the pylorus; as this occurs the tip is gently advanced into the duodenal bulb. The proximal duodenum is carefully evaluated. Thereafter, the endoscope is withdrawn into the stomach and the cardia, gastric fundus and upper portion of the lesser curve are viewed by reversing the tip in the moderately distended body of the stomach. If gastric varices or evidence of portal hypertensive gastropathy are present they are noted and documented.

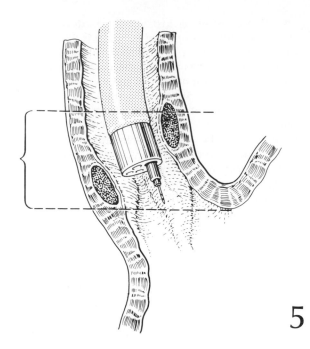

5 On completion of panendoscopy the endoscope is partially withdrawn and positioned above the gastro-oesophageal junction, and the varices in the lower 5 cm of the oesophagus are injected.

5

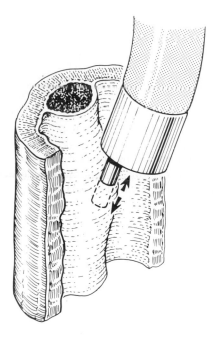

6

Injection technique

6 The endoscope tip is manoeuvred into position and the target varix identified. The endoscopist passes the injector through the channel into the field of view and the tip is positioned 2 cm beyond the end of the endoscope. Care should be taken to avoid inadvertent puncture of the plastic injector sheath and damage to the endoscope channel by the needle when advancing the injector. The injector should not be passed through the channel with the endoscope tip in a position of acute flexion. The needle should remain in the retracted position until the tip of the injector has passed through the endoscope and is visible to the endoscopist. All movements and manipulation of the injector are performed *only* by the endoscopist. A practice aiming pass with the needle retracted is useful to determine the direction of the advancing needle.

7 The assistant is instructed to advance the needle and a small volume of solution is discarded into the oesophageal lumen in order to fill the injector. The endoscopist inserts the needle directly into the centre and most prominent part of the varix by advancing the injector a further 5 mm: the length of the visible needle and the angle of insertion determine the depth of puncture. If the needle is well placed and appears intravariceal, the assistant is instructed to inject 1 ml of sclerosant. If this is achieved without resistance the assistant injects further sclerosant. With further injection of sclerosant the varix will be seen to distend above and below the injection site and become paler. This is the indication to stop the injection. A total volume of no more than 5 ml is usually required for a large varix: smaller varices require proportionately less sclerosant. On completing injection of the first varix, the remaining varices are injected. After a previous series of injections, varices will be smaller and less sclerosant is injected. During subsequent endoscopy, varices may be thrombosed and appear firm and cord-like. If increased resistance to insertion of the needle and injection of sclerosant with leakage around the needle is noted, confirming obliteration of the variceal channel, no further injection should be undertaken.

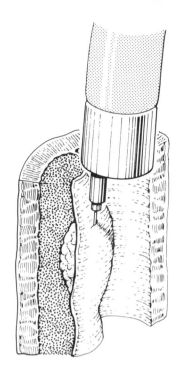

7

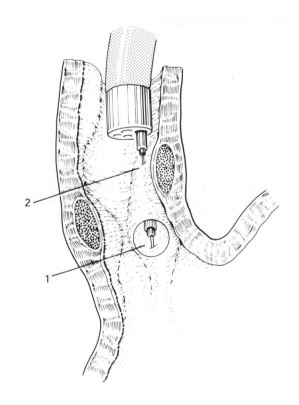

8

8 A second series of injections is performed at a higher level for large varices (site 2). The fibrescope is withdrawn 2–3 cm and the varices injected (usually 2–3 ml of sclerosant is sufficient). As the varices become smaller after several previous injections, they are injected only at the lower site (site 1).

9 Accurate placement of the needle is critical in obtaining effective delivery of sclerosant and avoiding complications which may follow incorrect injection. A tangential flat angle of insertion as shown in *Illustration 7* is preferable to avoid deep injection: a less acute angle with a perpendicular approach may transfix the varix and penetrate the oesophageal wall, resulting in an intramuscular injection. In this situation increased resistance to injection will be noted by the assistant and no blanching or distension of the varix will occur. The injector and needle should be withdrawn and a further injection performed after accurate placement of the needle.

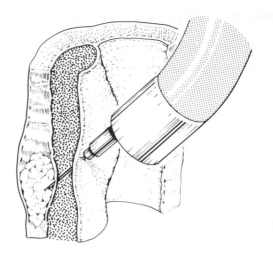

9

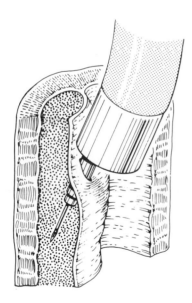

10

10 The needle should not be left protruding while selecting a further varix for injection because inadvertent laceration of a varix with accompanying bleeding may occur, especially with coughing or peristalsis. Needle insertion and variceal puncture requires a delicate wrist action by the endoscopist while manipulating the injector. This provides a limited controlled forward momentum of about 5 mm.

Injection by attempting to spear the varix or forceful jabbing of the varix with the needle may result in deep insertion and cannulation of the varix with entry of both needle and the hub of the catheter sheath and resultant bleeding from the varix on extraction.

EMERGENCY SCLEROTHERAPY

Initial measures

Urgent intravenous fluid resuscitation is started. The authors' group uses pharmacological therapy in patients with suspected variceal bleeding, although the efficacy remains controversial[4]. Vasopressin, its synthetic analogue terlipressin, and somatostatin have been used to lower portal pressure[4]. The most commonly used agent is vasopressin, which should be administered as a continuous intravenous infusion. Combination of glyceryl trinitrate with vasopressin reduces the side effects caused by vasopressin alone and potentiates the portal haemodynamic effects. The glyceryl trinitrate can be administered intravenously, sublingually, or transdermally. A combination of continuous intravenous vasopressin (0.4 units/min) and sublingual glyceryl trinitrate (one tablet every half hour for up to 6 hours) was used[4], but currently the authors, like others, have converted to using a continuous infusion of somatostatin or octreotide.

Endoscopy

Urgent endoscopy is essential. The patient is positioned as for elective sclerotherapy as shown in *Illustration 2*. One-third of patients with suspected variceal bleeding do not, in fact, have varices. Patients shown to have varices on endoscopy fall into one of three groups although the differentiation may be difficult during active bleeding: (1) those with actively bleeding varices; (2) those whose varices have stopped bleeding; (3) those who have varices but are bleeding from another lesion. At endoscopy, variceal bleeding that has stopped is diagnosed if adherent blood clots are noted on a varix, or when varices are present in a patient with upper gastrointestinal bleeding in whom panendoscopy demonstrates no other cause of bleeding.

Emergency endoscopy should be performed in the endoscopy unit where all the necessary equipment is available. Many units have a fully equipped emergency endoscopy trolley and if necessary this can be taken into the operating room or to the intensive care unit. It is imperative that full resuscitative facilities are available together with skilled staff experienced in dealing with emergencies. Two endoscopy assistants should be present throughout. Adequate monitoring is necessary during the procedure. Emergency endoscopy should not commence until satisfactory venous access and central venous pressure measurement are established and volume replacement and resuscitation procedures with blood transfusions are initiated to correct hypovolaemia. If bleeding is extensive, endotracheal intubation is essential before endoscopy to protect the airway and avoid aspiration.

Intravariceal injection

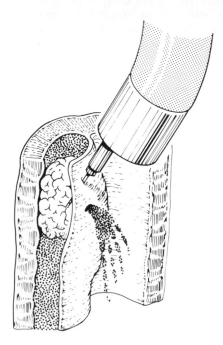

11 Active variceal bleeding with a jet of blood or rapid oozing is immediately dealt with by controlling the bleed with intravariceal sclerotherapy. Urgent control of bleeding with accurate placement of the needle and sclerosant should be performed without delay while there is adequate visibility. No attempt should be made to inject distal to the active bleeding site or to insert the needle into the bleeding point, because this may enlarge the hole and aggravate bleeding with extravasation and loss of sclerosant. A technique similar to elective intravariceal sclerotherapy is used with needle insertion proximal to the bleeding site. A total volume of 5 ml of sclerosant is usually sufficient. Distension and blanching of the varix indicate that the needle is in the correct position and that the appropriate volume of sclerosant has been injected. After the bleeding has been controlled, the other variceal channels are sclerosed. A second series of injections is usually performed at a higher level, as depicted in *Illustration 8*. Panendoscopy is undertaken on completion of sclerotherapy to exclude other lesions.

11

Combined paravariceal and intravariceal injection

12a–c The authors' group prefers this technique to control active variceal bleeding. The needle is inserted in a paravariceal position and sclerosant injected proximal to the bleeding point to compress the bleeding site by raising a weal (*Illustration 12a*). Sufficient sclerosant is injected to control the bleeding (*Illustration 12b*). If this does not completely control the acute bleeding, the paravariceal injection is repeated alongside the bleeding point. The procedure is completed by injecting the varix intravariceally (*Illustration 12c*). The volume injected paravariceally should not be more than 1 ml at each site to avoid ulceration of mucosa. The remaining variceal channels are then sclerosed. Panendoscopy is performed on completion of sclerotherapy to exclude other lesions.

If variceal bleeding is profuse, vigorous lavage through the endoscope channel and elevation of the head of the table to 30° may improve visibility and allow identification of the bleeding site. No blind attempts at injection should be used. The procedure is usually performed with the patient on his/her side as depicted in *Illustration 2*. With profuse bleeding the patient requires endotracheal intubation. The procedure may be facilitated by placing the patient on his/her back on the bed (or operating table) and adjusting the headpiece to an angle of 45°. If immediate sclerotherapy cannot be performed because of lack of expertise or inadequate visibility, bleeding should first be controlled by balloon tube tamponade before the patient is subjected to further sclerotherapy[4].

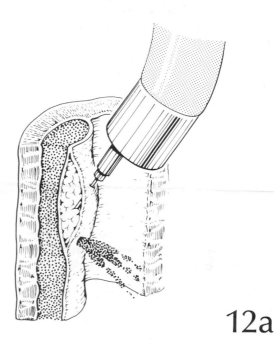

12a

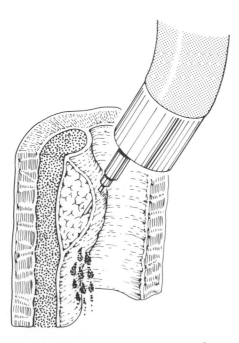

12b

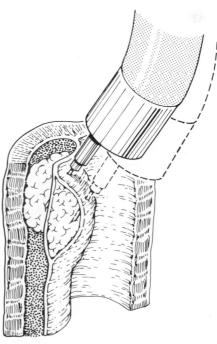

12c

Balloon tube tamponade

13 The four-lumen balloon tube (Minnesota tube) is effective in temporarily controlling variceal bleeding and gaining time for resuscitation and management planning[3,4]. Before inserting the balloon tube in stuporous or comatose patients, the airway should be protected by an endotracheal tube to prevent aspiration. A new tube should always be used and the inflated gastric and oesophageal balloons tested underwater to confirm a complete air seal. The deflated lubricated tube is passed through a bite guard via the mouth after adequate topical pharyngeal anaesthesia. Passage via the nose should not be used because of potential pressure necrosis of the nasal cartilage. The left index finger in the mouth facilitates initial passage of the tube by guiding the tip of the tube over the posterior tongue, through the cricopharynx and prevents coiling of the tube in the pharynx. If difficulty is encountered negotiating the cricopharynx, especially when an endotracheal tube is in place, a McGills forcep and laryngoscope are used to pass the tube under direct vision. The tube is inserted almost fully and the epigastrium auscultated to confirm that the gastric balloon is in the stomach by instilling air with a 50-ml syringe into the aspirating lumen. The gastric balloon is inflated with 50-ml increments of air to 200 ml. If the patient shows signs of discomfort, inflation *must* stop as the gastric balloon may be in the lower oesophagus and the position should be rechecked. When fully inflated, the tube is pulled back until the balloon engages the gastro-oesophageal junction and abuts on the cardia. A partially split tennis ball, secured over the tube, maintains firm traction against the bite guard and ensures constant compression on the cardia by the gastric balloon.

The oesophageal balloon is inflated only if bleeding continues after traction on the gastric balloon. The oesophageal balloon pressure should not exceed 40 mmHg or be maintained for more than 14 h. Thereafter, preferably within 6–12 h, sclerotherapy should be undertaken to achieve more lasting control because of the high rate of recurrence of bleeding (60%) after removal of the tube. If bleeding persists or recurs after the tube has been placed, the tube should be checked and, if found to be correctly situated, a further diagnostic endoscopy should be performed. A bleeding source that has been missed during the initial endoscopy may be the cause of continued bleeding. Because of associated dangers, a balloon tube should be used only when required to control endoscopically confirmed variceal bleeding[5,6].

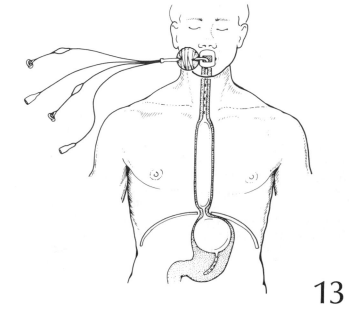

13

Postoperative care

Elective sclerotherapy

After elective outpatient sclerotherapy, patients are observed in the endoscopy suite recovery room for an hour before discharge. Bleeding following elective sclerotherapy is rare. Retrosternal discomfort is treated with antacids. After admission for acute variceal bleeding, the first two injection sclerotherapy sessions are performed in hospital. Further injection treatments are performed on an outpatient basis.

Injection sclerotherapy is repeated at weekly intervals until the varices have been eradicated. The first subsequent assessment is performed at 3 months and then repeated 6-monthly or yearly for life[7]. Any recurrent variceal channels noted during repeat endoscopy require a further course of injection sclerotherapy. If ulceration extending over more than one-quarter of the circumference of the oesophagus is present at the site of previous sclerotherapy, further injections are deferred for 2 weeks to allow the ulceration to heal. Minor ulceration or slough is usually ignored.

Emergency sclerotherapy

The patient is returned to an intensive care unit for 24 h after injection. Unless the patient is stuporous or comatose, oral fluids are allowed for the first 24 h and thereafter a regular diet is recommended. Prophylactic antibiotics are not administered routinely in uncomplicated cases. Hepatic encephalopathy and ascites are treated with standard therapy. Mild retrosternal discomfort and low-grade pyrexia may occur for 24 h after injection. If either is excessive or if the patient has dysphagia, a Gastrografin contrast swallow is obtained to exclude an injection site leak[6].

No further bleeding will occur in 70% of patients. If bleeding does recur, vasopressin or somatostatin is commenced and the patient re-endoscoped. Recurrent bleeding from oesophageal varices is treated by repeat injection similar to the initial procedures. If bleeding is massive and satisfactory control is not achieved by sclerotherapy, a balloon tube is placed for acute control and followed by sclerotherapy within 6–12 h. Bleeding from oesophageal ulceration or slough is treated conservatively with oral sucralfate. In the unusual event of persistent bleeding from injection ulceration, intravenous somatostatin is administered.

In patients who have continued acute variceal bleeding after two emergency sclerotherapy injection sessions during a single hospital admission, we recommend that bleeding be temporarily controlled with balloon tube tamponade followed by a surgical procedure[4,6,8]. Unfortunately, it is not possible to predict during initial evaluation and variceal injection which patients will not ultimately respond to sclerotherapy.

Outcome

Elective sclerotherapy

In the Cape Town 10-year prospective study evaluating the long-term management of patients after oesophageal variceal bleeding[7], oesophageal varices were eradicated in 123 of 140 patients. A median number of five injections were required to eradicate the oesophageal varices which remained eradicated for a mean of 19 months. Varices recurred in 37 patients after a mean of 15 months and were easily re-eradicated by further injection sclerotherapy. Recurrent variceal bleeding was unusual after the varices had been eradicated and occurred in only 13 of the 123 patients.

Acute variceal injection

The success rate of a single injection treatment is 70%[4,6]. The 30% of patients who have further bleeding after initial injection of sclerosant should have a second injection performed; in this group the success rate is more than 90%[4,6].

References

1. Wodak E. Akute gastrointestinale Blutung; Resultate der endoskopischen Sklerosierung von Osophagusvarizen. *Schweiz Med Wochenschr* 1979; 109: 591–4.

2. Paquet K-J, Oberhammer E. Sclerotherapy of bleeding oesophageal varices by means of endoscopy. *Endoscopy* 1978; 10: 7–12.

3. Terblanche J, Krige JE, Bornman PC. Endoscopic sclerotherapy. *Surg Clin North Am* 1990; 70: 341–59.

4. Terblanche J, Burroughs AK, Hobbs KE. Controversies in the management of bleeding oesophageal varices. *N Engl J Med* 1989; 320: 1393–8, 1469–75.

5. Burnett DA, Rikkers LF. Nonoperative emergency treatment of variceal haemorrhage. *Surg Clin North Am* 1990; 70: 291–306.

6. Kahn D, Bornman PC, Terblanche J. A 10-year prospective evaluation of balloon tube tamponade and emergency injection sclerotherapy for actively bleeding esophageal varices. *HPB Surg* 1989; 1: 207–19.

7. Terblanche J, Kahn D, Bornman PC. Long-term injection sclerotherapy treatment for oesophageal varices: a 10 year prospective evaluation. *Ann Surg* 1989; 210: 725–31.

8. Bornman PC, Terblanche J, Kahn D, Jonker MA, Kirsch RE. Limitations of multiple injection sclerotherapy sessions for acute variceal bleeding. *S Afr Med J* 1986; 70: 34–6.

Preoperative and postoperative management of patients undergoing major upper gastrointestinal surgery

Glyn G. Jamieson FRACS, FACS
Dorothy Mortlock Professor of Surgery, University of Adelaide, Department of Surgery, Royal Adelaide Hospital, Adelaide, Australia

Haile T. Debas MD
M. Galante Distinguished Professor of Surgery and Dean of the School of Medicine, University of California, San Francisco, California, USA

Modern surgery of the gastrointestinal tract is a very safe procedure in patients who are healthy, apart from the specific problem for which they are having their operation. Furthermore, whether a patient is generally fit can usually be ascertained simply from the history. Thus, regardless of age, if patients live an independent existence, do their own shopping and gardening and can walk up several flights of stairs without difficulty, the likelihood of a battery of preoperative tests turning up some abnormality critical to the outcome of an operation is remote.

However, because any major surgery can lead to problems where it may be helpful to know what the preoperative situation was, it is usual to carry out simple investigations in all such patients before surgery. These include determining the patient's blood group and haemoglobin level, obtaining a chest radiograph and, in older patients, an electrocardiogram, and general examination of renal function by measuring the blood creatinine level.

There are other tests which are appropriate to specific operations and these are considered below.

Oesophageal surgery

Preoperative

Diagnosis and operative planning

Today most patients have already had an endoscopy and biopsy by the time they present to the surgeon. If the diagnosis has been made from barium contrast studies, then endoscopy and biopsy should be carried out before surgery. If contrast studies have not been undertaken, they should be carried out as they are helpful in operative planning, giving an anatomical record for observation.

Before surgery all patients should undergo computed tomography to look for both lung and liver metastases, either of which might greatly alter a planned operative approach. Computed tomography may also give information about tumour size and its degree of invasiveness, although the latter is not a sufficiently reliable assessment upon which to base decisions about the operability of a tumour.

If a cervical operation is planned some surgeons advocate an assessment of vocal cord funtion before operation.

It is worth emphasizing at the outset that age is not a significant factor in oesophageal surgery: the major determinants of outcome are the patient's cardiovascular and respiratory fitness.

Cardiovascular fitness

An electrocardiogram is useful for showing any disturbances of cardiac rhythm and sometimes also to reflect past ischaemic events. An exercise electrocardiogram or stress test may uncover incipient ischaemia but the authors prefer to use the cardiac ejection fraction determined by a gated blood flow scan as a means of determining cardiac health. If the ejection fraction is less than 40% this is regarded as a significant risk factor for surgery, and in general terms is a contraindication to a major procedure.

Respiratory fitness

All patients should have an assessment of their lung function and blood gases. Values which should raise concern about a patient's ability to withstand major surgery are: (1) forced expiratory volume of gas less then 1 litre, (2) a vital capacity less that 70% of normal; and/or (3) an arterial oxygen tension of less than 70 mmHg. In patients with marginal lung function it is sometimes best to perform a tracheostomy at the same time as upper gastrointestinal surgery for optimal access to the patient's airways.

Nutrition

Patients with oesophageal cancer are often in a poor nutritional state. The measurement of serum albumin is a relatively crude test of the nutritional state but, taken with the patient's dietary history and evidence of weight loss, it is probably as accurate a measure as is available. Prolonged intravenous feeding is not indicated because any gains in terms of nutrition are usually lost by the complications from the intravenous line. Nevertheless it does seem sensible to commence nutritional support in such patients in the week before surgery and this can be done by a fine nasoenteric tube, an elemental diet or a feeding jejunostomy. The last technique may be used more often in the future with the development of laparoscopic jejunostomy.

Preoperative and perioperative therapy

Neomycin, 200 ml as a 1% solution, is given to the patient orally several hours before surgery in order to reduce oral and oesophageal flora. A broad-spectrum cephalosporin is also given intravenously immediately before surgery. This drug can be continued for 24 h but is then discontinued and subsequent antibiotics are given for specific indications only.

If a non-thoracotomy oesphagectomy is planned it is useful to digitalize the patient the day before surgery as there is a high incidence of cardiac arrhythmias when the surgeon's hands are dissecting behind the heart. Digitalis helps prevent such arrhythmias.

Antithrombotic measures such as intermittent calf compression should always be used, and some surgeons also use minidose subcutaneous heparin.

After the induction of anaesthesia various tubes are passed and monitors and lines established such as nasogastric tube, urinary catheter, intravenous lines, central venous lines and pulse oximetry for measuring oxygen saturation, intra-arterial line for monitoring blood pressure, epidural catheter for pain relief.

Postoperative care

There are few, if any, scientific studies examining the best way of caring for patients after major oesophageal surgery. Surgeons tend to develop their own beliefs, based on their own and others' experience, and sometimes hold to these beliefs as though they are established fact rather than surgical lore. The authors present here an approach which they believe is cautious and has proved effective.

The aim is always to extubate patients as soon as possible after surgery, and preferably while still in the operating theatre. The use of epidural anaesthesia has been very beneficial for pain relief, allowing early extubation. A chest radiograph is taken in the recovery area immediately after the operation, both to check the position of chest drains and particularly to make sure that there has been full lung expansion and that there is no pneumothorax.

Most patients spend their first few days in an intensive care or intensive nursing ward, during which time the patient's haemodynamic and respiratory status is carefully monitored and intensive chest physiotherapy is begun.

The epidural catheter is left in for as long as possible, and the urinary catheter for a further 24 h after the epidural catheter is removed (often on the third or fourth day after surgery).

It is unlikely that a nasogastric tube plays any useful role in these patients but, being creatures of habit and tradition, the authors still tend to leave it in for a few days after operation. It is usually removed some time after the third day.

Chest drains

Two chest drains are left, one anteriorly to remove air and one posteriorly to the region of the anastomosis (if in the chest) to drain blood and pleural fluid. The anterior drain may be clipped after 24 h and removed after a further 24 h. The posterior drain is left until after oral feeding is established, some time in the second week after surgery. Patients should be nursed in the semiupright position to help prevent gastro-oesophageal regurgitation.

Feeding

A feeding jejunostomy catheter is inserted in all patients and means that there is no urgency at all to recommence oral feeding.

Jejunostomy feeds are usually begun (initially with normal saline) on the third day after the operation and full-scale feeding is introduced slowly over the following week.

Patients are allowed to suck ice chips from the first night of their operation but are not given anything else by mouth until after a water-soluble contrast swallow examination has demonstrated anastomotic integrity. This investigation is carried out between the eighth and tenth days after surgery.

Patients then advance slowly through a liquid, to a sloppy to a soft diet. It is worth emphasizing that a normal contrast study 8 days after the operation does not mean that a leak may not become evident at a later time. Such an occurrence is, however, unusual.

Specific postoperative complications

Lung complications such as pneumonia and more severe problems such as adult respiratory distress syndrome may occur after major oesophageal operations and should be treated by antibiotics and respiratory support, as is appropriate (often prolonged ventilation with adult respiratory distress syndrome).

Bleeding from a small mediastinal vessel sometimes occurs in the immediate postoperative period. Frustratingly, even when bleeding is substantial much of the blood does not come out in a chest drain. If haemodynamic stability is easily maintained with fluids, and perhaps one or two units of blood, bleeding usually ceases. If there is haemodynamic instability, reoperation is indicated. With the 'in-between cases' it is often best to return the patient to the operating room, evacuate accumulated clotted blood and deal with any bleeding points (sometimes none are found).

Anastomotic leakage

Anastomotic leakage should never occur in the first few days after surgery as there is really no excuse for the surgeon not ensuring that the anastomosis is 'water tight' at the end of the procedure.

Leakage occurs when a portion of the anastomosis not only fails to heal but is actually ischaemic and the ensuing necrotic portion of the wall loses its integrity. This process takes several days to develop but is usually evident by the end of the first week. When leakage occurs it may be associated with one of two courses.

Subclinical leak
Sometimes a patient makes steady progress and when the contrast study is performed, about 8 days after surgery, a leak is revealed. If this is a minor leak, i.e. is not associated with a collection of fluid, then no action is taken other than to continue jejunal feeding and maintain ice chips only by mouth. Some surgeons allow fluids by mouth under these circumstances but it seems prudent to limit oesophageal and gastric motility as much as possible to promote healing of the defect. A contrast study is peformed again 5–7 days later, by which time most of these minor leaks will have healed.

If the leak is major, i.e. is associated with contrast medium passing into a fluid collection, then the only difference is that the help of radiological colleagues is sought in order to place a percutaneous drain into the collection. This not only drains the collection but establishes an external fistula, which is an important principle of treatment in leakage from any anastomosis.

Continuing leakage can be monitored partly by the nature of the fluid which is draining (saliva is usually easily recognized) and, if in doubt, a dye or brightly coloured cordial can be drunk to see if egress occurs. When the fistula is thought to have closed it should be checked by another contrast swallow before commencing oral intake.

Clinically evident leakage
'Clinically evident' is something of a catch-all phrase. It should be a maxim for the oesophageal surgeon that whenever a patient is not doing well, whatever the expression of the clinical decline (i.e. respiratory, cardiac, renal failure or combinations of system failure) a leak from the anastomosis should be considered as the primary cause until it is proved otherwise by a contrast swallow.

If a leak is found under these circumstances then percutaneous drainage should be established if possible. If this leads to stabilization and then improvement of the patient, as is usually the case, continued conservative management is pursued. Oral feeding is commenced only after a contrast study has demonstrated that the anastomosis has healed.

On the other hand, if sepsis is uncontrolled in spite of percutaneous drainage and the patient continues to deteriorate, a further operation is undertaken. It is important not to wait too long for this step, no longer then 48 h after insertion of percutaneous drainage for clear signs of improvement. If it does not occur, the patient is returned to the operating theatre. At this time it may occasionally be enough to drain any collection and establish adequate drainage of the anastomosis. On the other hand, it is often the surgeon's last shot at rectifying a disaster and it is therefore usually best to treat the situation as one would a patient presenting late with Boerhaave's syndrome, with drainage and oesophageal exclusion.

Thoracic duct injury

Injury to the thoracic duct usually becomes manifest when nutritional feeding commences on about the fourth or fifth day after operation. There is a fairly rapid increase in drain losses or in fluid accumulation in the chest. Once suspected, it can be verified by ceasing the jejunal feeds and the fluid loss usually diminishes greatly. Most surgeons undertake a trial of conservative management, which essentially means replacing the enteral with parenteral nutrition for 7–14 days. Occasionally a fistula will close spontaneously, which is why a trial is worthwhile, but usually operative closure of the fistula is required. At operation the use of a dry field and a sharp pair of eyes (which usually means the surgical resident!) is often all that is required to find the chylous leak point. It should be sutured closed without trying to dissect the thoracic duct free. The tissue in the region of the aortic hiatus, excluding the aorta, can also be ligated in continuity as an added means of ligating the thoracic duct.

If difficulty is encountered in finding the chylous leak, Intralipid is instilled into the jejunostomy and the chyle then turns milky, aiding identification of the point of leakage.

A chylous fistula in the neck is seen very infrequently, or perhaps more accurately nearly always resolves spontaneously, and so possibly it occurs more often than is recognized.

Recurrent laryngeal nerve injury

Whenever the cervical oesophagus is mobilized there is the potential for damage to the recurrent laryngeal nerves. This is best avoided by keeping dissection close to the oesophageal wall and using gentle retraction only of the trachea and thyroid gland. In spite of this, between 10% and 20% of patients develop some degree of temporary hoarseness after surgery. Permanent hoarseness occurs in only a very small percentage of patients.

Avulsion of the left recurrent nerve during blunt oesophagectomy is best avoided by allowing the cervical operator to define the plane of separation for the oesophagus down past the aortic arch.

If unilateral vocal cord paralysis proves to be a clinical problem in the postoperative period, injection of the cord with an absorbable material such as Gelfoam can be undertaken.

Gastric surgery

Preoperative

The preoperative management of patients undergoing elective gastric surgery is generally simple. This is particularly true in those operations in which the gastrointestinal tract is not entered, such as Nissen fundoplication and proximal gastric vagotomy. More complex preoperative management is required in the more major operations, particularly when preoperative derangement in nutrition, volume, electrolyte or acid–base status has occurred.

Elective duodenal ulcer surgery

The diagnosis is established from the history, endoscopy and/or upper gastrointestinal contrast studies. When the ulcer is in the stomach malignancy must be excluded with multiple biopsies and brush cytology. Gastric acid secretory studies are unnecessary in most patients because the results have little influence on the selection of operative technique. Two settings in which gastric acid secretory studies are useful include the patient with a recurrent ulcer after a previous ulcer operation and the patient in whom the diagnosis of gastrinoma is strongly suspected but unproven by the secretin test. In the former situation a modified sham feeding test or the measurement of basal acid secretion may provide strong evidence for incomplete vagotomy. In the latter, the demonstration that basal acid output is equal to or exceeds 60% of the maximal acid response to pentagastrin or histamine provides strong confirmatory evidence for the diagnosis of gastrinoma or Zollinger–Ellison syndrome.

Preoperative assessment of the patient being prepared for ulcer surgery is similar to that of any patient undergoing abdominal surgery. Little is required beyond the routine urine and blood tests and assessment of cardiac and renal function, unless an underlying illness necessitates a fuller evaluation. Patients on long-term H_2-receptor antagonist therapy or on omeprazole develop hypochlorhydria or achlorhydria and may have bacterial colonization of the stomach. Such patients have been shown to develop an increased incidence of wound infection after surgery. It is the authors' practice, therefore, to discontinue H_2-receptor antagonist therapy 48 h and omeprazole 5–7 days before surgery. Sequential compression boots are used during the operation in all obese patients and in those over 50 years of age. Low-dose heparin therapy is reserved for patients with a previous history of deep vein thrombosis or pulmonary embolism. A single dose of first or second generation cephalosporin is administered intravenously on transfer to the operating theatre. Some people consider this practice unnecessary in patients with duodenal ulcer, who are generally hypersecretors of acid. Others give prophylactic antibiotics for 24 h. A nasogastric tube is usually placed after the patient has been anaesthetized.

Urgent and emergency ulcer surgery

Complications of peptic ulcer may require urgent or emergency operations. Urgent operation may be required in the patient with gastric outlet obstruction. Preoperative management is directed at preventing aspiration, improving any underlying malnutrition, and correcting any abnormality of extracellular volume, electrolyte or acid–base balance. Nasogastric aspiration is instituted. Some advocate prolonged nasogastric suction in the hope that gastric tone will return before the operation. The value of this practice has not been proven. Treatment with H_2-receptor antagonists or omeprazole will reduce acid secretion and hence limit further fluid loss. Correction of extracellular volume deficit and of hypokalaemic, hypochlorhydric, metabolic alkalosis is generally accomplished by the administration of saline containing potassium chloride. It is exceedingly rare that administration of dilute hydrochloric acid or a solution of ammonium chloride will be required. Ammonium chloride should not be used in the presence of any liver disease. Unless very severe nutritional deficit exists, it is preferable not to institute total parenteral nutrition. Rather, a feeding jejunostomy may be placed at operation so that enteral feeding may be started early after surgery. The stomach is lavaged with saline the night before surgery. After the final wash, 1% neomycin, 200 ml, is inserted into the stomach and the nasogastric tube is clamped. Perioperative parenteral antibiotic therapy is important in patients with gastric outlet obstruction. Postoperative wound infection is significantly reduced with this regimen of antibiotic therapy.

In patients with a perforated ulcer, the essence of preoperative management is to make a prompt diagnosis, institute nasogastric suction and perform early abdominal exploration. It is best to use triple antibiotic intravenous therapy (ampicillin, aminoglycoside and metronidazole) because it is not always entirely clear which viscus has perforated.

The preoperative management of a patient with a bleeding ulcer is that of volume resuscitation with crystalloids and blood. Perioperative antibiotics have been shown to reduce wound infection significantly in patients with a bleeding ulcer.

Gastric malignancy

Once the diagnosis is established by biopsy, the surgeon needs to know the exact proximal extent of the tumour and whether it has metastasized to the liver and regional lymph nodes. The first goal is achieved by the surgeon personally performing or being present at the endoscopy. The second goal is best accomplished with computed tomography of the abdomen to look for hepatic or lymph node metastases. If the patient is nutritionally depleted, enteral nutritional supplement either orally or via nasogastric or nasoduodenal tube is preferable to total parenteral nutrition. Rarely is the latter form of nutritional support used because of the length of time required and the complications attending the procedure. More than 50% of patients with carcinoma of the stomach have hypochlorhydria or achlorhydria. As a result, the stomach tends to be colonized with bacteria and postoperative wound infection is high. In addition, at operation the surgeon may discover unsuspected invasion of the transverse mesocolon, necessitating colon resection. For all these reasons the patient with gastric cancer should undergo full mechanical and bacteriological preoperative preparation. Mechanical bowel preparation is best achieved with an isosmotic electrolyte solution or magnesium sulphate and enemas. Bacteriological preparation of the bowel is accomplished with a combination of oral neomycin and erythromycin base. Prophylaxis against thromboembolic disease is particularly important in patients with gastric malignancy because they may have a hypercoagulable state.

Postoperative care

Routine postoperative management in gastric surgery is also simple. The major issues revolve around prevention of respiratory complications, management of the nasogastric tube and the timing of oral intake. The general approach to respiratory care in the patient who has undergone surgery has been discussed earlier. The management of the nasogastric tube appears to follow no scientific guidelines and is largely the surgeon's choice. In general, it may be removed 24 h after antireflux operations and by the third day after proximal gastric vagotomy. After vagotomy and drainage or after gastric resection, the tendency is to keep the nasogastric tube in longer. It is generally removed after gastrointestinal function has returned, the 24-h volume of suction is less than 1000 ml, the patient can tolerate two successive 4-h periods of clamping of the nasogastric tube without nausea or fullness, and the residual volume is less than 200–300 ml. Clear fluids are started as soon as gastrointestinal function returns, as evidenced by the passage of flatus or faeces. The diet can then be advanced rapidly to full fluid, soft and normal diet.

After Nissen fundoplication, patients will feel full after a small amount of food and it is therefore preferable to give them six small meals a day for the first few weeks. Patients who have had gastric resection or vagotomy with drainage are susceptible to the dumping syndrome. They should therefore be instructed, at least for the early postoperative period, to take six small meals a day, to take their meals dry, to lie down for 20–30 min after the meal and drink their fluids after that. They should also avoid a high carbohydrate diet. All these patients should be told they may experience diarrhoea but that it is generally short-lived.

Delayed gastric emptying requiring prolonged nasogastric suction may occur after surgery for at least three reasons: a mechanical problem at the suture line such as a haematoma, small leak, too narrow an anastomosis; the development of postoperative pancreatitis; or gastric neurogenic or myogenic abnormality. The stomach should empty well within 4–6 days of a gastric operation. If there is failure of gastric emptying beyond this, the serum amylase should be measured to rule out pancreatitis. If the problem persists to 10 days, a water-soluble contrast study should be undertaken. The study will define the presence of any mechanical problem. If the problem persists for 14 days or longer, a careful endoscopic examination should be performed. Suture-line haematoma and oedema will resolve with time. A technical problem may require surgical revision at some time. If the anastomosis is widely patent and there has been no preoperative atony, computed tomography of the abdomen should be performed to rule out pancreatitis.

A special problem is posed by some patients who have had gastric atony secondary to long-standing gastric outlet obstruction. Such patients, especially if they have also undergone truncal vagotomy, may develop delayed gastric emptying which may sometimes persist for weeks. Such patients rarely respond to prokinetic agents such as metoclopramide. The surgeon must anticipate and prepare for this complication by performing a gastrostomy, if possible, and a feeding jejunostomy. If this is done, the patient can be discharged home in reasonable time and resolution of the problem can be awaited patiently.

Illustrations by T. Boraine and A. Mannell

Left thoracoabdominal approach for exposure of the oesophagus

Aylwyn Mannell FRACS, FRCS, MS
Specialist Surgeon, Rosebank and Linksfield Park Clinics and Consultant Surgeon, Baragwanath Hospital and University of Witwatersrand, Johannesburg, South Africa

Principles and justification

The left thoracoabdominal approach gives excellent exposure of the cardio-oesophageal junction, the distal thoracic oesophagus and the stomach.

Indications

The indications for this approach include adenocarcinoma of the cardia, squamous carcinoma of the distal oesophagus, connective tissue tumours adjacent to or involving the cardio-oesophageal junction, and gastric cancer involving the proximal half of the stomach.

The left thoracoabdominal approach is also used for the Leigh–Collis gastroplasty, the gastric fundal patch operation described by Thal and for oesophagogastrectomy in the management of early, uncontaminated perforation of the distal oesophagus.

Preoperative

Many patients with obstructing lesions near the cardio-oesophageal junction are in a state of semi-starvation, and preoperative nutritional rehabilitation is extremely important to ensure that wounds and anastomoses will heal. Oral or enteral feeding of a high-calorie, high-protein liquid diet is essential. If necessary, a malignant stricture may be partly dilated to allow passage of a nasogastric tube which, ideally, should be of small calibre and made from Silastic to decrease pharyngeal discomfort which would limit the patient's ability to cough effectively. The patient may also be fed intravenously but gastrostomy or jejunostomy should be avoided. These procedures are associated with a small but real risk of morbidity and mortality and can complicate subsequent major surgery.

Death following oesophagogastrectomy is usually due to pneumonia. Preparation of the patient for surgery is therefore aimed at preventing postoperative pulmonary complications, which are common after thoracotomy. Every effort must be made to improve pulmonary function: the patient must stop smoking and obvious wheezing on auscultation of the lungs is an indication for bronchodilator therapy. Chest physiotherapy is essential to train the patient to cough vigorously and to clear secretions. Incentive spirometry is of great value in preventing and treating atelectasis: training the patient to achieve maximal lung inflation with the incentive spirometer should begin as soon as the decision to operate has been made. Purulent sputum will require appropriate antibiotic treatment based on culture results.

Obvious deficits in hydration, haemoglobin levels and electrolyte balance must be corrected. In patients from countries in which tuberculosis is prevalent active pulmonary tuberculosis must be excluded, and careful assessment of cardiovascular status is required for elderly patients.

Antibiotic prophylaxis

To reduce debris in the oesophagus and stomach, oral or enteral intake should be stopped at least 12 h before surgery. Broad-spectrum parenteral antibiotic prophylaxis is given with the premedication and continued for 24 h after surgery.

Anaesthesia

Deflation of the left lung will improve surgical access for the left thoracoabdominal approach. With the patient supine, a double-lumen endobronchial tube is inserted after induction of anaesthesia and before the patient is positioned for the operation. Careful monitoring of the arterial blood gases is necessary: when the patient is placed in the right lateral position for a left thoracoabdominal procedure the dependent right lung is compressed by the weight of the mediastinum and arterial hypoxaemia, secondary to one-lung anaesthesia, can develop. Arterial hypoxaemia is exacerbated by pre-existing disease in the dependent lung, by significant blood loss and by a long operation. The surgeon must weigh the benefits of improved exposure against the risks of prolonged hypoxaemia and keep the time during which the left lung is deflated to a minimum.

Insertion of nasogastric tube

If not already in place, a nasogastric tube should be inserted after commencement of anaesthesia and before the operation begins. This facilitates rapid intraoperative identification of the intra-abdominal oesophagus and postoperative decompression of the stomach when required. Transanastomotic passage of the nasogastric tube allows enteral feeding to continue in the recovery phase.

Operation

Position of patient

1 The position of the patient on the table determines to a large extent the success of the left thoracoabdominal approach. A suitable table that can be easily rotated and fitted with chest attachments capable of fixing the patient firmly in position is essential.

The patient's left side is elevated with sandbags under the hip and shoulder to achieve an angle of 60° with the table. The left arm is drawn upwards and forwards, supported by a thoracic arm rest. To fix the patient in this position adhesive strapping is applied across the buttocks to the table and to the left arm in the thoracic arm rest. The operating table is turned to the left side for the abdominal phase and to the right side for the thoracic dissection.

The patient is prepared for abdominal and left thoracic incisions. Application of a clear adhesive drape helps to keep the sterile towels in position during movement of the table.

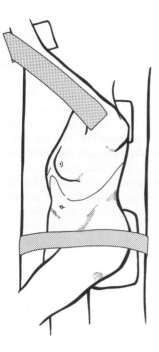

1

Incision

2a, b Several approaches may be selected. An oblique thoracoabdominal incision begins midway between the xiphisternum and umbilicus, extends across the costal margin over the desired intercostal space or rib and is continued to the inferior angle of the scapula up to the lateral edge of the erector spinae muscle (*Illustration 2a*). This incision is appropriate for the younger patient with good respiratory function.

The midline abdominal incision extends from the xiphisternum to below the umbilicus. The left thoracic incision follows the line of the seventh or eighth rib from the costal margin to the lateral edge of the erector spinae muscle (*Illustration 2b*). These incisions, which preserve the costal margin, are recommended for the frail elderly patient and those with poor respiratory function.

Postoperative instability of the costal margin and extensive incisions into the diaphragm can result in serious impairment of pulmonary mechanics, increasing the risk of postoperative pneumonia.

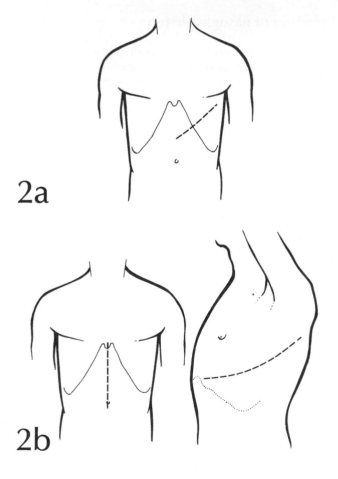

2a

2b

Exploration of abdomen

Using the oblique incision, the anterior lamina of the rectus sheath over the left rectus muscle is divided. The muscle is transected with electrocautery, the left superior epigastric vessels are ligated and divided and the peritoneum is opened in line with the incision up to the costal margin.

If a separate abdominal midline incision is used the linea alba and parietal peritoneum are divided.

In patients for whom the operation is undertaken for malignancy, a laparotomy is now performed before opening the chest. The liver, general peritoneal cavity and pelvic peritoneum are examined to identify metastatic spread. The coeliac nodes are palpated for evidence of involvement or extracapsular spread. The tumour is examined to assess local infiltration and spread into the diaphragm or stomach. Gross metastatic spread to suprapancreatic, splenic hilar, porta hepatis and para-aortic lymph nodes is excluded.

Thoracic incision

3 If no contraindication to operation is identified the oblique thoracoabdominal incision is continued over the costal margin along the course of the appropriate rib, which is usually the seventh or eighth rib. Serratus anterior and latissimus dorsi muscles are divided with electrocautery along the course of the rib. Bleeding points in the muscles are carefully controlled to limit blood loss.

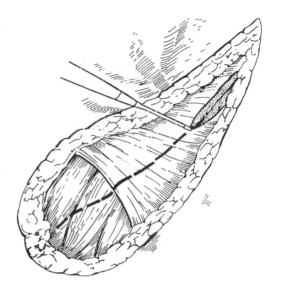

3

Division of intercostal muscles

4 The intercostal muscles are divided along the line of insertion into the superior margin of the rib below, avoiding injury to the intercostal vessels and nerve. This division is continued to the lateral border of the erector spinae muscle. The left lung is allowed to deflate and the pleural cavity opened.

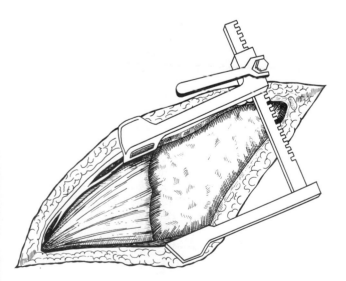

4

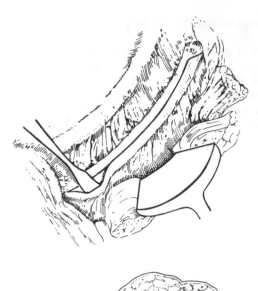

5a

Rib resection

5a–c If compliance of the chest wall is limited, a rib may be removed and the pleural cavity entered through the bed of that rib. When the rib is exposed, the periosteum is incised with electrocautery and separated from the rib using a periosteal elevator and Doyen's rasparatory. The rib is divided with a costotome and removed from behind the rib angle to its costal end, together with the costal cartilage and a small segment of the costal margin to prevent subsequent overriding on closure of the wound. At this stage, branches of the musculophrenic vessels will require ligation.

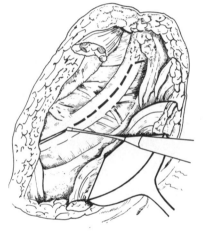

5b

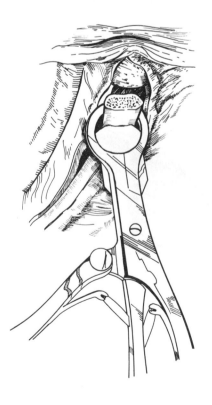

5c

Division of diaphragm

6 The diaphragm is cut from the point of division of the costal margin in line with the phrenic muscle fibres towards the oesophageal hiatus. Haemostasis in the cut edges of the diaphragm is secured by suture ligation, with particular care to ligate the branches of the inferior phrenic vessels near the hiatus. Each leaf of the divided diaphragm is attached to the cut edge of the chest wall muscles with sutures, which improves exposure. A Finochietto retractor is inserted between the ribs and opened widely.

Circumferential incision of the diaphragm may be performed to preserve the phrenic nerve and its branches. After division of the costal margin a Finochietto retractor is inserted to expose the diaphragm, which is then divided circumferentially 3 cm from its insertion into the thoracic margin. The incision should run parallel to the rib cage for about 15 cm.

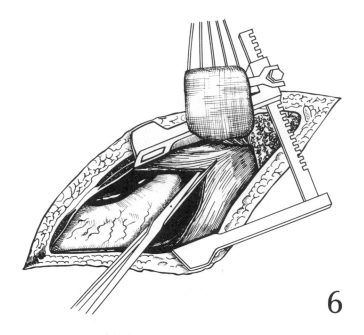

6

Thoracic exploration

7 Any adhesions to the base of the lung should be freed and the inferior part of the pulmonary ligament is divided to facilitate retraction of the lung. The left side of the posterior mediastinum is exposed and, if the operation is being performed for malignancy, it is essential to determine the palpable extent of tumour. The oesophagus must be divided 10 cm above the tumour to ensure complete microscopic clearance. If the upper resection margin is less than 10 cm, the specimen should be submitted to frozen section to confirm that the proximal line of resection is clear of tumour.

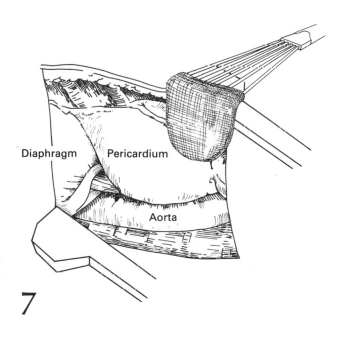

Diaphragm   Pericardium

Aorta

7

Thoracic dissection

8 With the left lung retracted anteromedially, incision of the pulmonary ligament is continued up to the inferior pulmonary vein. The mediastinal pleura overlying the oesophagus is incised and dissected away from the posterior mediastinal contents. The anterior aspect of the aorta is separated from the oesophagus, inferior mediastinal glands, fat and vagus nerves. Small oesophageal arteries arising from the aorta are ligated and divided. Any mediastinal pleura overlying a tumour should be resected with the lesion. Mobilization of the oesophagus is continued to the arch of the aorta; care must be taken to avoid opening the pericardium or injuring the thoracic duct, which may be identified during the dissection. A Jacques catheter is now passed around the mobilized oesophagus for retraction during the next phase of dissection and the vagal trunks are divided above the tumour.

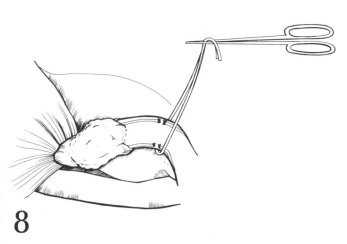

8

Abdominal dissection

9a–c In cases where the diaphragm has been incised in a radial direction, this is continued into the oesophageal hiatus. However, if a malignant lesion is close to the oesophageal hiatus a cuff of diaphragmatic muscle is removed. The peritoneum on the right aspect of the intra-abdominal oesophagus is incised and the incision continued distally, dividing the lesser omentum close to the liver as far as the gastric antrum. The right gastric vessels should be preserved if gastric reconstruction is planned. The left peritoneal reflection from the intra-abdominal oesophagus is incised, the vagal trunks exposed and divided. For benign lesions and for resection of squamous cancer of the distal oesophagus, where metastases and splenic hilar nodes are found in less than 5% of cases, the gastric fundus is mobilized by ligation and division of the short gastric and left gastroepiploic vessels, close to the splenic hilum. The spleen is carefully preserved to reduce the risk of infective and thromboembolic complications in the postoperative period. With ligation and division of the coronary vein and left gastric artery at its origin from the coeliac axis, mobilization of the distal thoracic and intra-abdominal oesophagus is now complete.

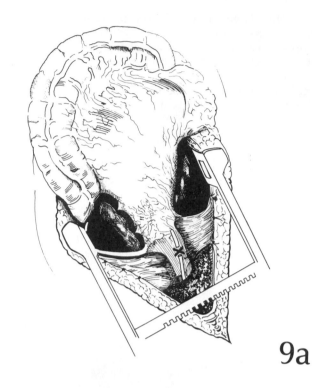

9a

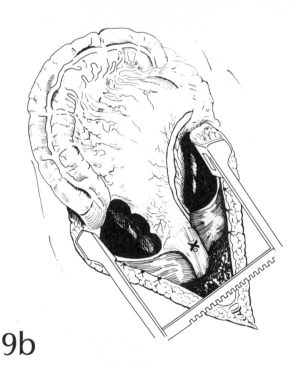

9b

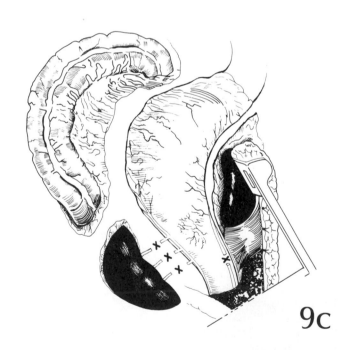

9c

Laparotomy and left thoracotomy

10 If separate abdominal and thoracic incisions have been used, the abdominal dissection should be completed before the abdomen is closed, and the thoracic dissection performed in part through the widened hiatus.

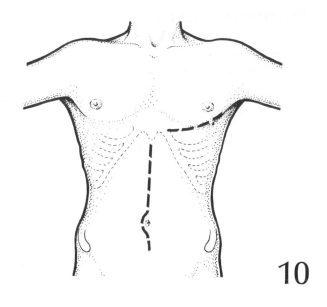

Division of left triangular ligaments

11 Following a separate abdominal midline incision the left triangular ligament of the liver is divided and the left lobe retracted to improve access to the cardio-oesophageal area.

Gastric mobilization

The gastrocolic ligament is divided up to the spleen, ligating and dividing the left gastroepiploic vessels and vasa brevia close to the hilum of the spleen. Care must be taken to secure accessory vasa brevia running on the posterior abdominal wall to the gastric fundus. The peritoneal reflection between stomach and diaphragm is divided to complete mobilization of the gastric fundus.

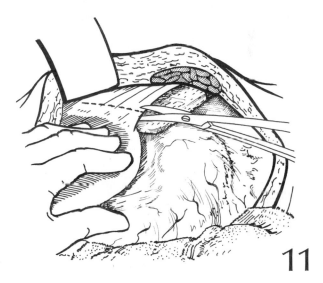

Mobilization of cardio-oesophageal junction

The lesser omentum is divided close to the liver, preserving the right gastroepiploic vessels. A branch of the left gastric artery to the left lobe of the liver may need to be ligated and divided. The peritoneum over the intra-abdominal oesophagus is incised and the vagal nerves identified, cauterized and divided. If the operation is performed for a malignancy in the cardio-oesophageal region, the coeliac nodes are gently stripped towards the stomach. The coronary vein and left gastric artery at its origin from the coeliac axis are ligated and divided. A cuff of diaphragmatic muscle may be removed. The left lobe of the liver is retracted and the hiatal musculature is divided, beginning at the left posterior aspect and continuing to the right side. The remainder of the abdominal dissection is determined by the pathology of the lesion and by selection of stomach, jejunum of colon for reconstruction.

Wound closure

Where the thoracoabdominal incision has been used, the diaphragm is now closed with interrupted mattress sutures of 0 Ethibond placed 2 cm from the cut edge. The finished suture line is reinforced with a continuous second layer to reduce the risk of diaphragmatic dehiscence. If the costal margin has been divided, the costal cartilage is repaired with wire sutures. The pleural cavity is irrigated with a warm saline antibiotic solution. Pericostal sutures of 2/0 Ethibond are inserted and an underwater basal drain is led out of the chest in the mid-axillary line. The left lung is allowed to reinflate and the pericostal sutures are tied. The muscles of the chest wall are repaired. The abdominal extension of the thoracoabdominal incision is closed and the skin is sutured.

Postoperative care

The most important aspects of the postoperative care include monitoring of intravenous fluid therapy and the prevention of pulmonary infection. The patient's fluid needs must be carefully titrated against the urine output and central venous pressure readings to avoid fluid overload.

The patient is nursed sitting upright and kept free of pain with regular doses of narcotic analgesics or patient-controlled analgesia. If the operation was prolonged, the patient frail and elderly or the postoperative arterial blood gases unsatisfactory, a nasotracheal tube should be left in place for 24–48 h for intermittent mandatory ventilation and regular tracheobronchial toilet.

Chest physiotherapy is essential to help the patient cough effectively and the preoperative incentive spirometry should be continued in the postoperative period. Prophylactic antibiotics should be continued until the left lung is fully re-expanded, there is no residual haemothorax and the intercostal drain can be removed.

Nasogastric aspirations will keep the stomach empty in patients in whom gastric reconstruction was performed. By the third postoperative day, when the patient has recovered from postoperative ileus, the nasogastric tube may be used for enteral feeding. After a Gastrografin swallow is performed on the sixth postoperative day to exclude anastomotic leakage, the nasogastric tube may be removed and the patient commenced on a graduated oral diet.

Abdominal incisions for approaching the abdominal oesophagus and stomach

P. G. Devitt FRACS, FRCS
Senior Lecturer in Surgery, Department of Surgery, Royal Adelaide Hospital, Adelaide, Australia

Principles and justification

The type of abdominal incision chosen and the way in which it is fashioned and closed is often a matter of personal preference, although some important principles can be stated. The most important is that the choice of incision should provide the best exposure of the area to be operated upon so that safe surgery can be performed with the minimum of difficulty. This principle is particularly important in upper abdominal surgery, where access under the costal margin and diaphragm can be difficult. Of secondary importance, the wound should be easy to fashion and close. While attention must be paid to the cosmetic effects of any incision, this is of lesser importance in upper abdominal surgery where the underlying condition is often life-threatening and priority must be given to ease and sometimes speed of access.

Choice of incision

Three types of abdominal incision are commonly used for operations on the stomach and lower oesophagus.

1 A midline incision provides good access for most procedures. The incision is easy to make and access to the abdominal cavity is gained quickly. Neither muscle fibres nor nerves are divided. The wound is easy to extend and easy to close.

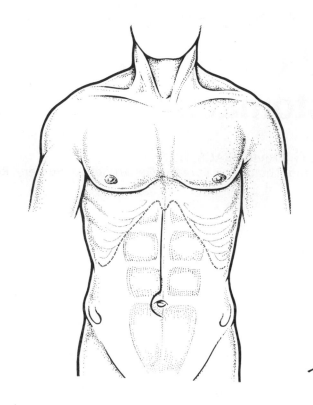

1

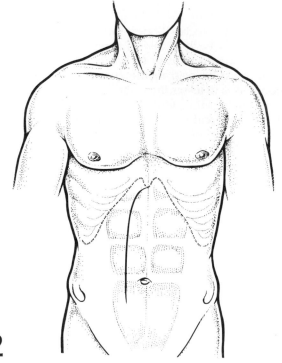

2

2 The paramedian incision is more time-consuming to make than the midline incision and if it is truly vertical may not give adequate exposure to the subdiaphragmatic region. Exposure can be improved by curving the upper extension of the incision towards the midline. This once popular incision is little used today.

3 A subcostal incision in a patient with a wide costal margin gives good access both to the proximal stomach and duodenum. In addition, the incision can easily be extended across the left costal margin and into the chest.

Method of incision

A scalpel is the instrument of choice for most surgeons, but diathermy can be used for the deeper layers. The skin is held on the stretch and a firm incision is made, the initial stroke going into the subcutaneous fat. All layers down to the peritoneum are usually incised with the knife. The peritoneum is grasped between two forceps and opened with either a knife or pair of scissors. Further extension of this incision in the peritoneum is performed with scissors; blood vessels are coagulated as they are encountered.

Haemostasis

Subcutaneous fat is prone to infection and every effort should be made to control bleeding, minimize trauma and reduce contamination. Many small bleeding points will stop bleeding of their own accord or with gentle pressure from a gauze pack for a few minutes; unnecessary cautery can be avoided in this way. Larger vessels may need to be ligated or cauterized. Excessive use of electrocoagulation increases tissue necrosis and the risk of infection. Despite this, some surgeons maintain that the chance of wound infection is no greater when cutting diathermy is used as the method of incision.

Wound protection/infection

Opening the gastrointestinal tract increases the risk of wound infection. Apart from preoperative preparation with prophylactic antibiotics and the use of bactericidal soaps, the risks of infection may be reduced by covering the edges of the wound with plastic sheeting or gauze packs. Probably of greater importance is meticulous haemostasis and minimization of tissue trauma. The latter is difficult to avoid if fixed retractors are used.

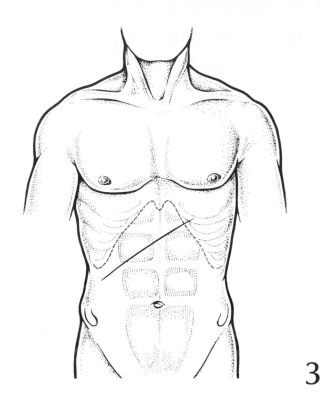

3

Preoperative

Even if it is anticipated that surgery will be performed wholly through the abdominal incision, it is prudent to prepare the patient for possible extension of the operation into the chest or the lower abdomen. This means that the patient should be placed on the operating table in a position which will allow the chest to be opened. In proximal gastric or lower oesophageal surgery this will usually be the left side of the chest and access may be easier if a sandbag or rolled-up towel is placed under the left side of the patient. The skin should be prepared up to the nipples and down to the pubic symphysis. Skin preparation should include the flanks so that drains and feeding tubes may be inserted if required.

Approaches to the upper abdomen

Midline incision

The length of the incision will depend on the shape of the patient and the procedure to be undertaken. It can be taken up to the xiphisternum and down to the pubic symphysis. The xiphisternum can be incised or excised with bone-cutting forceps. When dissecting in this region, terminal branches of the internal mammary artery which will bleed freely and require coagulation are encountered. Even for upper abdominal surgery, it is often necessary to extend the distal end of the incision beyond the umbilicus. If this is to be done, it is more aesthetically pleasing to make the incision around instead of through the umbilicus. The wound is also easier to close if some rectus sheath is left attached to the umbilicus.

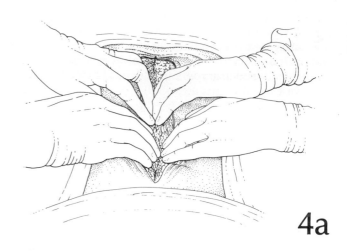

4a

4a, b The subcutaneous fat is usually incised, but in the obese patient it is easy to stray from the midline and to miss the linea alba. One way of avoiding this problem is to pull the subcutaneous fat away from the midline. There is a relatively bloodless plane of cleavage which can be developed by lateral traction. With the surgeon and his assistant retracting the skin at 180° to the line of the incision, the fat can be split down to the linea alba. The linea alba is then incised using either knife or cautery. The underlying peritoneum is opened to the left of the falciform ligament. To complete the exposure the falciform ligament is ligated and divided. Provided it is sewn up correctly, this incision is no more liable to dehiscence than a paramedian incision.

Paramedian incision

This is more laborious to fashion than the midline incision and involves incision into the right (or left) rectus sheath 2–3 cm from the median decussation. The tendinous intersections of the rectus muscle adhere to the sheath and several of these need to be divided before the belly of the muscle can be retracted laterally. The posterior rectus sheath is incised and the underlying peritoneum opened. The paramedian incision has been superseded by the midline incision, but the former approach should be used where there has been a previous paramedian incision. In such cases the wound is best opened by incising the rectus muscle and splitting it longitudinally. A more laterally placed incision has been described. The approach is the same

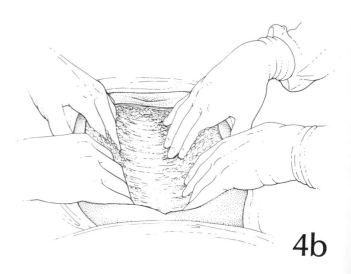

4b

as for the conventional paramedian incision, with lateral displacement of the rectus muscle, but with the incision through the anterior and posterior rectus sheaths placed over the lateral third of the belly of the muscle. This incision is claimed to have a negligible incidence of incisional hernia when compared with midline wounds[1].

Subcostal incision

This is the most time-consuming of the three types of incision. Rectus sheath and muscle must be cut, as well as the oblique and transverse muscles of the anterior abdominal wall. Bleeding is more substantial and difficult to control, as the vessels retract into the cut edges of the muscle. If this exposure is taken from the right flank and across the left rectus muscle, it gives good exposure to both the duodenum and the proximal stomach, and is useful in obese patients with wide costal margins. If necessary, the incision can be taken straight across the left rectus muscle, the costal margin and into the left chest.

The skin incision is made 2–3 cm below the costal margin; if made any less than this, there is insufficient muscle left attached to the costal margin to take sutures when closing the wound. When the rectus muscle is cut, branches of the superior epigastric artery are encountered and coagulated. At the lateral aspect of the wound the segmental dorsal nerves are encountered; the eighth is usually divided, but the ninth should be identified and preserved.

The cut rectus muscle heals to form a fibrous intersection, and as it is segmentally innervated (providing the ninth dorsal nerve has been left intact), it is unlikely that there will be any significant denervation or subsequent weakness.

Exposure

5 Even with an incision in the correct position and a wound of appropriate length, good access is frequently difficult to obtain in upper gastrointestinal surgery. Many different types of fixed retractor are available to improve exposure. Perhaps the simplest and most useful is the sternal retractor. The bridge is fixed as near to the head of the operating table as possible without impeding access for the anaesthetist. It is helpful if the operating table has a separate head section that can be lowered. The bridge should be low; with too steep an angle the blade of the retractor may slip from under the sternum. When the incision has been made, wound protectors (plastic sheeting or gauze packs) are positioned before the retractors; a self-retaining retractor is placed in the wound. If the surgeon operates standing on the right of the patient, the retractor should be placed so that the shaft sticks into the assistant's abdomen instead of his own! The blade of the sternal retractor is placed over a pack on the xiphisternum.

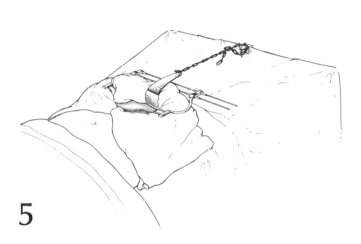

5

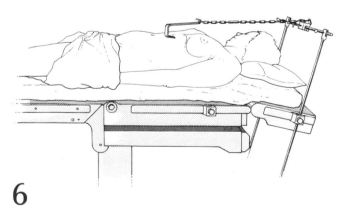

6

6 The retractor may be custom-made; alternatively, the middle blade of a self-retaining retractor may be sufficient. With the blade in position, a length of chain is used to haul the retractor towards the bridge. When the chain has been made fast, further retraction can be obtained by pivoting the bridge backwards by lowering the head section of the table.

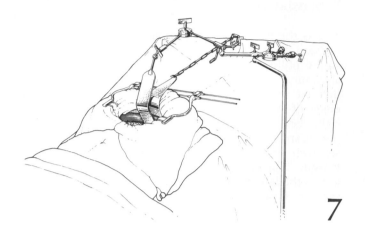

7,8 Other retractors are useful to hold up the liver. These can be fixed to the operating table. Once the retractors are in position, the table can be tilted feet-down (reverse Trendelenburg) so that the contents of the abdominal cavity fall downwards, increasing the access in the upper abdomen.

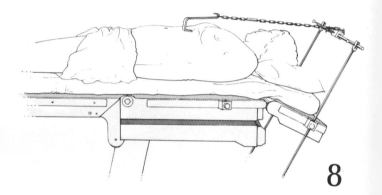

Wound closure

Wounds heal by formation of dense fibrous scar tissue across cut surfaces and not by re-establishment of the layers of the abdominal wall. The aim of wound closure is to produce apposition of the wound edges and splinting to allow the fibrous tissue to develop and mature. It is unnecessary to close the wound in layers and mass closure is sufficient. Material of sufficient tensile strength and durability must be chosen to keep the wound intact in the postoperative period and to allow fibrous healing to occur. Sutures should be placed at no more than 1-cm intervals and at least 1 cm of tissue away from the wound edge[2]. The sutures should loosely approximate the edges of the wound. If they are too tight, the local tissue oedema and increased intra-abdominal pressure that occurs after operation will cause the material to cut through the tissues. If the wound is closed in a continuous manner, bearing the

above principles in mind, the amount of suture material needed exceeds the length of the wound fourfold.

Early wound failure is usually the result of incorrectly placed sutures or inadequately tied knots. Late wound failure may result from poor choice of suture materials.

Knots

The first suture is placed at the upper end of the wound. Continuous suturing is the most common practice. The knot should be buried in the deep layers; if it is left in the subcutaneous fat it can become a source of sinus formation or irritation to the patient.

9 Alternatively, a loop of nylon swaged onto a needle can be used; this will obviate the need for a knot at the start of suturing.

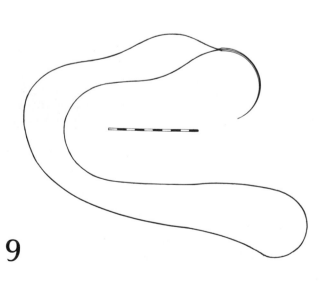

10 Most surgeons use the modified square or reef knot, in which two throws are put on the initial tie. This is followed by a single throw and a third throw which can be double. Coated and monofilament materials tend to slip and at least three throws should be placed.

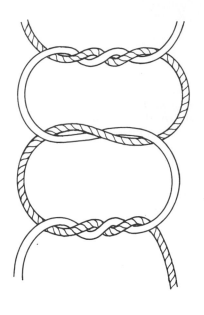

10

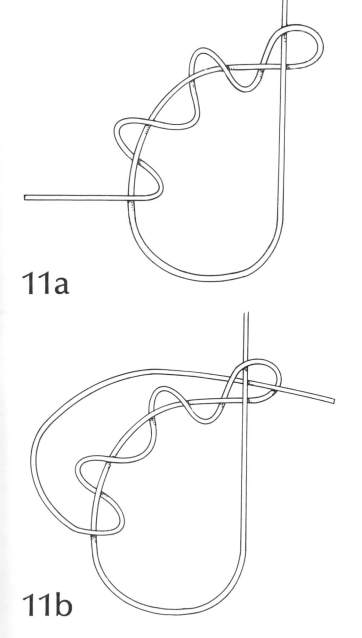

11a

11b

11a, b Used less often, the fisherman's knot is simple to execute and is reliable. It is particularly useful for monofilament materials. The assistant holds the long end of the suture taut and vertical, the surgeon wraps the short end once round the long end and then twists the short end on itself for six or seven turns. The tip of the suture is then passed through the wrap and pulled tight[3].

As each suture is placed, the tip of the needle must be in view to reduce the chance of underlying structures being damaged or caught up in the suture. This can either be done by placing a finger under the wound edge and guiding the needle out of the wound, or by placing forceps on the wound edge and lifting. The latter is safer practice, as most needlestick injuries occur during wound closure.

When the wound is half closed, another suture is started from the bottom end with the aim of making the final closure in the middle of the wound. In this way, what is often a difficult apposition around the umbilicus is made easier, and the final sutures are placed with greater safety by leaving the sutures loose until the last ones are in place. The final knot should be tied so that it can be buried in the deep layers.

12 The subcutaneous fat does not need to be sutured and a subcuticular stitch provides a cosmetic finish to the closure. Polypropylene on a straight or curved cutting needle is suitable. This material runs easily and excites little tissue reaction. Arguments have been made for the use of skin staples. These are expensive compared with sutures, but may reduce the chance of needlestick injury. It is certainly quicker to close wounds with staples, but the time saved in closing the wound is unlikely to defray much from the overall cost of the operation.

Suture materials

Suitable materials to close the deep layers of the anterior abdominal wall include nylon and polypropylene monofilament sutures and the newer synthetics polydioxanone and polyglyconate. These materials invoke little tissue reaction and maintain their tensile strength. Polydioxanone and polyglyconate have the advantage of dissolution after several months. These sutures should be used for the linea alba and the anterior rectus sheath. Catgut and the synthetics polyglycolic acid and polyglactin do not maintain sufficient tensile strength, with loss of strength by 4 weeks. These materials are unsatisfactory for the linea alba or the anterior rectus sheath, but can be used for the posterior rectus sheath and peritoneum. However, it is unnecessary to close the peritoneum as a separate layer. It does not contribute to the strength of the wound and may even increase adhesion formation.

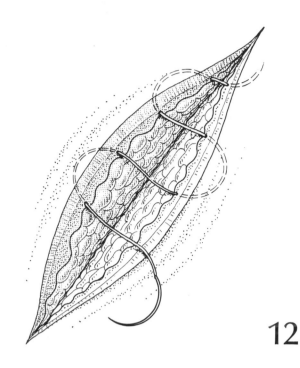

12

Single-layer or mass closures

Midline incisions are closed in a single layer. All layers except for the skin and subcutaneous fat are incorporated. If wound failure is a potential problem, such as in severe malnutrition, a 'near and far' technique can be used to close the wound (*see Illustration 15*).

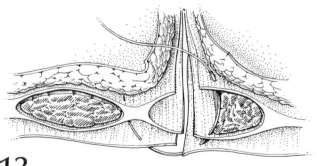

13

13 The paramedian incision can also be closed in a single layer. The suture is placed through the anterior and posterior rectus sheaths with the belly of the muscle displaced laterally. With the more laterally placed paramedian incision this type of mass closure is not practical and the wound should be closed in separate layers.

Two-layer closures

The paramedian wound is often closed in two layers, the posterior rectus sheath incorporating the peritoneum and being sewn with catgut or a rapidly absorbed synthetic. A monofilament or slowly absorbed synthetic (polydioxanone or polyglyconate) is used for the anterior rectus sheath. Similarly, the subcostal incision can be closed in two layers. A long incision may need two lengths of suture material, but a shorter subcostal wound can be closed with a continuous length of monofilament.

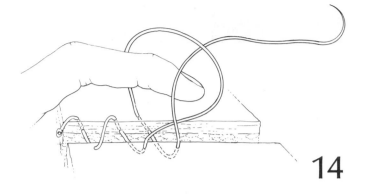

14

14 The knot is placed at the medial end of the wound and the short end held in an artery clip. The deep layer is closed in a continuous fashion and a grocer's knot is tied at the lateral end. With this type of knot the loose end of the suture is grasped through the last loop of suture material placed in the tissues and brought through as another loop. The second loop is pulled up and, in doing so, the first loop tightens down as the first throw of the knot. The process is repeated until several throws have been made and then all the free end of the suture material is passed through the loop and the knot pulled tight. The suture does not need to be cut, and the free end can be brought back, closing the anterior muscle layers and rectus sheath and tied with the original short end.

Tension sutures are mentioned only to be condemned. They are not needed for primary wound closure. Similarly, a dehisced wound can usually be brought together satisfactorily without recourse to these sutures. Tension sutures are painful, unsightly and cut into the tissues. Infection around the sutures and sinus formation is common. The patient is left with an ugly scar. If a wound does split open, it can usually be closed quite satisfactorily by undermining the subcutaneous fat and exposing 4–5 cm of abdominal wall muscle.

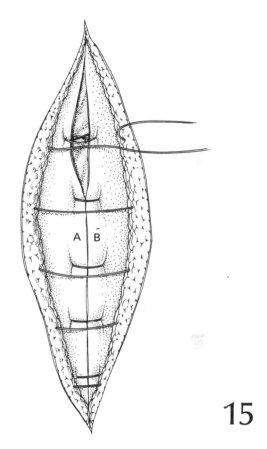

15

15 A 'near and far' technique can then be applied and combined with interrupted sutures to close the wound. Several lengths of monofilament suture material are needed and it is wise to use either nylon or polypropylene. Suturing is started as for a standard wound closure. The first suture is continuous and a 4-cm deep bite of tissue on one side (B) of the wound is married with a 1-cm deep bite on the opposite side (A) of the wound. At the same level the suture is now placed 1 cm from the edge of side B and taken over to be inserted 4 cm deep on side A. The two ends of the suture material are now tied over side B. The suture is now placed 1 cm *down* on side B and the process repeated. It is unlikely that more than two of these sutures will be made with each length of material and an interrupted suture is inserted for every third suture. This technique is laborious but produces a sound repair.

The skin may be closed over the repair. Drains and stomas should be brought out through separate incisions otherwise they may weaken the main laparotomy wound.

References

1. Kendall SWH, Brennan TG, Guillou PJ. Suture length to wound length ratio and the integrity of midline and lateral paramedian incisions. *Br J Surg* 1991; 78: 705–7.

2. Jenkins TPN. The burst abdomen: a mechanical approach. *Br J Surg* 1976; 63: 873–6.

3. Wattchow DA, Watts JMcK. The half blood knot for tying nylon in surgery. *Br J Surg* 1984; 71: 333.

Sutured oesophageal anastomosis

Anthony Watson MD, FRCS, FRCS(Ed), FRACS
Consultant Surgeon, The Wellington Hospital, London, UK

Principles and justification

The choice of sutured or stapled oesophageal anastomoses is dictated largely by personal preference. Such comparative studies as are available show no significant differences in the rates of anastomotic dehiscence[1,2]. Sutured anastomoses are marginally more time consuming to perform but are associated with a lower incidence of anastomotic stricture[3], particularly when the smaller staple heads are used. The author's preference has been for hand-sutured anastomoses using the technique described, which has produced reliable results over almost two decades.

The principles involved in the construction of oesophageal anastomoses are similar whether the anastomosis is to stomach, jejunum or colon, and whether the anastomosis is sited in the mediastinum or the neck. Gastro-oesophageal anastomosis is described,

as it is the most widely practised technique and the author's preference following oesophageal resection. Oesophageal anastomoses have a greater propensity for leakage than most gastrointestinal anastomoses, because of the relatively poor vascularity of the oesophagus, the absence of a serous layer, and the high intraluminal pressures generated on swallowing. Consequently, great care must be exercised in ensuring that vascularity is preserved and that the anastomosis is performed with adequate access and without tension. The anastomosis is performed using a single layer of 3/0 silk, as a non-absorbable or delayed absorption material is believed desirable, and the consistency of silk makes it less likely to cut through the fragile oesophagus than some of the newer, synthetic delayed absorption materials.

Operation

1 After construction of a greater curve gastric tube, a horizontal incision is made on the posterior aspect of the gastric tube about 3 cm from its apex, the length of the incision corresponding to the diameter of the transected oesophagus.

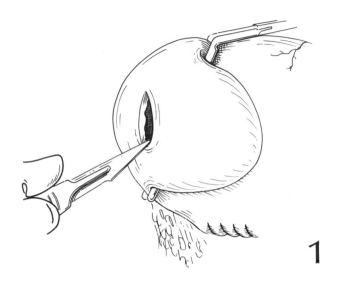

1

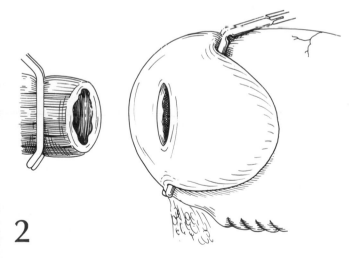

2

2 For mediastinal anastomoses, the proximal oesophagus has usually been divided just below the apex of the mediastinum and the gastric tube is held close to the inferior margin of the thoracotomy wound. The gastric tube and the proximal oesophagus are held in light, non-crushing clamps (such as Satinsky clamps), which are loosely applied about 1 cm proximal and distal to the proposed anastomotic margins. It is vitally important that the mucosa is clearly visible, particularly in the oesophagus where the mucosa and submucosa are the strongest layers and a tendency to retraction of the layers exists, particularly if transection is performed under tension.

3 The proximal oesophagus and the gastric tube are kept separate until the posterior layer of sutures has been placed. Stay sutures are first placed between each corner of the divided oesophagus and the respective corners of the posterior gastrotomy. These are introduced from the serosal aspect of the stomach through to the gastric mucosa, and from the oesophageal lumen through the mucosa and out through the muscular layers, ensuring that an adequate bite of oesophageal mucosa and submucosa is obtained. These sutures are held in the haemostats for later tying by the 'parachute' technique.

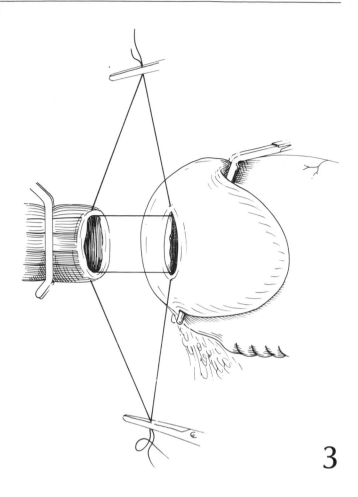

3

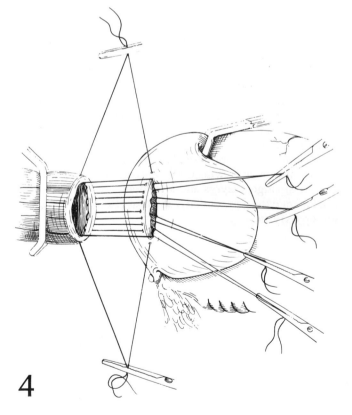

4

4 The posterior layer of sutures is then placed as a series of horizontal mattress sutures 3 mm in width and 3 mm apart. They are constructed as inverting sutures, traversing all layers from gastric mucosa through to gastric serosa, oesophageal muscle and through oesophageal mucosa. Each suture is then returned from oesophageal muscosa to muscle and from gastric serosa to mucosa. Each suture is held in a haemostat for later tying.

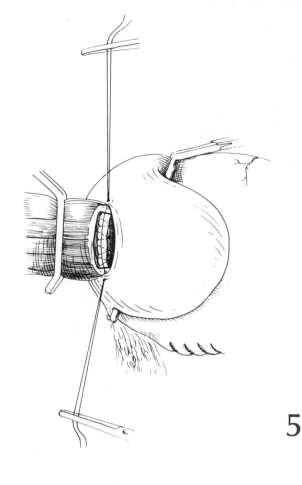

5 When an appropriate number of horizontal mattress sutures has been placed in the posterior layer (usually four or five), the luminal surfaces are approximated by bringing the gastric clamp close to the oesophageal clamp. Starting with the corner stay sutures, each suture is then tied sufficiently tightly to approximate the stomach and the oesophagus gently and to avoid undue tension which may cut through or devascularize the oesophagus.

5

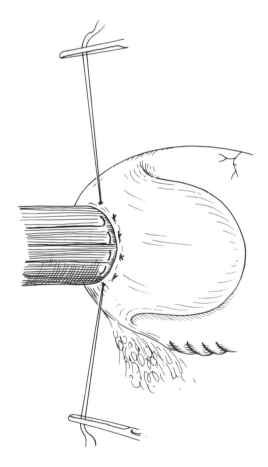

6 Once the posterior layer of sutures has been placed, the clamps are removed and the nasogastric tube is fcd through the anastomosis and sited in the gastric tube. A similar number of horizontal mattress sutures is placed in the anterior layer of the stomach and oesophagus, in identical fashion to the posterior layer, except that each suture may be tied and cut immediately after placement.

6

7 The part of the gastric tube proximal to the anastomosis is then placed over the suture line and fixed by two sutures superiorly to the apical mediastinal pleura and by one suture on each side to the posterior mediastinal pleura. This manoeuvre is performed to seal the anastomosis and to divert tension from the anastomotic line to the apex of the gastric tube during postural changes.

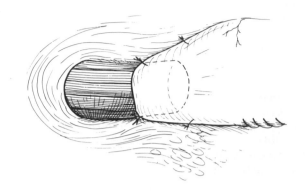

7

Postoperative care

Oral feeding is withheld and the nasogastric tube and basal chest drain are retained until the Gastrografin swallow on the fifth day after operation has confirmed anastomotic integrity. Nutritional status may be maintained by total parenteral nutrition through a peripheral line until the patient's oral intake is adequate, usually within 48 h of commencement of oral fluids.

It is the author's preference to maintain thoracic epidural analgesia during the postoperative period, which enables pain-free cooperation with chest physiotherapy without the need for systemic opiates[4].

Outcome

The technique described has been performed with a clinical anastomotic dehiscence rate of 2.3%, half of which were fatal. This compares favourably with the rates of 3.8% after sutured anastomosis reported by Paterson and Wong and 2.9% using stapled anastomosis[3]. The rate of other complications is low, with an 8% incidence of anastomotic stricture requiring endoscopic dilatation, compared with 13–25% following stapled anastomosis[1,2]. Overall hospital 30-day mortality is 8.6%, which has fallen to 6.6% in the last 6 years coinciding with the routine use of thoracic epidural analgesia[4,5].

References

1. Hopkins RA, Alexander JC, Postlethwait RW. Stapled esophago-gastric anastomosis. *Am J Surg* 1984; 147: 283–7.

2. Wong J. Esophageal resection for cancer: the rationale of current practice. *Am J Surg* 1987; 153: 18–24.

3. Paterson IM, Wong J. Anastomotic leakage: an avoidable complication of Lewis–Tanner oesophagectomy. *Br J Surg* 1989; 76: 127–9.

4. Watson A. Surgery for carcinoma of the oesophagus. *Postgrad Med J* 1988; 64: 860–4.

5. Watson A. Oesophageal neoplasms. *Curr Opin Gastroenterol* 1990; 6: 590–6.

Illustrations by Denise Smith

Hand-sewn techniques for gastric anastomoses

Z. H. Krukowski PhD, FRCS(Ed)
Consultant Surgeon, Aberdeen Royal Infirmary, and Honorary Senior Lecturer, University of Aberdeen, Aberdeen, UK

N. A. Matheson ChM, FRCS, FRCS(Ed)
Consultant Surgeon, Aberdeen Royal Infirmary, and Honorary Senior Lecturer, University of Aberdeen, Aberdeen, UK

Single-layer interrupted anastomosis is preferred to two-layer techniques because it achieves more anatomical realignment of the layers of the bowel, less luminal reduction and less interference with blood supply. It also has the important advantage of simplicity. Single-layer anastomosis is applicable with minor variations throughout the gastrointestinal tract. The standard method described is based on a single layer of interrupted appositional serosubmucosal sutures which consistently achieves satisfactory results[1,2]. Hand-sutured single layer anastomoses are preferred to stapled anastomoses because of their versatility, low complication rate and economy.

SINGLE-LAYER SEROSUBMUCOSAL APPOSITIONAL ANASTOMOTIC TECHNIQUE

1 The basic technique is that each suture incorporates the submucosa but avoids the mucosa. Minor modifications may be made at some sites, e.g. a continuous technique for gastrojejunostomy.

For many years braided polyamide (nylon) 3/0 (2-metric) sutures mounted on proprietary 'Control Release' atraumatic needles have been used. This non-absorbable material is preferred because of its combination of handling, knotting and tissue inertia properties which are presently unmatched by any synthetic absorbable material.

Knots are tied with three throws. The first throw is deliberately crossed, adjusted for tension on the second throw, and the knot locked with the third throw. The tension in the knots should be sufficient to appose the tissues snugly and without strangulation.

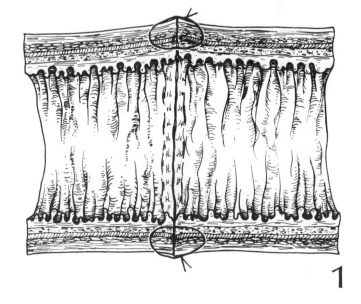

1

PREPARATION OF ROUX-EN-Y LOOP OF JEJUNUM

2 A Roux-en-Y loop is one of the most useful devices in reconstructive gastrointestinal surgery and the ability to fashion it correctly is fundamental. The first step in preparation of a Roux loop is vascular division so that by the time it is to be used for anastomosis any ischaemia at the proposed site of division should be apparent. The distance of jejunal division from the duodenojejunal junction is not critical and depends on the anatomy of the main jejunal vessels supplying the arcades. The first pedicle of sufficient length to permit easy ligation determines the site of division. Transillumination of the mesentery improves accurate identification of the main vessels of the appropriate arcade. The vessels are ligated in continuity after isolation by division of the overlying peritoneum on both sides of the mesentery. According to the vascular anatomy and required length it may or may not be necessary to divide more than one main vascular pedicle.

3 Care must be taken to avoid incorporation of the junctions of blood vessels in bulky ligatures.

4 The jejunum is cleared over a 2-cm length; one or two terminal branches of the jejunal vessels are divided close to the bowel wall to achieve this. After vascular isolation of the proposed loop the rest of the operation may proceed and division of the jejunum is postponed until it is required for anastomosis. The jejunum is cross-clamped at right angles with a Schumacher's clamp and divided distal to the clamp. The distal end is held in a pair of Babcock's forceps and mopped clean with a topical antiseptic.

The distal end is passed, usually in a retrocolic direction, through a convenient window in the transverse mesocolon for the proximal anastomosis to the stomach or oesophagus. This anastomosis is made first (*see* below) and the jejunojejunostomy is the final step in restoration of continuity.

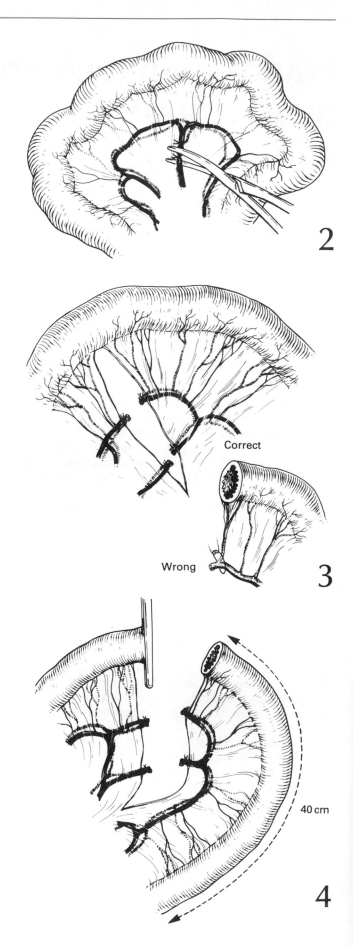

2

Correct

Wrong

3

40 cm

4

End-to-side jejunojejunostomy in a Roux loop

5 Angle sutures are passed horizontally through the proximal jejunum about 5 mm proximal to the Schumacher's clamp, and through the antimesenteric border of the distal jejunum about 40 cm distal to the end of the Roux loop. Care should be taken to place the distal sutures at the appropriate distance apart with the bowel under moderate tension. It is easy to make the enterotomy in the distal bowel too long.

The antimesenteric border of the distal jejunum between the angle sutures is incised with cutting diathermy and the lumen mopped with topical antiseptic.

The Schumacher's clamp is removed and the proximal bowel aspirated and mopped with topical antiseptic. Haemostasis is secured with fine diathermy coagulation. The angle stitches are tied.

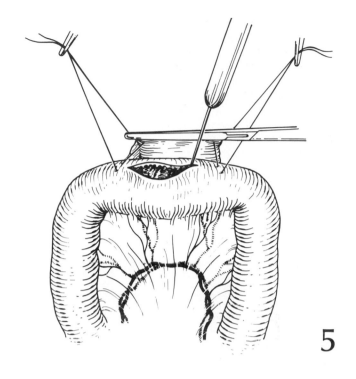

5

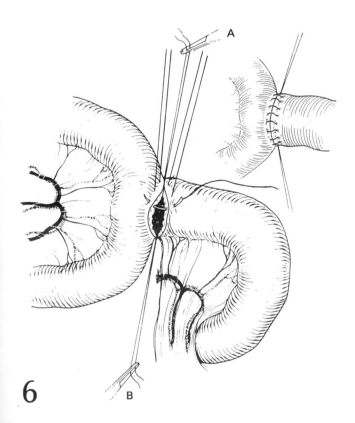

6 The anterior sutures are inserted serially into the submucosal plane of the proximal jejunum, piercing the serosa about 5 mm from, and emerging at, the cut edge, entering this part of the distal jejunum just superficial to the mucosa and emerging again about 5 mm from the edge. The sutures are placed about 5 mm apart. A mid point marking suture may be used to aid accurate placement of the whole series. The stitches are held one after the other between the finger and thumb of an assistant.

The anterior sutures are tied serially and cut.

6

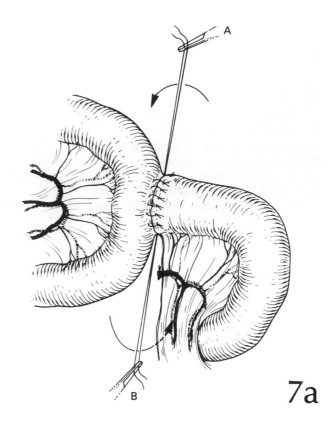

7a

7a, b The distal angle suture is passed behind the anastomosis which is rotated through 180° to expose the posterior aspect.

The posterior row of sutures is placed serially, tied and cut.

Rotation of the anastomosis through 180°, which permits all the knots to be placed on the serosal aspect, depends on mobility. If the site of the jejunal section is close to the duodenojejunal junction, sufficient mobility may be lacking. If this is the case, sutures may be inserted from the anterior aspect.

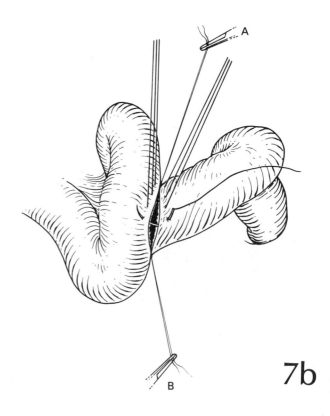

7b

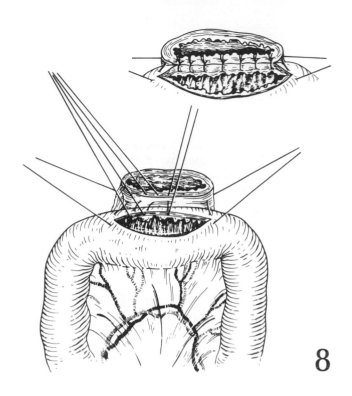

8 The angle stitches in this case are left untied until the first (posterior) layer has been placed. Sutures are inserted serially into the submucosa at the cut edge of the proximal jejunum and emerge at the cut edge of the distal jejunum. As before, about 5 mm of bowel is included on both sides and the sutures are placed about 5 mm apart. A mid point marking stitch may again be used.

The sutures are tied in series with knots on the luminal aspect and cut. The anterior layer is completed as in *Illustration 7a* and *b*.

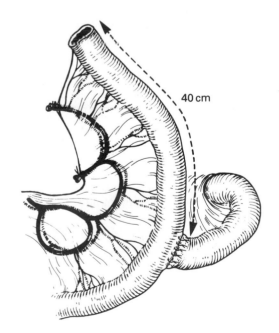

RECONSTRUCTION AFTER TOTAL GASTRECTOMY

9 Roux-en-Y oesophagojejunostomy by the abdominal route is the preferred reconstruction after total gastrectomy for malignant neoplasms of the body or antrum of the stomach. Oesophagogastrectomy for malignant tumours at the cardia is not described here.

10 The oesophagus is mobilized for 6 cm proximal to the cardia and two full thickness horizontal stay sutures are inserted 4 cm proximal to the cardia. A right-angled non-crushing clamp (Haughton's) is placed proximal to the stay sutures. The clamp is necessary to relieve undue traction on the subsequent anastomotic sutures. The oesophagus is transected with scissors 1.5 cm distal to the cross-clamp and the lumen mopped with a topical antiseptic.

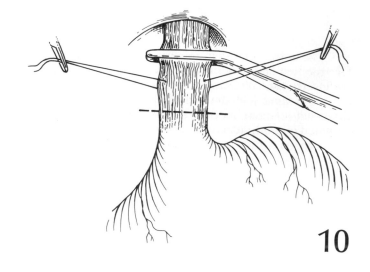

10

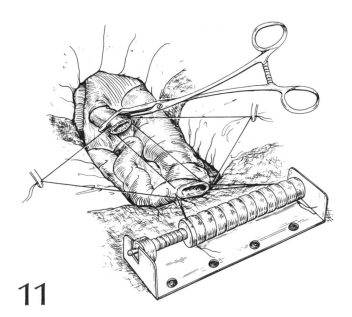

11

11 The previously prepared Roux loop is passed in a retrocolic direction and adequacy of the blood supply is confirmed. To prevent the jejunum slipping into the depths of the abdomen during placement of the posterior row of sutures, two short stay sutures are inserted transversely through the jejunum and are either clipped with artery forceps or held in a suture-holding clamp. A horizontal serosubmucosal angle suture is inserted into the antimesenteric border of the jejunum about 5 mm from the divided end. A corresponding bite of the right side of the oesophageal wall is taken and the suture held in a pair of artery forceps. A similar angle suture is placed on the mesenteric aspect of the jejunum and the other side of the oesophagus.

12 A series of serosubmucosal sutures is placed 5 mm apart on the oesophagus and up to 7 mm apart on the jejunum if there is significant discrepancy in diameter between the two. It is seldom necessary to use a mid point suture because of the relatively narrow diameter of the oesophagus. Care is taken not to pick up the anterior wall of the oesophagus. The sutures are inserted just beneath the mucosa on the cut edge of the jejunum and emerge in the same plane at the cut edge of the oesophagus. If the oesophageal mucosa retracts excessively it may be incorporated in a full-thickness suture. After insertion each suture is held untied in series in the suture-holding clamp.

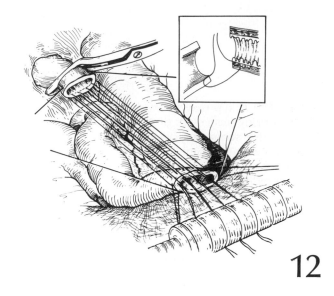

12

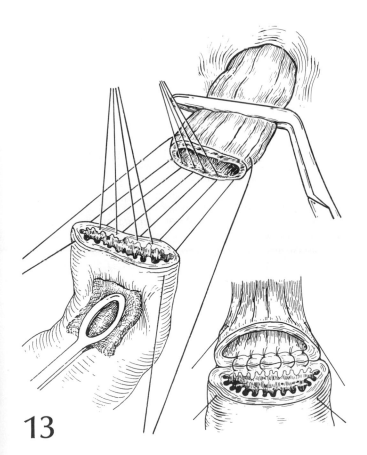

13

13 When all the sutures are in place the stay sutures on the jejunum are removed and the jejunum is pushed down the sutures with a swab mounted on a holder until the jejunum apposes the oesophagus.

The sutures are tied serially and cut. The oesophageal clamp is released and patency of the lumen confirmed.

14 The clamp may be reapplied to relieve tension during placement of the anterior row of sutures. The anterior serosubmucosal sutures are now inserted in series from jejunum to oesophagus and are held either in a series of artery forceps or in the suture-holding clamp.

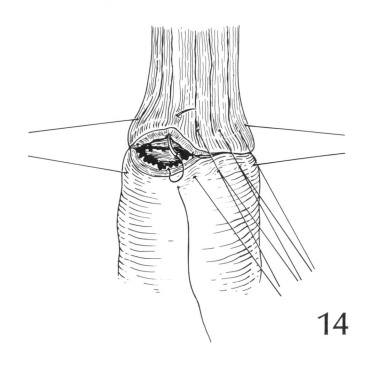

14

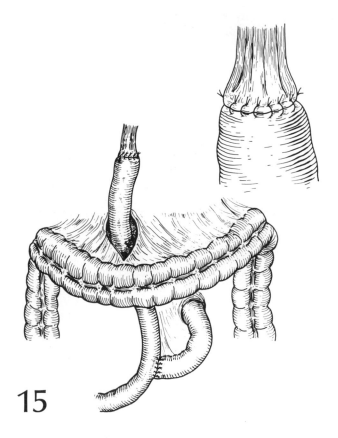

15

15 The angle sutures followed by the anterior row are tied serially and cut. There is no requirement for additional sutures and there must be no tension on the anastomosis. Drains are not used.

The end-to-side jejunojejunostomy is then made as previously described.

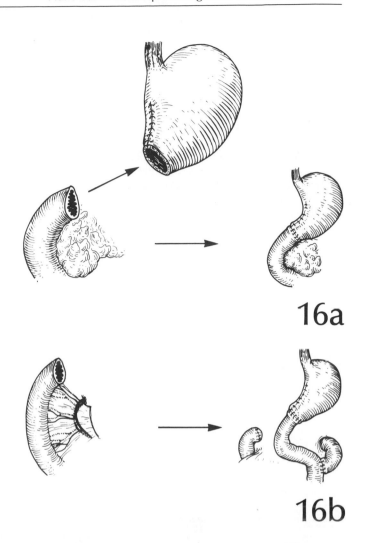

RECONSTRUCTION AFTER PARTIAL GASTRECTOMY

16a–d
The options for reconstruction after partial gastrectomy are: gastroduodenal (Billroth I) (*Illustration 16a*); gastrojejunal with a Roux loop (*Illustration 16b*); gastrojejunal with a loop of jejunum (Billroth II or Pólya (*Illustration 16c*)); or interposed jejunal loop between the gastric remnant and the duodenum (*Illustration 16d*).

After partial gastrectomy, a gastroduodenal anastomosis (Billroth I) is preferred but when there is residual malignant disease in the region of the proposed anastomosis with the possibility of later recurrence and obstruction, a gastrojejunal anastomosis (Billroth II/Pólya or Roux-en-Y) is preferred. In either event restoration of continuity is facilitated if the gastric remnant is first partially closed to reconstitute a 'lesser curve'.

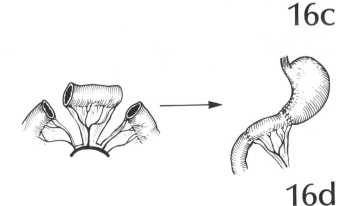

16d

Reconstitution of a 'lesser curve'

17 A pair of Schumacher clamps is placed in parallel at right angles to the greater curve of the stomach at the point of proposed division. About 4–5 cm of the stomach is incorporated and the diameter should exceed that of the duodenum for gastroduodenal anastomoses.

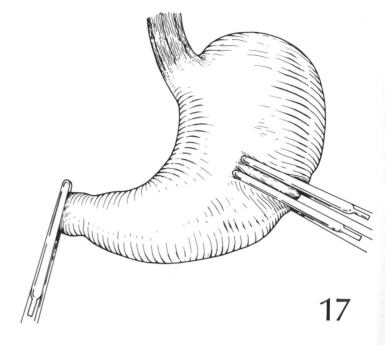

17

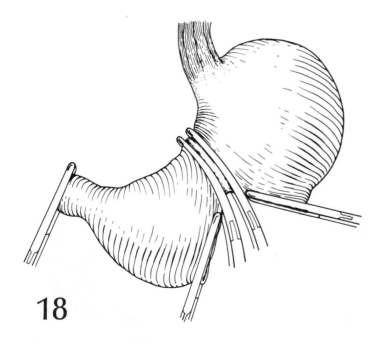

18

18 The stomach is divided between the Schumacher clamps. Two Parker–Kerr clamps are applied, extending from the tips of the Schumacher clamps across the lesser curve and angled towards the cardia. The Parker–Kerr clamps are applied with a gap of approximately 0.5 cm between them.

19 The stomach is divided distal to the Parker–Kerr clamps and the resected stomach removed.

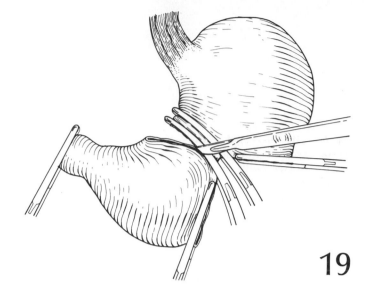

19

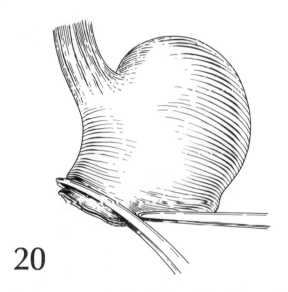

20

20 The distal Parker–Kerr clamp is released, leaving a cuff of crushed gastric tissue distal to the proximal clamp.

21 The proximal clamp is used to present the stomach for the insertion of a continuous layer of 3/0 (2-metric) all-coats polydioxanone.

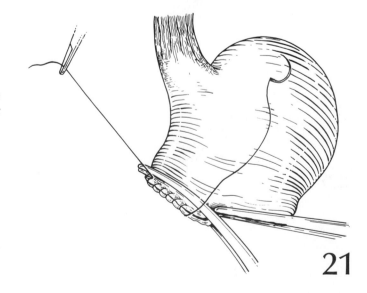

21

22 The proximal Parker–Kerr clamp is removed and the first layer of continuous polydioxanone suture buried with a second layer of continuous 3/0 (2-metric) serosubmucosal polydioxanone. Routine reconstitution of a 'lesser curve' simplifies subsequent gastroduodenal or gastrojejunal anastomosis, avoiding any valve or more complex reconstruction.

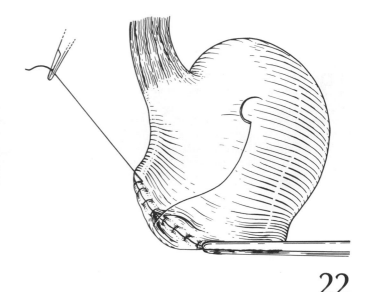

22

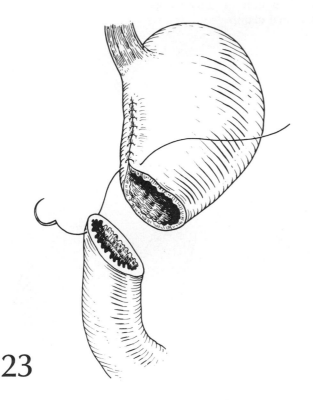

23

Gastroduodenal anastomosis

23 The most important suture in making a safe gastroduodenal anastomosis is the superior angle stitch which is inserted in the serosubmucosal plane on the anterior aspect of the stomach. This emerges near the oversewn edge of the reconstructed lesser curve and is reinserted in a similar fashion in the posterior aspect of the reconstructed lesser curve. It is then placed horizontally and serosubmucosally through the superior aspect of the divided duodenum and held in artery forceps. A similar horizontal angle suture is inserted through the greater curve aspect of the divided gastric remnant and correspondingly into the inferior border of the duodenum, and is held in artery forceps. These angle stitches are placed about 5 mm from the cut edge in each case. The divided ends of the stomach and duodenum should come together without tension but during placement of the sutures a gap of 2–3 cm should be maintained to allow accurate placement of the posterior layer.

24 The posterior row of serosubmucosal sutures is inserted serially. A mid point marking suture may be of help. The distance between the sutures is approximately 5 mm, but according to discrepancy in size this may be larger on the gastric side and smaller on the duodenum. In each case about 5 mm of tissue is incorporated. The sutures are placed serially and held by an assistant. When all have been placed they are tied and cut. The knots lie on the luminal aspect but are overlaid to a considerable extent by the mucosa.

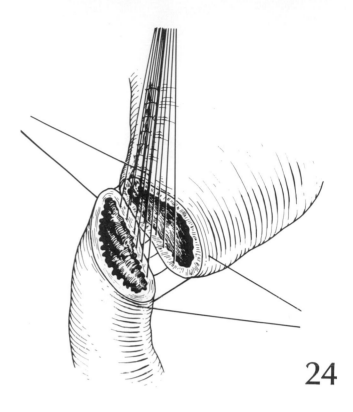

24

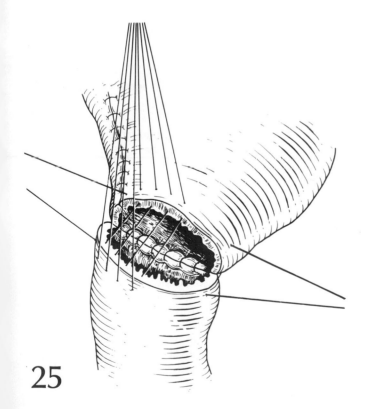

25

25 The anterior row of sutures is placed in a similar fashion in the serosubmucosal plane. A mid point marking suture is helpful in achieving accurate suture placement, particularly if the size of the lumen exceeds 3 cm. When the anterior sutures have been inserted, the angle sutures are tied and held. The anterior sutures are then tied serially and cut.

26   The angle sutures are cut and the anastomosis is complete.

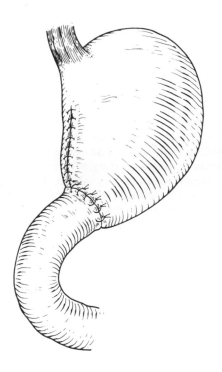

26

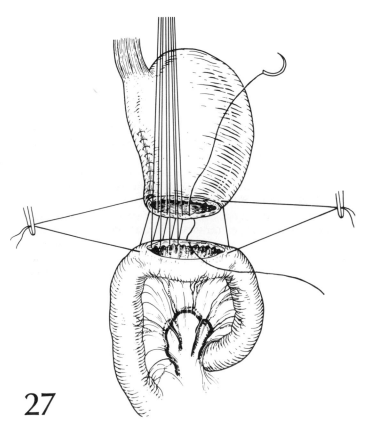

27

Gastrojejunal anastomosis with Roux loop

This is performed in the same way as a gastroduodenal anastomosis.

Gastrojejunal anastomosis to loop of jejunum (Pólya/Billroth II)

After identification of the duodenojejunal junction, a loop of proximal jejunum is brought in either a retrocolic or antecolic direction to lie in lax apposition with the distal stomach in an isoperistaltic direction.

27   An angle suture is placed through the corners of the reconstructed lesser curve as for a Billroth I anastomosis and inserted as a horizontal serosubmucosal suture through the jejunum on the antimesenteric border. A horizontal serosubmucosal angle suture is placed on the greater curve aspect of the gastric remnant and horizontally through the jejunum at the proximal end of the proposed enterotomy. A longitudinal enterotomy of 5–6 cm is made. The posterior row of interrupted serosubmucosal sutures is inserted serially, tied on the luminal aspect and cut. A mid point marking suture may be used to subdivide the anastomosis.

28 The anterior sutures are inserted serially. When the anterior sutures have been placed the angle sutures are tied and held.

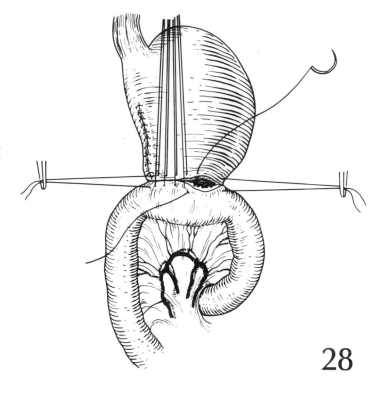

28

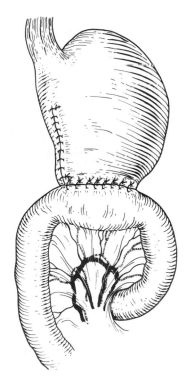

29

29 The anterior row of sutures is tied serially and cut, the angle sutures are cut and the anastomosis is complete.

Jejunal interposition

It is occasionally necessary in reconstructive gastric surgery to interpose a segment of proximal jejunum between the gastric remnant and the duodenum. The gastrojejunal anastomosis is made as shown in *Illustrations 23–26*, and the jejunoduodenal anastomosis is a straightforward end-to-end anastomosis.

GASTROJEJUNOSTOMY

30 The anastomosis to be described is retrocolic with a vertical stoma in the gastric antrum. Accessibility together with the profuse vascularity of the stomach makes a continuous single layer technique attractive.

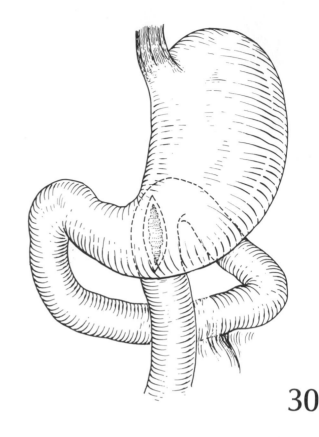

30

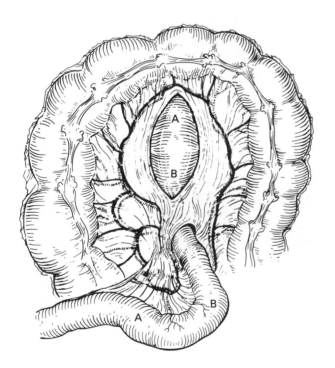

31

31 The greater omentum and transverse colon are raised to expose the posterior aspect of the transverse mesocolon. Both layers are incised vertically, taking care to avoid the middle colic vessels and tributaries, and to expose the posterior aspect of the gastric antrum. The greater curve is at A and the lesser at B. The alignment of the proposed anastomosis is shown by A and B on the jejunum.

32 The greater and lesser curves are lightly grasped with a pair of Babcock's tissue forceps and rotated to align the stomach with the proximal jejunum. The proximal jejunum is identified at the duodenojejunal flexure and a convenient segment isolated between the Babcock's forceps. The jejunum is disposed afferent end to lesser curve and should lie with laxity. The afferent loop need not be excessively short with the anastomosis close to the duodenojejunal junction.

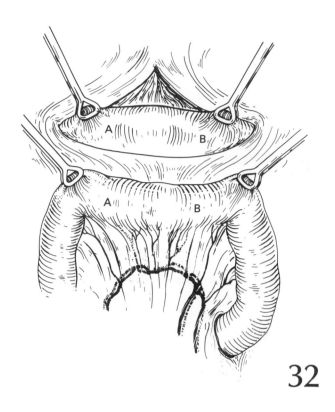

32

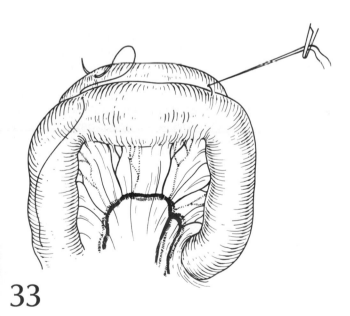

33

33 An angle suture is inserted serosubmucosally through the jejunum proximally and the posterior wall of the stomach close to the lesser curve. This is tied and held. A similar suture is inserted through the jejunum and close to the greater curve of the stomach. Strips soaked in topical antiseptic are laid round the anastomotic site.

34 The jejunum and then the stomach are opened with cutting diathermy. The gastric contents are aspirated with suction, taking care to avoid contamination. Haemostasis is secured with accurate diathermy of the submucosal vessels.

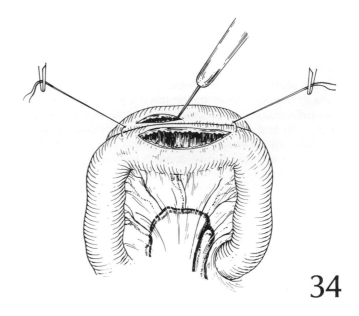

34

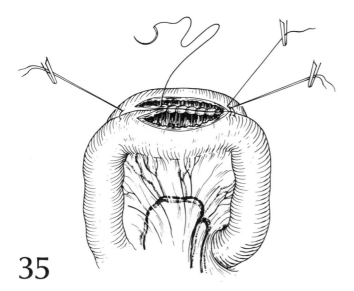

35

35 The anastomosis is started at the proximal end of the jejunotomy with a continuous 3/0 polydioxanone suture. The suture is passed from the serosal aspect of the jejunum to emerge on the gastric serosa and knotted on the outside; it is then passed through the gastric wall to emerge on the mucosal aspect. Continuous insertion then begins at approximately 5-mm intervals. The suture is place in the serosubmucosal plane on the jejunal side but may include the mucosa on the gastric side if necessary for complete haemostasis.

36 At the corner a loop of suture is held on the serosal aspect of the jejunum and the needle is passed through the stomach to emerge on the mucosal aspect. It is then passed through the jejunum from the mucosal aspect and the suture is locked at the corner by passing it through the loop on the serosal aspect.

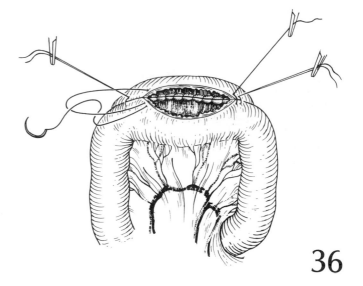

36

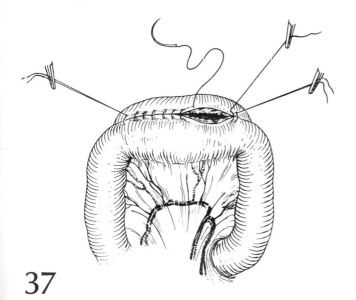

37

37 The direction of suturing is then reversed, passing back through the jejunum to the stomach on the anterior aspect of the anastomosis. Serosubmucosal placement eliminates mucosal pouting.

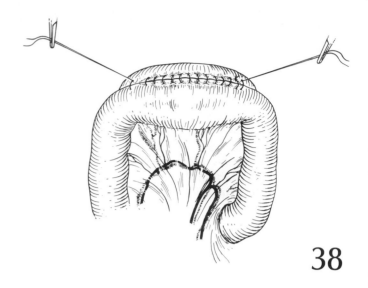

38 Once the final stitch has been placed the continuous suture is knotted close to its proximal end.

38

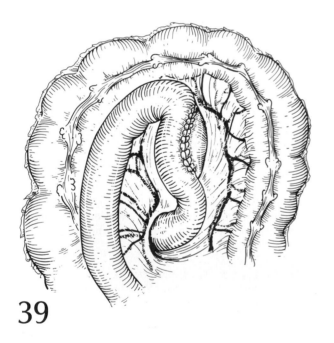

39

39 The angle sutures are cut and the stomach allowed to return to its normal position as shown in *Illustration 30*.

Postoperative care

Following total gastrectomy with oesophagojejunal anastomosis oral fluids are withheld for 7 days until a radiographic contrast study has shown an intact anastomosis. In contrast, oral fluids are commenced after 24 h following partial gastrectomy or revisional gastric surgery.

References

1. Irwin ST, Krukowski ZH, Matheson NA. Single layer anastomosis in the upper gastrointestinal tract. *Br J Surg* 1990; 77: 643–4.

2. Matheson NA, McIntosh CA, Krukowski ZH. Continuing experience with single layer appositional anastomosis in the large bowel. *Br J Surg* 1985; 72(Suppl): S104–6.

Illustrations by Angela Christie

Stapling techniques for gastric anastomoses

J. L. Chassin MD
Chairman, Department of Surgery, The New York Hospital Medical Center of Queens, New York, USA

STAPLED OESOPHAGOJEJUNAL ANASTOMOSIS AFTER TOTAL GASTRECTOMY

After total gastrectomy it is essential that an oesophago-jejunal anastomosis be constructed in the Roux-en-Y fashion. If the descending limb of the jejunum between the oesophagojejunostomy and the jejunojejunostomy measures 60–70 cm, the danger of bile refluxing into the oesophagus is eliminated. Reflux of bile produces a serious and painful oesophagitis. A side-to-end oesophagojejunal anastomosis can be constructed efficiently and safely using the EEA device if proper precautions are observed. Ideally, the cut end of the oesophagus will have a diameter sufficiently large to admit a 28-mm or 31-mm diameter EEA cartridge. If a 25-mm (EEA-25) cartridge is used, the anastomosis will be too small to accommodate passage of all of the foods generally consumed by 10–15% of patients on a regular diet. Correction requires postoperative dilatation of the stricture. In most patients, gentle dilatation of the oesophagus in the operating room will permit the passage of the EEA-28 cartridge. It is dangerous to perform vigorous dilatation as this may result in an occult tear in the lining of the oesophagus and possible postoperative leakage.

Preparation of oesophagus

After digital dilatation of the lumen of the oesophagus, the diameter of the lumen is measured using the sizer. Sizers are produced with diameters of 25, 28 and 31 mm. Lubricating jelly is used to facilitate the passage of the instrument into the oesophagus. This will determine which cartridge is to be used.

Insertion of EEA device

1 A 2/0 polypropylene (Prolene) purse-string suture
is inserted through the full thickness of the
oesophagus, starting at the top about 3–4 mm from the
cut end of the oesophagus. Bites of about 4 mm are
taken, and care is taken to ensure that the mucosal layer
is caught by each bite of suture material. Four guy
sutures are inserted for traction at 1, 4, 7 and 10 o'clock,
and a clamp is applied to each.

The cut end of the jejunum is gently dilated using
lubricated fingertips and the EEA sizers are inserted to
determine whether the lumen of the jejunum will in fact
admit the selected cartridge. The anvil of the EEA
cartridge is then removed and lubrication applied to the
instrument. The EEA device is passed gently into the
lumen of the jejunum. When the device has been
inserted about 6 cm, the wing-nut is rotated in a
counterclockwise fashion so that the central rod will
protrude from the cartridge and impinge on the
antimesenteric border of the jejunum. When this has
been confirmed by palpation, electrocautery is used to
make an incision over the rod that will be just large
enough to permit passage of the rod through the wall of
the jejunum. A small purse-string suture of polypropylene is inserted into the jejunum close to the rod and
the anvil is attached to the protruding rod. It is
important to ensure that the screw fastening the anvil to
the rod is tight. A serious error in construction of this
anastomosis can result if the mucosa at point Y is caught
by the advancing cartridge and taken to point X. If this
occurs, firing the stapler will occlude the efferent limb
of the jejunum and the anastomosis will be completely
obstructed.

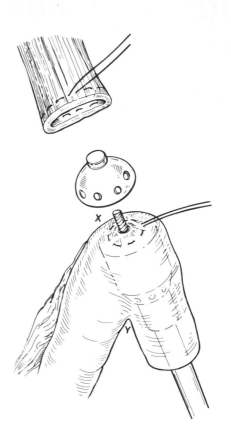

1

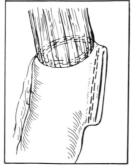

2

Passage of anvil into oesophagus

2 The lumen of the oesophagus is again gently dilated
with lubricated fingertips. The assistant grasps the
four clamps attached to the guy sutures to stabilize the
oesophagus and the anvil of the EEA device is gently
inserted into the oesophagus. When this has been
accomplished, the oesophageal purse-string suture is
tied snugly around the central rod of the EEA device and
the tails of this suture are cut. The guy sutures are then
removed.

Firing the EEA device

The wing-nut is turned in a clockwise direction until the space between the anvil and the cartridge has been properly closed. It is necessary to ascertain that no extraneous tissue has been trapped between the cartridge and the anvil before this closure, after which the EEA device is fired. The wing-nut is then turned in a counterclockwise direction for about seven half-turns. The instrument is rotated, the anvil disengaged from the anastomosis, and the EEA device removed from the operative field.

The anvil is detached from the cartridge and the two doughnuts of tissue removed. Both doughnuts should be demonstrated to form complete rings of tissue if the stapling device has performed properly.

Checking the integrity of the anastomosis

The index finger is inserted through the open end of the jejunum, through the anastomosis and into the ocsophagus. The anastomotic ring should be intact. The finger is then withdrawn just enough to allow insertion into the efferent segment of the jejunum. If the XY error described in *Illustration 1* has occurred, then entrance into the efferent segment is completely obstructed by an erroneously placed staple line. In this case, the anastomosed segment is excised and a new oesophagojejunal anastomosis is performed.

If no errors are detected by palpation, a TA 55 stapling device is applied to the blind segment of jejunum at a point about 1.5 cm proximal to the oesophagojejunostomy (*Illustration 2*). This is then closed and fired, and the surplus jejunum excised along the stapling device. The everted mucosa noted in the staple line is lightly electrocoagulated and the anastomosis inspected on all sides to detect any visible defect. An additional check of the integrity of the anastomosis can be conducted by asking the anaesthetist to inject 1–200 ml of methylene blue solution through the nasogastric tube into the oesophagus while the efferent limb of jejunum is occluded either by manual compression or a non-crushing Doyen clamp. Leakage of blue dye from the anastomosis or the stapled proximal end of jejunum may then be seen.

Construction of Roux-en-Y jejunojejunostomy

3 A point on the efferent segment of jejunum 60 cm distal to the oesophagojejunostomy is identified and a longitudinal 1.5-cm incision using either scalpel or electrocautery is made on the antimesenteric surface of the jejunum. The proximal cut end of jejunum is identified at point B and the open end of jejunum is aligned so that it points in a cephalad direction. This segment is then apposed to the antimesenteric border of the descending limb of jejunum adjacent to the incision at point A.

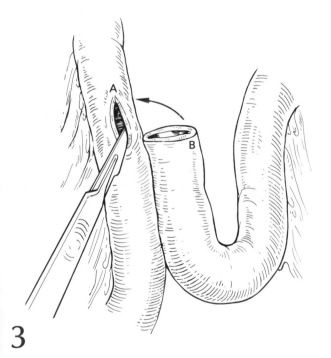

3

4 One fork of the GIA stapling device is inserted into the jejunal incision at point A (*Illustration 3*) and the other fork into the open end of the proximal jejunum. The device is closed, fired and removed.

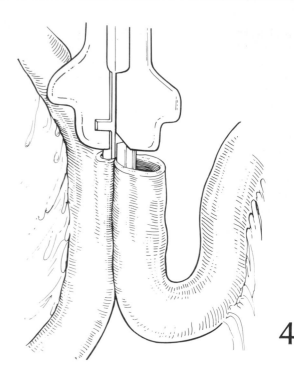

4

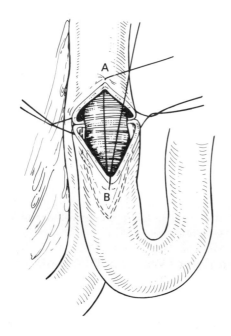

5

5 This stapling accomplishes the posterior layer of a front-to-back anastomosis between the proximal and efferent segments of jejunum. Guy sutures are placed to capture the ends of the GIA staple line at points C and D (*Illustration 6*). A third guy suture is inserted to bisect the anastomosis.

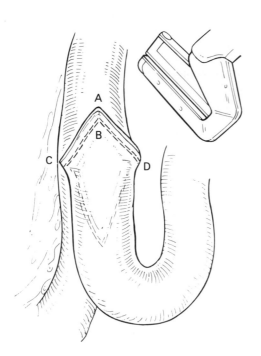

6

6 Tying this suture will approximate point A to point B. A clamp is attached to each of the three guy sutures and additional Allis' clamps are placed along the everted tissue from points A to C. A TA 55 stapler with 3.5-mm staples is then applied and this portion of the anastomosis is closed in eversion. The stapler should be placed deep to the guy sutures at points AB and C. The redundant tissue is excised but the guy suture is preserved at point AB. The stapling device is removed and the everted mucosa is lightly electrocoagulated. Several Allis clamps are applied to the everted jejunal tissue from point AB to point D. Again, the stapling device should be deep to the guy suture at point AB as well as point D. When the stapler has been properly positioned, the staples are fired and the surplus jejunal tissue is excised. The everted mucosa is lightly electrocoagulated and the stapling device removed.

All aspects of the anastomosis are inspected carefully. A large functional end-to-side anastomosis has been constructed. When properly performed this has proved to be a very effective, simple and safe anastomosis.

STAPLED GASTRO-OESOPHAGEAL ANASTOMOSIS AFTER OESOPHAGOGASTRECTOMY

A distressing long-term complication after anastomosis of the oesophagus to the gastric remnant following resection is the regurgitation into the oesophagus of bile and pancreatic secretions. This regurgitation frequently produces an ulcerative oesophagitis that is more painful even than the reflux of acid into the oesophagus. If more than half of the proximal stomach has been removed, end-to-end anastomosis of the oesophagus to a small gastric remnant is highly likely to produce a severe oesophagitis. (To avoid this complication, it may be preferable to perform a total gastrectomy with Roux-

en-Y oesophagojejunostomy which will avoid reflux oesophagitis.)

If a gastric remnant is to be retained, an extensive Kocher manoeuvre is performed after lesion resection, and the head of the pancreas and proximal duodenum are elevated in a cephalad direction. The cut end of the oesophagus is brought down over the anterior surface of the gastric remnant. If an end-to-side gastro-oesophageal anastomosis can be performed at a point at least 6 cm distal to the proximal cut end of the gastric remnant, gastro-oesophageal reflux will be minimized.

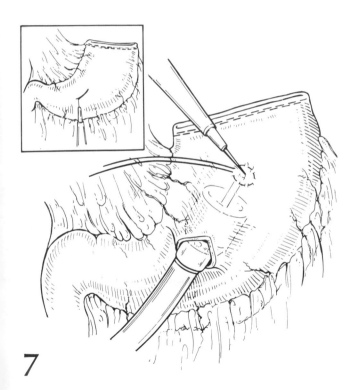

7

Construction of the EEA anastomosis

7 To insert the EEA stapling device into the gastric pouch, a 3-cm incision is required. If a Heincke–Mikulicz pyloroplasty is planned, the longitudinal incision is made across the pylorus using electrocautery at this time, and the EEA cartridge is inserted through this incision. Otherwise, electrocautery is used to make an incision of 3 cm in the anterior wall of the lower half of the gastric remnant.

The anvil is removed from the tip of the EEA device which is then inserted into the gastric incision. The wing-nut at the base of the stapling device is rotated in a counterclockwise direction so that the central rod protrudes from the cartridge. A 2/0 polypropylene purse-string suture is made in the stomach around the tip of the rod and electrocautery is used to make a stab wound directly over the central rod. The rod is pushed through this stab wound and the anvil reattached to the rod. The stab wound should be made at a point 5–6 cm distal to the proximal margin of the gastric remnant. The purse-string suture is tied around the central rod and the tails of this suture are cut.

8 A 2/0 polypropylene purse-string suture is placed in the distal end of the oesophagus. Each stitch should include the full thickness of the oesophagus, including the mucosa. The tails of this stitch are grasped with a haemostat and guy sutures are inserted just deep to the purse-string suture at 2, 5, 8 and 11 o'clock. A haemostat is attached to each of the guy sutures and the assistant positions these four sutures so that the lumen of the oesophagus is held wide open. It is helpful to dilate the oesophagus gently with lubricated Hegar dilators. Vigorous dilatation may induce tears in the mucosa. If a tear is undetected, it may contribute to a postoperative anastomotic leak.

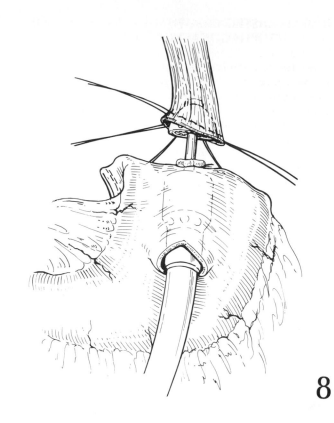

8

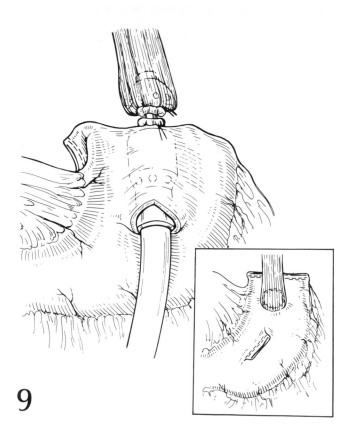

9

9 The lubricated anvil is inserted into the oesophagus, the purse-string suture tied and the guy sutures removed. The wing-nut on the stapling device is rotated so that the anvil is properly approximated to the cartridge, and the staples are fired. The wing-nut on the stapling device is then rotated to separate the anvil from the cartridge and the anvil is disengaged from the newly fashioned anastomosis. The stapling device is removed from the stomach. The two doughnuts of tissue are removed from the cartridge. If either of the doughnuts is not intact, there may be a defect in the anastomosis. If this possibility exists the anaesthetist should instil several hundred millilitres of methylene blue solution and the entire anastomosis should be observed to detect a possible leak. If there is a defect in the anastomosis, this is repaired with several sutures of 4/0 silk.

Closure of gastrotomy

Several Allis' clamps are applied to approximate the gastrotomy incision with the mucosa in eversion. A TA 55 stapler with 4.8-mm staples is placed beneath the Allis' clamps, closed and fired. The tissue protruding from the stapling device is excised using a scalpel and the everted mucosa is lightly electrocoagulated before removal of the stapling device.

In some cases this anastomosis can be expedited by using the CEEA stapling device. With the CEEA technique the anvil is detached from the cartridge and is then passed into the oesophagus. The purse-string suture is tied around the anvil and the cartridge is passed into the gastric remnant as described above. By rotating the wing-nut, a sharp spear can be made to protrude from the cartridge through the gastric wall. The anvil is then reattached to the cartridge. Otherwise, the technique is the same as described for the EEA device.

Anastomosis when the oesophagus is narrow

When the lumen of the oesophagus is too narrow to permit the passage of anything but an EEA-25 cartridge, the method of choice of constructing a gastro-oesophageal anastomosis is the GIA technique, as described below. Using this technique, a large anastomosis can be constructed in spite of the smaller lumen of the oesophagus. When a 25-mm cartridge is used, a significant number of patients will require postoperative dilatation of stricture.

Gastro-oesophageal anastomosis using the GIA technique[1]

10 Successful use of the GIA technique for gastro-oesophageal anastomosis requires that the distal end of the oesophagus reaches a point at least 6 cm caudal to the cephalad margin of the gastric remnant. A longitudinal incision of 1.5 cm is made in the anterior wall of the stomach just behind the distal margin of the oesophagus using electrocautery. The GIA stapling device is inserted for a distance of about 3.5 cm, with one fork in the gastric remnant and the other in the open lumen of the oesophagus. The device is locked and the staples fired. This manoeuvre accomplishes anastomosis between the back of the oesophagus and the front of the gastric remnant.

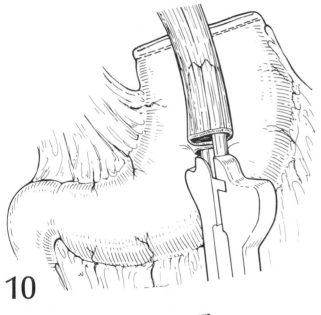

10

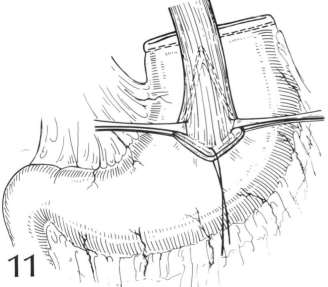

11

11 The right and left ends of the GIA staple line are grasped in Allis' clamps. The oesophagus and stomach are bisected midway between the two Allis' clamps with a 4/0 guy suture. The remaining defect between the oesophagus and stomach is then closed by triangulation with two applications of a TA 55 stapling device as now described.

12 Additional Allis' clamps are applied between the left Allis' clamp and the guy suture to approximate the oesophagus and stomach in eversion. A TA 55 stapling device is placed just deep to the Allis' clamp and the guy suture, closed and fired.

The redundant tissue protruding from the stapler is excised with Mayo scissors, but the guy suture is not cut. The everted mucosa is lightly electrocoagulated.

Additional Allis' clamps are applied to close the remaining defect between the stomach and the oesophagus. A TA 55 stapler is placed deep to the guy suture and the Allis' clamps. The stapling device is then fired and the protruding tissue excised with Mayo scissors together with the guy suture. The everted mucosa is lightly electrocoagulated and the stapling device removed.

Staples of 4.8 mm are used for these anastomoses unless the thickness of the stomach and oesophagus are significantly less than average.

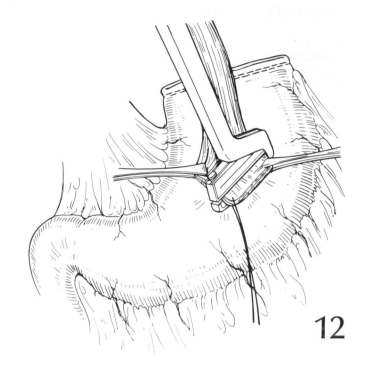

12

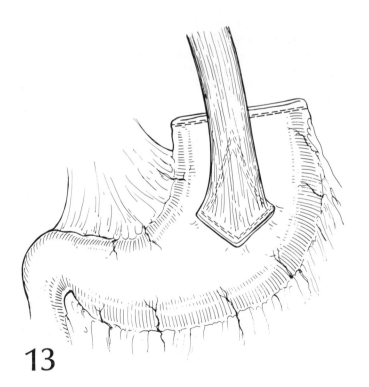

13

13 The completed back-to-front gastro-oesophageal anastomosis is checked for integrity by injection of several hundred millilitres of methylene blue solution into the stomach through the nasogastric tube.

After oesophagogastrectomy, 15% of patients experience persistent difficulty in gastric emptying, so most surgeons perform some type of drainage procedure. The author prefers a pyloromyotomy.

STAPLED GASTROJEJUNOSTOMY AFTER BILLROTH II GASTRECTOMY

Resection of stomach

14 The omentum is detached from the greater curvature of the stomach as described in the chapter on pp. 185–196. The desired point of transection of the stomach is determined, ensuring that the nasogastric tube is retracted by the anaesthetist above the line of transection. A Payr clamp is applied across the body of the stomach, and a TA90 stapler 1 cm cephalad to the Payr clamp. Using 4.8-mm staples, the stapler is closed and fired. The stomach is then incised flush with the staples and the stapler is removed. The everted gastric mucosa is lightly electrocoagulated.

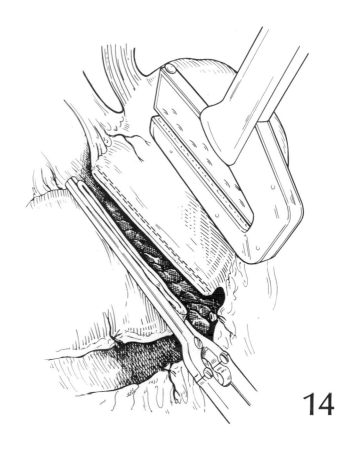

14

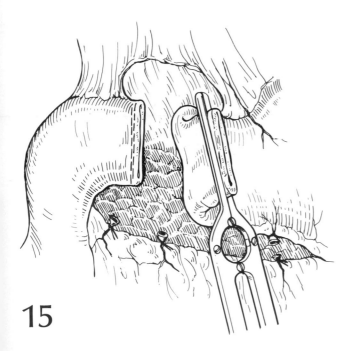

15

Duodenal closure

15 After dissection of the stomach and duodenum off the pancreas for a distance of 2–3 cm beyond the pylorus, a TA 55 stapler with 4.8-mm staples is applied to the duodenum beyond the pylorus. Although stapling a duodenum which is mildly or moderately thickened is a safe procedure, in some patients with chronic ulcer disease the duodenum is remarkably thickened, to the extent that a stapler will devitalize the tissue. In such rare cases, stapling is contraindicated. When the stapler has been applied and fired, a straight clamp is placed across the proximal duodenum or pylorus and the duodenum divided flush with the stapler. The stapler is then removed and the everted mucosa lightly electrocoagulated. It is not necessary to invert the staple line with a layer of sutures.

Stapled gastrojejunostomy

A 1-cm transverse stab wound is made with the electrocoagulator on the posterior surface of the gastric pouch 3 cm proximal to the gastric staple line. A second 1-cm stab wound is then made on the antimesenteric border of the jejunum.

16 The GIA stapler is inserted with one fork in the gastric stab wound and the other in the jejunal stab wound. The stapler is locked and a 4/0 atraumatic silk suture is inserted between the stomach and jejunum just beyond the tip of the stapling device. The stapler is fired. This will produce a side-to-side anastomosis between the gastric pouch and the jejunum about 5 cm in diameter. The stapling device is removed and the GIA staple line through the stab wound is carefully inspected. Bleeding points are controlled with careful electrocoagulation or with a 5/0 atraumatic polyglactin (Vicryl) suture. If there is diffuse bleeding along the entire staple line, the staple line can be oversewn with a continuous 5/0 polyglactin suture to achieve haemostasis. Significant bleeding is uncommon.

It is important that the anastomosis is constructed at a point no closer than 3 cm from the distal termination of the gastric pouch, otherwise the blood supply of a thin strip of stomach between the anastomosis and the gastric staple line will be inadequate.

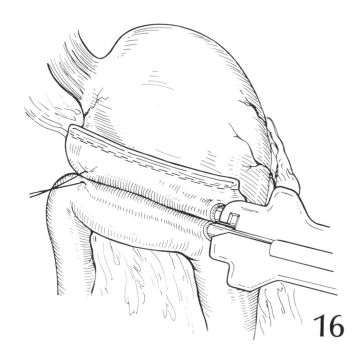

16

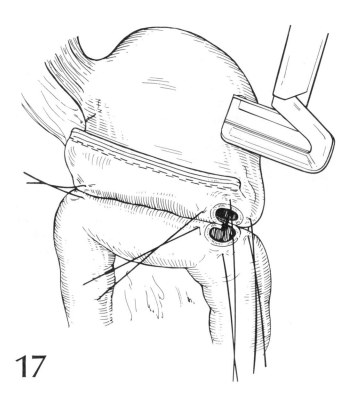

17

Closure of stab wound

17 The stab wound between the stomach and jejunum is closed with a TA 55 stapler, usually with 3.5-mm staples. To expedite this step it is necessary to identify both ends of the GIA staple line and to capture them either with silk stitches or Allis' clamps. One or two stitches or Allis' clamps are inserted to close the remaining defect with the mucosa in eversion. The TA 55 stapler is applied beneath either the guy sutures or the Allis' clamps, closed and fired. Redundant tissue protruding from the stapler is excised and the everted mucosa is lightly electrocoagulated. The stapling device is removed.

STAPLED HEINEKE–MIKULICZ PYLOROPLASTY

18 A 5–6-cm longitudinal incision is made on the anterior wall of the gastroduodenal junction using electrocautery. The incision should be centred over the pyloric muscle. Guy sutures encircling the cephalad cut end of the pyloric muscle and the caudal termination of the divided pyloric sphincter are inserted, and a third guy suture is placed through the full thickness of the gastric and duodenal walls at the midpoint between the two previously placed sutures. The middle guy suture approximating stomach and duodenum is tied, and additional Allis' clamps are applied to the full thicknesses of stomach and duodenum to close the defect with the mucosa in eversion.

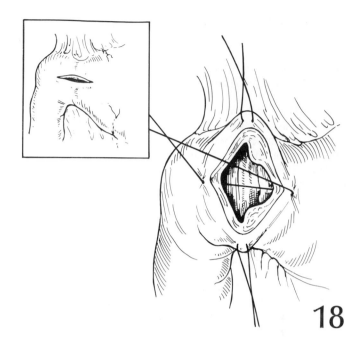

18

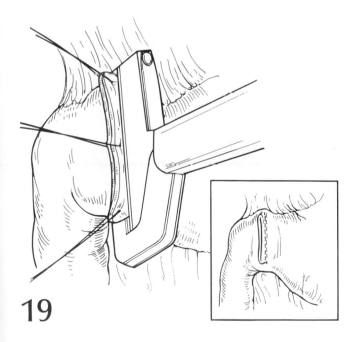

19

19 A TA 55 stapler is placed just deep to the Allis' clamps and the guy sutures. The stapler is closed and fired, and a scalpel is used to excise the redundant tissue flush with the stapler. The everted mucosa is lightly electrocoagulated and the stapling device removed.

STAPLED GASTROJEJUNOSTOMY

20 The transverse colon is elevated and the avascular portion to the left of the middle colic artery is identified. An 8–10-cm transverse incision is made through the avascular mesocolon and the posterior wall of the lower gastric antrum extracted through this incision.

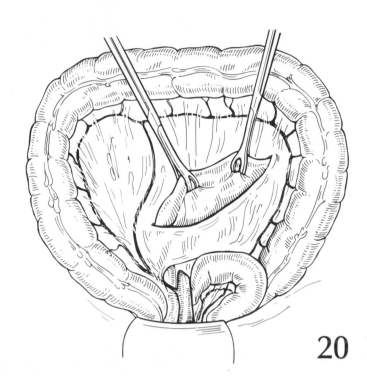

20

21 To fix the mesentery of the colon to the gastric wall throughout the circumference of the protruding stomach, 4/0 interrupted sutures are applied.

The ligament of Treitz is identified and a segment of proximal jejunum, 10–15-cm distal to this ligament, is placed adjacent to the stomach. A 1-cm longitudinal stab wound is made on the antimesenteric border of the jejunum using electrocautery, and a similar 1-cm stab wound is made through the wall of the adjacent stomach. The GIA stapling device is inserted with one fork in the stomach and the other in the jejunum. The stapling device is locked and a 4/0 silk suture is inserted to fix the stomach and jejunum near to the tip of the stapling device. The stapling device is fired, removed and the GIA staple line is inspected for bleeding.

Allis' clamps are applied to the left and right ends of the GIA staple line, along with one or two additional Allis' clamps, and the stab wound is closed with the mucosa in eversion. A TA 55 stapler is placed just deep to the Allis' clamps, the jaws of the stapler closed and the staples fired. The redundant tissue is excised flush with the stapler, and the everted mucosa is lightly electrocoagulated. The stapling device is then removed to complete construction of a large gastrojejunal anastomosis.

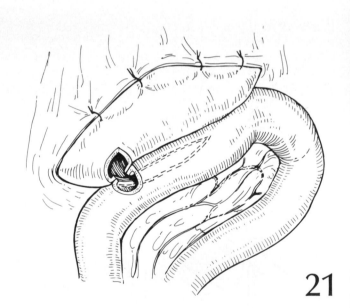

21

References

1. Chassin JL. Stapling technique for esophagogastrostomy after esophagogastric resection. *Am J Surg* 1978; 136: 399–404.

Further reading

Chassin JL. *Operative Strategy in General Surgery: An Expositive Atlas*. 2nd edn. New York: Springer-Verlag, 1993.

Illustrations by Antoine Barnaud

Abdominal and right thoracic subtotal oesophagectomy

Bernard Launois MD, FACS
Professor, Digestive and Transplantation Surgery, Hôpital Pontchaillou, Rennes, France

Guy J. Maddern PhD, MS, FRACS
Jepson Professor of Surgery, University of Adelaide, The Queen Elizabeth Hospital, Adelaide, Australia

History

Before 1946, the only widely practised approach to the thoracic oesophagus had been described by Sweet[1] using a left-sided thoracotomy. Although this operation permitted relatively good access to the lower third of the oesophagus, cancers of the middle and upper third of the oesophagus were dissected with greater difficulty because of the overlying aortic arch. In 1946 Lewis described the abdominal and right thoracic approach[2] for subtotal oesophagectomy. This operation was adopted by Tanner in the UK[3] (Lewis–Tanner operation) and by Santy[4] in France (Lewis–Santy operation), and has remained the favoured operation for an abdominal and right thoracic subtotal oesophagectomy.

Operations

ABDOMINAL APPROACH

The operation is usually commenced with the abdominal approach which enables the assessment of liver metastases, the involvement of draining lymph nodes and the performance of gastrolysis.

Incision

1a, b A midline incision is used, with the approach to the hiatus being facilitated by a substernal retractor. This provides improved access to the intra-abdominal oesophagus.

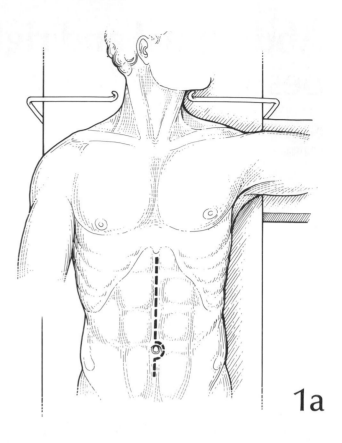

1a

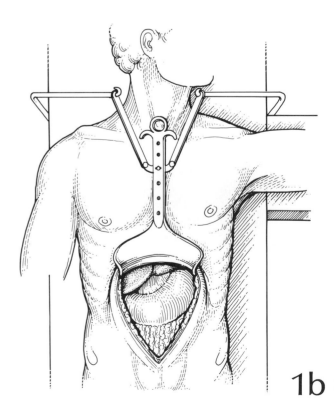

1b

2a, b

The first step is to tie and divide the vessels of the gastrocolic ligament and the short gastric vessels. It is important during the mobilization of the greater curve of the stomach to identify and preserve the right gastroepiploic vessels. The abdominal oesophagus is dissected next. The left triangular ligament of the liver is divided and the left lobe retracted to the right to reveal the oesophageal hiatus. This should be dissected with scissors under direct vision after dividing the peritoneum in front of the oesophagus. By opening the tissues to the left and right of the oesophagus a curved clamp can be introduced and a tape passed around the oesophagus. The tape can then be used to provide traction on the abdominal oesophagus which aids in the ligation and division of the remaining short gastric vessels.

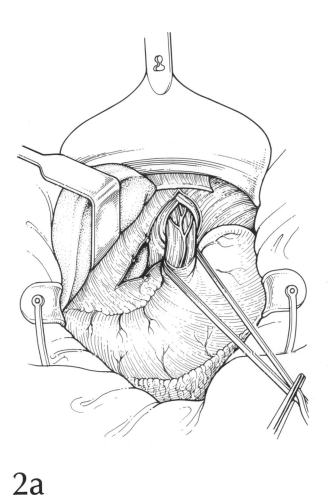

2a

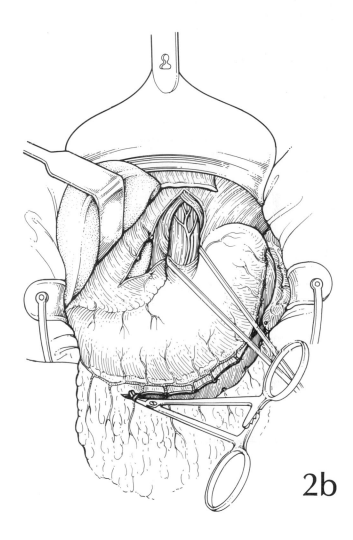

2b

3 From inside the lesser sac, with the mobilized greater curve of the stomach held upward and to the right, the left gastric vascular pedicle and its associated lymph nodes are dissected. The left gastric vein and artery are individually identified, ligated and divided.

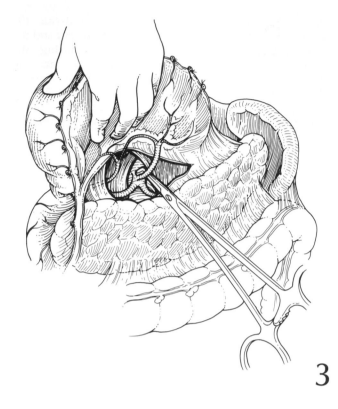

3

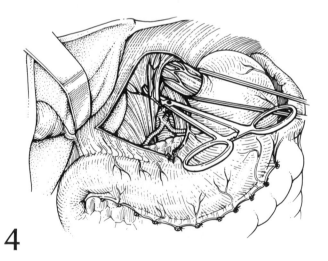

4

4 The lesser omentum is then ligated and divided from the hiatus down to the pylorus. Mobilization of the duodenum (Kocher manoeuvre) is not routinely performed for this operation but can be undertaken if increased gastric mobility is required.

A pyloroplasty or a pyloroclasia is performed to help prevent delay in gastric emptying, which sometimes occurs after this procedure. Pyloroclasia is usually performed using the thumb and middle finger as dilators which pass through the pylorus by invaginating the gastric or duodenal wall to disrupt the sphincteric mechanism.

The right crus is divided and the hiatus opened. The intra-abdominal oesophagus is then freed from all its hiatal attachments by a combination of blunt and sharp dissection.

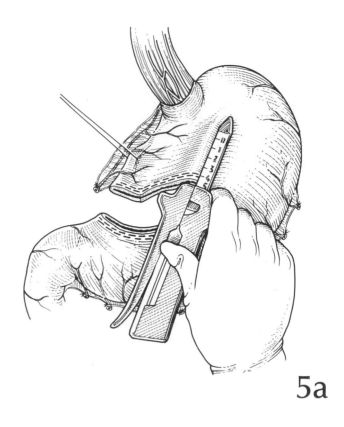

5a

5a, b A gastric tube can be constructed at this stage, although this can be delayed until the thoracic part of the operation. The gastric tube is constructed from below the 'crow's foot' on the antrum of the stomach up to the hiatus. This is most readily performed by using a surgical stapler (e.g. GIA) and leaving the last 5 cm at the cardia unstapled until the oesophagus and stomach have been successfully mobilized and delivered into the chest. The danger of completing the gastric tube at this stage is that, should the oesophageal cancer prove unresectable, then a complete obstruction has been created unnecessarily. The staple line is oversewn to ensure haemostasis and minimize the possibility of a leak.

A feeding jejunostomy can now be inserted to facilitate postoperative enteric nutrition.

Wound closure

A closed suction drain is placed behind the stomach up to the hiatus and the abdomen is closed.

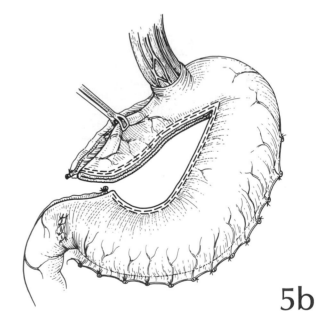

5b

THORACIC APPROACH

Position of patient

6 The patient is placed on the left side with a sandbag under the left ribs. Great care should be taken to ensure not only that the patient is well supported and secured, but that no unsupported pressure points exist. The right arm is most conveniently strapped to a padded overhead rail.

Incision

There are two possible thoracic incisions, one using a rib resection and the other passing through the intercostal space. The authors have found an unacceptable incidence of paradoxical respiration after rib resection and now recommend an intercostal approach through either the sixth intercostal space for lower third cancers or the fifth intercostal space for cancers of the middle and upper third. Gradual increase in the rib retraction at intervals during the procedure can produce adequate retraction without rib fracture even in elderly patients. The scapula, once freed from its muscular attachments inferiorly, should be retracted upwards. At this stage it is possible to confirm the location of the ribs by counting from the second rib, felt at the apex of the thorax, down to the desired interspace. The periosteum of the rib is lifted with a periosteal elevator and the intercostal space opened on the lower border of the rib. The pleura is then opened.

A Finochietto or Lortat–Jacob retractor is positioned and gently opened. Any pleural attachments are freed, and the lung mobilized to the hilus. The lung is retracted forwards and collapsed. It can be held in this position by fixing a broad blade attached to the rib retractor.

7 The right pulmonary triangular ligament is divided close to the posterior edge of the inferior lobe of the right lung, up to the right inferior pulmonary vein.

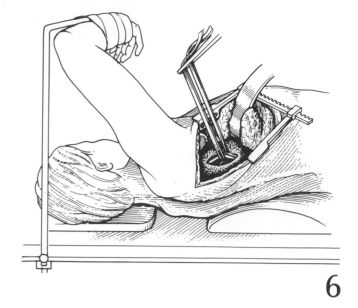

6

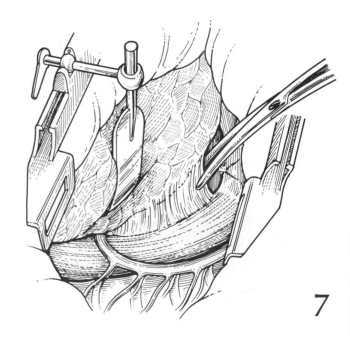

7

8 Scissors are introduced vertically between the pericardium and the posterior mediastinum. Opening the scissors reveals a plane close to the pericardium, and it is then possible to dissect upwards along this plane.

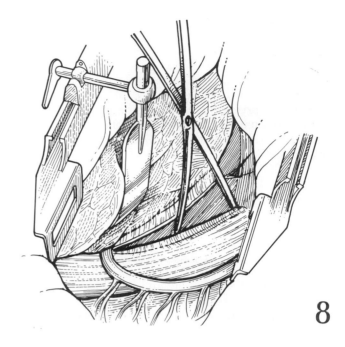

8

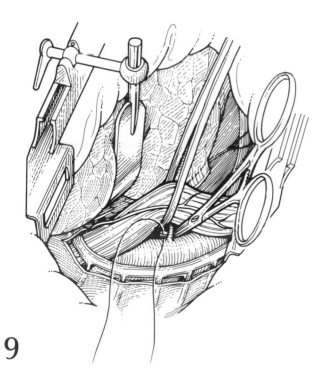

9

9 The fingers of the left hand can palpate the posterior aspect of the oesophagus and retract it from the posterior mediastinum. The pleura is then opened along the vertebral column. The scissors are opened horizontally, exposing the oesophageal arteries which are tied and divided.

10 The azygous vein is identified and ligated in continuity or transfixed and then divided.

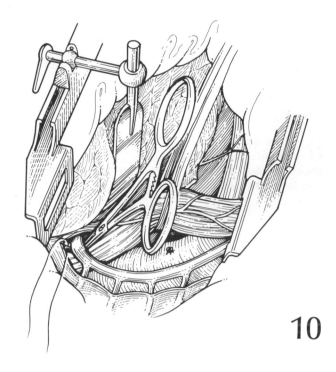

10

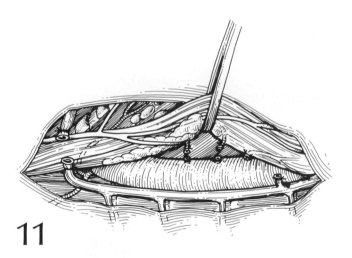

11

11 The oesophagus is mobilized above and below the tumour and tapes are passed around it to aid in retraction during the tumour dissection.

12 The oesophagus and tumour are now dissected from the surrounding structures, including the pericardium, the right and left main bronchi and the aorta. While it is desirable not to open into the tumour during the dissection, this is a preferable option to an unexpected aortic or bronchial laceration.

Difficulty in this dissection can occur at the pericardium, the trachea and/or the aorta. Extension of dissection into the pericardium is not a contraindication to resection, as a portion of pericardium can be excised safely. The pericardium is opened in front of the adhesions and then divided around the margin of the tumour. Dissection is almost never extended into the right inferior pulmonary vein.

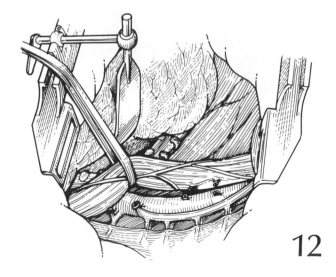

12

13 The aorta is sometimes involved by neoplastic spread. The technique used to free the cancer in these circumstances is to dissect between the intima and the adventitia of the aorta. It is important, however, to return outside the adventitia once the tumour is freed. The large oesophageal artery that arises from the aortic arch is best ligated and divided. Sometimes the artery is involved in the tumour. Ligation is not then possible, and the artery must be oversewn after the tumour is resected.

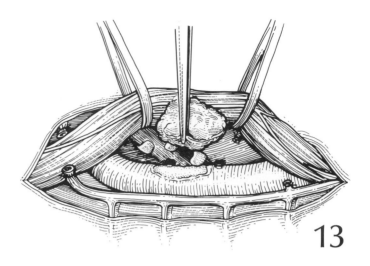

13

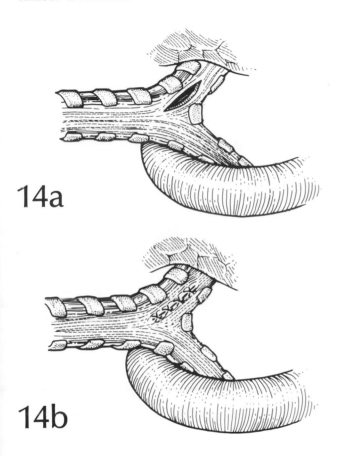

14a

14b

14a, b In some cases the most difficult part of the dissection is to detach the tumour from the trachea and the bronchus. When the neoplastic process involves the cartilaginous rings or the carina, there is little risk of opening the respiratory tree. However, when the membranous portion is involved, dissection is trickier. It is usually possible to find a plane between the trachea and a thin membrane covering it. This dissection should be directed to cutting only the neoplastic adhesions, otherwise a tracheal tear can occur. If such a tear appears, it is possible to repair it with interrupted stitches of 5/0 polypropylene (Prolene). This is relatively straightforward and usually successful.

15 The thoracic duct is found in the groove between the oesophagus and the vertebral bodies. It is important to ligate at least its inferior portion if a subsequent chylothorax is to be avoided.

Once the oesophagus and cancer are fully mobilized the stomach is delivered into the chest. Care should be taken to maintain the correct orientation and to avoid possible twists. The nasogastric tube is withdrawn into the cervical oesophagus.

A gastric tube can be formed at this stage either by using a GIA stapler or with a TA 90, which is easily manipulated in the thorax, leaving the last 5 cm at the cardia unstapled.

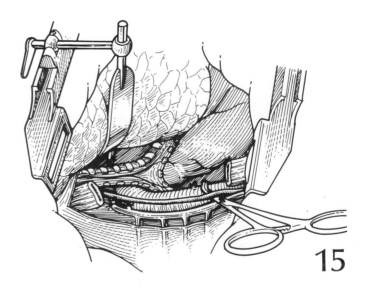

15

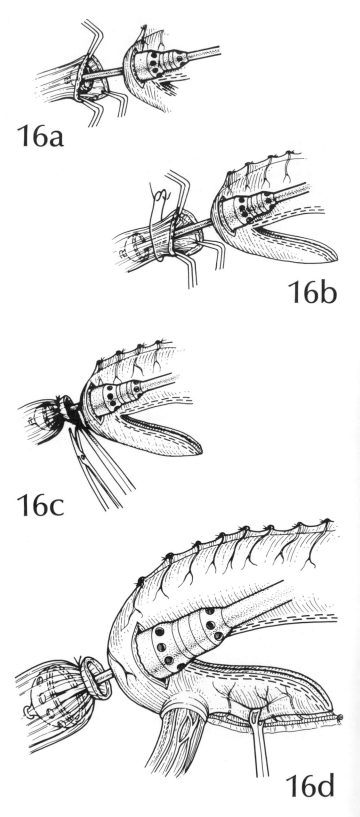

16a

16b

16c

16d

16a–d The proximal portion of oesophagus is grasped with a Satinsky clamp and divided below. Two methods can be used to tie a purse-string to the anvil of the stapler. The first is to place a tie around the anvil rod after it has been introduced into the oesophagus. This is done by placing three clamps on the oesophageal wall to hold open the lumen of the oesophagus and then the anvil is introduced into the lumen and a ligature is tied 'en masse' around the entire oesophageal wall[5]. Excess oesophagus distal to the ligature is then trimmed off. The second method is to place an over and over purse-string suture in the oesophageal stump (see chapter on pp. 148–152).

A gastrostomy is made below the apex of the gastric tube. Often it is convenient to make the gastrotomy in the portion of the stomach destined to be removed. The stapling device is introduced through the gastrotomy, into and through the stomach, the anvil is attached and secured and the anastomosis is performed by fitting the stapler.

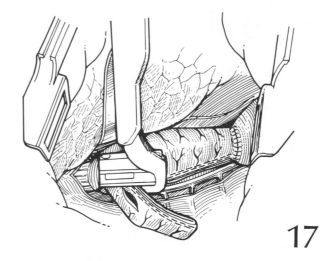

17 The remaining stomach is removed with the gastrotomy by stapling the remaining section of the tube and the staple lines are then oversewn. The nasogastric tube is passed down into the stomach and the thoracic drain inserted. The chest is then closed.

17

Postoperative care

A nasogastric tube is positioned below the anastomosis under visual control during thoracotomy and the thoracotomy is closed around a thoracic drain placed at the base of the thorax. Another drain is located at the apex in case of air leakage. The patient is then transferred to the intensive care unit and is intubated and ventilated for 24 h or more until the blood gases are satisfactory. The patient is then moved to the surgical ward. The drain is taken out after 3 or 4 days when there is less than 150 ml of clear effusion. Feeding by the jejunostomy is started as soon as bowel activity commences. The nasogastric tube is usually taken out after 7 days. Oral feeding is then progressively reinstated.

In case of an anastomotic leakage feeding is only performed via the jejunostomy and the anastomosis is not checked by a Gastrografin meal. If there is a suspicion of leakage (fever), the authors prefer to cease oral feeding and feed the patient by the jejunostomy.

References

1. Sweet RH. Surgical management of carcinoma of the midthoracic esophagus. *N Engl J Med* 1945; 223: 1–7.

2. Lewis I. The surgical treatment of carcinoma of the oesophagus with special reference to a new operation for growths of the middle third. *Br J Surg* 1946; 34: 18–31.

3. Tanner NC. The present position of carcinoma of the oesophagus. *Postgrad Med J* 1947; 23: 109–39.

4. Santy P, Mouchet A. Traitement chirurgical du cancer de l'oesophage thoracique. *J Chir* 1947; 63: 505–26.

5. Campion JP, Grossetti D, Launois B. Circular anastomosis stapler *Arch Surg* 1984; 119: 232–3.

Anatomy of the hiatus and abdominal oesophagus

Hiram C. Polk Jr MD
Ben A. Reid Sr Professor and Chairman, Department of Surgery, University of Louisville School of Medicine, Louisville, Kentucky, USA

Mark A. Malias MD
Resident Surgeon, Department of Surgery, University of Louisville School of Medicine, Louisville, Kentucky, USA

G. G. Jamieson MS, FRACS, FACS
Dorothy Mortlock Professor of Surgery, University of Adelaide, Department of Surgery, Royal Adelaide Hospital, Adelaide, Australia

Anatomical relations of distal oesophagus and fundus of the stomach

In the lower thorax, the oesophagus first lies anteriorly and then anteriorly and to the left of the aorta. It then passes further to the left as it passes through the oesophageal hiatus to join the stomach. The segment of oesophagus that lies in the abdomen during repose is about 3 cm long. However, there is appreciable shortening of the oesophagus during swallowing, belching and vomiting. The abdominal oesophagus is more or less retroperitoneal with peritoneum covering its anterior and left side only. Posteriorly the oesophagus lies on the left hiatal pillar of the left (or right) crus of the diaphragm, which separates it from the aorta. The left lobe of the liver lies anterior to the abdominal oesophagus and to its right lies the caudate lobe. The physical presence of these structures means that the most direct access to the abdominal oesophagus is anterior and left.

As in all surgical procedures, exposure is the key to a successful operation. Much has been written about the length of the left triangular ligament. However, experience has shown that the thickness of the left morphological lobe of the liver is more often a limiting factor for adequate exposure of the oesophagus than the length of the left triangular ligament.

Visualization of the oesophagus can be improved by retracting the left lobe of the liver orad and to the right. If necessary, access can be improved further by dividing the left triangular ligament and folding the left lobe inferiorly on itself before retracting it to the right.

If the left lobe of the liver is too thick to fold up on itself, exposure may be difficult. It is worth noting that some surgeons do not think it is necessary to mobilize the left lobe of the liver at all in approaching the abdominal oesophagus.

1   The angle of entry of the oesophagus into the stomach, termed the angle of His, varies between 30° and 70° in healthly subjects, and in the cadaver averages about 20° (*see Table 1*).

The gastro-oesophageal junction is often, somewhat loosely, referred to as the cardia. The fundus of the stomach can be arbitrarily defined as the segment of stomach above an imaginary line drawn horizontally through the point of the angle of His. The height of the fundus above this point is 2–5 cm and averages about 3.6 cm in the cadaver.

The configuration of the fundus is usually round but occasionally it is short and conical, which makes manipulations such as a fundoplication difficult.

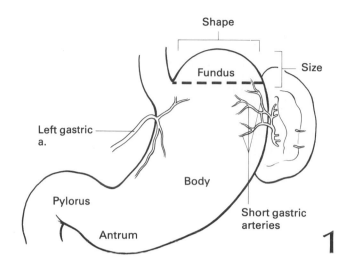

Table 1 Measurements made in fresh cadavers

	Mean (cm)
Length of triangular ligament	7.1
Thickness of sides of hiatus	
Left	0.3
Right	0.3
Distance apex hiatus to superior short gastric artery	8.8
Distance apex hiatus to superior left gastric artery	5.5
Height of fundus	3.6
Angle of His (cardiac notch) (°)	20.8
Distance between mucosal gastro-oesophageal junction and external gastro-oesophageal junction	1.6
Surface of bare area of stomach (cm^2)	18.1

Modified and reprinted from ref. 1 with permission of the publishers.

2   The fundus of the stomach is completely covered with peritoneum anteriorly, but posteriorly coverage is incomplete. The area above the upper reaches of the lesser omental sac is not covered by peritoneum and is known as the bare area of the stomach. This is most often a crescent-shaped area, with its greatest extent along the upper portion of the posterior lesser curvature and the right portion of the fundus. It then extends in an ever narrowing band towards the apex of the fundus. The extent of the bare area is 0–40 cm^2. A large bare area can be a limiting factor in mobilization of the fundus.

Posteriorly the fundus of the stomach lies directly on the diaphragm.

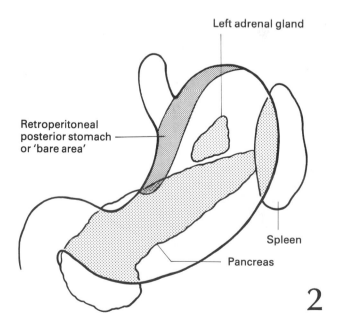

Musculature

3 As with the gastrointestinal tract in general, the oesophagus has an outer longitudinal layer and an inner circular layer of smooth muscle, the inner layer being the thicker of the two. Opinion is divided as to whether a morphological lower oesophageal sphincter exists. It is accepted that there is no thickening to correspond with the whole of the 2–3 cm of the manometrically measureable lower oesophageal sphincter. However, in the distal 1–2 cm of the oesophagus (and particularly on its left side) some thickening of the musculature has been described, which may represent the uppermost gastric sling fibres – oblique muscle fibres that sling around the gastro-oesophageal junction from the lesser curve.

The submucosa deep to the muscularis propria is composed of loose areolar tissue. Consequently the mucosa can be dissected away from the muscle easily. This laxity is useful in oesophagomyotomy for achalasia. Once a small incision has been made through the oesophageal muscle into the submucosa, a fine clamp can be inserted and gently opened and closed in order to separate the muscle from the mucosa. Division of the muscle overlying the jaws of the clamp is then simple.

Transection of the oesophagus at the level of the hiatus is followed by retraction of the proximal cut end into the posterior mediastinum as a result of contraction of the longitudinal layer which is fixed superiorly.

Contraction of the longitudinal muscle may also contribute to the development of sliding hiatus hernia.

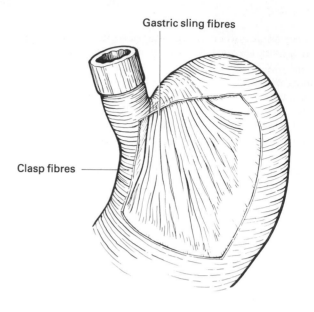

Gastric sling fibres

Clasp fibres

3

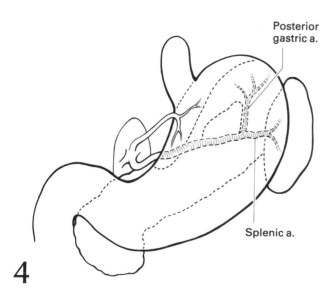

Posterior gastric a.

Splenic a.

4

Blood supply

4 The anterior and right sides of the cardia of the stomach and the lower oesophagus (directly above it) are supplied by one or more ascending branches of the left gastric artery, and the posterior and left sides by branches of the posterior gastric or fundal branches of the splenic artery. The left inferior phrenic artery rarely has any role in the blood supply, despite its proximity to the area. The lower thoracic oesophagus may also receive one or more small direct branches from the aorta. The oesophagus has a rich intramural arterial anastomosis in its submucosal layer, which is continous with a network in the submucosa of the stomach. This explains how, following a near-total gastrectomy, an upper gastric remnant retains its viability when its external blood supply has been completely divided.

Nerve supply

The distal oesophagus is autonomically innervated. Vagal inhibitory, non-cholinergic, non-adrenergic fibres are responsible for sphincteric relaxation associated with swallowing, belching, vomiting and at least some episodes of gastro-oesophageal reflux. There are also excitatory vagal cholinergic fibres responsible in part for basal sphincteric tone. The physiological role of the inhibitory sympathetic adrenergic innervation, which has been identified pharmacologically, remains to be defined. Vagal nerves innervating the distal oesophagus run a long downward course which is largely intramural after leaving the vagal trunks. This explains why skeletonization of up to 5 cm of the distal oesophagus, as practised in proximal gastric vagotomy, does not result in permanent dysfunction of the lower oesophageal sphincter.

Phreno-oesophageal ligament

This structure tends to be given greater prominence in surgical texts than in anatomy texts. It attaches the oesophagus anteriorly to the peritoneum and endo-abdominal fascia from the undersurface of the diaphragm. This fascia splits into two layers – a filmy layer that passes downwards to the gastro-oesophageal junction and a stronger superior layer that passes through the hiatus to blend with areolar tissue surrounding the oesophagus. When viewed from the thorax, the phreno-oesophageal ligament is the layer of tissue binding the oesophagus to the edges of the oesophageal hiatus. It is most easily demonstrated as a definite ligament or membrane from the abdomen. When the peritoneum in front of the hiatus is stretched by downward traction, the ligament can be seen to form a white line similar to that seen alongside the ascending and descending colon. Division of the peritoneum along the inferior aspect of the white line and the tissue immediately deep to it takes the surgeon into the mediastinum in front of the oesophagus.

Mobilization of the distal oesophagus

Mobilization of the distal oesophagus is achieved most simply by entering the lower mediastinum through the phreno-oesophageal ligament, allowing entry to the loose areolar tissue in front of the oesophagus. The normal oesophagus can then be encircled with the forefinger, passing from left to right behind the oesophagus. There is always fibroareolar tissue posteriorly, which must be broken through. The higher in the mediastinum the encirclement is undertaken, the weaker the posterior layer becomes. Mobilization posterior to the distal oesophagus should always be undertaken with great care, particularly when previous transmural peptic oesophagitis has resulted in perioesophageal inflammation and scarring. Under these circumstances it may be advisable to perform the mobilization using sharp dissection under direct vision, as the oesophageal wall (which is not robust) might otherwise be split by the mobilizing finger passing too anteriorly through the plane of least resistance.

When mobilized by blunt dissection, the encircling finger nearly always contains the anterior trunk of the vagus nerve and excludes the posterior trunk (which tends to lie between the pillar of the hiatus, posteriorly and to the right of the oesophagus). It is interesting that when the oesophagus is mobilized through a laparoscope, the posterior vagus nerve is often included with the oesophagus. This may be because the mobilization is undertaken from the right side of the oesophagus and is in a slightly deeper plane.

The amount of the oesophagus that can be mobilized upwards through the hiatus is limited by the dimensions of the oesophageal hiatus. If further mobilization is required, exposure can be improved either by dividing the right and left pillars of the hiatus or by dividing the hiatal opening vertically, anterior to the oesophagus, and extending forwards until the pericardium is reached. Care must be taken with such a median phrenicotomy, first because it is inadvisable to incise the pericardium and secondly because the anterior branch of the left inferior phrenic vein usually crosses in front of the oesophageal hiatus on its way to the inferior vena cava or left hepatic vein and thus must be ligated.

5 The distal mobilization of the oesophagus and upper stomach is limited at the cardia, or just below, by the left gastric trinity (the left gastric vein, the left gastric artery and the coeliac branch of the posterior vagal trunk). If mobilization distal to the cardia is required then the surgeon should commence to the right of the lesser curve about 3 cm below the gastro-oesophageal junction and cross obliquely below the cardia towards the angle of His. This should be done both anteriorly and posteriorly. Care must be taken not to damage the anterior vagal trunk in this dissection. The anterior vagal trunk, which is palpable as a thin cord when the region is stretched from below, is closely applied to the anterior surface of the oesophagus 5 cm above the cardia. As it passes inferiorly it crosses to the right of the oesophagus. At the level of the phreno-oesophageal ligament it is still close to the right side of the oesophagus; in the lesser omentum it is about 1 cm from the lesser curve. A similar mobilization to this is carried out during proximal gastric vagotomy and ensures that both vagal trunks are displaced to the right, away from the oesophagus.

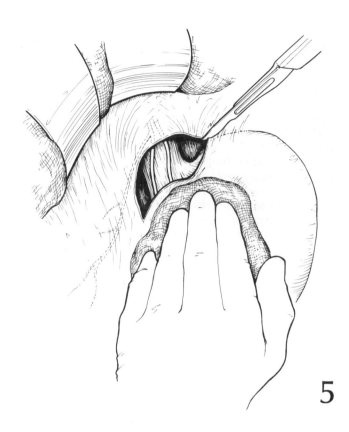

5

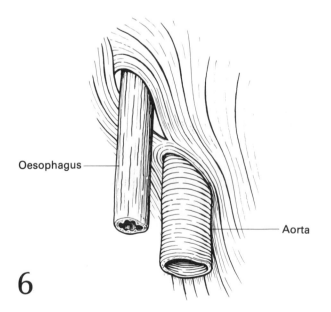

Oesophagus

Aorta

6

Oesophageal hiatus

6 The oesophageal hiatus is the opening in the diaphragm through which the oesophagus passes into the abdomen. The hiatus is at the level of T10 and lies to the left of the midline, with its anterior extent about 1 cm posterior to the central tendon of the diaphragm. The hiatus is formed from the left and right crura of the diaphragm. It is not only a somewhat longitudinal opening but also an oblique opening: its anterior and superior margins may lie more than 1 cm in front of its posterior and inferior margin. This obliquity adds to the difficulty of the radiologist when trying to define the level of the gastro-oesophageal junction relative to the hiatus. The tissue that forms the inferior margin of the oesophageal hiatus also forms the median arcuate ligament across the front of the aorta.

7 The crura of the diaphragm arise from the anterior surfaces and discs of L1–L3 as well as from the anterior longitudinal ligament of the spine. The right crus tends to reach slightly lower in its origin from the first three lumbar vertebrae, the left tending to arise from the first two lumbar vertebrae. Fibres arising from the right side of the lumbar vertebrae most commonly diverge and then reconverge to form the boundaries of the hiatus. Fibres on the right side of the hiatus are innervated by branches of the right phrenic nerve and those on its left side by branches of the left phrenic nerve.

The way in which the fibres of the crura cross each other is variable. The considerable debate over such variations probably has no surgical relevance. Two points, however, are relevant to antireflux surgery.

First, the tendinous tissue binding the right and left limbs of the hiatus together inferiorly, of which the median arcuate ligament is a part, is often poorly defined. Surgeons who use this structure to place anchoring sutures, in fact, use a variety of tissues lying in front of the aorta, including some of the neural tissue of the coeliac plexus. Nevertheless, these tissues hold sutures well.

Secondly, the limbs or pillars of the hiatus are musculotendinous structures, with their tendinous portions tending to lie posterior to the muscular portions. The tendinous portions are the most accessible portion of the pillars when operating from the chest, but for the surgeon operating from the abdomen they are the least accessible portions. From the abdomen the more tendinous portions are often best identified by palpation. When narrowing the hiatus, it is important to suture the tendinous portions: the hiatus is best narrowed behind and inferior to the oesophagus. This approach also maximizes the intra-abdominal length of the oesophagus. The hiatal pillars and the phreno-oesophageal ligament were previously thought to be important in maintaining gastro-oesophageal competence but at present their role is uncertain.

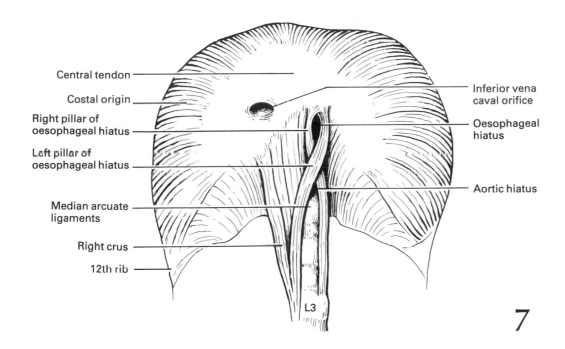

7

Acknowledgements

Table 1 and Figure 1 are reproduced from reference 1 with permission from J. B. Lippincott Co., Philadelphia, USA.

Reference

1. Wald H, Polk HC Jr. Anatomical variations in hiatal and upper gastric areas and their relationship to difficulties experienced in operations for reflux esophagitis. *Ann Surg* 1983; 197: 389–92.

Further reading

Hollinshead WH. *Anatomy for Surgeons,* 2nd edn, vols 1, 2, and 3. New York: Harper and Row, 1971.

Jamieson GG, Martin CJ. Antireflux surgery. The anatomy of the distal oesophagus and associated structures. In: Jamieson GG, ed. *The Anatomy of General Surgical Operations.* Edinburgh: Churchill Livingstone, 1992: 59–62.

Williams PL, Warrick R, Dyson M, Bannister LH, eds. *Gray's Anatomy,* 37th edn. Edinburgh: Churchill Livingstone, 1989.

Myotomy for achalasia: abdominal approach

Srdjan C. Rakić MD, PhD, FACS
Associate Professor of Surgery, Belgrade University School of Medicine, and Chief, Division of Oesophageal Surgery, Institute of Digestive Diseases, Belgrade, Yugoslavia*

History

Transabdominal oesophagomyotomy for achalasia was first described in 1914 by Heller, a German surgeon, and involved an extramucosal oesophagomyotomy on both the anterior and posterior walls of the gastro-oesophageal junction. Heller's operation was modified in 1918 by Groeneveldt of Holland who simplified the procedure to a single anterior myotomy. This modifica-tion was successfully popularized in continental Europe by Zaaijer in 1923 but its acceptance in the UK and North America took much longer. Numerous modifica-tions of this method have been introduced but an extramucosal myotomy remains the basis of surgical treatment for achalasia.

*Present address: Department of Surgery, Leyenburg Hospital, Postbus 40551, The Hague 2504 LN, The Netherlands.

Principles and justification

The management of patients with achalasia is directed toward disrupting the lower oesophageal sphincter, thereby facilitating gravity-induced swallowing and relieving dysphagia. This goal can be achieved either by forceful dilatation or by surgical oesophagomyotomy. While a prospective randomized trial has reported superior results for oesophagomyotomy, dilatation gives a good to excellent result in 65% of patients[1]. Oesophagomyotomy can be approached transthoracically or transabdominally; there is no convincing evidence that either approach is superior to the other. The distal extent of the oesophagomyotomy is debatable, as is the value of the addition of a concomitant antireflux procedure. The transabdominal approach to the distal oesophagus with hiatal dissection and, especially, gastric extension of the myotomy, disrupts the antireflux mechanism. Reconstruction of the gastro-oesophageal junction is thus important for preventing gastro-oesophageal reflux and its complications[2]. The author's preference is to perform an anterior partial fundoplication after completion of the oesophagomyotomy, extending 1 cm on to the stomach. The limited gastric extent of the myotomy assures its completeness, while a partial wrap around the myotomized distal oesophagus provides satisfactory control of gastro-oesophageal reflux without causing obstruction.

Indications

Assuming the absence of general contraindications, the operation can be performed either as the initial treatment for achalasia or after dilatation fails. The transabdominal approach is preferable in patients with compromised cardiopulmonary function, those who have undergone previous thoracic surgery and those who require a concomitant abdominal procedure. This approach may not be satisfactory if more than 10 cm of the distal oesophagus has to be incised. When in doubt, the transthoracic route is recommended. This approach is also better for extremely obese patients with associated oesophageal disease (diverticulum), or when dense abdominal adhesions are expected.

A challenging group of patients are those with either previous unsuccessful oesophagomyotomy or a sigmoid-shaped megaoesophagus. After a failed myotomy, the preoperative diagnosis must be accurate and the reason for failure identified. A clear distinction should be made between unsuccessful myotomy and other postoperative complications, especially reflux or dysphagia resulting from an antireflux procedure. Transabdominal repeat myotomy can be performed when symptoms are due to either an inadequate or a healed initial myotomy. After multiple failures, oesophagectomy with visceral reconstruction is a more reliable option[3]. The treatment of megaoesophagus is even more controversial. The results of oesophagomyotomy in these patients are not as good as in those with mild dilatation of the oesophagus, but which patient will have a poor result from this procedure is clinically unpredictable. Oesophageal resection has been recently recommended as the primary treatment for patients with megaoesophagus[3]. In the author's opinion, initial treatment by standard myotomy is justified. If failure then occurs, oesophageal resection is the best option.

Preoperative

Assessment

The characteristic symptoms in achalasia are dysphagia and regurgitation. The diagnosis is often first made from a barium swallow examination.

Endoscopy should be performed to rule out neoplasm or other lesions obstructing the oesophagus.

Manometry confirms the diagnosis of achalasia. The manometric criteria for achalasia are: (1) absence of peristalsis in the body of the oesophagus; and (2) incomplete relaxation of the lower oesophageal sphincter with swallowing. Elevated lower oesophageal sphincter and oesophageal baseline pressures are frequently present but their demonstration is not essential for the diagnosis.

Preparation of patient

Preoperative hyperalimentation because of weight loss is rarely needed. Although complications due to recurrent aspiration are unusual nowadays, the pulmonary status should be routinely evaluated and preoperative respiratory therapy carried out in selected cases. Before the operation it is particularly important to evacuate the oesophageal contents completely to prevent aspiration during induction of anaesthesia. This may require a liquid diet for a day or two, and oesophageal lavage through a nasal tube both the night before and the morning of the operation. The tube is kept under suction to empty the dilated oesophagus completely; it is left in place during the operation.

Anaesthesia

General endotracheal anaesthesia is used.

Operation

Incision

1 An upper midline incision beginning over the base of the xiphoid process and extending below the umbilicus on the left side provides the best exposure of the lower oesophagus and upper stomach. A table mounted, self-retaining upper hand two-bladed retractor is positioned.

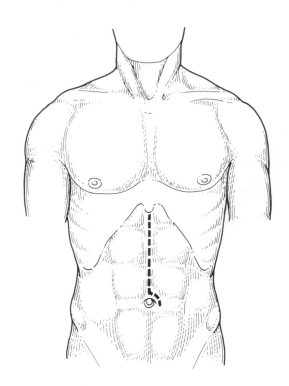

Mobilization of the left lobe of the liver

2 Mobilization of the left lobe of the liver is usually necessary for an adequate exposure. The left lobe is retracted by hand inferiorly to the right and the stretched left triangular ligament is divided with scissors or diathermy towards the midline (near the left hepatic vein). The mobilized left lobe is displaced downward and inward on itself and is retracted by a large S retractor which is placed over a saline-soaked pack. Bands extending between the stomach and the free edge of the spleen should be divided and a pack may be placed over the spleen.

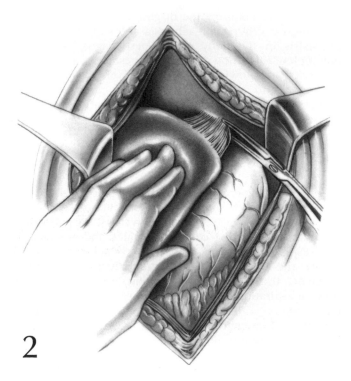

Exposure of the gastro-oesophageal junction

3 While the first assistant maintains downward traction on the stomach using a gauze pad or a pair of Babcock forceps, the peritoneum over the gastro-oesophageal junction is incised and the underlying oesophagus exposed. Care must be taken to preserve the anterior vagus nerve, which should be mobilized from the oesophagus and retracted gently to the right with a tape.

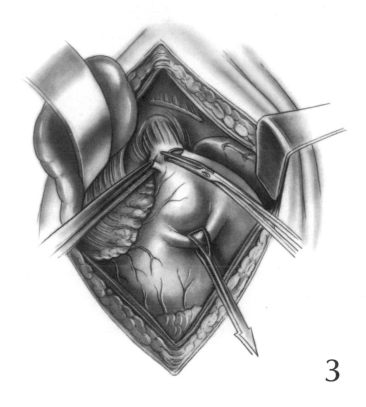

3

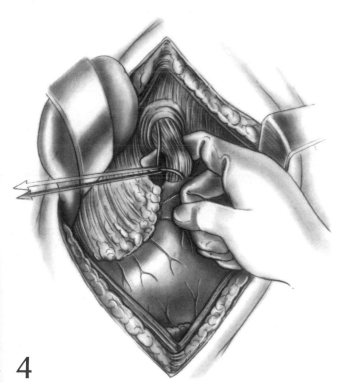

4

Mobilization of the oesophagus

4 Exposure of the anterior surface of the oesophagus is sufficient for a myotomy; however, mobilization of the whole oesophagus and downward traction provide better visibility of the oesophagus into the mediastinum, which is crucial for correct and safe performance of the myotomy. The oesophagus is mobilized by gently passing the right index finger around its distal end and it is encircled with a Penrose drain. Downward traction is applied while the phreno-oesophageal membrane is sectioned. A long, narrow, S retractor is inserted into the hiatus and the lower oesophagus is freed upwards from the adjacent structures using blunt and sharp dissection.

Myotomy

5 With the oesophagus under tension and gently elevated by the encircling Penrose drain, the incision is begun in the midline anteriorly and above the point of apparent constriction: the plane between the muscle and the mucosa is most easily identified at this level. The incision is deepened carefully through both the longitudinal and the circular muscles of the distal oesophagus down to the mucosa, which should remain intact.

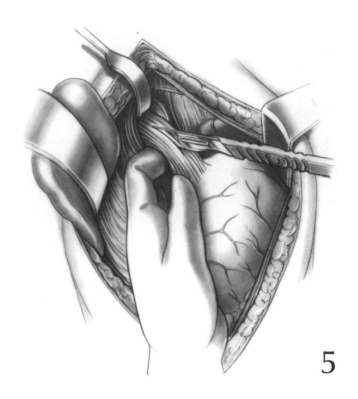

5

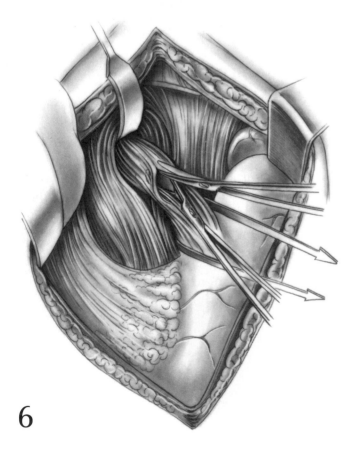

6

6 Once the oesophageal mucosa is exposed, further myotomy is carried out by following a cleavage plane between the overlying muscle layers and the mucosa. A right-angled clamp or a pair of blunt forceps is gently inserted into this plane and, by opening and closing the clamp, the muscle is separated from the mucosa. At the end of this manoeuvre, the tip of the semi-open clamp or forceps is gently elevated and the stretched muscle is cut with blunt-tipped scissors. Care should be taken not to cut the elevated muscle up to the very end of the clamp as tented mucosa may be perforated at this point. The sequence of division–elevation–cutting should be carried out at short intervals, not exceeding 1–1.5 cm in a single step. The oesophagus can be myotomized cranially in this manner for at least 10 cm, which is sufficient for achalasia. A metal clip is placed at the proximal corner of the myotomy to facilitate later radiographic evaluation.

7 After the myotomy is completed cranially, the incision is extended caudally. It is helpful to use a pair of right-angled forceps with the tips projecting caudally for this part of the myotomy. Ideally, the inferior boundary of the myotomy should be the stomach wall. A few small veins traversing the submucosa may help to identify the point when the stomach is reached but accurate identification of the gastro-oesophageal junction is usually difficult. The myotomy is therefore extended across the gastro-oesophageal junction for 0.5–1 cm over the anterior gastric wall. This limited incision on to the stomach assures an adequate caudal extent of the myotomy. Dense attachments make identification of the sub-mucosal plane in the area of the gastro-oesophageal junction difficult. Care is taken to avoid mucosal perforation, which is most likely to occur at this point. Any opening in the mucosa made inadvertently must be closed with fine sutures.

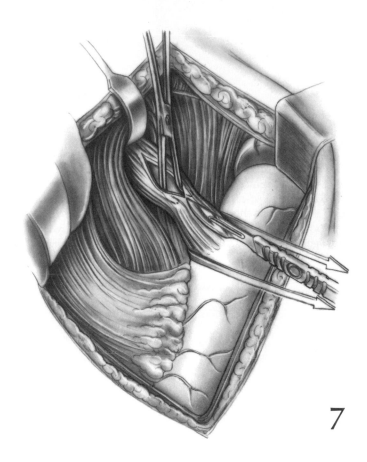

7

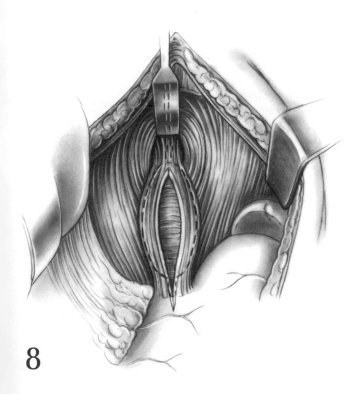

8

8 Care is taken to ensure that all muscular fibres are divided, at the same time avoiding perforation of the mucosa. It is helpful to insert a deflated oesophageal balloon dilator in the area of the myotomy with its distal end positioned across the gastro-oesophageal junction. The balloon dilator must be introduced carefully under manual and visual control in order to avoid the tip perforating the mucosa. The balloon is gently inflated, distending all constricting fibres, which are then divided.

9 The muscularis propria is dissected laterally and away from the oesophageal mucosa so that half of the mucosal circumference freely bulges through the myotomy. Haemostasis is secured using warm packs or fine ligatures. After the myotomy is completed, a metal clip is placed at the caudal margin of the myotomy. The balloon dilator is deflated and carefully replaced with a nasogastric tube. The anterior vagus nerve is released and returned to its normal position.

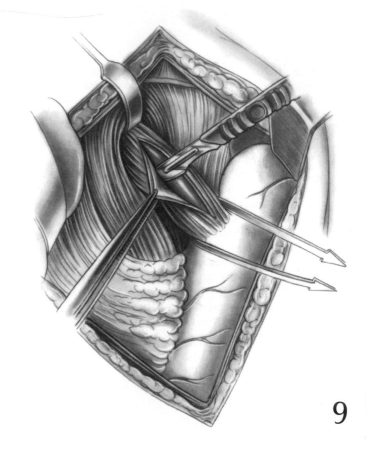

9

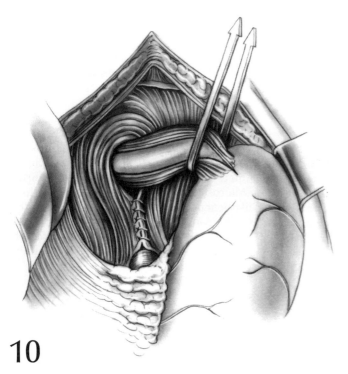

10

Approximation of crura

10 The crura of the diaphragm are reapproximated behind the oesophagus with interrupted 1/0 silk sutures placed 1 cm apart. After the sutures are tied, it should be possible easily to insert the index finger alongside the oesophagus through the hiatus.

Anterior partial fundoplication

11 To test whether mobilization of the gastric fundus is required, the fundus is rotated and its anterior surface laid over the myotomized oesophagus. Should any tension exist, division of the first few short gastric vessels is necessary. After the fundus is prepared for fundoplication, it is returned to its normal position. The serosa of the adjacent gastric fundus is now sutured to the left edge of the cut oesophageal muscle using 3/0 interrupted silk placed 1 cm apart or a 3/0 running polyethylene suture. The uppermost suture is placed first and includes the left diaphragmatic crus, fixing the fundoplication to the hiatus. The sutures must be seromuscular on the gastric side and include the full thickness of the cut muscle on the oesophageal side.

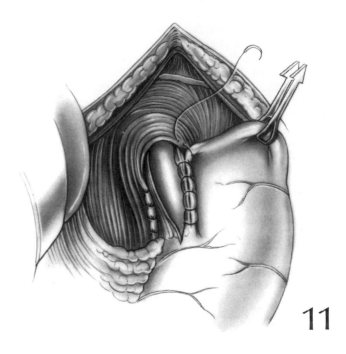

11

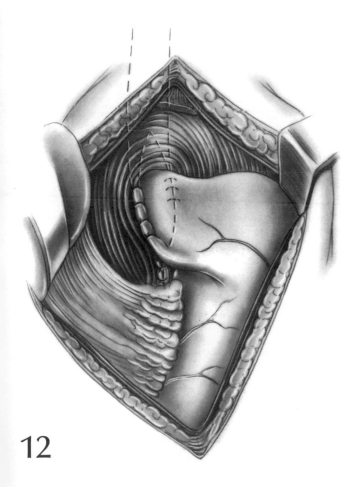

12

12 A flap of gastric fundus is placed anteriorly over the myotomy. The right edge of the gastric patch over the myotomy, which corresponds to the greater curvature of the stomach, is sutured to the right muscular border of the myotomy in the same manner as on the left side. The uppermost suture on this side should also be attached to the border of the hiatus. While suturing, care should be taken to avoid penetration into the oesophagus or the stomach, or damage to the vagi.

13 The total length of the gastric patch over the myotomy should be approximately 4 cm. A resulting partial anterior fundoplication of 180° does not add to the outflow resistance of the achalasic oesophagus and maintains the separation of muscular borders, thus preventing reunion of the myotomy. As it covers the exposed mucosa of the myotomized oesophagus, the anterior fundoplication also protects the suture line in case of inadvertent mucosal injury.

Wound closure

The wound is closed without drainage. The operation usually takes 60–70 min.

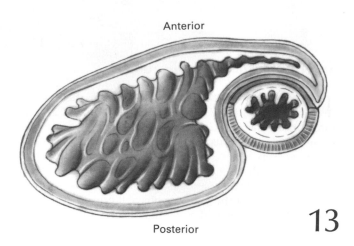

Anterior

Posterior

13

Postoperative care

The patient is ambulant on the evening of the operation. The nasogastric tube is removed on the morning after the operation, when sips of oral liquids are started. Diet is progressed to semisolid and then solid food by the third or fourth day after surgery. A barium swallow examination to demonstrate free passage of barium into the stomach is performed on the fifth day. The usual hospital stay is about 6–7 days.

If the oesophageal mucosa has been perforated and sutured the patient is kept on nasogastric suction for 3–4 days to prevent distension of the stomach and reflux during the healing period. Oral intake is suspended and fluids, antibiotics and gastric secretion blockers are administered intravenously. The suture line is tested for integrity by a water-soluble contrast study on the sixth day after operation. If no leaks are seen, oral liquids are started and the patient is gradually restored to solid food within a few days. A barium swallow examination is performed before discharge.

No significant morbidity has been recorded after this operation and potential complications are those that may follow any major abdominal surgical procedure. The single exception might be an unrecognized perforation of the oesophageal mucosa, which may lead to an oesophageal leak with development of an empyema or peritonitis. As the mucosal perforation, which is usually a pinpoint defect, is routinely covered by the fundic wrap, clinical evidence of perforation is exceptional.

Outcome

Good to excellent results have been reported following transabdominal Heller myotomy with a concomitant antireflux procedure in 85–95% of patients[1,4]. Failures are usually due to incomplete or healed myotomy and are more likely to occur in patients with previous unsuccessful myotomy or megaoesophagus. Severe gastro-oesophageal reflux and its complications are not likely after the procedure described here[1,4].

Between March 1970 and August 1991, 295 patients with oesophageal achalasia underwent a transabdominal myotomy with anterior fundoplication at the Institute of Digestive Diseases, Belgrade University Clinical Centre. There were 16 (5.4%) inadvertent injuries to the mucosa, all recognized during operation and managed by suture. Three inadvertent injuries to the spleen were managed by splenectomy. No significant postoperative morbidity was recorded. Excellent or good results were achieved in 89% of patients. Of the 24 unsatisfactory results, four patients (1.4%) had persistent symptoms due to inadequate or healed myotomy. Fourteen of the 52 patients with a preoperative oesophageal diameter larger than 6 cm and two of the seven patients who underwent repeat myotomy had a poor result. Four patients (1.4%) had severe gastro-oesophageal reflux. Three responded well to medical therapy, while one developed a stricture. The improvement rate was highest (94%) for those with a preoperative oesophageal diameter of less than 6 cm who underwent primary operation. It was, however, significantly lower for patients who underwent repeat myotomy (71%) or had an oesophageal diameter of more than 6 cm (73%).

References

1. Csendes A, Braghetto I, Henriques A, Cortes C. Late results of a prospective randomised study comparing forceful dilatation and oesophagomyotomy in patients with achalasia. *Gut* 1989; 30: 299–304.

2. Andreollo NA, Earlam RJ. Heller's myotomy for achalasia: is an added anti-reflux procedure necessary? *Br J Surg* 1987; 74: 765–9.

3. Orringer MB, Stirling MC. Esophageal resection for achalasia: indications and results. *Ann Thorac Surg* 1989; 47: 340–5.

4. Gerzić Z, Rakić S, Knežević J *et al*. Achalasia of the esophagus: treatment controversies and evaluation of primary abdominal repair in 250 consecutive patients. *Arch Gastroenterohepatol* 1988; 7: 69–72.

Illustrations by Susan Darrington

Abdominal fundoplication

Christopher J. Martin FRACS
Professor of Surgery, University of Sydney, and Head of Surgical Division, Nepean Hospital, Penrith, New South Wales, Australia

History

The operation of abdominal fundoplication for gastro-oesophageal reflux disease was first described by Rudolf Nissen in 1956[1]. Although there have been various modifications of technique since then, the common feature that has persisted is plication of the gastric fundus around the distal oesophagus and cardia, so that the term Nissen fundoplication has come to be used interchangeably with distal oesophageal fundoplication. Perhaps the most important modification of the operation over the past 30 years is the fashioning of the fundoplication short and loose as described by Donahue and Bombeck in 1977[2]. This has resulted in reduction of the problematic postoperative sequelae of postprandial epigastric bloating, dysphagia and inability to belch and vomit.

Principles and justification

Heartburn and acid regurgitation are the common symptoms of gastro-oesophageal reflux disease. They are extremely prevalent in Western societies. For the majority of sufferers, for whom the symptoms are occasional, avoidance of known precipitants and an occasional dose of antacid are all that are required. When medical advice is sought for more persistent symptoms, it is worthwhile to establish the diagnosis by flexible fibreoptic upper gastrointestinal endoscopy before commencing a medical programme which might include a combination of weight reduction, postural advice and dietary modification, as well as the use of agents that neutralize gastric acid, reduce gastric acid secretion and enhance oesophageal and gastric clearance.

Indications

Surgical treatment should be considered only after a concerted effort with medical treatment has been tried and has failed. What constitutes a concerted effort and failure will obviously vary from patient to patient and will be affected by other factors, such as age and fitness of the patient, tolerance of symptoms, rapidity of recurrence after reduction or withdrawal of medication, compliance with treatment and attitude to the concept of long-term drug therapy.

Preoperative

Fibreoptic endoscopy should always be performed before operation. The possibility that changes have occurred justifies repeating the procedure if the interval since diagnostic endoscopy is considerable. The preoperative endoscopy should specifically define the severity and extent of peptic oesophagitis, the presence and size of an associated hiatus hernia, and the presence and histological type of a segment of Barrett's oesophagus including the presence of dysplasia. A radiological contrast study of the oesophagus and gastro-oesophageal junction before surgery might demonstrate an associated hiatus hernia. More importantly from a planning point of view, it might demonstrate the presence of oesophageal stenosis, or definite or equivocal oesophageal shortening in conjunction with an irreducible hiatus hernia. In these cases consideration will need to be given to a thoracic rather than an abdominal approach.

Oesophageal manometry and oesophageal pH monitoring, although not mandatory, are recommended. Traditionally, oesophageal manometry has been performed in reflux disease to assess lower oesophageal sphincter tone and position. These measurements, however, are of limited use to the surgeon. Much more important is the recognition of the occasional patient with an unsuspected motility disorder of the oesophageal body, such as scleroderma or perhaps even achalasia, which will result in a change in clinical strategy. Lower oesophageal pH monitoring clearly defines the severity of oesophageal acidification. This is imperative in patients without ulcerative oesophagitis. This assessment is more sensitive and specific than other diagnostic criteria such as mucosal friability or erythema at endoscopy or abnormal morphometric scores of distal oesophageal mucosal biopsies, which have been used previously to establish the diagnosis of gastro-oesophageal reflux disease in the absence of ulcerative oesophagitis.

Counselling is also an important step in the preoperative preparation. As medical therapy can occasionally be as effective as surgical therapy, the patient should be aware that surgical control of reflux symptoms in the long term is not guaranteed and that there might be significant side effects of surgery, such as dysphagia (which is usually transient), early postprandial satiety and increased flatus production (which is universal). Other possible sequelae, which are now believed to be partly dependent on technique but which should be discussed, include difficulty with belching and vomiting, postprandial epigastric distension and borborygmus.

Operation

Incision

An upper midline incision from the xiphisternum to at least the umbilicus is required for good exposure. The incision can be extended below the umbilicus if necessary, as described in the chapter on pp. 139–147.

General exposure

Exposure can be optimized by: (1) displacing the mobile organs inferiorly by tilting the head of the operating table upwards; and (2) elevating the costal margins away from the operating table, as well as retracting them laterally and superiorly, using a retractor fixed to the operating table as described in the chapter on pp. 139–147.

Local exposure

1 Access to the gastro-oesophageal junction can be improved further by: (1) decompression of the stomach with a nasogastric tube; (2) retraction of the stomach inferiorly by the assistant using the nasogastric tube to achieve atraumatic purchase on the stomach (which also tends to reduce any hiatus hernia); (3) division of small peritoneal bands to the visceral surface of the spleen to prevent an inadvertent capsular tear; and (4) gentle retraction of the liver to the right after dividing the left triangular ligament and folding the left lobe inferiorly. This step is not regarded as necessary by some surgeons.

1

Initial mobilization of fundus

2 A small window is made in the peritoneum of the gastrosplenic ligament adjacent to the stomach at the level of the middle of the anterior border of the spleen. Individual leashes of vessels in this layer are ligated and divided progressively up as far as the angle of His, with division of the intervening peritoneum. Metal clips can be used to ligate the splenic ends of these cords as they are unlikely to become dislodged. This mobilization of the fundus allows progressively greater retraction of the stomach anteriorly, inferiorly and to the right.

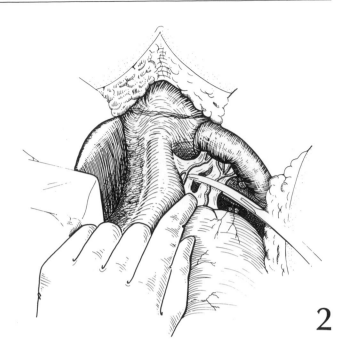

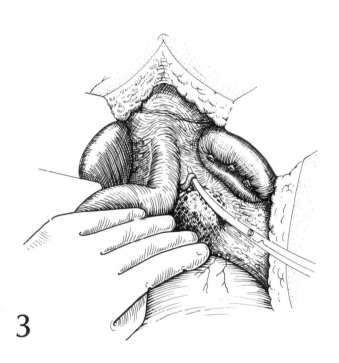

Further mobilization of fundus

3 The initial mobilization exposes further leashes of vessels entering the fundus from the bare area. These are progressively divided until the posterior branches of the left gastric artery on the lesser curve are reached. At the same time avascular adhesions that tend to obliterate the upper reaches of the lesser sac are divided.

Initial mobilization of distal oesophagus

4 The relatively avascular plane surrounding the oesophagus must be developed. This is best entered by dividing the peritoneal reflection of the phreno-oesophageal ligament to the left of the oesophagus and cauterizing and dividing small vessels to the left of the oesophagus.

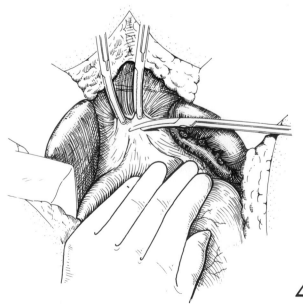

Identification and preservation of anterior and posterior vagal trunks

5 At this stage the anterior vagal trunk is visible and palpable as a cord just to the right and anterior to the oesophagus. This is best gently retracted with a fine rubber sling. The posterior vagal trunk is visible between the crura posterior to the plane of dissection.

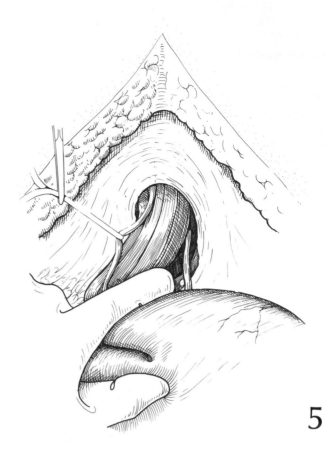

5

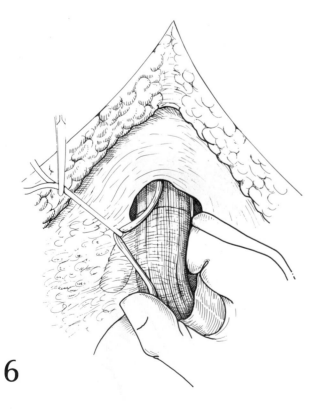

6

Encircling the oesophagus

6 The oesophagus is encircled from the left by passing the index finger behind it and the thumb between the anterior vagal trunk and the oesophageal wall to make a small window in the residual tissue anchoring the right side of the distal oesophagus. A narrow Penrose drain, passed through the window and around the oesophagus, thereafter acts as the principal oesophageal retractor.

Completion of distal oesophageal mobilization

7 With the oesophagus and anterior vagal trunk gently retracted to the left and right, respectively, the residual tissue anchoring the right side of the oesophagus can be mobilized, cauterized and divided under direct vision. At completion three fingers should be able to pass behind the oesophagus and through the window to the left of the anterior vagal trunk without tension. Any tension requires further mobilization in whichever is the appropriate direction.

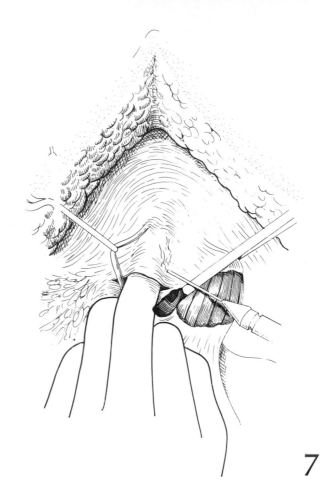

7

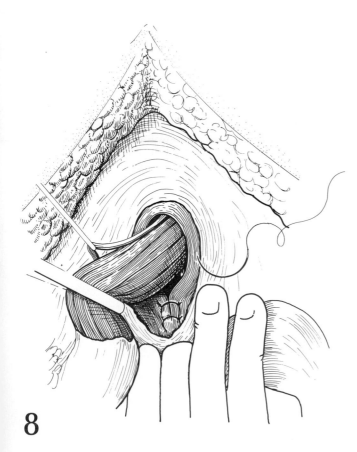

8

Crural plication

8 With the oesophagus retracted to the right, the margins of the hiatus are identified by a combination of sharp and blunt dissection and loosely plicated with one to three 0 polypropylene (Prolene) sutures, anterior to the posterior vagal trunk.

Testing the adequacy of fundal mobilization before fundoplication

9 The fundus is pushed behind the oesophagus into the window between the anterior vagal trunk and the oesophagus with the tips of the operator's right fingers. The ties on the short gastric vessels should appear at the leading edge. The leading edge is grasped with a pair of Babcock's forceps and approximated to the portion of anterior fundic wall to which it will be plicated, also grasped with Babcock's forceps. Tissue tension on the greater curve means that further mobilization is required.

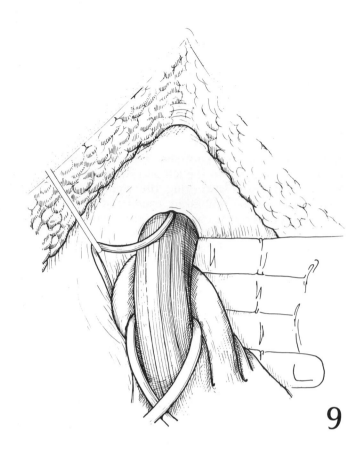

9

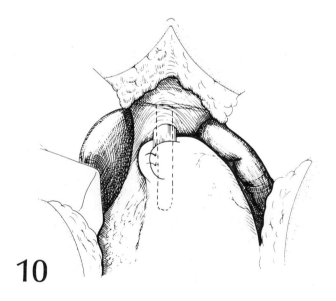

10

Fixing the fundoplication

10 The anaesthetist passes a 52–56-Fr Hurst mercury bougie orogastrically, which acts as a stent for the fundoplication. The fundoplication is secured with two or three 2/0 Prolene sutures. The oesophageal wall does not need to be incorporated in these sutures, as is commonly practised, as the fundoplication sits on the left gastric leash of vessels and cannot slip inferiorly. A single suture between the left wall of the oesophagus and the fundus prevents eversion of this aspect of the fundoplication.

Buttressing the fundoplication

11 The bougie is removed and the fundoplication may be overlaid by a 4 × 1 cm polytetrafluoroethylene (Teflon) felt patch secured at each corner by a 2/0 Prolene suture.

Wound closure

Haemostasis and the position of the nasogastric tube are checked and the abdomen is closed without drainage.

Postoperative care

Intravenous fluids and free nasogastric drainage are continued until peristaltic activity returns. The consistency of the food is progressively increased. The patient is warned first about the need to chew all foods carefully in order to avoid dysphagia, and second about the need to take small, frequent meals in the early postoperative period in the event of early satiety.

Complications

With careful attention to surgical technique, specific early complications of the operation should be extremely rare. These complications include oesophageal or fundic perforation (secondary to damage or ischaemia caused intraoperatively) and splenic haemorrhage.

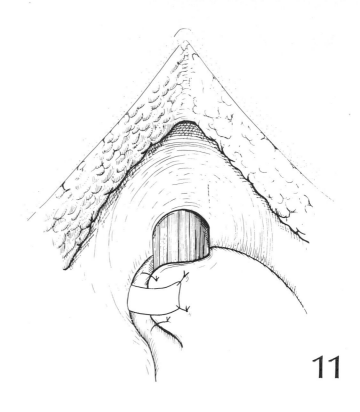

11

References

1. Nissen R. Eine einfache Operation zur Beeinflussung der Reflux-oesophagitis. *Schweiz Med Wochenschr* 1956; 86: 590–2.

2. Donahue PE, Bombeck CT. The modified Nissen fundoplication – reflux prevention without gas bloat. *Chir Gastroenterol (Surg Gastroenterol)* 1977; 11: 15–27.

Illustrations by Gillian Oliver

Surgical anatomy of the vagus nerves

Haile T. Debas MD
M. Galante Distinguished Professor of Surgery and Dean of the School of Medicine, University of California, San Francisco, California, USA

From the perspective of operative surgery of the upper gastrointestinal tract, the important aspects of vagal anatomy are relationships and distribution in the cervical and upper mediastinal regions and at and below the diaphragmatic hiatus. Central vagal anatomy, therefore, will not be dealt with in any detail. The importance of the cervical anatomy of the vagus relates to the need to protect the vagus and its laryngeal branches during surgery on the upper oesophagus. A thorough knowledge of vagal anatomy at the hiatus is essential for the performance of various types of vagotomy.

Besides meticulous anatomical dissection, the combination of anterograde and retrograde staining with horseradish peroxidase and immunocytochemistry has resulted in the definition, in great detail, of the central projections of the vagi as well as the type of neurones contained within them. This degree of detail will not be provided in this chapter, but the interested reader is referred to some excellent papers in the field[1,2].

Central vagus complex

The fibres of the vagus nerves that control secretion and motility of the gastrointestinal tract originate in the medulla oblongata from neurones of the dorsomotor nucleus of the vagus (DMNV), as well as the nucleus ambiguus (NA) and the nucleus tractus solitarius (NTS). Of the 60 000 fibres that constitute the abdominal vagi in humans, visceral efferents comprise approximately only 3%. Most secretory neurones arise from the DMNV, while most of the gastric motor efferents originate in the NA. Primary visceral sensory information is relayed to the DMNV via the tractus solitarius. General somatic afferent fibres of the vagus arise from the superior ganglion. The larger inferior ganglion (nodose ganglion) is the source of both general and special visceral afferent fibres. The vagus nerves issue from the cranium through the jugular foramen and the superior and inferior ganglia are outside the skull.

Functional anatomy of the vagus has been defined using central stimulation with electrical impulses or by hypoglycaemia. Electrical stimulation of the DMNV in cats leads to vigorous, prolonged gastric acid secretion. Hypoglycaemia stimulates the DMNV indirectly by acting on the lateral hypothalamus.

Cervical anatomy of vagus

1 After issuing from the skull via the jugular foramen, the right and left vagi enter the carotid sheath where they come to lie between and deep to the carotid artery and jugular vein.

The first surgically important branch of the vagus in the neck is the superior laryngeal nerve, which divides into the internal and external laryngeal nerves. The internal laryngeal nerve pierces the thyrohyoid membrane and is sensory to the larynx above the vocal cords. The external laryngeal nerve runs deep and parallel to the superior thyroid artery and is motor to the cricothyroid muscle (the tuning fork of the larynx) and the inferior constrictor.

Within the carotid sheath the vagus gives off cardiac branches, but the next surgically important branch of the cervical vagus is the right recurrent laryngeal nerve, which comes off the right vagus as the latter crosses the subclavian artery. The right recurrent nerve hooks around the vessel, and passes behind the common carotid to reach the groove between the trachea and the oesophagus. It runs up the tracheo-oesophageal groove, along the medial surface of the right lobe of the thyroid, and enters the larynx behind the right cricothyroid joint. The left recurrent laryngeal nerve comes off the left vagus behind the aortic arch, loops anteriorly around the vessel to go up the neck where it also travels in the tracheo-oesophageal groove. The recurrent laryngeal nerves are motor to all the intrinsic muscles of the larynx and are sensory to the larynx below the vocal cords.

Potential damage to the external laryngeal nerve occurs at the time of division of the superior thyroid artery during thyroidectomy. Damage to the recurrent laryngeal nerves can occur during cervical oesophagectomy, the excision of a pharyngo-oesophageal diverticulum or during gastro-oesophageal anastomosis in the neck following transhiatal oesophagectomy. In the last two procedures, neuropraxia of the left recurrent laryngeal nerve may result from pressure caused by retractors.

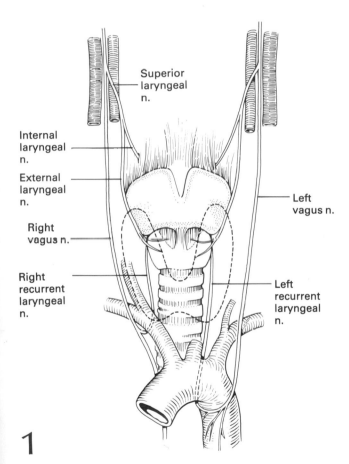

Superior laryngeal n.

Internal laryngeal n.

External laryngeal n.

Right vagus n.

Right recurrent laryngeal n.

Left vagus n.

Left recurrent laryngeal n.

1

Vagal anatomy within thorax

2   The vagus enters the thorax by crossing the first part of the subclavian artery on the right, and by passing anterior to the subclavian on the left. The superior cervical branches are given off in the neck within the carotid sheath and also enter the chest anterior to the subclavian artery. Within the chest, each vagus forms a network of nerves that surround the oesophagus. Although several small branches are given off to the tracheobronchial tree and lungs, pericardium, aorta and diaphragm, there are no major branches that the surgeon has to attempt to preserve during oesophagectomy.

Over the distal oesophagus, single anterior and posterior nerve trunks emerge from the neural reticulum around the oesophagus. Anatomists are in agreement that the left vagus forms the major portion of the anterior vagus but receives branches from the right vagus, and that the right vagus is mainly formed from the posterior vagus but receives branches from the left vagus[3, 4]. The right thoracic vagus lies mainly posterior to the oesophagus and usually to its left side. The two trunks are linked by several long and short communicating strands.

3   The vagal anatomy at the diaphragmatic hiatus is particularly important for the surgeon. The posterior vagus forms a single trunk 3–4 cm above the diphragm and remains a single trunk at the hiatus in 92% of cases, while the anterior vagus is a single trunk at the hiatus in only 66% of cases.

Abdominal vagus

A knowledge of the major divisions of the abdominal vagus is essential in the performance of vagotomy (see above). The anterior vagus trunk is usually found closely applied to the anterior surface of the abdominal oesophagus. The posterior vagus, on the other hand, is separated from the oesophagus by areolar tissue and may lie at any location from behind the oesophagus medially to the right crus of the diaphragm laterally. In about one-third of cases the posterior vagus runs along the right crus of the diaphragm at some distance from the oesophagus.

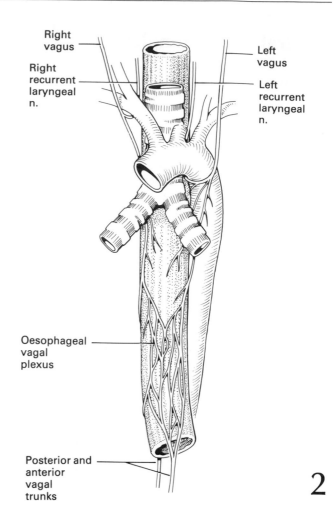

Right vagus

Right recurrent laryngeal n.

Left vagus

Left recurrent laryngeal n.

Oesophageal vagal plexus

Posterior and anterior vagal trunks

2

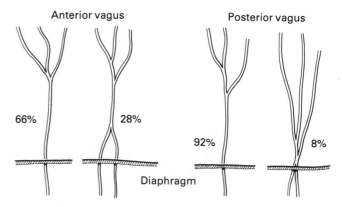

Anterior vagus

Posterior vagus

66%   28%

92%   8%

Diaphragm

3

Divisions of anterior vagus

4   The anterior vagus has three main divisions: hepatic gastric, and antral. In addition, it often gives off a communicating branch to the coeliac axis[4].

Hepatic branches

These are the first branches of the anterior vagus below the diaphragm and travel in the layers of the lesser omentum from the vagus towards the liver. These branches are multiple. When there is only one anterior vagal trunk in the abdomen, it gives two or more hepatic branches. When there are two or more anterior vagal trunks, usually each gives at least one hepatic branch.

On reaching the liver, the hepatic branches give off nerves to that organ before passing downward on the hepatic artery, forming a plexus from which branches are given off to the gallbladder, bile duct and pancreas. Besides these branches, a pyloric branch is given off that travels along the right gastric artery, and a deeper branch that travels along the gastroduodenal artery and subsequently along the right gastroepiploic artery to supply a small portion of the greater curvature of the stomach.

Gastric branches

A variable number of gastric branches comes off the anterior vagal trunk after it gives off the hepatic branches. The gastric branches arise as between five and ten thin twigs or as one to four main divisions which then subdivide to supply the anterior portion of the proximal stomach including the fundus[4]. At the lesser curvature these branches run in close relationship to the vessels of the stomach. The gastric branches penetrate the gastric wall at the lesser curvature and then travel between the serosa and muscle for a distance of 1–2 cm before penetrating to the submucosal and mucosal layers. Thus, these nerves can be effectively divided by anterior seromyotomy of the stomach.

The gastric branches innervate the parietal cell mass and the smooth muscle cells of the body and fundus. In highly selective vagotomy these branches are divided, leaving intact the hepatic branches and the innervation to the antropyloric region. When the gastric branches are divided basal acid secretion is reduced by about 70–80% and maximal acid output by about 50%. In addition to the division of the secretory fibres, motor nerve fibres that mediate receptive relaxation of the stomach during deglutition are also interrupted.

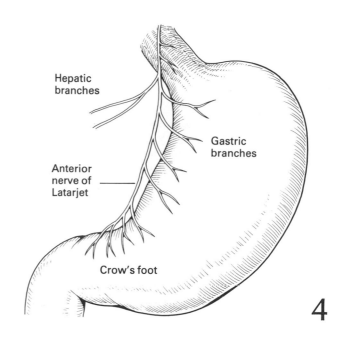

In some patients, one or more gastric branches may come off the anterior vagal trunk very high in the hiatus and travel in the peritoneal fold at the angle of His. It becomes necessary, therefore, that this peritoneal fold is completely divided towards the fundus to ensure completeness of highly selective vagotomy.

Anterior long nerve of antrum: anterior nerve of Latarjet

After giving off the hepatic and gastric branches, the anterior vagus continues distally towards the antrum about 1–2 cm from the lesser curvature. This nerve is often referred to as the anterior nerve of Latarjet, in honour of the French surgeon[5] who described it in 1921. It is also sometimes referred to as the greater anterior nerve of Mitchell. The anterior nerve of Latarjet passes onto the anterior wall of the stomach near the incisura. Over the antrum it fans out into branches akin to the digits of a crow's foot[6]. The most superior digit of the crow's foot is usually 7 cm from the pylorus.

The anterior nerve of Latarjet and its posterior counterpart supply the antropyloric mechanism which is responsible for antral 'milling' and pyloric sphincter functions. When performing proximal gastric vagotomy these nerves must be carefully preserved to avoid the need for pyloroplasty.

Divisions of posterior vagus

5   The divisions of the posterior vagus are analogous to those of the anterior vagus except that, instead of hepatic branches, the posterior vagus gives off coeliac branches. The divisions of the posterior vagus are, therefore, coeliac branches, gastric branches and the posterior long nerve to the antrum or the posterior nerve of Latarjet.

Coeliac branches

Coeliac branches originate from the posterior vagus below the diaphragm, although sometimes they may arise at the level of the diaphragm or even above. These branches join the left gastric artery 2–4 cm from the origin of the vessel and go to the coeliac axis. The exact distribution from there on has not been fully worked out but branches supply the pancreas, the small intestine and the right colon to the mid-transverse colon. As mentioned above, the coeliac branches of the posterior vagus not infrequently receive a communicating branch from the anterior vagus. They may also give fibres that join the hepatic plexus from the anterior vagus by coursing along the hepatic artery.

Gastric branches

On average, six gastric branches originate from the posterior vagus distal to the origin of the coeliac branches. They go to the posterior wall of the proximal stomach and are distributed in the stomach in a manner analogous to the gastric branches from the anterior vagus.

Posterior long nerve to antrum: posterior nerve of Latarjet

After giving off the coeliac and gastric branches, the posterior vagus courses towards the antrum as the posterior nerve of Latarjet. It is located within 1.5–2 cm of the lesser curvature of the stomach. Its distribution on the posterior surface of the antrum is similar to that of the anterior nerve of Latarjet on the anterior surface of the antrum. It, too, branches, giving the semblance of a crow's foot.

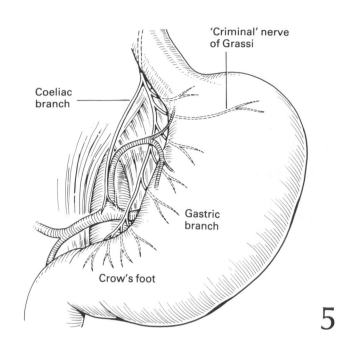

Anatomical points with special surgical significance

Distal oesophageal plexus

The gross anatomical distribution of the vagus has been described. What gross anatomy fails to show is that there is important vagal supply to the proximal stomach that is distributed over the distal 6–8 cm on the oesophagus. For most of this distance the oesophagus is usually abdominal. However, the proximal 2–3 cm may be at the hiatus or even above the diaphragm in many; the vagal trunks form 3–5 cm above the diaphragm. Hence the oesophageal fibres that supply the stomach derive either from high branches from the vagal trunks or from a residual neural plexus over the distal oesophagus. It is essential that the distal 7–8 cm of the oesophagus is skeletonized to achieve complete vagotomy of the parietal cell mass as described in the chapter on pp. 233–241. Hallenbeck *et al.* have quantified the difference that skeletonization of the distal 6–7 cm makes, and have shown significant reductions in acid response to hypoglycaemia and in the rate of ulcer recurrence when this is done[7].

Crow's foot of nerves of Latarjet

The distribution of the nerves of Latarjet resembles the digits of a crow's foot, the most proximal digit being about 7 cm from the pyloroduodenal junction. Amdrup and Jensen, who have defined the proximal limit of the antrum by intragastric pH probe, have indicated that the mucosal junction between the antrum and the body may be 3–4 cm higher up than the crow's foot[8]. On the basis of this, many surgeons have used as their starting point for proximal gastric vagotomy a point 3–4 cm proximal to the crow's foot, which would, therefore, be 10–11 cm from the pylorus. While the distal end of dissection may not be an important cause of incomplete vagotomy, the author believes the dissection should start at the crow's foot, or even one digit distal[9].

Angle of His

Vagal fibres that supply the fundus may be distributed within areolar tissue in the peritoneal fold to the left of the oesophagus at the angle of His. A special point should be made during the performance of proximal gastric vagotomy to ensure complete division of the tissue to the left of the oesophagus towards the most proximal short gastric artery.

'Criminal' nerve of Grassi

Grassi has called attention to an errant branch of the right vagus that crosses transversely behind the cardia to supply a portion of the fundus or proximal stomach. If this nerve is not cut, a portion of the stomach will remain innervated and test positive on pH probing during pentagastrin stimulation[10].

Gastroepiploic vagal innervation

A recurrent division of the hepatic vagal branches is distributed along the gastroduodenal and right gastro-epiploic arteries to the greater curvature of the stomach. Standard proximal gastric vagotomy leaves these vagal fibres intact, and some have suggested that this defect of the operation may add to ulcer recurrence. As a result, the so-called operation of 'extended proximal gastric vagotomy' has been suggested, in which division of these fibres at the junctions of the two gastroepiploic vessels at the greater curvature is added to the standard procedure of proximal gastric vagotomy[11]. However, Braghetto et al. have studied prospectively the effect of division of gastroepiploic nerves and could show no significant difference in postoperative gastric acid secretion beyond that achieved by standard proximal gastric vagotomy[9].

References

1. Fox EA, Powley TL. Longitudinal columnar organization within the dorsal motor nucleus represents separate branches of the abdominal vagus. *Brain Res* 1985; 341: 269–82.

2. Yamamoto T, Satomi H, Ise H, Takahashi K. Evidence of the dual innervation of the cat stomach by the vagal dorsal motor and medial solitary nuclei as demonstrated by the horseradish peroxidase method. *Brain Res* 1977; 122: 125–31.

3. Jackson RG. Anatomy of the vagus nerves in the region of the lower esophagus and the stomach. *Anat Rec* 1949; 103: 1–18.

4. Ruckley CV. A study of the variations of the abdominal vagi. *Br J Surg* 1964; 51: 569–73.

5. Latarjet CR. *C R Seanc Hebd Soc Biol* 1921; 84: 985.

6. Goligher JC. A technique for highly selective (parietal cell or proximal gastric) vagotomy for duodenal ulcer. *Br J Surg* 1974; 61: 337–45.

7. Hallenbeck GA, Gleysteen JJ, Aldrete JS, Slaughter RL. Proximal gastric vagotomy: effects of two operative techniques on clinical and gastric secretory results. *Ann Surg* 1976; 184: 435–42.

8. Amdrup E, Jensen HE. Selective vagotomy of the parietal cell mass preserving innervation of the undrained antrum. A preliminary report of results in patients with duodenal ulcer. *Gastroenterology* 1970; 59: 522–7.

9. Braghetto I, Lazo M, Leiva V et al. A prospective study of intraoperative histologic antrum and corpus boundary in patients undergoing highly selective vagotomy for duodenal ulcer. *Surg Gynecol Obstet* 1987; 164: 213–18.

10. Grassi G. A new test for complete nerve section during vagotomy. *Br J Surg* 1971; 58: 187–9.

11. Donohue PE, Bombeck CT, Yoshida Y, Nyhus LM. Endoscopic Congo red test during proximal gastric vagotomy. *Am J Surg* 1987; 153: 249–55.

Illustrations by Gillian Oliver

Total abdominal vagotomy and drainage

Haile T. Debas MD
M. Galante Distinguished Professor of Surgery and Dean of the School of Medicine, University of California, San Francisco, California, USA

History

Vagotomy has emerged as the cornerstone of surgical therapy in peptic ulcer. Total abdominal or truncal vagotomy not only denervates the acid-secreting part of the stomach but also the antropyloric mechanism that controls gastric emptying. Hence, truncal vagotomy causes significant impairment of gastric emptying. It must, therefore, be combined with a drainage procedure (pyloroplasty or gastroenterostomy) to obviate the problem of gastric stasis. Although truncal vagotomy and drainage can be performed transthoracically, the procedure is more easily accomplished through the abdominal route.

In the early 1940s Dragstedt popularized truncal vagotomy for the treatment of duodenal ulcer disease[1]. Initially, his operations were performed transthoracically and were not accompanied by a gastric drainage procedure. It soon became clear that two-thirds of the patients developed postoperative gastric stasis, and one-half of these patients eventually required a gastric drainage operation. In 1951 Dragstedt advised that a drainage procedure in the form of either a pyloroplasty or a gastrojejunostomy be added[2]. For nearly two decades truncal vagotomy and drainage enjoyed popularity as the operation of choice for peptic ulcer disease. Although the ulcer recurrence rate was acceptable at 6–10%, significant side effects, particularly the dumping syndrome and postvagotomy diarrhoea, led to a search for more selective operations. Now, in most parts of the world, proximal gastric or highly selective vagotomy has replaced vagotomy and pyloroplasty as the elective operation of choice for duodenal ulcer. Despite this, truncal vagotomy still remains an important operation in the armamentarium of the peptic ulcer surgeon.

Principles and justification

Indications

Truncal vagotomy and drainage is now used with decreasing frequency in the elective treatment of uncomplicated duodenal ulcer. Truncal vagotomy and pyloroplasty continues to be the procedure of choice, however, in the emergency treatment of patients with bleeding duodenal ulcers. Truncal vagotomy and drainage may also be the operation of choice in very old or very frail patients, particularly in the presence of gastric outlet obstruction. For most patients requiring an elective operation for duodenal ulcer, proximal gastric vagotomy is the procedure of choice. In the USA, many surgeons still favour truncal vagotomy and antrectomy with Billroth I anastomosis as the elective operation, mainly because of the very low rate of ulcer recurrence. Truncal vagotomy and pyloroplasty is sometimes employed in the treatment of frail patients with gastric ulcer. In this situation, the ulcer should be excised and submitted for frozen section. Life-threatening, uncontrollable bleeding from stress ulceration in critically ill patients is seldom seen nowadays. This is primarily because of aggressive control of gastric pH in postoperative patients and in those in intensive care units. Vagotomy and pyloroplasty combined with gastrotomy and suture control of the major bleeding sites may occasionally be useful in selected patients with uncontrollable bleeding from stress ulcers.

Operations

Position of patient

The patient is placed supine on the operating table with a least one arm secured to an armboard for venous access. A 15–20° reverse Trendelenburg position aids in displacing the intestine downwards away from the upper abdomen.

Incision

The abdomen is prepared and draped. The author routinely uses Steridrapes. A midline incision is employed extending from the umbilicus up to the left side of the xiphoid process and for 2–3 cm onto the sternum. It may often also be necessary to extend the incision below the umbilicus.

Exploration

Once the abdomen is opened, exploration is used to rule out unsuspected pathology. The supracolic compartment is first inspected, palpating the oesophageal

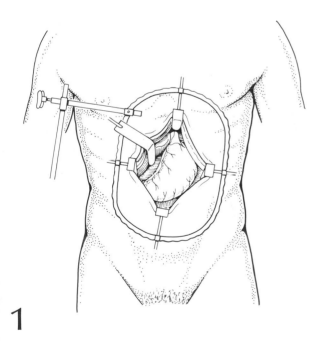

1

hiatus, both the left and the right lobes of the liver, the gallbladder and spleen. With the stomach retracted inferiorly, the body of the pancreas may be palpated through the lesser omentum. The stomach is palpated. The first portion of the duodenum is examined for scarring and ulceration. A gentle rubbing of the external surface of the duodenum with a damp sponge may result in the development of stippled erythema on the serosal surface characteristic of the presence of an active ulcer within the duodenum. It should be noted that an active ulcer will not always be present at the time of operation. Often, however, the first portion of the duodenum will be foreshortened, scarred and deformed as a result of repeated ulceration and healing.

The head of the pancreas is now palpated within the C loop of the duodenum. If there is some reason to suspect the presence of a gastrinoma, the duodenum should be mobilized thoroughly by a Kocher manoeuvre to palpate the head of the pancreas. The gastrocolic omentum should be divided to expose the entire length of the pancreas for careful examination and palpation. Intraoperative ultrasonographic examination of the pancreas, the liver and the upper retroperitoneum may even be necessary. The transverse colon is then delivered out of the abdomen and retracted superiorly to enable examination of the contents of the infracolic compartment and the pelvis.

Exposure

1 A decision must be made as to whether it is necessary to divide the left triangular ligament to aid in the retraction of the liver to expose the hiatus. This manoeuvre is seldom necessary if the modified technique described below (where the oesophagus is not mobilized) is used. The author prefers to use either the 'Iron Intern' or Bookwalter retractor. Both of these provide excellent elevation of the sternum and retraction of the liver using well padded body wall retractor and a modified Deaver retractor, respectively. If the Iron Intern is used a Balfour retractor is necessary to retract the wound edges. With the Bookwalter retractor, however, body wall retracting elements can be attached to the oblong ring of the instrument to retract the wound edges. An excellent exposure of the hiatus is thus obtained.

The surgeon can improve visibility further by wearing a head-mounted light and, extremely occasionally, by removing the xiphoid process.

Two techniques of vagotomy will be described. The first (the traditional one) mobilizes and encircles the oesophagus as a necessary step to identification of the vagus trunks. In so doing, however, a degree of disruption of the hiatus is caused. The second technique of vagotomy requires neither oesophageal mobilization nor extensive dissection[3].

TRADITIONAL TECHNIQUE OF TRUNCAL VAGOTOMY

2 With the stomach retracted downward, the region of the oesophagus is palpated. The nasogastric tube within the oesophagus greatly simplifies the identification of this organ. The peritoneal reflection over the abdominal oesophagus is divided transversely about 0.5 cm from the diaphragm. The incision is extended to the right towards the liver by dividing the uppermost part of the lesser omentum. Bleeding is controlled with electrocautery. Similarly, the incision is extended to the left towards the spleen.

It is seldom necessary to pack away the spleen. Should this be necessary, however, the left hand is passed between the diaphragm and the superior surface of the spleen. The spleen is gently retracted downward, and a moist laparotomy sponge is packed above and to the right of the spleen, displacing the organ inferiorly and to the left away from the oesophagus.

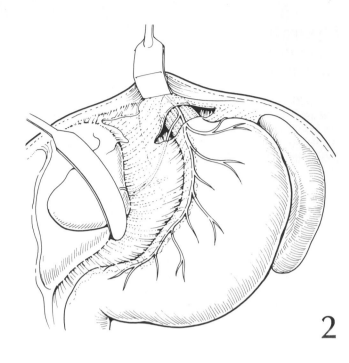

2

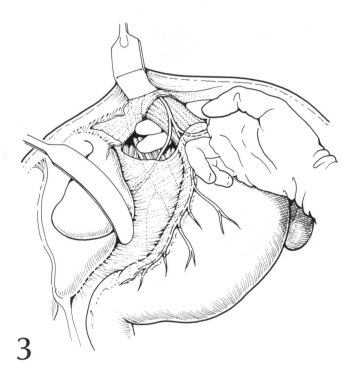

3

3 Next the oesophagus is mobilized bluntly. Two fingers are passed beneath the oesophagus on the left side. The aorta is readily palpable behind the oesophagus, and finger dissection proceeds to the right in the areolar tissue between the oesophagus and abdominal aorta. The posterior vagal trunk is often encountered at this stage. If so, it is mobilized with the oesophagus. As the dissecting finger passes to the right of the oesophagus, firm connective tissue, composed of portions of the phreno-oesophageal and the uppermost extension of the hepatogastric ligaments, is encountered. This has to be divided with curved scissors or with a cautery, often by the assistant, who is on the left side. Once this is done, the index finger can be passed clear around the oesophagus. The dissection behind the oesophagus is easily widened so that both the index and middle finger can be passed from the left side of the oesophagus to the right.

Using a long dissecting forceps, a 19 mm Penrose drain can now be passed to the fingers, grasped, and pulled around the oesophagus. A Kelly haemostat is used to clamp the two ends of the Penrose drain together. The drain can now be used to retract the oesophagus to the left, so that the area between the oesophagus to the left and the right crus of the diaphragm and caudate lobe of the liver can be dissected.

Anterior vagotomy

4 Anterior vagotomy is performed first. The trunk(s) of the anterior vagus is identified by palpation over the anterior surface of the oesophagus. The vagal trunk is raised off the oesophagus using the tips of a pair of right-angled forceps, or a nerve hook, and dissected up and down using the forceps so that about 2.5 cm of it is cleared. The nerve is doubly clamped with the right-angled forceps and divided. Another pair of forceps is applied about 1.25 cm below the distal forceps and the nerve segment between these clamps is excised and submitted for histological identification.

The author prefers to ligate the ends of the vagus with 2/0 silk sutures rather than apply haemoclips to them. A search for additional vagal fibres is made by palpation over the anterior surface of the oesophagus. In about 40% of patients, one or more additional trunks will be found and these must be divided between haemoclips or ligatures. A final inspection of the anterior surface of the oesophagus is made for small nerve fibres that need to be divided.

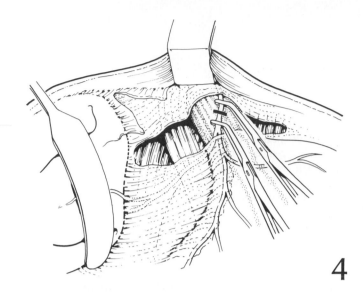

4

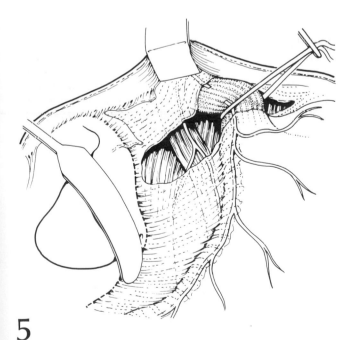

5

Posterior vagotomy

5 Posterior vagotomy begins by retracting the oesophagus to the left and exposing the interval between the oesophagus and the right crus of the diaphragm. The posterior vagus may have been identified earlier during oesophageal mobilization. If not, the surgeon uses palpation and direct visualization to identify the nerve. Most commonly, the nerve travels obliquely behind and to the right of the oesophagus to lie in the interval between the oesophagus itself and the right crus of the diaphragm. The nerve may lie, however, entirely behind the oesophagus, on the right crus at some distance from the oesophagus, or somewhere in between.

6 Once palpated, it is dissected under direct vision using a pair of right-angled forceps. It is handled in much the same way as the anterior vagus. A segment of it is also excised and sent for histological identification. The posterior vagus is usually larger than the anterior vagus and is found as a single nerve trunk in 95% of patients. Nevertheless, it is always wise to look for extra nerve fibres after the major trunk is divided. It is important to look for connecting branches from the anterior vagus above its division to either the posterior vagus below the point at which it is divided or the coeliac branch. If found, all communicating nerves must be divided. It should be noted that in most patients with ulcer recurrence after a previous incomplete truncal vagotomy, it is the posterior vagal trunk that is found intact.

Following completion of the vagotomy, the operative area is inspected for bleeding. If a laparotomy sponge had been used to displace the spleen, it is now removed carefully and the spleen is inspected for inadvertent damage. Next, a drainage procedure is performed.

Drainage procedure

The choice between pyloroplasty and gastroenterostomy as the drainage procedure depends on the status of the duodenal bulb. In most cases, a Heineke–Mikulicz pyloroplasty can be performed safely. If an inflammatory mass is associated with a severely distorted duodenal bulb, a gastrojejunostomy is a safer drainage procedure. Other types of drainage procedures that may be considered in the appropriate situations are the Finney and the Jaboulet pyloroplasties. The techniques for these types of pyloroplasty and for gastroenterostomy are described fully on pp. 242–250 and pp. 251–261.

Once the drainage procedure has been completed, the sponge from the subhepatic space is removed, as is the sponge at the hiatus. The operative sites are examined for haemostasis and the upper abdomen is irrigated with saline. The abdomen is closed without drains.

MODIFIED TECHNIQUES OF VAGOTOMY

The author prefers a simplified technique of vagotomy that does not require full mobilization of the oesophagus or extensive dissection at the hiatus. Following the traditional technique of truncal vagotomy, described above, a small percentage of patients develop a hiatus hernia and/or gastro-oesophageal reflux, presumably because of anatomic disruption caused by the operation.

The modified technique not only avoids extensive dissection but greatly simplifies the identification and sectioning of the vagal trunks.

Exposure is obtained as described above. It is seldom necessary to divide the left triangular ligament of the liver to perform this operation. The peritoneum over the abdominal oesophagus is incised transversely.

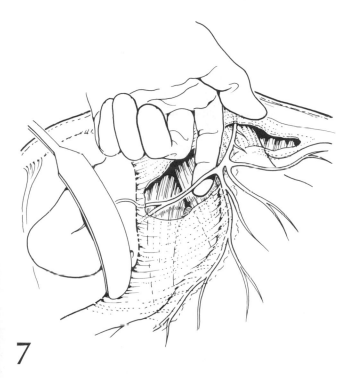

7

Anterior truncal vagotomy

7 The incision is carried to the right onto the lesser omentum short of the hepatic vagal branches within the lesser omentum. The hepatic branches, constant in their presence and location, are easily seen in most patients because the lesser omentum is not fatty at this level. Even when not clearly visible, the surgeon can place the left index finger above the incised edge of the lesser omentum. Gentle caudad retraction brings the hepatic branches taut. This manoeuvre brings the anterior vagal trunk into prominence and enables the surgeon to see or readily palpate it with the middle finger over the anterior surface of the oesophagus. The nerve trunk is then dissected with right-angled forceps for a distance of several centimetres. Two pairs of right-angled forceps are applied to the trunk and the nerve is divided between the forceps.

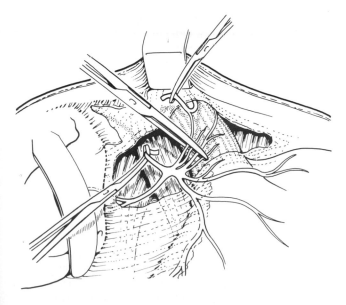

8

8 After division, the cut ends of the nerve are placed under traction sequentially to bring into prominence any other trunks of the anterior vagus and any branches originating at a point higher than the cut end of the trunk. A 2–3-cm section of the anterior trunk is sent for pathological identification.

Posterior truncal vagotomy

9 Exposure for the posterior truncal vagotomy is obtained by retraction of the oesophagus to the left and undertaking a minor degree of dissection between it and the right crus of the diaphragm. The key to identifying the posterior vagal trunk is its coeliac branch, which is constant in its course along the left gastric artery. If the index finger is placed on the aorta behind the oesophagus, and is then moved caudad along the anterior surface of the aorta, further distal progress of the index finger will be stopped by the left gastric artery as it comes off the coeliac axis. Gentle traction on the left gastric artery and the coeliac branch of the vagus with it will bring into prominence the posterior vagus, making it easily palpable. The posterior trunk is divided between right-angled forceps. Cephalad and caudad retraction of the proximal and distal cut ends of the vagus, respectively, will identify any additional branches or trunks that may need to be severed. A 2–3-cm piece of the trunk is removed and submitted for histological identification. The cut ends of the vagus are ligated with 2/0 silk sutures to prevent bleeding from any accompanying vessels. Secondary branches, if present, are divided between haemoclips.

The anterior and posterior surfaces of the oesophagus are then examined thoroughly for any uncut nerve twigs. Haemostasis is assured before pyloroplasty and closure.

Closure

The abdomen is closed, without drain, using continuous 0 Maxon sutures approximating the linea alba; several reinforcing, interrupted 0 Maxon sutures are also used. No subcutaneous sutures are necessary unless the patient is obese. Skin edges are approximated either with metal clips or with interrupted sutures of 3/0 silk.

Postoperative care

The postoperative management after abdominal vagotomy is described in the chapter on pp. 124–129.

Complications

Patients undergoing truncal vagotomy and drainage may develop the early complications that might occur in any patient undergoing an upper abdominal operation. Only specific complications and their management are discussed here.

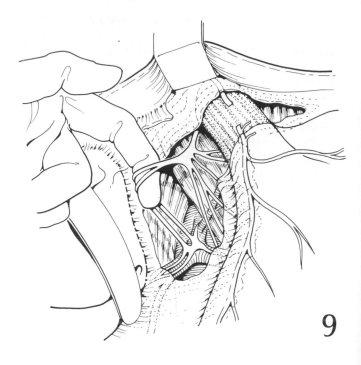

9

Oesophageal injury

A tear in the oesophagus may occur either as a result of the mobilization or dissection of nerve closely applied to the wall. When the injury is recognized, it is treated with direct suturing. The closure is reinforced further by pulling up some of the fundus and suturing it with 3/0 silk to the oesophagus or even performing a formal Nissen fundoplication. If an oesophageal injury has occurred, the perioesophageal area should be drained with a closed drainage system. A more serious problem arises when the oesophageal perforation is unrecognized at the time of operation. The patient will usually develop early signs and symptoms of sepsis and leucocytosis. Occasionally, these symptoms are delayed and appear only when the patient starts to take oral fluids. If other more common causes of sepsis are excluded, the patient should have a diatrizoate (Hypaque) swallow to locate any leak. If there is a leak, the patient is placed on triple antibiotics and taken back to the operating room. The goals of surgery are to repair the perforation, to reinforce it with a fundic wrap and to drain the area.

Splenic injury

Splenic injury is not uncommon. It is usually caused by medial retraction of the stomach, particularly when adhesions to the splenic capsule are present. The complication is more common in patients who have had a previous operation. It can be prevented by examination of the spleen for adhesions, early division of these adhesions and minimizing medial retraction of the stomach. Every effort should be made to conserve the spleen. If bleeding persists, however, the spleen should be removed.

Gastric outlet obstruction

This complication occurs as a result of suture line haematoma, technical problems with the pyloroplasty closure (inadvertent suturing of posterior wall to anterior wall; too much tissue inverted), oedema, or a minor suture line leak. The problem will resolve in most patients in 7–10 days. If not, a Hypaque swallow is required. If the obstruction has not resolved in 2 weeks, a careful endoscopic examination is necessary. In the meantime the patient is given total parenteral nutrition. If the obstruction is due to technical problems, the pyloroplasty should be revised as soon as possible. If the pyloroplasty is involved in an inflammatory mass, a retrocolic loop gastroenterostomy may be a safer procedure.

Postoperative pancreatitis

Fortunately this serious complication is uncommon after truncal vagotomy and drainage. The serum amylase concentration is often elevated, and no mechanical obstruction at the pyloroplasty is identifiable. The treatment is expectant, with the patient placed on total parenteral nutrition.

Postoperative jaundice

When postoperative obstruction jaundice occurs in a patient who has undergone suture control of a bleeding duodenal ulcer and vagotomy, the possibility of injury to the common bile duct should be seriously entertained. The diagnosis may be confirmed with ultrasonography, HIDA radionuclide scanning and/or transhepatic cholangiography. If obstruction of the common bile duct is identified, an operative approach will be required. The issue is the timing. It may be best to wait 3–4 weeks to allow for the bile duct to dilate. Also at that time, endoscopic retrograde cholangiography may be possible. It is unlikely, however, that the problem can be corrected endoscopically. Operative management will include cholecystectomy and Roux-en-Y choledochojejunostomy.

Leaking pyloroplasty

This is also an uncommon complication. The patient will either develop an acute abdomen or a subhepatic collection. In the former situation, an emergency operation will be required. In the latter, percutaneous drainage of the subhepatic collection may be possible.

The size of the leak can then be assessed by diatrizoate swallow and/or sinography. Further management depends on the findings. The patient should receive total parenteral nutrition, H_2-receptor antagonists to decrease gastric secretion and perhaps even the long-acting analogue of somatostatin. Eventually, however, surgical correction may be required.

The following late complications may also be encountered.

Recurrent ulcer disease

The incidence of recurrent ulcer after vagotomy and drainage for duodenal ulcer is 6–10%[4]. The causes of ulcer recurrence include:

1. Inadequate operation, usually because of incomplete vagotomy and occasionally because of inadequate drainage procedure. In about 70% of patients with incomplete vagotomy and ulcer recurrence, an intact posterior vagus is found at reoperation.
2. Zollinger–Ellison syndrome, a condition present in only 2% of patients with recurrent ulcer.
3. Excessive ingestion of ulcerogenic drugs, such as non-steroidal anti-inflammatory drugs.

If the recurrent ulcer is in the stomach, malignancy should always be excluded by endoscopy and biopsy.

The surgeon should have a well-formulated strategy for the diagnosis and treatment of recurrent ulcer. The diagnosis is usually suggested by recurrence of dyspeptic symptoms or by the development of complications: bleeding (overt or occult), perforation, or obstruction. The diagnosis is best established by endoscopy, although contrast studies of the upper gastrointestinal tract may also be useful. Having established the presence of recurrent ulcer, the next task is to establish the cause. The most important consideration is the possibility of incomplete vagotomy. This is best assessed by gastric secretory studies of acid. The basal acid output should be 2 mmol/h or lower. A basal acid output of 5 mmol/h or more is almost always indicative of incomplete vagotomy. The more direct way of testing completeness of vagotomy, however, is to stimulate the vagal centres in the brain either by insulin hypoglycaemia or by modified sham feeding (patient chews and spits without swallowing). The insulin test has been almost completely abandoned because of the risk of severe hypoglycaemia. Acid response to insulin hypoglycaemia or to sham feeding is evidence of incomplete vagotomy.

Zollinger–Ellison syndrome is ruled out by measuring plasma gastrin levels. It must be remembered, however, that vagotomy itself causes hypergastrinaemia. Hence, if a modestly elevated serum gastrin level is discovered, e.g. twice or three times normal, a provocative test with secretin should be performed. The intravenous administration of secretin, 2 units/kg, will cause a paradoxical increase of plasma gastrin (up to 100 pg/ml over basal) in Zollinger–Ellison syndrome, but will either have no effect or reduce plasma gastrin level in postvagotomy hypergastrinaemia. If a positive secretin test is obtained, a search for a gastrinoma should be initiated.

If the evidence suggests incomplete vagotomy, a decision must be made whether to treat the patient medically or to operate. Medical treatment requires a lifelong commitment to taking expensive medications. Except in the elderly, therefore, operative management will be necessary. The surgical options are to complete the vagotomy or to complete the vagotomy and perform antrectomy in addition. If at operation an intact vagal trunk, usually the posterior one, is found, completion vagotomy may suffice. If, on the other hand, the completion vagotomy is less than completely satisfactory, antrectomy with Billroth I anastomosis should be performed. If the primary operation included gastrojejunostomy, it is better to revise this and perform either a pyloroplasty or an antrectomy.

Dumping syndrome

This complication is seen in 10–15% of patients after vagotomy and pyloroplasty[5]. The symptoms may be mild and easily controllable with dietary measures. Occasionally, however, the symptoms can be quite severe. Two aspects of the syndrome are recognized. The early form, occurring within 30–60 min of eating, is manifested as abdominal pain, weakness, tachycardia with palpitation, and sometimes flushing and diarrhoea. The late dumping syndrome occurs 2 h or more after eating, and the symptoms are those of hypoglycaemia including lightheadedness, tachycardia, sweating and variable neuropsychiatric manifestations including seizure disorder or even coma. Early dumping syndrome is due to rapid entry of hyperosmolar chyme into the duodenum, leading to fluid shifts from the circulation into the gut lumen and to the release of a number of vasoactive substances from the gut, such as kinins, neurotensin and substance P. Late dumping syndrome is due to hyperinsulinism. The syndrome appears to be more common in slender women.

Most patients can be managed conservatively. Conservative measures include eating small dry meals, avoiding carbohydrates, lying down for 20–30 min after eating and drinking fluids about 30 min after eating. Severe symptoms can be effectively managed with the somatostatin analogue, octreotide; however, the drug has to be given by subcutaneous injection two or three times/day and long-term compliance of patients is poor. Surgical techniques to correct dumping include:
1. Pylorus reconstruction, a simple procedure that is 50–60% effective long-term.
2. Revision of gastroenterostomy with, or preferably without, pyloroplasty.
3. Antrectomy and Roux-en-Y gastrojejunostomy.
4. Insertion of a 10-cm antiperistaltic jejunal segment between the stomach and the duodenum.

The last procedure is seldom performed, because it tends to produce more problems than it solves.

The most important point to be made, therefore, is that it is easier to prevent than to treat dumping syndrome. In rare cases, dumping syndrome is a worse affliction for the patient than the primary peptic ulcer disease for which the operation was performed. Substituting proximal gastric vagotomy for truncal vagotomy as the primary elective operation for duodenal ulcer will prevent the development of this difficult side effect in almost all patients.

Postvagotomy diarrhoea

Diarrhoea develops in 10–20% of patients after truncal vagotomy and drainage[6]. The diarrhoea is usually mild, but in about 2% of patients it can be disabling. Typically, the diarrhoea is episodic and is associated with great urgency and the passage of much flatus with liquid stools. The exact pathophysiology of this complication is still unknown, and conservative measures to treat it are unsatisfactory. Interposition of a reversed segment of jejunum has been used to treat patients with the most severe postvagotomy diarrhoea. The results have been mixed and the operation is indicated only on very rare occasions.

Gallstone formation

An increased incidence of gallstone formation after truncal vagotomy has been reported on many occasions; the increase, however, is not significant[7]. Truncal vagotomy denervates the gallbladder and may also decrease the release of cholecystokinin from the duodenum. Both of these changes favour stasis in the gallbladder and stone formation.

References

1. Dragstedt LR, Owens FM Jr. Supradiaphragmatic section of the vagus nerves in the treatment of duodenal ulcer. *Proc Soc Exp Biol Med* 1943; 152–4.

2. Dragstedt LR, Woodward ER. Appraisal of vagotomy for peptic ulcer after 7 years. *JAMA* 1951; 145: 795–800.

3. Roberts JP, Debas HT. A simplified technique for rapid truncal vagotomy. *Surg Gynecol Obstet* 1989; 168: 539–41.

4. Stabile BE, Passaro E Jr. Recurrent peptic ulcer. *Gastroenterology* 1976; 70: 124–35.

5. Goligher JC, Pulvertaft CN, DeDombal FT, Conyers JH, Duthie HL, Feather DB *et al.* Five-to-eight-year results of Leeds/York controlled trial of elective surgery for duodenal ulcer. *BMJ* 1968; 2: 781–7.

6. Johnston D, Goligher JC. Selective, highly selective or truncal vagotomy? In 1976 – a clinical appraisal. *Surg Clin North Am* 1976; 56: 1313–34.

7. Thompson JC, Wiener I. Evaluation of surgical treatment of duodenal ulcer: short and long-term effects. *Clin Gastroenterol* 1984; 13: 569–600.

Illustrations by Gillian Oliver

Proximal gastric vagotomy

Haile T. Debas MD
M. Galante Distinguished Professor of Surgery and Dean of the School of Medicine, University of California, San Francisco, California, USA

Principles and justification

Proximal gastric vagotomy (PGV) selectively denervates the acid-producing part of the stomach (the body and fundus). The operation preserves the vagal innervation of the antrum and pylorus, making a gastric drainage procedure unnecessary. The operation is sometimes also referred to as highly selective vagotomy (HSV) or parietal cell vagotomy (PCV). Strictly speaking, the latter appellation should only by used when the operation is performed while the effect on parietal cell function is monitored either with an intragastric pH electrode or Congo red spray. PGV reduces both acid and pepsin secretion. Basal acid secretion is reduced by 80%, while maximal acid response to pentagastrin or to a meal is reduced by 50–60%. The rate of ulcer recurrence has varied from 2% to 22% among different surgeons, presumably because of variations in operative technique[1]. Although several potential sites of incomplete vagotomy are possible, the most important determinant of ulcer recurrence appears to be the thoroughness with which the distal 6–8 cm of the oesophagus is 'skeletonized' of vagal fibres. Hallenbeck *et al.* compared the results of PGV in which only the distal 1–2 cm was skeletonized with that in which distal 5–7 cm of the oesophagus was denervated[2]. The former operation was associated with a 15.4% incidence of proven recurrent ulceration and a 10.2% incidence of suspected recurrence. By comparison, when 5–7.5 cm of the distal oesophagus was skeletonized, only one of 14 patients developed a recurrent ulcer.

PGV requires meticulous operative technique, not only to accomplish complete vagotomy but also to preserve the innervation of the antropyloric mechanism, critically important in promoting normal gastric emptying postoperatively.

Indications

Worldwide, PGV is the choice for elective operation in duodenal ulcer disease. It is a safe operation with a rate of operative mortality of less than 0.3%[3]. It is also associated with the lowest incidence of such undesirable side effects as dumping and diarrhoea[4]. However, the incidence of ulcer recurrence after PGV (10–15%) is significantly higher than after vagotomy and antrectomy. Despite this, recurrent ulcer after PGV appears to be more responsive to H$_2$-receptor antagonists than does primary duodenal ulcer. In addition, should surgical management become necessary for ulcer recurrence, antrectomy with or without truncal vagotomy appears to be highly efficacious[5].

Prospective randomized clinical trials have established that patients with perforated duodenal ulcer should undergo PGV in addition to closure of the perforation[6]. Routine application of PGV in perforated duodenal ulcer is indicated unless the perforation has existed for longer than 24 h, is associated with significant peritoneal contamination, or the patient is unstable with severe cardiopulmonary, renal or other serious illness.

The application of PGV in the management of emergency or urgent complications of duodenal ulcer has not been unanimously accepted. When an emergency operation is performed to control bleeding, suture control of the bleeding ulcer can be accomplished via a duodenotomy that does not violate the pylorus[7]. The operation can then be completed with the performance of PGV providing the patient is stable, otherwise healthy and not old or frail. This approach is particularly appealing in women who are believed to be more susceptible than men to the development of dumping and other undesirable side effects following truncal vagotomy and pyloroplasty or vagotomy and antrectomy. The use of PGV and balloon dilatation of the pylorus in the surgical management of an ulcer that has caused gastric outlet obstruction appears unjustified. When this procedure was utilized in the past, acute pyloric perforation or postoperative obstruction occurred. Most surgeons in the USA prefer to treat duodenal ulcer with pyloric obstruction by vagotomy and antrectomy. The experience with PGV and pyloroplasty in this setting is insufficient to recommend the approach.

Some have advocated the use of PGV combined with ulcer excision in the treatment of benign gastric ulcer. Collected series from the literature show a rate of ulcer recurrence of 3–23% after follow-up of 2–12 years[8]. However, most surgeons prefer to treat gastric ulcer by antrectomy because it removes all the susceptible mucosa and results in a rate of ulcer recurrence of only 2%. At present, therefore, the prime indications for PGV are elective operation for duodenal ulcer, in perforated duodenal ulcer, and in good risk patients, particularly women, with bleeding from a duodenal ulcer.

Preoperative

Patients requiring PGV have the routine preoperative management of any patient of comparable age. Cardiopulmonary and renal evaluation is routine in patients over 40 years of age. Perioperative antibiotic use is probably unnecessary because the gastrointestinal tract is not entered and, even if it were, the stomach and duodenum in these patients are sterile because of the hypersecretion of acid. In practice, however, patients are given a second generation cephalosporin on arrival in the operating theatre and three more doses postoperatively, so that they receive antibiotic coverage for 24 h.

Immunoreactive plasma gastrin levels are measured routinely before surgery to rule out Zollinger–Ellison syndrome. The yield is small but the test is simple and relatively inexpensive. Although only one in 1000 patients with duodenal ulcer disease will have a gastrinoma, the incidence in those patients with severe enough disease to require an operation is unknown.

It is also advisable to discontinue H$_2$-receptor antagonists at least 24 h before operation and omeprazole 5–7 days preoperatively to restore acidity in the gastroduodenal lumen and to reverse any bacterial colonization that might have occurred over a long course of medical treatment. Again, this consideration is probably less important in PGV where the gastrointestinal tract is not entered than in vagotomy and drainage or gastric resection procedures.

Operation

General endotracheal anaesthesia is used. The patient is placed supine on the operating table and a nasogastric tube is inserted as soon as anaesthesia is induced. The abdomen is prepared and draped exposing the lower chest for 5–7 cm above the xiphisternal junction and the abdomen midway between the umbilicus and pubic symphysis. Tilting the operating table 15–20° in the reverse Trendelenburg position will allow the intestines to be displaced away from the upper abdomen. A midline incision is employed. Depending on the habitus of the patient, the incision may need to extend around the umbilicus. The upper limit of the incision should extend along the xiphoid process for 2–3 cm onto the sternum. Once the abdomen is entered, complete exploration is performed to rule out other unexpected pathology. The first portion of the duodenum is inspected for ulcer disease and the pyloric vein of Mayo, usually present, is identified. The first portion of the duodenum is often shortened, scarred and distorted. Sometimes the presence of an active ulcer is suggested by a characteristic stippling that develops when the serosal surface of the duodenum is gently rubbed with gauze.

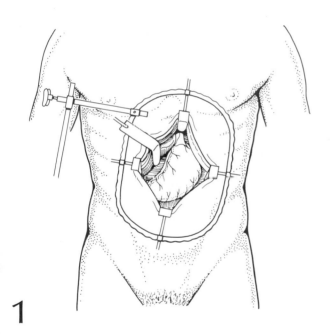

1

Exposure

1 The left triangular ligament of the liver is divided, taking care not to injure the inferior phrenic vein at the extreme right extent of the ligament. Once this ligament is divided, retractors can be used to expose the hiatus. The author prefers to use the Bookwalter retractor. Alternatively, the double-arm 'Iron Intern' may be used. One arm of the latter retractor is used to pull up the sternum, while a Deaver-type retractor is applied to the other arm to pull upwards and to the right the left lobe of the liver which frequently can be folded under the right lobe, protected with a moist laparotomy sponge and retracted.

With this retractor a self-retaining Balfour retractor needs to be used to keep the wound edges open. The advantage of the Bookwalter retractor, however, is that all the necessary blades to retract the sternum, the liver and the body wall can be attached to and optimally positioned on the oval ring of the instrument. If the above retractors are not available, the sternum can be retracted upwards using a Richardson retractor attached to a rope which can be tied to the rigid anaesthetic frame as originally suggested by Goligher. An excellent exposure is usually achieved with these retractors. A headlight significantly improves visibility.

It is now possible to retract the stomach downwards and to the left out of the abdomen and to examine the distribution of the anterior vagus nerve. Except in rare circumstances it is possible to visualize the hepatic branches within the lesser omentum near the gastro-oesophageal junction, and the anterior nerve of Latarjet as it courses along the lesser curvature 1.5–2 cm from the stomach. Distally, the nerve of Latarjet will cross the anterior surface of the stomach to divide into its terminal branches. Goligher has coined the term 'the crow's foot' to describe the appearance of the terminal branching of the anterior nerve of Latarjet.

Mobilization of oesophagus and vagal trunks

With the stomach retracted inferiorly, the oesophagus and the nasogastric tube within it are palpated. The peritoneal reflection over the abdominal oesophagus is incised and the incision carried to the right towards the hepatic branches in the lesser omentum. The oesophagus is then bluntly dissected with the finger.

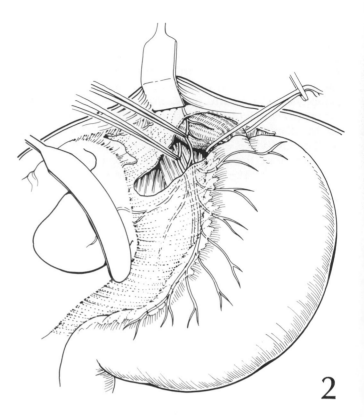

2 As the finger is passed behind the oesophagus, the posterior vagus nerve is often palpable. The oesophagus should be dissected leaving behind the posterior vagus nerve. Once the oesophagus is dissected circumferentially, a 0.75-inch Penrose drain is passed around it for retraction. Next, the anterior vagal trunk(s) is identified. This is best done by retracting the hepatic branches inferiorly with the right index finger while palpating with the middle finger over the anterior surface of the oesophagus. This manoeuvre brings the anterior vagal trunk(s) taut.

Using right-angled forceps, the anterior vagal trunk is dissected off the oesophagus and encircled with rubber vessel loops (or silk thread) for retraction to the right. The posterior vagus nerve is next identified. The oesophagus is retracted to the left and the areolar tissue between the oesophagus and the right diaphragmatic crus is dissected. The simplest way of locating the posterior vagal trunk is by retracting downwards its constant branch, the coeliac division. The coeliac division of the posterior vagus courses along the left gastric artery. The aorta below the diaphragm can be palpated with the right index finger. If the index finger is now drawn downwards over the anterior surface of the aorta, further downward progression of the finger will be stopped by the left gastric artery as it originates from the coeliac axis. Application of further traction on the left gastric artery, and hence on the coeliac division, will bring taut the posterior vagus wherever it is, thereby making it readily palpable. It is dissected and encircled with a vascular loop or silk ligature in a manner analogous to the anterior vagus nerve. The identification and dissection of the anterior and posterior vagal trunks at this stage is not always necessary, but this manoeuvre simplifies the subsequent steps of the operation. Having identified and gently retracted the anterior and posterior vagal trunks, the surgeon is now ready to start the vagotomy. Retraction of the stomach downwards and to the left, manually or with Babcock's clamps, is an essential manoeuvre.

Anterior vagotomy of the proximal stomach

PGV is started by identifying the distal limit of dissection. Frequently the crow's foot of the anterior vagus can be seen. If so, anterior vagotomy is started by taking the uppermost digit of the crow's foot. If the anatomy is not obvious, a point on the lesser curvature 7 cm from the pylorus (the pyloric vein of Mayo) is selected by ruler measurement and marked with a 3/0 suture on the antrum. Dissection will start here and proceed proximally.

Goligher has pointed out that there are three tissue layers at the lesser curvature where the lesser omentum inserts onto the stomach: an anterior layer in which vessels and the gastric branches of the anterior vagus are found; a middle areolar layer containing some vessels; and the posterior leaf of the omentum containing the gastric branches from the posterior vagus and vessels[9]. Taking these three layers individually greatly simplifies the operation.

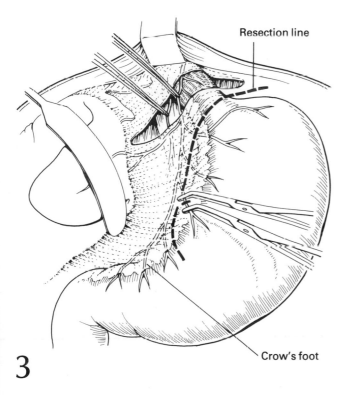

Resection line

Crow's foot

3

3 Starting at the selected distal point of dissection, a curved haemostat is passed under the vessels of the anterior layer. The vessels are clamped, divided and tied with 4/0 silk sutures very close to the gastric wall. The process is repeated serially up the lesser curvature, dividing the neurovascular structures in the anterior leaf, until the gastro-oesophageal junction is reached. Only small bites must be taken. Haemoclips should be avoided because they come off, causing annoying bleeding. Electrocautery must be avoided because the nerve branches being cut may transmit the current to the nerves of Latarjet.

The previously dissected anterior vagal trunk must be retracted and visualized. In the same manner, the middle layer is dissected and divided. It is easier at this point to proceed with division of the gastric branches from the posterior nerve of Latarjet and to leave the oesophageal dissection until later.

Posterior vagotomy of the proximal stomach

4   When PGV was first undertaken the author used to identify the posterior nerve of Latarjet by dividing the gastrocolic omentum to enter the lesser sac and by retracting the stomach superiorly. Now no attempt is made to identify the posterior nerve of Latarjet as an initial step, and the lesser curvature is dissected close to the stomach to divide the neurovascular structures in the posterior leaf of the lesser omentum. It is important to hug the lesser curvature but to take care to avoid including the wall of the stomach in the ligatures.

The first step in this posterior dissection is to enter the lesser sac with a curved haemostat at the distal point of dissection. Once a few vessels are divided, the anterior surface of the pancreas is clearly seen behind the stomach. Again, the devascularization–denervation procedure is carried up the lesser curve of the stomach towards the gastro-oesophageal junction. Near the cardia and behind it, the so-called 'criminal' nerve of Grassi may be seen coming off the posterior vagus nerve and coursing behind the stomach to the left. It must be divided.

At this stage it is often possible to visualize the posterior nerve of Latarjet on the posterior surface of the cut edge of the lesser omentum usually 1–1.5 cm from the edge.

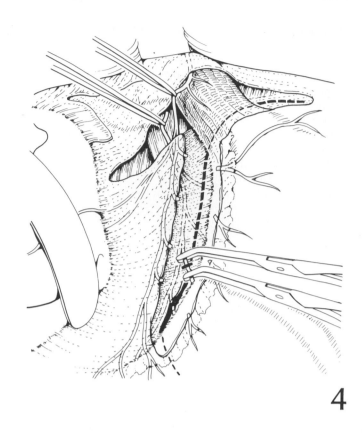

4

5

Oesophageal 'skeletonization'

5   The next task is to vagally denervate the distal 6–8 cm of the oesophagus, first anteriorly and then posteriorly. The anterior vagal trunk is gently retracted to the right and all neurovascular structures on the anterior surface of the oesophagus are divided. It is necessary to carry out this dissection carefully and meticulously. Some vagal fibres will be found embedded in the oesophageal muscle. These must be divided without injuring the oesophagus. The dissection must also extend beyond the oesophagus at the angle of His and all fibrous and areolar tissue in this location must be divided.

Next, the posterior surface of the distal oesophagus is skeletonized. The oesophagus is retracted to the left, and the posterior vagus to the right. The assistant can rotate the oesophagus with his fingers to expose the posterior surface to the surgeon. Again, meticulous division of all neural fibres over the distal 6–8 cm of the oesophagus is necessary. When this is done vagotomy is complete.

Inspection of completed vagotomy

6 It is now necessary to trace the anterior and posterior vagus nerves distally, following the nerves of Latarjet to the pylorus and ensuring that both these nerves are intact. The posterior surface of the oesophagus must be inspected and any undivided nerve fibres sought behind the cardia. Haemostasis must be adequate. The Penrose drain around the oesophagus and the vessel loops around the vagal trunks are removed.

At this point the surgeon has the option of imbricating the lesser curvature with 3/0 silk sutures that bury the dissected surface. Those who perform lesser curve imbrication cite two potential advantages; first, the procedure may minimize nerve regeneration, and secondly, it may help to prevent gastric perforation if lesser curve devascularization has occurred. It must be stated, however, that lesser curve necrosis is an extremely rare complication and probably occurs because the stomach wall is incorporated in a ligature.

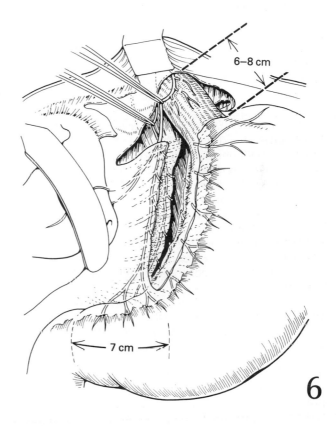

6

Potential pitfalls

7 The potential pitfalls in PGV are (1) inadequate margins of dissection resulting from a failure to denervate the distal 6–8 cm of the oesophagus or because of an inappropriate distal limit of denervation; and (2) secondary sites of incomplete vatogotomy, such as the angle of His fibres, the 'criminal' nerve of Grassi, or gastroepiploic nerves.

Of these, by far the most important is failure to skeletonize the distal 6–8 cm of the oesophagus. The study by Hallenbeck *et al.* showing the importance of this has already been cited[2]. Similar experience was reported by Liedberg and Oscarson[10]. These authors reported ulcer recurrence in four of 20 patients, and an 83% positive Hollander test when they performed PGV with limited denervation of the distal oesophagus. After modifying their procedure to include denervation of the distal 6–8 cm of the oesophagus, none of 60 patients developed ulcer recurrence and only 31% had a positive Hollander test.

The distal limit of denervation has not been found to be as critical as the proximal. For example, Johnston *et al.*, using anatomical landmarks, left only 6.5 cm of distal antrum innervated. By contrast, Amdrup *et al.*, employing either a pH electrode or Congo red spray to determine the antral–fundic junction, left an average of 9 cm of antrum innervated[9]. Despite these differences, both procedures were equally effective in inhibiting basal and maximal acid secretion. This type of comparison, however, gives little idea of long-term results with respect to ulcer recurrence. It has come to light, for instance, that ulcer recurrence in patients operated upon by the Copenhagen group was about 38% in a 25-year follow-up[11].

The results of incomplete vagotomy because of failure to divide the 'criminal' nerve, the nerves at the angle of His, or the gastroepiploic branches at the greater curve have not been quantified. However, on theoretical grounds the minor degree of incomplete vagotomy so caused may, with the passage of time, cause problems. Hypergastrinaemia develops after PGV. Any parietal mucosa left innervated will be chronically stimulated by the elevated levels of gastrin, not only to secrete acid but also to undergo hyperplasia. Because of these concerns, Braghetto *et al.* have proposed that the

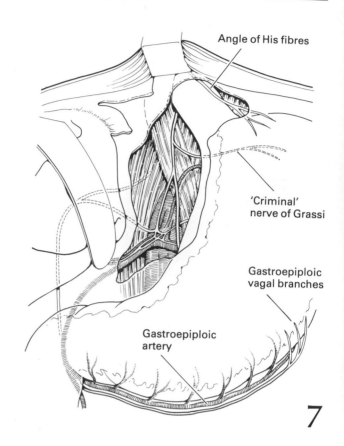

7

gastroepiploic fibres should be cut by dissection at the greater curvature at the junction of the left and right gastroepiploic arteries[12]. This procedure has been referred to as extended PGV.

Postoperative care

The nasogastric tube placed at the time of operation is kept on continuous low suction for 24 h and then removed. By the second or third postoperative day the patient may be started on clear fluids. Some surgeons prefer to wait until gastrointestinal motility returns as evidenced by the passage of flatus. If the patient tolerates clear fluid, the diet can be advanced quickly to a regular diet. The patient is typically discharged from the hospital any time between the fourth and sixth postoperative day. Because patients lose gastric accommodation after PGV, they are advised to eat smaller meals 4–6 times a day for 4–8 weeks. The author prefers to place the patient back on H_2-receptor antagonists for 2–3 weeks postoperatively, but this practice is based on preference and not on any documented evidence of advantage.

References

1. Jaffe BM. Parietal cell vagotomy: surgical technique, gastric acid secretion, and recurrence. *Surgery* 1977; 82: 284–6.

2. Hallenbeck GA, Gleysteen JJ, Aldrete JS, Slaughter RL. Proximal gastric vagotomy: effects of two operative techniques on clinical and gastric secretory results. *Ann Surg* 1976; 184: 435–42.

3. Johnston D. Operative mortality and postoperative morbidity of highly selective vagotomy. *BMJ* 1975; 4: 545–7.

4. Johnston D, Goligher JC. Selective, highly selective or truncal vagotomy? In 1976 – a clinical appraisal. *Surg Clin North Am* 1976; 56: 1313–34.

5. Herrington JL Jr, Bluett MK. The surgical management of recurrent ulceration. *Contemp Surg* 1986; 28: 15–24.

6. Boey J, Branick FJ, Alagaratnam TT *et al*. Proximal gastric vagotomy: the preferred operation for perforations in acute duodenal ulcer. *Ann Surg* 1988; 208: 169–74.

7. Johnston D, Lyndon PJ, Smith RB, Humphrey CS. Highly selective vagotomy without a drainage procedure in the treatment of haemorrhage, perforation and pyloric stenosis due to peptic ulcer. *Br J Surg* 1973; 60: 790–7.

8. Heberer G, Teichmann RK. Recurrence after proximal gastric vagotomy for gastric, pyloric and prepyloric ulcers. *World J Surg* 1987; 11: 283–8.

9. Goligher JC. A technique for highly selective (parietal cell or proximal gastric) vagotomy for duodenal ulcer. *Br J Surg* 1974; 61: 337–45.

10. Liedberg G, Oscarson J. Selective proximal vagotomy – short time follow-up of 80 patients. *Scand J Gastroenterol Suppl* 1973; 20: 12.

11. Hoffman J, Jensen H-E, Christiansen J, Olesen A, Loud FB, Hauch O. Prospective controlled vagotomy trial for duodenal ulcer. Results after 11–15 years. *Ann Surg* 1989; 209: 40–5.

12. Braghetto I, Csendes A, Lazo M *et al*. A prospective randomized study comparing highly selective vagotomy and extended highly selective vagotomy in patients with duodenal ulcer. *Am J Surg* 1988; 155: 443–6.

Pyloroplasty

Sean J. Mulvihill MD
Attending Surgeon, The Medical Center at the University of California, and Associate Professor of Surgery, Department of Surgery, University of California, San Francisco, California, USA

History

Pyloroplasty is used to promote gastric emptying following vagotomy or to relieve obstruction of the gastric outlet, usually due to peptic ulcer disease. Three main types of pyloroplasty have been described and are now known by the eponyms Heineke–Mikulicz, Finney and Jaboulay. Of these, the first is the most commonly used. Weinberg[1] contributed significantly to the popularity of the Heineke–Mikulicz pyloroplasty by demonstrating the safety and improved gastric emptying of a modified one-layer closure.

Principles and justification

In addition to inhibiting acid secretion, truncal vagotomy interferes with regulated motility of the antrum and pylorus and, consequently, gastric emptying. Dragstedt recognized early in his clinical experience with truncal vagotomy that an emptying procedure was required to prevent gastric retention. The surgeon has four main options in aiding gastric emptying following vagotomy: antrectomy, gastrojejunostomy, pyloroplasty and pyloromyotomy. The decision as to which procedure to undertake depends on the main indication for operation (i.e. bleeding, perforation, obstruction, or intractability), the degree of duodenal inflammation, the type of ulcer being treated, the overall condition of the patient and the training of the surgeon.

Of the three types of pyloroplasty, the Heineke–Mikulicz variation is simplest and satisfactory in most settings. Occasionally, chronic inflammation from duodenal ulceration produces retraction of the pylorus toward the liver hilum. In this situation, the Finney pyloroplasty may be preferred. There appear to be few long-term functional differences between the Heineke–Mikulicz and Finney variations[2]. It should be recognized that in the presence of severe inflammatory changes at the pylorus, gastrojejunostomy is a safer alternative emptying procedure.

Pyloromyotomy is mainly used for the management of infants with hypertrophic pyloric stenosis. Occasionally it is used to promote emptying following oesophago-gastrectomy. It is not recommended in the presence of pyloric inflammation such as in peptic ulcer disease.

Partial pylorectomy was initially used to excise anterior duodenal ulcers in an attempt to reduce recurrence rates; this was unsuccessful. Recently, partial pylorectomy has found a small role in conjunction with proximal gastric or truncal vagotomy in the management of duodenal ulcer complicated by pyloric stenosis[3].

Preoperative

Assessment and preparation

Upper gastrointestinal tract endoscopy is the most important diagnostic tool in patients with symptoms suggestive of peptic ulcer disease and should be performed before surgery. Specific information to be gained from endoscopy includes the nature of the peptic disease (duodenal, gastric, or prepyloric ulcers, or gastritis), the presence or absence of pyloric or postbulbar stenosis and, in the case of gastric ulcer, the benign or malignant nature of biopsied specimens. In the emergency setting of haemorrhage, endoscopy is valuable in excluding varices or diffuse gastritis. Endoscopy is unnecessary and potentially dangerous in patients with perforation.

Barium contrast studies are complementary to endoscopy and are particularly valuable when symptoms of gastric outlet obstruction are present, when malignancy is suspected, or in reoperative gastric surgery.

Prophylactic intravenous antibiotics (usually a first-generation cephalosporin) are indicated in operations for bleeding, perforation, or gastric ulcers, but are unnecessary in the elective setting for intractable duodenal ulcer. In patients with gastric outlet obstruction, bezoars should be removed by endoscopy or nasogastric tube lavage before operation. A final gastric lavage with 100–200 ml 1% neomycin sulphate solution may reduce the rate of postoperative wound infection.

Prophylaxis against deep vein thrombosis with sequential compression stockings or low-dose subcutaneous heparin is begun immediately after operation. Bladder and nasogastric catheters are placed following induction of anaesthesia.

Anaesthesia

In all but rare instances the operation is performed under general anaesthesia with adequate muscle relaxation.

Operations

HEINEKE–MIKULICZ PYLOROPLASTY

Position of patient

The patient is positioned supine 5–10° in the reverse Trendelenburg position. The right arm is tucked and padded. The left arm is secured to an armboard for venous access.

Incision

Exposure is best gained through an upper midline incision from the xiphoid process to near the umbilicus. A self-retaining retractor frees the assistant. Two blades are used on the abdominal wall, one retracts the liver cephalad, and a fourth retracts the hepatic flexure of the colon caudad. All blades must be well padded.

1 Stay sutures are placed in the pylorus on either side of the mid-axis. A longitudinal gastroduodenal incision is made, extending for 5–6 cm, centred on the pylorus, or in the case of gastric outlet obstruction, on the narrowest portion of the pyloroduodenal channel. Bleeding vessels in the incision are lightly electrocoagulated. The stay sutures are used to distract the edges of the incision, allowing inspection of the duodenal bulb.

In emergency operations for haemorrhage, haemostasis is rapidly achieved by digital pressure on the bleeding gastroduodenal artery in the posterior ulcer. Blood and clots are then aspirated from the stomach and duodenum, so that accurate oversewing of the bleeding artery can be undertaken in a dry field.

2 Oversewing of an actively bleeding posterior ulcer is accomplished with three interrupted sutures of 2/0 silk. Two figure-of-eight sutures are placed deeply in the cephalad and caudad extents of the ulcer bed with the intention of occluding feeding branches of the gastroduodenal artery proximal and distal to the bleeding point. A third U-stitch is placed at the bleeding site to occlude any transverse pancreatic branch[4]. Failure to control this small branch is an occasional cause of recurrent haemorrhage. The surgeon should be conscious of the location of the common bile duct 1.0–1.5 cm to the right of the gastroduodenal artery.

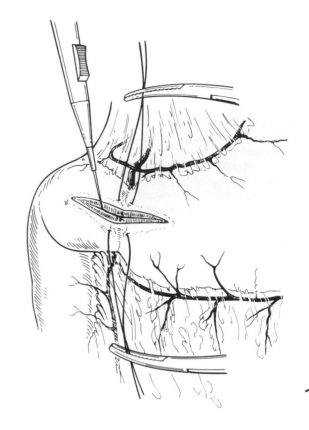

1

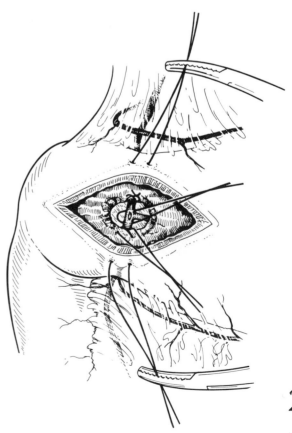

2

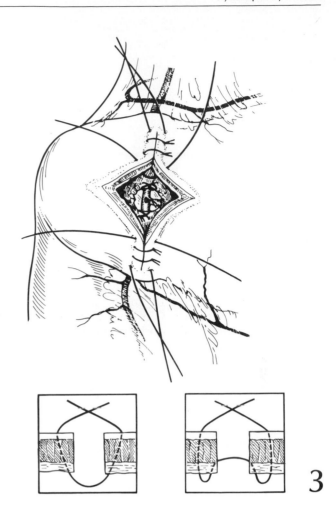

3 The pyloroplasty incision is closed transversely by distracting the stay sutures in cephalad and caudad directions. Interrupted 3/0 monofilament synthetic absorbable sutures of polyglycolate are placed at 4–5-mm intervals. Simple sutures may be alternated with Gambee sutures to ensure accurate approximation of all layers of the gastric and duodenal walls. The closure is begun at each end, working towards the middle.

Alternatively, a two-layer closure may be used, with an inner running, full-thickness 3/0 polyglycolate suture reinforced with outer, interrupted 3/0 silk Lembert sutures. Special care must be taken to avoid obstruction of the pyloric lumen from excessive infolding of tissue.

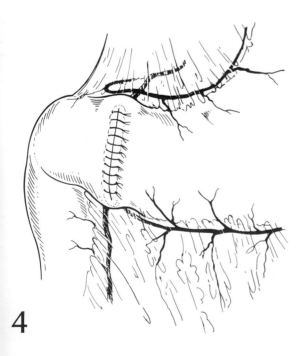

4 The completed pyloroplasty is widely patent. Omentum may be sutured over the closure if desired. A nasogastric tube is positioned along the greater curvature of the stomach before abdominal closure.

FINNEY PYLOROPLASTY

The abdominal incision and exposure for a Finney pyloroplasty are similar to those noted above.

5 Mobilization of the second part of the duodenum (Kocher manoeuvre) is required to relieve tension on the pyloroplasty closure. As the assistant provides traction on the second part of the duodenum towards the left, the surgeon divides the lateral peritoneal reflection with scissors or electrocautery. The duodenum is then swept anteriorly and to the left, exposing the vena cava posteriorly. Care must be taken to avoid injury to the bile duct superiorly and the hepatic flexure of the colon inferiorly.

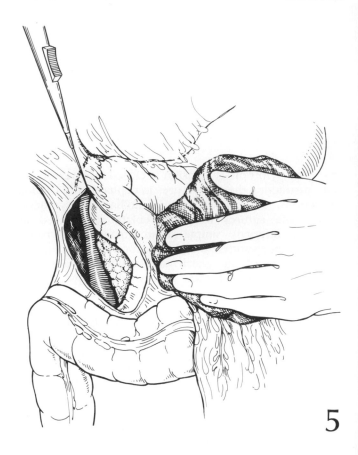

5

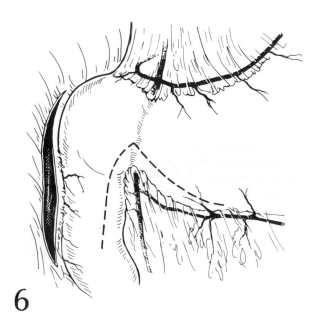

6

6 The gastroduodenal incision is made as an inverted U, close to the gastric greater curvature and medial duodenal wall. Placement of the incision closer to the gastric lesser curvature or lateral duodenal wall results in excessive tension on the anterior gastroduodenal closure. The incision extends for 10 cm, evenly divided between stomach and duodenum, and centred on the pylorus.

7 Three stay sutures are placed, one at each end of the incision and one at the apex of the inverted U.

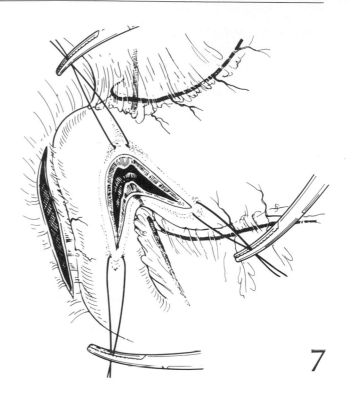

7

8 Closure is achieved with interrupted full-thickness simple sutures of 3/0 polyglycolate, beginning posteriorly between the stomach and duodenum. As the posterior layer progresses, the two stay sutures at the ends of the gastroduodenal incision are brought together.

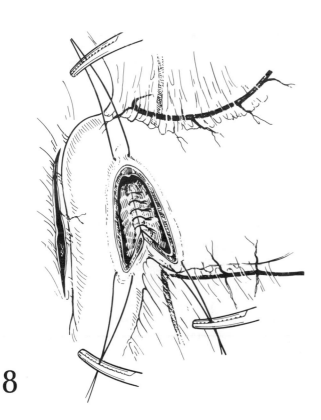

8

9 Closure is continued anteriorly and superiorly towards the third suture at the apex of the inverted U. Inversion of the mucosa is achieved by taking larger bites of serosa and smaller bites of mucosa. Gambee-type sutures may be used to aid this inversion and to provide accurate approximation of tissue layers.

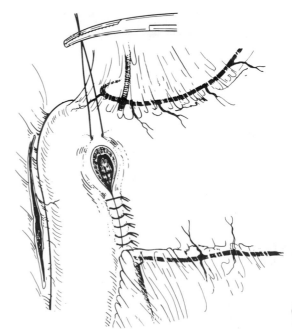

9

JABOULAY GASTRODUODENOSTOMY

Adequate mobilization of the duodenum with a wide Kocher manoeuvre is mandatory. If a tension-free anastomosis between the stomach and duodenum in non-inflamed tissue cannot be achieved, the surgeon should consider gastrojejunostomy as a safer alternative.

10a–c
A posterior layer of interrupted 3/0 silk sutures using seromuscular bites is placed over a distance of 6–7 cm. The end sutures are distracted as stays, the others may be cut. Longitudinal incisions are made in the stomach and duodenum. Small bleeding vessels are lightly coagulated. Closure of the anastomosis is in two layers. For the inner layer, full thickness bites of 3/0 polyglycolate are taken between the stomach and duodenum. Two strands are used, running in opposite directions, carried around each corner and tied to each other anteriorly. This is reinforced with anterior seromuscular 3/0 silk Lembert sutures.

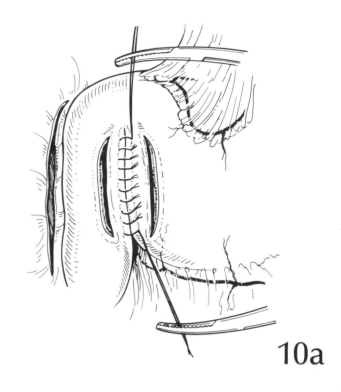

10a

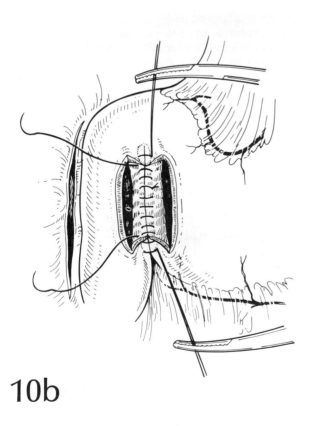

10b

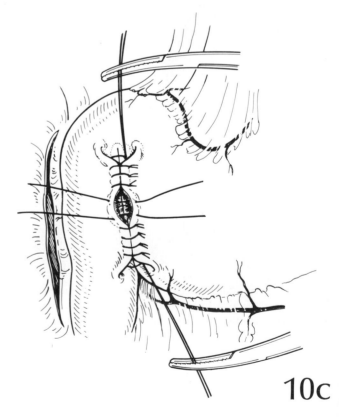

10c

PARTIAL PYLORECTOMY

11a–c The excision is planned to encompass the anterior half of the scarred pylorus. Stay sutures are placed at the cephalad and caudad aspects of the pyloric ring. Transverse incisions are made with cautery through the gastric and duodenal walls just proximal and distal to the pylorus. The anterior half of the pyloric ring is then excised. A gastroduodenal anastomosis with interrupted sutures of 3/0 polyglycolate is performed. Simple sutures may be interspersed with Gambee-type sutures to ensure accurate reapproximation of all layers. Occasionally, a discrepancy exists between the gastric and duodenal openings. Larger bites on the gastric side generally solve the problem. A Kocher manoeuvre may be necessary to relieve tension on the anastomosis.

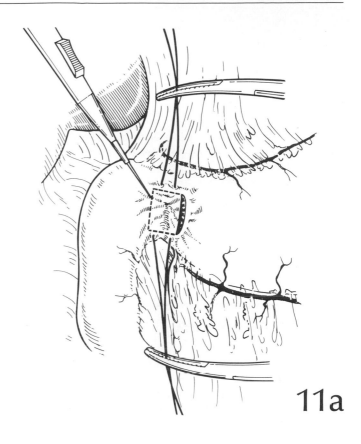

11a

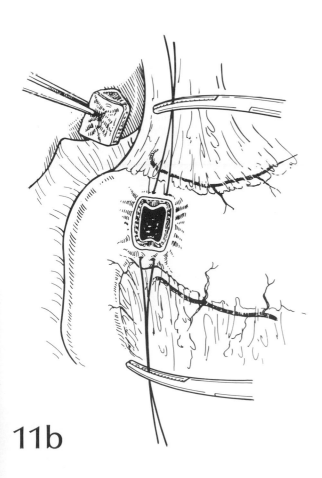

11b

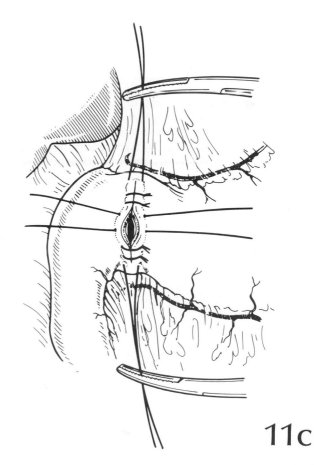

11c

PYLOROMYOTOMY

12 A longitudinal incision is made from the distal stomach to the first part of the duodenum across the pylorus, without opening the mucosa. A gentle spreading motion with a clamp opens the incision and facilitates identification of residual muscle fibres. Special care must be taken at the duodenal end of the incision to avoid inadvertent mucosal injury. As the muscle fibres are divided, the mucosa is encouraged to bulge outwards. This dissection is difficult in the setting of pyloric inflammation or scarring.

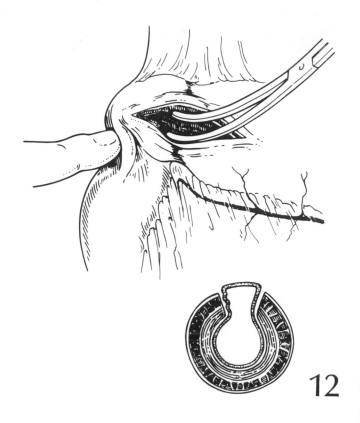

12

Postoperative care

Nasogastric tube decompression is usually used for 2–3 days after operation, although its benefits are debated. Intravenous fluids are required until satisfactory oral intake of liquids is present (usually the fourth day after operation). Analgesia is provided by patient-controlled intravenous injections of morphine via a dedicated infusion device.

Outcome

Suture line leakage is rare, unless the surgeon has unwisely attempted pyloroplasty in the face of marked acute pyloric inflammation. A gastrojejunostomy is the better option in this case. Delayed gastric emptying is uncommon following pyloroplasty and usually relates to oedema from excessive tissue infolding, as in a two-layer Heineke–Mikulicz closure, or to haematoma at the suture line in a one-layer closure. Generally, emptying improves with time. Significant symptoms of dumping or diarrhoea occur in about 15% of patients undergoing truncal vagotomy and pyloroplasty. In 1% the symptoms may be severe enough to consider remedial surgery such as pyloroplasty reversal[5].

References

1. Weinberg JA. Vagotomy and pyloroplasty in the treatment of duodenal ulcer. *Am J Surg* 1963; 105: 347–51.

2. Thompson BW, Read RC. Long-term randomized prospective comparison of Finney and Heineke–Mikulicz pyloroplasty in patients having vagotomy and peptic ulceration. *Am J Surg* 1975; 129: 78–81.

3. Donahue PE, Yoshida J, Richter HM, Liu K, Bombeck CT, Nyhus LM. Proximal gastric vagotomy with drainage for obstructing duodenal ulcer. *Surgery* 1988; 104: 757–64.

4. Berne CJ, Rosoff L. Peptic ulcer perforation of the gastroduodenal artery complex: clinical features and operative control. *Ann Surg* 1969; 169: 141–4.

5. Cheadle WG, Baker PR, Cuschieri A. Pyloric reconstruction for severe vasomotor dumping after vagotomy and pyloroplasty. *Ann Surg* 1985; 202: 568–72.

Illustrations by Gillian Oliver

Gastroenterostomy

Haile T. Debas MD
M. Galante Distinguished Professor of Surgery and Dean of the School of Medicine, University of California, San Francisco, California, USA

Gastroenterostomy is usually performed by the anastomosis of the stomach to the jejunum. Two types of anastomosis are possible: loop gastrojejunostomy and the Roux-en-Y gastrojejunostomy. In loop gastrojejunostomy no provision is made to exclude the regurgitation of bile, pancreatic and enteric secretions into the stomach. Roux-en-Y gastrojejunostomy, on the other hand, is designed to prevent the reflux of bile, pancreatic juice and succus entericus into the stomach. This is accomplished by creating a 40-cm long, isoperistaltic jejunal segment between the gastrojejunostomy and the jejunojejunostomy which returns bile and other secretions to the jejunum more distally. A Roux-en-Y gastrojejunostomy is performed to correct or prevent troublesome alkaline reflux gastritis and oesophagitis.

Indications

Anastomosis between the stomach and the small intestine is performed in four clinical settings: first, in surgery for peptic ulcer where gastrojejunostomy is used as a drainage procedure for truncal or selective gastric vagotomy or to restore gastrointestinal continuity after gastric resection (Billroth II anastomosis); secondly, in surgery for malignant disease either following palliative or curative subtotal gastrectomy or as a palliative bypass when the pylorus is obstructed and

resection is impossible; thirdly, when the duodenum is obstructed, traumatized or resected; and, fourthly, when gastric bypass is used as a treatment for morbid obesity.

Gastroenterostomy may be constructed as a side-to-side anastomosis, or as a Roux-en-Y procedure. It may also be antecolic or retrocolic depending on whether the anastomosis is made to lie anterior to the transverse colon or behind it. The choice of the type of gastroenterostomy depends primarily on the surgical problem.

Gastroenterostomy in peptic ulcer surgery

The preferred type of gastroenterostomy in ulcer surgery is usually a retrocolic hook-up in which the stomach is anastomosed to a loop of jejunum behind the transverse colon. Since the advent of stapling instruments, and in the era where elective truncal vagotomy and gastrectomy are becoming rare, surgeons are constructing antecolic gastroenterostomies with increasing frequency. However, retrocolic rather than antecolic gastroenterostomy is preferred because fewer complications ensue (poor gastric emptying, afferent loop syndrome and volvulus[1]). Roux-en-Y gastrojejunostomy is rarely used in primary surgery for peptic ulcer disease. It is, however, employed in the management of postgastrectomy problems, particularly alkaline reflux gastritis[2] and dumping syndrome[3].

251

Gastroenterostomy in surgery for gastric malignancy

When the pylorus is obstructed with malignant disease and when resection is impossible, gastroenterostomy is occasionally performed to provide palliation. In this case, antecolic gastroenterostomy is preferred because the mesocolon may already be, or may in the future become, invaded with tumour. Antecolic gastroenterostomy is also preferred when subtotal gastrectomy is performed for gastric carcinoma for the same reason. Occasionally, radical gastrectomy may require removal of more than 75% of the stomach. In such a circumstance the surgeon should seriously consider performing total gastrectomy. However, if a decision is made to retain a small gastric pouch, Roux-en-Y gastroenterostomy may be more appropriate since this reconstruction will prevent the complication of bile reflux which occurs more frequently after extensive gastric resection.

Gastroenterostomy in duodenal obstruction or trauma

Palliative gastroenterostomy is frequently performed for actual or impending duodenal obstruction in patients with carcinoma of the pancreas and, less frequently, the duodenum or colon. In these circumstances, antecolic loop gastroenterostomy is the most expedient choice. In severe duodenal or pancreaticoduodenal trauma, gastroenterostomy may be required either because the duodenum has been resected or the pylorus intentionally closed with absorbable sutures or stapled across to divert gastric chyme to protect duodenal repair (duodenal diverticulization). Here, too, antecolic anastomosis is frequently selected.

Gastroenterostomy in gastric bypass surgery

After partition of the stomach in surgery for morbid obesity, the small proximal pouch is anastomosed to a Roux-en-Y[4] limb. The Roux-en-Y limb is brought up to the stomach through a defect created in the mesocolon.

Operations

Incision

The incision used is determined by the requirements of the primary operation. In peptic ulcer surgery and gastric bypass operation the incision is usually midline. In pancreaticoduodenal operations, however, the incision may be midline, right subcostal or double subcostal. When the operation is specifically performed to construct a gastroenterostomy, a supraumbilical midline incision is employed.

LOOP GASTROENTEROSTOMY

Retrocolic gastroenterostomy in peptic ulcer surgery

When the intact stomach is to be used for anastomosis, e.g. after truncal vagotomy, the most dependent portion, preferably just proximal to the muscular antrum, should be selected. The principles of the operation are that after the completion of gastroenterostomy: (1) the most dependent portion of the posterior wall of the stomach is anastomosed to the jejunum; (2) the afferent limb is as short as is comfortably possible (5–8 cm); (3) the anastomosis is retrocolic; and (4) the completed anastomosis lies infracolic.

Technique

1   The lesser sac is entered by dividing the gastrocolic omentum and the posterior wall of the stomach is exposed. The transverse colon is retracted out of the wound and transilluminated to visualize the middle colic vessels and their branches. An avascular portion of the mesocolon is selected, usually to the left of the middle colic vessels, and is opened with a scalpel or pair of scissors for a distance of 6–7 cm.

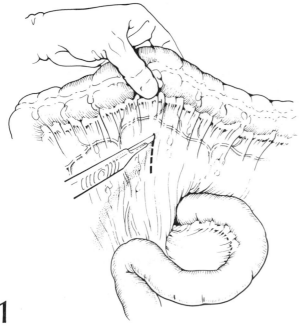

1

2 The site for anastomosis on the posterior wall of the stomach is selected and marked by applying two pairs of Babcock's forceps. Using several 3/0 silk sutures, the posterior edge of the window created in the mesocolon is approximated to the posterior wall of the stomach so that it lies at least 2 cm proximal to the gastrojejunostomy when it is completed. Next, a loop of jejunum is brought through the mesocolon for isoperistaltic anastomosis. The loop is selected so that the afferent limb is as short as possible, preferably no more than 5–8 cm.

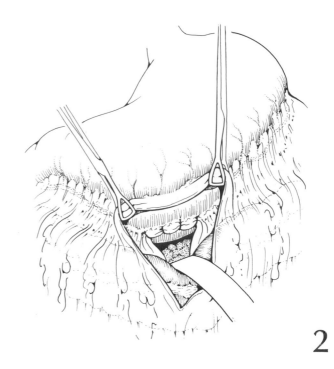

3 The anastomosis is begun by placing 3/0 silk sutures between the stomach and jejunum about 2 cm from the mesocolon previously sutured to the stomach. Corner sutures of 3/0 silk are first placed about 5–6 cm apart. The placement of these sutures will determine the size of the gastrojejunostomy. More interrupted sutures are then placed at 0.3–0.5-cm intervals. These seromuscular sutures must be deep enough to include the submucosa. This posterior row of sutures should be placed on the jejunum midway between the mesenteric and antimesenteric borders. All sutures are applied before they are tied. Once tied, the sutures are not cut until the openings on the stomach and jejunum are made. Before opening the stomach, nasogastric suction should be applied to empty it. The opening in the stomach is best made with cautery about 0.5 cm from the posterior row of silk sutures extending from one corner suture to the other. If large submucosal vessels are encountered, these are best secured by under-running them with 4/0 chromic catgut or Dexon sutures before cutting. As soon as the stomach is opened any fluid within it should be removed by suction. Next, the opening in the jejunum is made, again 0.5 cm from the previous suture line. Care must be taken not to damage the opposite wall of the jejunum. The jejunal opening should be slightly smaller than the gastric opening because the jejunal wall stretches and the opening gets larger during the performance of the anastomosis.

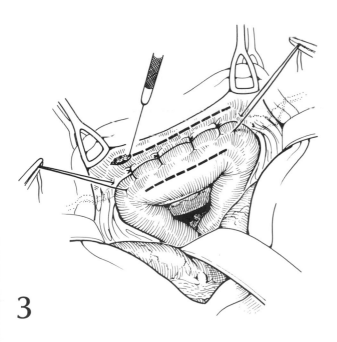

4 The posterior inner layer sutures can now be
applied. Continuous absorbable 3/0 or 4/0 sutures
(Dexon, Maxon or chromic catgut) are used, beginning
at the middle of the incision and progressing laterally in
both directions. These sutures are haemostatic and
should encompass the full wall of both the stomach and
jejunum. The suturing is carried onto the anterior wall,
bringing the edges of the stomach and jejunum
together. This suture will form the inner layer of the
anterior portion of the anastomosis. It is often
advantageous to use the Connell technique to simplify
inversion of the mucosa when the anterior wall of the
anastomosis is contructed.

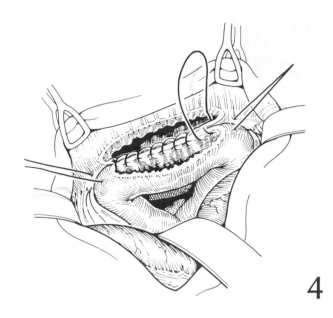

4

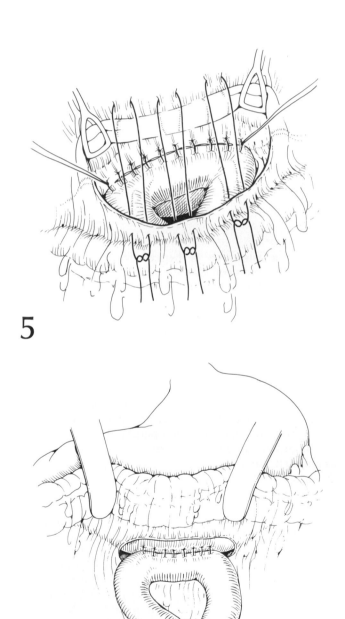

5

5, 6 Interrupted 3/0 silk sutures are next applied
to complete the outer wall of the anterior
portion of the gastroenterostomy. Finally, the anterior
edge of the mesocolon is approximated to the stomach
about 2 cm from the anastomosis. When these sutures
are tied, the gastrojejunal anastomosis will come to lie
in an infracolic position.

An alternative to the above approach where the
gastrojejunocolic anastomosis is performed in the
supracolic compartment and then reduced to the
infracolic position is to bring the posterior wall of the
stomach through the defect created in the mesocolon
and to perform the anastomosis below the mesocolon.

6

Antecolic gastrojejunostomy

The construction of an antecolic gastrojejunostomy is similar to that of the retrocolic variety. The main difference is that the anastomosis lies in front of the transverse colon, and because of this the afferent loop of the jejunum must, of necessity, be longer. A site for the anastomosis is selected so that there is adequate space behind the anastomosis when it is completed for the transverse colon to distend as necessary. This point is usually 20–30 cm from the ligament of Treitz.

The anastomosis is performed in an identical manner to the retrocolic gastrojejunostomy. Both retrocolic and antecolic anastomoses can also be made using a stapler such as a GIA stapler. Stapled anastomoses are being used with increasing frequency, particularly in antecolic gastroenterostomy.

7–9 The sites for anastomosis on the stomach and jejunum are determined and the two organs are held together with either Babcock's clamps or, preferably, 3/0 silk traction sutures. Using electrocautery, an opening is made in the stomach large enough to allow insertion of one fork of the GIA instrument. A similar opening is made in the jejunum adjacent to the opening in the stomach and the other fork of the instrument inserted. The two forks are brought together and closed. The site for anastomosis is again inspected to ensure the instrument is approximated properly and no extraneous tissue is caught. The instrument is then fired. It applies two rows of staples on either side and cuts in between. The instrument is removed and the newly formed anastomosis examined for integrity and haemostasis.

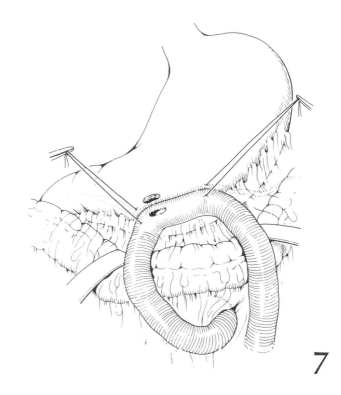

7

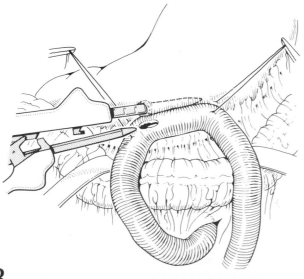

8

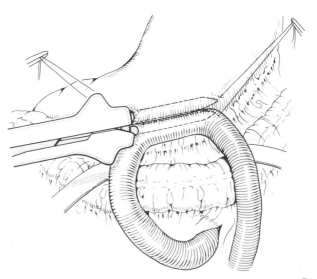

9

10 The stab wounds in the stomach and jejunum used to introduce the instrument are brought together with the application of the stapler and are closed using inverting sutures of 3/0 silk.

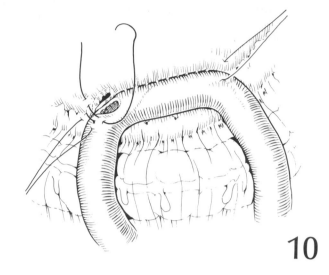

10

ROUX-EN-Y GASTROJEJUNOSTOMY

Indications

Roux-en-Y reconstruction is rarely used in primary surgery for peptic ulcer. It is employed in the following clinical situations: (1) following very high gastrectomy as may be required for a high-lying benign gastric ulcer or for gastric malignancy; (2) in patients with severe alkaline reflux following a previous gastrectomy; (3) in the treatment of dumping syndrome where a gastro-duodenal or a Billroth II anastomosis is converted to a Roux-en-Y gastrojejunostomy; and (4) in gastric bypass operation for morbid obesity[5].

Preoperative

When the indication is dumping syndrome or alkaline gastritis, the diagnosis must be firmly established. Dumping syndrome is diagnosed from typical clinical features including postcibal weakness, abdominal discomfort, tachycardia with palpitation, sweating and even flushing. These symptoms are frequently associated with urgent diarrhoea and constitute the 'early' dumping syndrome, occurring within the first 30–60 min of eating. The same patient may also have a 'late' dumping syndrome, where symptoms of hypoglycaemia occur 2–3 h after the ingestion of a meal. If necessary, the presence of dumping syndrome can be confirmed by showing rapid gastic emptying with radionuclide studies or by provoking the symptoms by asking the patient to drink 100 ml of 50% glucose in water. This will reproduce the early symptoms and, if the patient has late dumping syndrome, a fall of plasma glucose below 50 mg/100 ml with concomitant increase in immunoreactive plasma insulin levels will be found 2–3 h after the ingestion of the meal. Unfortunately, the Roux-en-Y procedure is not always successful and sometimes replaces symptoms of stasis for those of dumping. There is no way to determine before operation which patients will develop stasis, although the longer the Roux limb the higher the incidence of dumping.

When a Roux-en-Y procedure is being contemplated to treat alkaline reflux, a firm diagnosis is necessary. Unfortunately, the diagnosis is very difficult to make. Endoscopy and biopsy should show the presence of severe gastritis and the absence of other lesions such as recurrent ulcer. Severe weight loss is common, and iron deficiency anaemia is seen in 25% of patients. If vagotomy and/or gastrectomy have been performed for ulcer disease, the presence of complete or near complete achlorhydria must be documented by gastric secretory tests. Two important clues include the presence of bilious vomiting and of heartburn unrelieved by antacids. The occurrence of bile reflux may also be demonstrated by measuring high concentrations of bile salts in the gastric aspirate or by scintigraphic studies using an intravenously administered radiolabelled substance normally excreted in the bile. The accumulation of radiolabel in the area of the stomach is evidence of bile reflux. Again, it should be pointed out that, despite all the best efforts of the surgeon, the diagnosis is difficult to establish.

Technique

Take-down of previous anastomosis

The operation is usually remedial, following previous gastrectomy. If the initial operation was a Billroth I gastrectomy, the anastomosis must be taken down. If the initial operation was a Billroth II, however, the anastomosis need not be taken down. Instead, the afferent limb may be divided with the GIA stapler and moved 40–45 cm down for jejunojejunal anastomosis.

11, 12 Traction sutures (3/0 silk) are applied at either edge of the anastomosis both on the stomach and the duodenal side. The anastomosis is divided with electrocautery. The duodenal stump is closed securely in two layers, an inner continuous layer of 3/0 absorbable suture and an outer layer of interrupted 3/0 silk. The opening in the stomach, which has been marked with traction sutures, is usually suitable, after minor preparation, for end-to-side anastomosis with the Roux-en-Y limb.

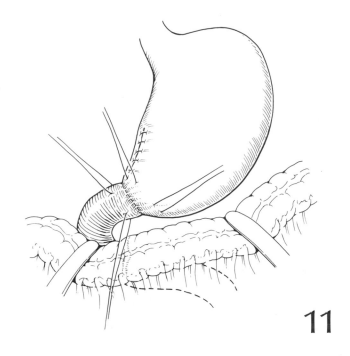

11

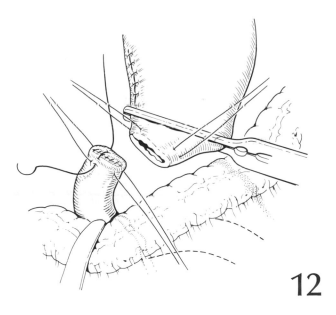

12

Division of jejunum

13 It is usually necessary to divide a few mesenteric vessels at the site of transection division and the adjacent avascular mesentery to the transverse arcade. The jejunum is divided with a GIA stapler (or clamps can be used). By always making this division distal to the previously placed 3/0 silk marking suture, the proximal end is never confused with the distal end. A row of 3/0 silk seromuscular sutures is used to invert the staple line on the distal end of the cut jejunum.

Selection of jejunal segment

14 A 40–45-cm Roux limb will be required. After delivering the transverse colon out of the abdominal wound, the jejunum is dissected free from any adhesions. The ligament of Treitz is identified and a point selected within 10–20 cm of the ligament for jejunal transection. Selection of this point depends on examination of the mesenteric vascular arcade, and the ease with which the distal resection line can be brought up to the stomach. This point is marked with a 3/0 silk suture on the antimesenteric side. Using a sterile ruler, 40–45 cm of the jejunum is measured distal to the suture. A second marking 3/0 silk suture is applied at this point.

By transilluminating the mesocolon an avascular area is selected to the left of the middle colic vessels. This is opened for a distance of 4–5 cm. The distal jejunum is now passed through the defect in the mesocolon for anastomosis with the stomach. Care must be taken not to twist the mesentery.

Anastomosis is made between the opening in the stomach and the side of the jejunum. Corner sutures of 3/0 silk are applied between the stomach and the jejunum such that the proximal suture is within 2 cm of the closed end of the jejunum to avoid creating a large blind pouch. A posterior row of 3/0 silk seromuscular sutures is applied and then tied.

The jejunum is now opened parallel to the gastric opening. The opening in the jejunum is made smaller than that in the stomach. The inner layer of continuous 3/0 Maxon (or other absorbable material) is started in the midpoint of the posterior wall using two sutures. The suturing is carried out towards each corner and onto the anterior wall. All layers of the jejunum and stomach are included. The anastomosis is completed with an anterior outer layer of inverting 3/0 silk sutures. The anastomosis should be 5–7 cm in width.

Closure of defect in mesocolon

If the gastrojejunal anastomosis has been made to lie infracolic, the technique described for the construction of a retrocolic loop gastrojejunostomy is employed.

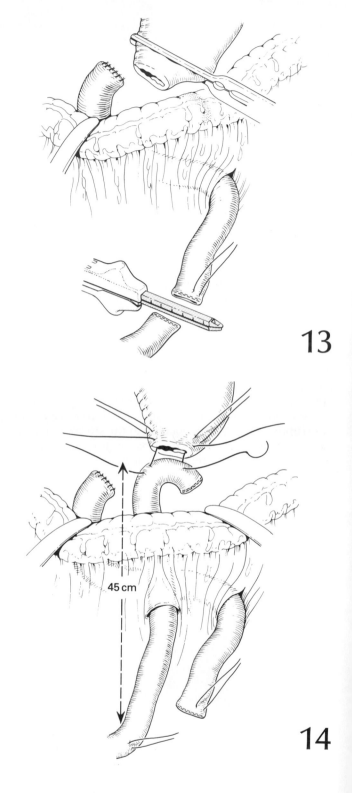

Often, however, the gastrojejunal anastomosis cannot be made to lie infracolic, either because the gastric remnant is small or adhesions prevent this from happening. In this case, the defect in the mesocolon is closed by interrupted sutures between the mesocolon and the Roux jejunal limb.

Jejunojejunal anastomosis

15 The proximal cut end of the jejunum is easily identified because of the traction suture on it. The second traction suture that marked a 40–50-cm segment is also identified. The proximal jejunum is anastomosed end-to-side to the jejunum at the level of the second traction suture. This creates effectively a 40–45-cm isoperistaltic Roux-en-Y limb of jejunum. The anastomosis is again performed in two layers with an inner layer of continuous absorbable suture and an interupted, inverting seromuscular layer of 3/0 silk. The posterior layer of interrupted silk sutures is first applied. The stapled end of the jejunum is then held with three Allis' clamps and, using electrocautery, the stapled edge is excised. The inner layer of continuous suture and the outer anterior layer of interrupted suture can then be inserted.

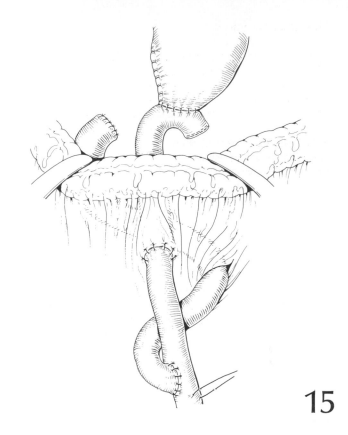

15

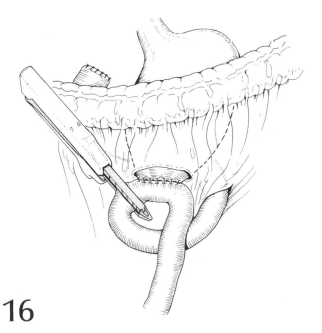

16

Creation of Roux-en-Y gastrojejunostomy after Billroth II gastrectomy

16 If the primary operation was a Billroth II gastrectomy, the original gastrojejunal anastomosis can be preserved. The anastomosis is identified and dissected so that the afferent and efferent limbs can be positively identified. The afferent limb is then transected with the GIA stapler just distal to the anastomosis. The gastric end of the transected jejunum is inspected and the staple line is inverted with interrupted 3/0 Lembert sutures.

17 Using a sterile ruler, a 40–45-cm length of jejunum is measured beyond the gastrojejunostomy and the point marked with a 3/0 suture. The divided end of the proximal jejunum (the afferent limb) is now anastomosed end-to-side to the jejunum at the previously selected site. The technique is identical to that described above.

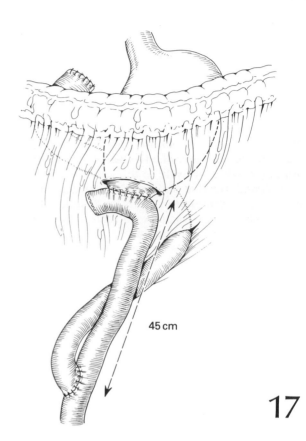

45 cm

17

Postoperative care

Postoperative care is described in the chapter on pp. 124–129.

Complications

Early complications

Gastroenterostomy is associated with few specific complications in the early postoperative period. Suture line haematoma causing delayed gastric emptying can occur. This complication tends to occur more frequently after a stapled anastomosis. It is effectively prevented by the continuous haemostatic suture in a two-layer anastomosis. Problems in gastric emptying can also occur if the mesentery has been twisted or the operation has resulted in severe kinking of the jejunum. If a retrocolic loop gastrojejunostomy is not made to lie infracolic, the jejunal limb can become obstructed as it crosses the defect in the mesocolon. Small bowel herniation through this defect is also theoretically possible.

Late complications

Afferent limb syndrome
An afferent limb that is too long may develop a motility disturbance, causing improper emptying of the segment. Large volumes of bile accumulate in this reservoir. The segment tends to empty at once from time to time, causing a large volume of bilious fluid to enter the stomach. The patient becomes nauseated and vomits the fluid. The vomiting typically occurs in the morning.

The afferent limb syndrome is prevented by using a short afferent limb (less than 10–15 cm) between the ligament of Treitz and the gastrojejunal anastomosis. The treatment of the established syndrome is either to convert the anastomosis to a gastroduodenal (Billroth I) anastomosis or to revise it so that the afferent limb is shortened to 10 cm or less.

Jejunogastric intussusception
This rare but serious complication is well described in the literature[6,7]. It occurs only in loop gastroenterostomy. Irons and Lipin collected 100 cases from the literature in 1955. Either the efferent or afferent limb may intussuscept into the stomach. In 80% of cases the efferent limb is the intussusceptum. In most of the rest the afferent limb intussuscepts, and in rare cases both limbs may do so. The condition may produce an acute abdomen with high small bowel obstruction. Occasionally, however, a more chronic form of intermittent obstruction and occult bleeding results. A barium swallow will establish the diagnosis by demonstrating a filling defect in the stomach made up of coils of intestine. Treatment is surgical. Occasionally the intussusceptum is gangrenous and requires resection. If the intussusception is viable and can be reduced, however, several options exist. These include conversion to Billroth I anastomosis, resection of the anastomosis and creation of a new anastomosis with a shortened afferent limb, which is retrocolic if possible.

Twisted gastrojejunostomy

This rare complication is seen with antecolic loop anastomoses where a twisting of the gastrojejunal anastomosis around the vertical axis causes obstruction. It is conveniently treated by conversion to a retrocolic anastomosis or to Billroth I.

Alkaline reflux gastritis

This condition has been discussed above as an indication for Roux-en-Y gastrojejunostomy. Its true incidence is difficult to establish and the creation of Roux-en-Y gastrojejunostomy is associated with significant late failures.

'Roux syndrome'

Following Roux-en-Y gastrojejunostomy, some 10–30% of patients develop the 'Roux syndrome'. The longer the Roux limb, the higher the incidence. These patients are unable to tolerate oral intake, particularly of solids, and progressively lose weight. They have distressing bilious vomiting. Upper gastrointestinal contrast study, as well as endoscopy, shows a patent anastomosis with no gross abnormalities. However, radionuclide gastric emptying studies show severe impairment of emptying of both solids and liquids. The Roux limb of the jejunum appears to have no functional peristaltic activity; instead it appears to serve as an effective barrier to gastric emptying. Prokinetic agents such as metoclopramide and cisapride are of little benefit.

Treatment is surgical and requires conversion to Billroth I or II anastomosis.

References

1. Bushkin FL, Woodward ER. Alkaline reflux gastritis. In: Ebert PA, ed. *Postgastrectomy Syndromes. Major Problems in Clinical Surgery*, Vol. 20. Philadelphia: Saunders, 1976: 49–63.

2. Ritchie WP. Alkaline reflux gastritis: a critical reappraisal. *Gut* 1984; 25: 975–87.

3. Miranda R, Steffes BC, O'Leary JP, Woodward ER. Surgical treatment of the postgastrectomy dumping syndrome. *Am J Surg* 1980; 139: 40–3.

4. Alden JF. Gastric and jejunoileal bypass: a comparison in the treatment of morbid obesity. *Arch Surg* 1977; 112: 799–806.

5. Griffen WO Jr, Young VL, Stevenson CC. A prospective comparison of gastric and jejunoileal bypass procedure for morbid obesity. *Ann Surg* 1977; 1986: 500–9.

6. Irons HS, Lipin RJ. Jejuno-gastric intussusception following gastroenterostomy and vagotomy. *Ann Surg* 1955; 141: 541 6.

7. Waits JO, Beart RW Jr, Charboneau JW. Jejunogastric intussusception. *Arch Surg* 1980; 115: 1449–52.

Partial gastrectomy (and antrectomy) with a gastroduodenal anastomosis: Billroth I gastrectomy

Glyn G. Jamieson FRACS, FACS
Dorothy Mortlock Professor of Surgery, University of Adelaide, Department of Surgery, Royal Adelaide Hospital, Adelaide, South Australia, Australia

Haile T. Debas MD
M. Galante Distinguished Professor of Surgery and Dean of the School of Medicine, University of California, San Francisco, California, USA

History

In 1881 Theodore Billroth performed the first successful gastrectomy in a patient with distal gastric cancer. The operation was an extended pylorectomy, with the duodenum being anastomosed to the lesser curve of the stomach. He repeated this technique in his second patient, and then changed the anastomosis to the greater curve in his next three patients. Although only the first patient survived the operation, it is the technique practised in the last three that has come to be known as a Billroth I gastrectomy. Early in the 20th century, Shoemaker extended the resection to include all the distal stomach and much of the lesser curve of the stomach, in the operation known today as a Billroth I gastrectomy. Precise removal of the antrum may have been first performed by Edwards and Herrington in 1953, and it was certainly this group who popularized the technique with truncal vagotomy for duodenal ulcer disease.

Principles and justification

Indications

This operation is carried out much less often today than even 20 years ago, because of the decline in the need for peptic ulcer surgery and the change in incidence and site of gastric cancers from the distal stomach to the cardia region.

Nevertheless, gastric ulcer remains the peptic ulcer least successfully treated by acid-suppressant drugs, and distal gastrectomy with removal of the ulcer and a gastroduodenal anastomosis remains the gold standard of surgical treatment for gastric ulcer. The authors, however, believe that antrectomy rather than partial gastrectomy is all that is required.

Partial gastrectomy with duodenal anastomosis is virtually never indicated in the treatment of duodenal ulcer today.

In relation to gastric cancer, the debate continues over the extent of gastrectomy and of accompanying lymph node resection that should be carried out. Suffice it to say that many surgeons undertake the least possible operation that encompasses the gastric cancer primary, and for those surgeons a distal gastrectomy is the operation of choice for an antral cancer. Even here, however, surgeons are divided as to whether the anastomosis should be to the duodenum or to the jejunum, with the majority favouring the latter.

Preoperative assessment is considered in the chapter on pp. 124–129.

Operation

Incision

1 A midline incision is used to approach the stomach. The lesser sac is entered to the left of the midline outside the gastro-omental (epiploic) arcade. The gastrocolic omentum is divided, proceeding from right to left, until the left gastro-omental (epiploic) artery and one or two short gastric pedicles have been divided. In due course if there is any hint of tension on the anastomosis, additional short gastric vessels can be divided.

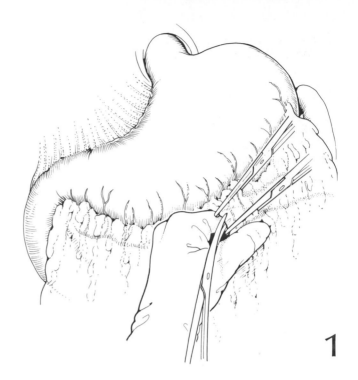

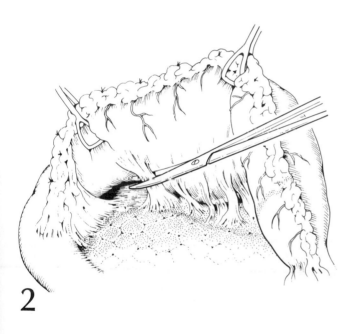

2 The gastrocolic omentum is now divided towards the duodenum; here the lesser sac is obliterated to a greater or lesser degree and it is necessary to recreate the separation between the gastrocolic ligament and the posterior wall of the lesser sac in order to remain separate from the middle colic vessels.

3 As the surgeon approaches the pylorus, the dissection is directed towards the duodenal wall so that the right gastro-omental (epiploic) artery is divided. The pylorus is recognized by a transverse vein running across it, and when picked up between finger and thumb, the pyloric ring of muscle is easily felt. The vessels between the head of the pancreas and the first part of the duodenum are small and easily torn and its is best to use fine artery forceps (mosquito forceps) to clip these vessels prior to division.

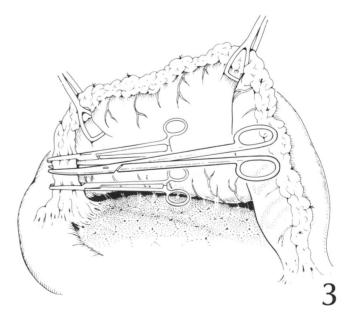

4 The first part of the duodenum immediately distal to the pylorus is completely mobilized and the right gastric artery is sought above and to the left of the pylorus. The right gastric artery is usually insubstantial, but occasionally can be of larger size. It is ligated and divided, and the filmy lesser omentum is divided up to the hepatic branch of the vagus, which is always easily identified as the structure limiting further cephalad dissection.

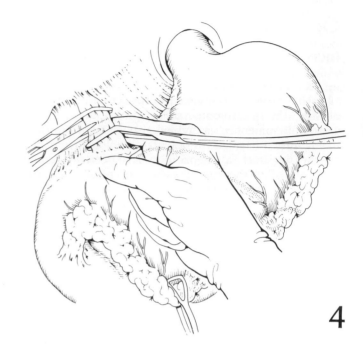

5 The duodenum is next divided between clamps applied immediately distal to the pylorus, with a crushing clamp on the gastric side and a soft bowel clamp applied several centimetres distally on the duodenal side. The division is performed with a scalpel to divide the intestine on the duodenal side of the crushing clamp.

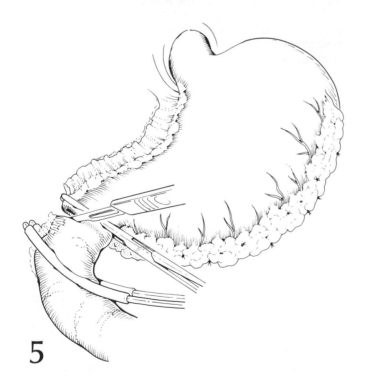

6 The distal portion of the stomach can now be held skywards and any adhesions to the posterior surface of the distal stomach are divided. If the operation is being performed for gastric ulcer the point of division of the stomach on the lesser curve should include the ulcer, even if this lies quite close to the cardia (A–A). It is important to gently dissect the lesser omentum away from the stomach, immediately proximal to the ulcer. In order to do this, a pair of fine curved forceps can be of help, gently opening and closing the forceps next to the gastric wall in order to find a way through to the lesser sac. When this has been achieved, all the remaining tissue in the lesser omentum is divided. The determining factor for how high the lesser curvature of the stomach is resected is always the site of the gastric ulcer. How much of the greater curve is taken depends on whether a classic partial gastrectomy is to be undertaken (B–B) (and in the authors' view the only indications for this today would be in order to encompass a distal gastric cancer in a palliative procedure) or whether an antrectomy only is being undertaken, which is preferable for a gastric ulcer.

If a gastric ulcer is sited high on the lesser curve, it may be necessary to make a gastric division at right angles to the lesser curve for 2–3 cm. The gastric division then proceeds more nearly parallel to the proximal part of the lesser curve, and crosses the stomach to reach the greater curve. This resection line leads to the removal of about 25% of the stomach.

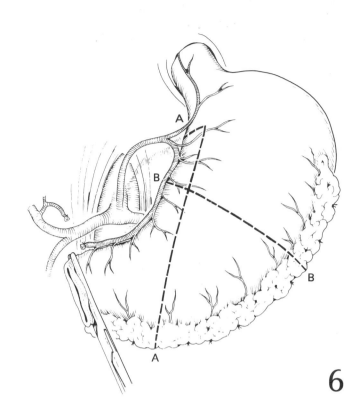

6

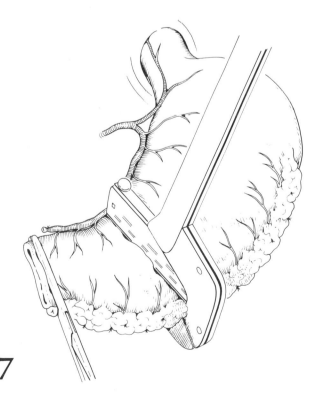

7

7 Removal can be accomplished by hand suturing of the divided stomach in two layers. This is time consuming, however, and the laxity of the gastric mucosa makes the suturing tedious at times. The authors prefer to use a transverse anastomotic stapler approximately 90 cm in length. If the resection is being carried out for a very distal tumour or ulcer, then the point of division is not much proximal to the 'crow's foot' on the lesser curve and vertically opposite this on the greater curve. There is no difficulty in encompassing the whole width of the stomach with a stapler at this point.

The staples on the greater curve side of this anastomosis are later excised in order to open a hole 3 cm in diameter for anastomosis of the stomach with the duodenum. If the ulcer is higher on the greater curve of the stomach, a transverse anastomotic stapler approximately 3.5 cm in length is used to make the right-angled limb and then the 90-cm stapler is used for the vertical limb.

8 On occasions the 90-cm stapler does not encompass the whole width of the stomach wall. In this instance the unstapled portion on the greater curve side is cut across and is later used for anastomosis with the duodenum.

It is a matter of preference whether the staple line is inverted by a running suture with one of the authors using this technique and the other not. The gastroduodenal anastomosis can be carried out in one layer, as described in the chapter on pp. 153–172, or in two layers as described below.

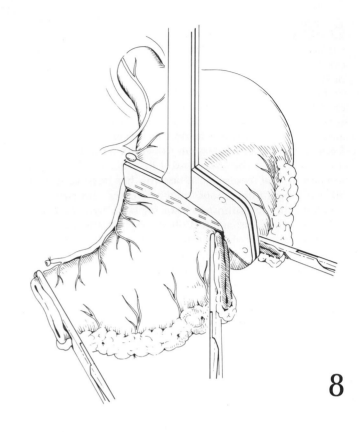

8

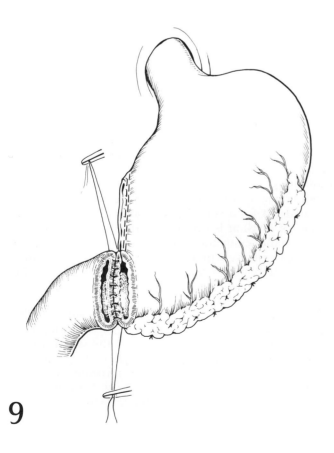

9

9 Stay sutures are placed at either end of the anastomosis and interrupted non-absorbable sutures, e.g. 3/0 silk or Prolene, are used to suture the posterior seromuscular layer of the stomach to the same layer of the duodenum.

10a, b A posterior all-coats running suture is then inserted using 3/0 polydioxanone or 3/0 chromic catgut. The authors begin this suture in the midline posteriorly, inserting two sutures – one to be brought clockwise and one to be brought anticlockwise. These sutures meet in the midline anteriorly. The anterior seromuscular coat is then closed using interrupted sutures as for the posterior wall. German surgeons at the turn of the century christened the three-way meeting point of the reconstructed lesser curve and the anterior and posterior wall of the gastroduodenal anastomosis as the *jammerecke* – the angle of sorrow! To prevent the angle of sorrow becoming a vale of tears, the authors insert a purse-string suture at the angle with the suture passing from the front wall of the anastomosis (stomach) to the front wall of the anastomosis (duodenum), to the back wall of the lesser curve (stomach), to the front wall of the lesser curve (stomach).

As mentioned previously, there should be no tension on the anastomosis; extra length for the stomach can always be obtained by further dividing short gastric vessels.

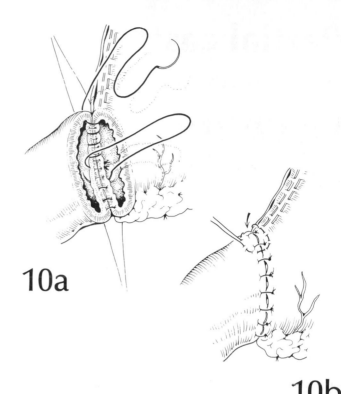

10a

10b

Wound closure

No drains are used and the wound is closed in a routine fashion.

Postoperative care

General postoperative care and the possible complications are considered in the chapter on pp. 124–129.

Partial gastrectomy with gastrojejunal anastomosis including Roux-en-Y reconstruction

Michael W. Mulholland MD
Associate Professor, Department of Surgery, University of Michigan, Ann Arbor, Michigan, USA

History

In 1881 Billroth performed the first successful partial gastrectomy for cancer. It was Shoemaker in 1911, however, who extended the indication for partial gastrectomy to include benign ulcer disease. For over 30 years thereafter subtotal gastrectomy became an important operation for peptic ulcer. Truncal vagotomy for peptic ulcer was reintroduced by Dragstedt in 1942, and truncal vagotomy with drainage or with partial gastrectomy became the most important ulcer operation in the 1950s and 1960s. In the subsequent three decades gastrectomy has been replaced by increasingly more selective types of vagotomy as the cornerstone in the treatment of duodenal ulcer. Gastric resection is now seldom employed as the sole operation for duodenal ulcer. Antrectomy combined with vagotomy is still a common procedure for duodenal ulcer in the USA. Gastric resection, however, is the standard procedure for benign gastric ulcers and gastric malignancies.

Principles and justification

Indications

Partial gastrectomy, performed so that the lesion is included, is utilized as treatment of benign gastric ulcer[1]. Partial gastrectomy in the form of antrectomy may be combined with truncal vagotomy in the operative treatment of duodenal ulcer disease, particularly when gastric outlet obstruction due to pyloric cicatrization has occurred[2]. Gastric malignancy confined to the distal stomach is another indication for partial gastrectomy. Occasionally, invasion of the stomach by malignant tumours originating in other organs, particularly the transverse colon, may require distal gastrectomy. Performance of gastrojejunal reconstruction in the form of a Roux-en-Y anastomosis is indicated in patients with alkaline reflux gastritis[3].

Preoperative

Preoperative preparation is dictated by the complication of the disease requiring gastrectomy for treatment. In the presence of pyloric obstruction, electrolyte abnormalities are common. Loss of gastric secretions high in hydrochloric acid through vomiting will lead to hypochloraemic alkalosis. Renal loss of potassium in attempts to retain hydrogen ions, together with potassium loss from vomiting, results in accompanying hypokalaemia. While prolonged preoperative nasogastric suction is not helpful in preventing postoperative gastric atony in patients with pyloric obstruction, vigorous attempts should be made to remove retained food and gastric bezoars before operation.

Anaemia and coagulation defects should be corrected before surgery. Because upper abdominal incisions may compromise pulmonary function, gastric surgery should not be performed in the presence of active pulmonary infection. Pulmonary physiotherapy and bronchodilators are often helpful; cigarette smoking should be stopped.

Patients undergoing gastric resection should receive preoperative systemic antibiotics. In the presence of pyloric obstruction or achlorhydria, the luminal flora of the stomach contains much higher numbers of enteric organisms and may resemble, qualitatively and quantitatively, the flora of the small intestine. A second or third generation cephalosporin usually provides sufficiently broad coverage.

Operation

Incision

1 A long vertical midline incision extending from the level of the xiphoid process to the umbilicus provides superior exposure of the upper abdomen for performance of partial gastrectomy.

Upon entering the peritoneal cavity, the round ligament may be divided to allow placement of retractors and to partially mobilize the left lobe of the liver.

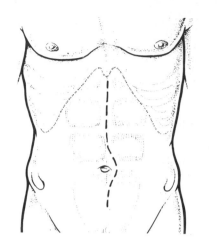

1

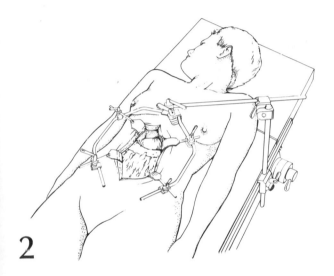

2

Retractors

2 Exposure of the upper abdomen is achieved using a Bookwalter retractor or other, similar, self-retaining device. The costal margins should be elevated and retracted superiorly. The left lateral segment of the liver does not need to be mobilized extensively; superior distraction with the retractor usually provides adequate exposure of the proximal stomach and the area of the left gastric artery. Placement of the patient in a mild degree of reverse Trendelenburg position is often helpful in improving exposure.

Anatomy

3 Performance of gastrectomy demands familiarity with the vascular anatomy of the stomach. Because of extensive intramural collateral vessels, the stomach may retain viability with only one major arterial supply intact. The first portion of the duodenum, in contrast, is much more susceptible to ischaemia produced by surgical devascularization. The vascular landmarks may be used to delineate various degrees of gastric resection. An approximately 50% resection of the stomach is achieved when the stomach is divided along a line from the mid point of the lesser curvature to a point half the distance from the pylorus to the gastro-oesophageal junction along the greater curvature. A 75% gastrectomy requires division of the stomach just distal to the first branch of the left gastric artery to the origin of the left gastroepiploic artery.

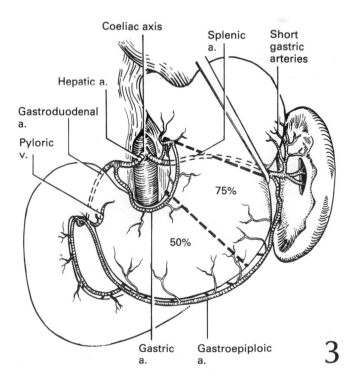

3

Division of gastrohepatic ligament

4 If the operation is performed for a neoplasm, possible posterior extension and fixation to the pancreas or to the middle colic vessels must be anticipated. The posterior wall of the stomach may be inspected by division of the relatively avascular superior portion of the gastrohepatic ligament.

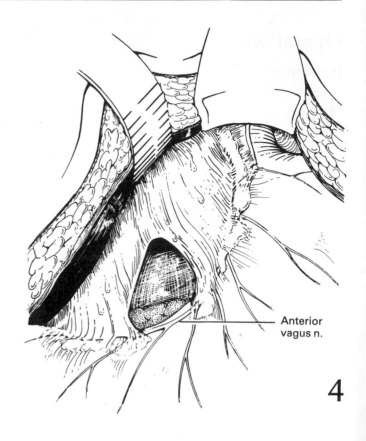

Anterior vagus n.

4

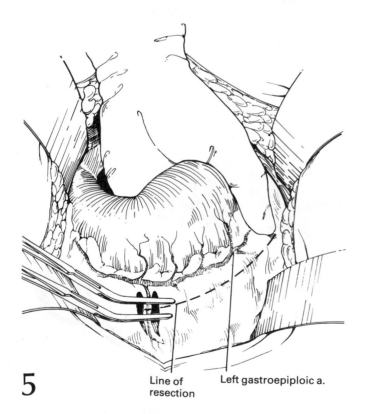

5

Line of resection

Left gastroepiploic a.

Mobilization of greater curvature

5 The gastrocolic ligament is divided, preserving the gastroepiploic vessels if the operation is performed for benign disease and omental resection is not required. Introduction of the surgeon's left hand through the incision in the gastrohepatic ligament can help to guide the dissection and to avoid damage to the middle colic vessels. The omentum receives its major blood supply from the right and left gastroepiploic vessels, and division of small vessels along the greater curvature will not lead to omental infarction.

Preparation of greater curvature

6 Division of the gastrocolic ligament for a 50% gastrectomy should proceed to a point midway between the pylorus and the gastro-oesophageal junction. This point often corresponds to the 'watershed' area between the right and left gastroepiploic vessels. The gastric wall should be cleared of adherent fat and areolar tissue in preparation for division and subsequent anastomosis. A suture, placed at the superior border of the cleared space, is helpful in marking the end of the dissection and as a means of applying traction to the proximal stomach after transection.

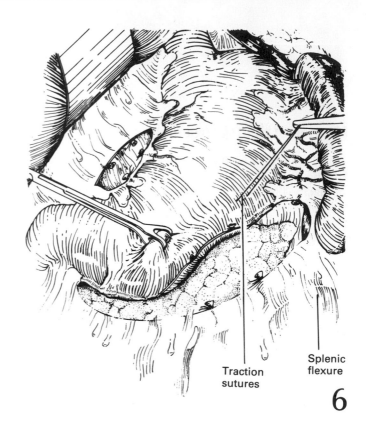

Traction
sutures

Splenic
flexure

6

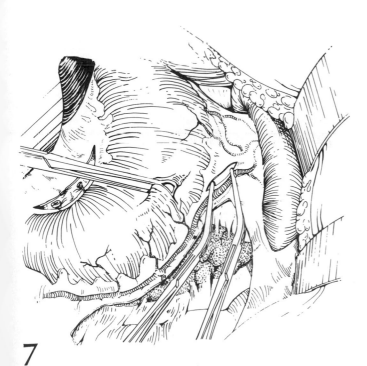

7

Division of left gastroepiploic vessels

7 Performance of a 75% gastrectomy may require division of the left gastroepiploic vessels or the lowermost short gastric vessels.

Ligation of right gastroepiploic vessels

8 Mobilization of the greater curvature is completed by division of the right gastroepiploic vessels. The stomach is retracted cephalad and the right gastro-epiploic artery is identified at its origin from the gastroduodenal artery. The gastroepiploic artery is divided close to its origin, along with adjacent fibrous tissue.

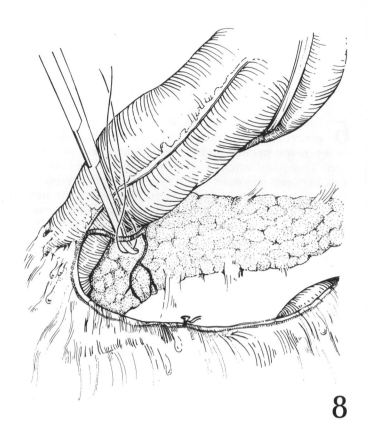

8

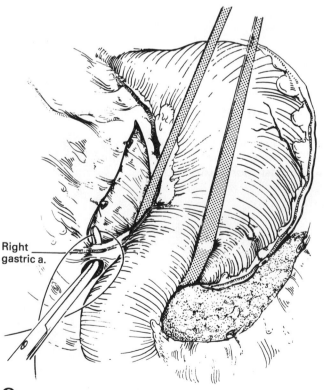

Right gastric a.

9

Ligation of right gastric vessels

9 As the dissection proceeds distally along the lesser curvature, the right gastric artery will be identified near the proximal duodenum. The artery should be ligated close to the duodenum. Care must be taken not to injure the common bile duct if inflammation caused by peptic ulceration has distorted the first portion of the duodenum.

Lesser curvature neurovascular arcade

10 The vascular arcade originating from the left gastric artery parallels the lesser curvature of the stomach. The left gastric vessels reach the stomach as paired branches supplying the anterior and posterior surfaces. The anterior and posterior arcades may be dissected separately; mass ligation, particularly in obese individuals, should be avoided.

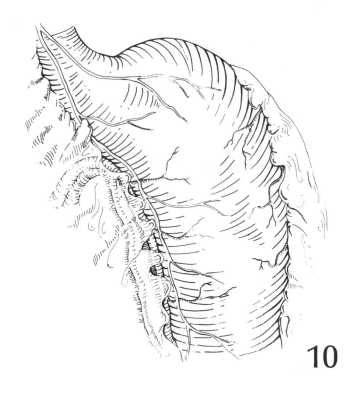

10

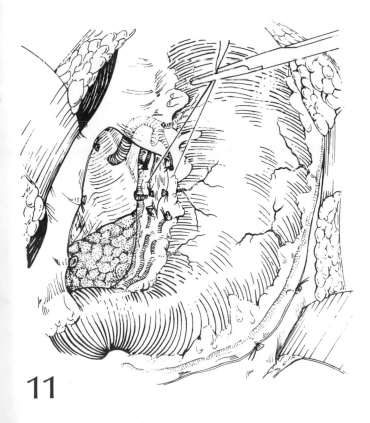

11

Preparation of lesser curvature

11 An area along the lesser curvature is prepared for division and subsequent closure analogous to the dissection performed along the greater curvature. A second traction suture should be placed to control the proximal stomach after transection.

Division of duodenum

12a–c Traction is applied to the stomach toward the patient's left. The duodenum is divided just distal to the pylorus and the ulcer, if present. Division may be accomplished either with a stapler or with clamps (*Illustration 12c*). Stapled transection has the advantages of ease and simultaneous closure of the duodenum.

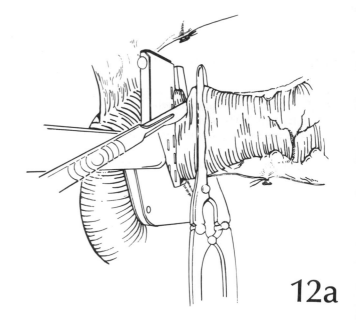

12a

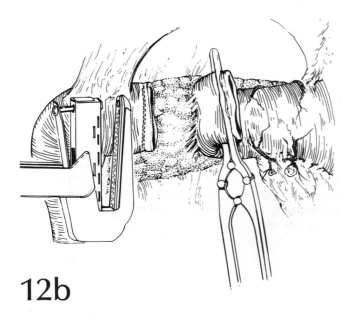

12b

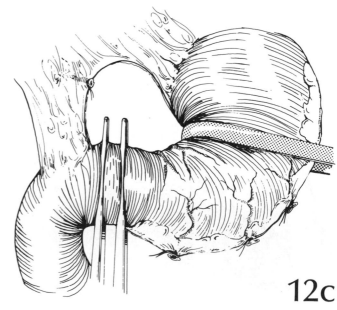

12c

Closure of duodenum

13a–d If the duodenum is divided using clamps, closure should be performed in two layers. The bowel clamp is replaced by Babcock's clamps, care being taken not to encompass an excessive amount of the duodenal wall. After placement of traction sutures superiorly and inferiorly, the cut edge of the duodenum is closed using interrupted absorbable sutures. Closure is completed by a second layer of interrupted seromuscular sutures, e.g. 3/0 silk. If the duodenum has been divided with a stapler the staple line is inverted with interrupted 3/0 silk sutures.

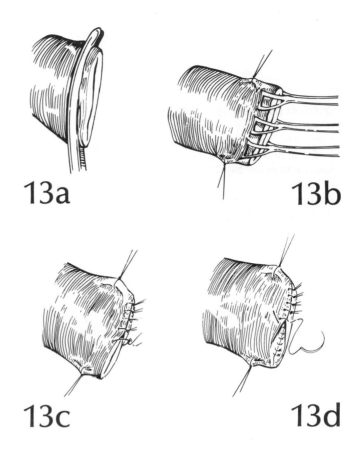

13a

13b

13c

13d

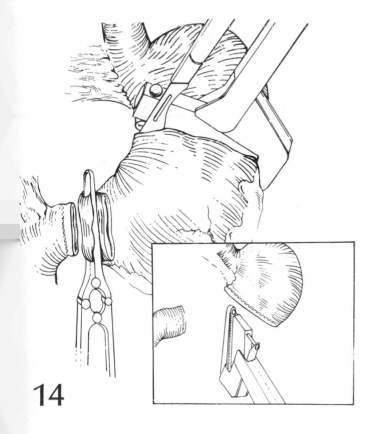

14

Proximal division of stomach

14 The use of surgical staplers greatly facilitates proximal division of the stomach. A TA-90 instrument can be used to close the proximal gastric pouch with a double row of staples: an occlusive clamp is placed distally to prevent escape of gastric contents during transection. Longer length GIA-type staplers may also be employed, using a second application if the stomach is too broad for division with a single load. Some oozing of blood may occur between staples. If this does not cease spontaneously, manual ligation should be performed or a running haemostatic suture applied.

Position of gastrojejunostomy

15 The gastrojejunal anastomosis may be constructed by bringing the jejunum to the gastric pouch either in front of the transverse colon or in a retrocolic position through the transverse mesocolon. In either case, a proximal loop of jejunum should be selected that will reach the stomach without tension and free of angulation. It is crucial that the afferent limb draining pancreatic and biliary secretions is not occluded due to excessive length or kinking.

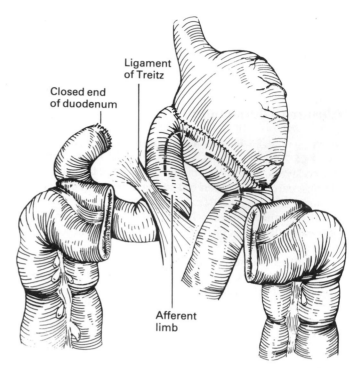

15

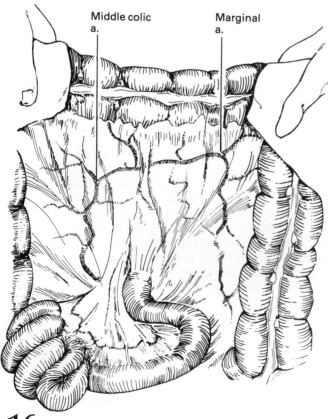

16

Incision in transverse mesocolon

16 If a retrocolic gastrojejunostomy is selected, an incision in the transverse mesocolon to the left of the middle colic vessels is performed. The transverse colon is placed on traction, exposing the course of the middle colic vessels and the marginal artery running parallel to the splenic flexure. The transverse mesocolon is incised in the clear area to the left of the middle colic vessels and an opening is created that will comfortably accommodate the jejunum.

Gastrojejunostomy: sutured technique

17 The gastrojejunal anastomosis may be performed with either a sutured or stapled technique. In the former, the staple line of the gastric transection is partially imbricated with interupted seromuscular sutures. The jejunal loop is delivered through the incision in the transverse mesocolon to approximate the gastric pouch. An appropriate length of stapled closure is excised with electrocautery after placement of interrupted sutures between the posterior gastric wall and the jejunum.

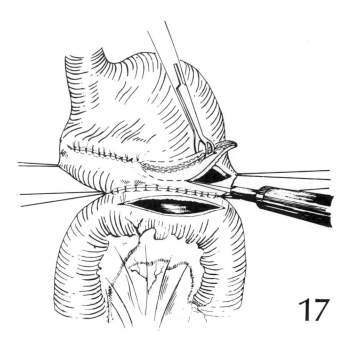

17

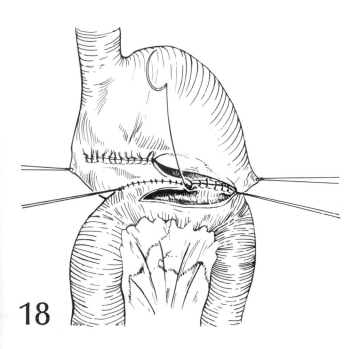

18

Posterior inner suture

18 The posterior layer of the anastomosis is reinforced with a running absorbable suture. The suture should include the full thickness of both the stomach and jejunum.

Anterior portion of anastomosis

19 The posterior running absorbable suture is continued anteriorly as a running Connell suture. The Connell stitch inverts the anastomosis in preparation for the second layer of interrupted seromuscular sutures.

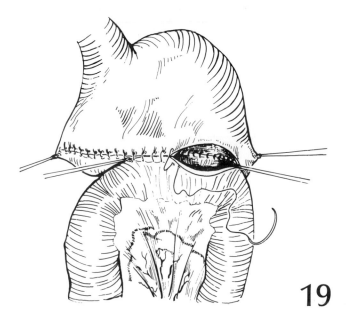

19

Completion of anastomosis

20 A second layer of non-absorbable interrupted sutures is placed to complete the anterior portion of the anastomosis.

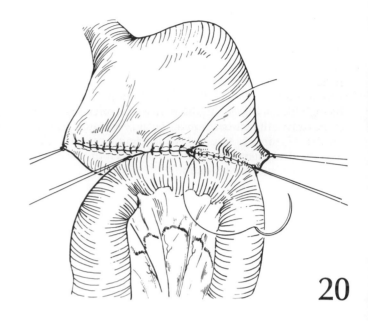

20

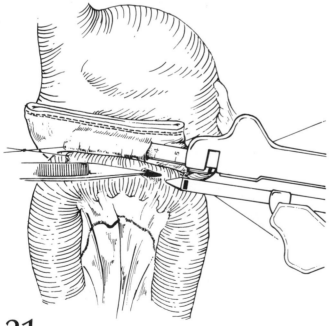

21

Stapled gastrojejunostomy

21 A stapled gastrojejunostomy may be performed with a GIA-type surgical stapler. The jejunum and stomach are approximated using traction sutures. A stab wound is made in the stomach using electrocautery so that an anastomosis will be created 2.5–3 cm from the line of gastric transection. Placement of the anastomosis in this position will ensure that the margin of gastric tissue between the anastomosis and the stapled closure has an adequate blood supply. A similar stab wound is made in the jejunum along its antimesenteric border, and both forks of the instrument are inserted.

Stapler application

22 The instrument is closed and fired, creating the anastomosis with two double, staggered, rows of staples. The instrument is removed and the staple line is inspected for haemostasis.

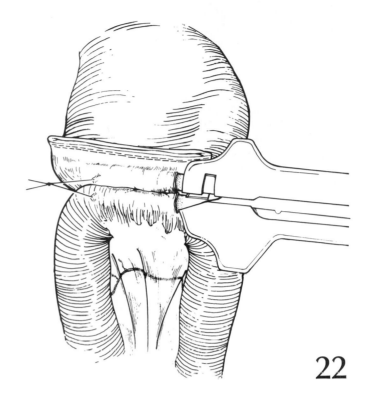

22

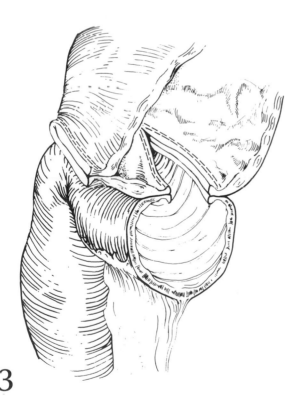

23

Anastomotic reconstruction

23 This view shows the geometry of the stapled gastrojejunal anastomosis.

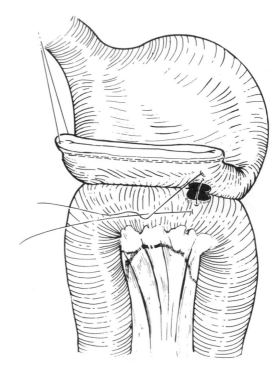

Closure of stapler defect

24 Removal of the stapler reveals the presence of a (now common) hole used to introduce the instrument. This may be closed simply by placement of interrupted, inverting seromuscular sutures.

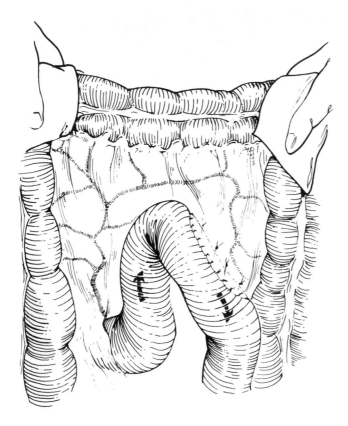

Closure of mesocolon

25 The potential hernia created by the incision in the transverse mesocolon should be repaired by sutures placed from the mesocolon to the gastric wall. The gastrojejunal anastomosis should lie inferior to the transverse mesocolon.

Roux-en-Y reconstruction

26 For a Roux-en-Y reconstruction, the stomach is mobilized and transected as previously described. The jejunum is transected distal to the ligament of Treitz so that the intestine distal to the transection may be approximated to the gastric remnant without tension. It is occasionally necessary to divide one of the jejunal arterial arcades to mobilize the intestine. The distal intestine is delivered through the incision in the transverse mesocolon and approximated to the posterior wall of the stomach using traction sutures.

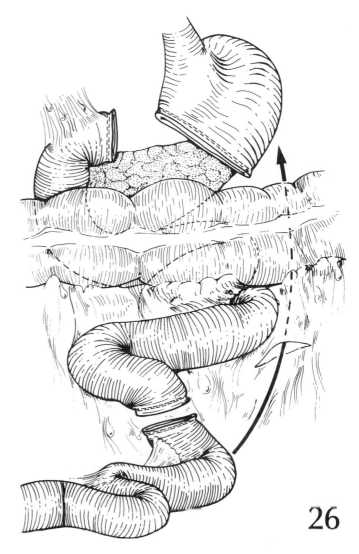

26

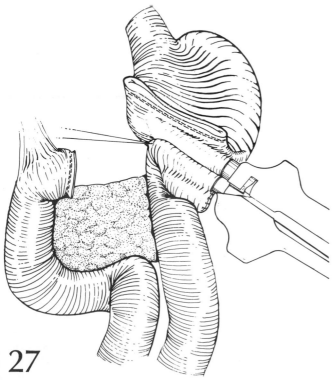

27

Gastrojejunal anastomosis

27 The gastrojejunal anastomosis may be performed in a manner analogous to that illustrated previously, using either staples or a sutured technique.

Enteroenterostomy

28 Intestinal continuity is restored by creation of an enteroenterostomy. In order to prevent reflux of biliary and pancreatic secretions into the gastric remnant, a jejunal limb of 40 cm is constructed. The small intestine should be measured along its antimesenteric border, with care not to unduly stretch it during this manoeuvre. As with the gastrojejunal anastomosis, the enteroenterostomy may be constructed by a sutured or stapled technique. For a stapled anastomosis, two small stab wounds are created in the antimesenteric borders of the small intestine. One fork of a GIA stapling device is placed in each intestinal lumen. The defect used for stapler introduction is closed with interrupted sutures after inspection of the staple line for haemostasis.

Postoperative care

Postoperative care following partial gastrectomy includes the standard intravenous fluids, wound care and pulmonary toilet for major laparotomy. Nasogastric suction should be continued until ileus resolves. Perioperative antibiotics are administered in the first 24 h after the operation.

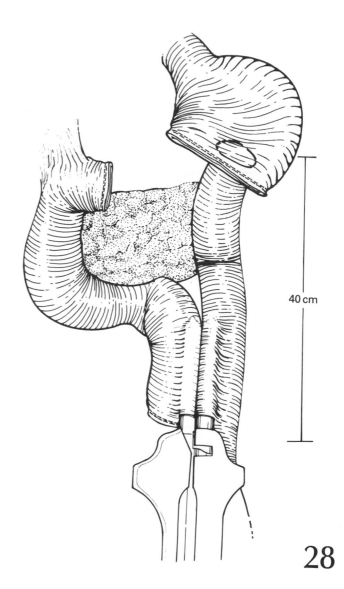

28

Complications

Haemorrhage may occur in the immediate postoperative period after partial gastrectomy, either into the peritoneal cavity or into the lumen of the intestine. Intraperitoneal haemorrhage can occur due to an improperly tied mesenteric, short gastric, or omental vessel, or because of an unrecognized injury to the spleen. Intraperitoneal haemorrhage, if rapid, presents as shock, and if less rapid as an unexplained fall in packed cell volume. Rapid haemorrhage requires immediate reoperation and control of the bleeding site.

Intraluminal haemorrhage occurs in the postoperative period in as many as 5% of cases of partial gastrectomy, most commonly from the operative suture line. Bleeding from the gastrojejunal suture line may be recognized intraoperatively by the anaesthetist if a properly functioning nasogastric tube is in place. Bleeding from the suture line that begins in the first few days after operation should be investigated endoscopically after evacuation of clots from the gastric remnant. Treatment of the bleeding vessel by endoscopic

electrocautery or heater probe application has greatly reduced the need for reoperation in this circumstance. Judicious application of insufflation and cautery must be performed, however, in the presence of fresh, partially healed suture lines.

Duodenal stump dehiscence is the most difficult complication following partial gastrectomy with gastrojejunal anastomosis, accounting for half of the operative deaths[4]. Duodenal dehiscence most commonly occurs within the first week after operation, with a peak incidence on the fifth day. Rapidly developing signs of peritonitis should alert the surgeon to this possibility.

Duodenal dehiscence may be caused by: (1) duodenal ischaemia caused by improper dissection of the first portion of the duodenum; (2) insecure closure of the duodenal stump due to technical error; (3) insecure closure of the duodenal stump due to scarring, oedema or tumour infiltration; (4) periduodenal infection or pancreatitis; or (5) duodenal distension caused by obstruction of the afferent limb of the gastrojejunostomy. Because prevention of duodenal dehiscence is preferable to its treatment, distal gastrectomy should be avoided when intraoperative assessment indicates that secure duodenal closure may not be possible. In these instances, an alternative operation, e.g. vagotomy and drainage, should be considered. If distal gastrectomy must be performed, protective decompressive duodenostomy may be used to avoid duodenal dehiscence or to establish a deliberate, controlled duodenal fistula rather than an uncontrolled leak[5]. A soft catheter (16-Fr Foley or Malecot) is inserted into the duodenal stump after placement of a purse-string suture. The area of the duodenal closure is drained with a closed drainage system (Jackson–Pratt drains).

Mechanical causes of gastric retention in the early postoperative period include anastomotic oedema or scarring, retrogastric hernia, hernia through the mesocolon and jejunogastric intussusception. Retrogastric hernia may occur after either antecolic or retrocolic gastrojejunal anastomosis. Because of greater length and mobility, the efferent limb usually herniates through the retrogastric hiatus created by formation of the anastomosis. This potential hernia can be eliminated by suturing either the efferent limb or the afferent limb to the posterior parietal peritoneum. Symptoms are not dramatic and include colicky abdominal pain and bilious vomiting. Contrast radiographic studies demonstrate the site of obstruction below the gastrojejunal stoma. Treatment is surgical.

Mechanical obstruction of the gastric outlet can also be caused by herniation of the gastrojejunostomy limbs through the mesocolonic defect created for a retrocolic anastomosis. The hernia occurs when either the mesocolon is not sutured to the gastric wall or when those sutures are disrupted. Symptoms are similar to those of retrocolic hernia, and upper gastrointestinal contrast studies are usually diagnostic. Prompt reoperation and reduction of the hernia is indicated because of the possibility of intestinal ischaemia. The mesocolon should be sutured circumferentially to the stomach above the gastrojejunostomy.

Jejunogastric intussusception involves the efferent loop in more than 75% of cases and presents in the early postoperative period with a syndrome of abdominal pain, nausea and vomiting. The complication may be diagnosed by contrast radiography or endoscopy. If spontaneous reduction is not prompt, operative repair should be undertaken because of the potential for small intestinal infarction.

References

1. Adkins RB, DeLozier JB, Scott HW, Sawyers JL. The management of gastric ulcers: a current review. *Ann Surg* 1985; 201: 741–51.

2. Mulholland MW, Debas HT. Chronic duodenal and gastric ulcer. *Surg Clin North Am* 1987; 67: 489–507.

3. Ritchie WP Jr. Alkaline reflux gastritis: late results of a controlled trial of diagnosis and treatment. *Ann Surg* 1986; 203: 537–44.

4. Ahmad W, Harbrecht PJ, Polk HC. Leaks and obstruction after gastric resection. *Am J Surg* 1986; 152: 301–7.

5. Rossi JA, Sollenberger LL, Rege RV, Glenn J, Joehl RJ. External duodenal fistula: causes, complications, and treatment. *Arch Surg* 1986; 121: 908–12.

Bleeding gastric or duodenal ulcer

John E. Meilahn MD
Assistant Professor of Surgery, Department of Surgery, Temple University School of Medicine, Philadelphia, Pennsylvania, USA

Wallace P. Ritchie Jr MD PhD
Professor and Chairman, Department of Surgery, Temple University School of Medicine, Philadelphia, Pennsylvania, USA

Of the estimated 4 000 000 people in the USA with peptic ulcer disease, about 100 000 bleed each year. The attendant mortality rate has remained relatively constant at 6–10% during the past 30 years, despite numerous advances in therapy. Predictors of increased chance of death from an episode of ulcer haemorrhage include an age of over 60 years, multiple organ system disease, transfusion of 5 or more units of whole blood or its equivalent, the recent stress of operation, trauma or sepsis, and the performance of emergency surgery to control haemorrhage (in these patients mortality rates range from 15 to 25%). The mortality rate in patients undergoing emergency surgery is twice as high for bleeding gastric ulcer as it is for bleeding duodenal ulcer.

Duodenal ulcer: background

Although the number of elective operations for duodenal ulcer disease has declined dramatically in recent years (due, at least in part, to the widespread use of H_2 antagonists and other agents), the rate of hospitalization for duodenal ulcer haemorrhage has been relatively stable over the past several decades (25 per 100 000 US population). It is important to note that nearly 70% of these patients will stop bleeding spontaneously without the need for surgical or endoscopic intervention.

Predictors of continued bleeding or rebleeding

A subset of patients with upper gastrointestinal haemorrhage carry a major risk for rebleeding, and therefore for emergency surgery. These include patients who present with shock and acute anaemia because of the magnitude of their blood loss, those with a documented coagulopathy, those in whom bleeding occurs while the patient is already hospitalized for a related or unrelated condition, those in whom endoscopy reveals active bleeding or oozing, and those in whom a visible vessel or sentinel clot is demonstrated, whether bleeding or not (50–100% rebleeding rate). The location of the ulcer also influences the risk of rebleeding, specifically ulcers located deep on the posterior and inferior wall of the duodenum in close proximity to the gastroduodenal artery, and those gastric ulcers which are high on the lesser curvature in close proximity to the left gastric artery.

Aims of surgery

Surgical intervention is used to arrest acute bleeding either by resecting the ulcer or by direct suture of the bleeding point to control the major arterial branches adjacent to the ulcer. In addition, a procedure designed to decrease gastric acid production should be added to allow healing of the ulcer and to prevent rebleeding. This usually involves some form of vagotomy to limit parietal cell innervation, or antrectomy to ablate gastrin production, or both. For gastric ulcer, control of the ulcer diathesis may require antrectomy to remove the portion of stomach at highest risk for ulcer formation.

Gastric ulcer: background

Gastric ulcer is a chronic disease characterized by cyclical exacerbations with significant recurrence rates even while the patient is receiving medical treatment. Unlike duodenal ulcer disease, it is not usually associated with hypersecretion of acid; rather its pathogenesis is probably multifactorial, including increased duodenogastric reflux, gastric stasis, decreased gastric mucosal blood flow, use of non-steroidal anti-inflammatory drugs, and hereditary factors. It is thought that the resistance of the gastric mucosa to injury is impaired so that subsequent exposure to both acid and pepsin results in ulceration. Hospital admissions for perforated gastric ulcers have been stable (one per 100 000 US population), but those for bleeding gastric ulcers have recently increased dramatically[1] (from 14 to 28 per 100 000 between 1980 and 1985).

While up to 70% of gastric ulcers may heal spontaneously at 12 weeks, healing may be enhanced by medical management, including the use of H_2 antagonists (up to 89% healing), antacids (up to 79% healed, but with significant side effects), sucralfate (up to 75% healing), omeprazole or misoprostol. However, relapse is common, even with intially successful therapy. Between 7 and 20% of patients on H_2 antagonists may experience recurrence at 1 year. Without maintenance therapy, up to 80% recur within the same time period.

Types of gastric ulcer

Type I gastric ulcers are the most common type of gastric ulcer with an incidence ranging from 60 to 70%. They are usually located in the antrum near the zone of transition between the proximal acid-secreting mucosa and the distal antrum, but are often located near the lesser curvature. This zone moves proximally with age. Acid secretion is usually low.

Type II gastric ulcers are those found with a simultaneous duodenal ulcer or scar. Pre-existence of the duodenal ulcer may have contributed to partial gastric outlet obstruction and to formation of the gastric ulcer. Acid production is higher than in type I ulcers and is more characteristic of typical duodenal ulcer disease. These ulcers account for 10–20% of all gastric ulcers.

Type III gastric ulcers (20% incidence) are located within 3 cm of the pylorus (prepyloric), and are almost always associated with increased acid production.

Csendes and colleagues[2] from Chile have proposed the existence of a fourth type of gastric ulcer (type IV) which is found in the upper third of the stomach less than 5 cm from the gastro-oesophageal junction. This type of ulcer was found in 27% of patients in the study and a 75% incidence of blood group O and a 64% incidence of presentation with haemorrhage was noted. Acid secretion was low, comparable to that found with type I ulcers. In the USA and Europe this group comprises less than 5% of all gastric ulcers.

Relationship to non-steroidal anti-inflammatory drugs

Since a single ingestion of aspirin can cause gastric subepithelial haemorrhage within 1 h, and regular intake can commonly cause gastric erosions, it is not surprising that chronic use of non-steroidal anti-inflammatory drugs leads to frank gastric ulceration in up to 25% of patients, with a special predilection for the antrum. The use of H_2 receptor antagonists along with non-steriodal anti-inflammatory drugs in arthritic patients does appear to reduce the incidence of duodenal ulcers in these individuals and also reduces the incidence of gastric mucosal haemorrhage. This latter effect is probably of minor clinical significance, and, in any case, H_2 antagonists have little effect on prevention of gastric ulcers in users of non-steroidal anti-inflammatory drugs. Sucralfate or omeprazole may be more effective in this setting.

Concurrent use of misoprostol, a prostaglandin analogue, has been shown to reduce gastric ulcer formation (from 22% to 6% in one recent prospective study). Since the complications of gastric ulcer, including bleeding, may present without significant warning, especially in elderly patients with arthritis or a history of peptic ulceration and who take non-steroidal anti inflammatory drugs, this group of patients should be considered for active prophylaxis.

Competing therapies

Surgeons have come to rely on preoperative oesophagogastroduodenoscopy to diagnose both the cause and location of an upper gastrointestinal bleed. The use of the endoscope has been extended to include immediate treatment of the bleeding ulcer in selected patients. As already noted, if successful, endoscopic haemostasis may allow avoidance of surgery altogether in high-risk patients, or may permit the performance of a definitive operation under elective conditions.

Endoscopic haemostasis is generally unsuccessful in those patients with ulcers which bleed massively or in those which are relatively inaccessible to the endoscopist because they are located in a scarred duodenal bulb or have thick overlying clot. If the ulcer is actively but not massively bleeding, or if it bears the stigmata of recent haemorrhage, including the presence of a visible vessel or clot, endoscopic haemostasis may be attempted provided that surgical back-up is promptly available if the attempt fails. Intervention is also justified in the non-bleeding ulcer in which a visible vessel is seen, because, in this setting, in-hospital rebleeding rates are as high as 50–80%. Ulcers which have a clean base, or which have a flat pigmented spot indicative of old haemorrhage, represent a low risk for rebleeding and do not require attempts at endoscopic haemostasis[3].

Endoscopic injection or sclerosis

This method was initially used to control variceal bleeding and its use has since been extended to control bleeding gastric and duodenal ulcers. Enthusiasm for the approach is due to its relatively low cost, ease of availability and application, and apparent effectiveness in several controlled trials. Absolute ethanol, polidocanol with adrenaline (epinephrine), or adrenaline alone have all been injected around the ulcer base, into a visible vessel if present. These treatments have been applied both to actively bleeding gastroduodenal ulcers and to those demonstrating the stigmata of recent haemorrhage. With the latter, the injection itself may cause immediate bleeding in up to 30% of cases; this is usually readily controlled by immediate continued injections.

Initial success in arresting haemorrhage has been reported in up to 90% or more of cases. Rebleeding may occur in 10–30% of these, with the higher rates observed when the ulcer is actively bleeding before therapy. It has been noted that injection therapy may be less efficacious in ulcers which are greater than 2 cm in size and in those which produce torrential bleeding, especially in the duodenum. The long-term effects of sclerosant injection on the gastroduodenal wall have not been well studied.

Endoscopic cautery

Monopolar electrocoagulation with or without simultaneous water irrigation has been used to achieve immediate haemostasis in patients with bleeding ulcers. However, the depth of tissue penetration and injury is difficult to control, and the end of the probe may require frequent cleaning, making this modality less attractive than injection.

On the other hand, bipolar electrocoagulation produces a well-defined current pathway and controlled subsequent tissue coagulation, minimizing the possibility of transmural injury. The current modification of this concept is the bipolar circumactive probe (BICAP), which uses six equally spaced electrodes, allowing coagulation independent of tip orientation. A central water channel enables irrigation of the bleeding area. The 50-W probe is pressed against the ulcer to coapt the underlying artery and current applied to coagulate the ulcer base and feeding vessel. The BICAP is available in two sizes (3.2 mm and 2.4 mm) to allow passage through the endoscope, and is both portable and relatively easy to use.

Recent prospective studies involving either actively bleeding gastric or duodenal ulcers or those with a non-bleeding visible vessel demonstrate initial immediate haemostasis with BICAP therapy in 91–100% of cases, with rebleeding rates of 6–20%. The large majority of rebleed episodes were treated with surgery.

It should be noted that delayed perforation of duodenal ulcers after treatment with the BICAP has been reported.

Endoscopic heater probe

The heater probe has an aluminium tip containing an internal heater coil which is controlled by an external power source which regulates both the amount of energy and the duration of the applied pulse. The tip of the probe is covered with polytetrafluoroethylene to minimize adherence to tissues and is heated to 250°C, thus transferring heat energy to tissues by thermal conduction. Heater probes are available in sizes 2.4 and 3.2 mm (10-Fr), and are used by pressing the probe firmly against the bleeding point with subsequent application of multiple pulses to a preset energy (20–40 J), producing coaptive coagulation. The probe may be applied around the ulcer base, and also to the bleeding point. It may be applied to the ulcer tangentially as well as *en face*.

The heater probe has been used successfully to control actively bleeding ulcers, although occasional difficulty has been noted in proper positioning of the probe in the duodenum, especially if scarring and deformity are present. A recent prospective trial with actively bleeding gastric and duodenal ulcers noted immediate haemostasis in 83% of patients, with the remainder requiring immediate surgery. In patients whose ulcers were initially controlled, 11% experienced a rebleed and also required surgery. Attempts to treat four rebleeding duodenal ulcers with a second heater probe application resulted in anterior duodenal perforation in two patients. Another prospective study, including non-bleeding ulcers with a visible vessel as well as actively bleeding gastric and duodenal ulcers, reported a rebleeding rate of 28%, with one duodenal perforation during initial heater probe treatment.

Laser

Both argon and neodymium–yttrium–aluminium–garnet (NdYAG) lasers are suitable for use with the flexible endoscope. The argon laser wavelength (440– 520 nm) corresponds to that of maximal absorption of haemoglobin, so that tissue penetration is low, achieving only superficial coagulation. Although immediate haemostasis can be achieved, rebleeding rates appear to be higher than those seen with the NdYAG laser, which has been widely investigated and has been shown to be effective. The NdYAG laser, with a wavelength of 1064 nm (near infrared), demonstrates deeper tissue penetration and coagulation than the argon laser, and has superior efficacy in preventing rebleeding. The equipment, however, is extremely expensive, immobile, not widely available and is relatively difficult to learn to use properly.

To control oozing or bleeding, the laser is manoeuvred as close to an *en face* position as possible, about 1–1.5 cm from the ulcer. Multiple pulses are applied circumferentially around the base of the ulcer, beginning at the periphery and then moving closer to the centre. A visible vessel is not directly coagulated since this may cause bleeding. Anatomical characteristics which may prevent laser use include duodenal deformity or a poorly accessible gastric ulcer high on the lesser curvature.

Controlled trials demonstrate that the NdYAG laser is effective in controlling both actively bleeding ulcers and those with the stigmata of recent haemorrhage, including a visible vessel. However, rebleeding rates have been reported to be high after treatment of actively bleeding ulcers with a visible vessel (up to 60%) and during the operator's learning phase (rebleeding rate of 57% compared with 14% after experience has been gained).

Principles and justification

Indications

Traditional indications for operation for bleeding gastric or duodenal ulcers include: massive bleeding. on presentation with exsanguination and hypotension; ulcers which continue to bleed over time so that frequent transfusion is necessary to maintain a stable haematocrit (generally the need for more than 1 unit of whole blood every 6–8 h constitutes an indication for surgery); and ulcers which, after initial cessation of bleeding, rebleed while the patient is still hospitalized. The advent of various endoscopic methods of treatment has changed the indications for surgery in those centres in which such expertise exists. This is particularly true in elderly patients in whom emergency surgery has a high mortality rate. Success in achieving haemostasis endoscopically may lead either to surgery in an elective setting or to no surgery at all if subsequent medical management is effective in healing the ulcer. The danger in relying exclusively on non-operative endoscopic therapy is that patients who fail then come to surgery in a more unstable state with a higher transfusion requirement, and hence a higher rate of surgical mortality.

Greater urgency is attached to modest bleeding in situations where blood availability for transfusion is limited, either because of local conditions or difficulty in cross-matching individual patients with preformed antibody. Transfusions may not be possible in the face of patient refusal because of religious beliefs. In these situations, early operation may be warranted.

Bleeding duodenal ulcers

The majority of bleeding duodenal ulcers are located along or near the posterior aspect of the duodenal bulb, where the gastroduodenal artery travels from the superior to the inferior border of the duodenum. The typical penetrating posterior ulcer erodes into a branch of this large artery or into the artery itself, with the vessel partially exposed at the ulcer base. The vessel acquires a hole in the side, resulting in either active bleeding through the hole or clot extrusion from the visible vessel.

Ulcers based posteriorly are fed by a rich gastroduodenal arterial supply, and direct suture control of both superior and inferior aspects is necessary. In addition, the transverse pancreatic artery connects to the medial aspect of the gastroduodenal artery behind the duodenum. Thus, suture control of the medial aspect of a duodenal ulcer is also frequently necessary.

Post-bulbar ulcers are located lateral to the gastroduodenal artery and may impinge closely upon the ampulla of Vater. In this instance, it is essential to appreciate the position of the common bile duct to avoid its compromise by improper suture placement.

Oversewing with truncal vagotomy and pyloroplasty

Control of bleeding from a duodenal bulb ulcer can often be accomplished quickly by longitudinal division of the anterior proximal duodenum with extension across the pylorus onto the stomach. This approach readily exposes the bleeding ulcer and permits digital compression of the bleeding point. The ulcer may then be oversewn superiorly, inferiorly and along its medial aspect. After haemostasis has been achieved, closure is performed using the Weinberg modification of the Heineke–Mikulicz pyloroplasty. Definitive control of the ulcer diathesis is accomplished by truncal vagotomy of both anterior and posterior branches, resulting in a decrease in acid production of about 50%. Since the procedure can be done relatively quickly, it has special applicability in elderly patients. Mortality rates are related to age and associated risk factors, ranging from 2% to 17%; the incidence of rebleeding ranges from 4% to 22% and may be reduced by the effective placement of multiple deep sutures during oversewing as described.

Oversewing with vagotomy and antrectomy

When bleeding has been controlled by direct pressure and suture through an anterior duodenotomy with extension onto the stomach, partial distal gastric resection, including the antrum, may be performed with reconstruction via a Billroth I gastroduodenostomy or, preferably in the author's opinion, as a Billroth II gastrojejunostomy. Anterior and posterior truncal vagotomy must be added to this procedure. Such an approach results in a decrease in acid production of about 90%, with ulcer recurrence rates as low as 1%. Mortality rates range from 11% to 21%, and are greatly influenced by the risk status of the patient. Using the APACHE II scoring system to stratify patients, it has been found that patients with a score of greater than 10 are at high risk compared with patients with a score of 10 or less. For these high-risk patients[4], truncal vagotomy with antrectomy for bleeding duodenal ulcer has a mortality rate of 33%, while truncal vagotomy with drainage has a significantly lower mortality rate of about 17%.

Oversewing with duodenotomy and parietal cell vagotomy

In selected young patients who are considered to be stable and at low risk, the bleeding duodenal ulcer may be visualized by a longitudinal duodenotomy and oversewn. The duodenotomy may then be closed longitudinally. If the pylorus is not divided and the patient remains haemodynamically stable, a parietal cell vagotomy may then be performed. The procedure generally requires a relatively prolonged operating time (up to, or more than, 3 h). In a recent retrospective review of 52 low-risk patients (median age 47 years, with mean preoperative transfusion requirement of 5 units and only two patients in shock), duodenotomy and parietal cell vagotomy was performed with no post-operative deaths[5]. It should be noted that only 12 of these patients were bleeding actively at the time of operation. Duodenal ulcer recurrence was reported to be 12% at 3 years, with half of these presenting with rebleeds.

Transection of the pylorus was not required in any of these patients to visualize the bleeding ulcer, and may be avoided altogether if ulcer location has been determined by adequate preoperative endoscopy. However, division of the pylorus for ulcer localization or for exposure to allow oversewing does not necessarily preclude subsequent parietal cell vagotomy as the pylorus may be reconstructed longitudinally in the line of the incision.

Giant duodenal ulcer

Patients with giant duodenal ulcers (diameter of 2 cm or more) present with bleeding as the most common indication for emergency operation. These ulcers are more likely to rebleed on medical therapy, and demonstrate higher mortality rates compared with smaller duodenal ulcers. Since they represent a more severe form of the ulcer diathesis, consideration should be given to a more extensive surgical procedure to prevent recurrence. If the intraoperative haemodynamic status permits, resection with antrectomy and truncal vagotomy should be performed.

Oversewing of the ulcer with truncal vagotomy and pyloroplasty may be performed in less stable patients. If the duodenum is heavily scarred and non-pliable, pyloroplasty may not be possible. Instead, antrectomy should be performed with reconstruction as a Billroth II gastrojejunostomy. Closure of the duodenal stump may be difficult if fibrosis is present. The anterior wall of the duodenum, if pliable, can be sutured onto the posterior wall and the distal edge of the ulcer crater using the Nissen method, avoiding suture placement into the common bile duct. Alternatively, if the anterior wall is too stiff to allow closure, a jejunal serosal patch may be fashioned to close the duodenal stump with either a loop of jejunum or a Roux-en-Y limb. It must be emphasized that attempts to resect the ulcer bed under these conditions are fraught with extreme hazard.

Procedure of choice

Although oversewing of the bleeding ulcer with subsequent vagotomy and antrectomy has been shown to be effective in the prevention of recurrent ulcer bleeding and may be undertaken with low mortality rates in the selected low-risk patient, most surgeons favour truncal vagotomy and pyloroplasty after suture control of bleeding for the usual duodenal bulb ulcer, despite a somewhat higher risk of rebleeding. The procedure is straightforward and can be speedily performed with lower mortality rates in elderly high-risk patients. However, when a giant duodenal ulcer is encountered or when extensive duodenal scarring and deformity is present, resection combined with antrectomy and vagotomy may be preferable.

Bleeding gastric ulcers

The lesser curvature of the stomach is supplied by both right and left gastric arteries, while the greater curvature is supplied by both right and left gastro-epiploic arteries and the short gastric vessels. Each artery divides into anterior and posterior branches which perforate the muscular layers to supply the submucosal plexus which serves as the blood supply for the gastric mucosa. Because of the rich collateral blood flow represented by the submucosal plexus, the stomach can have multiple feeding arteries ligated without compromising its viability. The submucosal plexus is more vestigial along the lesser curvature, so that mucosal ischaemia can occur in this area if the lesser curvature is extensively devascularized (as in parietal cell vagotomy). This is uncommonly seen clinically. Previous or concomitant splenectomy with sacrifice of the left gastroepiploic artery may place a proximal gastric remnant at risk of ischaemia if the left gastric artery is taken simultaneously. This situation is also rare. More common (10% of patients) is the aberrant left hepatic artery which arises from the left gastric artery. Care must be taken to preserve this hepatic blood supply when dissecting close to the lesser curvature.

Many bleeding gastric ulcers penetrate only to the submucosa and have little or no scar tissue in their base. Submucosal vessels found bleeding may have a diameter of the order of 0.5 mm and usually travel across the base of the ulcer. Larger more chronic ulcers have usually penetrated the muscularis propria. In these, a serosal artery, typically with a diameter of 0.9 mm or more, may loop up to the base of the ulcer. In both types, the bleeding vessel may protrude above the floor or be flush with it, with localized aneurysmal dilatation and rupture at the point of bleeding.

Oversewing alone

Simple oversewing for bleeding gastric ulcer has traditionally been performed only in very high-risk patients thought to be poorly suited for more definitive therapy. In non-randomized studies, a mortality rate of 10% and a recurrence rate of 14% has been noted. In actuality, recurrence rates are probably much higher. If this approach is elected, multiple intraoperative ulcer biopsies are essential to exclude carcinoma. Postoperative use of H_2 receptor antagonists is also recommended. In general, if patients develop a bleeding complication while on H_2 blockers or during concurrent use of non-steroidal anti-inflammatory agents which must be continued, this procedure should not be used. In the authors' opinion, it is rarely appropriate under any circumstances.

Oversewing or excising the ulcer with vagotomy and pyloroplasty

Because of the relatively high mortality rates (10–40%) for emergency partial gastrectomy in the elderly, some surgeons oversew the ulcer or resect it by wedge resection if anatomically possible. This approach is then combined with truncal vagotomy and pyloroplasty. Mortality depends on the underlying status of the patient. For high-risk patients (APACHE II score of over 10), the mortality rate from truncal vagotomy and drainage was 9% in a recent series compared with a 22% mortality rate for patients undergoing distal gastrectomy. Therefore, this procedure may be appropriate in the elderly high-risk patient, even though ulcer recurrence rates range from 8% to 25%.

Distal gastrectomy including the ulcer

Ulcer recurrence is minimized by distal gastrectomy to include the antrum and ulcer. This procedure removes the ulcer and enables thorough histological examination to rule out carcinoma. It also removes the gastric ulcer-prone antrum near the antral–corporal border and eliminates the antrum as a source of gastrin. Billroth I gastroduodenostomy is usually possible and is preferable to Billroth II reconstruction. Truncal vagotomy is not felt to be necessary for the usual type I gastric ulcer, since it may predispose to gastric stasis in about 10% of patients and to severe diarrhoea in about 1%. However, vagotomy should be added for a type II ulcer (those found in association with duodenal ulcer) or type III ulcer (prepyloric), since these are usually associated with acid hypersecretion.

For elective operations, mortality rates are as low as 1–2%, with recurrence rates of about 2%. Mortality rates increase to 10–40% in emergency cases, with higher rates found in elderly patients with multiple associated medical problems.

Gastric ulcer with non-steroidal anti-inflammatory drugs

Because the antrum is at risk for ulceration in patients taking non-steroidal anti-inflammatory drugs, distal gastrectomy including the bleeding ulcer should be performed. Gastric erosions are commonly present and should be resected with the ulcer and antrum if possible.

Giant gastric ulcer

These ulcers are defined as those with a diameter equal to, or greater than, 3 cm. Patients having this condition require emergency operation for haemorrhage more frequently than those with smaller ulcers, massive bleeding being present in up to 50% of instances. Additional gastric ulcers may coexist. Unusual complications such as gastrocolic or duodenal–gastric fistulae have been noted. Biopsy should always be performed, since up to 10% of these ulcers are malignant, especially those over 5 cm in diameter. Non-operative therapy for uncomplicated giant ulcer has been reported to be effective, but, as noted, bleeding occurs frequently. Under these conditions, partial gastrectomy including the ulcer with a Billroth I gastroduodenostomy is the procedure of choice.

High-lying gastric ulcer

Total gastrectomy or proximal partial gastrectomy are both associated with high mortality rates, and are completely inappropriate for these ulcers. Wedge resection alone carries a recurrence rate of 33–48% and is often difficult. Non-resective procedures for haemorrhage are followed by high rates of rebleeding. A reasonable approach to high-lying ulcers is as follows: bleeding is controlled by immediate gastrectomy and oversewing. If the ulcer is located high on the posterior wall, Pauchet's procedure can be used (a distal gastrectomy with excision of a tongue of the lesser curvature, including the ulcer). If the ulcer penetrates into adjacent organs and cannot be resected, bleeding is controlled, the ulcer base is biopsied, and if benign, left *in situ*. A distal gastrectomy (not including the ulcer) is then performed (the Kelling-Madlener procedure) and a Billroth I gastroduodenostomy is created. This procedure is associated with a very low recurrence rate (0% in two studies), but a mortality rate of up to 15% has been noted in the elderly. Oversewing or excision with vagotomy and pyloroplasty may be considered, but these procedures have been associated with a rebleeding rate of up to 18%. When the ulcer is less than 2 cm from the oesophagogastric junction, resection using Csendes' procedure (Roux-en-Y oesophagogastrojejunostomy) may be performed with very low recurrence rates (none reported by Csendes)[2], but with significant mortality rates in the elderly, bleeding patient.

Procedure of choice

Distal gastric resection including the ulcer with Billroth I gastroduodenostomy is the procedure of choice for the usual bleeding type I gastric ulcer located in the antrum or distal body. A truncal vagotomy should be added for coexistent duodenal ulcer disease or for prepyloric gastric ulcers. Ulcer oversewing with biopsy or excision in conjunction with truncal vagotomy and pyloroplasty should be used only in high-risk and unstable patients because of the risk of rebleeding.

Preoperative

When the patient presents with upper gastrointestinal haemorrhage, assessment and correction of hypovolaemia, shock and tachycardia should be performed urgently. Initial resuscitation includes maintenance of the airway and breathing with supplemental oxygen. Intubation should be considered for the severely compromised patient. Cardiac monitoring and a 12-lead electrocardiogram should be performed to assess rate, rhythm and ischaemia.

Volume resuscitation via two large-bore peripheral intravenous catheters should be started. In the elderly, a central venous catheter should be inserted for volume replacement and its position confirmed by chest radiography.

Immediate laboratory studies should include haemoglobin or haematocrit, platelet count, electrolytes, creatinine and coagulation factors, including prothrombin time and partial thromboplastin time. At least 6 units of blood should be typed and cross-matched, and the patient transfused to, and kept at, a haematocrit of at least 30% and checked frequently.

A large-bore nasogastric tube should be placed to assess ongoing bleeding and to enable lavage and clot evacuation for subsequent endoscopy. Urine output should be assessed frequently by continuous bladder catheterization as a guide to volume resuscitation. Unless immediate transport to surgery is required, upper endoscopy should be performed to locate the source of the bleeding, to achieve endoscopic haemostasis if available and appropriate, and to guide the surgeon should laparotomy be necessary. The patient should be monitored and cared for in the intensive care unit with continuous systemic arterial pressure monitoring. As laboratory studies become available, coagulopathy should be corrected with either fresh frozen plasma or platelets.

If the patient continues to bleed massively with hypotension, preoperative endoscopy may not be possible; immediate operation should be undertaken. Intravenous antibiotics should be given before operation (for example, a broad-spectrum cephalosporin), but aminoglycosides should be avoided because of potentially compromised renal blood flow.

Anaesthesia

The bleeding patient brought for operation as an emergency requires general anaesthesia with endotracheal tube placement. A nasogastric tube should be placed before induction of anaesthesia to empty the stomach. Cricoid pressure during paralysis and intubation should be performed to prevent aspiration of the gastric contents. A neuromuscular blocking agent should be given to allow complete relaxation of the abdominal wall for maximal exposure.

If the patient has been fully resuscitated and is stable, conventional anaesthetic induction may be possible with thiopentone and the subsequent use of inhalational agents. Both thiopentone and inhalational anaesthetic agents are vasodilatory and their use may be inadvisable in the unstable patient with active bleeding. Instead, induction can be accomplished with either ketamine or etomidate which lack hypotensive side effects. A neuromuscular blocking agent is essential, and amnesic effects can be realized with hyoscine (scopolamine) or a benzodiazepine. If the patient then becomes stable, either an inhalational agent can be started in low doses or narcotics can be used, with a synthetic agent such as fentanyl preferred over morphine because of its better amnesic effects and fewer haemodynamic side effects.

Operations

BLEEDING DUODENAL ULCER: OVERSEWING, TRUNCAL VAGOTOMY AND PYLOROPLASTY

Incision and exposure

The patient is placed supine with both arms extended on arm boards. Following a prescrub, a prep solution such as povidone-iodine 10% is applied from the nipples to the pubic symphysis and the abdomen is draped. An upper midline incision is preferred as it allows extension both upward beside the xiphoid and downward around the umbilicus to permit adequate exposure.

1 The round and falciform ligaments are divided between clamps. Retraction of both costal margins upward is readily accomplished with bilateral retractors mounted on an 'upper arm'; a Balfour retractor is then placed to open the bottom of the incision. Alternatively, a large ring-type retractor such as a Bookwalter also provides excellent exposure. Laparotomy pads are placed to pack the transverse colon downward and are held in place with retractors, exposing the stomach and duodenum.

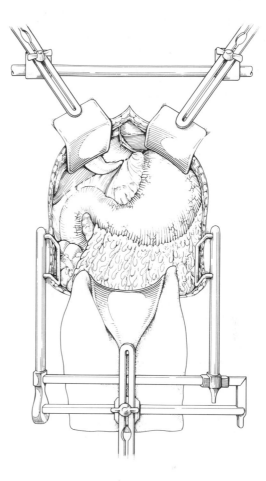

1

Duodenotomy

2 The pylorus is identified by inspection, using the prepyloric vein of Mayo running transversely on the anterior pylorus as a reference, and by palpation of its thickened ring. The approximate location of the common bile duct is noted so that injury during dissection can be avoided. Division of some of the lateral duodenal retroperitoneal attachments facilitates both duodenal exposure and the subsequent pyloroplasty. If the bleeding ulcer has been localized to the duodenal bulb by endoscopy, two 3/0 sutures are placed near the centre of the pylorus and held with haemostats for retraction. A longitudinal pylorotomy is made with electrocautery and extended onto the duodenum until the bleeding ulcer is visualized. Proximal extension onto the stomach for a total length of about 6 cm is then performed. Evacuation of blood and clot is performed with suction and manual extraction, avoiding mechanical injury to the duodenal mucosa.

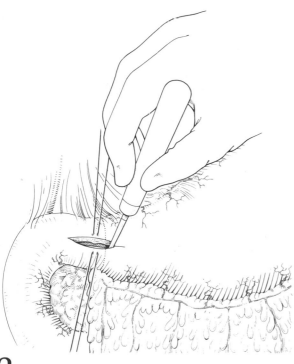

2

Suture ligation

3a, b
The ulcer base is examined to determine the location of vessels or the precise point of active bleeding. Immediate haemostasis can be effected by direct digital compression of the bleeding point. This also permits effective resuscitation by the anaesthetist. The bleeding point can be oversewn in a figure-of-eight manner using a 2/0 silk suture on a half-round needle. The gastroduodenal artery can then be suture-ligated both above and below the ulcer, and a U stitch placed to control bleeding from the medial aspect of the ulcer. In placing deep sutures, the location of the common bile duct should be noted and efforts made to ensure that it is not injured. After suture control of haemorrhage, irrigation and suction is used to clear the remaining duodenum and distal stomach of blood; a thorough search for other ulcers or causes of bleeding should be undertaken.

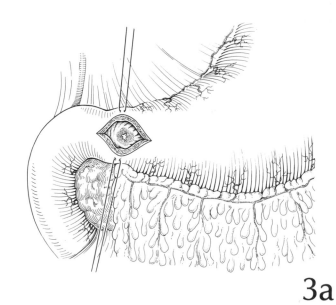

3a

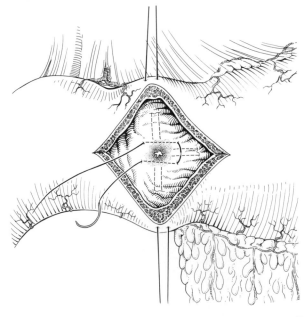

3b

Pyloroplasty

4 The longitudinal incision is then closed transversely as for a Heineke–Mikulicz pyloroplasty, with the previously placed pyloric sutures used for superior and inferior traction. Interrupted 3/0 silk sutures on a tapered needle are placed using a modified Gambee stitch. All sutures are placed before tying. The superior and inferior ends of the closure will 'dog ear' as the sutures are tied. Additional interrupted simple sutures may be placed to approximate the serosa closely, although few are usually needed. If the bleeding ulcer is located on the anterior wall, it may be excised as the duodenotomy is performed, and closure can also be performed as for a transverse pyloroplasty. If the ulcer is more distally located with a longer duodenotomy, or if duodenal stenosis is present distal to the pylorus because of scarring, closure utilizing a two-layer Finney pyloroplasty can be performed.

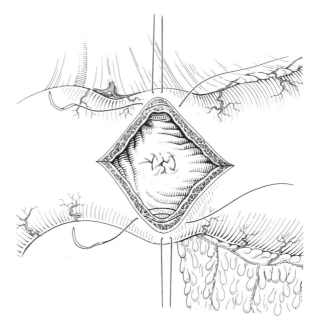

4

Oesophageal exposure

5 Attention is then turned to the distal oesophagus for truncal vagotomy. A long retractor is placed under the left lateral segment of the liver down to the diaphragm to elevate the liver anteriorly, exposing the distal oesophagus. The oesophagus is readily identified by palpation of the nasogastric tube. Downward traction of the stomach is maintained by pulling on the nasogastric tube along the greater curvature, taking care to avoid injury to the spleen. If the liver precludes adequate visualization of the oesophagus, the left triangular ligament may be divided and the left lateral segment can be folded to the right behind the retractor. The peritoneum to the right and left of the oesophagus is opened with scissors. With the surgeon standing on the right of the patient, the index finger of the right hand is passed behind and around the oesophagus from left to right using blunt dissection anterior to the aorta. The finger is passed out through the lesser omentum to the right of the oesophagus, using scissors to assist if necessary. A Penrose drain may be passed around the oesophagus at this point to assist with downward retraction.

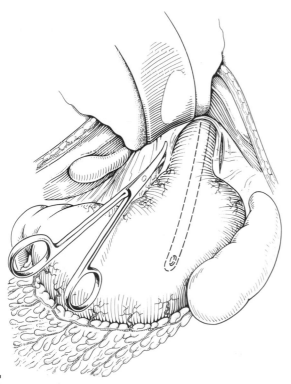

5

Posterior vagal trunk

6,7 The posterior (right) trunk of the vagus is identified as a cord behind the oesophagus which can be pushed by the finger to the right to allow visualization. Skeletonization with a nerve hook or right-angled clamp can verify its structure. The trunk should be clipped superiorly and inferiorly, and a section between clips should be removed for gross inspection and subsequent microscopic verification.

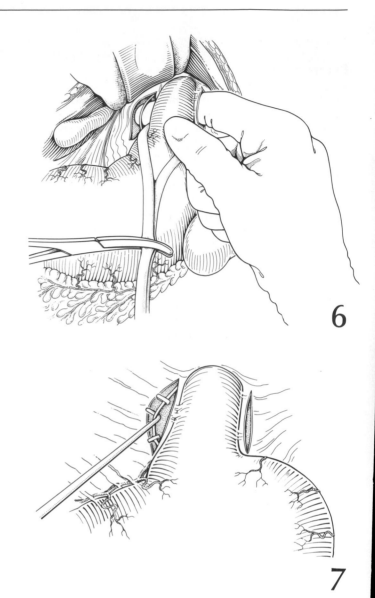

6

7

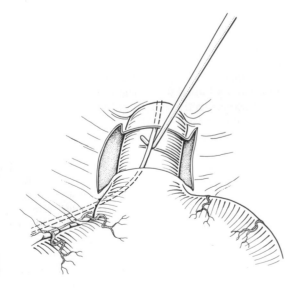

8

Anterior vagal trunk

8 The anterior (left) trunk should then be located in the areolar tissue anterior to the oesophagus by palpation for the cord and direct inspection. It may be necessary to divide this areolar tissue successively to identify the nerve, which should then be clipped and sectioned as for the posterior trunk. The oesophagus should be cleaned of tissue over a distance of 4 cm above the gastro-oesophageal junction to verify that no vagal branches persist.

BLEEDING GASTRIC ULCERS: DISTAL GASTRECTOMY WITH GASTRODUODENOSTOMY

Ulcer exposure

The patient is positioned and draped as described for bleeding duodenal ulcer, with the upper midline incision preferred. Details of retraction and placement of laparotomy packs are the same as shown in *Illustration 1*.

9 After exposure of the stomach, a longitudinal gastrotomy is made in the antrum using electrocautery and either narrow Deaver retractors or Babcock clamps are placed on each edge for elevation and exposure. Blood and clots within the stomach are evacuated with suction and manual extraction, and saline is used for irrigation. Narrow Deaver retractors may be placed within the gastrotomy to expose the gastric mucosa adequately in the search for the bleeding ulcer. Once located, haemostasis is achieved by direct digital compression and subsequent oversewing of the bleeding point using multiple 3/0 silk sutures. If malignancy is suspected, biopsy and frozen section should be performed. A thorough exploration of the abdominal cavity to exclude unsuspected disease should also be undertaken.

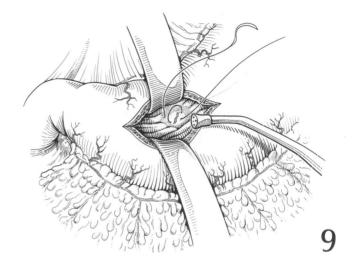

Gastric mobilization

10 The ulcer location is noted relative to the planned line of excision for antrectomy as the ulcer should be excised with the specimen. The antrum begins approximately 8–10 cm proximal to the pylorus along the lesser curvature, or at the incisura angularis. Along the greater curvature, it begins at a point about one-eighth the distance from the pylorus to the oesophagus. To ensure adequate distal resection, the line of gastric resection extends from the mid point of the greater curvature to a point on the lesser curvature just proximal to the incisura angularis. Silk sutures (3/0) are placed on both greater and lesser curvatures at these points and held on haemostats. The transverse colon is retracted inferiorly and the gastrocolic omentum is divided at the mid point of the greater curvature next to the stomach. Individual branches of the right gastroepiploic artery are taken between 3/0 silk ties, dissecting distally towards the pylorus. Dissection is kept close to the stomach to avoid injury to the middle colic vessels, which may be adherent. The posterior wall of the stomach is freed of adherent tissue to permit a finger to be placed under the stomach and to tent up the gastrohepatic ligament along the lesser curvature. If the ulcer has penetrated posteriorly, it may be adherent to the pancreas, and dissection will be proximal to this. If the stomach cannot be mobilized from the pancreas, then the posterior wall can be incised with electro-

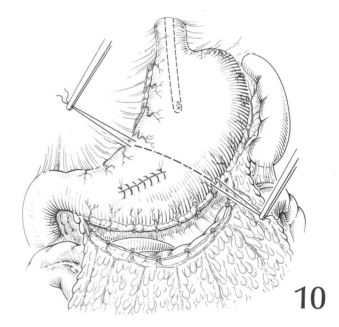

cautery around the ulcer base, leaving it *in situ*. The gastrohepatic omentum can then be divided distally, and the right gastric artery ligated between 2/0 silk ties. The left gastric artery need not be divided since the stomach is usually transected distal to it. If an aberrant left hepatic artery is present (10% incidence), it should be preserved.

Duodenal mobilization

11 Mobilization of the duodenum is necessary and is accomplished by the Kocher manoeuvre, in which the second portion of the duodenum is retracted medially and the lateral peritoneal and retroperitoneal attachments are divided. Blunt finger dissection behind the duodenum and head of pancreas is helpful in elevation. The duodenum should be mobilized from the area distal to the common bile duct down through the proximal third portion, taking care not to injure the superior mesenteric vein which travels across the anterior aspect of the third portion of the duodenum. As the Kocher manoeuvre is performed, the inferior vena cava, which lies posteriorly, should not be injured.

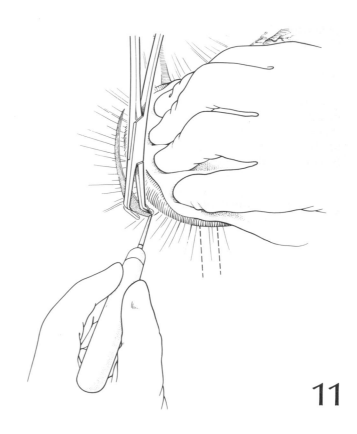

11

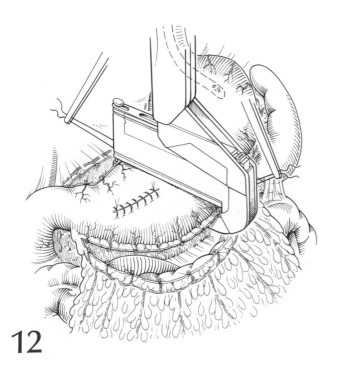

12

Division of stomach

12 The stomach may be transected at this point using a TA 55 or TA 90 stapler passed from the greater to the lesser curvature. Considerable embarrassment is avoided if the nasogastric tube is positioned proximal to the stapler before using it. Kocher clamps applied to the stomach distal to the stapler prevent gross spillage when a knife is used to divide the stomach along the distal side of the stapler.

Division of duodenum

13 Upward and medial traction on the distal stomach remnant allows dissection of the pylorus and proximal duodenum on their superior, posterior and inferior aspects. The duodenum should be mobilized to a point about 3 cm distal to the pylorus. The gastroduodenal artery should be preserved. A GIA stapler can then be passed from the inferior to superior aspect of the duodenum, and used to divide it just distal to the pylorus, allowing removal of the distal stomach and some proximal duodenum.

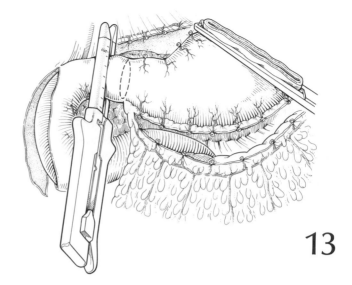

13

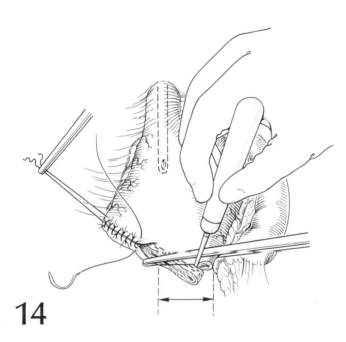

14

Preparation of gastric remnant

14 The proximal stomach and duodenal stump can then be approximated to assess the need for further dissection to remove tension from the anastomosis. If satisfactory, the width of the duodenum is superimposed on the distal stomach on a line at right angles to the greater curvature. The staple line superior to this anastomotic site is oversewn with interrupted 3/0 silk Lembert sutures. A bowel clamp is applied to the distal stomach, and electrocautery is used to resect the bottom corner of the stomach over the length corresponding to the width of the duodenum.

Gastroduodenal anastomosis: back row

15 The stomach and duodenal stump are approximated and 3/0 silk corner sutures are placed and held with haemostats. The corner suture at the superior aspect should be placed through both the front and back walls of the stomach as well as the duodenum. After turning both stomach and stump to expose their back walls, a back row of interrupted seromuscular 3/0 silk sutures is placed and tied. Electrocautery is used to resect the staple line across the duodenal stump, opening the lumen.

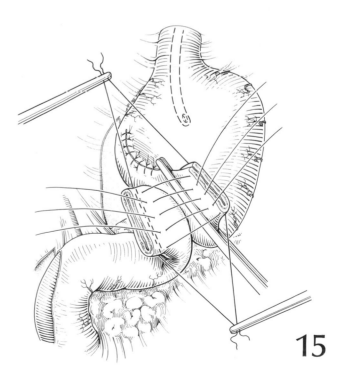

15

Anastomosis: inner layer

16 Beginning at the superior corner, a 3/0 polyglactin (Vicryl) suture is passed through the mucosa and serosa of both the stomach and the duodenum and tied. The short end is held on a haemostat, and the inner layer of the anastomosis is begun with a continuous, locking posterior suture. At the inferior corner the same suture is used to begin a Connell stitch to close the inferior half of the front wall. Before the front wall is completed, a second 3/0 polyglactin suture is placed adjacent to the first one at the back wall through the full thickness of stomach and duodenum and tied. It is then run as a Connell stitch along the remainder of the front wall to meet the first polyglactin suture and tied, thus inverting the front wall. The clamp is then removed from the stomach.

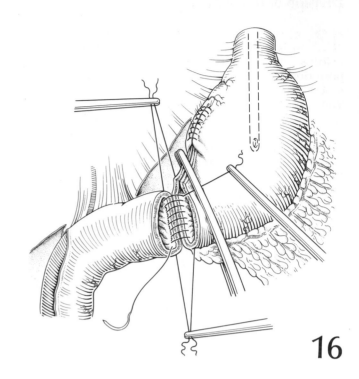

16

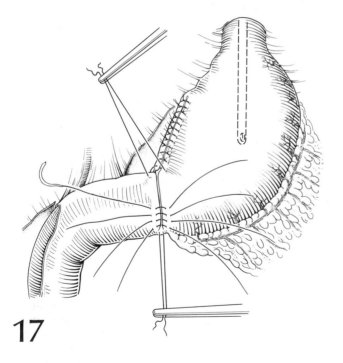

17

Anastomosis: front row

17 Both corner sutures are tied. A row of interrupted Lembert 3/0 silk sutures is placed to complete the outer layer of the front wall. The anastomosis is examined thoroughly to assess the need for additional Lembert sutures. The abdomen is irrigated with warm saline; some surgeons use an antibiotic such as cephazolin dissolved in the irrigant. Adjacent omentum can be placed over the anastomosis and tacked in place. If the gastric ulcer was either type II or III, truncal vagotomy should be added as in *Illustrations 5–8*.

Postoperative care

The patient may be cared for after operation in the intensive care unit or the recovery room with transfer to the ward determined by age, associated medical problems and intraoperative stability. Ventilatory support should be continued as necessary. Cardiac monitoring should be performed with a 12-lead electrocardiogram and compared with that obtained before operation. Serial creatine phosphokinase enzyme fractions should be obained if evidence of intraoperative or postoperative cardiac ischaemia exists. The haematocrit should be serially checked, with transfusions as necessary to maintain a level of at least 30. A full set of serum electrolyte levels should be measured. If dissection near the common bile duct has been performed, daily liver function tests should be done.

Nasogastric suction should be continued to monitor daily output, presence of blood, and to monitor and correct gastric pH to greater than 5.0. Administration of intravenous H_2 antagonists should be used to control gastric pH, with adjunctive use of antacids if necessary. Urinary catheterization should be continued to assess hourly urine output and to aid intravenous fluid therapy. In the elderly, a central venous catheter is advisable to monitor central venous pressure and to enable timely replacement of electrolytes such as potassium. If there is evidence of cardiac dysfunction, a Swan–Ganz catheter should be inserted to monitor cardiac output, left ventricular filling pressures, and systemic vascular resistance, and to guide the use of vasoactive agents if those are required.

Coagulation abnormalities or platelet deficiencies should be corrected as necessary. Several doses of antibiotics should be given after operation because of the clean-contaminated nature of the procedure with intragastric blood being an excellent culture medium.

Total parenteral nutrition should be considered for the high-risk patient. Subcutaneous heparin should be avoided, but sequential calf compression devices may be used to reduce the incidence of deep venous thrombosis.

Outcome

Acute complications

Complications following truncal vagotomy include ischaemia of the distal oesophagus when more than 4 cm has been skeletonized, or iatrogenic perforation if extensive dissection of vagal fibres has been undertaken with excessive enthusiasm. Left pneumothorax may result from finger dissection posterior to the oesophagus. Splenic injury may result from excessive traction on the stomach, omentum or splenic flexure of the colon. Complications of parietal cell vagotomy include ischaemia of the lesser curvature of the stomach after devascularization (incidence less than 1%) and postoperative intra-abdominal bleeding (about 1%).

If the ulcer has not been resected (as in vagotomy and pyloroplasty for bleeding posterior duodenal ulcer), early rebleeding may occur in 5–8% of patients[6]. Wound infections are more common after operation for gastrointestinal haemorrhage. Complications from gastroduodenostomy include gastric outlet obstruction from anastomotic narrowing, requiring anastomotic revision. Other complications include anastomotic leakage, bleeding from either intraluminal or extraluminal sources, and postoperative pancreatitis.

Postvagotomy and postgastrectomy syndromes

The dumping syndrome has been described either early or late after eating, but the early syndrome is much more common, occurring in up to 25% of patients after pyloroplasty or resection. With rapid travel of gastric contents into the duodenum, cramping and diarrhoea may result, with additional vasomotor symptoms of pallor, faintness and perspiration. Most patients can be managed with dietary changes.

Postvagotomy diarrhoea is often unassociated with eating and may occur at night. While cholestyramine may be helpful in the majority, truly refractory diarrhoea is found in only about 1% of patients.

Alkaline reflux gastritis with relatively constant epigastric pain and bilious emesis may be helped with H_2 antagonists or cholestyramine but, if these are unsuccessful, conversion to a Roux-en-Y gastrojejunostomy may be required to divert alkaline secretion from the stomach.

Options for patients with recurrence

Many patients with recurrences can be successfully managed medically; as with the original case, haemorrhage, perforation, obstruction or intractability may demand surgical correction. Recurrent ulcer disease should prompt investigation for gastrinoma, hyperparathyroidism, retained antrum in the case of a duodenal stump, or for antral gastric cell hyperplasia. Recurrent gastric ulcer should be biopsied to exclude a carcinoma. If no obvious cause is found and surgical intervention is deemed necessary, then antrectomy is usually performed if truncal vagotomy or parietal cell vagotomy was performed initially. If antrectomy was the initial procedure, then a subtotal gastrectomy with vagotomy or revagotomy should be considered.

References

1. Kurata JH, Corboy ED. Current peptic ulcer time trends: an epidemiologic profile. *J Clin Gastroenterol* 1988; 10: 259–68.

2. Csendes A, Braghetto I, Calvo F *et al.* Surgical treatment of high gastric ulcer. *Am J Surg* 1985; 149: 765–70.

3. Laurence BH, Cotton PB. Bleeding gastroduodenal ulcers: non-operative treatment. *World J Surg* 1987; 11: 295–303.

4. Schein M, Gecelter G. APACHE II score in massive upper gastrointestinal haemorrhage from peptic ulcer: prognostic value and potential clinical applications. *Br J Surg* 1989; 76: 733–6.

5. Miedema BW, Torres PR, Farnell MB, van Heerden JA, Kelly KA. Proximal gastric vagotomy in the emergency treatment of bleeding duodenal ulcer. *Am J Surg* 1991; 161: 64–8.

6. Hunt PS, McIntyre RLE. Choice of emergency operative procedure for bleeding duodenal ulcer. *Br J Surg* 1990; 77: 1004–6.

Bleeding oesophageal and gastric varices: stapling procedures

George W. Johnston MCh, FRCS
Honorary Professor, Queen's University Belfast, and Consultant Surgeon, Royal Victoria Hospital, Belfast, UK

History

Since Boerema and Crile first described direct ligation of oesophageal varices by a transthoracic approach there have been many modifications of the method. Japanese surgeons, disillusioned by the results of shunt surgery, employed transthoracic paraoesophageal de-vascularization and oesophageal transection combined with an abdominal component consisting of splenectomy and devascularization of the upper stomach together with vagotomy and pyloroplasty[1]. This extensive operation has never gained popularity in the West, and even in Japan thoracotomy is now included less frequently. The advent of mechanical staplers has renewed interest in the transection–devascularization procedures.

Principles and justification

Portal hypertension in itself does not require treatment and there is, as yet, insufficient evidence to support prophylactic therapy for oesophageal varices which have not bled. When varices do bleed the clinician is presented with a life-threatening situation, not only because of haemorrhage but because of the risk of liver failure in cirrhotic patients with limited liver reserve. Where efficient emergency sclerotherapy is available only a small proportion of patients require urgent surgery, either in the form of a portal systemic shunt or a devascularization–transection procedure. Burroughs and colleagues consider that if two attempts at sclerotherapy fail to control acute bleeding, one should proceed to emergency transection[2]. Where sclerotherapy is unavailable, emergency transection–devascularization is a viable alternative. Even if the initial bleeding episode is controlled by acute sclerotherapy, consideration has to be given to the prevention of recurrent bleeding whether by chronic injections, portal systemic shunt, or some form of oesophageal transection–devascularization procedure. Perhaps transection–devascularization is the preferred option in countries where compliance with a chronic injection programme is poor or where the risk of encephalopathy after the shunt procedure is high. A recent three-centre controlled trial demonstrated similar survival following either transection or repeated sclerotherapy[3].

Preoperative

Emergency oesophageal transection carries a high rate of mortality in these seriously ill patients and should be avoided in most patients with Child's grade C disease. Even in the elective situation the operation should probably be confined to those with Child's grade A and B disease. All patients should have documented varices which have bled. Where doubt exists about the source of bleeding, ultrasonographic examination is useful to assess splenic size when the organ is not palpable or percussible (one cannot have bleeding varices without splenomegaly). The aetiology of the liver disease should be established where possible by liver function tests, serological, immunological and histological examination. Coagulation studies are essential and replacement therapy should be employed where indicated. One dose of an intravenous cephalosporin is indicated at the time of surgery because of the necessary gastrotomy in these immunocompromised patients.

Anaesthesia

Halothane is probably best avoided for medicolegal rather than good scientific reasons. The volume distribution of most non-depolarizing muscle relaxants is increased, thereby giving rise to relative resistance but a longer duration of action. Obviously good hydration with adequate diuresis is desirable to reduce the risk of the hepatorenal syndrome, but overloading should be avoided in those patients with a high risk of postoperative ascites. Care is required with postoperative analgesia because of the impaired detoxication rate of the liver.

Operations

CONTROL OF OESPHAGEAL VARICES USING A CIRCULAR STAPLER

Position of patient and incision

The patient is placed supine on the operating table and a midline epigastric incision used in most patients. Where splenectomy is considered necessary because of hypersplenism a left subcostal incision gives better exposure. Exploration of the abdomen is carried out to confirm the diagnosis and exclude other disease. In portal hypertension the spleen is always enlarged and can be damaged by careless retraction. The hard, cirrhotic liver can also cause difficulties of access to the lower oesophagus.

Exposure of the left gastric pedicle

1 The most important route transmitting the high portal pressure to the oesophageal varices is the left gastric or coronary vein. This vessel requires ligation and can be approached either through the gastrohepatic omentum or via a window in the gastrocolic omentum. The latter route gives excellent access to the lesser sac and also to the splenic artery, should one wish to carry out a splenic artery ligation for hypersplenism in patients where the spleen is not being removed.

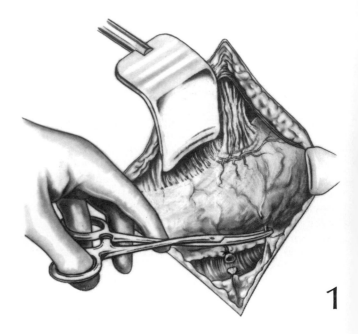

1

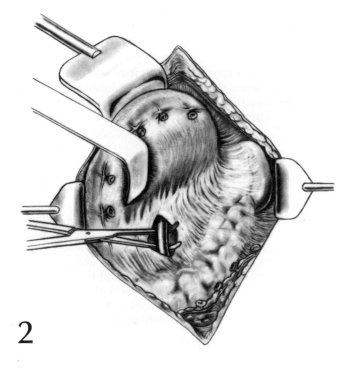

2

Ligation of the left gastric pedicle

2 The mobilized stomach is retracted upwards and adhesions in the lesser sac are divided until the left gastric pedicle is reached at the upper border of the pancreas. Even in portal hypertension these adhesions are generally not very vascular and diathermy is sufficient to control bleeding. The pedicle of the left gastric vessels is cleared sufficiently to allow vision of the main left gastric vein. It is not necessary to dissect out the individual vein, as this can give rise to unnecessary bleeding. The group of vessels present in the pedicle can be ligated in continuity using a non-absorbable suture placed by fine right-angled forceps. A number of ligatures should be applied. The largest size of metal Ligaclip should also be used as it provides a useful marker in later radiology.

Mobilization of the oesophagus

3 Attention is now turned to the region of the gastro-oesophageal junction. In portal hypertension the peritoneum on the front of the oesophagus generally contains multiple spidery venules. In spite of this extra vasculature it is usually possible to visualize the 'white line' underneath the peritoneum marking the position of the phreno-oesophageal ligament. A transverse incision is made in the peritoneum at this level, bleeding from the small peritoneal vessels being controlled by diathermy. When the phreno-oesophageal ligament has been exposed it is brushed upwards with a small gauze dissector. This exposes the oesophagus and the large perioesophageal collateral veins which lie deep to the peritoneum. The lateral and posterior aspects of the lower oesophagus are mobilized under direct vision using gauze dissection, bringing into view the large collateral channels which run with the posterior vagus nerve. This mobilization should not be done blindly, particularly if there is perioesophagitis as a result of previous injection sclerotherapy or secondary to previous reflux oesophagitis.

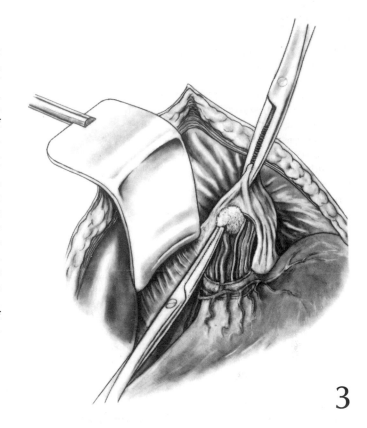

3

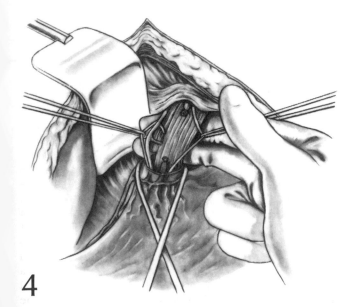

4

Devascularization of the lower oesophagus

4 There are usually one or two large collateral channels which run with the anterior vagus and a number of even larger vessels with the posterior vagus. It is usually possible to free these vessels from the vagal nerves which are then protected in Silastic slings. At this stage it is useful to place a rubber catheter sling around the oesophagus, excluding the vagal nerves. The anterior collateral veins are divided between ligatures. With the fingers of the right hand positioned behind the oesophagus the posterior veins are displaced forwards to facilitate their separation from the posterior vagus and subsequent division. It is permissible to sacrifice one of the vagi, usually the anterior, if there is significant difficulty in separating it from the venae comitantes. Some operators consider that these portoazygos collaterals should be preserved. In any case, it is essential to free the oesophagus from these large extrinsic vessels for a distance of about 6–8 cm.

Division of perforating veins

5 Perforating branches passing directly into the oesophagus from the venae comitantes require individual ligation or diathermy coagulation. Usually there are only one or two perforating branches on the front of the oesophagus but three or four such veins usually penetrate the oesophagus from the posterior vessels. It is often stated that dissection around the hiatus carries a high risk of serious haemorrhage in patients with portal hypertension but this is rarely the case. However, mobilization of the oesophagus can be more difficult in patients with perioesophagitis.

The extent of devascularization of the upper stomach depends on whether or not it is considered necessary to undertake a splenectomy. In Western society hypersplenism is not a major problem and splenectomy is indicated in a minority of patients only. If the spleen is not being removed, perhaps it is wiser not to divide the short gastric vessels since one can easily encounter troublesome bleeding, particularly if these vessels are very short.

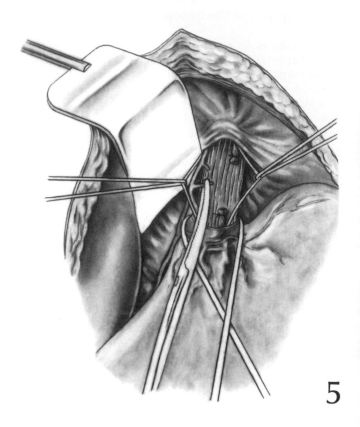

5

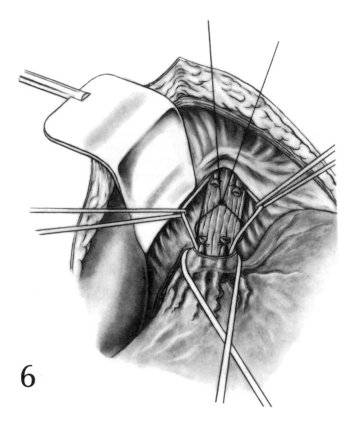

6

Placement of encircling ligature

6 A 0 linen or silk ligature is passed around the now cleared oesophagus and loosely tied. It is important to place this ligature in position before the insertion of the stapling device; with the rigid gun in position it is technically more difficult and increases the risk of damage to the oesophageal wall. Again it is important to ensure that both vagal nerves lie outside the encircling ligature.

Insertion of stapling gun

7 A small gastrotomy is made in a relatively avascular part of the anterior wall of the stomach and an obturator sizer is passed into the oesophagus to determine the largest size of gun head that can be slipped into the oesophagus without risk of damage. The correct size of EEA stapler (usually no. 28 or 31) or ILS stapler (usually 29 or 32) is selected. The closed gun is advanced via the gastrotomy into the lower oesophagus, making sure that neither the encircling ligature nor the sling around the oesophagus impede the passage of the gun up the lumen.

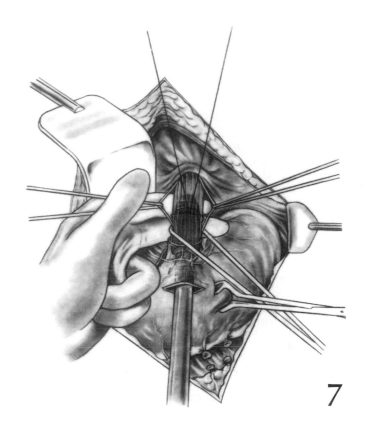

7

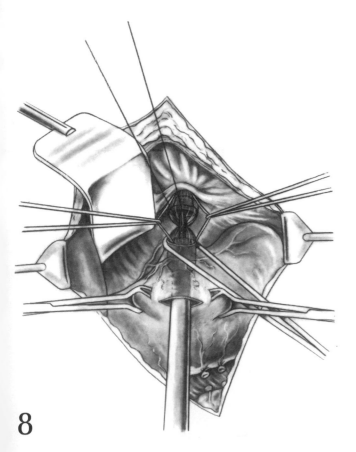

8

Technique of transection

8 When the gun has been advanced into the oesophagus for 5–6 cm, a 3-cm gap is opened up in the head and the instrument is drawn back down the oesophagus until the lowest part of the gap lies immediately above the gastro-oesophageal junction. Light traction is applied to the oesophageal sling while the assistant carefully maintains the gun in the correct position. The encircling ligature is tightened around the stem of the gun into the gap between the anvil-carrying nose cone and the staple-carrying cartridge immediately above the cardia. It is important to remove the rubber sling from around the oesophagus at this point before the head of the gun is tightened, otherwise one risks entrapment of the sling, thereby interfering with stapling. The head of the gun is closed and the trigger pulled to complete the anastomosis.

Confirmation of a satisfactory transection

9 The head of the gun is opened and the instrument drawn through the newly completed anastomosis. A complete 'doughnut' indicates a satisfactory transection. A finger is gently introduced through the gastrotomy to confirm a satisfactory suture line and to direct a nasogastric tube into the stomach for postoperative decompression. The gastrotomy wound is closed in two layers. Since a vagotomy has not been carried out, a gastric drainage procedure is not required. The abdomen is closed without drainage.

Modifications of circular stapler technique

Simple transection

In a patient with acute bleeding the operating time can be reduced by doing a simple transection alone without any devascularization. However, the risk of rebleeding may be greater although there is no controlled trial to prove this.

Addition of splenectomy

In Western society hypersplenism is rarely a significant problem. In areas where schistosomiasis is prevalent, however, massive splenomegaly is often present and splenectomy should therefore be considered almost as a routine. Splenic artery ligation alone can be useful in non-schistosomiasis patients in helping to lower portal pressure, at least on a temporary basis.

Addition of vagotomy and drainage

Although this is part of the Sugiura operation, there is no logical justification for the procedure as a routine. If there is a concomitant peptic ulcer, however, the gastrotomy for the introduction of the gun should be made in the most dependent part of the stomach and this opening subsequently used for a gastrojejunostomy in conjunction with vagotomy.

Transection of the mucosa only

Since full thickness oesophageal transection removes a portion of the lower oesophageal sphincter, Hirashima and colleagues[4] advocate mucosal transection only,

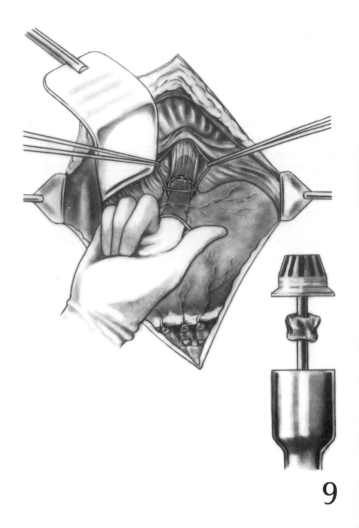

9

leaving the muscle intact. A longitudinal incision is made in the muscle layer of the distal oesophagus and a mucosal cuff isolated circumferentially using scissor dissection. A ligature is placed around the mucosa inside the oesophageal muscular tube. When the stapling gun is inserted only the mucosal flange is resected, leaving the muscular mechanism intact. The oesophageal muscle coat is then sutured over the mucosal staple line.

Addition of an antireflux procedure

Vankemmel advocates a cardioplasty using a linear stapler to provide a valvular flange in the fundus[5]. He claims that this 'gastro-oesophageal dam' minimizes gastro-oesophageal reflux. Some advocate the use of a Nissen fundoplication. This is technically easy if the spleen has been removed or the short gastric vessels divided, but is somewhat more difficult if the fundus has not been mobilized, since one cannot safely pull down on the recently sutured oesophagus.

CONTROL OF GASTRO-OESOPHAGEAL VARICES USING A LINEAR STAPLER

Transabdominal subcardiac linear stapling for oesophageal varices

Although the technique of managing bleeding varices using linear staplers is described in the literature supplied by the manufacturers of stapling instruments, very few patients have been reported and there is little evidence of the long-term effectiveness of the technique. Subcardiac linear stapling does not attack the site of bleeding in 90–95% of patients, i.e. the lower 3–5 cm of the oesophagus, and thus late rebleeding rates are high. The technique, however, has merit in a few well defined situations in patients with acutely bleeding varices:

1. Where there is a fixed hiatus hernia which causes difficulty in mobilization of the oesophagus.
2. Where the oesophagus is likely to be friable in a patient bleeding within a few days of recent sclerotherapy, particularly if there have been a number of episodes of sclerotherapy.
3. Where there is gross perioesophagitis related to previous repeated sclerotherapy, making mobilization of the oesophagus dangerous.

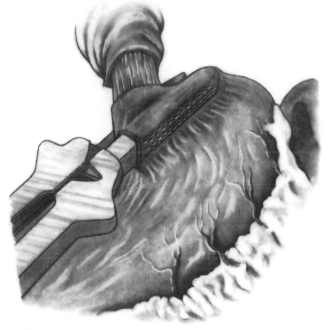

10 The stomach is exposed and the region of the gastro-oesophageal junction identified. A small gastrotomy is made on the lesser curvature of the stomach, 2 cm below the cardia, and the bleeding from the edges of the wound controlled. An SGIA 50 stapler, which contains no blade, is used. One limb is inserted inside the stomach via the gastrotomy and advanced to the top of the fundus. The second limb is placed on the anterior gastric wall on the serosal aspect and the gun closed and fired. Four lines of staples are inserted into the anterior gastric wall. The identical procedure is carried out on the posterior gastric wall and the gastrotomy closed. Nasogastric aspiration is advisable for a few days.

10

Cardiofundectomy for gastric varices

Although gastric varices account for well under 10% of all variceal bleeding, they are a particularly difficult problem. Sclerotherapy is technically difficult and often ineffectual. Direct suturing gives temporary control but rebleeding is common. Even portal systemic shunts do not always stop bleeding from gastric varices. Yu and colleagues have described an oblique cardiofundectomy for the control of bleeding gastric varices[6].

11 Initially the oesophagus and upper stomach are devascularized and Yu and colleagues also advise splenectomy. This gives easy access for the TA90 stapler, applied obliquely across the fundus of the stomach from halfway down the greater curvature to within about 2 cm of the gastro-oesophageal junction. The gun is fired and the redundant fundic area with its tortuous varices excised and the gun removed. It is wise to add a continuous seromuscular suture of 2/0 polyglactin (Vicryl) to ensure complete haemostasis. Nasogastric aspiration is advised for a few days.

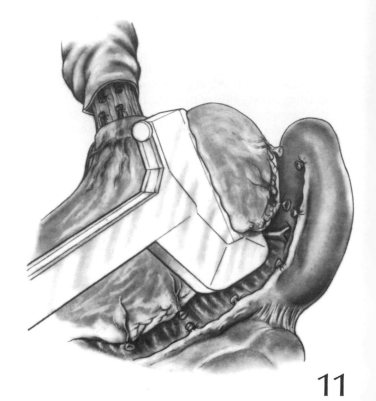

11

Postoperative care

Following transection nasogastric aspiration continues for 24–48 h after surgery and oral fluids are withheld until the 5th postoperative day. There is no indication for radiological studies before starting oral fluids. In some patients increasing ascites may be a problem postoperatively and the cautious use of diuretics is required. On returning to solid food the patients are warned that they may experience some temporary dysphagia. With modern staplers only about 5% require later oesophageal dilatation.

Outcome

Since January 1976 the author has performed 136 stapled oesophageal transections with devascularization. Only 27 were done as emergencies, the remainder being performed electively, often during the same hospital admission but usually within a few weeks of the onset of bleeding. In addition to oesophageal transection and subdiaphragmatic devascularization, 26 patients had splenectomy and 12 had splenic artery ligation because of hypersplenism. There were 22 operative deaths in the series, 10 of these occurring in patients with Child's grade C disease. There were eight deaths in the 27 patients undergoing emergency transection, giving an emergency mortality of 30%

compared with a 13% mortality rate for the 109 patients undergoing an elective procedure. No patient developed a suture line leak. However, two patients did have oesophageal leaks; both occurred about 2 cm above the anastomosis and were thought to be related to intraoperative dilatation before transection. One of these patients died from mediastinitis and the other survived following simple suture. Fifteen patients in the series required oesophageal dilatation because of stricture formation. Of the 114 patients who survived to leave hospital, 42 have had recurrent haemorrhage in a follow-up period extending from 3 months to 16 years. Often recurrent haemorrhage was of a minor nature and only 7 of the 42 patients died as a result of bleeding. Where recurrent varices were identified as the cause, post-transection sclerotherapy was used in 28 of the patients. The overall 5-year and 10-year cumulative survival rates for the whole series were 46% and 27%, respectively. Forty-seven patients remain alive at the time of review and the majority are well and free of jaundice, ascites or encephalopathy.

References

1. Sugiura M, Futagawa S. A new technique for treating oesophageal varices. *J Thorac Cardiovasc Surg* 1973; 66: 677–85.

2. Burroughs AK, Hamilton G, Phillips A, Mezzanotte G, McIntyre N, Hobbs KEF. A comparison of sclerotherapy with staple transection of the esophagus for the emergency control of bleeding from esophageal varices. *N Engl J Med* 1989; 321: 857–62.

3. Triger DR, Johnson AG, Spencer EFA *et al*. A controlled trial comparing endoscopic sclerothrapy with oesophagogastric devascularisation and transection in the long term management of bleeding esophageal varices. *Gut* 1990; 31: A592.

4. Hirashima T, Hara T, Benitani A, Juan I-K, Sato H. A new stapling technique in esophageal mucosal transection. *Jpn J Surg* 1982; 12: 160–2.

5. Vankemmel MH. Highly selective portal decompression for bleeding esophageal varices. *Int Surg* 1985; 70: 125–8.

6. Yu T-J, Cheng K-K, Lai S-T *et al*. A new operation for the management of gastric varix bleeding. *Chinese Med J (Taipei)* 1989; 43: 49–56.

Illustrations by Diane Kinton

Perforated peptic ulcer

F. J. Branicki DM, FRCS
Department of Surgery, University of Queensland, Royal Brisbane Hospital, Queensland, Australia

Principles and justification

Perforated peptic ulcer may be suspected following the sudden onset of abdominal pain in a patient presenting with signs of peritoneal irritation, even in the absence of a history of peptic ulceration. A diagnosis of visceral perforation may be substantiated by the presence of free gas on plain abdominal radiographic examination and this is evident in up to 92% of patients with perforated duodenal ulcer; it is possible to detect as little as 1 ml of free gas on scrutiny of erect and supine films. Voluminous free gas is usually evident following gastric perforation.

Conservative management

Prospective trials have shown that three risk factors merit consideration: (1) a history of concomitant medical illness (diabetes mellitus, cardiovascular disorders, pulmonary disease, etc.); (2) history of duration of perforation greater than 24 h; and (3) hypotension (systolic blood pressure < 100 mmHg) on presentation[1]. Any one risk factor militates against any form of definitive surgery for perforation in the absence of haemorrhage. In the presence of all three risk factors surgery is very often associated with a fatal outcome – open surgical intervention in such a patient is obviously inappropriate and conservative, non-operative management is advisable. The use of combination antibiotic therapy, total parenteral nutrition in the fasted patient undergoing continuous gastric decompression, and the possibility of percutaneous drainage under image guidance of intra-abdominal infected collections which may become apparent, hold the best prospects for survival in the moribund patient.

A perforated duodenal ulcer may seal spontaneously with fibrin, omentum or by contact with adjacent organs. Conservative management may be advocated[2], particularly if abdominal symptoms and signs on serial physical examination are improving. When conservative treatment is contemplated a Gastrografin swallow should be performed soon after admission to determine whether any free extravasation of contrast material is evident. A conservative management regimen, without resort to surgery for perforated duodenal ulcer, has been shown in a randomized trial to carry a mortality rate comparable with simple closure, although the subsequent duration of hospital stay was greater in the non-operated group[2]. If abdominal signs do not improve within 6 h of first assessment on admission, surgery is recommended.

It is unwise to adhere to a non-operative management plan if free leakage of contrast medium into the peritoneal cavity is seen, laparotomy then being advisable unless the patient has all three risk factors for mortality following simple closure of the perforation[1] and is moribund.

Surgical management

The consensus among general surgeons is that surgical intervention is necessary in most patients with gastroduodenal perforation, but there is less accord with regard to the desirability of definitive antiulcer surgery in an emergency setting. The advent of satisfactory medical therapy for peptic ulcer has led many surgeons to advocate simple closure with antiulcer medication and subsequent maintenance therapy and lifelong treatment may be sensible in patients with concurrent medical disorders. Simple closure is safe in even relatively inexperienced hands but carries the disadvantage that, in the absence of long-term antiulcer treatment, recurrence is a major cause of morbidity in patients with acute[3] or chronic[1] duodenal ulceration. There is evidence to support an individualized management policy, with definitive surgery in the form of highly selective vagotomy following simple closure and lavage being recommended for the low-risk patient[3].

Perforated duodenal ulcer

No human data have confirmed that mediastinitis is a cause for concern following mobilization of the oesophagus to facilitate vagotomy in a contaminated peritoneal cavity; nevertheless, a definitive antiulcer procedure is not recommended for the surgeon who lacks expertise in gastric surgery. There is, however, general agreement that perforation associated with overt gastric haemorrhage does require definitive antiulcer surgery rather than simple closure alone. Postoperative gastrointestinal haemorrhage may arise from a suture line, from the primary ulcer or from a second 'overlooked' lesion. Simple closure of a small anterior/superior perforation of a duodenal ulcer may not enable adequate inspection of the posteromedial duodenal wall. Postoperative haemorrhage is a well recognized risk in patients with so-called 'kissing' duodenal ulcers, subjected to simple closure of a perforated anterior ulcer without recognition of a second posterior lesion. Endoscopic documentation of antecedent ulceration at multiple sites is usually lacking and the operating surgeon usually has no knowledge of the likelihood of ulceration at several sites, before or even during laparotomy, when such a possibility is often not even considered. An awareness of ulcer disease previously diagnosed at endoscopy and the nature and extent of recent active lesions is of value when surgical strategy is under deliberation.

Occasionally at operation a duodenal ulcer may be found to have already spontaneously closed, being sealed by omentum or fibrin. In these circumstances, unless the site of the perforation is thoroughly inspected, it is impossible to determine the exact nature of the perforation and the strength of the fibrin seal, which may be very thin and tenuous. A greater degree of confidence as to outcome may be obtained by taking down the seal and closely inspecting the perforation site before proceeding with simple closure, with or without definitive surgery. In addition, real concerns exist as to the safety of omental patch repair for closure of a perforation greater than 2 cm in diameter, some form of excisional surgery being preferred. Options for excisional surgery include vagotomy and antrectomy with gastroduodenal or gastrojejunal reconstruction or Pólya gastrectomy. Simple closure of even small perforations is not generally recommended; sutures may cut out and the defect increase in size – omental patch repair is generally the procedure of choice, with or without definitive surgery.

In the author's experience, there has been no hospital fatality from definitive surgery in patients without any of the three identifiable risk factors already mentioned[1] who were managed by omental patch repair and highly selective vagotomy. The only major mobidity encountered, requiring a lengthy hospital stay, occurred in a patient who developed a biliary fistula, subsequently demonstrated to arise from the site of duodenal closure. This highlights the need to seal the leaking duodenum adequately.

Perforated gastric ulcer

When perforated gastric ulcer is encountered at laparotomy, there is always the concern that the ulcer may be malignant, because even frozen section may fail to confirm underlying malignant disease. Gastric ulcers are often larger than duodenal ulcers and simple closure may give rise to further leakage. With the exception of high-risk surgical candidates, perforated gastric ulcer is best managed by gastrectomy: there is little place for ulcer excision alone and suture closure of the defect. When operative and/or histological findings suggest that a gastric perforation is likely to be neoplastic in origin, it is preferable to perform a gastric resection along the lines practised for malignancy proven preoperatively at endoscopic biopsy. Despite the fact that perforation of a gastric neoplasm is associated with intraperitoneal seeding of malignant cells, a radical gland dissection is justifiable in the absence of disseminated macroscopic disease, provided that the patient's general condition is satisfactory. Gastric resection, deferred for 1 week following patch repair of a perforated gastric neoplasm, is preferred in the patient deemed to be unfit for the procedure at first presentation.

Perforated stomal ulcer

Simple closure alone is advisable in the high-risk surgical candidate with perforated stomal ulcer. In fit patients definitive treatment is recommended but complete vagotomy following an incomplete procedure in the past is not for the inexperienced surgeon. Indeed, a gastric resection may be accomplished with greater ease and safety. The choice of procedure will depend on the patient's general condition and the exact nature of previous surgery. Multiple sites of ulceration may be identified in a patient found at laparotomy to have perforation of a single ulcer. If the patient's general condition permits, some form of definitive therapy is advisable, particularly if the need for non-steroidal anti-inflammatory drugs (NSAIDs) is ongoing.

Preoperative

Once a diagnosis of perforated peptic ulcer has been made on clinical and/or radiological grounds, effective analgesia is prescribed. A vented nasogastric tube of large calibre is inserted to enable continuous decompression of the stomach. Shaving of the abdominal skin is unnecessary in many patients, and may be deferred until anaesthesia has been induced. An intravenous infusion is established and occasionally rapid correction of extracellular fluid deficit is necessary in the hypotensive patient. Although most patients are afebrile on admission, broad-spectrum antibiotic therapy (e.g. cephalosporin and metronidazole) is commenced before surgery if gross contamination is suspected. In patients presenting with hypotension, an indwelling urethral catheter is passed to enable urinary output to be monitored, preoperatively and at least hourly in the postoperative period. In most patients over 60 years of age preoperative prophylaxis against venous thromboembolism is wise (heparin, 5000 units twice daily) unless there is evidence of concomitant overt haemorrhage or if multiple sites of ulceration are suspected.

Anaesthesia

Surgery is usually performed under general anaesthesia. Thoracic epidural anaesthesia provides adequate analgesia in the immediate postoperative period, and is particularly useful for patients with pulmonary disease.

Operations

Incision

The incision of choice for upper abdominal emergency surgery is a midline incision. An upper midline incision gives adequate exposure for simple closure of a perforation and/or definitive surgery. Open operation for visceral perforation requires access sufficient to enable adequate peritoneal lavage with (preferably) Hartmann's solution which, in contrast to normal saline, does not interfere with macrophage function in the first 24 h after surgery.

In patients presenting late with a large perforation, gross contamination of the abdominal cavity often requires the removal of fluid collections and also of food debris. A decision to proceed with definitive surgery requires the midline skin incision to be extended superiorly. A paraxiphoid extension of the incision is particularly important in obese patients, in whom access to the oesophageal hiatus may be otherwise poor. In addition, it is sometimes necessary to continue the incision inferiorly beyond the umbilicus. This distal extension may be made during the course of the procedure should access prove inadequate. The author's preference is to use an Upper Hand (Hepco) retractor. With the use of self-retaining retractors for each costal margin it is usually unnecessary for an assistant to have to retract costal margin or liver during the performance of a highly selective vagotomy or gastric resection.

It is salutary to recall that patients presenting with features of perforated peptic ulcer may, at first sight, have no gross abnormality apparent on opening the abdominal cavity. It is particularly important to open the lesser sac, aspirate any contents in its deepest recesses in the left upper quadrant, and inspect with great care the posterior gastric wall superiorly. Unless such attention to detail is paid, a small perforation with minimal contamination in the lesser sac may be overlooked.

SIMPLE CLOSURE OF PERFORATED DUODENAL ULCER

At laparotomy the diagnosis is confirmed and free gastroduodenal contents are aspirated with a sump sucker inserted in subphrenic, subhepatic, paracolic, infracolic and pelvic compartments. Repeated peritoneal lavage is usually withheld until the perforation has been closed or the lesion excised.

The stomach can be retracted to the left in a gauze swab held by the assistant; in obese individuals the duodenum may be brought to a more accessible position by manipulating the nasogastric tube until it lies close to the anterior gastric wall adjacent to the greater curvature of the stomach and then holding the nasogastric tube by a Babcock's clamp, over a gauze swab, to facilitate safe gastric retraction without fear of slippage. The Babcock's clamp is sited just proximal to the pylorus. The position of the Babcock's clamp may be adjusted during the procedure to provide optimal access and avoid damage from prolonged application to the gastric wall.

1 Most duodenal perforations are less than 1 cm in size and are amenable to expeditious omental patch repair. Application of an omental patch requires prior placement of a series (three or four only for small ulcers) of interrupted absorbable sutures. For small perforations the sutures may be placed directly through the wall to the lumen of the duodenum to emerge on the far side of the ulcer for retrieval.

In larger ulcers, suture placement requires retrieval from within the site of perforation before passage within the lumen to the opposite side. This is cumbersome and is not recommended. Dissolution of absorbable sutures must also be borne in mind and it is advisable not to place the sutures through the open lumen but to take transverse seromuscular bites of the viscus on either side of the ulcer. Arterial haemostats may be placed on the end of each suture before tying each one over an omental patch. It is not usually necessary to fashion an omental frond as a redundant portion of omentum which does not need division is available.

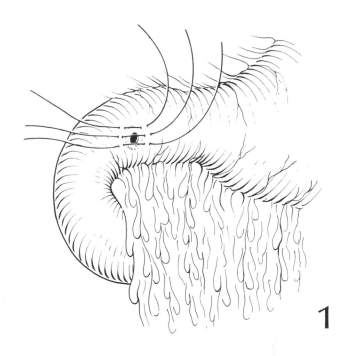

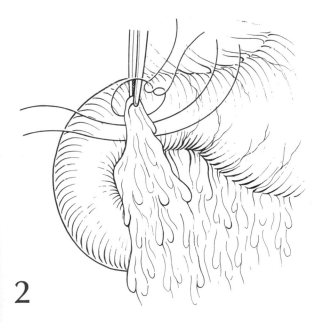

2 A seromuscular suture is placed through the duodenum superior to the perforation and is passed through the apex of the selected area of omentum. This suture is the first to be tied and fixes the apex of the omentum to a site beyond the ulcer, obscuring the site of perforation from view.

3 The sutures are released in turn from the haemostats and are then tied, without tension, to avoid the possibility of ischaemia in the patch or cutting out of the sutures.

Interrupted non-absorbable sutures are then placed to join the patch and the duodenal wall to isolate the site of perforation and make it watertight. This is particularly important when the perforation is larger than usual and excisional surgery is considered inadvisable in view of the patient's poor general condition.

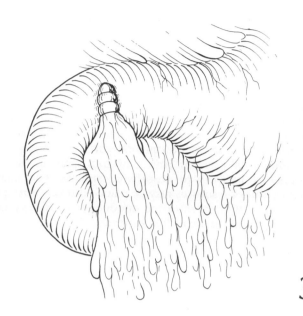

3

PERFORATED DUODENAL ULCER WITH OBSTRUCTION

A combination of significant duodenal obstruction and perforation is unusual. A chronically stenosed fibrotic duodenum is unlikely to perforate spontaneously at this stage in the natural history of the disease but occasionally, intraoperative concern is raised that omental patch repair will be followed by postoperative gastric outlet obstruction. However, oedema and inflammatory damage in the duodenal wall adjacent to a perforated ulcer are responsible for the appearances and these often subside in the postoperative period. Gastroenterostomy or gastric resection are usually unnecessary, except to treat the small perforation which occurs within ulceration which is almost circumferential in nature. In these circumstances a patch repair may be followed by progressive stenosis as ulceration heals postoperatively on medical management. If circumferential ulceration is suspected at the time of perforation then vagotomy and antrectomy are advocated, but the latter procedure should be avoided in patients over 60 years of age as it may be associated with functional gastric outlet obstruction, in the absence of mechanical hold-up, and may take up to 6 weeks to resolve. In the elderly, who tolerate prolonged hospitalization less well, a Pólya gastrectomy is preferable.

PERFORATED DUODENAL ULCER WITH HAEMORRHAGE

While posterior duodenal ulcers are more likely to bleed than anterior ulcers, large anterior ulcers may occasionally present with features of overt haematemesis and/or melaena and free perforation. Simple ulcer closure is inappropriate and some form of

definitive surgery is required. Plication following adequate luminal exposure and subsequent truncal vagotomy and pyloroplasty or gastroenterostomy is inappropriate for the large (>2 cm) anterior ulcer. Excisional surgery is advocated in these circumstances; truncal vagotomy and antrectomy are associated with the lowest rate of ulcer recurrence and provide for a larger gastric remnant, and therefore are advocated in preference to Pólya gastrectomy in younger patients.

In the patient with a combination of free perforation and haemorrhage arising from a small anterior ulcer of the duodenum, ulcer excision with subsequent pyloromyotomy to include the defect and pyloroplasty closure is recommended, followed by truncal vagotomy. Personal experience has led to the view that the more time-consuming procedure of highly selective vagotomy is not justifiable as definitive surgery in most patients presenting with bleeding peptic ulcer, particularly in the elderly if there has been evidence of shock on presentation. Patients presenting with haemorrhage often have concomitant medical illness in concert with haemorrhagic instability. Accordingly, the more expeditious procedure of truncal vagotomy and pyloroplasty is advised for bleeding duodenal ulcer with ulcer excision/plication, the use of highly selective vagotomy being confined to relatively fit younger patients[4].

DEFINITIVE OPERATION FOR PERFORATED DUODENAL ULCER

There is little doubt that, for the patient with a long history of protracted peptic ulcer disease or those in whom gastrointestinal bleeding/perforation has occurred in the past, definitive surgery is the preferred option. Experience in Hong Kong, where peptic ulcer disease reaches almost epidemic proportions, has shown that even patients with acute ulceration presenting with perforation fare better in the long term with definitive antiulcer surgery in the form of omental patch repair and highly selective vagotomy[3]. However, this report documents the results obtained by a small group of surgeons with particular experience of the procedure in an elective setting and it would be inappropriate to recommend highly selective vagotomy in combination with patch repair on a widespread basis to surgeons with little or infrequent practice of the technique.

Highly selective vagotomy has a greater role to play in the management of perforated duodenal ulcer than is currently promoted. This view implies a thorough training in operative technique, which can give good results even without intraoperative testing. In the absence of familiarity with the procedure, a truncal vagotomy and pyloroplasty with closure of the defect is advocated. Recurrent perforation with localized abdominal signs occurring in the days following patch repair may be treated conservatively in the absence of haemodynamic instability, but haemodynamic instability or generalized peritonitis merits surgical intervention, either further omental patch repair or gastric resection with truncal vagotomy and antrectomy or Pólya gastrectomy.

PERFORATED GASTRIC ULCER

Optimal treatment of a perforated benign gastric ulcer is dependent on its location. Prepyloric ulceration is amenable to truncal vagotomy and antrectomy in patients under 60 years. For patients with ulceration at the angulus incisura or on the lesser curvature, Billroth gastrectomy with gastroduodenal reconstruction is preferable. Gastric ulcers are often large, and closure is more difficult, with a propensity for early reperforation. Simple closure is advisable for patients presenting with risk factors previously described for duodenal ulcer[1] or when a small ulcer perforation is suspected to be drug related (e.g. NSAID ingestion). Simple closure of a gastric ulcer may be accomplished in much the same manner as for duodenal ulcer, although division of the gastrocolic or gastrohepatic omentum may be required to provide adequate access.

PERFORATED STOMAL ULCER

Stomal ulcer perforation is often dealt with by simple closure. Subsequently the acid secretory status of the patient may be investigated with appropriate decisions for management strategy. If, however, the patient is considered to be in a satisfactory condition, some form of definitive procedure is preferable, either omental patch repair combined with vagotomy or gastric resection. If the previous operation was a partial gastrectomy, truncal vagotomy is the procedure of choice and will obviate the hazards of a further gastric

resection. Perforation of stomal ulcer is rare following vagotomy and gastroenterostomy but the services of an accomplished gastric surgeon are required for completion of a previously inadequate vagotomy or, perhaps, gastric resection.

Postoperative care

Following simple closure of a perforated duodenal ulcer, peritoneal lavage with at least 3 litres of Hartmann's solution should be performed and should be continued until the aspirated intra-abdominal fluid is no longer turbid. Intra-abdominal drainage is unnecessary in the majority of patients: it is prudent, however, to drain the right subhepatic space with a large-bore drain, if closure of a large perforated ulcer has been performed in a patient unfit for excisional surgery. A drain should be chosen so that, should leakage around the patch occur, it will excite an inflammatory reaction to produce a conduit for a fistulous track on withdrawal. In this situation latex rubber is preferred.

Gastrointestinal haemorrhage should be investigated with upper endoscopy, which can be safely performed, despite suture lines and air insufflation, 2–3 days following surgery. The identification of a bleeding site suitable for therapeutic endoscopic measures with, for example, adrenaline 1:10 000 injection is the goal for the control of continued or recurrent haemorrhage. Endoscopic application of diathermy near a suture line is best avoided early in the postoperative period because of the possible risk of disruption with anastomotic leakage.

Future developments

The adoption of laparoscopic techniques for oversewing of duodenal ulcer perforation[5] is certain to become more widespread. The use of definitive laparoscopic antiulcer surgery, posterior truncal vagotomy and anterior seromyotomy has been described in an elective setting for the treatment of duodenal ulceration[6]. It is likely that definitive antiulcer laparoscopic surgery in combination with patch repair will be introduced in the immediate future. In the high-risk patient the use of laparoscopic techniques must be monitored with suitable randomized trials to evaluate long-term efficacy.

References

1. Boey J, Choi SKY, Poon A, Alagaratnam TT. Risk stratification in perforated duodenal ulcers: a prospective validation of predictive factors. *Ann Surg* 1987; 205: 22–6.

2. Crofts TJ, Park KG, Steele RJ, Chung SS, Li AK. A randomized trial of nonoperative treatment for perforated peptic ulcer. *N Engl J Med* 1989; 320: 970–3.

3. Boey J, Branicki FJ, Alagaratnam TT *et al.* Proximal gastric vagotomy. The preferred operation for perforations in acute duodenal ulcer. *Ann Surg* 1988; 208: 169–74.

4. Branicki FJ, Coleman SY, Fok PJ *et al.* Bleeding peptic ulcer: a prospective evaluation of risk factors for rebleeding and mortality. *World J Surg* 1990; 14: 262–70.

5. Nathanson LK, Easter DW, Cuschieri A. Laparoscopic repair/peritoneal toilet of perforated duodenal ulcer. *Surg Endosc* 1990; 4: 232–3.

6. Katkhouda N, Mouiel J. A new technique of surgical treatment of chronic duodenal ulcer without laparotomy by videocoelioscopy. *Am J Surg* 1991; 161: 361–4.

General techniques in abdominal laparoscopic surgery

Allan E. Siperstein MD
Department of Surgery, Mount Zion Medical Center of University of California, San Francisco, USA

Laparoscopic surgery promises to be a major revolution in the field of general surgery. It is now realized that the pain and other inflammatory mediators resulting from a large abdominal incision, rather than the intra-abdominal dissection, are the major determinants of speed of perioperative recuperation. The advantages of minimally invasive surgery are well known in other surgical disciplines such as gynaecology and orthopaedics, and general surgeons have been relatively slow in adopting this technology. Several years ago, laparoscopic cholecystectomy was considered to be a clinical curiosity and its acceptance by the surgical community was delayed, in part because of its radical departure from standard surgical practice and in part because it was developed outside major academic centres. A variety of complex general surgical procedures, including colonic resection, gastric resection, Nissen fundoplication, adrenalectomy and even Whipple procedures have now been successfully performed laparoscopically, and it is felt by many in the field that in the future the majority of cases will be performed laparoscopically, including operations such as hepatic resection and vascular anastomoses.

Factors driving the rapid advancement in laparoscopic surgery are rapid recovery and discharge of the patient from hospital. There appear to be fewer wound problems, especially with infection and dehiscence, as the small portals of entry result in far less tissue devascularization. There is also considerable drive from the patients to have their procedures performed laparoscopically because of the decreased perioperative pain, an earlier return to work and a better cosmetic result. Reports of higher complication rates with laparoscopic surgery, especially among surgeons with more limited experience, are cause for concern. As the surgeon's experience increases, the complication rate decreases significantly to the point where currently the rate of complications of laparoscopic cholecystectomy may be the same as, or lower than, that for open cholecystectomy.

This chapter will review the major techniques common to laparoscopic surgery. Previously, emphasis has been placed on reinventing operations so that they may be undertaken laparoscopically. Now there is more emphasis placed on applying the tried and established methods of open surgery to laparoscopic procedures. Although much of the instrumentation may be different, the honoured principles of gentle tissue handling, careful dissection, exposure and haemostasis apply equally to both open and laparoscopic surgery.

Equipment

Video cameras

1 The technical advance that made laparoscopic surgery practical, although it had been in theory possible for many decades, was the advent of the single chip camera. This was small enough to be used practically in the operating room.

Previously, laparoscopic procedures, mostly diagnostic, had been widely performed; however, the surgeon had to look directly through the laparoscope so that only one person at a time in the operating room could view the field. This made it possible for a single operator to perform only diagnostic laparoscopy and simple tissue manipulation and biopsy. Beam splitters were developed that allowed two surgeons to look through the same laparoscope simultaneously, but these were cumbersome and reduced the brightness of the field considerably. With the advent of the video camera attached to the end of the laparoscope, it is now possible for all personnel in the operating room to view the operative field comfortably.

Laparoscopic surgery also represents a new era of technical and electronic complexity in the operating room, requiring a variety of electronic equipment, including cameras, light sources, insufflators, television monitors and often video cassette recorders and video printers. This equipment is delicate, expensive and requires considerable training in its use and maintenance. As all personnel are able to view the operative field equally well, this has resulted in a different level of interaction between the surgeons and the nursing staff. Once the nurses are trained in the step-by-step conduct of the procedure, they are better able to anticipate the instrument needs of the surgeon.

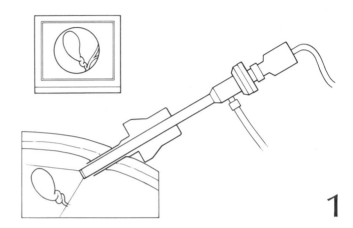

1

Instruments

2a–i Laparoscopic surgery presents several major limitations not present in open surgery. A more limited array of instruments is available, but new instrumentation is evolving rapidly, with many new and innovative products being brought to market. Currently there is a variety of instruments, such as straight and curved dissectors, scissors, cautery devices, bowel graspers, and more that are of a design very similar to that used in open surgery. A major limitation placed on the surgeon is the restricted degree of freedom of instrument movement imposed by working through ports placed through the abdominal wall. The surgeon is able to move the instrument in and out of the port, rotate it along the axis of the port and pivot it around its fixed point in the abdominal wall. This is considerably more limiting than the movements possible by the human arm and hand, and requires new skills so that instrument movement is not clumsy. The laparoscopic surgeon manipulates a three-dimensional world on a two-dimensional television monitor and therefore lacks binocular vision. Depth perception is considerably impaired, often resulting in repetitive motions of underpointing or pastpointing. As the surgeon's hands are no longer able to manipulate tissue directly, there is severely diminished tactile feedback. By probing the tissues with an instrument the surgeon is able to gain some idea as to how rigid or mobile a structure is but this sense is obviously severely impaired.

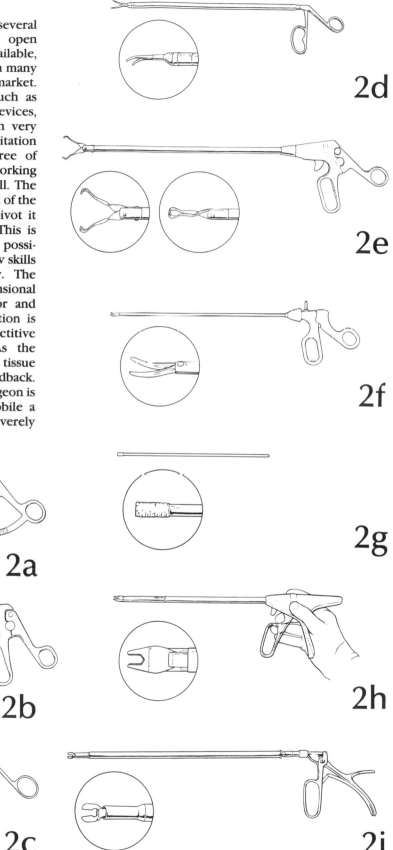

2d

2e

2f

2g

2h

2i

2a

2b

2c

Operative techniques

Abdominal procedures

3 A prerequisite for performing a laparoscopic procedure is creation of a potential working space within the abdominal cavity as well as the use of trochars to provide a portal for entry. This is most commonly done by insufflating the peritoneal cavity with carbon dioxide gas to a pressure of 15 mmHg. Insufflators now exist that automatically sense the intra-abdominal pressure and deliver carbon dioxide gas at a controlled rate until the desired pressure is established.

4 To create a pneumoperitoneum, the most common technique is to create an infraumbilical incision where the abdominal wall is thin. It is then important that the abdominal wall is pulled upwards, usually with towel clips, to create a negative intra-abdominal pressure so that a specially designed Veress needle can be passed into the abdominal cavity. The needle itself is designed with a spring-loaded blunt tip that retracts into the shaft of the needle when pushed against the tissues. This exposes the sharp tip of the needle which may be felt to pop twice as it crosses first the fascia and then the peritoneum. The spring-loaded blunt tip then slides forward, protecting the viscera from the sharp needle tip. The purpose of pulling up on the abdominal wall is both to put the fascia under tension and to create a negative intra-abdominal pressure so that when the needle enters the peritoneal cavity, air begins to enter the peritoneum through the needle, further helping to keep the needle tip away from the viscera.

Various methods have been described to try to improve the safety of this technique. The patient is placed in a Trendelenburg position so that the viscera moves cephalad and the needle is directed towards the pelvis to minimize the chance of entering the aorta or vena cava. It is most important, however, to appreciate the tactile feedback from the Veress needle such that advancement is stopped once the needle is felt to enter the peritoneal cavity. The major contraindication to use of the Veress needle is previous abdominal surgery in the area where the needle is to be placed, as the viscera may have adhered to the abdominal wall.

Once the tip of the needle is felt to be within the peritoneal cavity, it is essential to perform a saline drop test. A syringe with saline is affixed to the needle; the most important part of this test is actually drawing back on the syringe to make sure that neither the bowel nor a blood vessel has been entered. A small amount of saline is then gently injected, feeling that there is no undue resistance. Finally, the syringe is taken off the Veress needle and the small amount of saline left in the hub of the needle is seen to drop freely into the peritoneal cavity. At this point it is safe to attach the hose from the insufflator to the Veress needle and begin insufflation

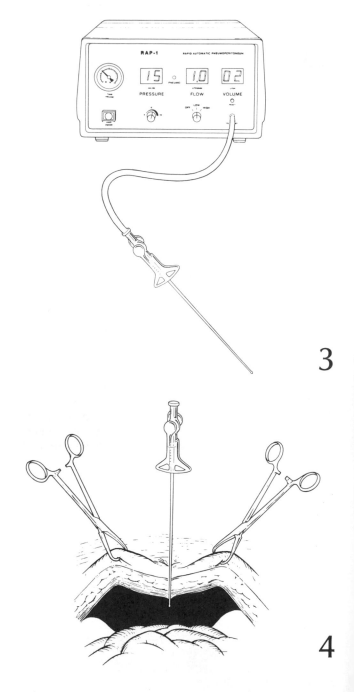

with carbon dioxide at a low rate for at least the first litre. The abdomen should be percussed at this point to ensure that a pneumoperitoneum is being established. While gas is being introduced, it is important to see that the abdomen is distending symmetrically, otherwise the tip of the needle may have inadvertently entered the viscera. To reduce potential complications further, all patients should have nasogastric tubes and Foley catheters placed before the beginning of the procedure so that these structures are maximally decompressed. During the process of insufflation it is best to keep the Veress needle still to minimize the chance of bowel laceration.

Placement of trocars

5 Once pneumoperitoneum has been established to 15 mm pressure, a 10-mm diameter laparoscopic trocar for the camera is placed through the infraumbilical incision. Most of the designs today consist of a sharp metal point for cutting through the abdominal wall and some mechanism to prevent the point from cutting the viscera once it has entered the abdominal cavity. After the Veress needle has been withdrawn, the trocar is pushed with constant pressure, sometimes with a slight twisting motion, to advance it through the abdominal wall. It is important to apply most of the force through the wrist rather than the shoulder. In addition, the other hand should grip the shaft of the trocar to prevent sudden overadvancement of the trocar into the underlying structures once it has cut through the abdominal wall. Again, tactile feedback is important to place these trocars safely. The sudden decrease in resistance as the trocar goes through the abdominal wall and the subtle click of the safety shield coming into place should alert the surgeon that the tip of the trocar has entered the peritoneal cavity. The centre core of the trocar is then removed, leaving a thin tube through the abdominal wall with some type of valve arrangement to retain the pneumoperitoneum when no instrument is in the trocar.

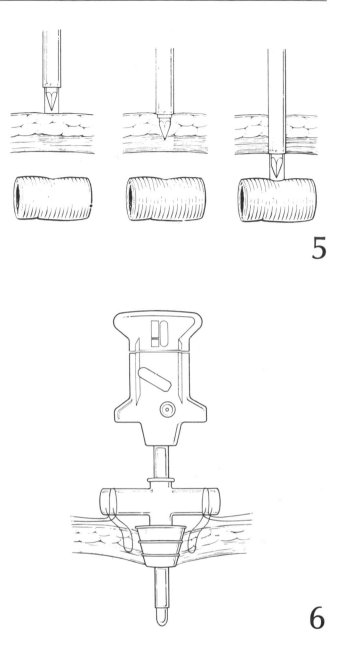

5

6

6 Alternative methods exist for obtaining access to the abdominal cavity. Hasson has developed a blunt-tipped trocar that bears his name.

It is inserted by performing a small, usually infraumbilical, cut down so that the peritoneal cavity can be entered directly. Once this has been done, the blunt-tipped trocar is passed under direct vision into the abdominal cavity, and as a slightly larger skin incision must be made, sutures are used to approximate tissue and to hold the trocar in place. The method is indicated in patients who have had previous surgical incisions near the intended site of trocar placement. In fact, this method offers several advantages and should be considered for routine use. As the abdominal cavity is entered directly and without sharp instruments, the risk of bowel or vessel injury is minimized. In addition, as the diameter of this trocar is much larger than that of the Veress needle, the pneumoperitoneum may be established much more rapidly, allowing the laparoscope to be introduced into the abdomen and the procedure started before the full pneumoperitoneum has been established. Many patients have a small umbilical hernia and this pre-existing fascial defect is easily and quickly entered with the Hasson trocar.

Other alternative methods to pneumoperitoneum establishment have been described using so-called gasless laparoscopy where the potential space in the peritoneal cavity is created by lifting up on the abdominal wall with a device placed within the peritoneal cavity. One potential advantage of such an approach is that there is no risk of gas embolization in the creation of the pneumoperitoneum. Another is that trocars may be used without the valves or reducers which are necessary for an airtight fit in conventional laparoscopy. What has limited the widespread acceptance of such devices is the fact that they create less space within the abdominal cavity. The technique may be suitable for more limited procedures.

To access the thoracic cavity, no gas needs to be instilled. In fact, this should in general be avoided because of the risk of gas embolism. A small incision is made between the ribs and a valveless trocar may be placed directly into the thoracic cavity. Double-lumen endotracheal tubes are used and the lung on the operated side is allowed to deflate.

Laparoscopes

7a–d The laparoscope consists of a metal rod usually 10 mm in diameter with a viewing port as well as another channel for illuminating the field via a fibreoptic cable connected to a light source. The camera is clipped to the back of the laparoscope, thus allowing the image to be displayed on a television monitor. The simplest laparoscopes to use are the 0° or end-viewing design in which the field of view is directly ahead of the scope. An alternative design is for the field of view to be angled at 30° or 45° from the axis of the laparoscope. The advantage of this configuration is that the laparoscope may be moved in an arc allowing two sides of a given structure to be observed. With the 0° laparoscope it is possible only to move nearer to or farther from an object but not to change the angle of view. With more complex laparoscopic procedures it is highly desirable to be able to view a given structure from different angles during the course of dissection. Although the field of view is generally small, it is highly magnified, allowing fine structures, even small blood vessels, to be identified.

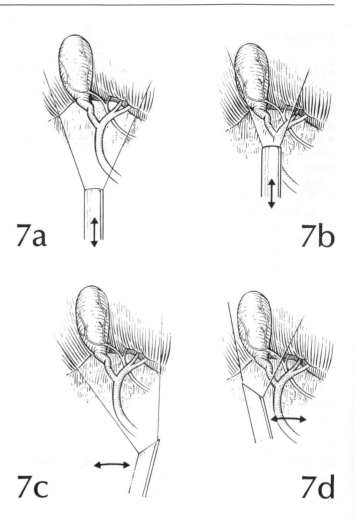

7a

7b

7c

7d

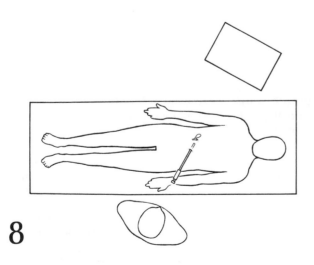

8

8 For the direction of instrument movement to correspond with what is seen on the television monitor, it is important for the surgeon to be positioned directly behind the laparoscope, with the instrument aimed directly toward the television monitor. This arrangement is important and is often not fully appreciated. When this position is not taken, the surgeon's movement to the right in the operating field will appear as a movement to the left on the monitor, making co-ordinated fine movements difficult.

This results in the placement of operative personnel differently from in open procedures. For example, in laparoscopic appendicectomies the surgeon should stand to the patient's left, with the laparoscope at the umbilicus pointing into the right lower quadrant with the monitor directly ahead of this to the right of the patient's feet. Given the length of the laparoscopic instruments, this also makes for a more comfortable working position for the surgeon.

Placement of additional ports

9a, b Once the viewing laparoscope is in place additional laparoscopic ports are almost always required. These are always placed under direct vision, viewing the peritoneal surface of the abdominal wall as the trocar is placed to avoid visceral injury. While viewing from the inside, the intended place of port placement is indented from the outside with the surgeon's finger. To plan more precisely for port placement, it is useful to use a 22-gauge needle with a local anaesthetic so that the intended path of port placement may be tested, especially when ports are placed near the epigastric vessels, the bladder or adhesions. Injection of local anaesthetic as the needle is slowly withdrawn also provides for excellent postoperative pain relief. An incision is then made in the skin in the direction of Langer's lines or in the direction of the surgical incision should conversion to an open procedure be required. As these ports are placed under direct vision, safety shields around the trocar point are not mandatory, but offer an added margin of safety. It should be emphasized that if difficulty is encountered in having an optimal angle of dissection or if more retraction is required, the surgeon should not hesitate to add additional ports as needed.

Retraction and exposure

Retraction and exposure are areas that pose some difficulty in laparoscopic surgery. The pneumoperitoneum tends to cause the colon and small bowel to fall more toward the side of the abdomen, helping particularly with exposure in the upper abdomen. The organ being removed may itself be grasped and used to help with the exposure. This is most commonly done in cholecystectomy where the fundus of the gallbladder is grasped and pushed as far as possible into the right upper abdomen, thereby rotating the liver cephalad and exposing the cystic and common duct. If atraumatic graspers are used, this technique of retracting the liver is particularly useful in upper abdominal surgery such as laparoscopic closure of a perforated duodenal ulcer or staging laparoscopy for patients with adenocarcinoma at the head of the pancreas. Particularly fragile organs, for example the inflamed appendix, may require more gentle means of retraction. It is useful to place a loop or snare of suture around the distal end of the appendix, tightening it to hold the tissue but not to cut into it. The free end of the suture may then be grasped and used to manipulate the appendix during the course of the dissection with minimal risk of perforation. Solid organs are often easily retracted with the use of specially designed fan retractors. These consist of a shaft that will fit through the laparoscopic trocar with broad deformable attachments that can be moved into position to retract the spleen or liver gently over a broad surface area.

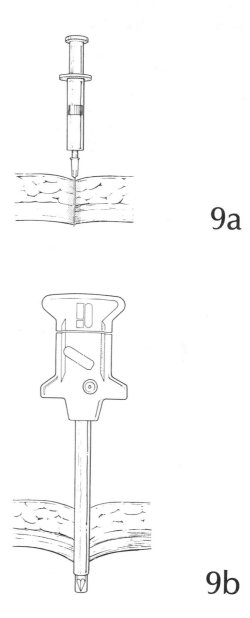

9a

9b

Positioning of the table is also important to allow gravity to assist as much as possible. This is employed to a much greater degree than is usually done in open surgery. The extreme angles used often require that the patient be especially well padded and secured to the operative table. The general principle is that the organ being dissected is elevated. For example, in laparoscopic cholecystectomy the patient is often put in the reverse Trendelenburg position with the right side up, causing the colon and small bowel to fall away from the area of dissection. In laparoscopic adrenalectomy where a medial visceral rotation may be used to gain access to the adrenal gland, the patient is often best positioned entirely on the side.

Principles of dissection

The principles of laparoscopic dissection do not differ fundamentally from methods used in open surgery. It is essential to maintain a dry field at all times, as the smallest oozing will obscure the field. Another important general principle is that dissection should be performed from inferior to superior to avoid blood running down and obscuring the field yet to be dissected. A variety of straight and curved dissectors is now available in configurations identical to those used in open surgery. Monopolar cautery is used quite extensively in an attempt to keep a dry field and a number of the dissecting instruments, including scissors and graspers, have attachments so that they may be used with the monopolar cautery.

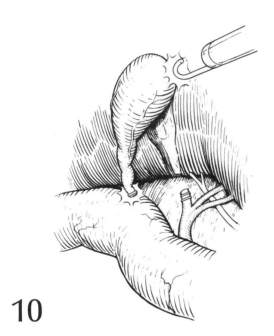

10

10 In addition, hooks with both L- and J-shaped tips are used to dissect gently small strands of tissue before they are cauterized.

Monopolar cautery represents a potential hazard because of the inadvertent conduction to adjacent viscera. This is more of a problem in laparoscopic than in open surgery as the entire length of the instrument may not be in the field of view and part of the instrument may inadvertently be in contact with an adjacent loop of bowel. In addition, the surgical field is generally kept quite dry, increasing the risk of conduction through the tissues themselves but decreasing conduction of current through surrounding fluid. For this reason, a number of bipolar instruments are being developed in which the current is conducted between the jaws of the instrument, minimizing the chance of such conduction injury. Use of laser energy for both cutting and cautery was popular earlier in the history of laparoscopic surgery and the term laser cholecystectomy was often used. Studies have shown that the laser is no more effective than electrocautery, and the cumbersome laser equipment and increased smoke generation within the abdomen make it less effective to use. Although there may be certain applications where laser energy is more effective, it has been abandoned by most general surgeons. Other technologies are being developed using ultrasound energy both to heat and mechanically disrupt tissue.

Suturing and stapling

Conventional suturing is less widely used in laparoscopic surgery as the refined movements to drive a needle through delicate tissue are more difficult to accomplish and continued improvements are being made in the needle holders themselves. For this reason surgeons turn to alternative means to achieve haemostasis or perform an anastomosis. Deformable metal clips, much like those used in open surgery, are widely used laparoscopically. These are available in self-reloading, multiple firing devices. Devices that fire a single staple to approximate two adjacent structures have been developed. These are similar in design to skin staplers and are used laparoscopically to, for example, attach a polypropylene mesh to the underlying fascia in a laparoscopic hernia repair.

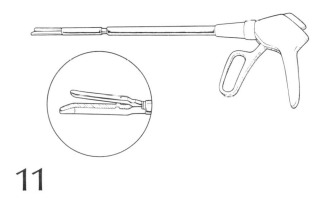

11

11 Stapling devices for performing gastrointestinal anastomoses have been miniaturized and adapted for laparoscopic use. This allows the division of bowel within the abdomen without the risk of stool lcakage as well as the creation of anastomoses entirely within the abdominal cavity.

It should be noted that in most laparoscopic bowel resections much of the dissection is performed laparoscopically, then the ends of the bowel to be anastomosed are exteriorized through a small incision and the anastomosis itself performed extracorporeally using more conventional staplers or a suturing technique. Similar laparoscopic stapling devices have been developed that are in fact haemostatic and are extremely useful for dividing bowel mesentery and lung while providing haemostasis. Such stapling devices have even been successfully used to divide and control the splenic artery and vein.

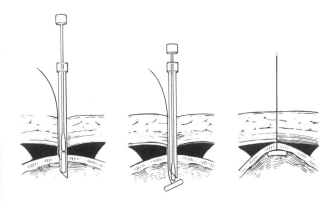

12

12 Other interesting means of suturing have been developed. One of the most novel is the T-fastener. This has been most widely used to secure the stomach or small bowel wall to the abdominal wall in the creation of a laparoscopic gastrostomy or jejunostomy. The device is analogous to that used to secure price tags to clothing: a needle containing a suture with a crossbar at the end is passed into the lumen of the viscus. The T-bar is then ejected within the lumen of the viscus and may be pulled up to secure the organ to the abdominal wall.

Retrieval of a specimen

Once the dissection of an organ has been completed in a laparoscopic procedure, the excised specimen must be removed from the abdomen. The specimen is often larger than the small incisions through the abdominal wall. The fascia around the umbilicus is easily stretched and may be incised with minimal additional discomfort to allow organ removal. In the case of the gallbladder, the neck is often exteriorized and the bile and stones removed to facilitate removal of the gallbladder wall through a 10-mm trocar site. Devices have also been developed to cut larger solid organs into smaller pieces, although in some cases this may interfere with adequate pathological staging of tumours. In laparoscopic hysterectomy the vagina is used to remove the specimen and in laparoscopic sigmoid colon resection the anus has been used for specimen removal, obviating the need for additional skin incisions.

Completion of procedure

At the completion of the procedure, it is important to inspect the operative field under reduced peritoneal pressure as the pneumoperitoneum may tamponade venous or portal bleeding. It is also important that the trocars are removed under direct vision with the laparoscope and the sites inspected to ensure that there is no bleeding. The camera is removed last. It is becoming increasingly recognized that it is important to close the fascia of trocar sites larger than 10 mm to avoid bowel herniation. In closing the fascia at the conclusion of an open surgical procedure, it would be unacceptable to leave a gap in the fascia that would admit a finger. The same principle applies to laparoscopic procedures. Hernation is probably less prevalent than it otherwise would be as many of the trocars are placed obliquely through the abdominal wall resulting in a flap valve effect once the trocars are removed. With the increasing use of ports up to 12–18 mm or even larger, the importance of fascial closure is becoming increasingly recognized. Long-acting local anaesthesia is injected at port site closures.

Postoperative care

If local anaesthesia has been used at the port sites, there is usually little discomfort after operation. Patients may exhibit referred shoulder pain, Kehr's sign, because of retained gas within the peritoneal cavity, although this rapidly resolves as the carbon dioxide is quickly resorbed. Postoperative pain may often be managed without the use of narcotics which may further minimize postoperative ileus. Laparoscopic procedures result in remarkably less ileus so that patients, even after colon resection, may be fed on the day of, or the day after, surgery. The reduced problem with ileus is thought to be due to less bowel manipulation, packing and tissue irritation. However, more recent studies have demonstrated that patients undergoing open procedures may be successfully fed much earlier than is the current practice. The decreased pain and diminished narcotic requirement after laparoscopic surgery makes the patient less anorexic immediately after surgery.

Although laparoscopic techniques are rapidly evolving with a plethora of new instrumentation and novel approaches to certain laparoscopic procedures, classic surgical techniques are valid. As opposed to operations being reinvented for laparoscopic techniques, the trend is toward laparoscopic technology evolving such that common surgical procedures, especially the more complex ones, may be performed using established techniques and principles.

Laparoscopic Nissen fundoplication

Glyn G. Jamieson FRACS, FACS
Dorothy Mortlock Professor of Surgery, University of Adelaide, Department of Surgery, Royal Adelaide Hospital, Adelaide, Australia

Robert Britten-Jones
Clinical Senior Lecturer and Senior Visiting Surgeon, Department of Surgery, Royal Adelaide Hospital, Adelaide, Australia

Operations which alter gastrointestinal function, but which do not require the removal of an organ or part of an organ, seem ideally suited to being undertaken laparoscopically. Fundoplication falls firmly into this category. The procedure was first reported in 1991 by Dallemagne who divided the short gastric vessels in performing the technique. The authors feel justified in calling their technique a Nissen fundoplication, as the anterior wall of the stomach is used without dividing the short gastric vessels as first described by Nissen.

Principles and justification

Indications

The indications for surgery and the objectives of the procedure are identical to the open technique. Whether the suturing which is achieved is as durable as the open technique is a question which will be answered only by long-term follow-up studies.

Contraindications

At present the relative contraindications to performing a fundoplication laparoscopically are a large fixed hiatus hernia and stricturing and shortened oesophagus. No doubt, with experience, these findings will be regarded as less of a problem.

Operation

A Veress needle is introduced immediately below the left costal margin in the mid-clavicular line and the abdomen is insufflated with CO_2 in the usual manner. The limit for intra-abdominal pressure is set at 10 mmHg as mediastinal emphysema can occur during this procedure. Although not usually a problem, patients can occasionally experience severe chest pain after surgery as a result of this complication.

1 A 10-mm port is introduced just to the left of the midline (to avoid the falciform ligament) approximately two-thirds of the way from the xiphisternum to the umbilicus. The telescope (0° or 30°) with attached camera is introduced through this port. Additional ports are placed in (1) the left anterior axillary line below the costal margin (10-mm port), (2) just below and to the left of the xiphisternum (5-mm port), (3) below the right costal margin in the mid-clavicular line (10-mm port or 5-mm port), and (4) about 5 cm below the left costal margin in the mid-clavicular line (12-mm port). The surgeon sits between the patient's legs, which are supported in stirrups, and the table is tilted to a 30° head-up position.

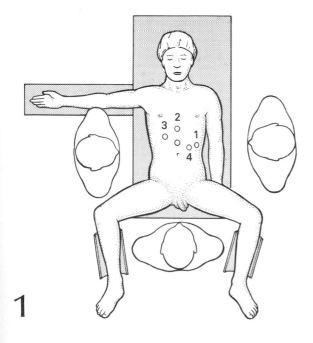

1

2 A 5-mm probe or pair of grasping forceps is inserted through port (3) and the second assistant, standing on the patient's right, uses it under the left lobe of the liver to elevate it and retract it away from the oesophageal hiatus. A grasping forceps is then placed through port (2) for the surgeon's left hand, and a hook diathermy or pair of curved diathermy scissors is placed through port (4) for the surgeon's right hand. A further Babcock type grasping forceps is placed through port (1) and the first assistant, standing on the patient's left, uses this to grasp the stomach below the cardia and pull it downwards. A nasogastric tube is passed to ensure that the stomach is deflated.

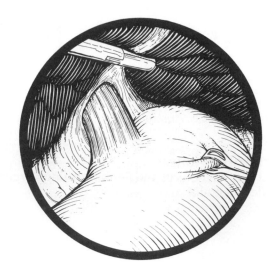

2

The position of the hiatus is most easily found by opening the lesser omentum over the caudate lobe which takes the surgeon to the right side of the hiatus. The peritoneum and fascia in front of the hiatus is divided transversely with the diathermy hook or diathermy scissors, taking care to avoid the anterior vagus nerve(s), and then vertically downwards on either side over the pillars of the oesophageal hiatus. It is not as easy initially to find the oesophagus as might be expected. In fact, when carrying out the procedure for the first few times it may be helpful if an endoscope is passed, as the light clearly demonstrates the position of the oesophagus.

Attention is turned to cleaning the right pillar of the hiatus. Two manoeuvres may help in demonstrating the crus. The first is to place the grasping forceps through port (2) in the hiatus superiorly and to lift it craniad. The second is to have the assistant pull the stomach in the direction of the left iliac fossa. The region between the oesophagus to the left and the crus to the right is now dissected vertically for about 4–5 cm. The pair of grasping forceps through port (2) is used to displace the oesophagus to the left to aid in this dissection. The posterior vagus may be seen during this dissection but it is not as obvious as is sometimes stated, particularly if the dissection is kept close to the right wall of the oesophagus. Attention is now turned to the left pillar of the hiatus. Once again the two helpful manoeuvres are carried out with the assistant this time pulling the stomach towards the right iliac fossa. This time the grasping forceps is used to displace the oesophagus to the right while cleaning the tissue between the oesophagus and the left pillar of the hiatus.

In undertaking this dissection there is a tendency to pass through the hiatus into the thorax and care must be taken to avoid the pleura. The authors have found that they must continually try to keep the dissection as distal as possible (where it is more difficult) and not up in the chest (where it is easier). This part of the dissection is not difficult, but making an opening behind the oesophagus does prove difficult on occasions. The problem is that the angle of entry of the various instruments means that when a pair of forceps is pushed behind the oesophagus, it tends to pass through the hiatus into the chest, or at least bury itself in the diaphragm.

Although port (1) is the most posteriorly placed port and in theory should be the best access for an instrument to pass behind the oesophagus, in practice the authors find that ports (2) or (3) are the best through which to carry out this manoeuvre. An instrument passed through the hiatus from port (1) will tend to be aimed at the heart, so it is also safer to proceed from right to left behind the oesophagus. Having an instrument with a curve or angle at the end facilitates this part of the procedure. When a passage has been created by an instrument behind the oesophagus, it is used to push the oesophagus anteriorly and the opening behind the oesophagus, the window, is gradually enlarged. Once again it must be emphasized that the dissection should be kept in the abdomen and not stray too much into the chest. It is important to dissect a moderately generous window behind the oesophagus of 4–5 cm in length, as this allows the stomach freer passage later in the operation. A nylon tape can be introduced percutaneously and slung around the oesophagus to emerge through the skin, or alongside one of the ports. Traction on this tape may help during passage of the stomach behind the oesophagus.

3 Attention is now turned to the stomach and a point is chosen on the anterior wall about 5 cm distal to the gastro-oesophageal junction and about halfway across towards the spleen. No dissection of the greater curvature or short gastric vessels is undertaken. The stomach is grasped with the forceps through port (1) and pushed upwards as high as possible to determine the mobility of the site chosen. If it appears tethered, then a trial and error process is used to find the most mobile part of the anterior wall of the stomach. This is then pushed to the left side of the oesophagus where grasping forceps with a ratchet are placed through port (3) and behind the oesophagus to pick up the anterior gastric wall.

As the stomach is drawn to the right, behind the oesophagus, the forceps through port (1) help to push the stomach from behind. It is this procedure which is made easier if a substantial window behind the ocsophagus has been constructed.

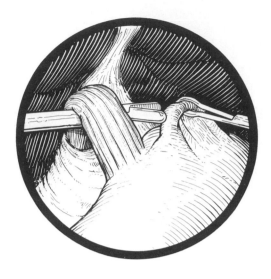

3

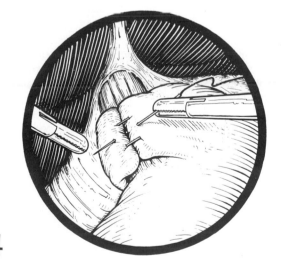

4

4 A pouch of anterior wall, approximately 3 cm in length, is brought behind the oesophagus and then the anterior wall to the left of the oesophagus is picked up and brought in apposition to the pouch. The nasogastric tube is removed and a 52-Fr bougie is passed down the oesophagus. Stitches can be inserted at this stage but early in their experience the authors found it helpful to insert staples to hold the two walls of the stomach together to facilitate subsequent insertion of sutures. A 12-mm port is introduced through port (2) and the stapler is introduced and two or three staples inserted. The stapler is removed and two needleholders are introduced. Three 3/0 polypropylene sutures are now inserted approximately 1 cm apart in order to create a wrap 2 cm in length. A mixture of intracorporeal and extracorporeal knot tying techniques are used. If staples have not been used to produce stomach wall apposition, it is easiest to insert the first suture and tie the knot extracorporeally. With the tissues held together, the remaining sutures can be placed and tied intracorporeally or extracorporeally.

The bougie is removed and replaced with a nasogastric tube. If there is any blood accumulation, the area is irrigated and the irrigating solution is sucked out. The ports are removed, the abdomen deflated and the skin incisions are closed.

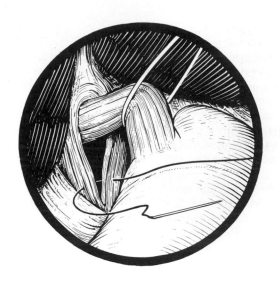

5 The introduction of a traction tape around the oesophagus (see earlier) also facilitates the use of sutures to close the hiatus behind the oesophagus if this is thought necessary. Closure of the hiatus should be done before drawing the stomach around behind the oesophagus. Once again, one or two extracorporeal or intracorporeal sutures can be used.

5

Postoperative care

Oral intake is commenced on the first postoperative day and patients are kept in hospital until the third or fourth postoperative day before discharge. It is likely that in future, with patients who can be instructed about the cautious introduction of a normal diet, discharge may occur earlier.

Outcome

The operation has been undertaken in 131 patients of ages ranging from 20 to 75 years, 74 of whom were men. The median operating time was 95 min (range 45–240 min). In 15 patients the procedure was converted to an open operation for technical reasons such as perioesophagitis and shortening, adiposity obscuring anatomy and large left lobe of the liver obscuring anatomy.

Follow-up in these patients is extremely short. Even so, there have been several poor results which would have been unlikely to have occurred had the technique been performed as an open operation, e.g. acute incarceration of a paraoesophageal hernia (two patients), acute oesophageal obstruction (one patient). One patient died following a straightforward procedure because of acute thrombosis of her coeliac axis and superior mesenteric artery.

Conclusions

This is a documentation of the authors' initial experience with laparoscopic Nissen fundoplication and results will probably improve as experience grows and instrumentation is developed which is more specific for the technique. It is as yet too early to say that laparoscopic fundoplication will produce comparable results to open fundoplication, but the authors believe that eventually this is likely to be the case, particularly if the procedure is reserved for the uncomplicated and non-obese patient.

Preoperative evaluation of the liver including imaging

A. N. Adam FRCP, FRCR
Professor, Department of Interventional Radiology, Guy's and St Thomas' Hospital, London, UK

I. S. Benjamin BSc, MD, FRCS
Professor, Academic Department of Surgery, King's College Hospital, London, UK

A number of diagnostic techniques are now available to the hepatobiliary surgeon. In addition to clinical assessment and biochemical and haematological measurements, many imaging modalities are making an increasing contribution to the preoperative evaluation of potentially resectable liver tumours. The choice of procedure for each case depends on the availability of individual investigative modalities in each centre. However, it is important that a systematic approach is developed, particularly for the common clinical syndromes, in order to optimize the use of diagnostic facilities and to strike a balance between the goal of accurate preoperative diagnosis and the overuse of investigations which are often invasive and expensive. Accurate planning and good liaison between the surgeon and the hepatobiliary radiologist avoids the performance of unnecessary invasive radiological procedures. For example, if a patient is being investigated by percutaneous transhepatic cholangiography (PTC) it is important that the radiologist communicates with the surgeon before the patient leaves the fluoroscopy suite so that a decision can be taken regarding further management. If this involves the percutaneous introduction of a biliary endoprosthesis, this is best carried out immediately after the diagnostic cholangiogram rather than subjecting the patient to a second avoidable and unnecessary PTC before stenting.

Accurate preoperative imaging can help to establish the precise location of masses within the liver and the extent of ductal and vascular involvement. In many cases radiological investigations will determine that a particular mass is irresectable, whereas in others they will enable accurate planning of the operative approach. In cases of biliary obstruction, radiology can frequently demonstrate the cause of the obstruction. The choice of treatment in patients with obstructive jaundice will depend on the diagnosis and the clinical state of the patient. If surgery seems appropriate, accurate preoperative imaging will help to determine the best approach.

Definition of the nature of the disease is not the sole objective of radiology. It is also important to define the extent of the disease, the condition of the liver, the presence or absence of cirrhosis (or the atrophy/hyperplasia complex), and the patient's general condition with regard to nutritional status, sepsis and other potential risk factors. This complete diagnostic assessment is essential before surgery is undertaken for major biliary and hepatic disease.

Two categories of diagnostic problems are considered here: (1) biliary tract obstruction and (2) the intrahepatic mass.

Biliary obstruction

A careful history and thorough clinical examination may suggest a diagnosis in a proportion of patients and may direct the sequence of radiological investigations. In the case of patients presenting for the first time with jaundice, it is well established that progressive painless jaundice is frequently associated with malignant biliary obstruction. However, pain is common both with pancreatic cancer and with hilar biliary tumours[1], and also occurs frequently in patients with carcinoma of the gallbladder. Conversely, obstruction due to previously undetected gallstones may be painless. Nevertheless, a long history of symptoms consistent with biliary tract pain before the onset of obstructive jaundice is still strongly suggestive of benign biliary tract disease.

Clinical examination may reveal signs of respiratory and cardiovascular disease which make the patient unsuitable for major surgery. Stigmata of chronic hepatocellular failure (such as palmar erythema or spider naevi) may suggest the secondary effects of prolonged and severe biliary tract obstruction, but should also raise the suspicion of unrelated intrinsic parenchymal liver disease.

Standard biochemical testing is routine whenever biliary disease is suspected. Such tests are non-specific and may be of more value in following the course of a disease after treatment than in providing diagnostic information. However, minor changes in the liver enzymes, and in particular alkaline phosphatase, should not be ignored as they may be the only clue to continuing biliary tract disease in the absence of jaundice or other biochemical abnormalities. More complex serological tests, such as autoantibody estimations, are usually unnecessary unless there is a strong suspicion of intrinsic liver disease, although it is the authors' practice to carry out hepatitis B and C antigen screening routinely in all new referrals. This is particularly important in patients from overseas, especially those from areas where hepatitis is endemic.

In the initial biochemical screen, the patient's general condition is assessed by measuring renal function (by means of creatinine clearance) and by determining nutritional status. Nutritional status can be crudely assessed by haemoglobin and albumin values and, if these are abnormal, more sophisticated assessment may be indicated.

It is important whenever possible to gain some initial assessment of the presence of infection. Any external drainage from a tube or fistula should be cultured immediately for both aerobic and anaerobic organisms. Patients who are febrile should also have culture of the blood before any investigation or treatment, and at every episode of invasive radiology involving the biliary system, bile should be aspirated and cultured. The importance of having bacteriological information in advance of any septic episodes which may complicate the patient's course cannot be too strongly emphasized.

This will allow an informed choice of antibiotics when indicated for prophylaxis or the treatment of infective complications.

If the possibility of malignant disease is entertained but unproven, any aspirated bile is also sent for cytological examination. This has been found to be valuable before surgery in patients with hilar cholangiocarcinoma. The place of direct fine needle aspiration cytology in relation to individual clinical problems is considered below.

The nature and sequence of biliary imaging techniques and the decision to use angiography depends on the nature of the presentation and the presumed site of the problem within the biliary tract. The procedures available will be considered separately.

Jaundice

In the majority of patients presenting initially with jaundice a combination of clinical history and physical examination may reveal the diagnosis. The distinction between 'medical' and 'surgical' jaundice may be obvious in most cases, but it is in the difficult case that a carefully ordered approach to diagnosis is important. Most algorithmic schemes[2,3] rely on ultrasonography to detect the existence of dilated intrahepatic or extrahepatic bile ducts. While the classical sign of 'surgical' jaundice has long been dilatation of the intrahepatic ducts, biliary obstruction without ductal dilatation may be found in a significant proportion of patients – 16% in one series[4]. Thus, when the history and physical findings strongly suggest one of the variants of biliary obstruction, the finding of non-dilated intrahepatic ducts on ultrasonography does not exclude extrahepatic biliary obstruction. It should, on the other hand, alert the clinician to the possibility of severe secondary biliary fibrosis or concomitant hepatic disease. Conversely, gross ductal dilatation may occur in the presence of intermittent gallstone obstruction. However, ductal dilatation should not be accepted as a normal finding, and a subtle or intermittent cause of obstruction should always be sought in such cases.

Ultrasonographic scanning has long been the investigation of first choice for determining the obstructive nature of jaundice and has an accuracy of more than 90%[5,6]. The level of obstruction can also be defined in most patients (*Figure 1*), in 95% of 65 patients with biliary obstruction in one prospective study[7]. This is at least as good and probably superior to the performance of computed tomographic (CT) scanning with a prediction level of 90%. Moreover, ultrasonography produced valuable diagnostic information in the majority of cases and was able to distinguish with 88% accuracy between benign and malignant aetiology, again somewhat better than the performance of CT scanning

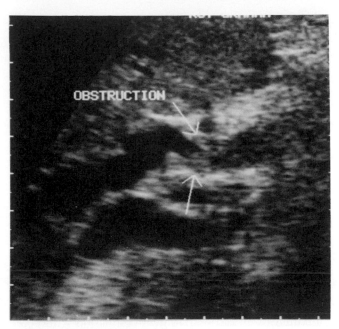

Figure 1   Ultrasonographic scan showing tapering of the common hepatic duct to the point of obstruction by a cholangiocarcinoma.

(63%). Ultrasonographic scanning is very reliable in the detection of cholelithiasis, although small bile duct stones, particularly those lying in the distal biliary tree, still pose difficulties.

Advances in ultrasonographic scanning techniques have raised the possibility that surgeons might be prepared to operate on the evidence of ultrasonography alone in the presence of obstructive jaundice. Eyre-Brook and colleagues[8] showed that the interpretation of ultrasonography was correct in 95% of 132 patients who underwent laparotomy for jaundice, concluding that it was safe to proceed directly to surgery only when an experienced ultrasonographer has demonstrated findings 'typical' of distal common bile duct obstruction due to gallstones or tumour. Duodenoscopy should also be performed before operation in order to detect unsuspected periampullary tumours. Full biliary imaging, particularly for cases of proximal obstruction, is of paramount importance. It is also important not to assume that biliary calculi demonstrated ultrasonographically are necessarily the cause of obstruction.

It is important to be cautious when assessing patients with possible obstruction of a surgically created biliary–enteric anastomosis. Wilson and Toi[9] suggested that ultrasonography accurately detects obstruction in such patients. In the authors' experience, ultrasonography usually shows dilated bile ducts in this setting but completely normal ultrasonographic scans have been seen by the authors in patients with significant anastomotic stenoses shown by cholangiography and proven at surgery (unpublished data).

If ultrasonography is unsatisfactory or incompletely diagnostic, the choice lies between endoscopic retrograde cholangiopancreatography (ERCP) and PTC as the next diagnostic test. PTC is generally preferred for cases of proximal bile duct obstruction and ERCP for cases with suspected distal obstruction. Controlled studies have compared the value of these two modalities[10,11], but such comparisons are not particularly helpful in clinical practice. The tests are complementary and the order in which they are performed is usually dictated by the experience and expertise of the institution. PTC is contraindicated in patients with severely deranged coagulation, although in the authors' experience this has not been a major problem and can usually be overcome by the use of fresh frozen plasma and platelet infusion at the time of the investigation. In an experimental study[12] it was found that when performing fine needle aspiration biopsy of the liver – a procedure similar to PTC in its traumatic effects – the level of anticoagulation had no effect on the amount of bleeding. Gross ascites is a more important contraindication, particularly in the presence of biliary peritonitis. ERCP, on the other hand, may fail to demonstrate the proximal intrahepatic biliary tree fully, particularly when there is asymmetrical stricturing at the hilum. Some operators have used balloon catheters to overcome this problem, but the authors prefer the percutaneous route to evaluate the intrahepatic biliary tree completely in this situation. The chief advantage of ERCP is that it allows visualization of the periampullary region and provides a pancreatogram in most cases. This is particularly helpful when periampullary tumours or iatrogenic choledochoduodenal fistulae are suspected, and also when obstruction may be due to adenocarcinoma of the pancreas or to chronic pancreatitis.

Although the choice of route of biliary intubation usually depends on local practice and experience, there are now many centres at which both interventional radiology and interventional endoscopy are practised and, in certain situations, one is clearly superior to the other. For example, endoscopic papillotomy is an option for patients with choledocholithiasis and so ERCP is preferred in cases of gallstone obstruction. On the other hand, in patients with extensive hilar tumours infiltrating both lobes of the liver and in whom both sides need to be drained to recruit sufficient hepatocytes for palliation, the success rate of percutaneous drainage is significantly higher than that of endoscopic intubation so that PTC is preferred (*Figure 2*).

Recently magnetic resonance (MR) cholangiography has become feasible using fast-spin echo techniques[13,14]. MR cholangiography can demonstrate both normal and dilated bile ducts but the anatomical detail provided is still inferior to that obtained by conventional cholangiographic techniques.

Angiography is of value in patients with biliary obstruction due to tumour. It is helpful in defining arterial anatomy and particularly in assessing tumour involvement, especially of the portal vein. Recent

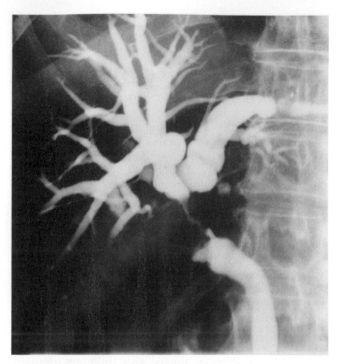

Figure 2   Tight stricture of the upper common hepatic duct in a patient with enlarged lymph nodes at the hilum of the liver shown on PTC.

advances have also made it possible to predict tumour involvement of the portal vein and its main branches by ultrasonography. Doppler ultrasound scanning allows positive identification of blood vessels and demonstrates the direction of blood flow. Colour-coded Doppler scanning has further increased the ability of radiologists to detect abnormalities of the hepatic and portal venous system[15]. In distally placed tumours, particularly those of the pancreatic head, irresectability may be inferred from arterial encasement as well as venous involvement[16]. Ultrasonography is less reliable at demonstrating tumour involvement of arteries than of large veins, so that arteriography may still be indicated.

Magnetic resonance angiography is making rapid advances as a means of assessing the portal venous system[17]. The presence or absence of portal vein occlusion, the direction of flow, and the presence of collateral vessels may be accurately demonstrated. This technique promises to replace angiography in many patients being considered for hepatic resection or transplantation.

In summary, in the authors' approach to the jaundiced patient detailed ultrasonography is the key to accurate diagnosis. When distal bile obstruction due to a clearly demonstrated pancreatic tumour or uncomplicated choledocholithiasis has been demonstrated, ultrasonography may be the only preoperative imaging required. However, this constitutes a minority of cases and direct biliary imaging is usually undertaken. The choice of

ERCP or PTC depends upon the probable site of the lesion, and on any contraindications that are present. If ultrasonography shows no evidence of biliary obstruction or any other suspicious pathology, and if the clinical history, physical examination and biochemical investigations are consistent with the possibility of a non-obstructive cause of the jaundice, percutaneous liver biopsy would then normally be performed. The use of needle biopsy of the liver without prior demonstration of non-dilated ducts on ultrasonography is regarded as a potentially hazardous procedure and is not recommended in this context[18, 19]

Hilar obstruction

Obstruction of the confluence of the hepatic ducts in the absence of previous surgery is commonly due to tumour arising in the bile ducts or gallbladder, or to tumour arising elsewhere within or outside the liver. When biliary obstruction at this level has been identified by ultrasonography, investigation is directed towards elucidating the nature and extent of a potentially malignant process. Ultrasonographic scanning defines adequately the level of the lesion and suggests its malignant nature in the majority of cases (*Figure 3*), but is not so effective in defining intrahepatic extension of tumour. Involvement of second order ducts in the intrahepatic biliary tree – an important indicator of irresectability – is frequently underestimated by ultrasonography[7, 20–22]. Thus, biliary contrast imaging is almost always required in hilar obstruction, and PTC is the preferred approach (*Figure 4*). When the obstruction is complete it may be necessary to use ERCP to define the lower end of the stricture, although in cases where ultrasonography has

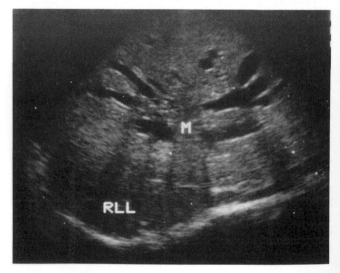

Figure 3   Cholangiocarcinoma of the hilum of the liver seen on ultrasonography. The mass (M) is slightly hypoechoic. Dilated intrahepatic ducts converge towards the lesion.

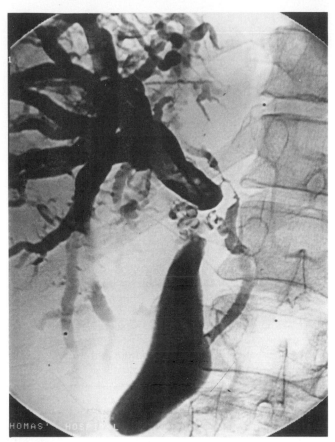

Figure 4   Hilar cholangiocarcinoma shown on PTC. Strictures of the right hepatic duct, left hepatic duct and the upper common hepatic duct are visible. The lower common hepatic duct and the common bile duct appear normal. The intrahepatic ducts are dilated.

been adequate this may not be essential. It is important to allow time to elapse and carry out delayed films with the patient tilted head up before accepting that there is a complete obstruction at the confluence. When there is no communication between the right and left hepatic ductal systems, separate punctures should be carried out to visualize the entire biliary tree.

In a significant number of patients with carcinoma of the gallbladder, neither CT nor ultrasonographic scanning reveal any abnormality of the gallbladder wall. The combination of these methods is more accurate than either alone and diffuse wall thickening or a mass is demonstrated in approximately 50% of patients. Carcinoma of the gallbladder causing hilar obstruction may produce specific subtle cholangiographic signs, particularly distortion of the intrahepatic bile ducts of segment V[23]. In patients with metastatic tumour or filling defects due to primary hepatocellular carcinoma, ultrasonographic scanning may demonstrate an extraductal hilar mass or loose tumour within the biliary system, while PTC may identify the rare cases of polypoid tumour within the hilar ductal system. The distinction may be important because of the possibility of local excision by

curettage with a relatively good prognosis[24]. At the time of PTC, bile should be aspirated for bacteriological and cytological examination. Exfoliative cytology is somewhat inferior to fine needle aspiration cytology (which yields positive results in 95% of cases, including both preoperative and operative specimens) and it may be valuable to perform PTC-guided or ultrasound-guided fine needle aspiration cytology in cases where a hilar mass is demonstrated[25].

Some workers, particularly in Japan, have made extensive use of cholangioscopy for diagnosis and staging of biliary tumours. This technique may be used following percutaneous transhepatic biliary drainage and has proved valuable in differentiating benign biliary strictures and polyps[26]. Nimura has used this technique in about two-thirds of patients undergoing diagnostic and staging procedures for hilar cholangiocarcinoma, and has used cholangioscopic biopsy following multiple segment percutaneous transhepatic biliary drainage to guide the extent of resection of intrahepatic ducts[27].

Angiography should be carried out in all cases of cholangiocarcinoma thought at initial ultrasonography and PTC to be potentially resectable. A combination of cholangiography and angiography is an accurate means of defining irresectability of hilar tumours. Preoperative diagnosis of tumour invasion of the portal venous wall would be extremely helpful in patients with hilar malignancy, but there is no completely satisfactory method for its detection. Although CT arterioportography (*Figure 5*) is routine in this situation, the technique delineates only the contrast medium-filled configuration of the vessel lumen and clarity is often poor. Also, given the anteroposterior projection of the ductal system, subtle infiltration or compression of the portal venous wall by cancer may not be defined. Similarly, other imaging modalities such as conventional ultrasonography, CT scanning and MRI do not reveal

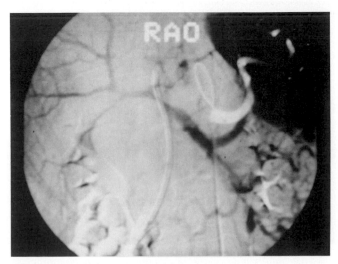

Figure 5   Indirect splenoportogram of hilar cholangiocarcinoma showing compression of the main portal vein at the liver hilum. An endoscopic stent can be seen in situ.

early invasion of the portal vein. Intraportal ultrasonography has recently been used to detect invasion of the portal vein wall. This involves inserting a catheter into an ileocolic venous branch exposed through a right lower pararectal incision. Under fluoroscopic guidance the catheter is advanced into the right or left portal vein through the main portal trunk. Real-time images are recorded on video tape using 20 MHz and 30 MHz transducers. As an alternative, percutaneous insertion of the catheter is possible using a transjugular or transhepatic approach. Preliminary results suggest that intraportal ultrasonography is helpful in detecting or excluding early invasion of the portal vein by bile duct cancer and may be useful when CT scanning or angiography fails to provide sufficient discrimination[28].

Another approach to portal venous imaging is percutaneous transhepatic portography, which some authors use in combination with PTC and biliary drainage. Nimura has also used transhepatic portal venous embolization in order to reduce the functional capacity of the hepatic parenchyma which will be resected, and so encourage contralateral hyperplasia in an effort to prevent postoperative hepatic failure[29].

In patients with hilar cholangiocarcinoma, CT scanning is valuable for demonstrating lobar or segmental atrophy of the liver (*Figure 6*), although this is often suggested on cholangiography. CT scanning is not as good as ultrasonography in demonstrating the cause and level of biliary obstruction. Contrast-enhanced CT scanning can define portal venous involvement by tumour but is less useful in demonstrating hepatic arterial encasement and cannot therefore replace angiography in the preoperative assessment of cholangiocarcinoma. Assessment of tumour involvement of the caudate lobe can be difficult. Intravascular ultrasonography via a probe mounted on a catheter

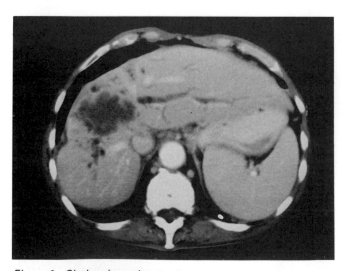

Figure 6   Cholangiocarcinoma shown on CT scan infiltrating mainly segment IV (the quadrate lobe) of the liver. Dilated intrahepatic ducts are evident in the right and left lobes. The right lobe is significantly atrophic.

inserted in the inferior vena cava may help to resolve this problem (LH Blumgart *et al.*, 1992, personal communication).

Laparoscopy (and laparoscopic ultrasonography) is used increasingly in the diagnosis and staging of liver lesions. In the diagnosis of hepatocellular carcinoma it allows safe biopsy under direct vision, including biopsy of the non-tumorous liver, and there is evidence that this offers some advantage over 'blind' biopsies[30]. Although laparoscopy only allows visualization of about two-thirds of the liver surface, the assessment can now be extended by the use of laparoscopic ultrasonography[31]. Experience with the technique is limited and its true value is still being determined.

In summary, ultrasonographic scanning should be the first investigation in patients with hilar biliary obstruction, followed by PTC unless ultrasonography has demonstrated unequivocal evidence of irresectability. The whole of the biliary tree should be visualized, even if this requires several separate punctures. Bile must be obtained for culture and cytology and, in patients with hilar masses that are potentially resectable, fine needle aspiration cytology should be carried out. The presence or absence of vascular involvement should be established; if this cannot be achieved by high quality ultrasonography or contrast-enhanced CT scanning, angiography is indicated. It is important to be aware that a benign stricture may present as a possible hilar malignancy.

Distal obstruction

The first line investigation should be ultrasonography; this usually defines the level of obstruction although duodenal gas may limit the technical quality of the investigation. ERCP should be performed unless contraindicated on anatomical grounds or because or recent incompletely resolved pancreatitis. The ampulla of Vater should be inspected carefully, and biopsies and both brush and aspiration cytology (possibly after intravenous secretin administration) should be carried out if there is any suspicion of periampullary or pancreatic malignancy. Cholangiography should be as complete as possible, and a balloon catheter may be needed if the obstruction is higher than originally suspected. Pancreatography is obtained whenever possible as this is an accurate means of demonstrating pancreatic carcinoma or pancreatitis.

Ultrasonographic scanning and ERCP may adequately define a malignant obstruction of the common bile duct or may demonstrate clearly a benign cause such as cholelithiasis. Further investigation is indicated if the presence of malignancy cannot be confirmed or excluded, or when a malignant lesion has been shown which is potentially resectable. In such situations CT scanning is very valuable as it can demonstrate pancreatic carcinoma with an accuracy greater than 90%. CT-guided fine needle aspiration biopsy is very useful in providing cytological proof of malignancy. Ultrasonography, ERCP and angiography are now most commonly used as adjunctive modalities when the CT diagnosis as equivocal[32]. Angiography may be valuable in demonstrating portal venous occlusion (which is non-specific and may occur with chronic pancreatitis) and arterial encasement (which rarely occurs in benign disease). It is not always possible to exclude malignancy with certainty, but if the history is consistent with obstruction due to chronic pancreatitis then a period of observation may be warranted provided any jaundice is resolving.

The assessment of resectability of pancreatic carcinoma depends on evidence of spread beyond the limits of normal resection margins or on the invasion of local structures, particularly the portal vein. A combination of ultrasonography, CT scanning and angiography will define the majority of such cases. In future intraportal ultrasonography may also be used if further information is needed. In patients with periampullary carcinoma, angiography is not normally performed since portal venous involvement is very rare.

The use of laparoscopy and laparoscopic ultrasonography has already been mentioned. It has proved valuable in the staging and planning of treatment for pancreatic cancer with distal bile duct obstruction[31, 33]. Laparoscopy is certainly of benefit in demonstrating small peritoneal nodules which elude detection by ultrasonography and CT scanning and unnecessary laparotomy can be avoided in a number of patients.

In summary, ERCP is the preferred investigation in patients with distal biliary obstruction, and the objective is to define the presence of malignancy, preferably with cytological diagnosis. CT scanning is frequently sufficient for the definition of irresectability but, in selected cases, angiography may be required.

After cholecystectomy

Approximately 10–40% of patients have symptoms after cholecystectomy. In many cases these are unrelated to the biliary tract and only a few patients have symptoms caused by biliary tract obstruction. However, unless a positive diagnosis is achieved and implicates factors outside the biliary tract, the possibility of retained common bile duct stones, benign stricture formation, biliary–enteric fistula, one of the many periampullary problems, or an undisclosed biliary or periampullary tumour must be sought.

Ultrasonographic scanning should be the first investigation as it can rapidly provide information about the biliary tree and surrounding structures. If fistulae or indwelling biliary tubes are present, these should be used to obtain fistulograms or tubograms. Endoscopy is mandatory in the investigation of patients after cholecystectomy since a large proportion may have a lesion which can be identified by endoscopy alone. ERCP is the most useful investigation in this group of patients. Care must be taken to exclude iatrogenic biliary–enteric fistula which may be responsible for persistent late symptoms[34]. If a benign iatrogenic bile duct stricture is encountered at ERCP, it may also be necessary to undertake PTC to obtain full cholangiography, although this is needed less frequently than in cases of biliary tumour.

Benign iatrogenic biliary injuries

Some patients present early in the postoperative phase after cholecystectomy with evidence of biliary injuries. The major modes of presentation are biliary peritonitis (either generalized or as a local collection of bile in the subhepatic space), an external biliary fistula with leakage of bile through a drain or through the abdominal wound, and early obstructive jaundice. The initial investigation in each case is ultrasonography, and in the case of a localized collection, percutaneous drainage under ultrasound guidance is often useful for diagnosis and as a temporizing measure. It may occasionally provide definitive management if the biliary leak has come from a small radicle in the gallbladder bed or from a slipped clip on the cystic duct. Early ERCP may be indicated, and may allow the placement of an endoscopic stent in cases of minor ductal leak or a leakage from the cystic duct stump.

However, many patients present some time after cholecystectomy and in such cases ERCP is performed early in the investigation. High strictures are not fully delineated by ERCP if there is a major disruption of the common bile duct and in such patients PTC should be carried out. All separately obstructed segments should be identified at PTC. Ultrasonography and CT scanning may be helpful in demonstrating the presence of lobar atrophy (*Figure* 7) or segmental obstruction over-

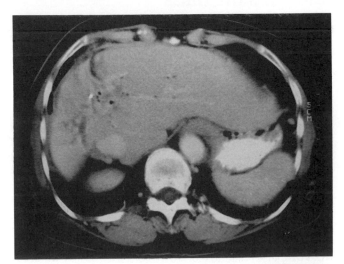

Figure 7   CT scan of a patient who had separate anastomoses of the right and left hepatic ducts to jejunum to repair a benign biliary stricture following cholecystectomy. Marked atrophy of the right lobe caused by longstanding obstruction is evident. Dilated intrahepatic ducts are seen in the atrophic lobe.

looked at PTC. These investigations will also help to demonstrate the portal vein and its branches. Portal venous collaterals and splenomegaly are usually obvious on the CT scan.

The use of angiography in patients with benign hilar strictures is restricted to the following groups of patients:

1. those with a history of major bleeding at the time of the initial operation, suggestive of vascular damage;
2. those with a history of gastrointestinal haemorrhage suggestive of portal hypertension with oesophageal varices;
3. patients with splenomegaly detected clinically or on scanning, or those with oesophagogastric varices seen on routine endoscopy;
4. those with established lobar atrophy on cholangiography or on ultrasonographic or CT scanning.

If there is any doubt regarding vascular injury and, in particular, if there is evidence of the atrophy/hypertrophy complex with rotation of the liver, angiography may be essential both for full diagnosis and as a guide to the best surgical approach. In a series of 130 patients in whom biliary strictures developed after cholecystectomy, angiography was performed selectively according to these criteria in 41 cases; vascular damage was unidentified in 28 of these (68%)[35].

Some patients with chronic incomplete bile duct strictures may also merit needle biopsy of the liver to define the degree of hepatic damage before undertaking surgery.

Intrahepatic mass

Patients may present with a mass in the epigastrium or right upper quadrant which is thought to arise from the liver. The mass may be the initial presenting feature but quite commonly it is found during investigation of known or suspected malignant disease elsewhere, and particularly in the gastrointestinal tract. As with the investigation of biliary tract obstruction, the diagnosis is evident in the majority of cases at an early stage, but there are numerous pitfalls and exceptions so that an ordered approach to investigation is advised. It is important to state at the outset that percutaneous needle biopsy of the liver mass is not recommended at an early stage of investigation. This point will be justified and emphasized below. In many non-specialist units, biopsy may be considered the most direct route to complete diagnosis. However, the biopsy of focal liver lesions is not only often unhelpful in the management, but carries the risk of serious and sometimes life-threatening complications and may jeopardize subsequent curative surgery.

Clinical assessment

Abdominal palpation will normally have already revealed the liver mass. The clinician should direct particular attention to the following points: jaundice, signs of hepatocellular insufficiency and collateral circulation, nutritional impairment, lymphadenopathy, abnormal chest signs, cutaneous or anorectal malignancies, or mucocutaneous angiomata. In the abdomen attention should be paid to the mass itself, determining whether it is regular or irregular, whether there is a palpable or ballottable gallbladder, separate masses within the abdomen, splenomegaly or ascites. A bruit may be audible in some cases of haemangioma, arteriovenous malformation or malignant liver tumour. It must be remembered that not all masses suspected of being intrahepatic on presentation and even on initial investigation prove to have arisen from the liver. We have seen duodenal, renal and adrenal tumours, as well as retroperitoneal sarcomas and leiomyosarcoma of the inferior vena cava, present in this manner. While it may not always be possible to identify these tumours clinically, a plane of cleavage can sometimes be palpated between the mass and the liver which moves with respiration. However, some masses which appear to be separate are, in fact, pedunculated liver tumours and arise from the lower margin of the liver (e.g. from the quadrate lobe, i.e. segment IV).

Biochemistry

Full initial screening of haematological and biochemical parameters is normally performed. Hepatitis B and C antigen screening is carried out as a routine, particularly in view of the association between primary hepatocellular carcinoma and hepatitis. More specialized tests reflect the previous experience and referral pattern of an individual unit. Serum tumour markers, including alpha-fetoprotein, carcinoembryonic antigen and CA19-9 are routinely measured. In appropriate cases, blood samples are also taken for hydatid serological testing, and fasting blood samples are obtained for measurement of hormone levels in case the lesion is a primary or secondary endocrine tumour. In addition, plasma neurotensin levels and serum vitamin B_{12} binding capacity are measured because these are useful tumour markers for the fibrolamellar variant of hepatocellular carcinoma[36]. It is not, of course, necessary to await the results of these specialized investigations before proceeding with further diagnostic evaluation.

Imaging investigations

Further investigation of the liver mass most usefully follows an algorithmic approach as illustrated in *Figures 8* and *9*. The procedures adopted depend on whether hepatic lesions are thought to be focal or multicentric,

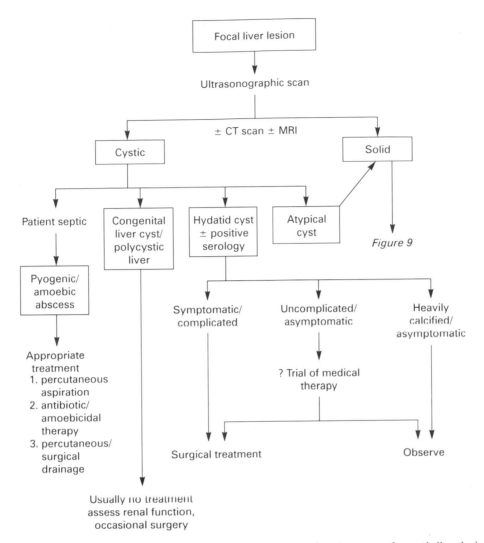

Focal liver lesion

Ultrasonographic scan

± CT scan ± MRI

Cystic

Solid

Patient septic

Congenital
liver cyst/
polycystic
liver

Hydatid cyst
± positive
serology

Atypical
cyst

Figure 9

Pyogenic/
amoebic
abscess

Symptomatic/
complicated

Uncomplicated/
asymptomatic

Heavily
calcified/
asymptomatic

Appropriate
treatment
1. percutaneous
   aspiration
2. antibiotic/
   amoebicidal
   therapy
3. percutaneous/
   surgical
   drainage

? Trial of medical
therapy

Surgical treatment

Observe

Usually no treatment
assess renal function,
occasional surgery

Figure 8   Algorithm of imaging procedures used in diagnosing the cause of a cystic liver lesion.

and whether they are cystic or solid (*Figure 10*). Thus, the first investigation is normally ultrasonography to allow early separation of cystic and solid lesions and also to exclude large bile duct obstruction. If ultrasonography shows multiple solid lesions suggesting tumour not amenable to surgical cure, a biopsy may be performed during the same session to obtain a pathological diagnosis. However, in most cases with solitary lesions the patient should have a CT scan. CT scanning performed with dynamic incremental bolus techniques is the acknowledged gold standard for liver tumour imaging[37,38]. Hepatic parenchymal enhancement reaches a plateau approximately 40 s after a bolus injection of contrast medium. Most metastases are hypovascular and appear as low attenuation lesions within the opacified parenchyma (*Figure 11*). Tumours that may be hypervascular in relation to normal hepatic parenchyma (e.g. primary hepatoma and metastases from pancreatic islet cell tumour, carcinoid and renal

cell carcinoma) may become isodense during the non-equilibrium phase of maximum hepatic enhancement. Patients with suspected hypervascular tumours should have both a non-contrast and a dynamic contrast study.

Bolus dynamic contrast CT scanning ensures positive enhancement of the hepatic veins in addition to the portal veins, so that detected lesions can be located with respect to specific hepatic lobes and segments (*Figure 12*). Hepatic CT scanning usually requires 12–20 contiguous sections (average 16) and can almost always be achieved in less than 2 min when using a modern fast CT scanner.

Unfortunately, many centres still use infusion techniques in CT scanning of the liver. With these methods significant portions of the liver may not be examined until 5–10 min after the beginning of the infusion of contrast medium, and metastases may appear isodense with normal liver. In other cases the increase in

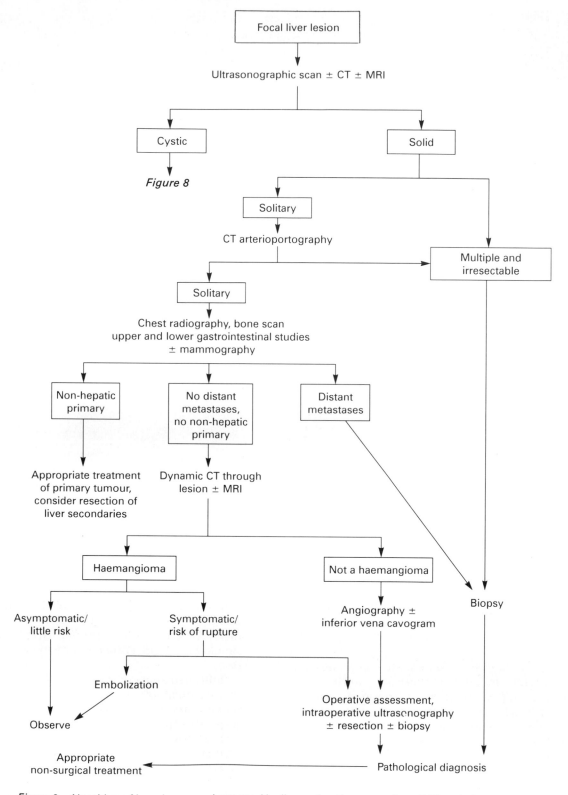

Figure 9   *Algorithm of imaging procedures used in diagnosing the cause of a solid liver lesion.*

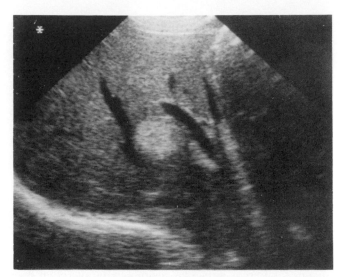

Figure 10   *Echogenic rounded mass in the right lobe of the liver seen on ultrasonography. This was a metastasis from a colonic carcinoma.*

attenuation of the hepatic parenchyma may be insufficient to reveal small lesions. Dynamic CT scanning of the liver should be the routine method. Compared with unenhanced CT scanning, dynamic sequential hepatic CT scanning does not markedly increase the number of patients correctly diagnosed as having liver metastases, but the number of lesions detected can be increased by as much as 40% and this is an important consideration in patients being considered for partial hepatic resection.

Helical CT scanning is an excellent method of dynamic CT scanning. Contrast medium (150 ml) is injected intravenously at the rate of 3 ml/s. Scanning begins 17 s after starting the injection. For routine evaluation of the liver 7 mm collimation is used and the entire liver is covered in approximately 21–25 s. Even if

5 mm collimation is used the entire liver can be scanned in 30 s in most patients. Because helical data are continuous, the location in which slices are reconstructed can be selected retrospectively by the radiologist. For small lesions in the liver it may be useful to reconstruct 10 mm 'thick' slices every 5 mm to reduce partial volume averaging. Reconstructing overlapping slices should make small haemangiomas and metastases more apparent.

Delayed hepatic CT scanning is a technique that uses contrast medium contained within hepatocytes and interstitial spaces some 4–6 h after the initial injection[39,40]. This represents the small percentage of contrast medium 'vicariously' taken up and excreted by the liver, as well as contrast medium that remains in equilibrium with that circulating intravascularly. Provided that an adequate iodine load (at least 60 g) has been used initially, an increase of hepatic CT number of some 20 Hounsfield units (HU) is seen at 4–6 h. Delayed hepatic CT scanning is a very sensitive technique in the detection of hepatic metastases but few centres use it routinely because of the inconvenience of scheduling examinations 4–6 h after the initial injection of contrast medium.

CT arterioportography (CTAP) is the most sensitive preoperative method of investigation of a liver mass. It is a 'super' intravenous bolus contrast-enhanced CT study in which the contrast medium is delivered selectively into the portal venous supply without prior systemic distribution and dilution. This is achieved by selective catheterization of the superior mesenteric artery. The technique results in greater hepatic parenchymal enhancement and contrast differentiation between focal lesions and background. The basic principle of CTAP is that normal liver parenchyma is enhanced by contrast medium delivered selectively via the portal vein, whereas liver neoplasms receive their blood supply mainly from the hepatic artery and remain unenhanced

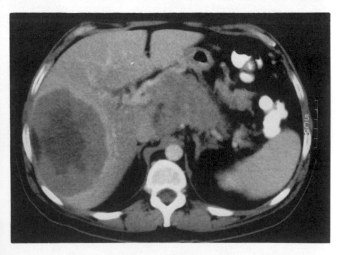

Figure 11   *CT scan showing metastases from carcinoma of the colon. A large mass can be seen in the right lobe of the liver containing necrotic areas.*

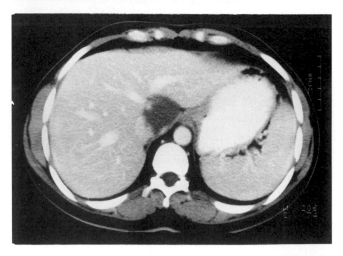

Figure 12   *Metastatic tumour in segment I (caudate lobe). Note the clear demonstration of the right, middle and left hepatic veins converging towards the inferior vena cava.*

during the portal and parenchymal phase of contrast distribution[30]. A recent study established that optimum parenchymal enhancement is achieved 18–67 s after injection of contrast material into the superior mesenteric artery[41]. To scan the liver within such a narrow time window a spiral technique is necessary. The authors use 150 ml of 60% contrast medium administered at a rate of 3 ml/s; the spiral CT sequence is started 20 s after the beginning of the injection. Parenchymal enhancement of 80–100 HU can be achieved compared with 50–70 HU after intravenous bolus injections. CTAP is an exquisitely sensitive technique for the detection of hepatic metastases[39, 42–44].

During CTAP perfusion, defects may be observed due to incomplete mixing of enhanced blood in the superior mesenteric vein with unenhanced blood in the splenic vein, resulting in hypoperfusion of the left hepatic lobe. In addition, central metastases may compress central portal vein branches resulting in hypoperfusion defects (*Figure 13*). Although non-tumorous attenuation differences are significantly more frequent with CTAP than with dynamic CT scanning, they are seldom a diagnostic problem because of their geographical pattern. In patients in whom it is unclear whether there is a hypoperfusion defect or a true focal lesion, it is advisable to perform a delayed hepatic CT study 4–6 h after CTAP. However, lesions may be missed in areas which have not opacified sufficiently and it is important not to interpret CTAP in isolation from a conventional dynamic study and, if appropriate, other examinations such as ultrasonography and MRI.

Lipiodol CT scanning has been advocated as a method of preoperative investigation, especially in patients with vascular tumours (*Figure 14*). Lipiodol injected selectively into the hepatic artery is taken up by tumours in a variety of patterns. Normal hepatic parenchyma also takes up lipiodol, but the contrast medium is cleared from the normal liver within approximately 1 week, whereas it is retained in tumours. In general, vascular tumours such as hepatomas take up lipiodol in a diffuse manner, whereas avascular lesions may not retain it or may demonstrate only peripheral uptake. It is thought that some abnormality of neoplastic vasculature encourages leakage of contrast medium into the tumour. Another explanation is that Kupffer cells clear lipiodol from the normal hepatic parenchyma, but these cells do

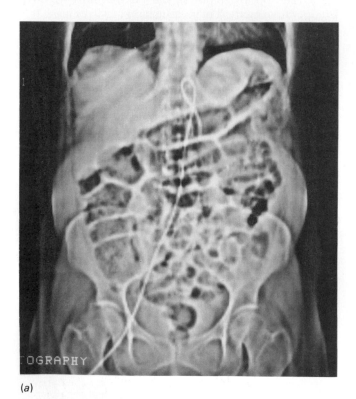

(a)

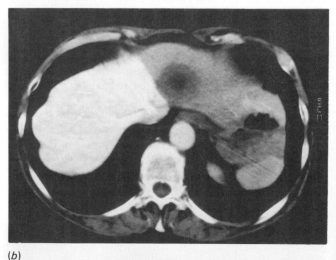

(b)

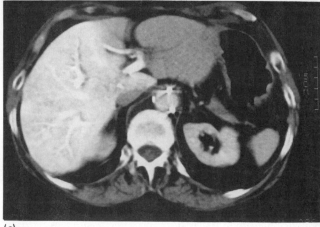

(c)

Figure 13 CT arterioportography. *(a) Scout view showing a catheter in position; the tip of the catheter is in the superior mesenteric artery. (b) Metastasis in the left lobe of the liver. The right lobe is perfused whereas no perfusion is seen in the left lateral segments. (c) Lack of opacification of portal vein branches in the lateral segments (compressed by the metastasis shown in b).*

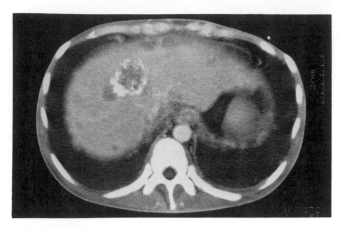

Figure 14   CT scan showing rim uptake of lipiodol around a metastasis from colorectal carcinoma. The lipiodol injection has been made several months before the CT examination. New metastases appear as low attenuation lesions without lipiodol uptake.

not exist within neoplastic tissue and lipiodol is retained within the latter. Usually about 10 ml lipiodol emulsion is injected into the hepatic artery and the CT scan is performed 7–10 days later, but both the contrast volume and the timing vary considerably from centre to centre. Residual lipiodol, particularly in the left lobe of the liver, may make it difficult to distinguish normal from diseased liver and, in one study, the technique did not contribute to decisions about surgical management in any of the 20 cases studied[45].

Magnetic resonance imaging (MRI) is a powerful tool in the evaluation of primary liver neoplasms. Determination of tumour extent and tissue characterization is provided with standard spin-echo T1- and T2-weighted imaging and is enhanced by the gradient-echo, fast spin-echo and fat suppression techniques. Intravenously administered contrast agents such as gadopentetate dimeglumine and superparamagnetic iron oxide provide additional opportunities for lesion characterization[46]. The major problem with the use of MRI in the upper abdomen is physiological movements, but this appears to have been solved by newly introduced fast-sequence and timing-parameter strategies. Short-TR/TE spin-echo sequences with extensive signal averaging and heavy T1 weighting produce images with exceptional anatomical detail and contrast differences between the liver tissue and tumour. MRI identified 14% more individual metastases and 3% more patients with liver cancer than CT scanning in a blinded comparative study of 142 patients undergoing both examinations. It also showed greater specificity (98%) than CT scanning (91%) in distinguishing patients without liver metastases. Differentiation of haemangioma from metastases was possible with more than 98% specificity by using heavily T2-weighted sequences[47]. On T2-weighted spin-echo images, intensity ratios between the lesion and liver tissue can be used

to distinguish hepatic cavernous haemangioma from malignant lesions with accuracy. However, since patients with focal liver lesions may also have diffuse liver disease, this relationship can be misleading. In doubtful cases the use of the intensity ratio between the lesion and fat tissue improves accuracy in the diagnosis of liver lesions. The combination of both ratios into a single diagnostic index in one study gave a correct classification of malignancy versus haemangioma in 92.3% of cases[48]. Superparamagnetic iron particles can be used as a tissue-specific MR contrast medium for the reticuloendothelial system. Contrast enhanced spin-echo sequences provide a marked contrast between the liver tissue and tumour, greater than the contrast values of T1- and T2-weighted images[49].

Despite advances in MRI of the liver, CT scanning remains the screening method of choice for focal liver lesions because (1) CT scanning is superior to MRI in the detection of extrahepatic disease; and (2) CTAP has a higher sensitivity than MRI in assessing liver lesions before surgery[39, 40]. However, accurate interpretation of CTAP requires the availability of a 'standard' bolus dynamic CT scan. If MRI is to replace CT as the routine screening method, a bolus dynamic CT study would have to be carried out before CTAP, thus increasing the cost and complexity of preoperative investigations.

Contact ultrasonography at the time of surgery is a very sensitive technique for detecting small lesions with a resolution of less than 0.5 cm. Used in combination with palpation, a hand-held probe in direct contact with the liver capsule allows both lobes of the liver to be fully assessed. Furthermore, the relationship of metastases to hepatic veins and bile ducts can be seen. This may influence the extent of the final resection at operation[50].

The use of preoperative laparoscopy and ultrasonography has already been mentioned[31]. There is early evidence that the technique may avoid unnecessary laparotomy in some patients with metastatic disease.

Patients must be routinely assessed for evidence of extrahepatic secondary tumours by clinical examination, chest radiography and, where appropriate, a radioisotopic bone scan. Upper and lower gastro-intestinal endoscopy or barium studies, intravenous urography and mammography (in female patients) may be valuable in patients with a single liver secondary of unknown origin.

The major indication for angiography is a proven solitary solid lesion with no evidence of primary tumour elsewhere and no other sites of secondary spread. However, this is only necessary if the general condition of the patient suggests suitability for hepatic resection. In patients who proceed to angiography, multiple tumours not detected on ultrasonographic or CT scanning are occasionally found, or a mass may have the characteristic appearance of a haemangioma. In some patients with lesions close to the inferior vena cava, inferior vena cavography may also be performed at the time of angiography, since compression or invasion of the vena cava may be found. This information is of value at operation. However, MR angiography or contrast-enhanced spiral CT scanning with subsequent coronal and sagittal or three-dimensional reconstructions obviate the need for inferior vena cavography in most patients.

Biopsy

If a solitary liver lesion is amenable to surgical resection in an eligible patient, it is not normally necessary to obtain the formal tissue diagnosis before laparotomy. However, in certain circumstances with resectable lesions and where pathological confirmation is necessary in patients with a contraindication to resection, the choice lies between percutaneous fine needle aspiration cytology or Tru-Cut needle biopsy. These procedures are best performed under ultrasound or CT guidance, although in the case of obstructing biliary tumours fluoroscopic guidance during cholangiography is a rapid and accurate method (*Figure 15*). In patients with primary hepatocellular carcinoma it may be valuable to take a biopsy sample of the uninvolved liver to detect and determine the severity of parenchymal liver disease such as chronic hepatitis or cirrhosis, as this is a relative contraindication to major hepatic resection. There may be some advantages to taking a biopsy during angiography, since immediate embolization is then possible if major haemorrhage occurs. It is also now possible to perform direct embolization of a needle biopsy track[51,52]. New automated biopsy devices utilizing relatively small calibre needles with a Tru-Cut action provide excellent specimens and probably reduce the risk of haemorrhage.

The complication rate of percutaneous liver biopsy varies from centre to centre and reflects the type of patients undergoing investigation. Complications are more frequent in biopsies performed for focal lesions than in those done predominantly for elucidation of cirrhosis or hepatocellular disorders, although it is difficult to acquire evidence from the literature to support this assumption. Biopsy is obviously contraindicated in those with an audible bruit and those who have highly vascular tumours on investigation, and in suspected hydatid disease. The risk of tumour dissemination by liver biopsy is small but finite[53]. Fine needle aspiration cytology appears to carry less risk than cutting needle biopsy[54], and the latter method should probably be used only when fine needle aspiration has failed to provide a diagnosis. False negatives may occur in up to one-third of cases of fine needle aspiration for focal liver lesion[55], and an experienced cytologist is required.

There are some potential benefits to performing a preoperative cytological and histological biopsy. Laparotomy may occasionally be avoided because of a firm diagnosis of a benign lesion such as focal nodular hyperplasia or liver cell adenoma, although even for these benign tumours direct inspection is often indicated and resection may sometimes be required.

Assessment of resectability

The criteria for resectability of solid hepatic tumours must be very carefully defined. Size alone is rarely a contraindication to attempted resection of a solitary primary or secondary liver tumour. Moreover, multiple colonic secondary deposits confined to one lobe do not contraindicate resection, and the criteria for potentially curative surgery have to be considered carefully in this light.

The management plans outlined in the algorithms in *Figures 8* and *9* have proved useful in a unit where the principal referral practice consists of potentially resectable tumours. The key to rational and successful management of these lesions is a complete and accurate preoperative assessment.

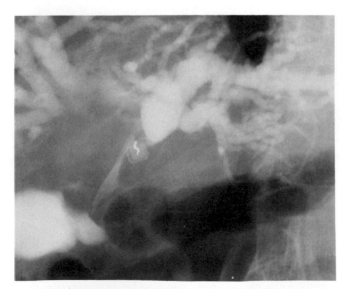

Figure 15   Fluoroscopically-guided biopsy of a hilar cholangiocarcinoma. A fine needle is guided immediately below the level of obstruction of the common hepatic duct.

References

1. Blumgart LH, Hadjis NS, Benjamin IS, Beazley RM. Surgical approaches to cholangiocarcinoma at the confluence of hepatic ducts. *Lancet* 1984; i: 66–70.

2. Benjamin IS, Allison ME, Moule B, Blumgart LH. The early use of fine needle percutaneous transhepatic cholangiography in an approach to the diagnosis of jaundice in a surgical unit. *Br J Surg* 1978; 65: 92–8.

3. Karran S, Dewbury KC, Wright R. Investigation of the jaundiced patient. In: Wright R, Alberti KGMM, Karran S, Milward-Sadler GDT, eds. *Liver and Biliary Disease: Pathophysiology, Diagnosis, Management.* 2nd edn. London: Baillière Tindall, 1994: 647–58.

4. Beinart C, Efremedis S, Cohen B, Mitty HA. Obstruction without dilation. Importance in evaluating jaundice. *JAMA* 1981; 245: 353–6.

5. Koenigsberg M, Wiener SN, Walzer A. The accuracy of sonography in the differential diagnosis of obstructive jaundice: a comparison with cholangiography. *Radiology* 1979; 133: 157–65.

6. Ferrucci JT, Adson MA, Mueller PR, Stanley RJ, Stewart ET. Advances in the radiology of jaundice: a symposium and review. *AJR* 1983; 141; 1–20.

7. Gibson RN, Yeung E, Thompson JN *et al*. Bile duct obstruction: radiologic evaluation of level, cause and tumour resectability. *Radiology* 1986; 160: 43–7.

8. Eyre-Brook IA, Ross, B, Johnson AG. Should surgeons operate on the evidence of ultrasound alone in jaundiced patients? *Br J Surg* 1983; 70: 587–9.

9. Wilson SR, Toi A. Sonography accurately detects biliary obstruction in patients with surgically created biliary-enteric anastomosis. *AJR* 1990; 155: 789–94.

10. Elias E, Hamlyn AN, Jain S *et al*. A randomized trial of percutaneous transhepatic cholangiography with the Chiba needle versus endoscopic retrograde cholangiography for bile duct visualization in jaundice. *Gastroenterology* 1976; 71: 439–43.

11. Matzen P, Malchow-Moller A, Lejerstofte J, Stage P, Juhl E. Endoscopic retrograde cholangiopancreatography and transhepatic cholangiography in patients with suspected obstructive jaundice. A randomized study. *Scand J Gastroenterol* 1982; 17: 731–5.

12. Gazelle GS, Haaga JR. Effect of needle gauge and level of anticoagulation on bleeding associated with biopsy of the liver. *Radiology* 1989; 173(P): 427.

13. Holland GH, Meakem TJ, Baeum RA, Schnall MD, Cope C, Kressell HY. MR cholangiography performed with fast SE technique. *Radiology* 1993; 189(P): 415.

14. Takehara Y, Ichijo K, Tooyama N *et al*. Breath-hold MR cholangiopancreatography performed with long-echo train, fast SE sequence and a surface coil in chronic pancreatitis. *Radiology* 1994; 192: 73–8.

15. Ralls PW. Color Doppler sonography of the hepatic artery and portal venous system. *AJR* 1990; 155: 517–25.

16. Appleton GV, Bathurst NC, Virjee J *et al*. The value of angiography in the surgical management of pancreatic disease. *Ann R Coll Surg Engl* 1989; 71: 92–6.

17. Finn JP, Eldelman RR, Longmaid HE, Jenkins RL, Lewis D. MR angiography. Prospective, blinded study with surgical validation in liver transplantation. *Radiology* 1990; 177(P): 92.

18. Benjamin IS, Imrie CW, Blumgart LH. Liver biopsy in 'difficult' jaundice. *BMJ* 1977; ii: 578.

19. Conn HO. Liver biopsies in extrahepatic biliary obstruction and other 'contraindicated' disorders. *Gastroenterology* 1975; 68: 817–21.

20. Smout JL, Bellemans MA, vanHerreweghe W. Klatskin tumours: radiological and imaging findings in eleven patients. *J Belge Radiol* 1991; 74: 177–81.

21. Looser C, Stain SC, Baer HU, Friller J, Blumgart LH. Staging of hilar cholangiocarcinoma by ultrasound and duplex sonography; a comparison with angiography and operative findings. *Br J Radiol* 1993; 65: 871–7.

22. Adam A, Benjamin IS. The staging of cholangiocarcinoma. *Clin Radiol* 1992; 46: 299–303.

23. Collier NA, Carr D, Hemmingway A, Blumgart LH. Preoperative diagnosis and its effect on the treatment of carcinoma of the gallbladder. *Surg Gynecol Obstet* 1984; 159: 465–70.

24. Gouma DJ, Mutum SS, Benjamin IS, Blumgart LH. Intrahepatic biliary papillomatosis. *Br J Surg* 1984; 71: 72–4.

25. Desa LA, Akosa AB, Lazzara S, Domizio P, Krausz T, Benjamin IS. Cytodiagnosis in the management of extrahepatic biliary stricture. *Gut* 1991; 32: 1188–91.

26. Nimura Y, Kamiya J, Hayakawa N, Shionoya S. Cholangioscopic differentiation of biliary strictures and polyps. *Endoscopy* 1989; 21 (Suppl 1): 351–6.

27. Nimura Y. Staging of biliary carcinoma: cholangiography and cholangioscopy. *Endoscopy* 1993; 25: 76–80.

28. Kaneko T, Nakoa A, Inoue S *et al*. Portal venous invasion by pancreatobiliary carcinoma: diagnosis by intraportal endovascular US. *Radiology* 1994; 192: 681–6.

29. Nagino M, Hayakawa N, Nimura Y, Dohke M, Kitagawa S. Percutaneous transheptic biliary drainage in patients with malignant biliary obstruction of the hepatic confluence. *Hepatogastroenterology* 1992; 39: 296–300.

30. Pagliaro L, Rinaldi F, Craxi A *et al*. Percutaneous blind biopsy versus laparoscopy with guided biopsy in diagnosis or cirrhosis. A prospective, randomized trial. *Dig Dis Sci* 1983; 28: 39–43.

31. Cuesta MA, Meijer S, Borgstein PJ *et al*. Laparoscopic ultrasonography for hepatobiliary and pancreatic malignancy. *Br J Surg* 1993; 80: 1571–4.

32. Freeny PC, Lunderquist A. The pancreas. In: Grainger RG, Allison DJ, eds. *Diagnostic Radiology*. Edinburgh: Churchill Livingstone, 1992: 1129–47.

33. Warshaw AL, Tepper JE, Shipley WU. Laparoscopy in the staging and planning of therapy for pancreatic cancer. *Am J Surg* 1986; 151: 76–80.

34. Hunt DR, Blumgart LH. Iatrogenic choledochoduodenal fistula: an unsuspected cause of postcholecystectomy symptoms. *Br J Surg* 1980; 67: 10–13.

35. Chapman WC, Halevy A, Blumgart LH, Benjamin IS. Postcholecystectomy bile duct strictures: management and outcome in 130 patients. *Arch Surg* 1995; 130 (in press).

36. Collier NA, Weinbren K, Bloom SR, Lee YC, Hodgson HJF, Blumgart LH. Neurotensin secretion by fibrolamellar carcinoma of the liver. *Lancet* 1984; i: 538–40.

37. Foley WD. Dynamic hepatic CT. *Radiology* 1989; 170: 617–22.

38. Ferrucci JT. Liver tumour imaging: current concepts. *AJR* 1990; 155: 472–84.

39. Nelson RC, Chezmar JL, Sugarbaker PH, Murray DR, Bernadino ME. Preoperative localization of focal liver lesions to specific liver segments: utility of CT during arterial portography. *Radiology* 1990; 176: 89–94.

40. Heiken JP, Weyman PJ, Lee JLT et al. Detection of focal hepatic masses: prospective evaluation with CT, delayed CT, CT during arterial portography, and MR imaging. *Radiology* 1989; 171: 47–51.

41. Graf O, Dock WI, Lammer J et al. Determination of optimal time window for liver scanning with CT during arterial portography. *Radiology* 1994; 190: 43–7.

42. Matsui O, Takashima T, Kodoya M et al. Liver metastases from colorectal cancers: detection with CT during arterial portography. *Radiology* 1987; 165: 65–9.

43. Soyer P, Roche A, Gad M et al. Preoperative segmental localization of hepatic masses: utility of three-dimensional CT during arterial portography. *Radiology* 1991; 180: 653–8.

44. Soyer P, Levesque M, Elias D, Zeitoun G, Roche A. Preoperative assessment of resectability of hepatic metastases from colonic carcinoma: CT portography vs sonography and dynamic CT. *AJR* 1992; 159: 741–4.

45. Dawson P, Adam A, Banks L. Diagnostic iodized oil embolization of liver tumours – the Hammersmith experience. *Eur J Radiol* 1993; 16: 201–6.

46. Power C, Ros PR, Stoupis C, Johnson WK, Segel KH. Primary liver neoplasms: MR imaging with pathological correlation. *Radiographics* 1994; 14: 459–82.

47. Ferrucci JT. MR Imaging of the liver. *AJR* 1986; 147: 1103–16.

48. Marti-Bonmati L, Torrijo C, Vilar J, Ronchera C, Paniagua JC, Talens A. Lesion/fat intensity ratio in MR characterization of hepatic masses. *J Comput Assist Tomogr* 1991; 15: 539–41.

49. Ham B, Reichel M, Vogl T, Taupitz, Wolf KJ. Superparamagnetische eisenpartikel. Klinische ergebnisse in der MR-diagnostik von Lebermetastasen. *Rofo Fortschr Geb Rontgenstr Neuen Bildgeb Verfahr* 1994; 160: 52–8.

50. Hartley MN, Poston GJ. Treatment strategies for the patient with colorectal liver metastases. *Surgery* 1994; 12: 256–60.

51. Allison DJ, Adam A. Percutaneous liver biopsy and track embolization with steel coils. *Radiology* 1988; 169: 261–3.

52. Dawson P, Adam A, Edwards R. Technique for steel coil embolisation of liver biopsy tract for use with the 'Biopty' needle. *Br J Radiol* 1992; 65: 538–40.

53. Quaghebeur G, Thompson JN, Blumgart LH, Benjamin IS. Implantation of hepatocellular carcinoma after percutaneous needle biopsy. *J R Coll Surg Edinb* 1991; 36: 127.

54. Ferrucci JT, Wittenberg J, Mueller PR et al. Diagnosis of abdominal malignancy by radiologic fine-needle aspiration biopsy. *AJR* 1980; 134: 323–30.

55. Zornoza J, Wallace S, Ordonez N, Lukeman J. Fine-needle aspiration biopsy of the liver. *AJR* 1980; 134: 331–4.

Perioperative care of patients with hepatobiliary disease

O. James Garden BSc, MD, FRCS(Ed), FRCS(Glas)
Senior Lecturer and Honorary Consultant Hepatobiliary Surgeon, University Department of Surgery and Scottish Liver Transplantation Unit, Royal Infirmary, Edinburgh, UK

Perioperative care of patients with hepatobiliary disease should include assessment of risk to ensure that the patient receives the most appropriate management. If surgery is indicated, it is essential to identify factors that may be improved prior to surgical intervention so that operative risk may be reduced and outcome improved. Extensive hepatic resection may be well tolerated when the remaining liver has normal function, but even minor resection in cirrhotic patients may be poorly tolerated[1]. Surgical intervention directed at the obstructed biliary tree, and the increased blood loss associated with portal hypertension, carry a particularly high risk of hepatic decompensation in the postoperative period.

Preoperative evaluation

Existing liver disease and current medication

The patient with liver disease presenting for surgical intervention may benefit from specific medical manage-ment of the underlying liver disease. Surgery in the presence of active alcoholic hepatitis carries a substan-tial risk and abstinence for as little as 3 months will reduce this risk. The development of alcohol withdraw-al syndrome during the perioperative period is best managed by the administration of alcohol rather than excessive doses of sedative drugs. Patients with active hepatitis who are on long-term steroid therapy may require an increase in steroid cover during the perioperative period.

Modified Child's grading

The use of clinical and biochemical parameters in the assessment of surgical risk in cirrhotic patients is well established (*Table 1*). The modified Child's classifica-tion correlates well with surgical risk and only the most urgent surgery should be contemplated in patients with modified Child's class C, in whom surgical mortality can exceed 50%[2-4].

Table 1 Modified Child's classification used to assess severity of liver disease in patients undergoing surgery (after Pugh *et al.*[2])

	1	2	3
Encephalopathy	Absent	Mild	Moderate to severe
Ascites	Absent	Minimal to moderate	Severe
Serum bilirubin (µmol/l)	< 34	34–51	> 51
Serum albumin (g/l)	> 35	28–35	< 28
Prolonged prothrombin time (s)	1–3	4–6	> 6

Child's grade A, 5 or 6 points; grade B, 7–9 points; grade C, 10–15 points.

Encephalopathy

The presence of even mild encephalopathy in the perioperative period is a significant adverse event and a number of factors, including the administration of sedative drugs, sepsis, bleeding and hypoxia can precipitate decompensation. Restriction of protein intake and the administration of enemas and lactulose in the preoperative period are required.

Ascites

Ascites increases the risk of wound breakdown and the development of incisional herniae. Spontaneous bacterial peritonitis should be excluded by diagnostic paracentesis and treated by prescribing appropriate antibiotics. Ascites should be controlled preoperatively by salt restriction and diuretic therapy (spironolactone). Aggressive paracentesis and intravenous administration of salt-poor albumin may be helpful in resistant ascites, but the need for such measures signifies the presence of severe hepatic disease.

Jaundice

Surgery for obstructive jaundice secondary to malignancy carries an increased risk of renal failure and has a high mortality when associated with preoperative anaemia. Preoperative relief of obstructive jaundice by endoscopic or percutaneous means may reduce operative risk but such manoeuvres may introduce infection and the benefit of preoperative stenting is now questioned. Renal failure is most likely to be prevented by adequate hydration throughout the perioperative period, but the precise role of mannitol and renal doses of dopamine remains uncertain.

Nutrition

It is extremely difficult to counter nutritional depletion in patients with severe liver disease. In the presence of ascites, weight may be a poor indicator of nutritional status and, since aggressive feeding may precipitate encephalopathy, suboptimal nutritional status may have to be accepted.

Coagulation

Preoperative administration of parenteral vitamin K should improve coagulation disorders secondary to poor nutrition and absence of luminal bile salts due to obstructive jaundice, but will not reverse coagulopathy secondary to hepatocellular dysfunction. Fresh frozen plasma should be administered to correct the prothrombin time to within 2 seconds of control before surgery if possible. Thrombocytopenia may not respond well to perioperative platelet transfusion, since this is usually secondary to hypersplenism, but platelet transfusion is indicated when the platelet count is less than $50 \times 10^9/l$. It should, however, be borne in mind that platelet function may be deranged and a normal platelet count does not preclude difficulties in controlling haemorrhage. Patients receiving aspirin therapy should have this discontinued for at least 3 weeks before surgical intervention.

Renal failure

Central venous pressure monitoring in the preoperative period may help to differentiate prerenal failure from the hepatorenal syndrome, since the former can be improved by appropriate fluid resuscitation. Associated hypoxia, sepsis, fluid imbalance, blood loss and drugs can contribute to renal failure in patients with liver dysfunction.

Intraoperative management

The quality of general anaesthesia and provision of intraoperative monitoring is crucially important in hepatic resectional surgery. Both hypocapnia and hypoxaemia reduce hepatic arterial flow and should be avoided during anaesthesia. Portal venous flow is sensitive to decreases in blood pressure and cardiac output, while spinal and epidural blocks are associated with a decrease in liver blood flow if hypotension occurs. Poor patient positioning on the operating table, increased intra-abdominal pressure, excessive surgical retraction and positive pressure ventilation can all reduce liver blood flow. These mechanical factors can be offset by increasing circulating blood volume.

Anaesthesia

Premedication

In the presence of severe liver disease, premedication is best omitted. Ranitidine may reduce the risk of gastric aspiration, but can reduce liver blood flow and is best avoided.

Induction and maintenance

All intravenous agents used to induce and maintain anaesthesia may lead to hypotension, but the risk is theoretically diminished if propofol is used.

All volatile anaesthetic agents reduce portal venous blood flow secondary to a decrease in cardiac output.

Isoflurane is the volatile agent of choice, since it is associated with preservation or an increase in hepatic arterial blood flow and carries a reduced risk of postoperative hepatic dysfunction. The efficacy of the neuromuscular blocking agents atracurium and rocuronium is not influenced by hepatic and renal failure.

The elimination of fentanyl is unchanged in cirrhosis and it is a suitable opioid analgesic. Regional analgesic techniques are commonly used after major surgery and may reduce the need for opioids. Regional anaesthesia can reduce the risk of precipitating encephalopathy, but coagulopathy is regarded as a contraindication to spinal and epidural anaesthesia.

Fluid replacement

Fluid losses should be replaced appropriately, with the proviso that large quantities of sodium-containing fluids may contribute to ascites in the postoperative period. Albumin solutions are useful in maintaining circulating volume and conserving liver and renal blood flow. Plasma volume is best maintained by giving fresh frozen plasma at an early stage. The development of significant coagulopathy in patients with liver disease who require blood transfusion should be anticipated, and aggressive maintenance of coagulation status will reduce postoperative bleeding complications and the need for blood products after surgery.

Monitoring

Monitoring and maintenance of body temperature is of prime importance during hepatobiliary surgery, since coagulopathy is compounded by hypothermia[5]. Body temperature can be maintained by adequate warming of all intravenous fluids, warming of inspired gases, provision of an adequate ambient temperature and the use of an effective warming blanket. In major hepatic resectional surgery it is the author's practice to site intra-arterial and internal jugular catheters to monitor arterial and central venous pressures.

Postoperative care

In the postoperative period, high dependency nursing or intensive care will be required to provide adequate observation of vital signs and conscious level and to detect ongoing blood losses. Monitoring includes regular measurement of heart rate, blood pressure, oxygen saturation, urine output, central venous pressure and conscious level, judged using a simple sedative scoring system combined with an assessment of pain control.

Patients undergoing major hepatic resection and those with poor preoperative liver function are at particular risk of developing postoperative hepatic decompensation. Maintenance of adequate liver function can be judged by regular assessment of conscious level, acid base status, blood glucose levels, blood lactate concentrations and prothrombin time.

References

1. Friedman LS. When patients with liver disease need surgery. *Int Med* 1993; 14: 25–34.

2. Pugh RN, Murray-Lyon IM, Dawson JL, Pictroni MC, Williams R. Transection of the oesophagus for bleeding oesophageal varices. *Br J Surg* 1973; 60: 646–9.

3. Garden OJ, Motyl H, Gilmour WH, Utley RJ, Carter DC. Prediction of outcome following acute variceal haemorrhage. *Br J Surg* 1985; 72: 91–5.

4. Brown RB. Anesthesia considerations in patients with liver disease. *Anesth Rev* 1993; 20: 213–20.

5. Rohrer MJ, Natale AM. Effect of hypothermia on the coagulation cascade. *Crit Care Med* 1992; 20: 1402–5.

Hepatic resection

O. James Garden BSc, MD, FRCS(Ed), FRCS(Glas)
Senior Lecturer and Honorary Consultant Hepatobiliary Surgeon, University Department of Surgery and Scottish Liver Transplantation Unit, Royal Infirmary, Edinburgh, UK

Henri Bismuth MD, FACS, FRCS(Ed)
Professor of Surgery, Unité de Chirurgie Hepatobiliaire et Transplantation Hepatique, Hôpital Paul Brousse, Villejuif, France

History

Although surgical removal of portions of the human liver was recorded in the 18th and 19th centuries, the first successful elective hepatic resection is credited to Langenbuch[1]. However, regular and extended hepatectomies to remove well defined anatomical portions of the liver have only been undertaken in the last few decades. Lortat-Jacob[2] and Tung and Quang[3] were among the pioneers of modern hepatic resection and were largely responsible for the evolution of classical hepatic resection techniques. The improved understanding of the segmental liver anatomy as described by Couinaud[4] subsequently provided the basis for the technique of segmental resection[5].

Principles and justification

Indications

The main indication for hepatic resection is primary or secondary hepatic malignancy, but the presence of benign lesions may also be an indication (*Table 1*).

Preoperative

Preoperative evaluation is aimed at determining the nature of the hepatic lesion and the potential for its resection. Patients with malignant hepatic tumours should be screened for extrahepatic metastases by chest radiography, and an abdominal and thoracic computed tomographic (CT) scan. Such preoperative evaluation may well require more advanced scanning techniques such as CT portography and nuclear magnetic resonance (NMR) imaging. The information obtained from such investigations is of paramount importance in planning the type of hepatic resection. The use of intraoperative ultrasonography is essential in defining intrahepatic anatomy and the boundaries of the tumours, and in facilitating resection.

Table 1   Indications for hepatic resection

Benign hepatic lesions:	Liver trauma
	Hepatic cyst
	Haemangioma
	Adenoma
	Fibronodular hyperplasia
Malignant hepatic lesions:	
Primary	Hepatocellular carcinoma (cirrhotic and non-cirrhotic liver)
	Cholangiocellular carinoma
	Haemangiosarcoma
Metastases	Colorectal
	Leiomyosaroma
Contiguous tumour	Gallbladder carcinoma
	Cholangiocarcinoma involving extrahepatic biliary tree
	Adrenal carcinoma

Operations

Perioperative morbidity and mortality can be kept to a minimum by adhering to a number of basic principles (*see* chapter on pp. 347–349). The key to successful hepatic resectional surgery is to undertake the procedure with adequate exposure and following full and appropriate mobilization of the liver. Before the hepatic parenchyma is transected, control of the appropriate supplying and draining vessels must be considered. Postoperative morbidity and mortality are diminished if the segmental anatomy of the liver is respected.

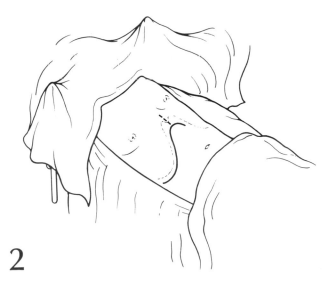

Position of the patient

1 The patient is positioned supine with the left arm extended at right angles to the body. The authors prefer to secure the patient's right arm to the side by means of a folded towel. This provides full access to the right hand side of the patient for the surgeon and assistant(s). It is unnecessary to place the patient in a lateral position, although placement of small sandbags or pillows beneath the right shoulder and right hip may improve access in patients undergoing resection of right-sided hepatic lesions. Tilting of the table can be used to improve exposure. ECG and monitoring leads should be kept clear of the lower chest and presternal area.

The abdomen and lower chest are prepared and draped, taking care to apply the drapes on the right side to the posterior axillary line. Two adjustable poles may be positioned beneath the upper drapes to facilitate attachment of subcostal retractors.

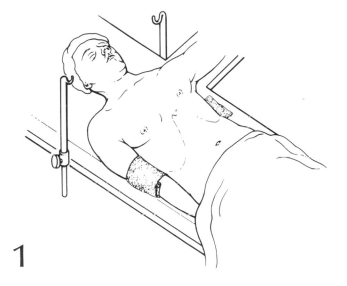

Incision

2 The initial incision depends upon the nature of the resection, but the surgeon should not hesitate to extend the wound to improve access. Although a midline incision may be employed for exploration of the abdomen in trauma patients, practice in elective resection a long S-shaped incision which follows the costal margin on the right side and can be extended on the left as appropriate. Exposure may be further improved in some patients with a narrow costal margin by extending the incision in the midline upwards to the xiphoid process. The authors have not found it necessary to extend the incision into the chest.

3 Once the abdomen is opened and a preliminary laparotomy has been undertaken, the ligamentum teres is divided between ties, one of which is left on the ligamentum teres and secured with a small forceps. The falciform ligament is incised using diathermy and separated from the anterior abdominal wall to facilitate placement of two large subcostal retractors. These are secured, in turn, by stout tapes applied to the two adjacent poles. The traction on the right subcostal retractor is best applied at the same height as the costal margin, although access to the liver is improved if traction to the left subcostal retractor is applied more vertically, approximately 8 cm above the level of the costal margin. Further retraction of intra-abdominal organs may be undertaken with carefully applied retractors, but the use of an additional fixed retractor system (Omnitract) frees the hands of the surgeon's assistant.

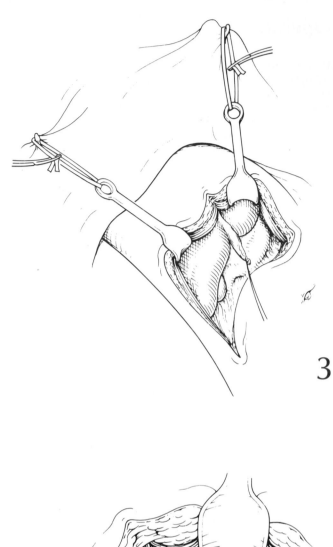

3

Exploration of the abdomen

In patients with hepatic malignancy, a thorough search is made of the peritoneum and regional lymph nodes to exclude extrahepatic dissemination of malignancy. The liver is carefully palpated and intraoperative ultrasonography is undertaken to confirm the position of the tumour and to assess its relationship with adjacent vascular structures. The presence of further lesions can be excluded using this technique. It may be necessary to take down any inflammatory adhesions, excising the parietal peritoneum if this is adherent to the hepatic tumour.

4 The right and left lobes are mobilized by first taking down any obvious capsular adhesions with diathermy. The falciform ligament is further incised using diathermy while gently retracting the liver inferiorly. Care is taken not to damage the suprahepatic cava and the hepatic veins which are identified by a combination of blunt and sharp dissection.

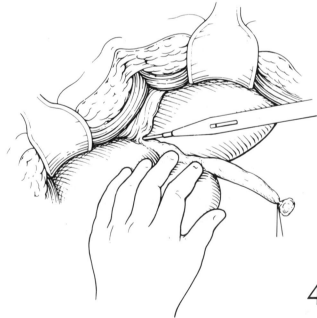

4

5 For left-sided lesions the left triangular ligament is incised with the diathermy, having previously placed a large pack over the stomach and oesophagus and beneath the left lobe of the liver. In this way the peritoneal attachment of the liver can be incised with diathermy, cutting down onto the pack below and so avoiding damage to the stomach and spleen. Care must be taken to avoid damage to the left hepatic vein as the left triangular ligament is freed close to the vena cava.

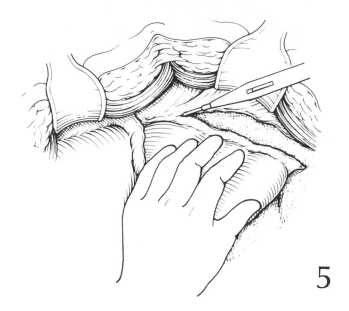

5

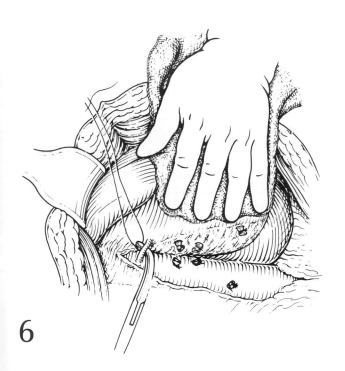

6

6 The right lobe can be similarly mobilized using diathermy to incise the anterior leaf of the coronary ligament and right triangular ligament as the liver is displaced inferiorly and across to the left of the abdomen by the assistant, whose hand retracts the right lobe of the liver using a gauze swab or pack. The dissection can be continued posteriorly, carefully separating the adhesions between the right adrenal gland and the bare area of the liver. In this way, the retrohepatic vena cava can be cleared downwards from its suprahepatic portion. When a lesion in the right liver is to be excised, it is useful to secure the short hepatic veins between the liver and vena cava. The authors prefer to divide these veins between Absolok clips or fine ties. In those patients with an accessory inferior right hepatic vein, formal ligature or oversewing of this vessel may be required. The short caudate veins can be similarly dealt with if excision of the caudate lobe is being considered.

7 As the vena cava is freed from the liver, the resection can continue superiorly to free the right hepatic vein from the overlying fibrous band of tissue which often tethers the right lobe to the vena cava superiorly. In this way, the right hepatic vein can be identified and encircled by means of a right angle forceps and Silastic sling. Any further attempts to secure this vessel are deferred until the inflow to the liver is secured. If troublesome bleeding is encountered at any stage during the freeing of the vena cava, a small swab or pack can be applied and the liver returned to the abdomen.

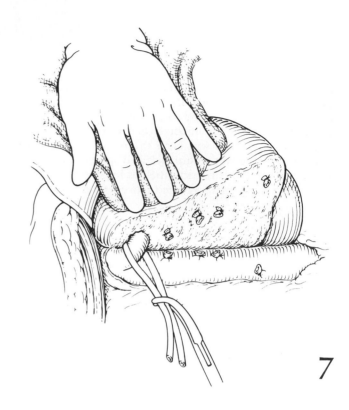

7

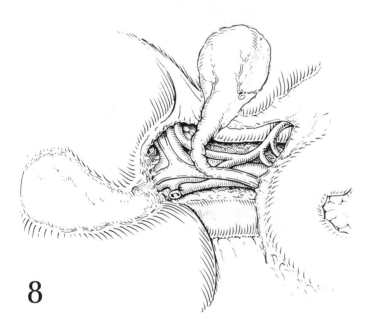

8

RIGHT HEPATECTOMY

8 Following thorough mobilization of the right lobe of the liver, the gallbladder is taken down from its bed using diathermy. The cystic duct and artery are exposed, ligated and divided. Division of the peritoneal reflection along the free edge of the lesser omentum and behind the common bile duct exposes the lateral side of the portal vein.

9 The portal vein is dissected free from the surrounding adventitial tissue by blunt dissection and, when traced upwards, its bifurcation is identified. The right branch of the portal vein is freed posteriorly, taking care to avoid inadvertent damage to any small caudate branches passing posteriorly. The right branch of the portal vein is secured with a Silastic sling.

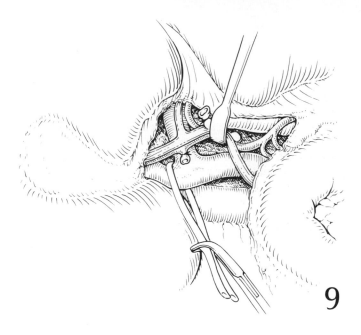

9

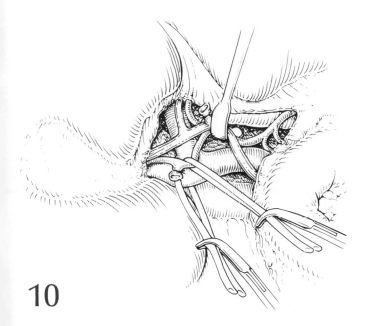

10

10 The right branch of the hepatic artery will normally be identified as it passes behind the common hepatic duct. This vessel is isolated and secured with a fine Silastic sling. No attempt is made at this stage to secure the right hepatic duct. Prolonged attempts at encircling the short right duct risk devascularizing it or ensnaring the left hepatic duct as it passes towards the midline.

11 The right branch of the portal vein is occluded by means of a straight bladed vascular clamp and the right hepatic artery is secured with a small bulldog clamp as the artery lies to the right or medial to the duct. A clear line of demarcation develops on the liver surface, running from the gallbladder fossa to the vena cava in the principal vascular plane. The capsule of the liver is incised with diathermy approximately 1 cm to the right of this line of demarcation. This avoids inadvertent dissection of the middle hepatic vein which is to be left intact on the residual liver. It is useful if the first assistant holds the quadrate lobe of the liver with a gauze swab secured in the left hand. Compression of the liver tissue will minimize blood loss.

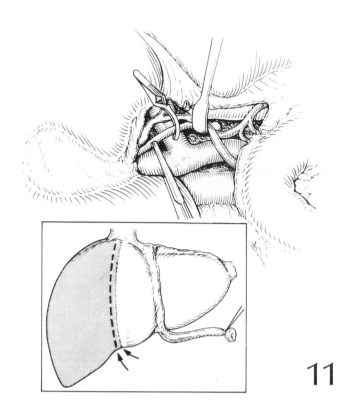

11

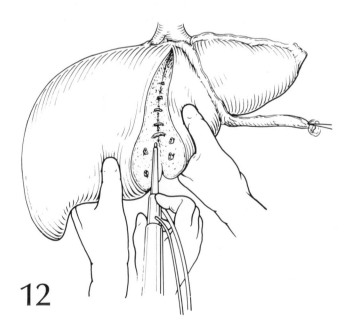

12

12 The liver dissection can be undertaken in a number of ways, but it is the authors' preference to employ a Cavitron ultrasonic surgical aspirator (CUSA) which skeletonizes the vessels within the hepatic parenchyma, allowing their identification before they are damaged and giving them an opportunity to retract into the liver substance. Small vessels (less than 2 mm) can be secured by diathermy before division with sharp scissors, although larger vessels and branches of the middle hepatic vein are best secured by ligation or application of Absolok clips.

13 The dissection is continued posteriorly along the entire length of the transected surface of the liver, taking care to avoid damage to the middle hepatic vein. The dissection is continued inferiorly, and the right portal pedicles are identified and dissected down onto the hilar plate using the Cavitron. The sectoral pedicles are isolated and divided between strong ligatures. In this way, the intrahepatic ducts are secured well away from the main confluence of the ducts at the hilus of the liver.

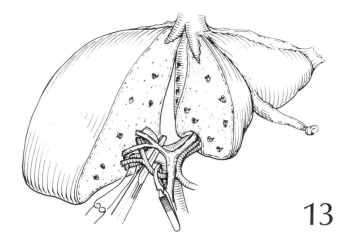

13

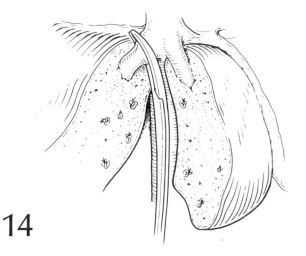

14

14 The dissection is continued posteriorly towards the vena cava. The dissection through the liver is better directed if the parenchyma to the right of the caudate lobe is opened inferiorly onto the vena cava which is protected by placement of the surgeon's left hand behind the right lobe of the liver. The dissection is continued superiorly to the right hepatic vein which, having previously been secured, is clamped and divided.

On delivery of the specimen from the operating field, the transected liver, vena cava and retroperitoneum are inspected carefully for bleeding points. These can be controlled by diathermy and an argon beam coagulator can be used to avoid removal of the coagulum which may be dislodged by conventional diathermy.

15 The right hepatic vein is secured by a running 4/0 polypropylene (Prolene) suture before removal of the clamp. The clamps on the right branch of the portal vein and right hepatic artery can be removed before confirming haemostasis at the porta hepatis. Bile leaks should be secured by careful placement of interrupted 4/0 polydioxanone (PDS) sutures. The transected surface of the liver can be sprayed with thrombin glue. Although this may not significantly reduce postoperative loss of blood, there is some evidence that it reduces the incidence of postoperative bile leakage. Large liver sutures or liver buffers should not be used to improve haemostasis since this is likely to promote necrosis of the liver and may risk damaging the intrahepatic ducts.

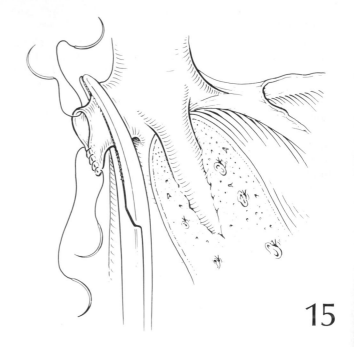

15

Wound closure and drainage

16 Two large bore drains are placed through separate stab incisions and connected to a closed drainage system. The tips of the drains are placed into the right subphrenic space and to the porta hepatis.

The wound is closed in layers using looped 1/0 polydioxanone sutures to the muscle layers and staples to the skin.

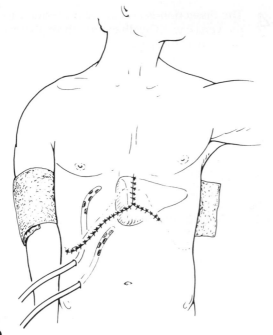

16

LEFT HEPATECTOMY

Access to the liver is the same as for a right hepatectomy. The left lobe is freed by dividing the falciform ligament towards the vena cava posteriorly and by dividing the left triangular ligament.

17 At the porta hepatis the left branch of the hepatic artery is identified and the left branch of the portal vein cleared at its bifurcation from the main portal vein trunk. When this vessel is encircled, care must be taken to avoid damage to the short posteriorly situated caudate branches. If the caudate lobe is to be left intact, the left branch of the portal vein is encircled distal to their origin. The left hepatic artery and left branch of the portal vein are secured with vascular clamps and this produces a clear line of demarcation between the right and left hemilivers. The gallbladder is normally dissected free from its bed by diathermy and the cystic duct and artery are divided between ties.

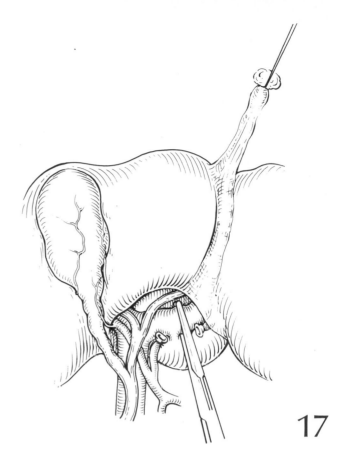

17

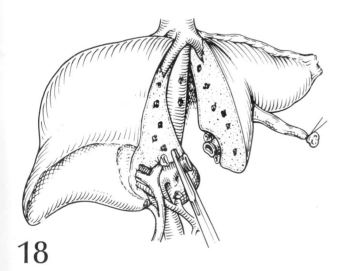

18

18 The capsule of the liver is incised about 0.5 cm to the left of the main scissura, running from the left border of the vena cava down to the gallbladder bed and hilus of the liver. The hepatic parenchyma is dissected with the Cavitron aspirator as for a right hepatectomy, but the middle hepatic vein on the right hemiliver is preserved. Once the dissection proceeds to the hilus, the left branch of the hepatic artery and the left hepatic ducts are ligated and divided distal to the hilar clamp. The anterior aspect of the hilus is then opened and the left branch of the portal vein is exposed, divided and oversewn with continuous 4/0 polypropylene. The left branch is generally smaller than the right branch of the portal vein, but it is still preferable to clamp and suture the divided vessel.

19 The liver transection is continued posteriorly, preserving the caudate lobe (segment I) along the well defined plane that extends from the left of the liver hilus. As the inferior vena cava is reached, the left hepatic vein is identified and secured with a vascular clamp within the liver substance. This vein is divided and the specimen delivered before oversewing the left branch of the portal vein with continuous 4/0 polypropylene.

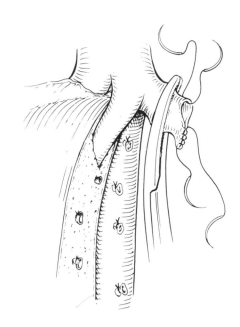

19

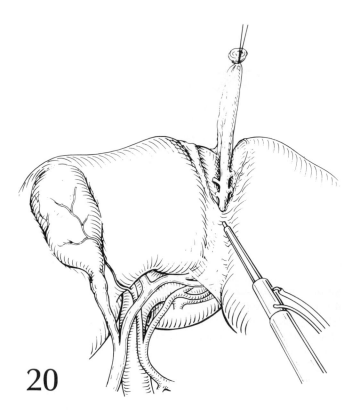

20

LEFT LOBECTOMY

Left lobectomy is the most straightforward of the classic hepatic resections since the left lobe is morphologically separate from the rest of the liver parenchyma. The positioning of the patient and the incision are as for the previously described hepatectomies, although this is one of the few hepatic resections that can be safely undertaken through an upper midline incision.

20 The left lobe is freed by division of the falciform and left triangular ligaments. The lesser omentum is opened with diathermy, taking care to identify any aberrant left hepatic artery. The falciform ligament and obliterated umbilical vein are retracted upwards by a secured tie and any bridge of liver parenchyma between the right and left lobes of the liver is divided by diathermy and the Cavitron aspirator.

21 The arterial and portal venous branches to segments II and III are easily identified and can be encircled following incision of the overlying peritoneum. These vessels are divided between ligatures. The pedicle to segment II is situated more posteriorly at the junction of the vertical portion of the round ligament and the horizontal left hilar branches. These vessels are similarly divided between ligatures, although it may be necessary to oversew any more substantial vessels to avoid bleeding following further mobilization of the left lobe.

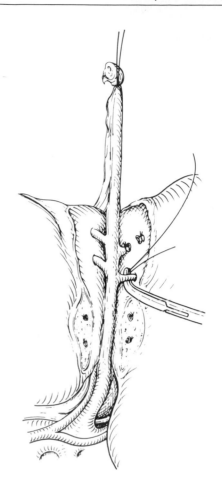

21

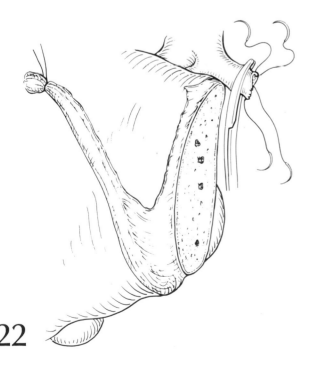

22

22 A clear line of demarcation will be observed to the left of the falciform ligament and the liver capsule is incised on its superior aspect about 0.5 cm to the left of the falciform ligament. The hepatic parenchyma is opened along its bloodless plane using the Cavitron aspirator and any further small vascular or biliary pedicles can be secured by fine ligatures. The left hepatic vein is identified posteriorly, clamped at its origin, divided and oversewn with continuous 4/0 polypropylene.

On delivery of the specimen, the transected liver surface is examined for bleeding or bile leakage. A single tube drain is normally passed through a separate stab incision down to the resected margin.

EXTENDED RIGHT HEPATECTOMY

The principles of extended right hepatectomy are drawn from those of right hepatectomy and left lobectomy.

23 The initial mobilization of the right liver and the preliminary hilar dissection are identical to those of right hepatectomy. The portal and arterial pedicles to segment IV are identified to the right of the round ligament following division of the overlying bridge of hepatic parenchyma if this is present. As the divided ligamentum teres is retracted upwards, the pedicles to segment IV are visualized and will require division between ligatures.

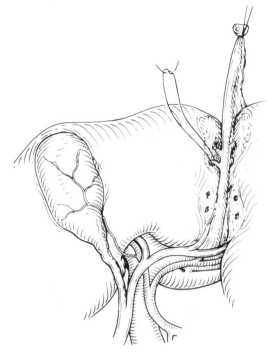

23

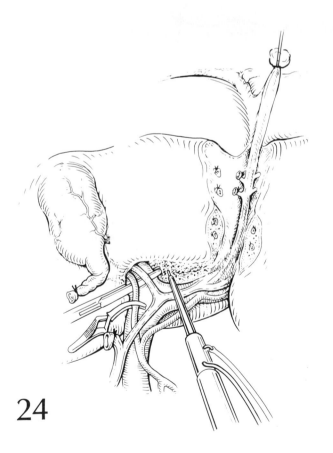

24

24 As the pedicles to segment IV are divided, the dissection proceeds with the Cavitron beneath the retracted undersurface of segment IV (quadrate lobe) and the left hepatic duct. There are often one or two small arterial branches present which may require division between ligatures. The dissection is continued to the cystic duct and artery which are divided between ligatures. This manoeuvre exposes the right hepatic artery and right branch of the portal vein which are dealt with in the same manner as for right hepatectomy. With the division of the segment IV branches and placement of clamps on the right hepatic artery and right portal pedicle, a clear line of demarcation develops between the devascularized right lobe of the liver and the left lobe to the right of the falciform ligament.

25 The hepatic parenchyma is incised approximately 0.5 cm to the left of this line of demarcation and the dissection is continued into the hepatic parenchyma using the Cavitron. Any further small vessels can be divided between ties, but the absence of substantial hepatic venous branches in the plane of dissection ensures a relatively bloodless operating field. Once the liver has been opened to the hilus of the liver and the posterior border of the quadrate lobe has been raised, the portal pedicle can be approached in the same way as for a right hepatectomy. The vessels are ligated and divided distal to the clamps and the dissection can continue posteriorly in the direction of the inferior vena cava, skirting and preserving the caudate lobe. The plane of this dissection passes to the right border of the inferior vena cava. The middle hepatic vein is clamped before being divided and oversewn with continuous 4/0 polypropylene. If the right hepatic vein has not previously been secured, the dissection continues onto the vena cava and the right hepatic vein is dealt with in the same manner as for the right hepatectomy.

If segment I is to be removed with this resection, the small vascular pedicles that pass from the portal vein are ligated. It is preferable for the small caudate veins which drain into the vena cava to have been divided between ties during the preliminary mobilization of the liver, but if this has not been possible, the posterior dissection should continue following division of the middle hepatic vein to the left border of the inferior vena cava. When this is done, the small caudate vessels can be isolated and divided between ligatures.

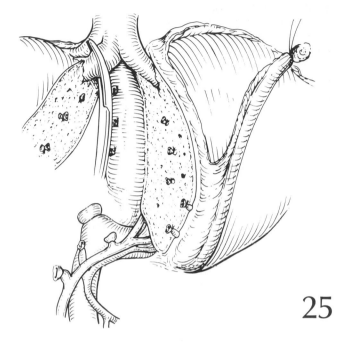

25

EXTENDED LEFT HEPATECTOMY

Left hepatectomy can be extended to include resection of segments I, V and VIII. The liver is mobilized from its peritoneal attachments as described for left hepatectomy. The boundary between the anterior and posterior sectors of the right hemiliver is situated along a plane 4 cm to the right and parallel to the main hepatic scissura, but peroperative ultrasonography may be used to localize the right hepatic vein and the right anterior sectoral vessels.

26 The liver is mobilized from its peritoneal attachments as described for left hepatectomy. The gallbladder is dissected from the liver bed and the left hepatic artery and left branch of the portal vein are isolated at the porta hepatis. In this resection, the left hepatic duct is best divided at an early stage and this facilitates mobilization of segment IV from the porta hepatis. The Cavitron is used to skeletonize the right portal pedicle which is traced along its length to enable the anterior sectoral pedicle to be encircled with a Silastic sling. This pedicle is clamped to produce a line of demarction between the right posterior sector and the anterior sector. The liver capsule is incised with diathermy approximately 1 cm anterior to this line of demarcation and the Cavitron is used to open up the plane of dissection, preserving the right hepatic vein on the posterior sector.

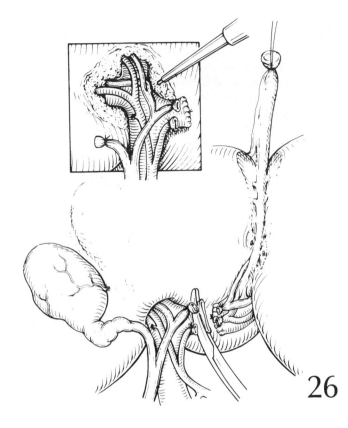

26

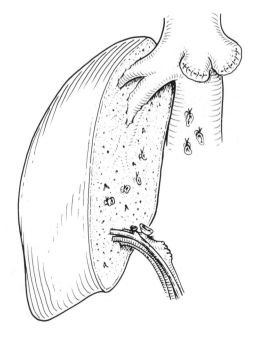

27

27 The resection is continued superiorly and enables isolation of the confluence of the middle and left hepatic veins which are divided once secured by a vascular clamp. These vessels are oversewn with 4/0 continuous polypropylene.

On delivering the specimen, haemostasis is secured and the absence of a bile leak confirmed. The right anterior sectoral pedicle is suture ligated.

Postoperative care

In the recovery room the blood pressure, pulse, temperature and urinary output are monitored continuously. If the central venous pressure has been maintained at a low level peroperatively to minimize venous bleeding, the patient may require an additional infusion of colloid or crystalloid solution. Serum concentrations of urea, electrolytes, potassium and blood sugar are measured immediately in the postoperative period and 6-hourly BMstix are undertaken in the first 48 h until it is clear that hypoglycaemia no longer poses a risk.

Complications

If haemostasis was satisfactory during operation it is unlikely that postoperative bleeding will be a significant problem, but drainage should be monitored for excessive blood loss and/or bile leakage. Disordered liver function tests are inevitable following major hepatic resection, but jaundice is usually mild if blood replacement has not been required and if a less major resection has been undertaken. In major liver resection, monitoring of serum lactate concentration, blood gases and prothrombin time will better reflect liver function. Correction of coagulation defects should only be undertaken by administration of blood products and vitamin K if there is evidence of haemorrhage. The major complications relating to hepatic resection are the development of jaundice and liver failure. The latter complication is more likely to arise if there has been hypoperfusion of the liver during surgery or extensive resection of normal liver. The risk is greatest in the cirrhotic patient and can only be minimized by careful preoperative selection.

Wound infection and intra-abdominal sepsis are now rare complications of major hepatic resectional surgery. Such collections can be managed by percutaneous drainage techniques and re-exploration is not usually required. More general complications inlcude atelectasis and chest infection.

References

1. Langenbuch C. Einfall von resection eines linksseitigen schnurlappens der leber. *Berl Klin Wochenschr* 1888; 25: 37–8.

2. Lortat-Jacob JL, Robert HG. Hépatectomie droit réglée. *Presse Med* 1952; 60: 549–51.

3. Ton That Tung, Nguyen Duorg Quang. A new technique for operation on the liver. *Lancet* 1963; i: 192–3.

4. Couinaud C. *Le Foie: Etudes Anatomiques et Chirurgicales*. Paris: Masson, 1957.

5. Bismuth H, Houissan D, Castaing D. Major and minor segmentomies "réglées" in liver surgery. *World J Surg* 1982; 6: 10–24.

Further reading

Bismuth H, Garden OJ. Regular and extended right and left hepatectomy for cancer. In: Nyhus LM, Baker RJ, eds. *Mastery of Surgery*. 2nd edn. Boston: Little Brown, 1992: 864–72.
Starzl TE, Iwatsuki S, Shaw BW. Left hepatic trisegmentectomy. *Surg Gynecol Obstet* 1982; 155: 21–7.

Liver abscess

I. S. Benjamin BSc, MD, FRCS
Professor, Academic Department of Surgery, King's College Hospital, London, UK

History

The first description of liver abscess is generally attributed to Bright of Guy's Hospital and was published in 1836. One of the earliest modern series was that of Ochsner et al. (1938)[1] who reported a series of 47 pyogenic abscesses of the liver. This was said to represent an incidence of about 1% of post-mortem examinations, and 0.008% of hospitalized patients. The peak age incidence was in the third and fourth decades, a different spectrum from the present situation in which the peak is in the sixth to eighth decades of life. In the pre-antibiotic era, open drainage was the only management option, but as long ago as 1900, percutaneous drainage of liver abscesses was described by Laurent using a specially designed long trocar and cannula.

Principles

The principles of management of hepatic abscesses do not differ fundamentally from the principles of abscess management elsewhere in the body, nor from the general principles governing surgery of the liver. Broadly, the presence of the abscess is established initially on clinical grounds and subsequently on imaging supported by generalized evidence of infection (such as leucocytosis) and, as a general rule, pus within a closed cavity must be released. The causative organism should be established whenever possible, either from blood culture or from direct aspiration of the abscess contents. Finally, the predisposing cause should be identified and, if necessary, eradicated. According to the general principles of liver surgery, the abscess can be localized within the hepatic segmental anatomy and an appropriate method of drainage selected which will cause least damage to normal liver tissue. If the underlying cause of the abscess is thought to be neoplastic, then consideration should be given to radical resection if possible, and if due to biliary disease then free drainage of as much of the intrahepatic biliary tree as possible should be secured by appropriate means. Other general principles of liver surgery such as attention to coagulation and support of impaired hepatocyte function should also form a part of the general management.

Aetiology

Liver abscesses are generally classified according to the nature of the infecting organism i.e. pyogenic, specific bacterial infection (such as tuberculosis), amoebic, parasitic and fungal. Both amoebic abscesses and hydatid cysts may contain only the primary infecting organism or parasite, or may be secondarily infected with pyogenic organisms. Pyogenic abscesses per primum are generally also subdivided according to the underlying cause. The most common varieties are taken into account in the classification shown in *Table 1*.

The frequency of these various causes displays distinct geographical variations. Pyogenic abscesses are by far the most common type of abscess in Western series, whereas in Eastern countries and in much of the Third World a liver abscess may be assumed to be of amoebic origin until proven otherwise.

Pyogenic abscess

The source of infection may be classified as in *Table 1*. In earlier series infection within the gastrointestinal tract was the commonest cause of pyogenic liver abscess, and most frequently appendicitis was responsible. The decreasing frequency of severe untreated appendicitis probably accounts for much of the shift in age spectrum from the third to the fifth decade with the passage of time. Complicated diverticular disease is now more common than appendicitis as a portal source. Umbilical sepsis remains common in Third World countries, particularly where it is the custom to dress the umbilical cord with infected materials. Portal blood is usually sterile, but chronic sepsis anywhere within the gastrointestinal tract may produce transient episodes of portal bacteraemia. This may be enhanced by obstructive jaundice, and there is also evidence that translocation of bacteria across the mucosa of the gastrointestinal tract is enhanced by starvation and by associated alterations in gastrointestinal microbial flora[2]. Sepsis associated with diverticular disease and thrombosed haemorrhoids may also be sources of portal pyaemia. Liver abscesses are rare in association with Crohn's disease, despite the bacteraemia which may occur in that condition. Benhidjeb *et al.*[3] reported a case of Crohn's disease which presented initially with a hepatic abscess. Pyogenic abscesses of gastrointestinal tract origin are frequently multiple.

Organisms of biliary origin now give rise to almost one-third of all pyogenic liver abscesses, usually as part of a syndrome of cholangitis and biliary obstruction. Garrison and Polk[4] reported that 22% of pyogenic hepatic abscesses arose from sepsis within the portal venous drainage region, compared with 32% of biliary origin. Cholangitis due to choledocholithiasis (or rarely other foreign bodies within the biliary tract), benign or malignant biliary strictures, congenital disorders of the biliary tree and primary sclerosing cholangitis may all be sources of such infection. Direct spread from acute cholecystitis or empyema of the gallbladder may also be included in this category.

1 Patients with chronic incomplete biliary tract obstruction, such as those with primary sclerosing cholangitis, recurrent biliary strictures after previous surgical repair, or occluded biliary stents are particularly prone to forming multiple small intrahepatic abscesses, initially in communication with the peripheral biliary radicals. The endoscopic retrograde cholangio-pancreatogram shown is of a woman with a malignant bile duct stricture and an abscess can be seen in communication with a right sectoral hepatic duct.

Table 1   Aetiology of liver abscess

Pyogenic
   Biliary tract origin
      'Ascending' cholangitis
      Stent occlusion
      Primary sclerosing cholangitis
   Portal origin
      Appendicitis
      Diverticular disease
      Inflammatory bowel disease
      Umbilical sepsis
   Traumatic
      Iatrogenic (e.g., biliary surgery, liver biopsy, post-embolization)
      Penetrating injuries
      Blunt liver trauma
   Neoplastic
      Degeneration
      Post-embolization
   Infected cysts
      Simple
      Choledochal
      Parasitic
   Contiguous spread
      Gallbladder
      Gastrointestinal perforation
   Metastatic from systemic sepsis (especially in immunocompromised hosts)
   'Cryptogenic'

Specific bacterial infections
   Tuberculosis

Fungal

Parasitic
   Amoebic
   Hydatid
   Clonorchis sinensis
   Ascaris lumbricoides

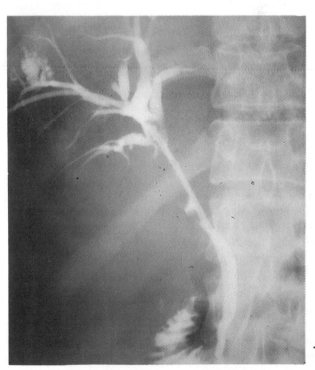

1

The symptoms of pyogenic abscess may be difficult to distinguish from those of the underlying suppurative cholangitis and, indeed, the principles of management may be similar, with the primary objective of securing good biliary drainage.

Asiatic pyogenic cholangitis is a separate category in which there is gross dilatation of the intrahepatic ductal system in association with intrahepatic stone formation, multiple strictures, and invasive sepsis which may partially destroy one or more segments of liver. This syndrome is frequently associated with parasitic infestation of the biliary tract. Such abscesses may not respond to drainage and may require partial liver resection for their eradication.

Chronic pancreatitis is said to produce biliary tract obstruction in about 15% of cases, but liver abscesses in this condition remain uncommon[5]. The combination of long-standing biliary obstruction and sepsis with impaired hepatic blood supply may be a potent cause of liver abscess; the author has seen one such patient in whom an indolent *Streptococcus milleri* liver abscess occurred following an otherwise uncomplicated pancreatoduodenectomy for chronic pancreatitis.

Haematogenous abscesses arising from systemic infection are much more common in immunocompromised patients. They constitute about 9% of all liver abscesses, and drug abusers, patients with leukaemia, diabetes or HIV infection, and those with other systemic infections such as subacute bacterial endocarditis may be at particular risk.

Iatrogenic causes (other than those associated with benign biliary strictures) are responsible for an increasing number of cases. Liver infection may follow percutaneous biopsy, percutaneous transhepatic cholangiography, or biliary stenting, when the stents become occluded (*Illustration 1*). Cases have also been reported following ethanol injection for hepatocellular carcinoma[6]. Embolization of large liver tumours may also result in a liver abscess, occasionally with gas-forming organisms.

Trauma (other than iatrogenic injury) is responsible for about 6% of pyogenic abscesses and this includes blunt injuries causing subcapsular haematomas which subsequently become infected. Contiguous spread from subhepatic, pleural or perinephric sepsis gave rise to the liver abscess in about 10% of patients in the series reported by Garrison and Polk[4].

The number of pyogenic abscesses described as 'cryptogenic' has diminished with improved investigation. In the series reported by Ochsner *et al.*[1] cryptogenic abscesses constituted 55–60% of the total, while in the series of Garrison and Polk[4] no cause could be found in only 15% of cases.

Amoebic abscess

This is caused by the organism *Entamoeba histolytica* which, while not indigenous to most Western countries, is found much more commonly with the increase of foreign travel. It has become indigenous in some immigrant populations such as the Hispanic population in the south and west of the United States. This may be particularly important because the organism may have a long latent period, occasionally up to 20 years. While amoebic abscesses classically contain the primary infecting organism, secondary infection with pyogenic organisms may also occur and can follow intervention.

Fungal abscess

These abscesses are found primarily in immunocompromised patients and may have a characteristic radiological appearance[7].

Tuberculous abscess

This form of abscess is extremely rare. Multiple small abscesses may be present in miliary tuberculosis or a single large granuloma (tuberculoma) can develop in the absence of any evidence of systemic tuberculosis. Organisms are rarely isolated from the lesion and treatment with antituberculous drugs may have to be empirical. The author has seen one case in which liver resection was required for a left-sided tuberculoma, the differential diagnosis being that of necrosis and superinfection within a primary liver tumour.

Parasitic disease

Hydatid disease
Although the diagnosis of hydatid disease of the liver is usually readily made on scanning, supported by positive serology, there may be confusion with other forms of liver abscess, especially if there is secondary infection. Bacterial infection may follow previous surgical treatment or may be spontaneous. Infection within simple cysts or hydatid cysts constituted 4% of all cases of pyogenic hepatic abscess in the series of Garrison and Polk[4].

Other parasites
Rare in Western medical practice, infestation of the biliary tree with *Ascaris lumbricoides* or with *Clonorchis sinensis* is extremely common in Asia, Africa and Central and South America. The biliary tract becomes secondarily infected, resulting in suppurative cholangitis, following which nests of worms within the liver parenchyma may cause pyogenic cholangitic liver abscesses. Chronic suppurative cholangitis (pyogenic Asiatic cholangitis) is a common sequel of infestation with *Clonorchis sinensis*.

Microbiology of pyogenic liver abscesses

In early reports, 38% of abscesses were reported to be sterile on culture[1] but this would now be uncommon. Bowers et al.[8] in a series of 34 patients reported a single organism in 15, polymicrobial growth in 11, and no positive culture in seven (material for culture was not obtained from one patient). The organisms found are usually of enteric origin. *Escherichia coli* and other organisms predominated in the 38 abscesses analysed by Barnes et al.[9] (*Table 2*). Staphylococcal infection was more common in earlier series but has now diminished in importance.

Anaerobic species are more commonly identified in recent times, the commonest being *Bacteroides fragilis*. More sensitive methods such as estimation of volatile and non-volatile fatty acids by gas liquid chromatography in the pus from abscesses allowed demonstration of the presence of anaerobic or microaerophilic bacteria in 14% of cases in one series[10]. However, *Streptococcus milleri* has also often been reported[11].

Lactobacilli have been found in an abscess following ethanol injection for hepatocellular carcinoma, and *Listeria* and *Yersinia* have also been reported. The responsible mycobacterium is only rarely cultured in cases of tuberculous infection[12], although infection with tubercle bacilli has been reported in association with HIV infection[13].

Pathology

Pyogenic liver abscesses are multiple in 50% of cases. There is a predilection for the right lobe rather than the left. Abscesses are frequently related to the portal venous radicals or to biliary radicals, in which case they may be bile-stained. The wall of the abscess may display characteristic features according to the infecting organism, but the common finding is of inflammatory infiltration of the surrounding liver. This may wall off the abscess so that in most cases it loses its communication with the biliary tree. The purulent contents may be foul smelling and contain gas, and the smell may be suggestive of a mixed aerobic/anaerobic infection.

Ameobic abscesses frequently reach a large size but are usually solitary. While 75% are on the right, those on the left side may be prone to intrapericardial rupture. The content of amoebic abscesses has the characteristic 'anchovy sauce' appearance and contains few pus cells but a great deal of debris.

Presentation and diagnosis

The presentation is characteristically one of pyrexia of unknown origin[14]. The classic constellation of signs includes sweating, anorexia, malaise, vomiting and

Table 2 Pathogenic aerobic organisms in 38 cases of liver abscess. Data from Barnes. et al.[9].

Organism	n
Escherichia coli	16
Klebsiella pneumoniae	6
Streptococcus sp.	6
Enterococcus	4
Proteus sp.	4
Enterobacteriaceae	3
Other Gram-negative rods (*Pseudomonas aeruginosa* 1)	3
Staphylococcus aureus	1

weight loss, often associated with pain in the upper abdomen. Although swinging fever is described as classical, an analysis of clinical features in 58 cases revealed this feature in only 25% of cases[15]. Ameobic abscesses may have an insidious onset with hepatomegaly, abdominal pain and fever; diarrhoea occurs in less than 20% of patients. Evidence of atelectasis or pleural effusion may be found in any case of hepatic abscess, with occasional pain referred to the shoulder tips, but this is a non-specific finding. Haemobilia has been reported in one child secondary to liver abscess, treated by selective arterial embolization[16]. Khan et al.[17] reported obstructive jaundice secondary to an amoebic liver abscess.

Choice of treatment

There are essentially three forms of treatment: antibiotic therapy without any invasive treatment, radiological aspiration or drainage, and open surgical drainage.

Long courses of high dose antibiotics may be used in some patients with multiple small hepatic abscesses when the underlying cause is unknown or has been eradicated but, in general, drainage is also necessary. While open drainage used to be the standard treatment for all liver abscesses, in recent years it has been overtaken by percutaneous drainage techniques on the grounds of equal efficacy and greater safety. The changing practice over the last decade or two has paralleled the increased use of percutaneous drainage for other intra-abdominal collections. During the years 1979–1988 the author encountered 36 such collections in a specialist hepatobiliary unit; prior to 1984, surgical drainage was the norm. Following the adoption of percutaneous drainage methods for intra-abdominal collections there was a significant fall in overall mortality from serious postoperative sepsis[18]. Others have also reported the increasing use of percutaneous drainage[19, 20].

Table 3 Retrospective comparison of surgical *versus* percutaneous tube drainage. Data from Bertel *et al.*[21].

	Surgical	Percutaneous
Number of patients	23	16*
Morbidity (%)	48	69
Hospital stay (days)	26	46

* Three required surgery.

The issue does not readily lend itself to controlled trial because of the differing circumstances surrounding liver abscesses in individual patients. A retrospective study of patients treated at the Mayo Clinic from 1977 to 1984[21] suggested that non-surgical drainage has significant disadvantages (*Table 3*). However, much of the morbidity in this series was associated with dislodged catheters and several patients undergoing percutaneous drainage required surgery because of inadequate aspiration of viscous abscess contents.

2a–f It has been the author's recent experience that it is rarely necessary to abandon percutaneous drainage because of viscous contents and frequent tube changes, regular flushing, and even breaking down of the walls between loculi by manipulating the catheter allows continued effective use of drainage techniques. A sequence of CT scans in a patient with a pyogenic abscess of unknown aetiology treated by percutaneous drainage is shown. *Illustration 2c* shows a contrast study performed after insertion of the catheter and reveals the complex abscess contents. The catheter was used to break down loculi within the cavity, and drainage and antibiotics continued for several weeks was followed by complete resolution without recurrence.

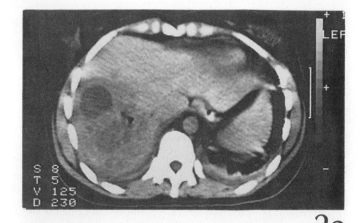

2a

2b

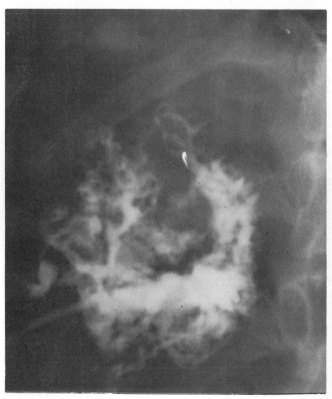

2c

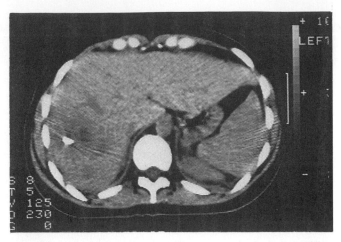

2d

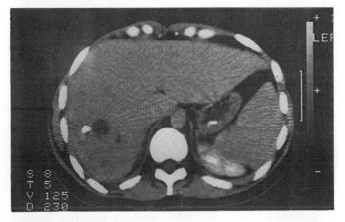

2e

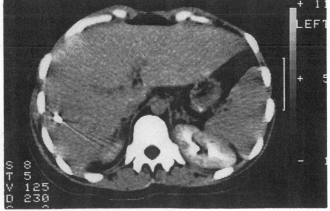

2f

Failure of drainage may, however, still result from technical factors or multiple abscesses. In such cases a combination of external drainage with prolonged systemic antibiotics is indicated. Attar *et al.*[22] used CT-guided drainage in 15 patients with abscesses of 5–1000 ml in volume, including some with multiple abscesses; only one patient required surgical drainage because of a true failure to respond. Enormous abscesses with a thick wall are unlikely to collapse completely, and may leave the problem of a residual cavity. It may be that such patients should be selected for surgical drainage.

For amoebic abscesses the issue of whether to aspirate or not remains controversial. De La Rey Nel *et al.*[23] prospectively randomized 80 patients to undergo aspiration or non-aspiration along with metronidazole treatment. This series, pursued over a period of 1 year in Durban, South Africa, suggested that aspiration did influence the course and outcome of treatment and the authors suggested a number of criteria for selection.

It should be emphasized again that it is important to consider the possibility of hydatid disease when considering aspiration, since percutaneous puncture of hydatid cysts with intraperitoneal leakage may both disseminate the disease and produce a potentially fatal anaphylactic reaction. Increasing experience suggests that percutaneous aspiration and instillation of alcohol or other scolicidal agent may be safe[24], but the author would still urge caution.

Preoperative

Clinical

Liver abscess should be considered in any case of pyrexia of unknown origin, especially in the presence of known biliary disease or when there has been biliary surgery, intervention or trauma. General examination is aimed at eliciting signs of systemic sepsis and multi-organ failure. Careful assessment of renal and hepatic function is undertaken, particularly in patients with associated jaundice. It is important to consider causes of immune deficiency in patients with otherwise unexplained liver abscesses. The abdomen is examined with a view to identifying localizing signs in the liver or elsewhere, with particular reference to other pathology within the gastrointestinal tract.

Haematological investigation is vital. Haemoglobin levels may fall precipitously in the presence of hepatic abscess (often in association with haemolysis and a raised ESR) and a neutrophil leucocytosis is typical of pyogenic abscess. Coagulation should be checked as a preliminary to surgical or radiological intervention. Biochemical testing usually shows an increased serum alkaline phosphatase concentration even in the absence of biliary obstruction. Aspartate aminotransferase (AST) levels may remain normal except in advanced disease. The albumin levels may fall precipitously in the presence of continuing liver sepsis, and this may also be predictive of a poor outcome. Where relevant, serological tests such as the ELISA test should be performed for amoebic or hydatid disease. IgG ELISA is a sensitive and specific test for invasive amoebiasis in comparison with evidence of previous exposure[25].

The importance of microbiology has already been mentioned. Blood cultures must be performed, though these are frequently negative. The question of aspiration of suspected abscesses is controversial because, although valuable for microbiological diagnosis of pyogenic abscesses, it may be unnecessary or unhelpful in amoebiasis and many would regard it as positively contraindicated in hydatid disease.

Imaging

The imaging results in 100 liver abscesses from two different geographical areas have been reviewed recently[26] and showed a preponderance, respectively, of amoebic and pyogenic or fungal abscesses. Plain abdominal radiography may give useful indicators such as elevation of the diaphragm, associated pleural effusion or consolidation of the underlying lung. Chest radiography may suggest extension of the infective process into the lung tissue or the formation of a bronchopleural fistula. An air/fluid level may be seen in some cases. However, ultrasonography has become the investigation of first choice and has, to a large extent, displaced colloidal liver scans in this role. Overall, ultrasonography will reach a correct diagnosis in 93% of cases[9]. Computed tomographic (CT) scanning may offer some increase in diagnostic accuracy as lesions as small as 2 cm can be identified. Because the pus in some abscesses is very thick, distinction between a solid lesion and an abscess is not always straightforward. In the case of multiple abscesses, other forms of diffuse parenchymal liver disease such as fatty infiltration, cirrhosis and multiple metastases have to be considered. Nevertheless, with CT scanning the diagnostic accuracy should approach 100%. Labelled white cell scanning or gallium scanning may be of complementary value. The value of magnetic resonance imaging (MRI) relative to CT scanning has yet to be established.

It should not be forgotten that the majority of liver abscesses are now of biliary origin, so that imaging of the biliary tract (usually by ERCP but occasionally by PTC) may form a critical part of the evaluation of liver abscesses.

Operations

OPEN SURGICAL DRAINAGE

It is important to appreciate the surgical anatomy of the liver. The most important surgical implication for patients with liver abscesses is the relationship between cavities and the major vessels, particularly the hepatic veins. An expanding liver abscess will push segmental vessels aside, so that the wall of an abscess cavity may be partially formed by displaced and compressed major vessels and biliary radicals. In the case of large abscesses (those usually treated surgically) the use of intraoperative ultrasonography may help to define these margins. If there is any suspicion of underlying malignancy then multiple biopsies should be performed. If this is strongly suspected and the general condition of the patient and anatomy of the lesion allows, immediate resection with a clearance margin should be considered.

Incision

3 The usual approach is transperitoneal, and a long right subcostal incision is recommended. This can be extended well across the midline to the left side and into the right flank if extensive mobilization of the liver is required. The disadvantage of this incision is the inaccessibility of the lower abdomen to palpation, particularly if a source of sepsis in the colon is considered likely. Nevertheless, a full laparotomy is indicated as far as is possible. The alternative retroperitoneal approach is no longer recommended. Although this minimizes the risk of peritoneal contamination, it is impossible to assess or to deal with other pathology, and careful packing and antibiotic therapy will avoid generalized peritonitis in any event.

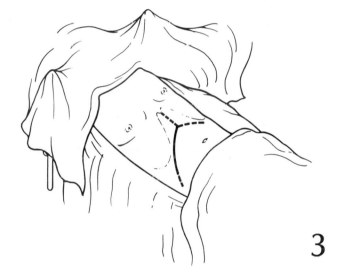

3

Localization of the abscess

4a,b The abscess can usually be localized by inspection and palpation. If the liver is greatly enlarged it may initially prove difficult to mobilize the right lobe of the liver, or even to insert a hand between the liver and the costal margin. Vigorous retraction of the costal margin using a fixed retractor system is recommended (*Illustration 4a*) but, in the case of a large abscess with risk of rupture, an initial aspiration using a trocar and cannula may be valuable (*Illustration 4b*). A large-bore needle may help to identify the site of an abscess, and samples are immediately taken for aerobic and anaerobic culture. Intraoperative ultrasonography is helpful in defining the extent of the abscess and its relationship to the major vessels and ducts.

A decision must also be taken on how to deal with any other abdominal pathology that is found. There is no absolute contraindication to resection of diverticular disease, for example, in combination with drainage of a liver abscess, but the general principles guiding multiple operative procedures at one laparotomy should be observed. The chief aim of the procedure is to deal with the liver abscess, and other pathology may be better dealt with through a different incision at a different time.

Once the site of the abscess has been identified, packs are used to wall off the rest of the abdominal cavity. If hydatid disease is thought to be a possibility then packs soaked in an appropriate scolicidal agent such as aqueous povidone-iodine (Betadine) should be used.

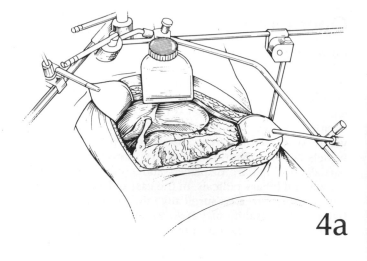

4a

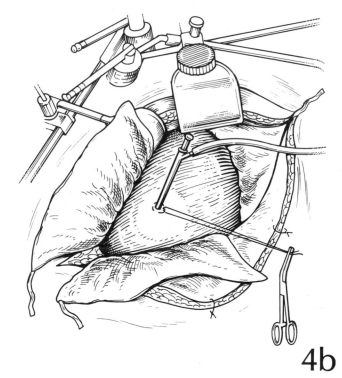

4b

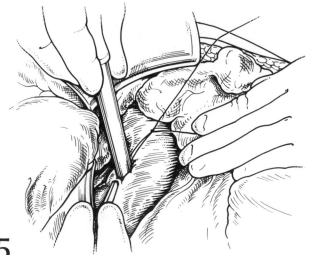

5

Aspiration of abscess

5 Following trocar aspiration an incision is made over the most superficial part of the abscess. If the liver parenchyma is thick at this level the incision can be made with the diathermy point. A large bore sucker is inserted into the cavity and the contents fully aspirated. A finger can then be inserted to assess the extent of the cavity and to help break down any internal loculi.

6a,b Although the simplest procedure is then to insert some form of large-bore drainage tube, deroofing is more likely to speed the resolution of large cavities. Deroofing is performed using the diathermy point, but care must be taken not to enter deeply into the liver parenchyma, since this may be the site of compressed segmental vesels and bile ducts which should not be disrupted. There is almost invariably some bleeding from the cut edges of the liver, and this is controlled by suturing small individual vessels (paying particular attention to small bile radicals which should be sutured separately) and then, if necessary, by controlling the cut rim of the deroofed cavity with a continuous locking mattress suture.

At the conclusion of this procedure it should be possible to inspect the lining of the cavity. The cavity should be carefully washed out and then packed for a few minutes to check for haemostasis and for bile leaks. Any small leaking bile radicals should be evident on removal of the packs and are carefully closed with a fine suture. If in doubt, radiological screening after injection of contrast medium into the biliary tree (via the gallbladder or bile duct) may reveal leaks. Injections of saline or diluted methylene blue dye may be used as a simpler alternative. In practice, it is less common to use these techniques for pyogenic abscess than for hydatid disease.

Consideration is now given to the type of tube drainage. Simple tube drains of the largest size available may be adequate and should be brought out through a separate stab wound. Suction drains become blocked and are usually unhelpful. Sump drains, particularly those of the irrigating variety, may be helpful for large cavities. The drains should be placed so that they exit in a dependent position and they must be securely fixed to the abdominal wall. Finally, if a flap of omentum is easily raised and can be laid into the cavity, this may also be helpful.

The abdominal cavity is finally washed out thoroughly with saline and closed in the usual fashion.

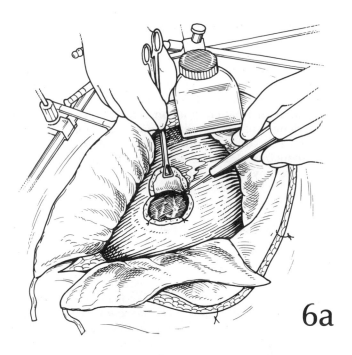

6a

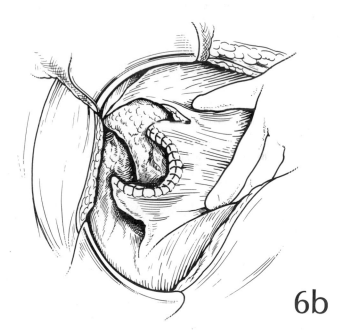

6b

LAPAROSCOPIC DRAINAGE

Cappuccino et al.[27] described the use of laparoscopy to guide and place intrahepatic and perihepatic drains in a patient in whom CT-guided drainage had failed to produce resolution. Robles et al.[28] described the technique in a patient with amoebic abscess. Extensive experience of these techniques has not yet been reported in the literature, and any advantages over percutaneous drainage with laparotomy in selected cases are as yet uncertain.

Postoperative care

Following open surgery a closed system of drainage is preferred to avoid ascending infection by exogenous organisms. If irrigation is to be used, a dilute antiseptic solution (such as aqueous povidone-iodine) is acceptable. A rate of 1 litre/24 h is usually adequate. The presence of drains is helpful since, in addition to postoperative ultrasonography, contrast medium can be instilled to determine whether the cavity is closing. Any postoperative bile leakage can be managed conservatively since the tube effectively functions as a controlled external biliary fistula. This drainage normally ceases spontaneously but, if not, a combination of ERCP and contrast tubography will identify the site and nature of the leak and determine whether any further action is needed. The tubes are removed when they have ceased to drain any significant amount of fluid and when the cavity is seen to be closing down around the tubes and a track is well established.

Antibiotics are usually continued for several weeks and follow-up antibiotics for a longer period are often used in the case of multiple abscesses. The choice of antibiotics, initially blind, can now be directed according to the microbiology and sensitivities determined on the operative samples.

Outcome

Until 1968 a mortality rate of 80–90% was regularly reported for liver abscesses, but overall mortality is now less than 10%. Factors which will determine outcome are age, multiplicity of lesions, associated biliary disease and malignancy. Adverse prognostic features include a raised serum AST level, low serum albumin level, persistently high white cell count and other complicating pathology. If a liver abscess fails to respond to treatment (whether conservative, percutaneous, or surgical) one should suspect continued obstruction to the biliary tree, a foreign body, or underlying malignancy.

References

1. Ochsner A, De Bakey M, Murray S. Pyogenic abscess of the liver. An analysis of 47 cases with review of the literature. *Am J Surg* 1938; 40: 292–319.

2. Ding JW, Andersson R, Soltesz V, Willen R, Bengmark S. Obstructive jaundice impairs reticuloendothelial function and promotes bacterial translocation in the rat. *J Surg Res* 1994; 57: 238–45.

3. Benhidjeb T, Ridwelski K, Wolff H, Gellert K, Luning M, Perschy J. Lover abscess as a first manifestation of Crohn's disease. *Dig Surg* 1992; 9: 288–92.

4. Garrison RN, Polk HC. Liver abscess and subphrenic abscess. In: Blumgart LH, ed. *Surgery of the Liver and Biliary Tract*. Edinburgh: Churchill Livingstone, 1994: 1091–102.

5. Reddy KR, Jeffers L, Livingstone AS, Gluck CA, Schiff ER. Pyogenic liver abscess complicating common bile duct stenosis secondary to chronic calcific pancreatitis. A rare presentation. *Gastroenterology* 1984; 86: 953–7.

6. Okada S, Aoki K, Okazaki N et al. Liver abscess after percutaneous ethanol injection (PEI) therapy for hepatocellular carcinoma. A case report. *Hepatogastroenterology* 1993; 40: 496–8.

7. Pastakia B, Shawker TH, Thaler M, O'Leary T, Pizzo PA. Hepatosplenic candidiasis: wheels within wheels. *Radiology* 1988; 166: 417–21.

8. Bowers ED, Robison DJ, Doberneck RC. Pyogenic liver abscess. *World J Surg* 1990; 14: 128–32.

9. Barnes PF, DeCock KM, Reynolds TN, Ralls PW. A comparison of amebic and pyogenic abscess of the liver. *Medicine* 1987; 66: 472–83.

10. Gupta U, Sharma MP. Etiology of liver abscess with special reference to anaerobic bacteria. *Indian J Med Res* 1990; 91: 21–3.

11. De Mestier P, Gujez C, Chakkour K, Khayat M, Chevalier T. Liver abscess caused by *Streptococcus milleri*. *Gastroenterol Clin Biol* 1992; 16: 1007–8.

12. Goh KL, Pathmanathan R, Chang KW, Wong NW. Tuberculous liver abscess. *J Trop Med Hyg* 1987; 90: 255–7.

13. Weinberg JJ, Cohen P, Malhotra R. Primary tuberculous liver abscess associated with the human immunodeficiency virus. *Tubercle* 1988; 69: 145–7.

14. Cohen JL, Martin FM, Rossi RL, Schoetz DJ Jr. Liver abscess. The need for complete gastrointestinal evaluation. *Arch Surg* 1989; 124: 561–4.

15. Ahmed L, el-Rooby A, Kassem MI, Salama ZA, Strickland GT. Ultrasonography in the diagnosis and management of 52 patients with amebic liver abscess in Cairo. *Rev Infect Dis* 1990; 12: 330–7.

16. Khalil A, Chadha V, Mandapati R *et al.* Hemobilia in a child with liver abscess. *J Pediatr Gastroenterol Nutr* 1995; 12: 136–8.

17. Khan JA, Jafri SMW, Khan MA. Obstructive jaundice: an unusual presentation of amebic liver abscess. *J Trop Med Hyg* 1990; 93: 194–6.

18. Pace RF, Blenkharn JI, Edwards WJ, Orloff M, Blumgart LH, Benjamin IS. Intra-abdominal sepsis after hepatic resection. *Ann Surg* 1989; 209: 302–6.

19. Falk KA, Angeras UJ, Friman VZ, Gamklou GR, Lukes PJ. Pyogenic liver abscesses: have changes in management improved the outcome? *Acta Chir Scand* 1987; 153: 661–4.

20. Farges O, Leese T, Bismuth H. Pyogenic liver abscess: an improvement in prognosis. *Br J Surg* 1988; 75: 862–5.

21. Bertel CK, Van Heerden JA, Sheedy PF. Treatment of pyogenic hepatic abscesses: surgical vs percutaneous drainage. *Arch Surg* 1986; 121: 554–8.

22. Attar B, Levendoglu H, Cuasay NS. CT-guided percutaneous aspiration and catheter drainage of pyogenic liver abscesses. *Am J Gastroenterol* 1986; 81: 550–5.

23. De La Rey Nel J, Simjee AE, Patel A. Indications for aspiration of amoebic liver abscess. *S Afr Med J* 1989; 75: 373–6.

24. Bastid C, Azar C, Doyer M, Sahel J. Percutaneous treatment of hydatid cysts under sonographic guidance. *Dig Dis Sci* 1994; 39: 1576–80.

25. Sathar MA, Simjee AE, De La Rey Nel J, Bredenkamp BLF, Gathiram V, Jackson TFHG. Evaluation of an enzyme-linked immunosorbent assay in the serodiagnosis of amoebic liver abscess. *S Afr Med J* 1988; 74: 625–8.

26. Barreda R, Ros PR. Diagnostic imaging of liver abscess. *Crit Rev Diagn Imaging* 1991; 33: 29–58.

27. Cappuccino H, Campanile F, Knecht J. Laparoscopy-guided drainage of hepatic abscess. *Surg Laparosc Endosc* 1994; 4: 234–7.

28. Robles PJ, Lara JG, Lancaster B. Drainage of hepatic amebic abscess successfully treated by laparoscopy. *J Laparoendosc Surg* 1994; 4: 451–4.

Illustrations by Peter Cox and Richard Neave

Splenectomy, partial splenectomy and laparoscopic splenectomy

Miles Irving MD, ChM, FRCS
Professor of Surgery, University Department of Surgery, Hope Hospital, Salford, UK

Stephen Attwood MCh, FRCS, FRCS(I)
Consultant Surgeon, Department of Surgery, Hope Hospital, Salford, UK

David Gough FRCS, FRCS(Ed), FRACS, DCH
Consultant Paediatric Surgeon, Department of Surgery, Royal Manchester Children's Hospital, Salford, UK

Principles and justification

The principal indications for splenectomy are trauma, hereditary spherocytosis, immune thrombocytopenia (idiopathic thrombocytopenic purpura), cysts and tumours, and as part of radical upper abdominal surgery such as total gastrectomy. The operation is also selectively used in the management of patients with chronic lymphocytic leukaemia, chronic granulocytic (myeloid) leukaemia, the lymphomas and hypersplenism due to a variety of causes.

In parallel with the recognition of the benefits of splenectomy has come an awareness of the danger from serious infection (particularly pneumococcal) that may follow, even years later, in children and adults[1,2]. As a consequence, in those cases where splenectomy is not essential every effort should be made to conserve part or all the spleen. Whether this advice is always sensible in adults is a matter of judgement in the individual case. It may well be decided that the potential benefit of preventing death from overwhelming septicaemia is outweighed by the postoperative mortality and morbidity of attempts at splenic preservation. If total removal is unavoidable, prophylactic antibiotic treatment and vaccination are advisable (*see* below).

Indications

Trauma

Where the spleen is avulsed or fragmented, splenectomy is the only feasible treatment. However, where it is lacerated or only a segment is avulsed, conservative treatment or partial splenectomy should be attempted, even if splenectomy has to be resorted to in the end. Unrecognized traumatic splenic injury of mild degree has probably gone untreated for years without harm. Recent diagnostic methods have established that a planned non-operative approach for selected cases of traumatic splenic rupture is both safe and effective[3].

1   The relatively non-invasive investigations of ultra-sonography and computed tomographic (CT) scanning have a high degree of sensitivity in revealing the presence of splenic injury and the associated haemoperitoneum. This allows a positive decision to be made to manage specific splenic injuries conservatively, such as that shown in the illustration of a patient who had major upper abdominal trauma with liver and splenic injury. The CT scan in *Illustration 1* shows a large fluid density collection in the left lobe of the liver consistent with a haematoma in the spleen which is displacing the stomach, filled with contrast medium to the left. A small amount of fluid is also seen lateral to the liver consistent with blood in the peritoneal cavity. The spleen is enlarged and is very heterogenous, particularly on its lateral aspect, consistent with splenic haematoma.

Because delayed splenic rupture is almost unknown in children, and in this age group the spleen is often the only organ injured, a policy of conservative management has always had considerable support among paediatric surgeons. With better imaging now available, increasing numbers of surgeons are adopting this policy in adults.

Autotransplantation of splenic fragments as free grafts can occur naturally after injury but is of no proven benefit as a planned surgical procedure.

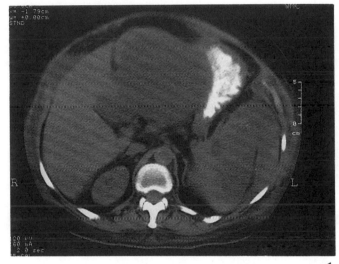

1

Hypersplenism

In this state the spleen, which usually is enlarged, is destroying one or more components of the blood (e.g. erythrocytes, leucocytes and platelets) at a rate which exceeds the ability of the marrow to produce them. This may be the result of abnormalities of the cells which make them more easily destroyed than normally, or of enlargement of the spleen resulting in stagnation of blood cells and their premature destruction. Hereditary spherocytosis, sickle cell anaemia, immune thrombocytopenia, splenic anaemia due to portal hypertension and lymphomatous infiltration of the spleen can be classified as forms of hypersplenism.

A form of immune thrombocytopenia occurs in 5–10% of patients with the acquired immune deficiency syndrome (AIDS). With its rising prevalence, AIDS has become a more frequent indication for splenectomy.

Leukaemias

Haematologists now consider that certain cases of chronic lymphocytic leukaemia, chronic granulocytic leukaemia and variants such as hairy cell leukaemia can be treated more effectively if the spleen is removed. The operation has to be performed when the patient is in good condition and free from infection. It is contraindicated in acute leukaemias, blast crises, and when the patient is deteriorating and/or infected.

Upper abdominal surgery

Splenectomy is often necessary during major upper abdominal operation, such as total gastrectomy or pancreatectomy, although when it is not essential for technical reasons the spleen should be left *in situ*.

Malignancy

While the nodes in the splenic hilum lie in the lymphatic drainage pathway from tumours of the lower oesophagus, stomach and pancreas, the benefits of splenectomy as part of a radical resection for these tumours has not been proven. The role of the spleen in immunity to malignancy is not known while, conversely, if lymph nodes in the splenic hilum are involved, the disease is at an advanced stage and carries a poor prognosis. It is therefore advisable to preserve the spleen in these operations as long as conservation does not compromise the clearance of overt malignant disease.

Giant splenomegaly

In some diseases such as myelofibrosis the spleen grows so large that its weight becomes unbearable and it becomes prone to repeated painful infarction. In these circumstances splenectomy is worthwhile.

Cysts, tumours, abscess, torsion, splenic artery aneurysm

In these rare conditions, splenectomy is necessary to establish the diagnosis as well as to treat the disease.

Staging laparotomy

Improvements in imaging and more effective treatment regimens mean that staging laparotomy, once an integral part of the effective treatment of Hodgkin's disease, is now redundant in most centres.

Preoperative

Close consultation with the haematologist and medical oncologist is essential in patients undergoing splenectomy for lymphoma or a haematological disorder. The surgeon should ensure that the haemoglobin, white cell and platelet counts have been measured recently and that the bone marrow has been assessed. Anaemia, leucopenia and thrombocytopenia are not in themselves contraindications to operation as long as the bone marrow shows evidence of its ability to produce these cells. There is rarely any benefit to be obtained from splenectomy for hypersplenism if the marrow is aplastic or totally replaced by tumour. If there is doubt about the role of the spleen in red cell or platelet destruction, survival studies with ^{51}Cr-labelled cells can be informative. In cases of haemolytic anaemia the gallbladder should be scanned with ultrasonography and, if gallstones are present, cholecystectomy is advisable at the time of splenectomy.

The surgeon should encourage colleagues to refer patients for splenectomy before the underlying disease and the associated cytopenias have progressed to the point where the patient is subject to serious infections. Splenectomy in infected hypersplenic patients almost never succeeds in improving their condition.

Before operation for uncomplicated splenectomy, two units of blood should be cross-matched. For large spleens, where there is a possibility of multiple vascular adhesions, up to six units of blood should be available. Platelet infusions should be ordered for severely thrombocytopenic patients but should not be given until the splenic artery has been tied. In cases of traumatic rupture of the spleen, preoperative colloid and blood transfusion is mandatory to resuscitate the patient.

The patient should be shaved from nipples to mid thigh and a nasogastric tube passed.

Anaesthesia

An endotracheal tube and muscle relaxation are essential. The anaesthetist should be warned that it may be necessary to divide the left costal margin and to open the thorax in difficult cases. Prophylaxis against venous thrombosis should be commenced before operation by prescribing subcutaneous heparin and is supplemented during operation by intermittent calf compression with pneumatic leg cuffs.

Operations

ELECTIVE SPLENECTOMY FOR NORMAL-SIZED OR SLIGHTLY ENLARGED SPLEEN

Incision

2 The patient is positioned supine on the operating table with a sandbag under the left lower ribs. A long midline or left subcostal muscle cutting incision is used.

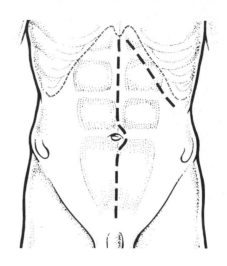

Exploration

General exploration commences with examination of the spleen, taking care not to tear any adhesions. The splenic hilum is palpated for lymph node enlargement and the liver examined for the presence of cirrhosis and tumour infiltration. The gallbladder is palpated and removed if it contains stones, a common finding in haemolytic anaemia.

The presence of accessory spleens is excluded by careful examination, paying particular attention to the gastrosplenic ligament, mesocolon and upper border of the pancreas.

Splenectomy

The operator's right hand is slid gently over the convex diaphragmatic surface of the spleen. In most cases it will slide without obstruction down to the lienorenal ligament. If adhesions are encountered they should not be broken down but dealt with in the manner described later.

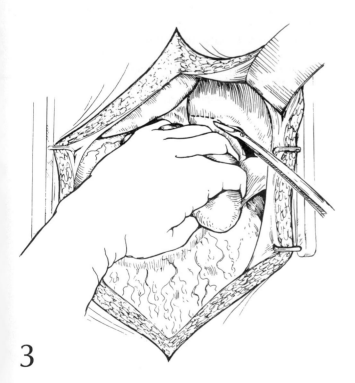

Mobilization of the spleen

3 The operator now substitutes his left hand for his right and gently pulls the spleen up towards the abdominal incision so that the taut posterior leaf of the lienorenal ligament is clearly demonstrated. This ligament is then incised with scissors along its full length allowing the posterior surface of the spleen and the contents of the hilum to be drawn up into the wound.

Division of vessels

4 At this stage a band of short gastric vessels passing to the upper pole of the spleen in the upper part of the gastrosplenic ligament may limit mobilization. These vessels are divided between artery forceps and ligated with 0 polyglactin (Vicryl) absorbable ligatures. Care must be taken not to include any of the stomach wall in the ligatures as this can lead to a gastric fistula. If difficulty is encountered because of the shortness of the ligament, it is often better to transfix and ligate the vessels on the gastric wall than to risk inclusion of gastric wall in the ligature.

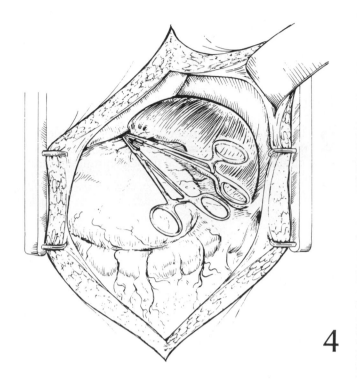

4

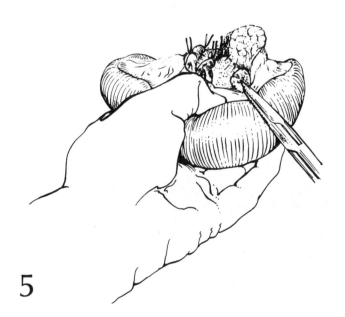

5

5 Attention is then turned to the posterior aspect of the splenic hilum. The tail of the pancreas is identified and carefully dissected from the hilum using scissors and gauze pledgets. Bleeding from small vessels can be arrested by diathermy coagulation or ligaclips. The splenic artery and vein become visible and can be dissected out and ligated in continuity with strong absorbable ligatures. The artery should be ligated before the vein. The vessels are then divided between the ligatures. In thrombocytopenic patients, platelet infusions should be given at this stage.

Division of the gastrosplenic ligament

6 The spleen is then turned over to demonstrate the gastrosplenic ligament and the attachments of the lower pole of the spleen to the splenic flexure of the colon, which are divided piecemeal between ligatures. This exposes the thin anterior leaf of the lienorenal ligament which, apart from a few small vessels, should be avascular. It is divided by dissection with the scissors, continued care being taken not to damage the pancreas. The spleen can now be removed. Haemostasis is secured by diathermy or suture ligation of any bleeding vessels in the splenic pedicle. If there has been extensive dissection in the left hypochondrium a low pressure suction drain should be placed in the subdiaphragmatic space.

The abdominal wall is then closed in layers.

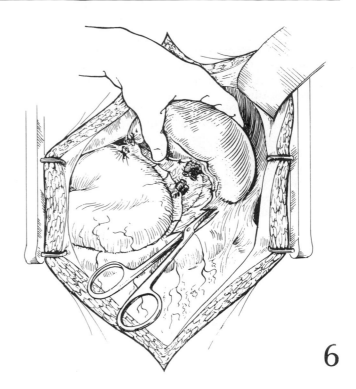

6

LAPAROSCOPIC SPLENECTOMY

Laparoscopic splenectomy is indicated for conditions such as immune thrombocytopenia or hereditary spherocytosis in which the spleen is usually of normal size or only slightly enlarged and where perisplenic adhesions are not a problem.

7 The patient is positioned head-up (anti-Trendelenburg) on the operating table in a partly chaired position and rotated 25–30° to the right. This allows gravity to assist with the retraction of the omentum and colon from the spleen. The patient's legs may be positioned in Lloyd-Davis supports. Some surgeons prefer to stand between the patient's legs while others prefer to stand on the patient's right side.

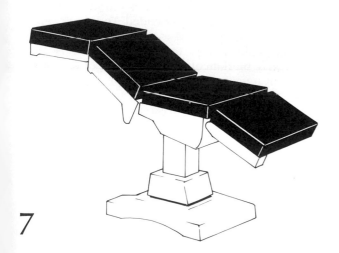

7

8 Port placements vary with the size of the spleen, the size of the patient and the view obtained at laparoscopy. A 10-mm port is first inserted above the umbilicus using a blunt entry technique to avoid damaging a large spleen. The peritoneum and spleen are assessed following insertion of the laparoscope and the degree of adhesion formation is evaluated. Two 12-mm ports are then inserted in the left side of the abdomen in the anterior axillary line below the costal margin, the other in the mid clavicular line at or above the level of the umbilicus. Two 10-mm ports are then inserted in the epigastrium and right upper quadrant.

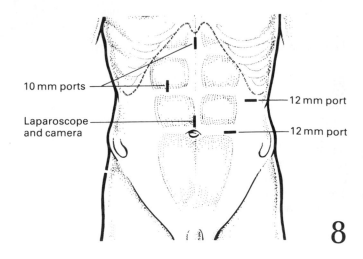

10 mm ports

12 mm port

Laparoscope and camera

12 mm port

8

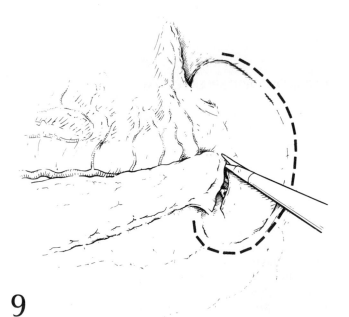

9

9 The anatomy of the upper abdomen is fully assessed using soft grasping instruments (Babcock forceps) to retract the stomach and lift the greater omentum. The splenic flexure of the colon and the spleen itself are assessed for adhesions posteriorly and accessibility to the splenic hilum is determined.

The operation commences with division of the attachments of the spleen to the splenic flexure of the colon, following which the spleen is retracted medially and the lienorenal ligament is divided. The use of clips is avoided if possible as these may interfere with subsequent application of the stapler. With very large spleens it may be difficult to see the upper half of the lienorenal ligament and a 30° telescope may help. The ligament is divided only as far as it can be clearly seen, leaving the rest until after division of the vessels in the splenic hilum.

10 A 12-mm blunt probe such as the Endogauge is used to lift the splenic hilum forwards. A pair of dissecting forceps is used to clear any adhesions posteriorly and so create a space for a laparoscopic stapling device to be placed across the hilum.

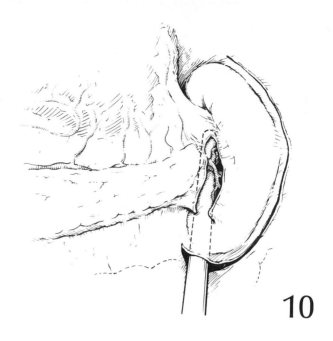

10

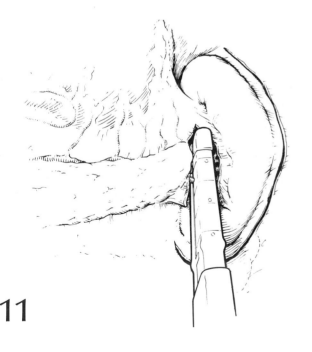

11

11 Vascular staples must be used and the stapler is fired two or three times until the hilum is fully divided.

12 Adhesions at the apex of the spleen and the upper remnants of the gastrosplenic and lieno-renal ligaments are then divided between clips or ties and the spleen is finally freed from all attachments.

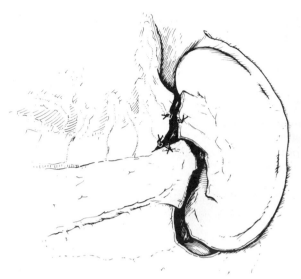

12

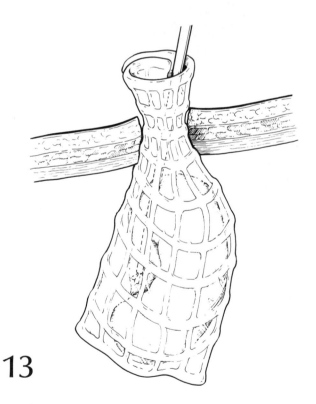

13

13 A sterile bag (Endobag) large enough to accommodate the whole spleen is introduced, the spleen is placed within it, and then macerated and aspirated. Maceration may be achieved with a liquidizing instrument, or by inserting the surgeon's finger into the bag, methodically fragmenting the spleen, and aspirating it with a large suction tube.

Haemostasis is checked, the presence of splenunculi is excluded, and the ports are removed.

MODIFICATION OF THE STANDARD OPEN
TECHNIQUE FOR RUPTURED SPLEEN

The principles of the operation are the same as for elective splenectomy, with the additional problems of the initial control of haemorrhage, the detection of associated injuries, and the desirability of conserving the spleen where possible.

Incision

This should always be a long midline incision which allows free and rapid access to other viscera that may be damaged.

Control of bleeding

14 It is first necessary to remove blood and clot from the left hypochordrium by scooping, mopping and suction. The left costal margin is lifted with a retractor by the assistant and the surgeon's right hand is thrust down to the splenic hilum where, in cases of continuing vigorous bleeding, the vessels are grasped between finger and thumb.

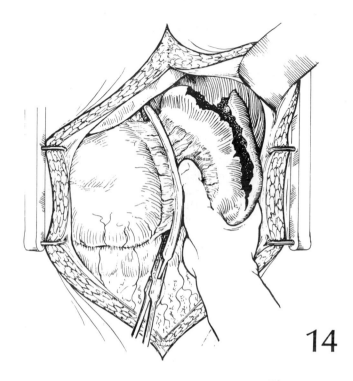

14

If at this stage the patient is grossly shocked, compression should be maintained until the anaesthetist has corrected the hypovolaemia. Where prolonged compression is necessary it may be achieved by occluding all of the hilar structures with a non-crushing intestinal clamp.

Once the situation has stabilized and it is ascertained that the spleen is so badly damaged that no form of conservation or repair is possible, splenectomy is carried out in a manner as near as possible to that described for elective splenectomy. The surgeon should avoid the temptation to apply forceps in a blind fashion and to mass-ligature structures in the splenic hilum, as this may damage the gastric wall and pancreatic tail. However, in certain cases it can be very difficult to isolate and ligate the major vessels and in such cases the clamped tissues can be transfixed and ligated with strong sutures.

CONSERVATION, REPAIR AND PARTIAL SPLENECTOMY FOR RUPTURED SPLEEN

Conservative treatment

Although non-operative treatment of patients with splenic injury is well established, and it is now evident that, with careful observation and transfusion support, certain ruptured spleens can be left *in situ* to heal, it remains a difficult policy to adopt in patients with abdominal trauma. The hazards are obvious in that other injuries can be missed, bleeding can recur, and delayed rupture may occur. Splenic conservation does not simplify the treatment of injured patients but makes it more complex, and the policy must be abandoned where continuous bleeding is evident and other injuries are suspected.

15a, b The decision to leave the spleen to heal spontaneously can also be taken at operation. Where a minor splenic injury is seen and bleeding has ceased, the area can be inspected carefully by retraction and without dividing the lienorenal ligament. The lesser sac is entered to allow examination of the splenic hilum, pancreas and retroperitoneal tissues. If these areas are free from damage and haematoma, the spleen can be left *in situ* and the abdomen closed with low pressure suction drainage to the area. In some cases, persistent oozing of blood from the torn splenic substance may be controlled by the local application of dry microfibrillar collagen (Avitene) or calcium alginate (Kaltostat).

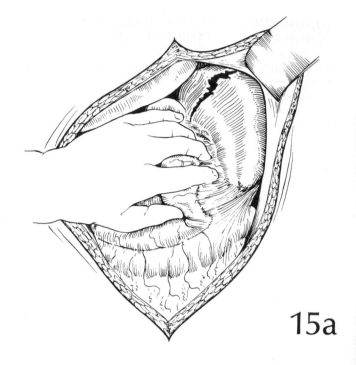

15a

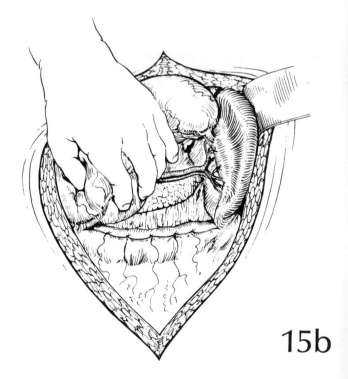

15b

Splenorrhaphy

16 Suture of splenic lacerations is advocated by some authorities, but where haemorrhage has ceased it is probably unnecessary and may even provoke rebleeding. However, bleeding from an easily accessible laceration in the lower pole of the spleen may be controlled by insertion of 0 polyglycolic acid sutures combined with ligation in continuity of the relevant polar artery. If active bleeding persists it is advisable to discontinue suturing and to perform total or partial splenectomy.

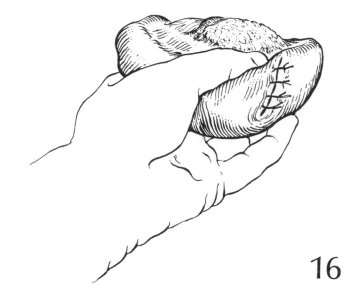

16

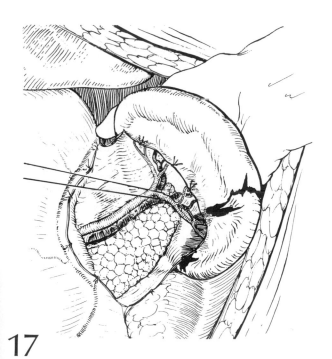

17

Partial splenectomy

If a fragment of spleen is completely or partially avulsed, usually at the upper or lower pole, then a different policy can be adopted. The main splenic artery usually divides before entering the splenic substance and the fact that these branches are end arteries allows partial splenic resection to be undertaken safely[1].

17 The spleen is fully mobilized as previously described by dividing the lienorenal and gastro-splenic attachments. The splenic pedicle is grasped by the assistant and compressed while the tail of the pancreas is dissected bluntly from the hilum and the vessels are exposed. Dissection close to the capsule exposes the relevant polar artery which is encircl ed and doubly ligated with a strong absorbable suture or occluded with metal clips.

18 Wedge resection is accomplished using cutting diathermy. Mattress sutures of an absorbable material such as 0 polyglactin are used to control oozing from the open edge. If the tissues are very friable the sutures can be inserted through collagen buttresses. After satisfactory haemostasis is obtained the abdomen is closed with suction drainage to the splenic area.

This procedure is probably only of value if more than half of the spleen is preserved.

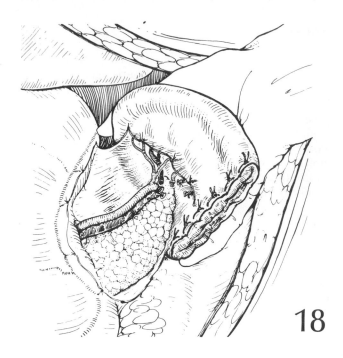

Splenic wrapping procedures

19 Major decapsulating injuries of the spleen are typically encountered in patients who present with delayed bleeding. In such individuals there is frequently a large subcapsular haematoma which, when evacuated, leaves an extensive area of denuded splenic pulp. Woven polyglycolic acid mesh is particularly helpful in achieving secure haemostasis in these cases. Topical haemostatic agents are applied to the bleeding areas and the entire spleen is encased in the mesh. The spleen is completely mobilized, attached only by its hilar vessels.

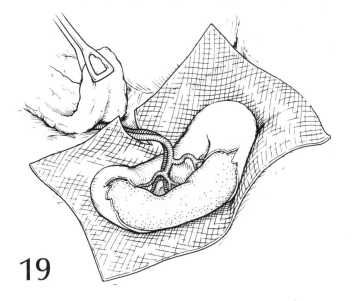

20 A window is fashioned in the mesh to accommodate the splenic artery and vein, and the spleen is enveloped by approximating the free edges of the mesh with polyglycolic acid sutures.

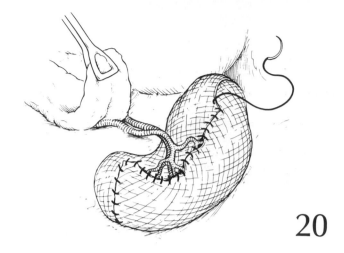

20

MODIFICATION OF OPEN TECHNIQUE FOR GIANT SPLEEN AND THE MANAGEMENT OF SPLENIC ADHESIONS

Providing they are mobile, huge spleens such as are found in myelofibrosis, chronic granulocytic leukaemia and the tropical splenomegalies are often easier to remove than small ones.

Incision

21 An oblique incision is made in the line of the ninth rib from the costal margin to the right iliac fossa. The incision may have to be very long to permit mobilization and delivery of the spleen.

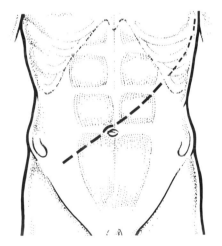

21

Mobilization

22 The abdominal section of the incision is opened and the surface of the spleen exposed. If the spleen is mobile and there are no adhesions the organ can usually be easily delivered from the abdomen because all the ligaments have been stretched. The technique of removal is then essentially the same as that already described for elective removal of A normal sized spleen.

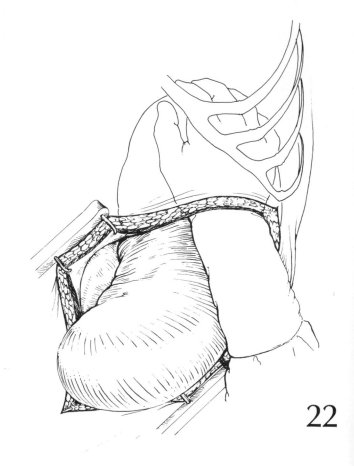

22

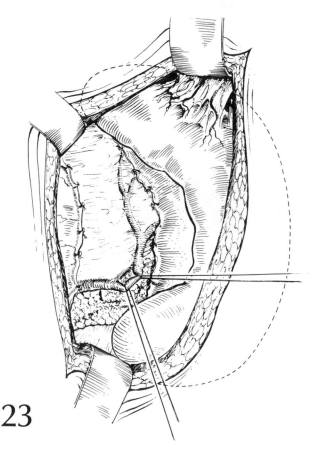

23

Management of splenic adhesions

Problems arise when the spleen is covered with vascular adhesions connecting it to the diaphragm and parietal peritoneum. In such circumstances the surgeon should not try to deliver the organ from the abdomen nor to break down the adhesions by blunt dissection.

23 The first step is to divide the gastrosplenic ligament, enter the lesser sac and expose the splenic artery at the upper border of the pancreas. The artery should be tied in continuity at the apex of one of its convolutions with strong linen thread ligatures (2 gauge) passed round it on an aneurysm needle.

24 The adhesions are then carefully assessed. If they are few and can be divided easily by electro-coagulation, laser, or between clamps under direct vision and without opening the chest, it is permissible to proceed.

If, however, there are many adhesions and they are thick and vascular, the incision should be extended, the costal margin divided, and the thorax opened through the bed of the ninth rib. The diaphragm is divided as far as is necessary to allow good access to the adhesions. The adhesions are divided and ligated individually until the lienorenal ligament is reached. Thereafter the operation proceeds as described above for elective splenectomy.

If such thick vascular adhesions are found at laparoscopic surgery they may be divided with diathermy scissors under vision. If this is difficult or the operative view poor, conversion to open surgery is indicated.

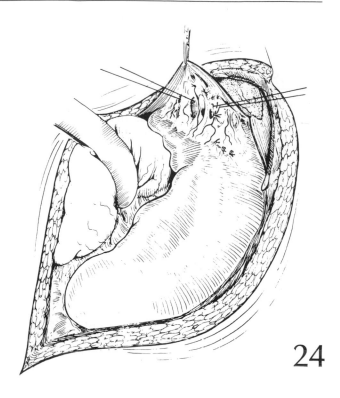

24

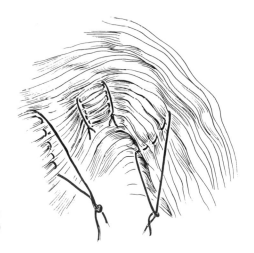

25

25 When a giant spleen with multiple adhesions is removed the surgeon may occasionally be left with a huge bed consisting of a large floppy diaphragm covered with raw oozing areas. This situation can be difficult to deal with and is virtually never completely controllable by diathermy coagulation, suction drains or haemostatic gauze. The most effective technique to control oozing is plication of the diaphragm with a series of firmly tied parallel 0 polyglactin sutures inserted at 5-cm intervals until bleeding is controlled.

Postoperative care

Most patients have an uncomplicated postoperative course following splenectomy or partial splenectomy. Suction drainage from the splenic bed usually diminishes to the point where the drains can be removed on the second postoperative day. A nasogastric tube is passed if the rare complication of acute dilatation occurs.

Intravenous infusion of crystalloids to maintain hydration is usually necessary for about 48 h and nasogastric suction can be discontinued after 24 h unless aspirates remain high. Skin sutures can be removed on the seventh day. Thrombocytopenic patients may develop considerable bruising of the skin around the wound, but this is usually of little consequence and resolves spontaneously. The thrombocytosis that follows splenectomy is no cause for alarm although, if the count goes above 1 million, it is reasonable to give aspirin by mouth until the count falls. Many patients develop some effusion and collapse of the left lower lobe of the lung which usually responds to physiotherapy.

It is now recognized that, even in adults, there is an increased risk of late systemic infection following splenectomy. Prophylaxis consists of vaccination against *Streptococcus pneumoniae* (and probably against *Haemophilus influenzae* type b and meningococcal strains A and C) as soon as is practicable after operation. Amoxycillin (250 mg daily) or phenoxymethy penicillin (250 mg twice daily) is advisable although opinions are divided as to whether this should be prescribed for life or for periods of up to 5 years. Post-splenectomy patients are advised to seek medical advice promptly whenever infection is contracted or seems likely, and should avoid areas where malaria is endemic. The risks of overwhelming post-splenectomy infection are particularly high in children and young adults.

References

1. Singer DB. Post splenectomy sepsis. In: Rosenberg HS, Bolande RP, eds. *Perspectives in Pediatric Pathology.* Vol. 1. Chicago: Year Book Medical Publishers, 1973: 285–311.

2. Robinette CD, Fraumeni JF. Splenectomy and subsequent mortality in veterans of the 1939–45 war. *Lancet* 1977; 2: 127–9.

3. Shandling B. Splenectomy for trauma, a second look. *Arch Surg* 1976; 3: 1325–6.

4. Redmond HP, Redmond JM, Rooney BP, Duignan JP, Bouchier-Hayes DJ. Surgical anatomy of the human spleen. *Br J Surg* 1989; 76: 198–201.

Preoperative assessment and preparation for biliary tract surgery

Attila Nakeeb MD
Surgical Resident, Department of Surgery, The Johns Hopkins Medical Institutions, Baltimore, Maryland, USA

Henry A. Pitt MD
Professor and Vice Chairman, Department of Surgery, The Johns Hopkins Medical Institutions, Baltimore, Maryland, USA

Historically, the surgical treatment of biliary tract diseases has been associated with significant morbidity and mortality. This increased risk is often related to biliary tract obstruction, and a direct correlation between operative mortality and the degree of jaundice has been documented (*Table 1*). In recent years a better understanding of the pathophysiology of obstructive jaundice has led to advances in preoperative management that have resulted in improved operative survival[1]. This chapter will briefly review the pathophysiology of obstructive jaundice, the preoperative assessment of these patients, and the important factors in the preparation for surgery on the biliary tract.

Table 1 Correlation of serum bilirubin levels with postoperative mortality

Bilirubin (mg/dl)	Patients (no.)	Mortality (%)
< 1.5	61	3.3
1.5–5	40	2.5
5–10	23	8.7
10–20	22	18.2*
> 20	9	33.3*

Modified from Pitt *et al. Am J Surg* 1981; 141: 66.
*p < 0.01 *vs* patients with bilirubin < 5 mg/dl ($\equiv$ 85.5 µmol/l).

Pathophysiology of jaundice

Biliary obstruction produces local effects on the bile duct that lead to derangement of hepatic function and, ultimately, to widespread systemic effects. Patients who are jaundiced are at increased risk for developing hepatic dysfunction, renal failure, cardiovascular impairment, bleeding problems, infections, wound complications and nutritional deficits. Each of these abnormalities will be discussed in more detail.

Hepatobiliary dysfunction

The biliary system normally has a low pressure. In patients with complete or partial biliary obstruction the biliary pressure rises and the secretory, metabolic and synthetic functions of hepatocytes are altered. Raised biliary pressure results in diminished bile secretion. Similarly, jaundiced patients have a decreased capacity to excrete drugs, such as antibiotics, that are normally secreted into bile. The increased concentration of bile acids associated with obstructive jaundice results in inhibition of the hepatic cytochrome P450 enzymes and, therefore, in a decrease in the rate of oxidative metabolism in the liver. The synthetic function of the hepatocyte is also decreased with obstructive jaundice, as evidenced by decreased plasma levels of albumin, clotting factors and secretory immunoglobulins.

Renal failure

The association between jaundice and postoperative renal failure has been known for many years[1,2]. The incidence of postoperative acute renal failure in jaundiced patients is approximately 10%. Moreover, the mortality rate in jaundiced patients developing renal failure has been reported to be as high as 75%. Endotoxins probably play a significant role in the renal failure associated with jaundice. They are present in the peripheral blood of approximately 50% of patients with obstructive jaundice, probably because of a lack of bile salts in the gut lumen that normally prevent absorption of endotoxins and inhibit anaerobic bacterial growth. Endotoxin causes renal vasoconstriction, redistribution of renal blood flow away from the cortex, and activation of complement, macrophages, leukocytes and platelets. As a result, glomerular and peritubular fibrin is deposited. This factor, in combination with reduced renal cortical blood flow, results in the tubular and cortical necrosis observed in jaundiced patients with renal failure.

Cardiovascular impairment

In addition to the hepatic dysfunction and increased propensity to develop renal failure, obstructive jaundice is known to cause severe haemodynamic disturbances including (1) decreased cardiac contractility, (2) reduced left ventricular pressures, and (3) impaired response to β agonist drugs such as isoprenaline (isoproterenol) and noradrenaline[1,2]. The effect of obstructive jaundice on the peripheral vasculature is to cause a decrease in total peripheral resistance. In addition to the direct effects on the heart and peripheral vasculature, jaundice results in hypovolaemia. The increased serum levels of bile acids associated with obstructive jaundice have both a diuretic and natriuretic effect on the kidney. The combination of hypovolaemia, depressed cardiac function, and decreased total peripheral resistance probably accounts for the susceptibility of jaundiced patients to develop shock in the perioperative period.

Coagulation

Disturbances of blood coagulation are also commonly present in jaundiced patients[1]. The most frequently observed clotting defect in patients with biliary obstruction is prolongation of the prothrombin time. This defect results from impaired vitamin K absorption from the gut, secondary to a lack of intestinal bile. This coagulopathy is usually reversible by parenteral administration of vitamin K. Moreover, endotoxin release in jaundiced patients results in a low-grade disseminated intravascular coagulation with increased fibrin degradation products. Jaundiced patients with circulating endotoxin or increased levels of fibrin degradation product before surgery are at increased risk of developing haemorrhagic complications. In addition to problems with endotoxaemia, cirrhotic patients may have even more complicated clotting abnormalities such as problems with thrombocytopenia from hypersplenism and fibrinolysis.

Immune system

Surgery in the jaundiced patient is associated with a significant rate of septic complications[1]. Jaundiced patients have a number of defects in cellular immunity that make them more prone to infection. Several authors have demonstrated impaired T cell proliferation, decreased neutrophil chemotaxis, defective bacterial phagocytosis and altered delayed hypersensitivity in these patients. The ability of hepatic Kupffer cells to clear bacteria and endotoxin from the circulation is also reduced in obstructive jaundice. In addition, the absence of bile from the intestinal tract plays a role in the infectious complications seen in patients with obstructive jaundice. Bacterial translocation from the gut has been shown to be increased in the setting of bile duct obstruction. Obstruction causes a disruption of the enterohepatic circulation and results in the loss of the emulsifying anti-endotoxin effect of bile acids. A larger pool of endotoxin is therefore available within the intestine for absorption into the portal circulation. The combination of a lack of bile in the intestine and the impairment of cellular immunity and reticuloendothelial cell function is probably responsible for the observed increase in septic and infectious complications in jaundiced patients.

Wound healing

Delayed wound healing and a high incidence of wound dehiscence and incisional hernias have been observed in patients undergoing surgery for the relief of obstructive jaundice[1]. Patients with bile duct obstruction have decreased activity of the enzyme propylhydroxylase in their skin. Propylhydroxylase is necessary for the incorporation of proline amino acid residues into collagen. Thus, the rate of collagen formation is decreased and wound strength is diminished. An increased incidence of wound infection also contributes to the frequent wound problems observed in these patients.

Nutrition

Other problems that face jaundiced patients are anorexia, weight loss and resultant malnutrition[1]. Appetite is adversely influenced by the lack of bile salts in the intestinal tract. In addition, patients with pancreatic or periampullary malignant lesions may have partial duodenal obstruction or abnormal gastric emptying, perhaps secondary to tumour infiltration of the coeliac nerve plexus. Patients with pancreatic or periampullary tumours may also have pancreatic endocrine and exocrine insufficiency. This latter problem may further compound other nutritional defects that, in turn, may multiply the immune deficits of the jaundiced patient.

Preoperative assessment

When a patient presents with jaundice, the objective is to identify any potentially treatable causes. The most important distinction is whether the jaundice is caused by intrahepatic cholestasis or extraheaptic obstruction. Fortunately, the differentiation between 'medical' and 'surgical' jaundice can be made relatively easily with a careful history, physical examination, review of serum biochemistry and radiological evaluation[1]. An algorithm for the evaluation of the jaundiced patient is shown in *Figure 1*. The following discussion will present an approach to the jaundiced patient that will allow an accurate diagnosis to be made without subjecting the patient to needless risk, discomfort or expense.

Clinical

The first and most important step in the preparation of the patient who is to undergo biliary tract surgery is to obtain a careful history. Important historical points to consider include occupational exposure, travel history or contact with anyone who has had hepatitis or jaundice. Similarly, any exposure to transfusions, blood, tattoos or body fluids should be noted. The patient also

needs to be questioned about drug ingestion, with special attention to alcohol and other hepatotoxins. A family history with respect to haemolytic anaemias or congenital hyperbilirubinaemias may also be helpful. Previous surgery, especially biliary, raises the suspicion of a benign biliary stricture or retained common duct stones. Hepatitis following transfusion or drug toxicity may also appear after a surgical procedure.

In the jaundiced patient the time of onset and progression should be determined and can often give a clue to the diagnosis. Viral hepatitis might be suspected if the jaundice presented with a rapid onset and was associated with nausea and anorexia. A history of biliary colic, on the other hand, suggests choledocholithiasis. Pancreatic cancer is more likely to present with progressive, painless jaundice and weight loss. A history of fever, chills and upper abdominal pain in addition to jaundice (Charcot's triad) is suggestive of cholangitis, which occurs more often in patients with choledocholithiasis than in those with malignant obstruction. Sepsis in patients with perihilar cholangiocarcinoma, underlying cirrhosis, liver abscesses and, especially, renal failure is associated with a very high perioperative mortality[3].

The colour of the patient's urine and stool should also be carefully noted. Total obstruction of the biliary tract results in acholic pale stools, increased amounts of

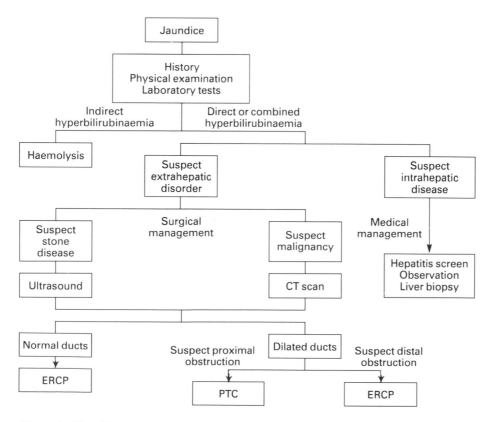

Figure 1   Algorithm for the management of the jaundiced patient. Reprinted with permission from Nakeeb and Pitt[1].

bilirubin in the urine, and absence of urine urobilinogen. If the urine is positive for bilirubin, then serum levels of conjugated bilirubin are usually raised. Stools that are black or silver suggest the presence of blood, which may indicate a periampullary lesion that is both bleeding and obstructing the distal bile duct.

On physical examination the abdomen should be carefully inspected, auscultated, percussed and palpated. A small liver may be discovered in patients with severe cirrhosis or hepatitis, a tender liver edge may be observed in those with hepatitis, congestive heart failure or alcoholic hepatitis, while a palpable, nontender gallbladder may be seen in patients with pancreatic or periampullary carcinoma (Courvoisier's sign). A tender gallbladder, on the other hand, may be palpated in cases of choledocholithiasis with associated cholecystitis (Murphy's sign). The stigmata of cirrhosis, such as ascites, spider naevi or periumbilical venous enlargement, should also be noted.

Biochemical assessment

In addition to the history and physical examination, biochemical evaluation is an integral part of the initial examination of the patient with biliary tract disease. The level of bilirubin can indicate the severity of the disease process, and bilirubin levels can be used to follow disease progression. The routine laboratory tests that should be performed on all jaundiced patients include direct (conjugated) and indirect (unconjugated) bilirubin, alkaline phosphatase, serum transaminases, albumin and amylase determinations. The urine also should be tested for bilirubin and urobilinogen, and coagulation studies should be performed.

Patients with haemolysis have an increase in the indirect (unconjugated) fraction of bilirubin, whereas the direct (conjugated) bilirubin level is normal (*Table 2*). The total bilirubin concentration in haemolysis rarely exceeds 4–5 mg/dl (68–85 μmol/l). Since unconjugated bilirubin is not excreted by the kidney, bilirubin is absent in the urine of patients with haemolysis.. If haemolysis is suspected, further laboratory tests should include a complete blood count, a blood smear, reticulocyte count, erythrocyte fragility test and a

Coombs test. The amino acid transaminases aspartate aminotransferase (AST) and alanine aminotransferase (ALT) are serum markers for hepatocyte damage. AST is found in liver, heart, kidney, skeletal muscle and brain tissue while ALT is found predominantly within hepatocytes, making it more specific for identifying liver injury.

Broad derangements of liver function tests are seen in patients with hepatic parenchymal disease (*Table 2*). The concentrations of both conjugated and unconjugated fractions of bilirubin are increased. With the increased level of conjugated bilirubin in the serum, bilirubinuria develops. In patients with acute hepatitis, serum levels of ALT and AST are markedly increased while alkaline phosphatase and bilirubin levels may be only slightly raised, and the serum amylase level is usually normal. The serum transaminases are also raised in alcoholic liver disease, with serum AST levels usually being more than twice the serum ALT levels. In the cirrhotic patient, serum bilirubin levels increase in proportion to the degree of parenchymal damage. Albumin and the coagulation factors V, VII, IX, X, prothrombin, and fibrinogen are all synthesized in the liver. The measurement of serum albumin levels and prothrombin time may therefore be helpful in assessing the degree of parenchymal liver injury.

In extrahepatic obstruction the fraction of direct bilirubin is significantly raised and the indirect bilirubin concentration is also moderately increased (*Table 2*). The highest elevations of bilirubin levels are usually found in patients with malignant extrahepatic obstruction where bilirubin levels may exceed 20 mg/dl (342 μmol/l). With malignant obstruction the alkaline phosphatase level is also increased to the same degree. Other liver function tests are usually normal or only slightly raised, and the amylase concentration is usually normal. Stones in the common bile duct, on the other hand, rarely cause an increase in the bilirubin level of more than 10–12 mg/dl (171–205 μmol/l). With choledocholithiasis, alkaline phosphatase levels are also usually increased to a moderate degree. As a gallstone passes through and momentarily obstructs the ampulla of Vater, serum transaminase levels may rise transiently. In this setting, hyperamylasaemia may also develop. I longstanding partial extrahepatic obstruction is present

Table 2 Laboratory tests in the diagnosis of hepatobiliary disease

Cause of jaundice	Serum bilirubin		Serum alkaline phosphatase	Serum transaminases	Urine	
	Conjugated	Unconjugated			Bilirubin	Urobilinoge
Haemolysis	↔	↑↑↑	↔	↔	0	↑↑
Hepatocellular dysfunction	↑↑	↑↑	↑	↑↑↑	↑↑	↑
Intrahepatic cholestasis	↑↑↑	↑↑	↑↑	↑↑	↑↑↑	0 or ↓
Extrahepatic obstruction	↑↑↑	↑↑	↑↑↑	↑	↑↑↑	0 or ↓

0, none; ↓, decreased; ↔, no change; ↑, mild elevation; ↑↑, moderate elevation; ↑↑↑, marked elevation.

liver damage and fibrosis can occur, resulting in a combined intrahepatic and extrahepatic biochemical profile.

Serum alkaline phosphatase is often a more sensitive indicator of obstruction, and levels may be increased when the bilirubin level is normal. This circumstance occurs most commonly with incomplete or partial obstruction. However, increased levels of alkaline phosphatase activity may also result from bone disease. If this possibility is suspected, serum 5'-nucleotidase or serum γ-glutamyl transpeptidase levels should be measured, since they both parallel changes in alkaline phosphatase from a hepatobiliary source and are not found in bone.

Radiological evaluation

The goals of the radiological evaluation of the jaundiced patient include (1) the confirmation of clinically suspected biliary obstruction by the demonstration of a dilated biliary tree, (2) the identification of the level and cause of extrahepatic biliary obstruction, (3) the selection of patients in whom surgical or interventional radiological or endoscopic treatment is indicated, and (4) the use of tests in a cost effective manner.

Abdominal plain radiographs

The likelihood of a plain abdominal radiograph providing diagnostic information in the patient with biliary obstruction is low. Abdominal radiography may reveal gallstones, a calcified gallbladder wall, or the outline of a distended gallbladder. Approximately 15–20% of gallstones are radio-opaque and can be visualized by radiography. However, cholangiography will still be necessary to determine whether common duct stones are present and to rule out other causes of jaundice such as hepatic parenchymal disease or an obstructing tumour. Plain radiographs may also be diagnostic of a spontaneous biliary fistula when air is present in the biliary tree or of emphysematous cholecystitis when air is noted in the gallbladder lumen or wall.

Ultrasonography

Ultrasonography (US) is commonly performed as the initial screening procedure in patients with biliary tract disease. It is non-invasive, inexpensive and widely available. Dilated intrahepatic bile ducts are a reliable sign of biliary obstruction, and most series report that ultrasonography can detect dilatation of the intrahepatic or proximal extrahepatic bile ducts with at least an 80% accuracy rate[1]. The normal extrahepatic bile duct diameter is less than 10 mm and normal intrahepatic ducts are less than 4 mm in diameter. Dilated ducts are easily detectable by ultrasonography and can often be identified before the onset of clinical jaundice.

Failure of ultrasonography to detect dilated ducts usually indicates a hepatic parenchymal source of jaundice. In this setting continued observation, screening tests for hepatitis, or liver biopsy may be indicated. However, the absence of ductal dilatation does not entirely rule out extrahepatic obstruction. In intermittent or partial obstruction the biliary tree may not be dilated. Likewise, in longstanding obstruction, especially if secondary biliary fibrosis or cirrhosis is present, dilated ducts may not be observed. In cases where extrahepatic obstruction is suspected despite negative ultrasonography findings, direct cholangiography, usually by the endoscopic route, may be indicated.

Ultrasonography can differentiate between extrahepatic obstruction and hepatocellular causes of jaundice in almost all cases[1], but it is limited in its ability to identify the cause and exact location of an obstructing lesion because it cannot visualize the entire common bile duct, especially the distal third, and it is unable to detect consistently stones in the common bile duct. Although ultrasonography is a valuable initial step in the evaluation of the jaundiced patient, further diagnostic studies such as computed tomographic scanning or direct cholangiography are therefore frequently necessary to identify the cause and exact location of the obstruction.

Computed tomography

1a,b Computed tomographic (CT) scanning can also be used to differentiate between intrahepatic disease and non-dilated ducts from extrahepatic obstruction[1], and it is more than 90% accurate in detecting the presence of ductal dilatation (*Illustration 1a*). The slightly higher success rate than with ultrasonography is because CT scanning provides better definition of anatomical structures and contrast media can be used to enhance delineations (*Illustration 1b*). CT portography or angiography and newer spiral or helical techniques have further improved the accuracy of this investigation in establishing the site and cause of biliary obstruction. In addition, CT scanning, especially with newer spiral techniques, can also provide highly accurate information regarding retroperitoneal extension, vascular invasion and spread to the liver in malignant causes of biliary obstruction.

CT scanning and ultrasonography therefore have similar utility in the diagnosis of biliary ductal dilatation. CT scanning may be the preferred initial screening procedure in obese patients, and most authorities agree that it is slightly more accurate in detecting the nature and anatomical level of obstruction. CT also has the advantage of being able to visualize the pancreas routinely and is therefore probably the screening procedure of choice if a pancreatic or periampullary malignancy is suspected. On the other hand, ultrasonography is less expensive, more widely available, and does not expose the patient to radiation; therefore, it should be performed initially if the clinical history suggests stone disease.

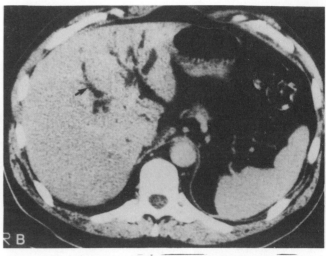

Figure 1(a)   CT scan in a patient with a perihilar cholangiocarcinoma demonstrating dilated intrahepatic ducts. The tumour cannot be differentiated from the liver parenchyma or portal vein in this scan with intravenous contrast medium.

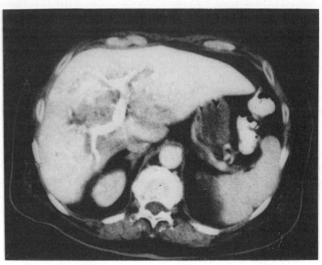

Figure 1(b)   CT angiogram in another patient with a perihilar cholangiocarcinoma. The tumour is clearly demarcated (dark) and the portal venous system is clearly visualized (white).

Magnetic resonance imaging

2a,b The use of magnetic resonance imaging (MRI) in the evaluation of the patient with biliary tract disease is relatively recent and the technique is still undergoing evaluation[1]. MRI is capable of detecting intrahepatic and extrahepatic biliary dilatation, but its sensitivity has not yet been compared with ultrasonography or CT scanning to determine its clinical usefulness. T2-weighted images in the coronal and sagittal planes may also be used to obtain a magnetic resonance cholangiogram. Initial studies suggest that MRI will identify a dilated biliary tree in approximately 85% of patients with obstructive jaundice, with the cause of obstruction being determined in approximately 60% of these patients. A more prominent role for MRI may be in its ability to define venous anatomy and identify the parenchymal extent of perihilar cholangiocarcinomas.

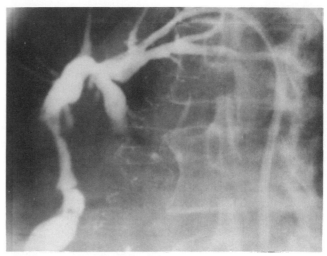

Figure 2(a)   Cholangiogram demonstrating a perihilar cholangiocarcinoma.

Biliary scintigraphy

Technetium-99^m labelled iminodiacetic acid derivatives (HIDA, DISIDA, PIPIDA) are injected intravenously, rapidly extracted from the blood and excreted into the bile. These radionuclide scans provide functional information about the patient's ability to excrete radiolabelled substances from the liver into a non-obstructed biliary tree. Biliary scintigraphy is useful in the management of neonatal jaundice, the detection of bile leaks, and the diagnosis of acute cholecystitis. Cholescintigraphy also provides a non-invasive method with which to evaluate the patency and function of biliary-enteric anastomoses and to study the kinetics of bile flow when disordered biliary motility is suspected.

In comparison with ultrasonography, CT scanning and MRI, biliary scintigraphy plays only a limited role in the evaluation of a patient with jaundice[1]. The technique has been used to diagnose common bile duct obstruction. In this setting any appearance of the nucleotide in the gastrointestinal tract indicates patency of bile flow into the duodenum. However, other available non-invasive tests such as ultrasonography or CT scanning have generally been shown to be more accurate and are therefore preferred.

Percutaneous transhepatic cholangiography

Direct cholangiography is indicated if dilated bile ducts are visualized by ultrasonography or CT scanning, or if the clinical suspicion of biliary obstruction remains high despite a negative ultrasonographic or CT scan. Cholangiography may be performed percutaneously or endoscopically. With percutaneous transhepatic cholangiography (PTC) the intrahepatic bile ducts are cannulated with a thin, flexible Chiba needle under radiographic control, and contrast material is injected to

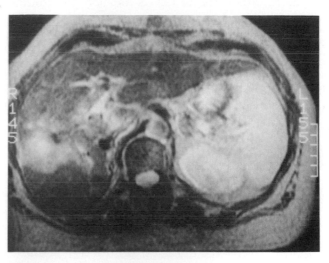

Figure 2(b)   MRI T2 image demonstrating the cholangiocarcinoma (white) in an atrophied right lobe in the same patient.

outline the bile ducts. PTC is successful in differentiating intrahepatic from extrahepatic obstruction in up to 96% of cases[1].

Percutaneous cholangiography can define the site of an obstructing lesion in approximately 95% of patients and the cause of the obstruction in nearly 90% of cases (*Table 3*). Diagnostic cholangiography can also be combined with a series of therapeutic manoeuvres such as the insertion of biliary stents or endoprostheses, percutaneous stone extraction, biliary dilatation and cholangioscopy. In addition, cholangiography provides an anatomical road map of the biliary tree that is useful during surgical procedures. Thus, in the management of the jaundiced patient the advantages of PTC are the ability to (1) establish a diagnosis, (2) determine the site and cause of obstruction, and (3) provide specific anatomical detail.

Endoscopic retrograde cholangiography

Endoscopic retrograde cholangiography (ERC) is another option for direct visualization of the biliary system. The technique requires a skilled endoscopist who is capable of cannulating the sphincter of Oddi with a side viewing duodenoscope. The success rate is approximately 85–90% and improves with the experience of the endoscopist. ERC is able to define the site and cause of extrahepatic obstructive jaundice in 75–90% of patients[1]. As with PTC, the complication and mortality rates of ERC are acceptably low. The major complications of the procedure are sepsis, acute pancreatitis and duodenal perforation. Prophylactic antibiotics should be administered before either PTC or ERC if biliary obstruction is suspected.

In the patient with jaundice who has dilated ducts on ultrasonography or CT scanning, direct cholangiography by either PTC or ERC is the next procedure to be used. PTC is less expensive, more widely available, requires less expertise than ERC, and has a higher success rate if dilated ducts are present (*Table 3*). In patients with complete biliary obstruction, PTC provides the surgeon with information about the proximal biliary tree, whereas ERC frequently can only delineate the anatomy of the distal bile duct. PTC is the preferred

Table 3 Comparison of percutaneous transhepatic and endoscopic cholangiography

Criterion	Transhepatic cholangiography	Endoscopic cholangiography
Success rate	>90% with dilated ducts, 70% with non-dilated ducts	80–90% with both dilated and non-dilated ducts
Identification of cause	90–100%	75–90%
Complications	5% (range 3–10%)	5% (range 2–7%)
Mortality	0.2–0.9%	0.1–0.2%
Expense	Less	More
Skill required	Less	More
Patient selection	Proximal lesions, altered gastroduodenal anatomy, failed endoscopic cholangiography	Distal lesions, pancreatic pathology, coagulopathy, ascites, failed transhepatic cholangiography

procedure for perihilar lesions if therapeutic manipulations such as biliary drainage, balloon dilatation or endoprosthesis placement are necessary. However, percutaneous cholangiography is contraindicated in patients with an incorrectable coagulopathy or with significant ascites.

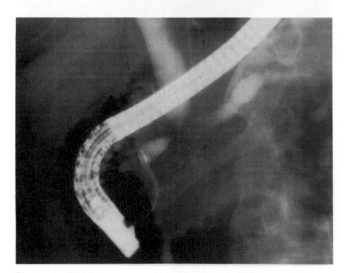

Figure 3   ERCP demonstrating obstruction of the bile duct and the pancreatic duct, 'double duct sign', in a patient with pancreatic cancer.

3 On the other hand, ERC is preferable to PTC in several instances. ERC allows endoscopic visualization of the upper gastrointestinal tract and ampullary region. Lesions can be biopsied and varices can be identified. Moreover, cannulation and injection of the pancreatic duct with contrast medium is often helpful in patients suspected of having pancreatic disease.

In patients with postcholecystectomy symptoms or sphincter of Oddi dyskinesia, ERC enables visualization and cannulation of the ampulla and manometric pressure recordings. As with PTC, therapeutic manipulations such as endoscopic sphincterotomy and stenting may be carried out in conjunction with ERC. However, ERC may be difficult or impossible to perform in patients with ampullary stenosis or in those who have altered gastrointestinal anatomy secondary to previous surgery.

The method of direct cholangiography should therefore be individualized in each case. In certain situations such as totally obstructing proximal lesions, PTC may be the procedure of choice. On the other hand, when non-invasive studies suggest periampullary or pancreatic pathology, ERC provides additional useful information. However, the final choice between these two procedures may ultimately be decided by the expertise of the radiologists and endoscopists at an individual institution.

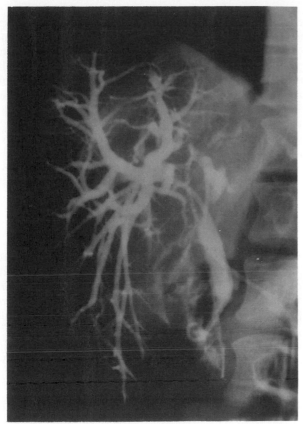

Figure 4(a)   Cholangiogram demonstrating a perihilar cholangiocarcinoma with extensive involvement of the right intrahepatic ducts and the common hepatic duct.

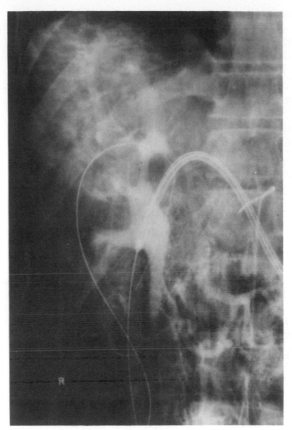

Figure 4(b)   Mesenteric angiogram demonstrating a patent main and left, but occluded right, portal vein branch in the same patient.

Angiography

4a,b   Coeliac and superior mesenteric angiography is not a routine investigative procedure in the patient with biliary tract disease. Angiography is performed in cirrhotic patients with bleeding oesophageal varices prior to portosystemic or transhepatic shunts or for therapeutic infusion of intra-arterial vasopressin. In jaundiced patients with active gastrointestinal bleeding, haemobilia can be diagnosed and treated with selective embolization by skilled invasive radiologists. Angiography may also be of benefit in predicting resectability in patients with periampullary or perihilar neoplasms.

With a pancreatic or periampullary neoplasm a normal angiogram indicates that the tumour will be resectable in approximately 75% of patients[1]. If the angiogram suggests vascular encasement, approximately one-third of the tumours will still be resectable. However, if the mesenteric veins are occluded by the

tumour, resection is usually not possible. Thus, major vessel occlusion rules out resection, and major vessel encasement makes resection less likely. However, angiography increases hospital cost and exposes the jaundiced patient, who is already at an increased risk of renal failure, to an additional contrast dye load. Angiography should therefore be used selectively.

Endoscopic ultrasonography

Endoscopic ultrasonography (EUS) is a relatively new investigation that may be of some benefit in the evaluation of the patient with biliary tract disease. A potential use is in the assessment of patients with malignant jaundice. Some reports suggest that endoscopic ultrasonography is able to predict resectability accurately in 85–90% of patients with pancreatic cancer[1]. A potential limitation of this technique, however, is that it may not be able to differentiate tumour infiltration of a vessel from simple compression. The addition of a pulsed Doppler may aid in this differentiation.

Advocates of endoscopic ultrasonography also claim that it can differentiate normal lymph nodes from those containing metastatic tumour. Normal lymph nodes are hyperechoic with indistinct margins, whereas lymph nodes containing cancer are hypoechoic with well defined margins. Preliminary studies suggest that endoscopic ultrasonography is 70–75% accurate in diagnosing lymph node metastasis[1]. Advocates further claim that, in patients with pancreatic cancer, it is superior to conventional ultrasonography, CT scanning and angiography in predicting resectability. Although promising, the ultimate role of endoscopic ultrasonography in the evaluation of patients with biliary tract disease must await further analysis.

Laparoscopy

Laparoscopy has recently been proposed as a useful technique for the staging of patients with suspected hepatobiliary and pancreatic tumours. Small liver and peritoneal metastases not detected by CT scanning or ultrasonography can be identified by direct examination. The addition of laparoscopic ultrasonography adds to the ability to assess mesenteric or portal vessel involvement as well as deeper liver lesions. Laparoscopy has been shown to be 65% accurate in predicting resectability (sensitivity 100%, specificity 50%) in patients with a pancreatic or periampullary malignancy without distant metastases. The addition of laparoscopic ultrasonography increased the accuracy of predicting resectability to almost 90%[1]. Thus, the combination of laparoscopy and laparoscopic ultrasonography is a valuable technique in staging patients with suspected pancreatic and periampullary malignancies. Whether it is as effective as the combination of CT scanning and angiography or spiral CT scanning in successfully predicting resectability has yet to be determined. Moreover, concerns about tumour implantation in port sites remains.

Liver biopsy

The application of ultrasonography and CT scanning has made percutaneous liver biopsy unnecessary in most cases of jaundice caused by extrahepatic obstruction. However, numerous indications for liver biopsy remain. If clinical and laboratory data indicate intrahepatic cholestasis and if dilated bile ducts are not present on ultrasonographic or CT scans, a liver biopsy is usually indicated. Liver biopsy may be useful if diagnostic studies are negative or equivocal or if parenchymal disease is suspected with extrahepatic obstruction.

Liver biopsy is relatively safe and reviews of very large series have reported mortality rates of 0.01–0.02% and a serious complication rate of 0.2–0.4%[1]. The most frequent complications of liver biopsy are haemorrhage and bacteraemia. This latter problem occurs most frequently in patients with chronic bile duct infections. Percutaneous liver biopsy is contraindicated if the patient is uncooperative or has an uncorrectable coagulation defect. If the patient has a prolonged prothrombin time or partial thromboplastin time or a diminished platelet count, attempts should be made to correct these abnormalities with vitamin K, fresh frozen plasma or specific component therapy. If the coagulopathy persists and liver biopsy is essential, laparoscopic or open liver biopsy may be indicated.

Assessment of risk

The morbidity associated with surgery in patients with biliary tract obstruction ranges from 30% to 60%, and the operative mortality varies between 2% and 15%[1]. Infectious complications including cholangitis, wound infections and intra-abdominal abscesses are the most common problems. Renal failure is a constant threat in the jaundiced patient. However, circulating endotoxin may also affect cardiac, pulmonary and hepatic function. As a result, multiple organ system failure is the most common cause of death in these patients.

A number of investigators have attempted to identify risk factors that may be associated with a poor prognosis. In various studies the risk factors that have been associated with increased mortality include: age greater than 60 years, malignant biliary obstruction, fever, haematocrit less than 30%, increased white blood cell count, hypoalbuminaemia, and elevations of serum bilirubin, alkaline phosphatase, blood urea nitrogen and creatinine levels. In multivariate analyses the assessment of nutritional status, renal function and underlying sepsis have been shown to be the most important factors in predicting which patients have a high operative risk[1]. Little[4] has devised a 'mortality index' which employs these factors to predict operative mortality in jaundiced patients (*Table 4*).

Table 4   Little's mortality index

Mortality index =

$$0.0016 \times \text{serum creatinine } (\mu\text{mol/l})$$
$$- 0.0227 \times \text{albumin } (\text{g/l})$$
$$+ 0.0641 \times \text{cholangitis score}$$
$$+ 0.6935$$

Cholangitis score:

0	if afebrile
1	if temperature <37.5°C
2	if >37.5°C without rigors
3	if >37.5°C with rigors, right upper quadrant pain
4	if fever with shock and/or mental changes

An index of 0.4 or greater is associated with a high risk of death.

Preoperative preparation

Patients with obstructive jaundice and those with hepatocellular disease severe enough to cause jaundice are prone to develop many secondary problems. Jaundiced patients are at increased risk for the development of renal failure, gastrointestinal bleeding, infections and wound complications. Cardiac, pulmonary and renal function must be considered in every patient undergoing major abdominal surgery. In addition, special attention must be focused on the nutritional status, coagulability, immune function and presence or absence of biliary sepsis in the jaundiced patient. Patients with chronic liver disease and cirrhosis may also develop ascites and encephalopathy which may require specific treatment.

Cardiopulmonary

In assessing cardiopulmonary status, the patient's age, history of recent myocardial infarction, presence of congestive heart failure, significant valvular aortic stenosis, or a disturbance of normal cardiac rhythm have all been correlated with increased operative risk[1]. Patients with significant cardiac disease should have a complete evaluation before surgery. The examination may include an electrocardiogram, echocardiography, and/or stress testing. Efforts should be made to maximize cardiac function before surgery by treating heart failure and arrhythmias and optimizing fluid status. In addition, patients with severe pulmonary disease may not be candidates for extensive abdominal surgery. Pulmonary function tests which reveal values of forced vital capacity or forced expiratory volume in one second which are less than 50% of predicted indicate significant lung disease, and these patients are at high risk for developing complications. Preoperative pulmonary preparation should include cessation of smoking, instruction in deep breathing and incentive spirometry, and the administration of bronchodilators if indicated. If bronchitis is a problem, oral antibiotics may also be indicated.

Renal

Jaundiced patients, especially those with cirrhosis and cholangitis, are at increased risk of developing renal insufficiency[1,2]. The maintenance of adequate blood volume is extremely important if renal complications are to be avoided. However, fluid management can be quite complex in jaundiced patients. These patients often benefit from invasive haemodynamic monitoring with central venous catheters and, in some cases, pulmonary artery catheters to assist in assessing intravascular volume. Several trials with a small number of patients suggest that the preoperative administration of oral bile salts may be efficacious in preventing the development of postoperative renal dysfunction[1,2]. The perioperative use of mannitol, which results in an osmotic diuresis, and intravenous fluid have also been successful in protecting the kidneys in cases of obstructive jaundice.

Nutrition

Perioperative hyperalimentation has been shown to be of benefit in reducing morbidity and mortality rates associated with surgery in patients with severe malnutrition[1]. Characteristics of patients at risk include (1) serum albumin less than 30 g/l, (2) weight loss of 10–20% over several months, (3) serum transferrin levels of less than 200 mg/dl, (4) anergy to injected skin antigens, and (5) a history of functional impairment. Patients with these characteristics may benefit from nutritional repletion through either parenteral or enteral nutrition prior to surgery. Although most patients with benign biliary problems are adequately nourished, various degrees of malnutrition are frequently present in patients with malignant obstruction. Patients with malignant obstructive jaundice should therefore be evaluated for evidence of malnutrition, and nutritional support should be instituted if necessary.

Coagulation

Patients with obstructive jaundice, cholangitis, or cirrhosis are all prone to excessive intraoperative bleeding. The most common clotting defect in patients with obstructive jaundice is prolongation of the prothrombin time (PT), which is usually reversible by parenteral vitamin K. Patients with severe jaundice and/or cholangitis may also develop disseminated intravascular coagulation (DIC) which may require infusion of platelets and fresh frozen plasma. Reversal of DIC also requires control of the underlying sepsis, which usually is due to cholangitis and requires biliary drainage and systemic antibiotics. In cirrhotic patients clotting abnormalities may be more complicated and include (1) thrombocytopenia secondary to hypersplenism, (2) prolongation of PT and partial thromboplastin time (PTT), and (3) fibrinolysis. Vitamin K should be administered if the PT is prolonged. If no effect is seen and/or the PTT is also prolonged, fresh frozen plasma should be given. Thrombocytopenia can usually be managed by intraoperative platelet infusions. If the patient has a shortened clot lysis time and hypofibrinogenaemia, ϵ-aminocaproic acid may be indicated.

Cholangitis

Biliary sepsis has also been identified as a major risk factor in the jaundiced patient[1,3]. Cholangitis may occur with either partial or complete obstruction of the bile duct, resulting in increased intraluminal pressure and infected bile behind the obstruction. Patients with uncomplicated cholangitis can usually be treated conservatively with appropriate antibiotics and fluid resuscitation. A subset of patients, however, will develop 'toxic' cholangitis (cholangitis plus hypotension and mental status changes). Patients with 'toxic' cholangitis have significant mortality when treated with antibiotic therapy alone and therefore require urgent biliary decompression.

Urgent surgical treatment is associated with significant morbidity and mortality. Both percutaneous and endoscopic biliary drainage have been proposed as effective treatment for the 5–10% of patients with 'toxic' cholangitis who are unresponsive to conservative treatment[1]. In patients with 'toxic' cholangitis and perihilar obstruction, percutaneous drainage by a skilled interventional radiologist is the procedure of choice, while in those with 'toxic' cholangitis due to distal obstruction by common duct stones, endoscopic sphincterotomy is the procedure of choice if an expert endoscopist is available.

Antibiotic coverage

Because of the depressed immune system that accompanies jaundice, adequate antibiotic coverage needs to be provided before any manipulation of the biliary tree as well as for the treatment of cholangitis. Under normal conditions, bile, the biliary tree and the liver are sterile. However, biliary stasis, obstruction, biliary-enteric anastomoses and foreign bodies predispose the biliary system to infection. The organisms most commonly isolated from the biliary tree include *Escherichia coli*, *Klebsiella pneumoniae*, enterococcus and, with increasing frequency, the anaerobe *Bacteroides fragilis*. Approximately two-thirds of patients with bactibilia will have Gram-negative aerobes, and 25–30% will have enterococci in their bile. Anaerobes are found in the bile of older patients, those with cholangitis and those with complex biliary problems and indwelling tubes[1].

Four factors must be considered when choosing antibiotics for the jaundiced patient: (1) the antibacterial spectrum of the antibiotic, (2) serum and liver concentrations, (3) biliary excretion and (4) toxicity. For many years the combination of a penicillin and an aminoglycoside has been recommended to cover the Gram-negative aerobes and enterococcus. However, concern about the nephrotoxicity of the aminoglycosides, especially in jaundiced patients, has led to a search for less toxic agents. Options include ureidopenicillins, third-generation cephalosporins and monobactams. The ureidopenicillins, such as piperacillin, have been shown to be effective in patients with cholangitis[1,5]. In a prospective, randomized study of 96 patients piperacillin was found to be as effective as the combination of tobramycin and ampicillin[5].

In patients with biliary obstruction and cholangitis serum levels of antibiotics are more important than

biliary excretion. The biliary excretion of antibiotics is significantly reduced in biliary obstruction, making it difficult to achieve high bile levels of antibiotics in the situations where they are most needed. Antibacterial specificity and toxicity are therefore the most important factors to consider in the selection of antibiotic therapy.

Prophylactic antibiotics should be administered in all patients undergoing operative or non-operative manipulations of the biliary tree including cholangiography and sphincterotomy. In uncomplicated cases a broad-spectrum first-generation cephalosporin such as cefazolin usually provides adequate coverage. If bile culture data are available, antibiotics that are specific for the organisms present in the bile should be chosen. In more complicated cases where multiple organisms are likely to be present but have not been identified, broader antibiotic coverage may be indicated. In this setting the ureidopenicillins, which cover the Gram-negative aerobes, enterococci and, to some degree, the anaerobes, may be a good choice in the non-allergenic patient.

Preoperative biliary drainage

During the 1970s the surgical relief of biliary obstruction in severely jaundiced patients was associated with postoperative morbidity in 40–60% and mortality in 15–20% of patients[1,6]. During this same period, numerous authors reported that percutaneous transhepatic drainage could be performed with little morbidity[6]. For this reason, preoperative percutaneous transhepatic drainage was recommended and supported by retrospective and non-randomized studies. However, prospective randomized studies failed to demonstrate any advantage of preoperative biliary drainage by either the percutaneous or endoscopic technique (*Table 5*). Moreover, preoperative biliary tract drainage has been shown significantly to lengthen the hospital stay for

Table 5　Results of randomized trials comparing preoperative biliary drainage

Authors	No. of patients	Type of drainage	Postoperative mortality (%)	
			No drainage	Preoperative drainage
Hatfield et al. (*Lancet* 1982; 2: 896–9)	55	Transhepatic	15	14
McPherson *et al.* (*Br J Surg* 1984; 71: 371–5)	65	Transhepatic	19	32
Pitt *et al.* (*Ann Surg* 1985; 201: 545–53)	75	Transhepatic	5	8
Lai *et al.* (*Br J Surg* 1994; 81: 1195–8)	85	Endoscopic	14	15

these patients. Thus, although retrospective analyses suggested that preoperative drainage might be beneficial, prospective randomized studies have not supported this finding.

Although these data suggest that preoperative biliary drainage may not be of any benefit in the routine patient, this manoeuvre may have some value in selected patients. The combination of preoperative percutaneous biliary drainage and hyperalimentation in patients with advanced malnutrition has been shown to reduce the morbidity and mortality associated with surgery in the jaundiced patient. Patients with 'toxic' cholangitis should also undergo endoscopic or percutaneous decompression of the biliary tree prior to surgery. Preoperatively placed catheters are also of value in the operating theatre during difficult hilar dissections as well as in aiding in the placement of long-term transhepatic stents.

Summary

Biliary surgery, especially in the jaundiced patient, has been and continues to be associated with high postoperative morbidity and mortality. This phenomenon is due to a multitude of metabolic abnormalities that occur when the bile duct becomes obstructed. As a result, these patients are prone to sepsis with associated hepatic, renal, cardiac and pulmonary organ failure. In addition, their immune system is depressed, they are frequently malnourished, they often have coagulopathies, and their wounds do not heal normally. Preoperative assessment includes a careful history and physical examination, a complete biochemical evaluation, and a number or radiological studies. Laparoscopy and liver biopsy may also be indicated in selected cases. Preoperative preparation must include treatment of underlying cardiac or pulmonary disease, maintenance of adequate blood volume, correction of coagulopathies and treatment of biliary sepsis. Antibiotic regimens that are not nephrotoxic are preferred, and non-operative biliary drainage may be required in patients with 'toxic' cholangitis. Selected patients with underlying renal disease and/or malnutrition may also benefit from a period of preoperative biliary drainage and hyperalimentation, preferably by an enteral route. Percutaneous transhepatic biliary drainage may be indicated before surgery in selected patients with perihilar obstruction in whom large-bore Silastic stents are to be placed intraoperatively.

References

1. Nakeeb A, Pitt HA. Jaundice. In: Polk HC, Gardner B, Stone HH, eds. *Basic Surgery.* 5th edn. St. Louis: Quality Medical Publishing, 1995: 558–78.

2. Green J, Better OS. Circulatory disturbance and renal dysfunction in liver disease and in obstructive jaundice. *Isr J Med Sci* 1994; 30: 48–65.

3. Gigot JF, Leese T, Dereme T, Coutinho J, Castaing D, Bismuth H. Acute cholangitis: Multivariate analysis of risk factors *Ann Surg* 1989; 209: 435–8.

4. Little JM. A prospective evaluation of computerized estimates of risk in the management of obstructive jaundice. *Surgery* 1987; 102: 473–6.

5. Thompson JE, Pitt HA, Doty JE, Coleman J, Irving C, Manchester B. Broad spectrum penicillin as an adequate therapy for acute cholangitis. *Surg Gynecol Obstet* 1990; 171: 275–82.

6. Nakeeb A, Pitt HA. The role of preoperative biliary decompression in obstructive jaundice. *Hepatogastroenterology* 1995; 42: 332–7.

Cholecystectomy, cholecystostomy and exploration of the bile duct

David C. Carter MD, FRCS(Ed), FRSC(Glas), FRCS, FRSE
Regius Professor of Clinical Surgery, Royal Infirmary, Edinburgh, UK

S. Paterson-Brown MS. MPhil, FRCS(Ed), FRCS
Consultant Surgeon, University Department of Surgery, Royal Infirmary, Edinburgh, UK

Principles and justification

Open cholecystectomy was until recently the commonest major general surgical operation and approximately 500 000 operations were undertaken annually in the USA and some 40 000 in the UK. The reported incidence of common bile duct stones in these patients varied from 6% to 19% with a mean incidence of just over 10%[1]. Large series of patients undergoing open cholecystectomy without mortality have been reported[2], but it is well recognized that patients undergoing emergency surgery are at greater risk, as are those having concurrent exploration of the common bile duct. Experience in specialist centres may fail to reflect national or regional experience. In the decade up to 1989, the annual mortality rate for cholecystectomy alone in the Lothian region of Scotland fell consistently below 1%, averaging some 0.6%, while the mortality of cholecystectomy with bile duct exploration fell from around 3% to fluctuate around 1%. In some years, cholecystectomy with bile duct exploration incurred no mortality, and this undoubtedly reflected the increasing use of endoscopic papillotomy in high-risk patients with choledocholithiasis, jaundice and cholangitis.

Since the advent of laparoscopic cholecystectomy in 1987 the number of patients undergoing open cholecystectomy has fallen sharply. In one large study involving seven European centres, only 4% of patients scheduled for laparoscopic cholecystectomy required conversion to open operation[3]. However, it is clear that the ability to perform open cholecystectomy is still an essential part of the surgeon's armamentarium and, in many areas of the world, lack of resources means that this is still the standard method of removing the gallbladder.

Indications for cholecystectomy

The indications for cholecystectomy have not changed substantially with the advent of laparoscopic cholecystectomy.

Gallstone disease

Cholecystectomy is indicated in patients with biliary colic or acute cholecystitis and can be undertaken early in the acute admission or as an elective procedure in patients who have had previous attacks. While the basis of pain in biliary colic and acute cholecystitis is relatively easy to understand, there is less certainty about the association between flatulent dyspepsia and gallstones and whether this symptom complex is in itself a sufficient basis for cholecystectomy. In general, the prevalence of flatulent dyspeptic symptoms is similar when individuals with and without gallstones are compared[4]. Cholecystectomy does not always relieve symptoms, and about one-third of patients consult their general practitioner because of recurrent pain in the year following cholecystectomy. Asymptomatic gallstones are no longer regarded as an indication for cholecystectomy as they remain asymptomatic in the great majority of cases; exceptions may be made in the case of younger patients with multiple small stones (and a potential risk of gallstone pancreatitis), diabetics (who are more liable to life-threatening complications if cholecystitis develops), patients receiving immuno-suppression, and those receiving long-term parenteral nutrition.

Acute acalculous cholecystitis

This relatively rare condition accounts for up to 5% of all cases of acute cholecystitis; it is usually associated with critical and prolonged illness such as that seen with multiple trauma, major burns and sepsis, and may be commoner in patients having multiple transfusions and/or total parenteral nutrition. Emergency cholecys-tectomy is indicated as the condition frequently progresses to gangrenous cholecystitis.

Acalculous biliary pain

There is greater uncertainty about the role of cholecys-tectomy in patients thought to have acalculous biliary pain. The pain is similar to that found in symptomatic gallstone disease but occurs in the absence of gallstones or proven gallbladder disease. The patients are predomi-nantly young or middle-aged women. The decision to undertake cholecystectomy is a matter for clinical judgement in individual patients, although some con-sider that a positive response to a cholecystokinin provocation test may help to identify patients likely to benefit from cholecystectomy. Cholecystectomy fails to relieve symptoms in about 50% of patients, and not all accept that a functional disorder of the gallbladder is a satisfactory explanation for pain. It is conceivable that a functional disorder of the sphincter of Oddi causes pain in some patients and that cholecystectomy is in-appropriate if sphincter dysfunction is proven at manometry.

'Prophylactic' cholecystectomy

On rare occasions, cholecystectomy is undertaken 'prophylactically' in patients having a catheter inserted into the hepatic artery for hepatic perfusion chemo-therapy.

Gallbladder cancer

Cholecystectomy for gallbladder cancer is discussed elsewhere.

Preoperative

Many patients undergoing cholecystectomy are elderly and have intercurrent diseases that require full assess-ment and may benefit from preoperative management. Many are obese and weight reduction is advisable whenever possible to minimize the difficulty of surgery and risk of complications.

Postoperative wound infection is largely preventable by prescribing perioperative antibiotics such as tazobac-tam. Up to one-third of patients have infected bile, and the risk of infective complications in such individuals is increased. Risk factors include age over 50 years, history of jaundice, tender palpable gallbladder with fever or leucocytosis, a non-functioning gallbladder on cholecystography, abnormal liver function tests, and abnormalities of the common bile duct (notably ductal stones). When three or more of these factors are present or the patient has obvious infection, antibiotic therapy may be advisable for 5–7 days. The common infecting organisms are *Escherichia coli* and *Streptococcus faecalis* and appropriate antibiotics are tazobactam or cefotaxime and amoxycillin, the objective being to produce high blood and tissue levels rather than high levels in the bile.

The patient's blood should be grouped and a sample saved so that compatible blood can be released quickly if transfusion is necessary. An intravenous line is established before anaesthesia, and a catheter is advisable in jaundiced patients to monitor hourly urine output. A nasogastric tube is not inserted routinely.

Anaesthesia

General anaesthesia is employed, the objective being to render the patient unconscious and provide adequate analgesia and good muscle relaxation. If a nasogastric tube has been passed, its tip should be withdrawn well into the stomach so that it does not obscure the bile duct and affect the interpretation of operative cholangiograms.

Operations

CHOLECYSTECOMY

Position of patient

1 A C-arm to allow fluoroscopy is highly desirable. If fluoroscopy facilities are not available, the patient is placed supine on a cassette changer top so that the tip of the ninth costal cartilage is opposite the centre of the grid. Foam wedges or small bolsters are placed under the lower left rib cage and left buttock so that the common bile duct is not superimposed on the lumbar spine during cholangiography. The plane of the grid remains at right angles to the X-ray beam in order to give clear definition. A foam pillow or water-filled balloon (or gloves) is placed under the ankles to avoid calf compression during surgery. Subcutaneous heparin is used to reduce the risk of deep venous thrombosis.

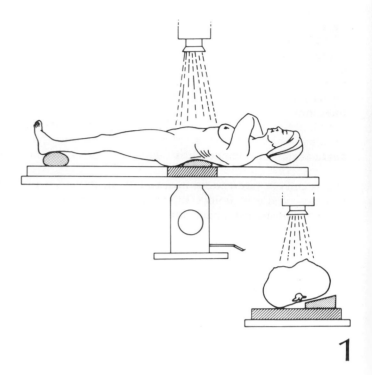

1

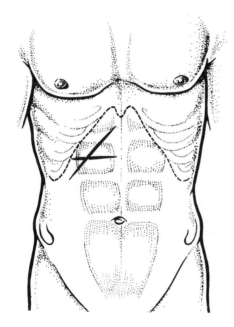

2

Incision

2 A Kocher's right subcostal or upper right transverse incision is used in preference to a vertical midline or right paramedian incision. Incision length is dictated by the patient's habitus and by the exposure needed once the peritoneal cavity has been entered and the findings assessed. Although incisions as small as 5 cm have been advocated for 'minicholecystectomy' and may provide adequate exposure in thin patients, failure to provide adequate access remains one of the major risk factors in cholecystectomy. The skin incision should be as long as is necessary for safe surgery. In the following description, a subcostal incision has been employed.

The surgeon normally stands on the patient's right with his assistant on the other side. The abdomen and lower chest is prepared and draped in the usual manner, but towel clips are avoided as they can obscure operative cholangiography. An adhesive skin drape is desirable to minimize wound infection. The subcostal incision is placed 4 cm below and parallel to the right costal margin and usually extends from close to the midline to the eighth or ninth costal cartilage.

3a–c Once the skin and subcutaneous tissue have been incised, the anterior rectus sheath is divided with a scalpel in the line of the skin incision. Diathermy is then used to cut through the rectus abdominis, coagulating or ligating any vessels. A Mayo or Roberts forceps can be passed behind the muscle so that it is placed on a slight stretch to facilitate the identification of vessels and their formal coagulation or ligation before they retract into the muscle. The peritoneum is next opened with a knife between forceps. The incision can then be lengthened with scissors or diathermy; if exposure is inadequate the muscle layers can be divided laterally with diathermy taking care to avoid damaging the ninth intercostal nerve.

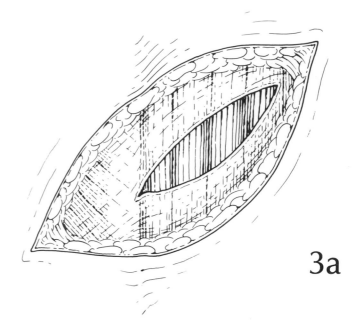

3a

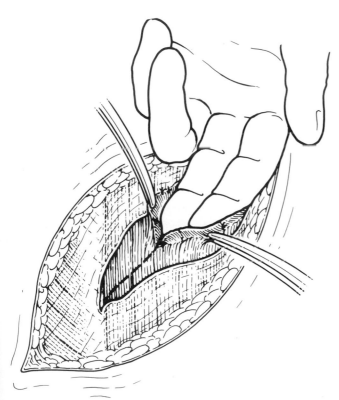

3b

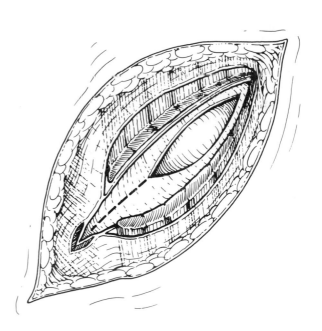

3c

Exploration

The peritoneal cavity is explored systematically paying particular attention to the oesophageal hiatus, stomach, duodenum, liver, gallbladder, small bowel and colon. The pancreas, spleen, kidneys, uterus and ovaries are not normally visualized but are palpated to detect any abnormality.

Exposure

The right hand is passed over the liver to introduce air so that the liver can descend into the wound. The gallbladder is grasped with two pairs of Mayo forceps or sponge-holding forceps, one pair being applied to the fundus and the other to Hartmann's pouch. This enables the gallbladder to be retracted downwards and laterally. Any adhesions are divided using dissecting scissors, taking care to avoid damage to the hepatic flexure of the colon or duodenum. Vascular adhesions involving the omentum may require ligature or diathermy.

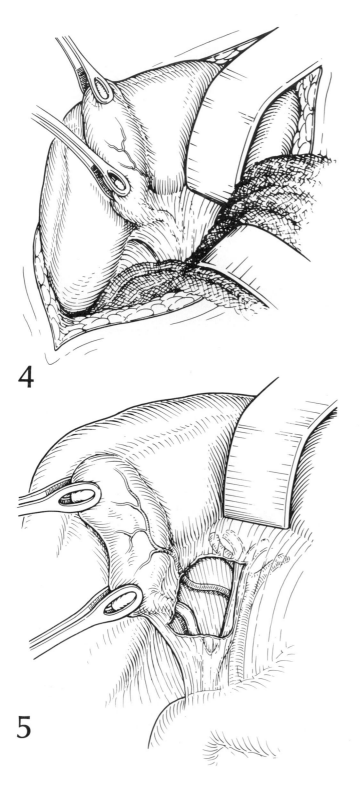

4 Two moist packs are then inserted. The first packs the colon downwards and prevents bowel from entering the operative field. The second is placed so that the duodenum, stomach and free edge of the lesser omentum can be retracted to the left throughout the operation. These packs can be kept in place by Deever's retractors fixed to a retraction system such as an Omnitract or ring system, or held by assistants. In the past, a third assistant was often used to retract the costal margin upwards, but this can now be achieved by a short-bladed retractor fixed to a retractor system or taped under tension to a vertical pole attached to the table and hidden beneath the drapes. If only one assistant is available, his left hand may be used instead of a Deever retractor to retract the lesser omentum to the left.

4

5 The peritoneum overlying the cystic duct is then incised using dissecting scissors, the incision being extended into the peritoneum overlying the common hepatic duct. The anatomy of the biliary tree is assessed carefully, noting the diameter of the cystic duct and common hepatic/common bile duct. A pledget held in a pair of Mayo or Robert's forceps is used to sweep adventitial tissues carefully away from the cystic duct and so display the triangle bounded by the cystic duct, common hepatic duct and inferior edge of the liver. This manoeuvre usually brings the cystic artery into view.

5

6 At every stage, one must remember that variations in the anatomy of the bile ducts and hepatic arteries are common. Common pitfalls are to mistake a small calibre common bile duct for the cystic duct (a potentially catastrophic cause of bile duct injury which is a particular problem in young slim women), failure to appreciate a low junction of the right and left hepatic ducts (the cystic duct in such cases may enter the right hepatic duct or one of its sectoral branches and the junction of right hepatic duct and left hepatic duct may be mistaken for the junction of the cystic duct and common hepatic duct), and failure to appreciate that the cystic duct is absent or very short. A common problem with arterial anatomy is posed by a right hepatic artery which swings far to the right before giving off a short cystic artery and multiple cystic arteries. The surgeon must have a clear picture of the anatomy before dividing any arterial or ductal structure; failure to appreciate the anatomy is the major cause of injury to the biliary tree or hepatic arterial supply.

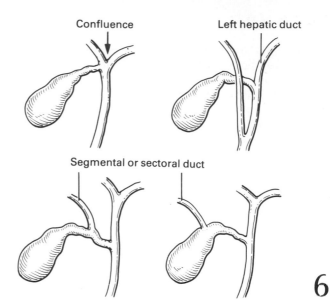

Confluence   Left hepatic duct

Segmental or sectoral duct

6

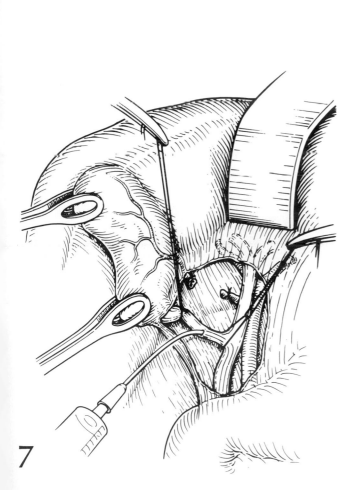

7

Operative cholangiography

There has always been (and probably always will be) controversy about the need for routine operative cholangiography. The authors undertake operative cholangiography routinely as a means of confirming ductal anatomy, avoiding ductal injury and detecting ductal stones.

Insertion of catheter

7 Many methods are available for operative cholangiography. The authors prefer to clear a length of cystic duct, tying a ligature around it just after it leaves the gallbladder and loosely encircling it with another ligature as it courses to join the common hepatic duct. A small scalpel (blade size No. 15) is used to incise, but not transect, the duct between these ligatures. A sample of bile is sent for bacteriological culture, and a fine cannula (e.g. Stoke or Trent cannula or ureteric catheter) is passed into the cystic duct and on into the common bile duct. Adhesions or mucosal valves which prevent ready passage can be broken down gently with a fine probe. It is important not to insert so much cannula that it passes into the duodenum and fails to provide a cholangiogram. A syringe of isotonic saline is used to flush all air from the cannula before its insertion to avoid air bubbles being mistaken for gallstones on the operative cholangiogram.

Once the cannula has been inserted and its patency confirmed by aspirating bile, the loose ligature around the cystic duct is tied to prevent leakage of contrast during cholangiography. Alternatively, metal clips (Ligaclips) can be used to occlude the cystic duct.

Exposure of films

All instruments and packs are removed from the abdomen and the wound is covered with a sterile towel. As indicated earlier, the patient lies on a cassette exchanger unless facilities for fluoroscopy and image intensification are available. If the patient has not been positioned with the left side raised by about 10–15°, the table can be tilted to make sure that the image of the bile duct is not obscured by being superimposed on the vertebral column. The saline-filled syringe is replaced by one containing 25% Hypaque or similar solution, again taking meticulous care to avoid introducing air bubbles during the exchange. Three films are then taken after introducing 2–3 ml, 4–6 ml and 7–10 ml of contrast medium respectively, the amount being influenced by the size of the duct system. The theatre is cleared momentarily of all personnel during exposure of the films, and the anaesthetist arrests ventilatory movement while the films are being exposed.

8 There are five criteria for a normal cholangiogram and these should be documented: (1) no filling defects in the biliary tree; (2) normal width of the common bile duct (opinions vary as to whether a diameter of up to 8 or 10 mm is normal at the level of insertion of the cystic duct); (3) gentle tapering of the common bile duct as it comes into proximity with the duodenum and enters its lumen; (4) free flow of contrast medium into the duodenum; and (5) normal filling of both the left and right hepatic ducts.

Once a cholangiogram has been obtained, the surgeon has three options: (1) to proceed with the operation if the cholangiogram is of acceptable quality and normal; (2) to proceed with duct exploration if a filling defect(s) is seen; and (3) to repeat the cholangiogram if the films are inadequate.

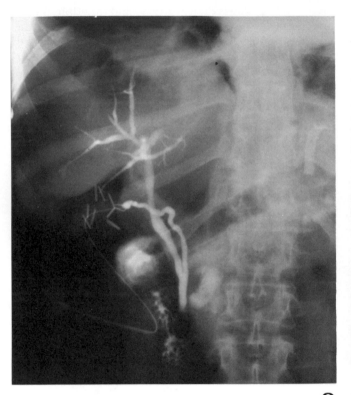

8

Removal of the gallbladder

9 Assuming that the cholangiogram is normal, the cannula is removed and the cystic duct is then securely tied with an absorbable ligature. The cystic artery is also doubly ligated and both structures are then divided.

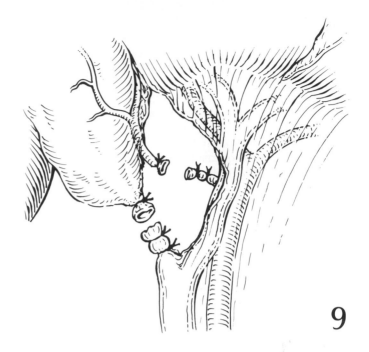

9

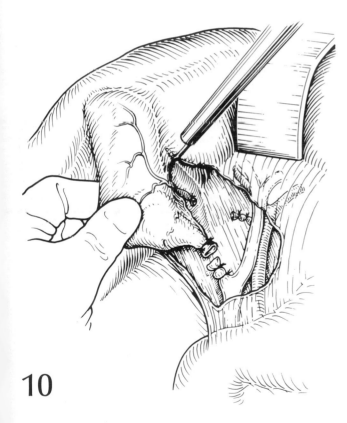

10

10 The gallbladder is kept under tension by gentle traction from the surgeon's left hand, and the fold of peritoneum attaching the gallbladder to the liver is divided using a combination of sharp dissection and electrocoagulation.

11a,b On occasion, it may be safer to remove the gallbladder using a 'fundus first' approach, particularly when inflammation or adhesion formation makes it difficult to display the common bile duct, cystic duct and cystic artery. If the 'fundus first' approach is adopted it is important to establish the correct plane between the gallbladder and its bed; dissecting too deeply will enter the liver parenchyma, while dissecting too superficially risks entering the gallbladder lumen. Dissecting too close to the gallbladder is the lesser of the two evils. A combination of sharp dissection, diathermy dissection and blunt dissection with a pledget is often needed, and the suction apparatus is often a surprisingly useful tool for blunt dissection. Care must be taken as the dissection approaches the main biliary tree and when displaying the cystic duct and cystic artery. It may be safer to leave a small oversewn cuff of Hartmann's pouch rather than to attempt hazardous dissection to free an adherent gallbladder and cystic duct from the common hepatic duct.

Partial cholecystectomy is also a sensible option in patients with cirrhosis and/or portal hypertension.

Regardless of whether the gallbladder is removed fundus first or by the more conventional method, a small swab is placed in the gallbladder bed to control oozing. Any small bleeding vessels are coagulated, and if bleeding is troublesome and persists, a gauze swab or small pack is left in the gallbladder bed for 3–5 min. If this does not produce adequate haemostasis, underrunning of the bleeding points with a fine absorbable suture may be needed.

Once haemostasis is achieved, the right upper quadrant is lavaged with warm saline which is then removed. A drain is not inserted routinely, although many surgeons use a small suction drain (e.g. Redivac) if there are lingering anxieties about haemostasis. The incision is closed using a mass suture technique, and the skin edges are approximated with metal clips.

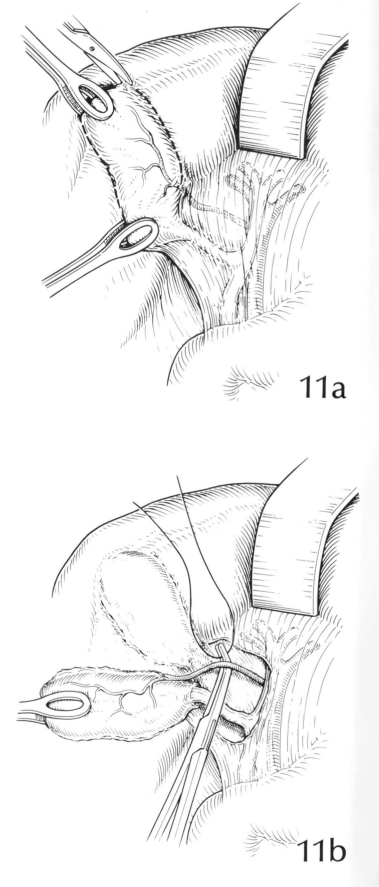

11a

11b

CHOLECYSTOSTOMY

Drainage of the gallbladder is occasionally indicated when cholecystectomy proves unduly difficult and potentially hazardous, and may be undertaken by an open or percutaneous technique. Open cholecystostomy will be described here.

12 If trial dissection indicates that cholecystectomy is impractical, the fundus of the gallbladder should be packed off from the surrounding tissues. The fundus is then incised between stay sutures or within a purse-string suture so that the lumen is entered and its contents evacuated. Alternatively, a trocar and cannula can be used with suction applied to the side arm of the cannula to empty the gallbladder of its contents. Large stones are sometimes difficult to extract, but every effort must be made to ensure that the gallbladder is emptied completely.

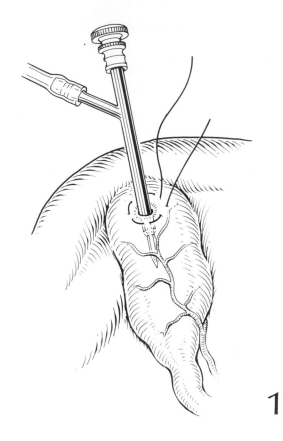

12

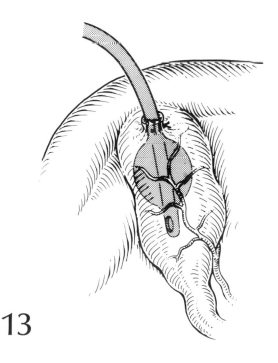

13

13 The cholecystotomy is next closed around a Foley catheter of appropriate size, after first passing the catheter through a small stab incision to one side of the main wound. The gallbladder wall is snugged around the emerging catheter using resorbable suture material, and most surgeons prefer to use a purse-string suture rather than interrupted sutures.

If possible, up to four interrupted sutures are then used to approximate the gallbladder wall to the peritoneum around the site of the stab incision. However, this may not be feasible if the gallbladder is not of sufficient size to lie comfortably against the peritoneum of the anterior abdominal wall.

EXPLORATION OF THE COMMON BILE DUCT

The decision to explore the common bile duct rests on the demonstration of stones on operative cholangiography or on palpation. Postoperative endoscopic retrieval of stones now offers an alternative approach which may be considered in a younger patient with a small calibre common bile duct and small stones. On the other hand, an elderly patient with large stones in a distended common bile duct is best served by operative exploration at the time of cholecystectomy. In general, a good reason is required not to proceed to explore the duct if stones have been demonstrated, and it should be borne in mind that endoscopic removal is not always successful and is not without risks.

14 Having removed the gallbladder and made the decision to explore the common bile duct, the second part of the duodenum is then mobilized by division of the lateral leaf of its peritoneal covering (Kocher manoeuvre). This allows the surgeon's hand to pass behind the duodenum and head of the pancreas to palpate the lower common bile duct. The anterior surface of the common duct is then cleared of its peritoneal covering and needled to obtain a specimen of bile for bacteriological examination.

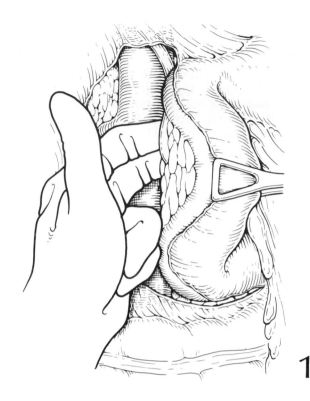

14

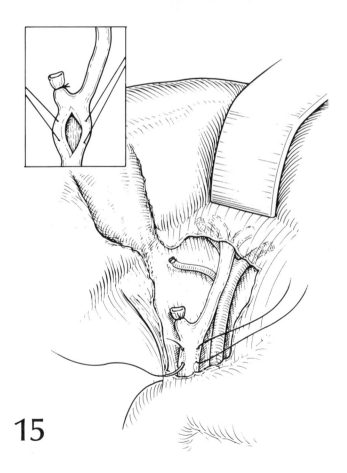

15

15 The duct is then incised between stay sutures using a size 15 blade and the longitudinal choledochotomy is enlarged using angled dissection scissors. The size of the opening is dictated by the size of the stones but it is usually about 15–20 mm long. Care must be taken when extending the incision upwards not to damage the hepatic arterial tree, and the right hepatic artery is often at particular risk as it loops in front of the bile duct. Similarly, care should be taken when extending the choledochotomy downwards not to damage the numerous small veins running on to the duodenum and so encounter troublesome bleeding.

16a–d

A fine catheter may be inserted into the bile duct at this stage and warm saline is used to try to flush out any small stones and debris. A flexible choledochoscope then offers the ideal method of inspecting the biliary tree from within and it should be passed down as far as the ampulla and upwards as far as the right and left hepatic ducts. Any residual stones are removed by further flushing with warm saline or by using a biliary Fogarty balloon catheter. The catheter is first passed into the duodenum and the balloon is carefully inflated. The catheter is then gently withdrawn allowing the balloon to deflate so that it passes through the papilla of Vater and sphincter of Oddi without undue force. Once above the sphincter region, the balloon is reinflated so that stones can be seen in the choledochotomy and withdrawn from the duct. A similar manoeuvre is used to extract any residual stones from the upper reaches of the biliary tree.

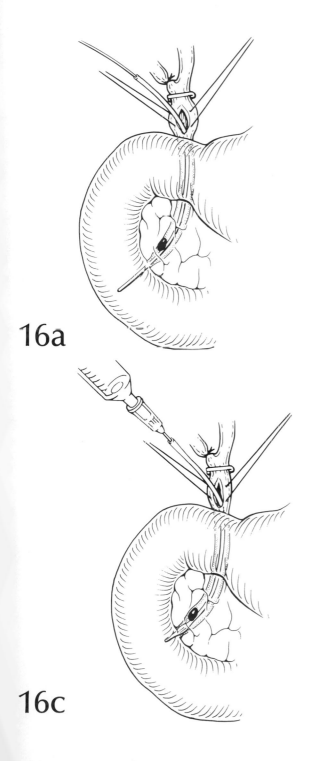

16a

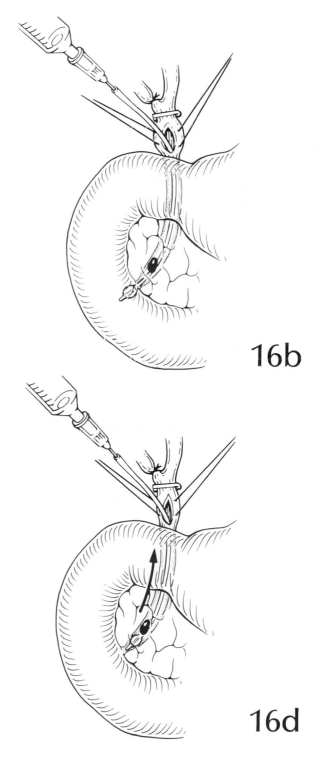

16b

16c

16d

17 If these measures fail, Desjardin's forceps can be inserted into the duct system to grasp any stones that are visible. Repeated attempts to grasp stones 'blindly' with Desjardin's forceps can damage the duct and should be avoided.

Stones which have not been retrieved at this stage can sometimes be recovered under choledochoscopic guidance using a Dormia basket.

A stone which is trapped at the lower end of the bile duct and cannot be dislodged can pose particular difficulties. Large stones can sometimes be retrieved if the choledochotomy is extended a little more distally so that the stone comes into view. Failing this, the surgeon can elect to open the duodenum and remove the stone following sphincterotomy, or to carry out a choledocho-duodenostomy leaving the stone in place. Simply closing the duct and relying on postoperative endo-scopic retrieval is not an option as the chances of successful endoscopic extraction are poor when the stone has been found to be impacted at open operation. Transduodenal extraction is the method of choice provided the surgeon is sufficiently experienced and the general condition of the patient permits, and a sphincteroplasty should be performed once the offend-ing stone has been removed.

Confirmation that the bile ducts have been cleared is obtained by choledochoscopy. If a choledochoscope is not available, post-explorative cholangiography can be performed using a Fogarty catheter with its balloon inflated to prevent leakage of dye while films are taken first of the upper reaches of the bile duct and then of its lower portion.

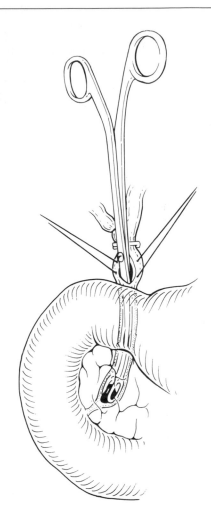

17

18 Once duct clearance has been confirmed, a rubber T tube (size 14–16 Fr depending on duct size) is inserted after trimming the ends of its short arm to an appropriate length and guttering this part of the tube. The choledochotomy is closed snugly around the T tube using interrupted 3/0 absorbable sutures such as polydioxanone (PDS). The T tube is brought out through the abdominal wall at a convenient point away from the main wound, taking care to ensure that it runs perpendicular to the axis of the bile duct. An anchoring suture to the skin is used to prevent the T tube from falling out prematurely.

Some surgeons do not insert a T tube after exploring the bile duct, but the authors insert one routinely and use it to obtain a check cholangiogram 5–7 days after the operation. Premature removal of the T tube may allow biliary leakage and biliary peritonitis and most surgeons do not remove the tube for at least 7–10 days.

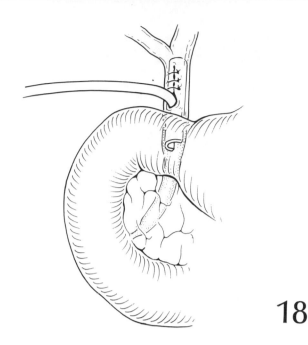

18

Postoperative care

Following cholecystectomy, patients are maintained on intravenous fluids for the first 12 h. Oral intake is resumed on the first postoperative day according to the clinical condition of the patient, and early mobilization is encouraged. After uneventful elective cholecystectomy, many patients are ready for discharge from hospital within a few days.

References

1. Menzies D, Motson RW. Choledocholithiasis – detection and open management. In: Paterson-Brown S, Garden OJ, eds. *Principles and Practice of Surgical Laparoscopy*. Philadelphia: WB Saunders, 1994: 81–104.

2. Clavien PA, Sanabria JR, Mentha G *et al*. Recent results of elective open cholecystectomy in a North American and a European center. Comparison of complications and risk factors. *Ann Surg* 1992; 216: 618–26.

3. Cuschieri A, Dubois F, Mouiel J *et al*. The European experience with laparoscopic cholecystectomy. *Am J Surg* 1991; 161: 385–7.

4. Banting S, Carter DC. Expectations of cholecystectomy. In: Paterson-Brown S, Garden OJ, eds. *Principles and Practice of Surgical Laparoscopy*. Philadelphia: WB Saunders, 1994: 53–66.

Minimally invasive surgery for gallstone disease: laparoscopic cholecystectomy

A. Cuschieri MD, MCh, FRCS, FRCS (Ed)
Professor and Head of Department, Department of Surgery, University of Dundee, Ninewells Hospital and Medical School, Dundee, UK

History

Some debate exists as to who performed the first laparoscopic cholecystectomy. Muehe was the first to describe the use of an operating proctoscope and carbon dioxide insufflation. The first series using dedicated laparoscopic instrumentation and ancillary equipment including a videocamera attached to the laparoscope was reported by Dubois *et al.* in 1989[1], while the first large retrospective series from a number of European centres was reported by Cuschieri *et al.* in 1991[2]. This report was soon followed by the prospective series reported by the Southern Surgeons Club[3]. Since then, laparoscopic cholecystectomy has become the standard surgical treatment for patients with symptomatic gallstone disease and can be used in over 95% of such patients.

Preoperative

Anaesthesia

Laparoscopic cholecystectomy is carried out under general anaesthesia. The patients are most commonly premedicated with benzodiazepines and some anaesthetists also give a long-acting 5-HT$_3$ antagonist to reduce the incidence of postoperative vomiting. Induction is carried out with thiopentone, and neuromuscular blockade is established using alcuronium or vercuronium in patients with hypertension. All patients are intubated with a cuffed endotracheal tube and ventilated mechanically. Nitrous oxide (66%), oxygen and enflurane are used to maintain anaesthesia with increments of alcuronium and fentanyl as required.

Monitoring during anaesthesia includes electrocardiography and measurement of blood pressure, oxygen saturation and end-tidal carbon dioxide (which is maintained at 30 mmHg). Fluid losses are replaced using Hartmann's solution. An intravenous injection of a cephalosporin (e.g. cephuroxime) is given at the start of the operation.

At the end of the procedure, neuromuscular blockade is reversed with neostigmine and atropine. Oxygen is administered for the first 3 h. Although potent opioid analgesics such as fentanyl are still used extensively to treat postoperative pain in the recovery room, increasingly many anaesthetists favour non-steroidal anti-inflammatory drugs, such as intravenous ketorolac, to minimize respiratory depression, nausea and sedation.

Operation

Laparoscopic cholecystectomy can be performed with the patient lying supine in either the classical or leg abduction position.

Leg abduction position

1 This position is favoured by many European surgeons. The patient is positioned supine on the operating table and the legs are abducted, preferably in the limb extension position and without the use of Lloyd-Davies stirrups. This position allows the surgeon to operate facing the patient's abdomen. The table is tilted 30° head up (reverse Trendelenburg position). The neutral electrosurgical pad is placed underneath the buttocks and connected to the electrosurgical generator. The assistant stands on the patient's right and the scrub nurse on the same side. The insufflator, suction/irrigation system, telescope heater, electrocautery unit and xenon light source are positioned on the right of the surgeon. The instrument trolley is placed on the left of the surgeon between him and the scrub nurse. The television monitor is placed on the right side of the patient such that the assistant and scrub nurse can clearly see the progress of the operation. Dual monitors are an advantage.

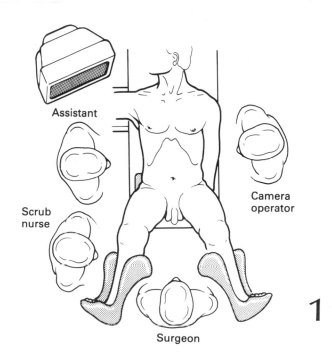

Classical supine position

2 This position is popular in North America and the United Kingdom. The patient is placed in the ordinary supine position with the table given a 30° reverse Trendelenburg tilt with the surgeon on the left and the assistant on the right of the patient. The classical supine position is less likely to cause compression trauma to the calf veins but two television monitors are required, one facing the surgeon and the other facing his assistant.

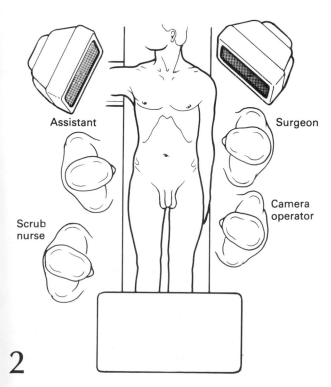

Nasogastric intubation and emptying of the bladder

A nasogastric tube is used to ensure complete gastric deflation during the procedure since a distended stomach and duodenal cap can obscure the operative field. The urinary bladder is emptied by a catheter (which is then removed) prior to the insertion of a Veress needle and creating a pneumoperitoneum. If catheterization is not practised routinely, it is important to percuss the suprapubic region to exclude a distended urinary bladder before inserting the Veress needle. The nasogastric tube is removed at the end of the operation.

Skin preparation and draping

The skin of the abdomen from the level of the nipple line to the pubic region is prepared with chlorhexidine soap followed by chlorhexidine-alcohol antiseptic solution (or suitable alternative). Standard drapes are used as for open cholecystectomy and some surgeons prefer to use disposable drapes. The edges of the drapes are sutured temporarily to the skin and skin clips should be avoided because of the anticipated need for intraoperative cholangiography.

Access to the peritoneal cavity

Two techniques are available: (1) closed peritoneal insufflation followed by the insertion of the optical port (blind or visually guided); and (2) open laparoscopy using the modified Hasson's cannula.

Closed pneumoperitoneum followed by insertion of optical port

This technique entails the initial creation of a carbon dioxide pneumoperitoneum using a Veress needle and electronic insufflator. The function of the spring loaded snap mechanism of the Veress needle should be confirmed before initial insertion, as should its patency by checking gas flow through it. The Veress needle is most often inserted at the subumbilical site where the optical port will be introduced. A different site is chosen if subumbilical adhesions are suspected.

After the checks on the Veress needle, the palpation test is performed. This test provides the surgeon with a clear mental idea of the depth required for insertion of the needle tip and is achieved by finger pressure depression of the abdominal wall down to the aorta. This distance can be alarmingly short in thin individuals.

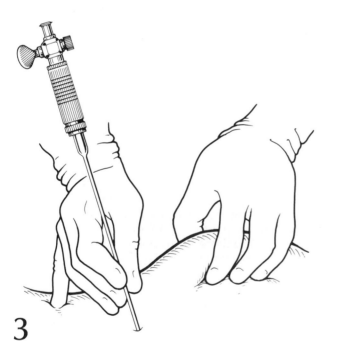

3

3 A small skin stab wound is made, with a pointed scalpel and the Veress needle is inserted. The safest technique involves holding the Veress needle along its shaft at a distance from its tip which is roughly equal to the estimated abdominal wall thickness in the individual patient. Held in this manner, the needle is 'threaded through' the parietes as the abdominal wall is lifted up by hand. A definite click is felt as the anterior rectus sheath is penetrated. With care, a second click should be felt by the surgeon when the posterior sheath and peritoneum are breached.

At this point clues to safe and free penetration of the peritoneal cavity may be obtained as follows:

(i) *Syringe aspiration test*: isotonic saline (5 ml) is instilled into the peritoneal cavity via the Veress needle. If the needle tip lies freely, it should not be possible to aspirate the injected fluid; if the fluid can be aspirated, incorrect needle tip placement is likely. Aspiration of yellowish fluid (signifying contamination with bowel contents) or bloodstained fluid indicates needle misplacement.

(ii) *Drop test*: The tap on the Veress needle is closed, and its terminal hub is filled with saline which forms a convex droplet due to its surface tension. This drop disappears down the shaft as soon as the tap is opened if the needle tip is unobstructed.

(iii) *Negative pressure test*: the tubing leading from the insufflator is next connected to the Veress needle in order to measure peritoneal pressure prior to insufflation. This manoeuvre should reveal a slight negative pressure which is accentuated by elevation of the abdominal wall.

(iv) *Early insufflation pressures*: the next clue to correct positioning is the insufflation pressure (which should not exceed 8 mmHg at 1 l/min gas insufflation). The more recent electronic insufflators incorporate an automatic sensor system which gives an alarm when the tip of the needle is obstructed during insufflation.

Insufflation of the peritoneal cavity is then continued at an initial inflow rate of about 1 l/min. If this process proceeds smoothly without significant cardiovascular changes, the insufflator can be switched to high flow to allow complete filling of the peritoneal cavity to a pressure of approximately 10–15 mmHg. At this point the Veress needle is withdrawn. During the insufflation process, all quadrants of the abdomen are percussed to confirm uniform as distinct from localized distension.

If, during induction of the initial pneumoperitoneum, the needle tip is thought to be incorrectly positioned, the needle is simply withdrawn and reinserted. The number of passes required should be recorded in the operation note. If blood is aspirated, simple withdrawal of the needle and reinsertion is reasonable. However, if blood fountains back up the Veress needle, major vessel injury is likely, and laparotomy should be performed with the Veress needle *in situ*. If bowel content is aspirated, the needle is withdrawn and reinserted in another site. In this event, it is important to inspect the area of bowel injury when the laparoscope is first introduced. If the hole in the bowel consists of a simple puncture, the administration of antibiotics and local lavage/suction followed by careful postoperative observation may be all that is required. More extensive injuries, e.g. when bowel has been lacerated, require immediate suture repair (laparoscopically or at open operation).

Blind insertion of optical port

The cannula used for insertion of the videolaparoscope should have an external diameter of 11 mm (in preference to 10 mm) and can be reusable or disposable. The larger port, when used with a 10.5 mm reducer, results in a bigger space between the telescope and the inner surface of the cannula and so ensures larger gas flows and maintenance of the pneumoperitoneum during the operation. Although many types of disposable ports have outer protective shields to minimize the risk of visceral injury by the trocar during insertion, this risk is not abolished, especially if the technique of insertion is faulty. If a non-disposable cannula is used, the flap valve (trap door) variety rather than the trumpet valve variety should be used as the latter restricts movement of the telescope. The non-disposable metal trocars are hollow and have a hole near the pointed tip. This design provides an important safety feature during insertion.

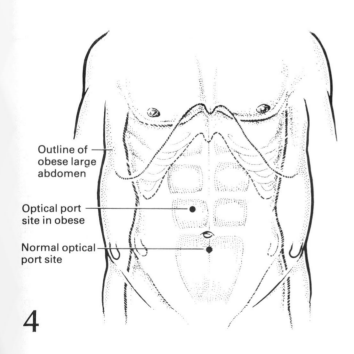

Outline of obese large abdomen

Optical port site in obese

Normal optical port site

4 The optimal site for insertion is the immediate subumbilical region. However, in large or obese individuals with a long distance between the umbilicus and the xiphoid process, the optical port should be sited at a higher level on either side of the umbilicus. If the subumbilical site is chosen, the skin incision used for insertion of the Veress needle is extended vertically or transversely to 1.5 cm and deepened to include the aponeurotic layer until the hiss of escaping gas is heard.

4

5   The trocar/cannula is held in the right hand with the butt firmly pressed against the palm and the index finger alongside the long axis of the shaft some 2.5 cm away from the tip. The periumbilical region is pulled firmly up by the left hand so that the abdominal wall is tented upwards, and the trocar/cannula is introduced through the subumbilical incision parallel to the axis of the aorta and pointing to the centre of the pelvis. Alternatively, two Littlewood's forceps are applied to the edges of the skin wound, and the abdominal wall is pulled upwards. Pressure from the wrist accompanied by to-and-fro rotational movement is used to 'ream' the trocar/cannula through the parietes. Pressure against the palm of the hand prevents the trocar from riding inside the cannula as it encounters the resistance provided by the abdominal wall. The tip of the index finger against the long shaft of the assembly acts as a safety stop in case of sudden give. With the disposable sheathed cannulae, a click is heard due to snapping of the sheath over the trocar point as soon as the peritoneal lining is breached. By contrast, with the non-disposable type, the perforation near the tip of the trocar leads to a sudden escape of gas with a resultant audible hiss as soon as complete penetration of the abdominal wall is achieved. The trocar is withdrawn before the cannula is advanced further. The gas line is then connected to the side port of the cannula, and the tap is opened to maintain insufflation of the peritoneal cavity.

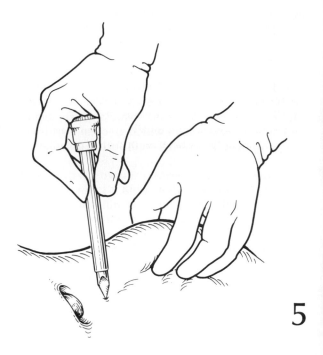

5

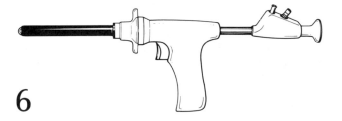

6

Visually guided insertion of the optical port

6   In this method the optical cannula is inserted under vision once the pneumoperitoneum has been created. This technique is possible using reusable or disposable equipment. The reusable device is known as the optical scalpel and is manufactured by Olympus (Japan). The disposable equipment is manufactured by United States Surgical Corporation (Norwalk, Connecticut, USA) or Ethicon (Cincinnati, USA).

All of the systems work on the same principle – an integral blade can be deployed to cut the abdominal layers under visual control until a safe window of parietal peritoneum (transparent as opposed to opaque) is created. These visual systems are undoubtedly safer and are recommended in difficult cases (obese patients and those with scars from previous surgery).

Open laparoscopy

Open laparoscopy dispenses with prior insufflation of the peritoneal cavity. The cannula is introduced through a small wound into the peritoneal cavity. After the cannula is fixed to the parietes with sutures to ensure an air tight seal, insufflation of the peritoneal cavity is commenced through the gas inlet of the cannula. Although open laparoscopy can be performed using an ordinary reusable or disposable port, the Hasson's cannula designed specifically for this purpose (initially for gynaecological laparoscopy) is better.

7 The modern versions of this device have three components: (1) a sliding olive which allows for variation in the length of the cannula inside the peritoneal cavity; (2) fixation suture wings attached to the olive; and (3) a blunt obturator.

Open laparoscopy virtually abolishes the risk of major vascular injury although injuries to the bowel may still occur.

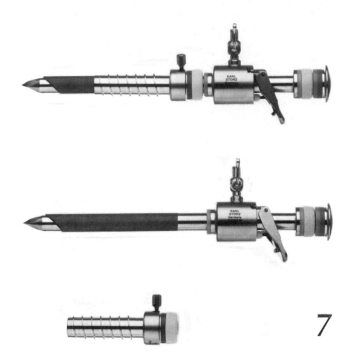

7

Insertion of the telescope

The previously heated 10 mm laparoscope (0° or 30°) is attached to the endocamera (sterile or inside transparent sterile plastic sleeve), the light cable is attached to the telescope, and the system is 'white balanced'. The telescope is then inserted down the optic port.

Insertion of operating and assisting ports

These ports are all placed under vision. If reusable cannulae are used, they should be equipped with flap valves in preference to trumpet valves as the latter require depression before instruments can be moved inside the cannula. Jamming of instruments inside the port not only slows down the procedure but carries the risk of stab injuries as increased force is needed to advance the instrument. Cannulae with trumpet valves damage the insulation of instruments used for electro-surgery and, for this reason, should not be used with these instruments. Another occurrence which is encountered frequently with both disposable and reusable cannulae is dislocation of the access port during instrument manipulation due either to valve sticking or the presence of congealed blood between the instrument and the cannula. With reusable cannulae, an external spiral screw relief can minimize this problem. Plastic cannulae fixation outer screws must not be used if the port consists of electroconductive material, since this results in electric isolation of the port from the abdominal parietes. In this situation, capacitance current from the electrode (each time this is activated) accumulates in the cannula as it cannot discharge to the abdominal wall. The cannula effectively becomes a charged electric capacitor and, if its tip then touches any tissue inside the abdomen, a high density current is discharged at the point of contact causing a burn.

In the majority of patients undergoing laparoscopic cholecystectomy, three accessory cannulae are needed. The location of these ports depends on the technique used to expose the triangle of Calot; North American or French. The North American exposure is easier provided the right lobe of the liver is not rigid and the quadrate lobe is not hypertrophied. Otherwise, the French exposure provides more adequate access.

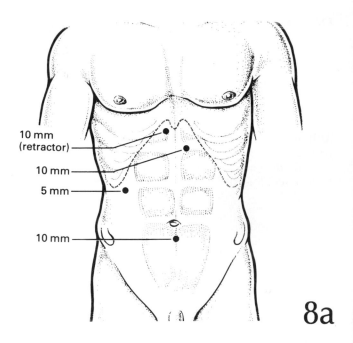

10 mm
(retractor)

10 mm

5 mm

10 mm

8a

French approach

8a,b The liver is retracted upwards by a medially placed retractor. The port sites for this technique are 10 mm upper left paramedian (for electrosurgical hook knife, scissors, etc.), 10 mm upper medial subcostal (for retraction, suction/irrigation) and 5 mm lower right hypochondrial just lateral to linea semilunaris (for grasping forceps).

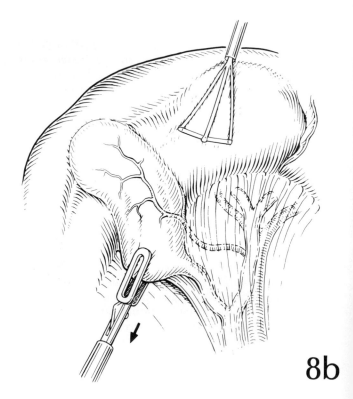

8b

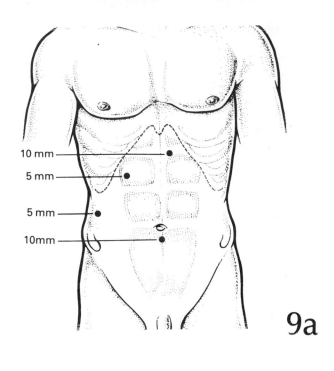

9a

North American approach

9a,b The cystic pedicle is exposed by grasping the gallbladder fundus which is then lifted together with the right lobe and rotated backwards. The following placements are used with this technique: 10 mm left upper paramedian (or just to the right of the midline avoiding the falciform ligament), 5 mm right upper midclavicular and 5 mm right lower axillary. The left upper paramedian cannula is placed about 1 cm lateral to the linea alba and 3 cm below the left costal margin. Some prefer to insert this cannula just to the right of the falciform ligament to obviate any entanglement in this structure. However, this position may result in crowding of instruments in the subhepatic pouch. The right upper cannula is best sited by reference to the gallbladder fundus using the finger depression technique for precise localization. This port must enter the parietes just below the liver edge. The right lower cannula is more laterally situated along the anterior axillary line some 4 cm below the costal margin. This cannula just skims the hepatic flexure and must be introduced with great care to avoid colonic injury.

With either the French or American approach the prescribed positions need to be adjusted in accordance with the build of the patient and, in particular, with the anatomy of the liver. An important consideration is the avoidance of placement of the ports above the inferior margin of the liver.

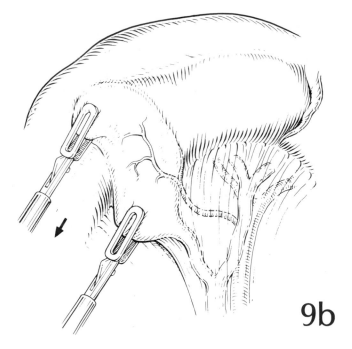

9b

Laparoscopic inspection

The initial laparoscopic inspection has three objectives: (1) detection of inadvertent injuries caused during insufflation and insertion of the main trocar/cannula; (2) exclusion of additional unsuspected intra-abdominal pathology; and (3) assessment of the feasibility of laparoscopic cholecystectomy.

A systematic inspection of the contents of the four quadrants and pelvis is undertaken. This step is equivalent to exploratory laparotomy during open cholecystectomy. Apart from excluding unsuspected disease, this inspection should rule out any significant trauma perpetrated during creation of the pneumoperitoneum or insertion of the first cannula.

To a large extent, the decision on the technical feasibility of the procedure is influenced by the experience of the surgeon in laparoscopic surgery. The situations which may be encountered are 'easy' cases, 'more difficult' cases, cases of 'uncertain feasibility' and unsuitable cases

'Easy' cases

10 There is minimal intraperitoneal fat and the gallbladder is floppy and non-adherent. When the gallbladder is lifted and retracted upwards by a pair of grasping forceps, the cystic pedicle (fold of peritoneum covering the cystic artery, duct and lymph node) is readily identified as a smooth triangular fold between Hartmann's pouch and the common bile duct.

'More difficult' cases

These include obese patients in whom the cystic pedicle is fat-laden. A gallbladder containing a large stone load may be difficult to grasp and this causes problems with retraction and exposure. The gallbladder may be distended due to cholecystitis or because of a stone impacted in the neck or Hartmann's pouch. Difficulties may also be encountered due to adhesions from previous surgery or abnormal anatomy of the hepatic arteries or extrahepatic biliary system. Provided the surgeon is experienced and is prepared to proceed slowly, these patients can undergo laparoscopic cholecystectomy with safety and a good outcome.

Cases of 'uncertain feasibility'

Trial dissection is indicated in such cases. This group includes patients with dense adhesions, those in whom the cystic pedicle cannot be visualized and patients with contracted fibrotic organs where the neck or Hartmann's pouch appears to be adherent to the common bile duct. In all these situations, the feasibility of the procedure becomes apparent as a careful trial dissection

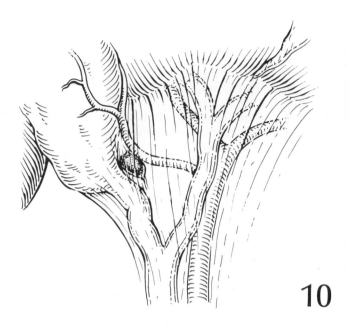

10

proceeds. In adopting this approach, common sense must prevail, and trial dissection should not be equated with a long hazardous procedure. If the surgeon cannot for any reason clearly identify and expose the structures of the cystic pedicle in the triangle of Calot in reasonable time, the case is converted to open surgery. Elective conversion must not be equated with surgical failure, and results in a much better clinical outcome than persistence with the laparoscopic approach in the presence of technical difficulties, which often result in iatrogenic injury and enforced conversion with enhanced morbidity.

Unsuitable cases

These include patients with severe acute cholecystitis with gangrenous patches or gross inflammatory phlegmon obscuring the structures of the porta hepatis, a chronically inflamed gallbladder with its neck adherent to the common bile duct (indicative of Mirizzi syndrome), and patients with advanced cirrhosis and established portal hypertension who have large high pressure varices surrounding the gallbladder and cystic pedicle.

In patients with severe acute cholecystitis which precludes safe dissection, a laparoscopic cholecystostomy may be performed with interval cholecystectomy at a later date.

Exposure of the subhepatic region and cystic pedicle

In the French technique a retractor is inserted through the upper medial right subcostal cannula and used to elevate the quadrate lobe. With an atraumatic grasper, introduced through the lower right port, the neck of the gallbladder is grasped and pulled anteriorly and downwards to display the cystic pedicle and the contents of the triangle of Calot (*see Illustration 8b*).

In the North American technique a gallbladder holding forceps is introduced through the right lower assisting port and is used to grasp the gallbladder fundus which is lifted in a lateral direction and rolled backwards to expose the subhepatic pouch. A second atraumatic grasper, inserted through the right upper cannula, is applied to the neck which is lifted upwards and anteriorly (*see Illustration 9b*). Although capture and retraction of the floppy non-inflamed gallbladder presents no problems, this step may be difficult in patients with a contracted fibrotic organ or if the gallbladder is distended or tightly packed with stones. Aspiration of the gallbladder by reducing the distension will permit a better grasp. A stone impacted in Hartmann's pouch may render capture of the neck of the organ very difficult. Attempts to dislodge the stone into the body of the organ, if successful, will greatly facilitate the dissection.

Dissection of the cystic pedicle

With both techniques, the cystic pedicle is inspected by advancing the telescope to obtain a closer view. In thin patients, this pedicle appears as a triangular fold between the neck of the gallbladder and the common bile duct which is often readily identified, especially if a forward oblique (30°) viewing telescope is used. The cystic pedicle outlines the margins of the triangle of Calot and contains between its superior and inferior leaves the cystic duct (usually anteriorly), the cystic artery (above and behind the duct) and the cystic lymph node which is closely applied to the neck of the gallbladder between the duct and the artery. The prominent anterior free edge of the cystic pedicle is formed as the peritoneum folds over the cystic duct. Dissection will prove difficult if the cystic pedicle is foreshortened or fat-laden.

The dissection of the cystic pedicle can be performed with scissors, electrosurgical hook knife or by teasing with fine pointed atraumatic graspers. In practice a combination of these techniques is often employed. Irrespective of the technique used, the first step consists of division of the superior leaf of the cystic pedicle.

The blunt teasing technique consists of stripping the peritoneum covering the cystic duct and artery in a medial direction towards the common duct against countertraction provided by a grasping forceps on the neck of the gallbladder. Oozing is controlled by soft coagulation, and the area is irrigated to maintain a clear view of the anatomy.

11a,b With the scissors technique, favoured by the author, the gallbladder is held retracted by an atraumatic grasper applied to its neck. The superior leaf of the cystic pedicle is divided from its free edge along the base of the triangle of Calot, keeping close to the medial aspect of the gallbladder as far as the liver. The dissection is kept superficial, dividing only the peritoneal covering and teasing it from the underlying structures. When the dissection has been completed, the cystic duct and artery become obvious, and dissection is then continued close to the cystic duct, mobilizing its posterior aspect with division of the inferior leaf of the cystic pedicle. The curved dissecting grasper is then employed to open the window between the cystic duct and the cystic artery. The tip of the instrument is placed in the cleft, and its jaws are opened gently and parallel to the two structures to commence the separation. This procedure has to be repeated several times until sufficient posterior mobilization has been achieved and a clear window is obtained. A fairly constant branch of the cystic artery traverses this window to supply the gallbladder neck. If identified, this branch is coagulated before division by the scissors. If oozing is sufficient to obscure the view at this stage, the area is irrigated, and minor bleeders are coagulated. When this has been completed, a gap becomes visible between the cystic duct in front and the artery behind. This gap is opened further by grasping and lifting the cystic duct anteriorly. A few fibrous attachments on either side of the gap are divided. Finally, the cystic duct is cleared of any residual extraneous tissues. In most patients, it is possible to isolate a 1.5–2·cm segment of the cystic duct. It is much safer to gain length by extending the dissection towards the gallbladder neck than extending medially.

The electrosurgical hook dissection is favoured by many surgeons. The instrument consists of a hollow insulated probe with a hook (J- or L-shaped) at the functional end. The other end is connected to the diathermy leads and also incorporates a suction/irrigation port which is controlled by a trumpet valve at the external end to release smoke and permit irrigation.

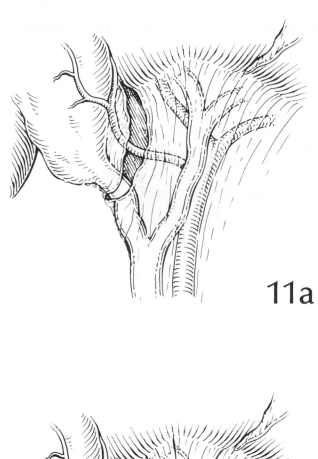

11a

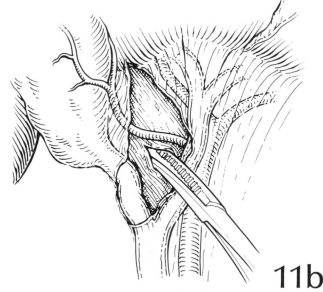

11b

12 The technique entails lifting the peritoneum of the cystic pedicle from the underlying structures with the hook and then applying blended current to cut the lifted peritoneal covering. Tenting of the tissue is essential before activating the current for three reasons: (1) it limits the electrosurgical burn to the tissue constricted by the hook; (2) the cut is facilitated by the tension on the tissue; and (3) the gap between the tissue and the underlying structures increases the safety margin against collateral thermal injury.

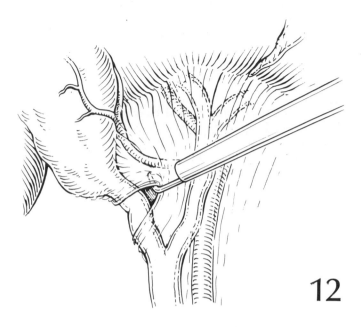

12

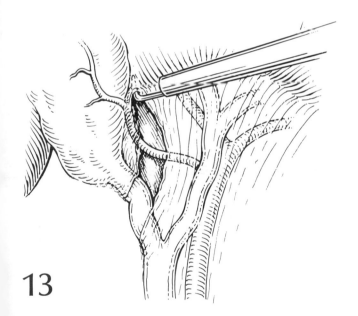

13

13 The dissection starts on the superior leaf of the cystic pedicle, proceeds laterally towards the neck of the gallbladder, and then curves upwards to the liver. The gap between the cystic duct and artery is identified.

14 Thereafter, the heel of the hook is inserted into this space and pushed backwards and medially before it is elevated in a forward direction to pick up the intervening tissue which is then cut by blender current. The inferior peritoneum of the cystic pedicle is divided using the same technique, keeping close to the neck of the gallbladder.

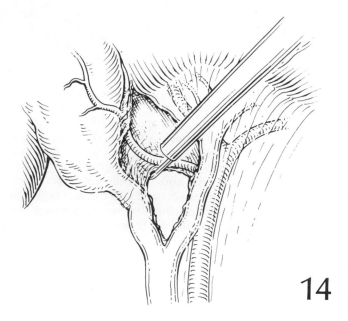

14

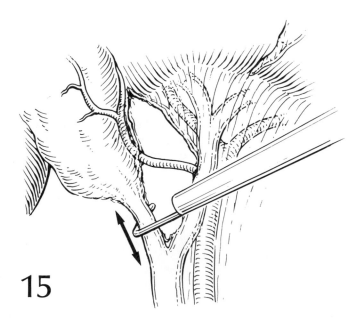

15

15 Eventually, it should be possible to place the hook around the mobilized cystic duct and to slide it up and down to separate any residual loose fibrous attachments.

The main disadvantage of electrosurgical dissection is the excess smoke generation. In addition, this technique causes considerable charring and some contraction of tissue planes.

The mobilized cystic duct must be clearly shown to be continuous with the neck of the gallbladder. Sometimes, an anomalous anterior cystic artery may be mistaken for the cystic duct and, as the cystic pedicle is under tension as a result of retraction of the gallbladder, pulsation may not be detected. Whenever this suspicion is raised, the telescope is advanced closer to the structure, and the retraction on the gallbladder is relaxed. This simple manoeuvre may restore obvious pulsations and help to resolve the problem.

Ligature/clipping and division of the cystic artery

16 The dissected cystic artery should be well displayed and shown to be terminating in the gallbladder. Anomalies of the cystic artery are common and have to be identified or excluded in every case. The most common anatomical arrangement is for the cystic artery to originate from the right hepatic artery as a single branch.

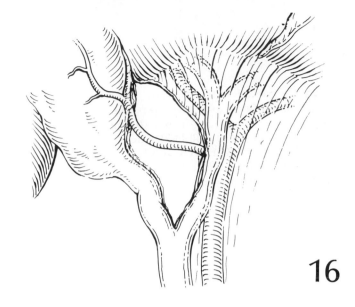

16

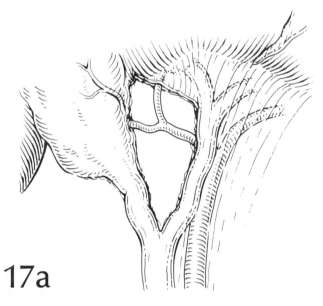

17a

17a,b The most dangerous variant is a looped right hepatic artery which can easily be mistaken for the cystic artery. Other important anomalies include early division of the cystic artery and aberrant origin of the right hepatic artery from the superior mesenteric artery.

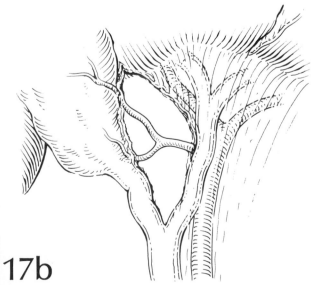

17b

18 A good length of cystic artery, at least 1 cm, should be mobilized if possible. Again, it is safer to gain the desired length by extending the dissection laterally towards the gallbladder neck. Most commonly, the fully mobilized artery is doubly clipped proximally. Although it is an end artery, its distal end should also be clipped before division by hook scissors at a safe distance from the proximal double clipped end.

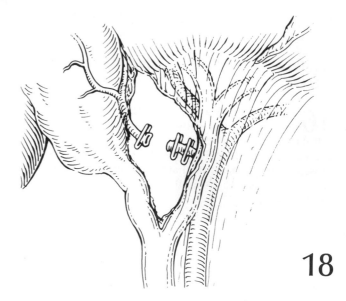

18

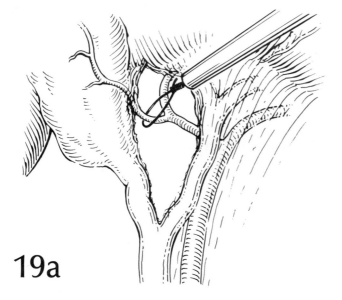

19a

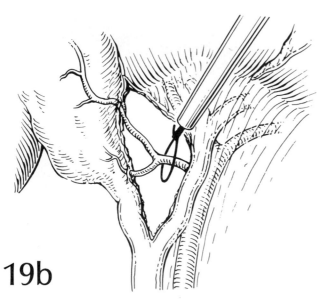

19b

19a,b Sufficient length of cystic artery for secure clipping may not be obtained when the artery divides early into anterior and posterior branches or when a short cystic artery arises from a looped right hepatic artery. In these situations, the safest technique is proximal ligature in continuity using 2/0 chromic catgut and a Roeder slip knot[4]. The distal end(s) may be secured by clipping.

Cholangiography

The need for operative cholangiography during laparoscopic cholecystectomy remains controversial. Some dispense with it altogether and others advocate a selective policy. The consensus view has changed in recent years in favour of routine intraoperative cholangiography for the following reasons:

1. Cholangiography provides a road map that identifies anomalies of the biliary tract which are especially relevant to safe ligature/clipping and division of the cystic duct.
2. Regular usage results in proficiency of cannulation of the cystic duct and in optimal interpretation of cholangiographic appearances. In this respect, the selective policy is counterproductive because the surgeon has difficulty in executing the procedure when he needs it most.
3. Cholangiography detects associated pathology including unsuspected stones.
4. Experience with and proficient use of intraoperative cholangiography is essential if a surgeon intends to progress to laparoscopic treatment of ductal calculi.

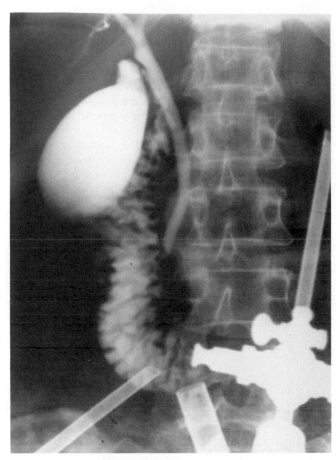

20a

20a,b Laparoscopic cholangiography can be performed either by injecting contrast medium into the gallbladder (cholecystocholangiogram) or into the cystic duct using a modern C-arm image intensifier to allow detailed fluoroscopy. This technique is far preferable to the use of portable X-ray machines with blind exposure of three films after successive injections of contrast medium[5]. Unless the cystic duct anatomy is grossly disturbed (e.g. suspicion of a Mirizzi syndrome), a cystic duct cholangiogram is usually preferred.

The gallbladder end of the cystic duct is clipped but not the medial end. A cut is made on the anterior wall of the cystic duct by fine pointed curved microscissors and deepened until the lumen is entered.

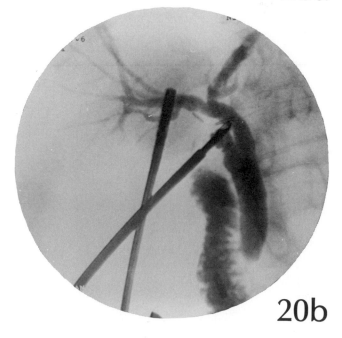

20b

21 Cannulation of the cystic duct (most commonly with a Cook ureteric catheter, 4–5 Fr) is considerably simplified by the use of a carrier device such as the cholangiograsper. The catheter is connected via a three-way tap to saline- and contrast-filled syringes (20 ml), and is inserted inside the cholangiograsper. The cholangiograsper loaded with the ureteric catheter is then introduced into the peritoneal cavity through the right upper port. With the jaws of the instrument open, the catheter is threaded inside the cystic duct. This step is greatly facilitated by steady injection of saline through the catheter to lift up the mucosal folds of the cystic duct.

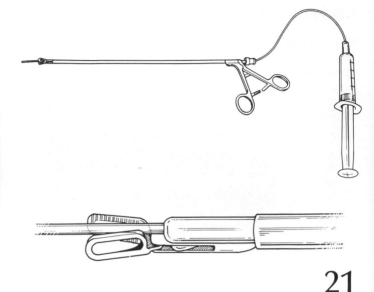

21

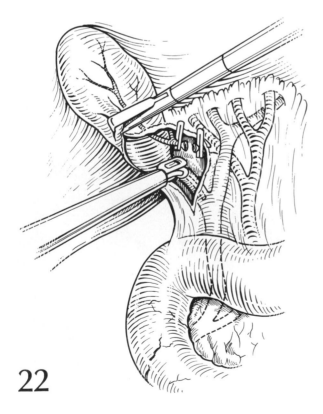

22

22 Once an adequate length is in place, the cholangiograsper is tilted medially and its jaws closed over the cystic duct and catheter. Contrast is injected slowly during image intensification to record the early phases of the duct filling.

On completion of the cholangiogram, the jaws are released, and the cholangiograsper and catheter are withdrawn. Fluorocholangiography performed in this manner should be completed within 10 minutes.

Closure and division of the cystic duct

Four techniques are available for securing the medial end of the cystic duct: (1) it can be clipped (metal or polydioxanone), (2) ligated in continuity, (3) secured by a preformed endoloop, or (4) closed by suture.

Medial clipping of the cystic duct

23 Most commonly, metal clips (titanium), usually double, are used although absorbable polydioxanone (Absolok, Ethicon) are preferred by some and do not carry the risk of stone formation. Both types of clip require specific applicators. It is important to apply the clips at right angles to the long axis of the duct and to ensure that the lateral wall of the common bile duct is not included in the clip. This problem may easily arise as upward and lateral displacement of the gallbladder often leads to tenting of the junction of the cystic and common bile duct. Although clipping of the cystic duct is the most popular method, this technique has certain disadvantages. In the first instance, clipping requires more duct length than ligature in continuity. Unless clips are applied at right angles to the axis of the duct, they are prone to slip and bile leakage postoperatively has a median reported incidence of 3%. Metal clips also may become internalized in the bile duct and form calculi.

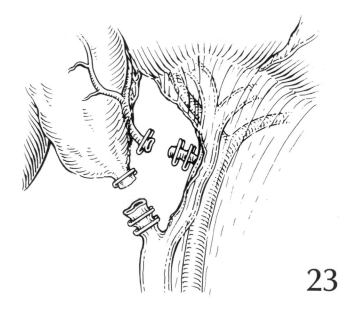

23

Medial ligature in continuity

24a–d This method involves ligature with an external Roeder slip knot after passing a 2/0 catgut around the cystic duct. The knot is fashioned externally and then slipped down and locked on the cystic duct close to the common bile duct. Dry chromic catgut (1.5 m in length) is best and is available commercially already mounted in a push rod. Alternatively, alcohol-packed material of suitable length is wiped clear of alcohol and left exposed on the sterile trolley to dry for at least 10 min. Ideally, this should be done by the scrub nurse at the start of the procedure.

The end of the catgut projecting beyond the bevelled tip of the push rod is grasped in a 3 mm needle holder and inserted inside a suture applicator passed through the left upper paramedian cannula. The end of the ligature is passed around the back of the cystic duct from above (*Illustration 24a*). The ligature is then grasped by the 5 mm needle holder (inserted through the right upper port) below the duct and transferred back to the 3 mm needle which is used to externalize the ligature (*Illustration 24b*). In order to prevent the ligature serrating the duct, closed forceps are inserted inside the loop to take up the tension (*Illustration 24c*). The Roeder knot is fashioned once the end of the ligature is exteriorized, and the knot is then slipped inside the abdomen by the push rod.

The resulting 'noose' is placed by the push rod a few millimetres medial to the opening of the cystic duct before it is locked tightly in place (*Illustration 24d*). The push rod is then withdrawn a few centimetres and the knot and its position on the duct are inspected.

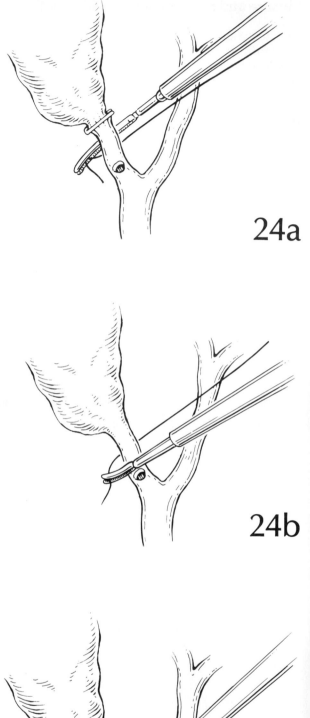

24a

24b

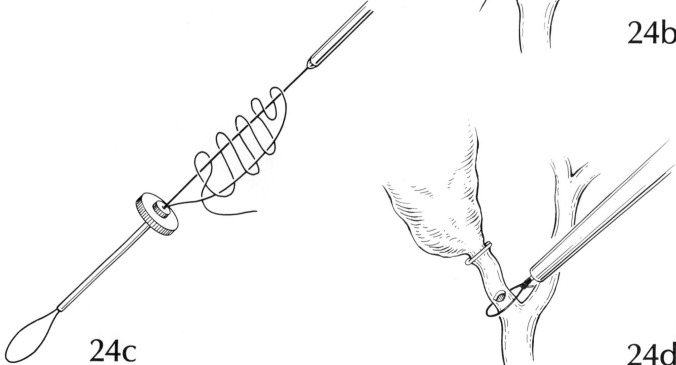

24c

24d

25 If considered satisfactory, the duct is then cut by claw scissors, and the excess suture, push rod and suture applicator are removed.

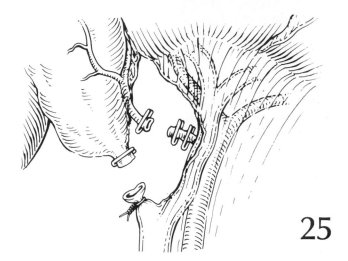

25

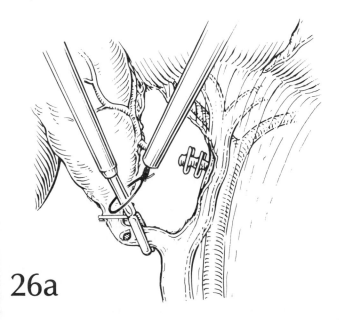

26a

Ligature by endoloop

26a,b An atraumatic grasper is passed through a preformed endoloop and used to grasp the cystic duct. The cystic duct is then divided just lateral to where it is grasped. The loop is threaded beyond the grasper, and the knot is tightened medial to the instrument before this is released.

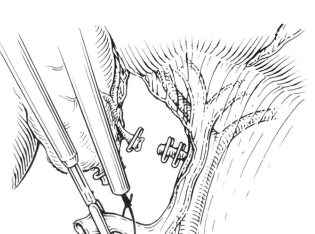

26b

27 After clipping and dividing the cystic duct, some surgeons apply an endoloop just medial to the proximal clip.

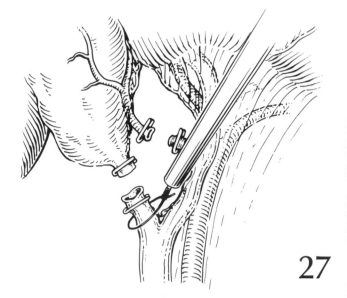

27

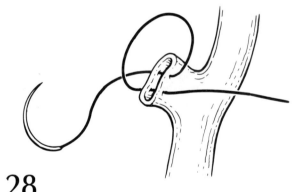

28

Suture closure of the cystic duct

28 This technique is necessary when the cystic duct is very short, and the opening is close to the common bile duct. A 3/0 catgut or synthetic absorbable atraumatic suture (Polysorb or coated Vicryl) is used to close the duct by a Z suture with intracorporeal knotting using a surgeon's knot. Closure and cutting of the cystic duct completes the detachment of the gallbladder from the structures of the porta hepatis.

Separation of the gallbladder from the liver bed

The plane of dissection is in the loose fibrous layer which separates the gallbladder from the subjacent fascia covering the liver bed. This plane is easy to find and follow in non-inflamed gallbladders, but can be difficult in cases with fibrous contracture. In any event, the dissection must not be carried through the superficial layers of the hepatic parenchyma as this causes excessive bleeding and may damage superficial bile ductules (including the ducts of Luschka) with the likelihood of postoperative bile leakage[6].

In non-fibrotic cases separation of the gallbladder from the liver can be carried out with electrosurgical, scissor or laser dissection.

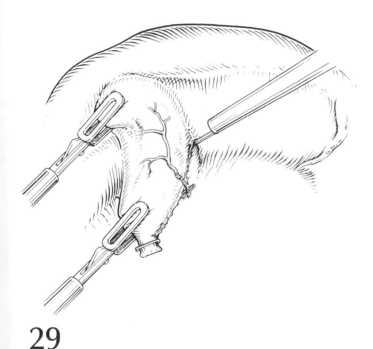

29 The detachment starts by separation of the gallbladder neck and infundibulum as the organ is held by an atraumatic grasper by the cut cystic duct. In non-adherent cases, this step should open up the loose areolar tissue plane between the gallbladder and the subjacent hepatic fascia. The gallbladder is held on the stretch by two grasping forceps, one on the fundus (assistant) and the other on the detached neck (surgeon's left hand). A pledget swab mounted on the appropriate laparoscopic holder is then used to separate, by blunt dissection, the undersurface of the gallbladder from the liver. This very efficient procedure mobilizes about 70% of the gallbladder in suitable cases and leaves only the lateral margins and the fundus still attached by their peritoneal reflections. These are then best divided by the electrosurgical hook.

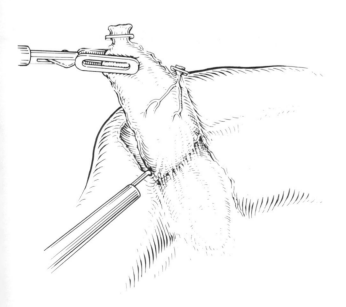

30 Following mobilization of the neck of the organ, the serosal lining on either side is divided with the electrosurgical hook-knife a few millimetres from the liver margin until the fundus is reached. Thereafter, with the gallbladder lifted upwards and held on the stretch in this position, the central dense fibrovascular attachments between the inferior surface of the gallbladder and the liver are divided with coagulation of any bleeding points. In these cases, particular attention is needed to ensure that the line of separation is not carried too deeply into the hepatic parenchyma. This problem should be suspected if excessive bleeding is encountered. Once separation of the gallbladder is complete, the fundus is grasped by the assistant until the organ is extracted.

31 When the fundal attachments are reached, reversal of the hold on the gallbladder facilitates the final separation. A grasper is placed on the fibrous tissue layer on the edge of the right lobe, just above the fundus, and used to elevate the liver as the gallbladder is allowed to hang down. It is steadied in this position by the other grasper held by the surgeon. The residual fundal attachments are then divided.

This technique is unsuitable for adherent contracted gallbladders or those which are deeply embedded in the liver substance.

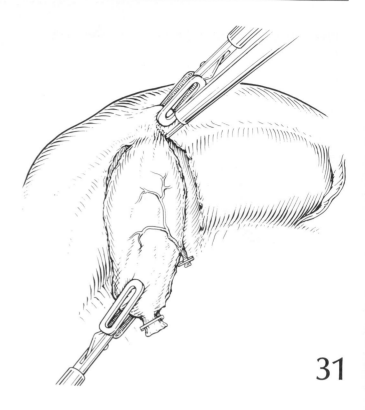

31

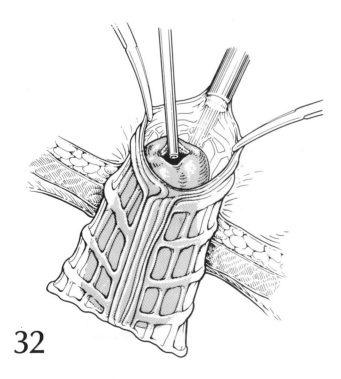

32

Extraction of the gallbladder

The gallbladder may be extracted through the left upper paramedian or umbilical incision. If the latter site is chosen, the telescope is removed from the umbilical port and reinserted through the left upper paramedian port.

32 Several instances of tumour implantation have now been reported in the exit wound in patients with unsuspected gallbladder cancer undergoing laparoscopic cholecystectomy for symptomatic gallstones[7]. For this reason, unprotected extraction is ill advised, and every gallbladder should be extracted inside a rip proof bag. Several types of bag are available, but the easiest to deploy is that marketed by Advanced Surgical which opens up following insufflation of its two constituent layers and, moreover, closes completely by means of a drawstring once the gallbladder is placed inside it.

A rip proof bag also solves the problem of extraction in the presence of a large stone load. When the neck is exteriorized, the bag is opened, and the edges are held up above the wound. The fluid contents of the gallbladder are aspirated through a small opening which is enlarged to crush and remove the stones by means of a Desjardin forceps. This technique has replaced all others, including ultrasonic or electromechanical rotary lithotripsy.

Inspection, suction/irrigation and haemostasis

Any clots are evacuated. The subhepatic region and the gallbladder bed are irrigated and sucked dry. Any bleeding points in the gallbladder fossa are electro-coagulated to ensure a dry operative field. The liver surface is closely inspected for any accidental stab wounds or minor lacerations. The suphrenic space and the right paracolic gutter are next irrigated and aspirated until the fluid is clear and any debris and clots have been evacuated. Finally, the rest of the peritoneal cavity including the pelvis is inspected. A subhepatic drain is not needed after routine laparoscopic cholecystectomy unless the dissection has proved difficult with oozing and some bile leakage, in which case a silicon subhepatic drain attached to a closed suction system is inserted.

Desufflation and removal of ports

It is important that the access cannulae are removed under vision to ensure that there is no abdominal wall bleeding from any of the wounds. Unless recognized and dealt with, this problem may result in significant postoperative morbidity. The desufflation of the pneumoperitoneum must be as complete as possible to reduce the amount of postoperative shoulder pain.

Suture of the stab wounds

The wounds are infiltrated with long acting local anaesthetic (bupivacaine) before closure. All 10 mm (or larger) wounds require closure of the aponeurotic layers because of the risk of hernia formation. Smaller wounds require superficial approximation only (sub-cuticular absorbable sutures or skin tapes).

Postoperative care

Following reversal of neuromuscular blackade and extubation, an oropharyngeal airway is inserted, and oxygen is administered by mask for the first 3 h. The patient is nursed on the side. Analgesia is administered as required. The majority of patients are ready for discharge the next day. Although day-case laparoscopic cholecystectomy is practised in some centres, this practice must be backed up with effective nursing care.

Acknowledgement

Illustrations 2 and *4* have been reproduced with permission from Cuschieri *et al* (ed.) *Laparoscopic Biliary Surgery*, 2nd edn, published by Blackwell Science Ltd, Oxford.

References

1. Dubois, F, Berthelot G, Levard H. Cholecystectomy by coelioscopy. *Presse Med* 1989; 18: 980–2.

2. Cuschieri A, Dubois F, Mouiel J *et al.* The European experience with laparoscopic cholecystectomy. *Am J Surg* 1991; 161: 385–7.

3. The Southern Surgeons Club. A prospective analysis of 1518 laparoscopic cholecystectomies. *N Engl J Med* 1991; 324: 1073–8.

4. Nathanson LK, Easter DW, Cuschieri A. Ligation of the structures of the cystic pedicle during laparoscopic cholecystectomy. *Am J Surg* 1991; 161: 350–4.

5. Cuschieri A, Shimi S, Banting S, Nathanson LK, Pietrabissa A. Intraoperative cholangiography during laparoscopic cholecystectomy. Routine versus selective policy. *Surg Endosc* 1994; 8: 302–5.

6. Deziel DJ, Millikan KW, Economou SG, Doolas A, Ko ST, Airan MC. Complications of laparoscopic cholecystectomy: a national survey of 4292 hospitals and an analysis of 77 604 cases. *Am J Surg* 1993; 165: 9–14.

7. Clair DG, Lautz DB, Brooks DC. Rapid development of umbilical metastases after laparoscopic cholecystectomy for unsuspected gallbladder carcinoma. *Surgery* 1993; 113: 355–8.

Illustrations by Gillian Oliver

Choledochoduodenostomy

R. C. G. Russell MS, FRCS
Consultant Surgeon, The Middlesex Hospital, London, UK

History

This operation was introduced in 1892 by Riedel, and since then has waxed and waned in popularity as a result of its potential for stenosis with consequent infection within the pancreatic portion of the bile duct. Its significant advantage now is that it provides access to the biliary tree for the endoscopist.

Principles and justification

Choledochoduodenostomy is indicated in the management of both benign and malignant disease, but only if the common bile duct is dilated to 12 mm or more. This operation should never be performed if the duct is small. For benign disease, the indications are now rare as the majority of common bile ducts can be cleared endoscopically or by combination with an operation. The only indication for stone disease is in elderly patients who do not have endoscopic access to the biliary tree because of a previous partial gastrectomy or a diverticulum at the ampulla of Vater which may make sphincterotomy difficult or dangerous. In the presence of stone disease and poor drainage a choledochoduodenostomy is ideal in the older person, but in the younger patient an end-to-side choledochojejunostomy is preferable.

In patients with oriental cholangitis or multiple intrahepatic stones, a choledochoduodenostomy can provide good drainage and direct access to the biliary tree for the endoscopist. However, it is rarely required as the percutaneous approach to the intrahepatic ducts is easier and more successful for clearing stones from the biliary tree, especially with the development of improved choledochoscopes.

The commonest indication for choledochoduodenostomy is malignant obstruction by pancreatic tumours. Provided the anastomosis is performed in the mid bile duct, recurrence of jaundice is rare (less than 10% in a series reported by Smith et al.[1]).

Preoperative

These patients are usually ill, infected and jaundiced, so they require careful preoperative preparation. Coagulation must be checked and corrected and vitamin K should be given. An intravenous infusion should be commenced the previous evening to ensure adequate hydration and a good urine output. The bladder is catheterized preoperatively. If the patient has malignant disease thrombolic prophylaxis with TED stockings and low-dose subcutaneous heparin should be instituted. Antibiotics are given as appropriate. It is presumed that endoscopy and, if malignancy is suspected, spiral computed tomographic scanning has defined the disease preoperatively and the operation plan is clear.

Operation

Incision

This is a minimally invasive procedure and thus the principles for such operations should be followed. A transverse 6-cm incision is adequate both to undertake a cholecystectomy and to perform the procedure, together with a gastrojejunostomy if required.

Exposure

The gallbladder is assessed as for a mini-cholecystectomy and removed both to increase exposure and prevent late sepsis subsequent to blockage of the cystic duct by tumour. The nature of the pathology is determined, and the preoperative findings are confirmed. To expose the bile duct and the duodenum the fascia which binds the hepatic flexure to the duodenum is divided to enable adequate exposure of the subhepatic space, the bile duct and duodenum. Mobilization of the duodenum is unnecessary. A stabilized ring retractor is used to facilitate the exposure.

Dissection

1 The cystic duct stump is followed to the bile duct, and the peritoneum over the bile duct is dissected to explore the wall of the duct and ensure that there is no tumour involvement. The first part of the duodenum is mobilized by dividing the branches of the right gastric artery and the adjacent peritoneum. These vessels are usually small and can be cauterized safely. This manoeuvre enables the first part of the duodenum to be brought up to the mid position of the bile duct without tension.

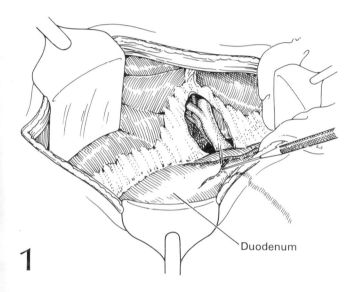

Duodenum

1

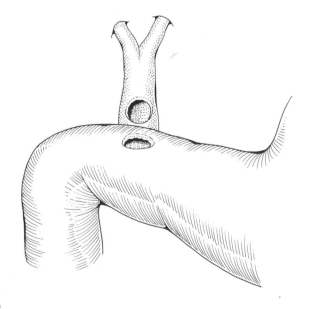

2

Formation of stoma

2 A disc of mid common bile duct, 1 cm in diameter, is removed from the anterior surface of the bile duct and a similar disc, 1 cm in diameter, is removed from the superior surface of the duodenum.

Anastomosis

3a–c The two holes are approximated and sutured with interrupted 3/0 polyglactin (Vicryl) or 4/0 polydioxanone (PDS) sutures incorporating all layers. It is easiest to start laterally and then to place the posterior suture. Sutures should be placed 3 mm apart and 3 mm deep to ensure an even closure. The sutures are tied after all the posterior layer has been completed. The anterior layer is then completed, and the sutures are tied at the end. An outer or covering layer is not necessary.

Closure

Meticulous haemostasis is ascertained, and the wound is closed without drainage as for a mini-cholecystectomy. Again, the muscle is infiltrated with 20–30 ml bupivicaine and adrenaline. The skin is closed with a subcuticular suture of 3/0 polydioxanone. A diclofenac suppository (100 mg) is given at the end of the procedure.

Postoperative care

These patients are ill and often have extensive malignant disease. They are thus prone to complications. Renal failure must be avoided by measurement of urine putput on an hourly basis, and appropriate action should be taken if the output falls below 30 ml/h. If there was evidence of biliary infection, appropriate antibiotics should be administered while the results of bile culture are awaited.

Oral fluids may be commenced the following day, and the intravenous infusion can be discontinued as soon as there is an adequate oral intake. Mobilization should start immediately, and care must be taken to avoid chest infection.

Outcome

For benign disease the morbidity should be less than 10% and the mortality below 1%, but for malignant disease the outcome is less good with a 30-day mortality of 15% and a significant morbidity of 30%. Unfortunately these patients are often regarded as having a terminal malignancy and do not receive the care they require, with the result that the ideal results achieved by some are not attained by many.

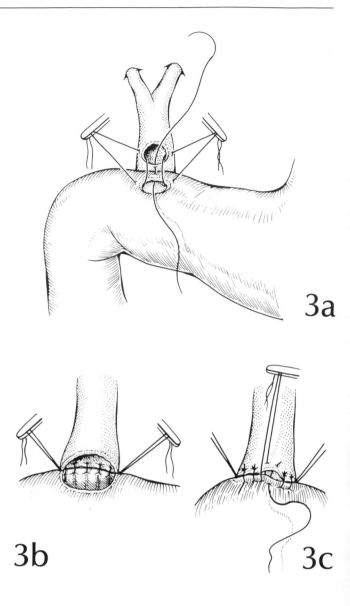

3a

3b

3c

References

1. Smith AC, Dowsett JF, Russell RC, Hatfield AR, Cotton PB. Randomised trial of endoscopic stenting versus surgical bypass in malignant low bile duct obstruction. *Lancet* 1994; 344: 1655–60.

Further reading

Bramhall SR, Allum WH, Jones AG, Allwood A, Cummins C, Neoptolemos JP. Treatment and survival in 13560 patients with pancreatic cancer, and incidence of the disease in the West Midlands: an epidemiological study. *Br J Surg* 1995; 82: 111–15.

Lillemoe KD, Sauter PK, Pitt HA, Yeo CJ, Cameron JL. Current status of surgical palliation of periampullary carcinoma. *Surg Gynecol Obstet* 1993; 176: 1–10.

Illustrations by Gillian Lee Illustrations

Bile duct cancer: resection

O. James Garden BSc, MD, FRCS(Ed), FRCS(Glas)
Senior Lecturer and Honorary Consultant Hepatobiliary Surgeon, University Department of Surgery and Scottish Liver Transplantation Unit, Royal Infirmary, Edinburgh, UK

Henri Bismuth MD, FACS, FRCS(Ed)
Professor of Surgery and Chairman of the Hepatobiliary Centre, Paul Brousse Hospital, Villejuif, France

Tumours involving the bile ducts pose a considerable challenge in biliary surgery. They may involve the ducts primarily or by extension from the liver, gallbladder, pancreas, the ampulla, duodenum or adjacent lymph nodes. Primary tumours of the biliary tract involving the gallbladder, ampulla and pancreas are dealt with elsewhere in this volume and this chapter is concerned only with cholangiocarcinoma involving the supraduodenal portion of the biliary tree up to and involving the confluence of the hepatic ducts. Early descriptions of bile duct tumours highlighted the difficulties of diagnosis and management given that these tumours characteristically invade locally with vascular, perineural and lymphatic involvement[1-3]. Subepithelial spread of tumour cells is of special importance in their management, and multiple lesions may arise from field change[4]. Although an increasingly aggressive approach to management has been advocated, only a minority of patients have potentially resectable disease at the time of presentation and 5-year survival following resection rarely exceeds 25%[5-7].

Principles and justification

Resection of the bile duct tumour has been shown to be the most effective way of achieving satisfactory long-term decompression of the biliary tree and clearly offers the only prospect of long-term survival. The pathological characteristics of this tumour and the absence of satisfactory imaging modalities to determine resectability may frustrate the surgeon, but mounting evidence now exists suggesting that resection can be undertaken with relatively low morbidity and mortality rates. Several studies have reported improved quality of life in patients who undergo tumour resection compared with those who have a biliary-enteric anastomosis[5,7]. The potential for improved quality of life and the long-term survival advantage require that patients who might benefit from resection be carefully identified.

The type of resection depends on the extent of the tumour within the biliary tree and its vascular involvement. For tumours that extend behind the duodenum to the pancreas, excision of the biliary tree with pancreaticoduodenectomy will be required. For lesions that extend into either the right or left duct, hepatic resection will be necessary. For the remaining tumours, wide excision of the entire supraduodenal biliary tree, cystic duct, gallbladder and related lymph nodes should be undertaken.

Preoperative

Confirmation of obstruction of the biliary tree will normally be achieved by abdominal ultrasonography. This investigation may localize accurately the level of obstruction, or this information can be inferred from the presence or absence of gallbladder distension. Advances in Doppler ultrasound imaging have enabled more accurate assessment of bile duct tumours, including the degree of vascular invasion. In many centres, endoscopic retrograde cholangiography will be undertaken to determine the nature of the obstruction, but this procedure rarely provides sufficient information about ductal involvement above the tumour. Percutaneous transhepatic cholangiography will overcome these deficiencies but, by introducing infection into the obstructed biliary tree, may compromise subsequent management if resection is not feasible.

1a–c Contrast enhanced computed tomographic (CT) scanning and nuclear magnetic resonance (NMR) imaging may allow detailed assessment of the biliary tree and tumour by non-invasive means. The CT scan shown in *Illustration 1a* demonstrates dilatation of the intrahepatic biliary tree which is more pronounced in the left hemiliver. A mass lesion is evident, predominantly involving the left hepatic duct and clearly obstructing the caudate ducts (arrowed). Long-standing obstruction above the confluence of the left and right hepatic ducts or associated vascular invasion may result in atrophy of one side of the liver. Selective hepatic arteriography with portal venous phase imaging is helpful in detecting vascular anomalies and tumour invasion. The mesenteric angiogram shown in *Illustration 1b* demonstrates an aberrant proper hepatic artery arising from the superior mesenteric artery. There is poor filling of the left hepatic artery, thought to be due to infiltration from a hilar cholangiocarcinoma which has been previously stented. The portovenous phase radiograph shown in *Illustration 1c* demonstrates tumour invasion of the left branch of the portal vein (arrowed).

These investigations indicate irresectability if there is: (1) multifocal or bilateral intrahepatic bile duct spread of tumour, (2) involvement of the portal vein, (3) bilateral invasion of the hepatic arterial and/or portal venous branches, or (4) evidence of unilateral vascular involvement with extensive contralateral invasion.

Although these criteria provide a useful guide to the radiologist and surgeon, it may be difficult to establish whether there is peritoneal dissemination of tumour, lymph node invasion or local extension into hepatic segment I. Laparoscopy and laparoscopic ultrasonography may be helpful in detecting such occult spread, but in the otherwise fit patient it may be more appropriate to contemplate operative decompression of the biliary tree rather than rely on endoscopic or percutaneous stent insertion. Furthermore, it should be borne in mind that submucosal, perineural and lymphatic spread of tumour may not be apparent before resection is attempted. Although frozen section biopsy of the bile duct may be used at the time of resection, it is unlikely that the surgeon would be able to undertake a more radical resection than that already being proposed.

Immediate preoperative assessment and preparation includes attention to the jaundiced patient's hydration and renal function, control of infection and assessment of coagulation status. The authors' practice is to undertake surgery under general anaesthesia with epidural blockade. Continuous monitoring is undertaken following placement of arterial, central venous pressure and urinary catheters.

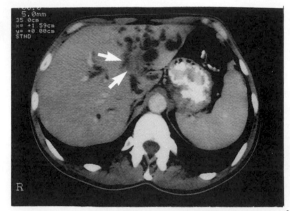

1a

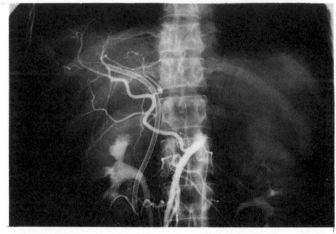

1b

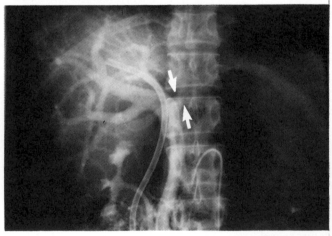

1c

Operation

2 The patient is positioned on the operating table with the right arm held beside the body by a folded towel and with the left arm extended. The abdomen is explored through a bilateral subcostal incision extended to the xiphisternum if necessary. Retraction of the costal margins is achieved by means of two large subcostal retractors secured by tapes to draped posts.

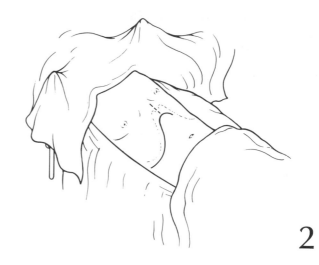

2

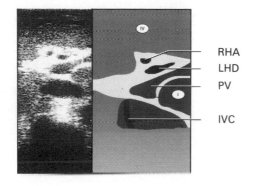

3a

RHA
LHD
PV

IVC

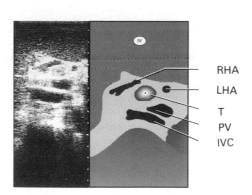

3b

RHA
LHA
T
PV
IVC

3a,b The peritoneal cavity is examined to exclude peritoneal tumour deposits and hepatic and nodal metastases. Intraoperative ultrasonography is undertaken to confirm the absence of hepatic dissemination of tumour and to assess the precise level of obstruction. Vascular anomalies and invasion can also be assessed in this way. The scan depicted shows the right hepatic artery (RHA) arching over a tumour involving the common hepatic duct just below the confluence of the right and left hepatic ducts (LHD). The left hepatic artery (LHA) is visible and the portal vein (PV) and inferior vena cava (IVC) are shown posteriorly. No evidence of vascular invasion is present.

Tumours at or below the hepatic confluence

Skeletonization of the biliary tree and lymphatics from the vessels is best achieved by commencing the dissection at the level of the first part of the duodenum. When preoperative investigations and operative assessment have confirmed that it is not necessary to sacrifice liver tissue, it is necessary to free the tumour above by taking down the gallbladder, lowering the hilar plate and freeing the base of the umbilical fissure.

The ligamentum teres is divided between ties, one of which is retained on the ligament to aid exposure of the hilus of the liver. The falciform ligament is divided with diathermy towards the vena cava, but the liver is not freed from its remaining peritoneal attachments.

4 With the liver retracted upwards and with the antrum of the stomach and first part of the duodenum displaced downwards, the peritoneum at the level of the first part of the duodenum is incised towards the free edge of the lesser omentum. In some patients it may be necessary to mobilize the second part of the duodenum and to free the hepatic flexure of the colon to gain adequate exposure behind the first part of the duodenum. Lymphatic and other vessels are divided (between ties or following diathermy) down to the common bile duct as it passes through or behind the head of the pancreas. A careful search is made for an accessory hepatic artery in the free edge of the lesser omentum as the dissection is carried posteroinferiorly to the exposed portal vein. Care should be taken to avoid damage to the pancreas at this level. The dissection is continued medially towards the gastroduodenal vessel which is skeletonized of its lymphatics as one moves towards the proper hepatic artery.

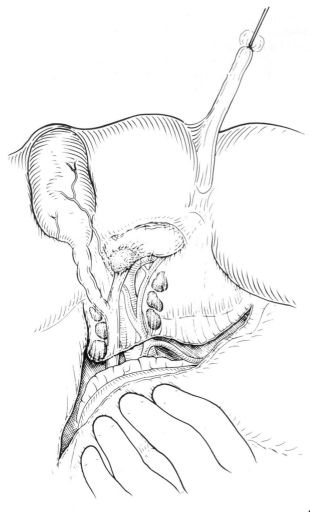

4

5 The common bile duct is freed from the underlying structures and secured above with a stout ligature, before being divided just above the pancreas. Bleeding from the two marginal arteries is controlled by suture ligation. The divided end of the bile duct is oversewn with continuous 4/0 polydioxanone (PDS). If the patient has previously been stented, to avoid delivering the intact stent through the divided duct it is transected with a pair of heavy scissors, delivering the lower end through the divided bile duct and displacing the upper end into the common bile duct, the lower end of which is ligated. In this way, contamination of the operating field by tumour cells is minimized.

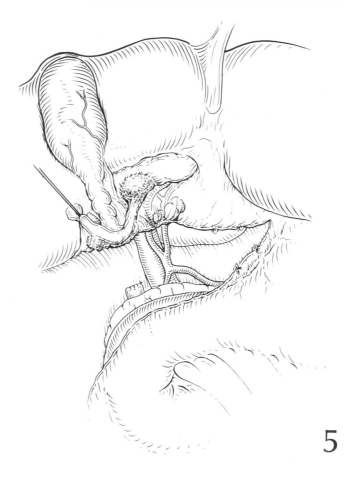

5

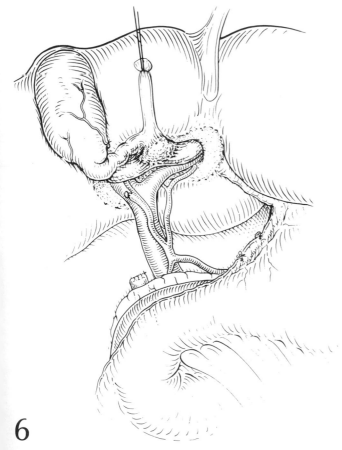

6 With the portal vein now exposed, the lymphatics can be cleared upwards and medially. The common and proper hepatic arteries are cleared of their associated lymph nodes as these are swept from the lesser omentum and upwards to the hilus of the liver.

6

7 The gallbladder is then dissected free from the liver using diathermy and retracted downwards to expose the cystic artery and the right branch of the portal vein behind. The cystic artery is divided between ties and this allows the lymphatics on the free edge of the lesser omentum to be swept from the right hepatic duct and right hepatic artery. The resected duct should now be entirely free of the skeletonized vessels posteriorly.

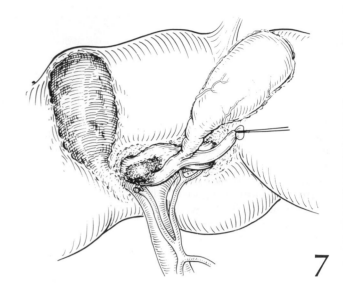

7

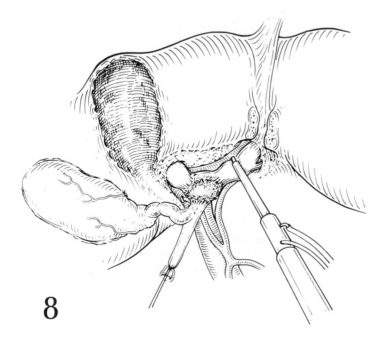

8

8 If a bridge of liver tissue is present between the quadrate and left lobes of the liver, its capsule is opened using diathermy coagulation. The Cavitron ultrasonic dissector can be used to skeletonize any intrahepatic vessels before they are coagulated and divided. By retracting the ligamentum teres upwards, the undersurface of the quadrate lobe of the liver is exposed. The peritoneum above the hepatic duct confluence is incised with diathermy and the hilar plate is lowered using the Cavitron dissector. In this way, the entire extrahepatic biliary tree and its associated lymphatics are freed from the portal vein and hepatic artery.

9 The left hepatic duct is divided as far proximally as possible, and the tumour and ductal confluence are displaced to the right to ascertain whether the main right hepatic duct can be divided or whether these should be divided at the level of the right sectoral ducts. A separate duct invariably drains the caudate lobe, and this and other adjacent ducts can be sutured together to create one or two separate orifices for anastomosis. The ducts should only be opposed without tension, and three or four interrupted 4/0 polydioxanone sutures will usually suffice.

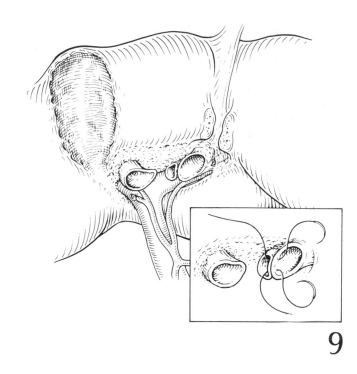

9

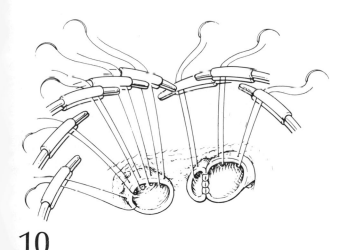

10

10 A 70-cm Roux-en-Y limb of jejunum is prepared, intestinal continuity being restored in two layers of continuous 3/0 polydioxanone sutures. The Roux-en-Y limb is delivered through the transverse mesocolon to which it is secured with several interrupted sutures. There should be no tension in the limb as it is drawn up to the hilus of the liver.

A hepaticojejunal anastomosis is undertaken in an end-to-side fashion between the ducts and the antimesenteric border of the jejunal limb. A conventional biliary anastomosis is undertaken, placing a single layer of 3/0 or 4/0 interrupted polydioxanone sutures into the anterior wall of the bile duct, passing the sutures from outside in. The needles are retained on shod clamps.

11 Although more than one biliary orifice may be present, it is preferable to undertake the anastomosis as if there was only one orifice. The anterior row of sutures is placed under tension and this enables precise placement of the posterior layer of sutures which are introduced from inside to outside on the jejunum and from outside to inside on the bile duct. The sutures are placed approximately 3 mm apart and secured with clamps. The jejunal limb is then 'rail-roaded' to the bile duct and the posterior layer of sutures is tied on the inside. The two corner sutures are retained on shod clamps while the others are cut.

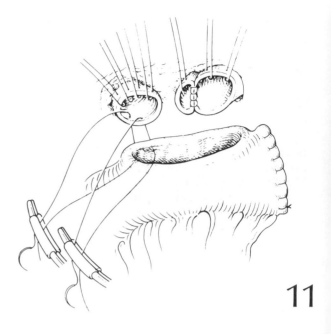

11

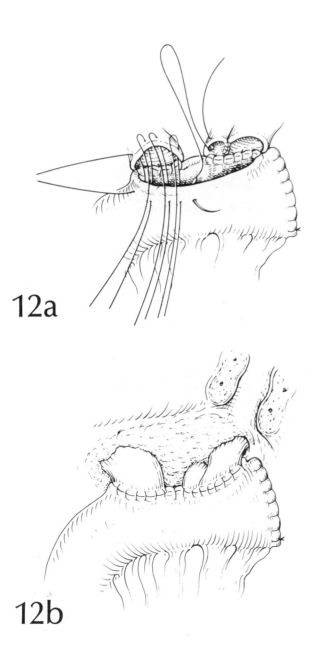

12a

12b

12a,b The anterior layer of anastomosis is now completed by passing the needles through the jejunal wall from the mucosal side outwards. Once the sutures have been placed, the stay sutures are cut and the anterior layer of sutures tied with the knots lying anteriorly. A transanastomotic stenting tube is not normally necessary.

Once haemostasis has been confirmed, a 24-Fr silicone tube drain is passed through a separate stab incision down to the anastomosis. The wound is closed in layers using looped polydioxanone to muscle and skin staples.

Excision of bile duct tumour and hepatic resection

For tumours which unilaterally invade the secondary biliary confluence or the vessels supplying one side of the liver, it is necessary to undertake a hepatic resection employing the techniques described above.

13 The initial dissection of the bile duct and tumour proceeds as described above. For a tumour predominantly affecting the left hepatic duct or vessels supplying the left liver, the left hepatic artery is divided between silk ligatures at its origin and swept upwards along with the adventitial and lymphatic tissue. In this way, the portal vein and its right and left branches are identified as they enter the liver. The left branch of the portal vein is secured between clamps at its origin. Care must be taken not to traumatize any caudate branches passing posteriorly, although the left hepatectomy will normally include excision of the caudate lobe.

The falciform and the left triangular ligaments are divided and the lesser omentum is freed from the lesser curve of the stomach. As the caudate lobe is freed from the vena cava, the line of demarcation between the left and right hemilivers will be evident.

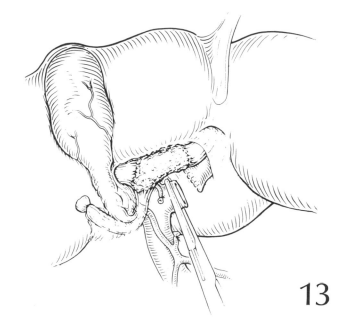

13

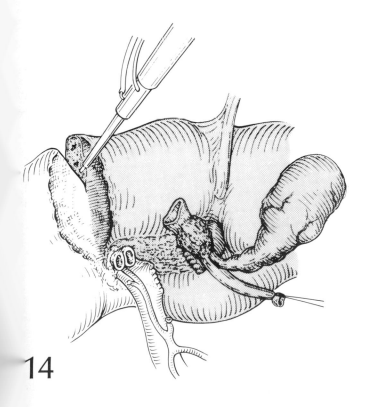

14

14 The right hepatic duct or sectoral ducts are divided well clear of the tumour, and the capsule of the liver is incised approximately 5 mm to the patient's left of the line of demarcation. The dissection into the liver is undertaken with the Cavitron dissector, skeletonizing small vessels and dividing these between ligatures. The middle hepatic vein is preserved on the right hemiliver as the dissection proceeds posteriorly and upwards. The vena cava is reached to the right of the caudate lobe.

The left hepatic vein is cleared and secured with a vascular clamp before being divided. Once the specimen is delivered from the wound, the left hepatic vein and left branch of the portal vein are oversewn using continuous 5/0 polypropylene (Prolene).

Haemostatis is secured and, if necessary, the anterior and posterior sectoral ducts are opposed with several interrupted polydioxanone sutures. The biliary anastomosis is fashioned to a 70-cm Roux-en-Y limb of jejunum as previously described.

Postoperative care and outcome

The principal source of morbidity following surgery in the jaundiced patient is the result of the development of hepatorenal failure and sepsis. A better understanding and use of prophylactic measures in the preoperative period have greatly reduced these risks. Preoperative biliary drainage remains a contentious issue and is addressed elsewhere. Peptic ulceration can develop in up to 5% of patients following Roux-en-Y hepatico-jejunostomy but, again, this risk is greatly minimized by the prophylactic administration of H_2 receptor antagonists. Most recent series report operative mortality rates of less than 5% with a 5-year survival of 5–20%.

References

1. Klatskin G. Adenocarcinoma of the hepatic duct at its bifurcation within the porta hepatis: an unusual tumour with distinctive clinical and pathological features. *Am J Med* 1965; 38: 241–56.

2. Altemeier WA, Gall EA, Culbertson WR, Inge WW Sclerosing carcinoma of the intrahepatic (hilar) bile ducts. *Surgery* 1966; 60: 191–200.

3. Longmire WP Jr, MacArthur MS, Bastounis EA, Hiatt J. Carcinoma of the extrahepatic biliary tract. *Ann Surg* 1973; 178: 333–45.

4. Gertsch P, Thomas P, Baer H, Lerut J, Zimmerman A, Blumgart LH. Multiple tumours of the biliary tract. *Am J Surg* 1990; 158: 386–8.

5. Baer HU, Stain SC, Dennison AR, Eggers B, Blumgart LH. Improvements in survival by aggressive resection of hilar cholangiocarcinoma. *Ann Surg* 1993; 217: 20–7.

6. Cameron JL, Pitt HA, Zinner MJ, Kaufman SL, Coleman J. Management of proximal cholangiocarcinomas by surgical resection and radiotherapy. *Am J Surg* 1990; 159: 91–8.

7. Guthrie CM, Haddock G, de Beaux AC, Garden OJ. Carter DC. Changing trends in the management of extrahepatic cholangiocarcinoma. *Br J Surg* 1993; 80: 1434–9.

Necrotizing pancreatitis

Hans G. Beger MD, FACS
Professor of Surgery, Chairman and Head of the Department of General Surgery, University of Ulm, Ulm, Germany

Michael H. Schoenberg MD
Department of General Surgery, University of Ulm, Ulm, Germany

Principles and justification

Natural course of acute pancreatitis

In most patients acute pancreatitis takes the course of an oedematous interstitial inflammation, characterized by periacinar and interstitial oedema. Mild acute pancreatitis generally causes low morbidity and conservative treatment results in a rapid improvement of symptoms with a complete cure in a matter of weeks (*Table 1*). In 10–20% of patients a necrotizing acute pancreatitis develops, identified morphologically by acute inflammation of the tissue with necrosis of the exocrine and endocrine pancreatic parenchyma and fatty tissue in and around the pancreas; moderate to severe clinical symptoms develop as a result of local and systemic complications. Bacterial contamination of the pancreatic and retroperitoneal necrotic tissue occurs in about 40% of patients with necrotizing pancreatitis. The subgroup of patients with infected necrosis may develop multisystem organ failure caused by vasoactive and toxic substances released from the pancreatic, peripancreatic and retroperitoneal inflammatory tissue. After the acute phase of the disease, a pancreatic abscess may develop in the third to sixth week as a result of bacteria within the inflamed, often necrotic, tissue. This abscess is liquified and surrounded by a fibrous wall which then forms a pseudocapsule. Pancreatic abscess and infected pancreatic necrosis are two different entities according to morphological, clinical, and laboratory criteria because, in patients with a pancreatic abscess, signs and symptoms of acute pancreatitis have generally subsided when pain, fever and leucocytosis reappear. Pseudocyst after acute pancreatitis represents either collections of peripancreatic fluid with or without connection to the pancreatic duct system. These fluid collections are surrounded by a capsule of fibrous tissue. An infected pseudocyst leads to clinical symptoms that are identical to those of a pancreatic abscess (*Table 2*).

Table 1 Classification of acute pancreatitis based on clinical, morphological, radiological and bacteriological criteria

	Frequency (%)
Interstitial oedematous pancreatitis	75
Necrotizing pancreatitis	
Sterile necrosis (60%)	10–20
Infected necrosis (40%)	
Pancreatic abscess	3
Pseudocyst after acute pancreatitis	5–7

Table 2 Incidence of infection in acute pancreatitis

	Necrotizing pancreatitis (%)	Acute pancreatitis (%)
Infected necrosis	30–40	5–8
Pancreatic abscess	~5	2
Infected pseudocyst	<2	<0.5
Total	35–45	7–10

Preoperative staging of the severity of the disease

Clinical management of patients with necrotizing pancreatitis should be based on clinical and radiological criteria and on bacteriological investigations. To evaluate the prognosis of patients with acute pancreatitis within 48 h after admission the Ranson criteria are the most widely accepted. However, the important clinical decision during the course of acute pancreatitis is related to the identification of patients suffering from interstitial oedematous or necrotizing pancreatitis; accurate identification is achieved by the use of biochemical data and computed tomographic (CT) scans. C reactive protein, lactate dehydrogenase and phospholipase A_2 are highly sensitive biochemical markers of occurrence of a necrotizing process during the course of acute pancreatitis (*Table 3*). Ultrasonography is much less useful in the staging of the severity of acute pancreatitis because of a low sensitivity for pancreatic and retroperitoneal necrosis.

Table 3   Criteria for diagnosis of a necrotizing pancreatitis

	Cut-off point	Detection rate (%)
C reactive protein	> 150 mg/l	93
Lactate dehydrogenase	> 5 U/l	87
Phospholipase A_2	> 5 U/l	84
Dynamic contrast CT scans	Non-perfused area	88

Medical management of necrotizing pancreatitis

The primary treatment for all patients with necrotizing pancreatitis ought to be conservative. Medical treatment follows the generally accepted guidelines of analgesia, maintenance of parenteral volume, energy supply and interruption of pancreatic secretion. Decompression of the stomach with a tube is important as is bladder drainage. Medical treatment with atropine, glucagon, calcitonin, somatostatin and the enzyme inhibitor aprotinin has not found general approval after controlled clinical studies failed to confirm their value. The use of albumin is essential in most patients for adequate volume replacement. An arterial oxygen pressure below 60 mmHg indicates the need for supplemental nasal oxygen or mechanical ventilation. Antibiotics should be used in patients with necrotizing pancreatitis, with imipenem or mezlocillin being the most effective drugs against the Gram-positive and Gram-negative bacteria found in pancreatic necrotic tissue. Intensive medical therapy is mandatory for patients with necrotizing pancreatitis.

Surgical treatment of necrotizing pancreatitis

Surgical treatment of necrotizing pancreatitis is based on the experience that patients who do not undergo surgery have a mortality rate exceeding 60% despite maximum intensive care treatment. The surgical treatment of necrotizing pancreatitis is indicated in patients who develop signs of an acute surgical abdomen, suffer from shock, sepsis or organ failure (*Table 4*). Persisting organ failure, such as pulmonary insufficiency, renal insufficiency and gastrointestinal bleeding, or severe metabolic insufficiency are criteria for surgical treatment if these complications persist or deteriorate in spite of maximum intensive care treatment. Patients who develop infected necrosis, based on ultrasound or CT-guided fine-needle puncture, are candidates for surgical treatment.

In patients suffering from a sterile pancreatic necrosis, surgical management has not been proved by controlled trials to be superior to non-surgical management. Sterile pancreatic necroses are therefore not an indication for surgical management.

Surgical treatment of necrotizing pancreatitis involves removal of devitalized tissue from the pancreas and retroperitoneal fatty tissue spaces and evacuation of fluid collections containing vasoactive and toxic substances and bacteria. Careful surgical treatment of pancreatic necrosis preserves functional pancreatic tissue between or below areas of devitalized tissue to minimize late functional impairment.

Table 4   Criteria for surgical treatment of necrotizing pancreatitis

Surgical acute abdomen
Sepsis persisting > 48 h
Shock
Severe local and/or persisting systemic complications:
   in spite of maximum intensive care treatment
   increasing pulmonary insufficiency
   persisting renal insufficiency
   infected necrosis
Severe local bleeding
Increasing adynamic ileus
Stenosis of gastrointestinal tract segments causing ileus

An algorithm which may be used to decide the best method of treatment is shown in *Figure 1*.

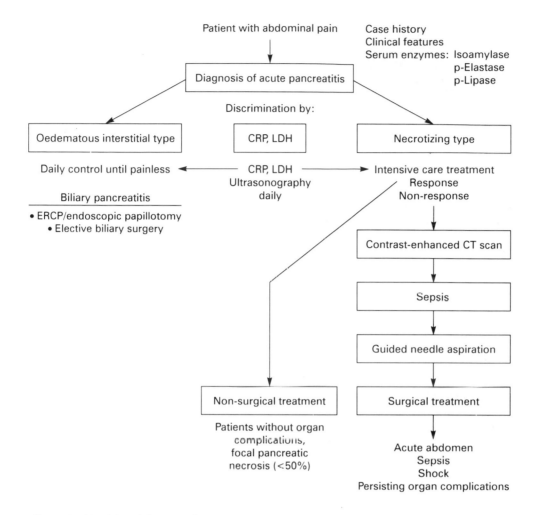

Figure 1   Algorithm defining pathways in acute pancreatitis. CRP, C-reactive protein; LDH, lactate dehydrogenase; ERCP, endoscopic retrograde cholangiopancreatography.

Operations

Surgical debridement and local lavage

An upper abdominal midline incision is used; in cases with body and tail necrosis and retroperitoneal necrosis, an upper abdominal transverse incision might be advantageous. After entering the lesser sac, devitalized haemorrhagic tissue is easily identified. Necrosectomy or debridement means dissection without a knife. A combination of necrosis debridement with the finger and intraoperative and postoperative local lavage of the lesser sac provides an atraumatic and continuous evacuation of devitalized tissue as well as removal of bacterially contaminated dead tissue and biologically active substances.

In order to preserve macroscopically normal tissue any *en bloc* resection should be avoided. Surgical haemostasis of bleeding vessels is of major importance for the patient's survival.

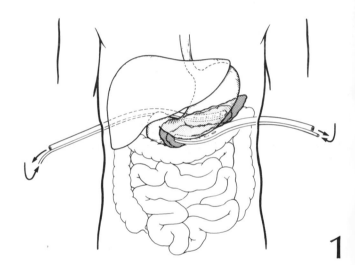

1   For postoperative continuous local lavage of the area of necrotic cavities, at least two large double lumen silicon rubber tubes are inserted (28–34 Fr). In cases of large extrapancreatic retroperitoneal necrosis, additional tubes are placed as required for complete evacuation of devitalized tissue and exudate. The gastrocolic and duodenocolic ligaments are used to create a closed retroperitoneal lesser sac lavage cavity.

The advantage of local lavage of the lesser sac and the cavities containing necrotic tissue is the atraumatic continuous removal of devitalized tissue in the weeks after the operation with removal of bacteria. The rate of flow of the lavage fluid in the first 48 h is 1–2 l/h of a continuous ambulatory peritoneal dialysis solution through the lesser sac to cleanse mechanically the inflamed areas and provide an antipyretic effect.

It is generally found that the inflammatory process after debridement continues to be active up to the second or third week of the disease. Short-term continuous local lavage for the first five postoperative days has many advantages. The criteria for discontinuing lavage are absence of any sign of acute pancreatitis and complete cleansing of the cavity confirmed by measuring endotoxins and enzymes and assessing the amount of bacteria in the lavage fluid.

It is well documented that surgical debridement and local lavage, even in the first 2–5 postoperative days, reduces the severity of the disease immediately in terms of an improvement of pulmonary function and of the Apache II scoring system.

The frequency of reoperation is 25–35%, mainly due to persistent sepsis; other causes of reoperation are massive diffuse local bleeding and appearance of progressive necrosis or development of a colonic fistula leading to an intra-abdominal abscess. Pancreatic fistulas are observed in about 10% of patients after surgical debridement, but usually close spontaneously. The occurrence of local complications is proportional to the extent of intraperitoneal and retroperitoneal parenchymal necrosis. The overall time spent in hospital by surviving patients is about 60 days; this length of stay is almost always related to uncontrollable local and systemic sepsis. Hospital mortality after surgical debridement and local lavage is between 10% and 20%.

Open packing

The use of open packing with multiple redressing reduces the risk of life-threatening complications caused by prolonged inflammation, even after surgery. An open abdomen with multiple redressing tends to remove the necrosis and can be carried out in combination with intraoperative lavage. However, multiple redressing entails many reoperations and a prolonged phase of intensive care; intestinal fistula, stomach outlet syndrome, mechanical ileus and incisional hernias as well as severe local bleeding into cavities are not infrequent complications of the technique. Hospital mortality after open packing is similar to that following debridement and local lavage.

Surgical treatment of pancreatic abscess

Pus collection in the area of the pancreas or in peripancreatic retroperitoneal spaces may occur after acute pancreatitis. Treatment with interventional ultrasound-guided drainage is the first choice. Drainage in connection with local lavage of the abscess cavity interrupts the septic reaction. A transabdominal surgical procedure is indicated if ultrasound-guided drainage of pancreatic abscess fails to interrupt the sepsis syndrome. A small incision in the upper abdomen is

Table 5 Principles of surgical management of acute pancreatitis

	Treatment
Interstitial oedematous pancreatitis	Non-surgical*
Necrotizing pancreatitis	
Sterile necrosis	Non-surgical; surgery if no response to ICU treatment
Infected necrosis	Surgical debridement
Pancreatic abscess	Interventional drainage; surgical drainage in cases of persisting sepsis
Postacute pseudocyst	Interventional drainage; surgical drainage is second choice

*Except biliary tract surgery in biliary pancreatitis.

mandatory to maintain direct access to the abscess cavity.

The principles of the surgical management of acute pancreatitis are shown in *Table 5*.

Further reading

Beger HG, Bittner R, Block S, Büchler M. Bacterial contamination of pancreatic necrosis: a prospective clinical study. *Gastroenterology* 1986; 91: 433–8.

Beger HG, Bittner R, Büchler M, Hess W, Schmitz JE. Hemodynamic data pattern in patients with acute pancreatitis. *Gastroenterology* 1986; 90: 74–9.

Beger HG, Krautzberger W, Bittner R, Block S, Büchler M. Results of surgical treatment of necrotizing pancreatitis. *World J Surg* 1985; 9: 972–9.

Beger HG, Büchler M, Bittner R, Block S, Nevalainen T, Roscher R. Necrosectomy and postoperative local lavage in necrotizing pancreatitis. *Br J Surg* 1988; 75: 207–12.

Beger HG, Büchler M, Bittner R, Oettinger W, Block S, Nevalainen T. Necrosectomy and postoperative local lavage in patients with necrotizing pancreatitis: results of a prospective clinical trial. *World J Surg* 1988; 12: 255–62.

Bittner R, Block S, Büchler M, Beger H. Pancreatic abscess and infected pancreatic necrosis: different local septic complications in acute pancreatitis. *Dig Dis Sci* 1987; 32: 1082–7.

Ranson JH, Rifkind KM, Roses DF, Fink SD, Eng K, Localio SA. Objective early identification of severe acute pancreatitis. *Am J Gastroenterol* 1974; 61: 443–51.

Warshaw AL, Richter JM. A practical guide to pancreatitis. *Curr Probl Surg* 1984; 21: 1–79.

Illustrations by Gillian Lee Illustrations

Drainage procedures in chronic pancreatitis

David C. Carter MD, FRCS(Ed), FRCS(Glas), FRCS, FRSE
Regius Professor of Clinical Surgery, Royal Infirmary, Edinburgh, UK

Kelvin R. Palmer MD, FRCP(Ed)
Consultant Physician, Western General Hospital, Edinburgh, UK

Principles and justification

Drainage operations in chronic pancreatitis have been based on the premise that relief of ductal obstruction and distension would relieve pain and might at least arrest the decline in pancreatic endocrine and exocrine function associated with the disease. However, there is an extremely variable relationship between duct size, histological evidence of pancreatitis, ductal pressure and pain, and the explanation for the relief afforded to the majority of patients by pancreaticojejunostomy remains uncertain.

1 Early attempts at pancreatic drainage such as the DuVal procedure involved retrograde drainage of the gland into a Roux loop of jejunum after amputation of the tail of the pancreas and splenectomy. It was soon appreciated that pain relief was short-lived and that more extensive pancreatic drainage was needed to deal with multiple duct strictures and ensure long-term patency of the pancreaticojejunal anastomosis.

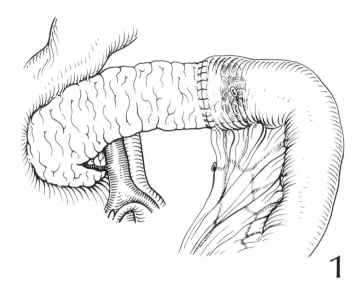

1

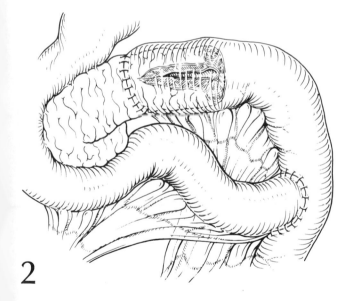

2

2 In the Puestow and Gillespie operation, the pancreatic duct was derooted from the tail to the neck of the pancreas, and the body and tail were then implanted into a Roux loop.

In the modern operation developed by Partington and Rochelle, a side-to-side anastomosis is created between the opened pancreatic duct and the side of a Roux loop of jejunum, the tip of the pancreas is not amputated, and the spleen is not removed. In the Partington–Rochelle operation the opened jejunum was simply sutured to the pancreatic capsule, whereas emphasis is now often placed on creating a mucosa-to-mucosa anastomosis between the duct and the jejunum. Alternative methods of duct drainage include the endoscopic insertion of stents to overcome obstruction of the pancreatic duct in the head of the gland (*see* page 474) and surgical drainage of the pancreatic duct into the back of the stomach (pancreaticogastrostomy) rather than the jejunum. Although pancreaticogastrostomy has advocates, the window created is small and most surgeons still regard pancreaticojejunostomy as the drainage operation of choice.

Preoperative

The diagnosis of chronic pancreatitis is not in itself an indication for operation as many patients can be managed conservatively. Pain which cannot be controlled by medical means is usually the cardinal indication for elective surgery and, as will be discussed, additional factors favouring surgical intervention are the presence of a pseudocyst (common), biliary tract obstruction (less common) and duodenal obstruction (rare). Most surgeons consider that pancreaticojejunostomy should only be performed if the pancreatic duct system is distended to a diameter of more than 7–8 mm (normal 2–4 mm), and the operation is easiest in patients with greatly distended ducts. On the other hand, there have been recent suggestions that duct distention is not the crucial determinant and that incising the chronically inflamed pancreas down to a non-distended duct may still allow pain relief, possibly by serving as a permanent 'fasciotomy' when the opened gland is anastomosed to the jejunum.

Ultrasonography and/or computed tomography can provide useful information about the pancreas and its duct system, the liver and biliary tree, and neighbouring vascular structures such as the splenic vein. It is now appreciated that splenic vein thrombosis is a not infrequent complication of chronic pancreatitis and the surgeon is best to be forewarned about the presence of large varices and splenomegaly.

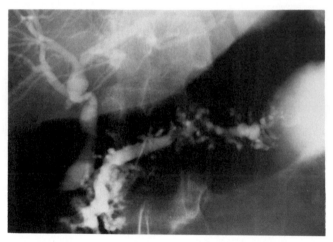

3

3   Endoscopic retrograde cholangiopancreatography (ERCP) provides the most valuable information about pancreatic duct size, presence of strictures and calculi, communicating pseudocysts, and biliary tract morphology. If a pancreatogram cannot be obtained endoscopically, percutaneous antegrade pancreatography is possible in skilled hands under ultrasound guidance or a pancreatogram can be obtained by direct puncture of the duct at operation. Intraoperative ultrasonography now offers an alternative means of defining pancreatic morphology, including duct morphology, if a pancreatogram has not been obtained before operation.

It must always be borne in mind that pancreatic cancer may be difficult clinically and at operation to distinguish from chronic pancreatitis, and operative biopsy may not always detect underlying malignancy. Calcification does not exclude cancer, the two conditions frequently coexist, and there is now some evidence that chronic pancreatitis is potentially a premalignant condition. Particular suspicion should be aroused if there is an isolated stricture of the pancreatic duct or a 'double duct sign' at ERCP with neighbouring strictures of the common bile duct and main pancreatic duct. Anxieties about malignancy are particularly important when pancreaticojejunostomy is being contemplated for chronic pancreatitis, given that the gland is left *in situ*, and most large series of patients treated by pancreaticojejunostomy include individuals in whom pancreatic cancer was overlooked at the time of surgery or developed subsequently. At the same time, the fact that pancreaticojejunostomy conserves the gland may avoid or defer the critical deterioration in pancreatic exocrine and endocrine function which is commonly precipitated by pancreatic resection in this disease.

Operations

PANCREATICOJEJUNOSTOMY

Pancreaticojejunostomy is carried out under general anaesthesia with the patient positioned supine and flat on the operating table. The availability of intraoperative ultrasonography means that intraoperative radiography can now be avoided. Although the operation can be performed through a vertical incision, a transverse or bilateral subcostal incision gives optimal exposure and can be reused if pancreatic resection is required subsequently.

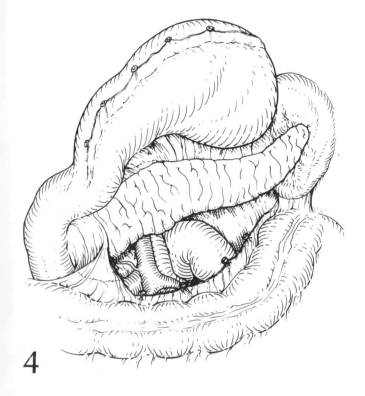

4

4 The lesser sac is opened widely by dividing the gastrocolic ligament between ligatures. The entire anterior surface of the pancreas must be exposed so that a large window is created which extends from the short gastric vessels on the left to divide the origin of the gastroepiploic vein on the right as it passes down to join the superior mesenteric vein just beneath the neck of the pancreas. It is also important to expose the front of the head of the pancreas and uncinate process by dividing the connective tissue which tethers the transverse mesocolon to the gland. It is safer and easier to begin this part of the dissection by dividing the tissue between the transverse mesocolon and the third part of the duodenum so that the superior mesenteric vein can be seen and safeguarded during the rest of the dissection. Avascular adhesions between the posterior aspect of the stomach and the front of the pancreas are divided fully with dissecting scissors to expose the front of the body and tail of the pancreas.

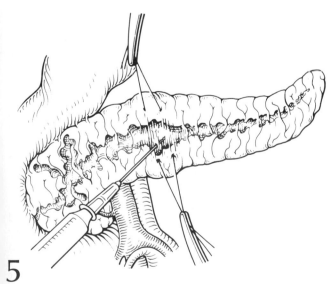

5

5 The pancreatic duct may be palpable when it is grossly distended and it is then a simple undertaking to enter it by a small longitudinal incision in the anterior aspect of the body of the gland. It is often helpful to locate the duct by needle puncture and a pair of stay sutures are then inserted above and below it at a convenient point in the body of the gland. The parenchyma is incised longitudinally between the stay sutures.

In patients with smaller ducts it is easy to pass above or below the duct and care must be taken not to cut through the entire thickness of the pancreas and enter the underlying splenic vein. Further needle puncture may be helpful in such cases and, if entry is still not achieved, a small transverse incision will locate the duct.

Once the duct has been opened a specimen of fluid is sent for cytological examination and a piece of parenchymal tissue is incised from the edge of the opened pancreas for histological examination. Some surgeons routinely measure intraduct pressure by inserting a needle attached to a manometer before incising the duct, while others insert a fine needle into the parenchyma to measure interstitial pressure.

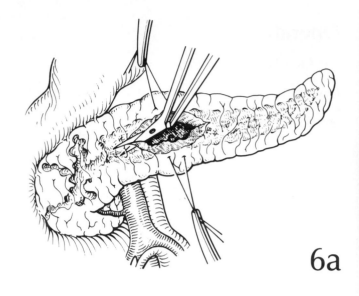

6a

6a, b The pancreatic duct system is then incised widely along its entire length and any calculi are picked out. The length of this incision is critical to the long-term success of the operation, and it must extend from just within the anterior pancreatico-duodenal arcade on the right to the tail of the pancreas on the left. Extensions may be necessary to deroof the accessory pancreatic duct and significant branches of the duct system in the uncinate process must be opened.

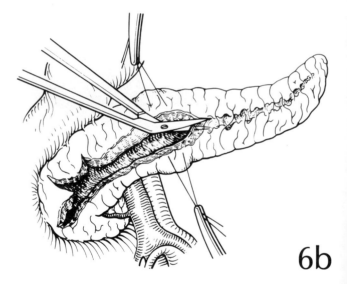

6b

7 In the operation described by Frey, the conventional operation of pancreaticojejunostomy is augmented by excising pancreatic tissue from the front of the head of the pancreas and uncinate process so that the entire duct system is laid fully open.

Dissecting scissors may be suitable for opening the duct but if there is calcification it is better to tent its anterior wall between stay sutures or the jaws of artery forceps and incise the pancreas with a scalpel.

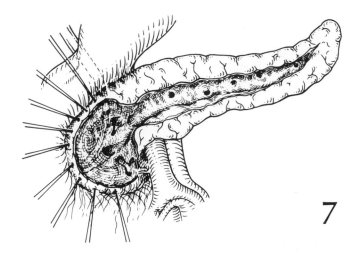

7

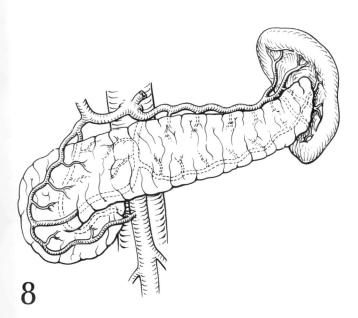

8

8 The arterial circulation is normally so disposed that there are no major vessels running on the anterior surface of the pancreas until the pancreaticoduodenal arcade is reached.

Occasionally the gastroduodenal artery gives off a significant branch to the transverse colon but this can usually be sacrificed with impunity given the collateral supply. If there is any doubt, the vessel can be occluded temporarily with a bulldog clamp while the mesocolon and greater omentum are inspected for pulsation. Bleeding points encountered while the duct system is being opened are best dealt with by suture-ligation and excessive diathermy should be avoided.

9a, b A Roux loop of jejunum is now prepared, dividing the arterial arcade, mesentery and jejunum at a convenient point in the proximal small bowel. A linear stapler allows the jejunum to be divided quickly, but the staple line is not haemostatic and it is advisable to oversew the transected distal staple line with a continuous 3/0 resorbable suture of polydioxanone (PDS). A window is now created in the transverse mesocolon and the distal end of the jejunum is passed through into the lesser sac.

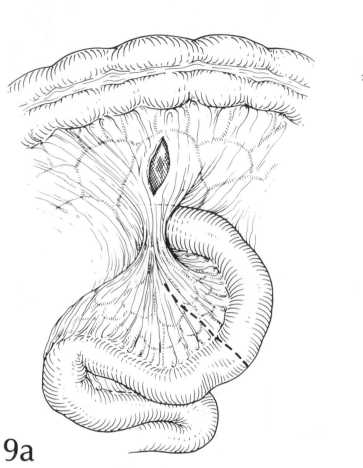

9a

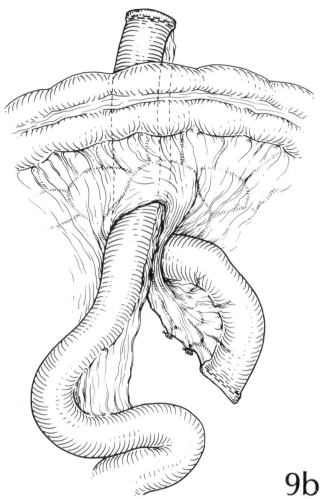

9b

10 The Roux loop is orientated so that its blind end is placed on the tail of the pancreas. This is usually the most 'comfortable' way for the jejunum to lie, and has the added advantage that more jejunum can be brought through the window in the mesocolon if biliary bypass is also needed.

Some surgeons have used 'triple bypass' in which the jejunal loop is used for anastomosis to the pancreas, biliary system and stomach. In the authors' view, patients who might be considered for triple bypass usually have such severe disease in the head of the pancreas that they are better served by resection of the head of the pancreas with formal restoration of pancreatico-enteric, biliary-enteric and gastro-enteric continuity. In patients with a communicating pseudocyst, the Roux loop can be used to drain the pseudocyst as well as the pancreatic duct.

Classical descriptions of longitudinal side-to-side pancreaticojejunostomy usually employed two layers of sutures for the anastomosis, but one layer of interrupted 2/0 or 3/0 delayed resorbable sutures is sufficient.

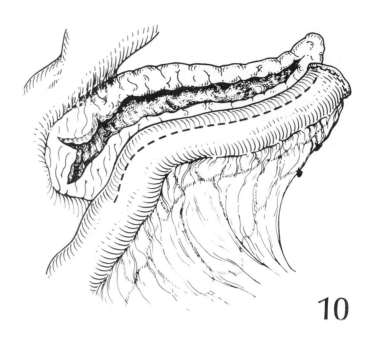

10

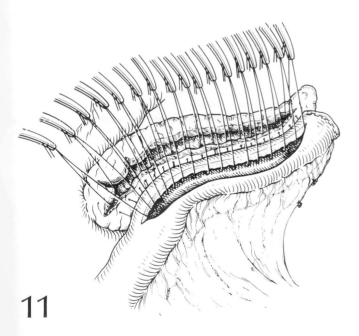

11

11 The jejunum is incised longitudinally along its antimesenteric border over a length equal to that of the pancreatic incision. The interrupted sutures are first inserted to create the inferior border of the anastomosis and it is often simpler to insert the entire layer before beginning to tie them. The sutures pick up the entire thickness of the jejunum and are inserted so that the knots will be on the inside of the anastomosis.

One school of thought holds that the pancreatic sutures should not be inserted so that they pass into the lumen in case they occlude side branches of the pancreatic duct system. However, the authors' usual practice is to create a mucosa-to-mucosa anastomosis, taking care not to occlude obvious side branches of the duct during suture insertion. The pancreatic tissue in chronic pancreatitis is usually much more fibrous than normal and is not friable. Once the sutures forming the inferior margin of the anastomosis have all been inserted and tied, they are cut short, retaining the two end sutures as stays.

12 The superior margin of the anastomosis is then performed, the sutures being inserted so that the knots are on the outside of this part of the anastomosis. It is good practice to insert the corner sutures first and to tie and retain them so that the stay sutures retained at the ends of the inferior margin can be cut. Once again it is usually easiest to insert all of the sutures and then to tie them, rather than tie each suture once it has been inserted.

Access is usually good but, on occasions, it is simpler to insert the superior row of sutures into the upper margin of the pancreatic incision, retaining their needles before commencing the inferior margin of the anastomosis. If this manoeuvre is adopted, the superior margin of the anastomosis is completed by picking up the jejunum as the final step.

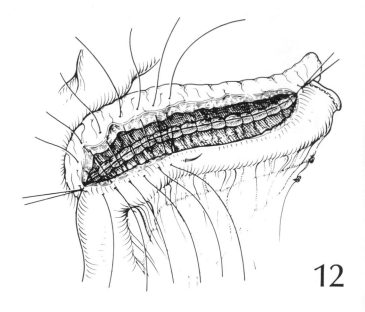

12

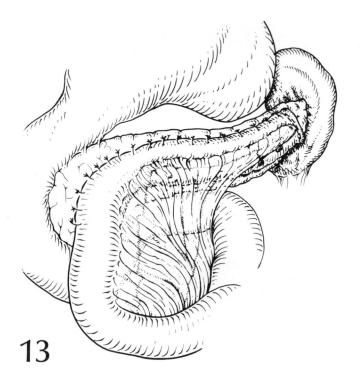

13

13 Whichever technique is adopted, the completed anastomosis should lie without tension in the lesser sac, and there should be no kinks in the Roux loop. One or two 'tacking' sutures can be inserted between the Roux loop and anterior surface of the pancreas to ensure that there are no kinks.

14 Intestinal continuity is now restored beneath the mesocolon by an end-to-side anastomosis between the cut proximal end of the jejunum and the side of the Roux loop. A twin occlusion clamp such as a Lane's clamp is ideal for the purpose and the anastomosis is created using two layers of continuous 2/0 resorbable material such as polydioxanone (PDS). Whereas the length of Roux loop used in gastric and biliary surgery is critical to avoid biliary reflux into the stomach or reflux of intestinal content into the biliary system respectively, the length of Roux loop in pancreaticojejunostomy does not appear to be vital. In general, the entero-enteric anastomosis is created at the most convenient point after the Roux loop emerges from the mesocolon into the infracolic compartment. Once the anastomosis is complete, defects in the mesocolon and small bowel mesentery are closed with interrupted sutures inserted carefully to avoid damaging blood vessels. If biliary enteric bypass is also to be performed, the anastomosis is created at this stage using one layer of interrupted 3/0 resorbable sutures to anastomose the side of the opened bile duct or the cut end of the transected bile duct to the side of the jejunum as it bends inferiorly from the pancreatico-jejunal anastomosis.

Haemostasis is checked and the abdomen is normally closed without drainage.

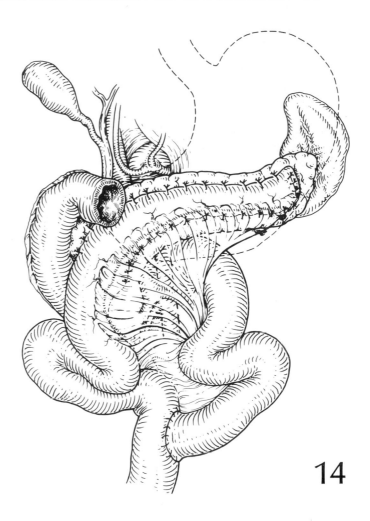

14

Outcome

Longitudinal pancreaticojejunostomy is a safe procedure which should carry no operative mortality and minimal morbidity. Patients must not be encouraged to believe that the operation will banish all of the problems associated with chronic pancreatitis, and a reasonable guideline is that about 70% of patients are pain-free or significantly improved when assessed 5 years after the operation. The procedure may prevent or defer the onset of troublesome exocrine pancreatic insufficiency and insulin-dependent diabetes, but cannot be expected to reverse existing insufficiencies. Much depends on the adequacy of drainage of the pancreatic duct system, on continuing wide patency of the anastomosis, and in the case of patients with alcoholic chronic pancreatitis, whether they abstain from alcohol consumption. Recurrence of pain is an indication to carry out ERCP and computed tomographic scanning to reassess the pancreas. In some cases it may be worthwhile attempting to provide more effective pancreatic drainage if the original pancreaticojejunostomy has been inadequate, and consideration should also be given to the Frey procedure as a means of eradicating ongoing inflammation in the head of the pancreas without exposing the patient to the risks and consequences of formal resection. However, many patients who experience major difficulties with pain after pancreaticojejunostomy become candidates for some form of partial, subtotal or total pancreatectomy.

ENDOSCOPIC DRAINAGE OF THE PANCREATIC DUCT

Endoscopic retrograde cholangiopancreatography (ERCP) and endoscopic ultrasonography now have a defined role in the investigation of pancreatic disease. Endoscopic sphincterotomy and stone retrieval are used widely to deal with choledocholithiasis, and endoscopic biliary stenting has an established place in the management of malignant low bile duct obstruction. However, the role of therapeutic endoscopic techniques in the management of chronic pancreatitis and its complications is much less clear. While it is technically possible to perform a wide range of procedures endoscopically, the results are often imperfect and these approaches should only be undertaken after full consideration of other options, and in centres with a full range of facilities and experience in imaging and pancreatic surgery.

Indications

(1) Patients with painful chronic pancreatitis with calculi or a stricture obstructing the main duct can be considered for endoscopic therapy with pancreatic sphincterotomy, stone extraction (with or without extracorporeal lithotripsy) and stent insertion (see below). A chronic pancreatic fistula or pseudocyst which persists because of a distal duct stricture can often be dealt with by endoscopic stenting of the stricture, although the procedure is often technically demanding, particularly if the duct system is disrupted and a guidewire cannot be passed readily through the narrowed area.

(2) Pseudocysts complicating chronic pancreatitis can be dealt with endoscopically, but only after the relative merits of the approach have been compared with those of conventional surgery or percutaneous drainage techniques. Large pseudocysts indenting the stomach or duodenum can be drained directly into the lumen of the gastrointestinal tract using a diathermy 'needle knife' followed by insertion of a double pigtail stent.

(3) Gastric varices which develop following splenic vein thrombosis can be dealt with endoscopically by injection of thrombin to stop bleeding or prevent rebleeding, although splenectomy and interruption of the short gastric vessels is often still needed for definitive treatment of this problem.

(4) Obstruction of the bile duct from chronic pancreatitis may be dealt with by endoscopic stenting as a temporary expedient but surgery is usually needed for definitive management.

(5) Pancreas divisum has been dealt with on occasions by endoscopic stenting or sphincterotomy of the accessory ampulla in patients troubled by persistent pain and recurrent attacks of pancreatic inflammation. The results of treatment are unpredictable and are often poor; patients with dilatation and slow emptying of the dorsal pancreatic duct are most likely to derive benefit from this approach. Even if long-term relief of symptoms is not afforded, the endoscopic approach at least allows rational decisions to be made regarding the likelihood of success following surgical attempts to improve duct drainage.

Technique

If therapeutic intervention is considered likely in patients undergoing diagnostic ERCP, the patient should receive prophylactic antibiotics, blood clotting is checked and blood is taken for grouping and cross-matching. ERP is first performed using standard technique and if endoscopic stenting of the pancreatic duct is indicated, pancreatic sphincterotomy is undertaken using a sphincterotome with a guidewire and following deep cannulation of the duct. The technique is identical to that used for biliary sphincterotomy, but the size of the opening created is more modest. It is sometimes difficult to insert the sphincterotome into the pancreas, and 'needle knife' sphincterotomy can be undertaken to facilitate its introduction (or, in some cases, to serve as a definitive procedure).

Balloon dilatation can be used as an alternative to minimize the risk of bleeding, to allow extraction of small calculi and to facilitate stent insertion. A Gruntzig type low profile balloon is inserted over a guidewire placed across the sphincter and dilated for 1–2 min to the pressures defined by the manufacturers. Overdilatation must be avoided as it can cause undue trauma and the development of severe pancreatitis.

If a sphincterotomy has been performed, calculi can be extracted using a conventional Dormia basket or occlusion balloons. In some cases, the small size of the pancreatic duct prevents these instruments passing beyond or capturing stones, and extracorporeal lithotripsy has been used in some centres to overcome this problem.

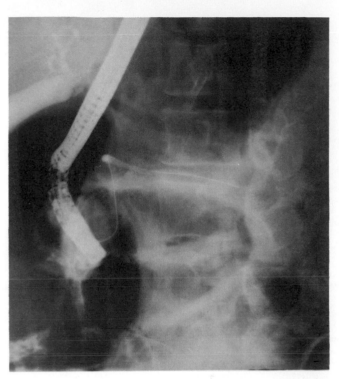

15 A hydrophilic catheter is next inserted deeply across the stricture. To achieve this it is first necessary to pass the guidewire through a stiff Teflon overtube and the assembly is then passed through the biopsy channel of the duodenoscope. The overtube is necessary to prevent kinking of the catheter in the duodenum. The stricture is intubated using a combination of guidewire insertion followed by forward movement of the overtube as the guidewire is slowly withdrawn. Once the guidewire is appropriately positioned the overtube is removed and a double barbed 3-Fr or 4-Fr plastic stent is railroaded across the stricture using the overtube as a 'pusher'. The objective is to leave the distal end of the stent protruding into the duodenum so that it can be removed easily if this becomes necessary.

15

Further reading

Carter DC. Surgical drainage procedures. In: Trede M, Carter DC, eds. *Surgery of the Pancreas*. Edinburgh. Churchill Livingstone, 1993, 309–19.

Ebbehoj N, Klaaborg KE, Kronberg O, Madsen P. Pancreaticogastrostomy for chronic pancreatitis. *Am J Surg* 1989; 157: 315–7.

Frey CF, Smith GJ. Description and rationale for a new operation for chronic pancreatitis. *Pancreas* 1987; 2: 701–5.

Prinz RA, Greenlee HB. Pancreatic duct drainage in 100 patients with chronic pancreatitis. *Ann Surg* 1981; 194: 313–20.

Prinz RA, Aranha GV, Greenlee HB. Redrainage of the pancreatic duct in chronic pancreatitis. *Am J Surg* 1986; 151: 150–6.

Chronic pancreatitis: distal pancreatectomy

R. C. G. Russell MS, FRCS
Consultant Surgeon, The Middlesex Hospital, London, UK

Principles and justification

All who undertake a distal pancreatectomy for benign disease must ask themselves if they are undertaking the right operation. So often the manifestations of the disease may be most obvious in the body and tail of the pancreas, but the cause of these manifestations lies in the head of the pancreas. In other words, much of the problem in the body of the pancreas is related to obstruction of the duct and, if that obstruction lies in the head or ampulla, a distal pancreatectomy will not resolve the situation. The common indication for resection of the body and tail of the pancreas is disruption of the duct at the neck of the pancreas due to trauma or an episode of severe acute pancreatitis with or without cyst formation. Occasionally, it is associated with duct strictures secondary to chronic pancreatitis, but this is rare and more usually the whole of the pancreas is involved.

Preoperative

Preoperative investigation

The essential investigation is contrast enhanced computed tomographic scanning using a spiral scanner to obtain good views of the arterial and venous phases. It is appropriate to undertake endoscopic retrograde cholangiopancreatography (ERCP) to ensure that the papilla is normal and the head of the pancreas has a normal duct system. The objective is to select patients who have a normal head of pancreas with disease confined to the body and tail of the pancreas. A Puestow-type procedure is not appropriate in these patients as the duct in the head of the gland is normal.

1a, b The ERCP shows a normal duct system in the head of the pancreas with complete obstruction at the level of the neck of the pancreas. There is no calcification in the head of the pancreas.

The computed tomographic scan confirms the presence of a normal pancreatic head with disease in the body and tail of the pancreas. In the scan shown in *Illustration 1b* there is complete transection at the level of the neck giving rise to a cyst and a dilated duct in the tail of the pancreas.

Preoperative preparation

Distal pancreatectomy for chronic pancreatitis is a major operation and, indeed, the procedure can be technically more demanding than a pancreato-duodenectomy because of the increased number of adhesions encountered which may result in a much greater blood loss. It is therefore appropriate to approach this operation circumspectly and, if there is much inflammation and the patient is in pain from that inflammation, a period of pancreatic rest with parenteral nutrition and nil orally can enable the inflammation to resolve and ease the operative procedure.

The immediate concern is to ensure that the patient is fit for surgery with a stable cardiovascular system, and is well hydrated with an infusion commenced the evening before the operation. The patient is catheterized and given preoperative antibiotics and thromboembolic prophylaxis with subcutaneous heparin and TED stockings. Because infection is a problem in these patients, invasive monitoring is avoided apart from an arterial line.

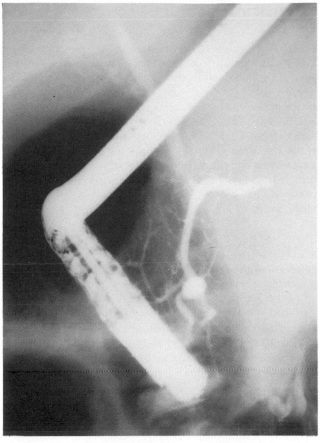

1a

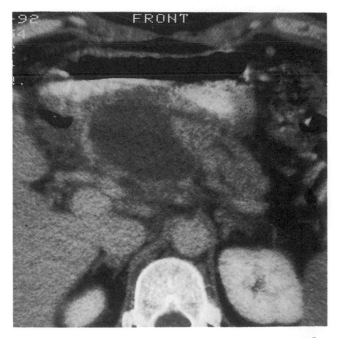

1b

Operation

There is a series of defined steps in this procedure which do much to ease the performance of the operation. First, the lesser sac is opened, then the splenic artery is tied near the coeliac axis, the short gastric arteries are tied, the colon is separated from the spleen and the mesocolon from the body of the pancreas, and finally the spleen is mobilized with the tail of the pancreas. There is a vogue for splenic-preserving pancreatectomy, but this is more suited to resection of benign tumours because the spleen is often intimately involved in the inflammatory process in chronic pancreatitis.

Incision

A straight transverse incision is suitable, starting at the tip of the 12th rib and extending to the right as far as is required. A bilateral subcostal or midline incision can be used, but the advantages of one over the other are minimal. After opening the abdomen a full laparotomy is performed to assess the extent of the disease.

Exposure of the pancreas

2 The body of the pancreas is best exposed by mobilizing the omentum from the greater curve of the stomach within the epiploic arch, and displacing the omentum and the colon with its mesocolon inferiorly away from the front of the pancreas.

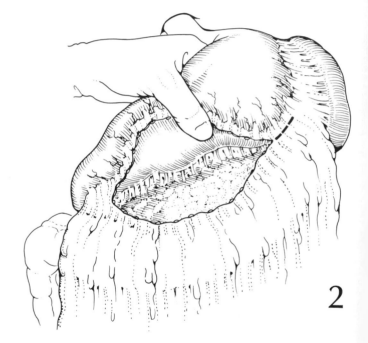

2

Divison of the gastrosplenic ligament

3 The dissection is continued up the greater curve, dividing the short gastric vessels near the stomach up to the uppermost short gastric artery level with the upper pole of the spleen, which should then fall away from the stomach with division of adhesions between the posterior wall of the stomach and pancreas.

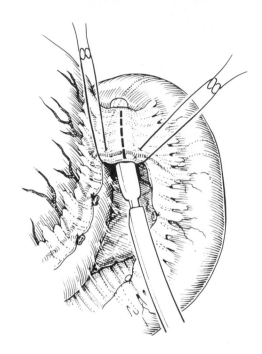

3

Ligation of the splenic artery

4 Using a stabilized ring retractor (Buchwalter) the stomach is retracted superiorly and the colon displaced downwards. The borders of the pancreas are defined from tail to neck above and below the pancreas. Attention is next turned to the trifurcation of the coeliac axis at the upper border of the neck of the pancreas. The hepatic artery is identified and freed from the superior margin of the pancreas. This artery is then followed towards the left until it merges with the splenic artery at its origin from the coeliac axis. The splenic artery is now tied to reduce the vascularity of the organs to be removed. As this dissection proceeds the upper border of the neck of the pancreas is displayed with the portal vein beneath. A little time spent dissecting the portal vein from the neck of the pancreas will be advantageous later in the operation. A tape is passed around the neck of the pancreas.

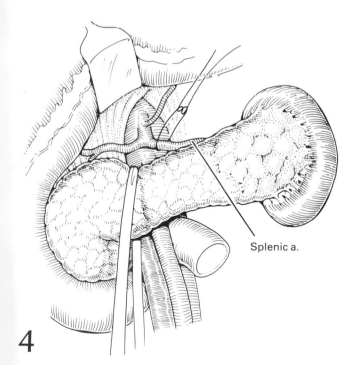

Splenic a.

4

Mobilization of the splenic flexure

5 The left gastroepiploic artery is traced down to the hilum of the spleen and there ligated. The remaining part of the omentum between the splenic hilum and the colon is divided, and the peritoneum which tethers the splenic flexure to the splenic hilum, the front of the kidney and the paracolic gutter is divided to enable the splenic flexure and its mesentery to be mobilized inferiorly. This enables the inferior border of the pancreas to be further exposed.

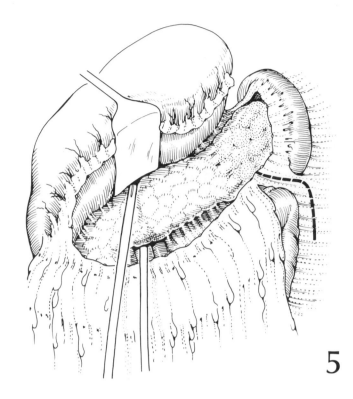

5

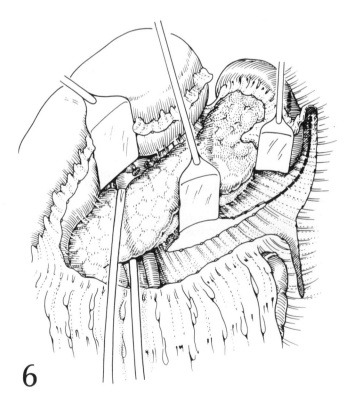

6

Mobilization of the spleen

6 The dissection of the inferior border of the pancreas is continued and extended beneath the pancreas where there is often an avascular plane, uninvolved by the inflammation of the pancreatitis. The plane is developed and extended laterally beneath the spleen where the lienorenal and lienophrenic ligaments are divided, so mobilizing the spleen upwards and anteriorly away from the posterior abdominal wall.

Dislocation of the spleen

7 In chronic pancreatitis there is often severe inflammatory change around the spleen. Careless hand mobilization of the spleen can cause much blood loss. This can be avoided by carefully dissecting the spleen away from the diaphragm with meticulous attention to haemostasis. The spleen so mobilized is now free from the diaphragm and can be dislocated to the right, enabling the plane of dissection developed posteriorly to be extended to the upper border of the pancreas. At the upper border of the pancreas care should be taken to avoid the adrenal gland which can be involved in the inflammatory process.

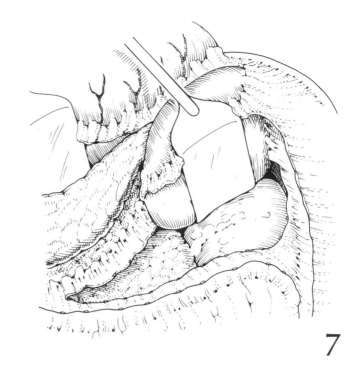

7

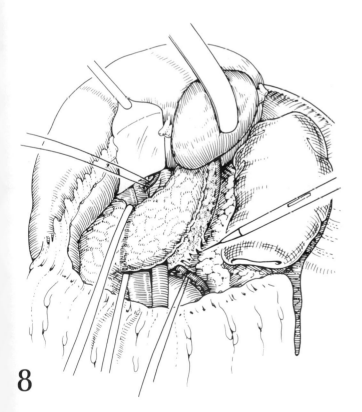

8

Dissection of the body of the pancreas

8 With the spleen and tail of the pancreas mobilized, care is required to dissect the body of the pancreas away from the posterior abdominal wall, avoiding deep dissection with damage to the renal vein and adhering closely to the posterior surface of the pancreas. Inferiorly, the inferior mesenteric vein should be avoided or tied if it joins the splenic vein, and superiorly the left gastric vein is tied and the coeliac axis avoided. As the dissection extends to the right, the position of the tape on the neck of the pancreas should be watched. To aid haemostasis, packing of the large exposed raw area reduces blood loss.

Control of the splenic vein

9 With the pancreas and spleen fully mobilized and brought over to the right side of the patient, the splenic vein is dissected onto the portal vein. With the tape around the neck of the pancreas as a guide, the splenic vein can be dissected, clamped and oversewn with 4/0 polypropylene (Prolene) on the portal vein.

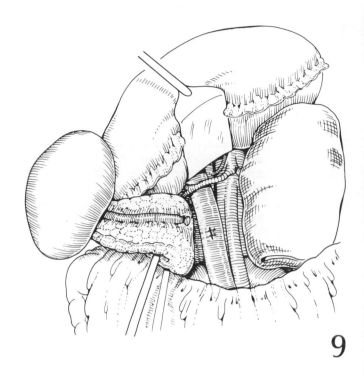

9

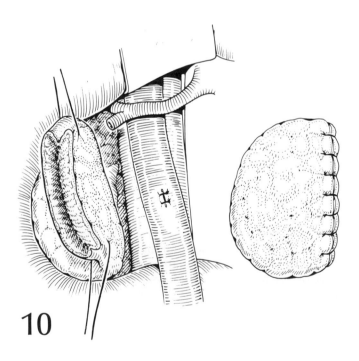

10

Division of the pancreas

10 The pancreas is now attached to the head by a narrow neck of tissue, which is divided cleanly with a knife with the head side controlled with stay sutures. Bleeding is controlled by sutures. The duct is carefully identified and closed with 4/0 polypropylene sutures. There is no advantage in draining the duct into a Roux loop. The pancreas is carefully closed with interrupted 2/0 sutures. Occasionally this closure is made easier by cutting with a 'fish mouth', but this can make the duct more difficult to find.

Closure

Careful haemostasis is essential before closure. A single closed tube drain is passed down to the bed of the pancreas and the wound is closed by the preferred method.

Postoperative care

The patient is maintained on intravenous infusion and nasogastric drainage until gastric emptying resumes a normal pattern. Occasionally gastric stasis may be prolonged, but it always resolves and patience is all that is required. The main complication of this operation is sepsis, either in the pancreatic bed or a left lower lobe atelectasis with secondary infection. Both resolve with conservative management. A fistula from the pancreatic duct is uncommon.

Approximately 70% of the pancreas has been removed, and as a consequence diabetes mellitus will occur in one-third of patients. Similarly, enzyme deficiency may be present requiring treatment by enzyme replacement therapy.

The overall mortality of this procedure should be 1–2%, and the morbidity 30% at most. Approximately 80% of patients have a good long-term result. The outcome in the remainder depends to a large degree on the success of the removal of the underlying cause of the chronic pancreatitis.

Further reading

Aldridge MC, Williamson RC. Distal pancreatectomy with and without splenectomy. *Br J Surg* 1991; 78: 976–9.

Geghardt C. Left resection in chronic pancreatitis. In: Beger H, Büchler M, Malfertheiner P, eds. *Standards in Pancreatic Surgery.* Berlin: Springer-Verlag, 1993: 392–5.

Konishi T, Hiraishi M, Kubota K, Bandai Y, Makuuchi M, Idezuki Y. Segmental occlusion of the pancreatic duct with prolamine to prevent fistula formation after distal pancreatectomy. *Ann Surg* 1995; 221: 165–70.

Sawyer R, Frey CF. Is there still a role for distal pancreatectomy in surgery for chronic pancreatitis? *Am J Surg* 1994; 168: 6–9.

Shankar S, Theis B, Russell RC. Management of the stump of the pancreas after distal pancreatic resection. *Br J Surg* 1990; 77: 541–4.

Warshaw AL. Conservation of the spleen with distal pancreatectomy. *Arch Surg* 1988; 123: 550–3.

Pancreaticoduodenectomy: pylorus preservation

Henry A. Pitt MD
Professor and Vice Chairman, Department of Surgery, The Johns Hopkins Medical Institutions, Baltimore, Maryland, USA

History

Pancreaticoduodenectomy was popularized by Whipple and his colleagues in the 1930s[1]. Numerous modifications of the original two-stage operation were introduced in the 1940s and 1950s and, by the 1960s, the 'standard Whipple procedure' was a one-stage operation that included a partial pancreatic resection and an antrectomy. During the 1970s, a trend evolved towards more radical operations including total pancreatectomy, portal vein resection and extensive retroperitoneal lymph node dissection. However, concerns about increased postoperative morbidity and mortality as well as a poorer quality of life with these more radical operations led Traverso and Longmire[2] to introduce the pylorus-preserving pancreaticoduodenectomy in 1978.

Principles and justification

Pylorus-preserving pancreaticoduodenectomy was originally described by Traverso and Longmire for the management of patients with chronic pancreatitis. Many pancreatic surgeons believe that it is the procedure of choice when the pancreatitis is most severe in the head and uncinate process and the pancreatic duct is not dilated. In this situation a Puestow procedure cannot be performed, and a distal pancreatectomy is less likely to relieve the pain that is usually the primary indication for surgery. In addition, many of these patients also have relative or significant narrowing of the distal bile duct which is also easily dealt with by pylorus-preserving pancreaticoduodenectomy.

The operation may also be indicated for a variety of other benign as well as malignant diseases. At present the most common indication for pylorus-preserving pancreaticoduodenectomy is a tumour arising in the periampullary region[3-5]. These tumours include adenocarcinomas that arise in the head of the pancreas, the ampulla of Vater, the distal bile duct and the duodenum. Pylorus-preserving pancreaticoduodenectomy is also indicated for the other less common neoplasms that may arise in the head of the pancreas. These tumours include the cystic neoplasms, both cystadenomas and cystadenocarcinomas, the islet cell tumours which may be either benign or malignant, and cystic and papillary (Hamoudi) tumours as well as a variety of very rare lesions.

Some surgeons have expressed concern that pylorus-preserving pancreaticoduodenectomy may not be an adequate operation for pancreatic cancer. However, at The Johns Hopkins Hospital and at several other institutions it is performed in more than 80% of these patients[4,5]. For those who express concern about the pylorus-preserving procedure, recurrence at the duodenal margin and the adequacy of the lymph node dissection are the major issues. On the other hand, those who are advocates of pylorus-preserving pancreatico-duodenectomy point out that frozen section of the duodenal margin prevents local recurrence, and they also report excellent survival data[3-5]. In addition, the quality of survival has been reported to be better with pylorus preservation than with either the standard Whipple procedure (which includes an antrectomy) or with more radical operations including total pancreatectomy and extensive retroperitoneal lymph node resection[6].

Preoperative

Regardless of the underlying pathology, the most likely presenting symptoms for patients who will require pancreaticoduodenectomy are pain and jaundice. A history of excess alcohol intake and chronic pain in middle-aged patients are most suggestive of chronic pancreatitis. On the other hand, the onset of relatively painless jaundice in an elderly patient makes an obstructing carcinoma the most likely diagnosis. In these jaundiced patients, the presence on physical examination of a non-tender, palpable gallbladder almost confirms the diagnosis of a malignancy. By the time these patients present, they may be severely jaundiced and may have lost considerable weight. Thus, the decision of whether or when to operate cannot be taken lightly.

In deciding whether to perform surgery, several patient and disease characteristics must be considered. The patient's age in itself should not be a factor in this decision. Most carefully selected elderly patients will tolerate pancreaticoduodenectomy without difficulty[3], while a younger patient with severe cardiac, pulmonary or renal disease may not fare so well. Similarly, underlying cirrhosis, especially if the patient also has portal hypertension, may significantly increase the risk of surgery. Patients who present with obstructive jaundice experience a myriad of physiological abnormalities which alter cardiac, pulmonary, hepatic, renal and immune function. In addition, these patients frequently have coagulation defects, impaired wound healing and a moderate degree of malnutrition.

As a result, a number of experts have recommended preoperative biliary drainage. However, the routine use of preoperative drainage remains controversial, but most authorities agree that jaundice should be relieved and surgery should be delayed in patients who are severely malnourished, have underlying renal disease and/or biliary sepsis. Abnormal laboratory data will provide information about sepsis, nutrition, renal function, the degree of biliary obstruction and coagulation.

1a,b In addition to deciding whether the patient can withstand surgery, in those with a malignancy it is necessary to determine whether the tumour is resectable. Percutaneous ultrasonography will demonstrate dilated bile ducts, a distended gallbladder and larger liver metastases. However, ultrasonography is not the best way to evaluate the pancreas or mesenteric vasculature and does not usually detect small liver metastases. Computed tomographic (CT) scanning is better at visualizing the pancreas, and newer spiral or helical techniques provide good information about the mesenteric vessels as well as detecting small liver metastases (*Illustration 1a*). Magnetic resonance imaging has not proved to be better than current CT techniques in staging these patients. Some experts have recommended the routine use of mesenteric angiography to assess vascular involvement by a pancreatic tumour (*Illustration 1b*), but the newer CT techniques may obviate the need for routine angiography.

Having information about the anatomy of the biliary tree prior to surgery is also usually helpful. An ultrasonogram or CT scan normally determines the level of obstruction. However, a cholangiogram will define the exact anatomy and is also very accurate in determining the specific diagnosis. The cholangiogram can be obtained by either the percutaneous transhepatic or the endoscopic retrograde (ERCP) technique. In patients with disease in the periampullary area, ERCP is usually preferred because the duodenum and ampulla can be visualized. In addition, biopsies can be taken and, if the diagnosis is in doubt, a pancreatogram can also be obtained. Moreover, in some patients who have not developed jaundice, the pancreatogram may detect a malignant stricture in the pancreatic neck or uncinate process or may suggest chronic pancreatitis.

A newer technique that may also be helpful in staging these patients is endoscopic ultrasonography. This investigation will usually detect obstruction of the bile and pancreatic ducts and visualize the tumour. Vascular involvement and lymph node metastases may also be detected with this technique. However, its accuracy in comparison with CT scanning and angiography or spiral CT scanning in determining resectability has yet to be determined. Another approach for staging these patients is laparoscopy. Laparoscopic examination will usually detect metastases on the surface of the liver and on the peritoneum. The addition of ultrasonography to laparoscopy increases its ability to determine resectability. However, laparoscopy is considered to be unnecessary by those who believe that operative palliation has advantages over non-operative palliation and that the decision with respect to resectability can only be made by the operating surgeon.

Another issue that must be considered is the need for a tissue diagnosis. In patients with obvious liver metastasis whose jaundice can be relieved with an endoprosthesis, needle biopsy of a liver lesion will

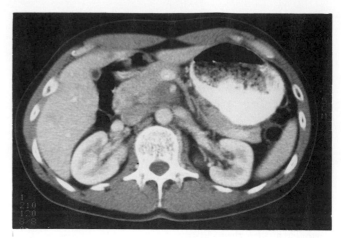

1a

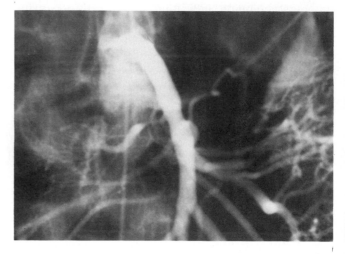

1b

usually provide the diagnosis. Similarly, in patients with large, unresectable lesions of the body or tail of the pancreas who do not require palliation of jaundice or duodenal obstruction, needle biopsy will avoid the need for a laparoscopy or laparotomy. However, if the CT scan demonstrates a potentially resectable mass in the periampullary area in a fit patient, preoperative biopsy is not indicated because the results of the biopsy will not alter the decision to operate. Moreover, some concern exists that the biopsy may spread tumour cells and adversely affect outcome. Additional issues to consider in preoperative preparation such as the perioperative use of prophylactic antibiotics and fluid management in these jaundiced patients are discussed in the chapter on pp. 395–407.

Anaesthesia

ERCP, endoscopic ultrasonography, percutaneous or endoscopic placement of biliary stents and angiography can usually be performed with intravenous sedation and analgesia. On the other hand, laparoscopy usually requires a general anaesthetic. Similarly, laparotomy to determine resectability and undertake a pancreatico-duodenectomy is also performed under a general endotracheal anaesthesia. In choosing an anaesthetic regimen, agents which can cause cholestasis or hepato-toxicity should be avoided in these jaundiced patients.

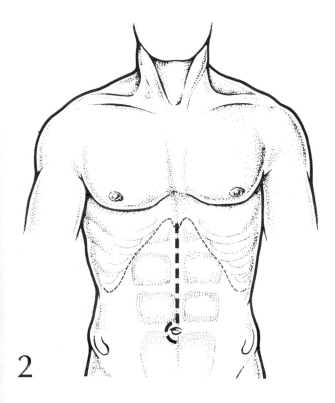

2

Operation

Incision and exploration

2 A pylorus-preserving pancreaticoduodenectomy may be performed through either a midline or a right and partial left subcostal incision. However, the midline incision allows more flexibility in tube and drain placement and avoids wound problems that commonly occur in the right flank.

Once the abdomen is open, a thorough exploration is undertaken. The liver and all peritoneal surfaces are carefully inspected for any sign of metastatic disease. Any suspicious lesions are biopsied, and the presence of liver or peritoneal metastases is generally taken as a contraindication to resection. On the other hand, tumour involvement of lymph nodes within the boundary of resection is not a contraindication to resection. However, spread of tumour to lymph nodes outside the usual areas of resection may be a reason to forgo resection. Most tumours that require pancreatico-duodenectomy are localized to the head, uncinate and/or neck of the pancreas. Spread throughout the body and tail of the gland is present in some cases, and the decision to undertake resection in such cases requires considerable judgement.

Kocher manoeuvre

3a,b If tumour spread has been excluded, an extensive Kocher manoeuvre is performed. The incision along the lateral border of the duodenum should also be carried to the right to free some of the attachments of the hepatic flexure of the colon from the retroperitoneum. The duodenum, head of the pancreas and the tumour can usually be easily separated from the inferior vena cava and aorta. However, extension of tumour into these structures occasionally precludes resection. Extensive mobilization of the head of the pancreas is also important to determine the extent of tumour spread into the uncinate process. The tumour may extend behind the superior mesenteric or portal vein and still be resectable. However, encasement of the superior mesenteric artery is usually regarded as a contraindication to resection.

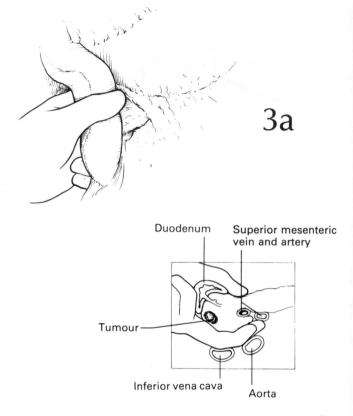

3a

Duodenum

Superior mesenteric vein and artery

Tumour

Inferior vena cava

Aorta

3b

Cholecystectomy and division of the bile duct

4a,b The next step in deciding on resectability is to expose the portal and superior mesenteric veins. Detachment of the gallbladder from the liver and division of the bile duct facilitates determination of the relationship between the portal vein and the tumour.

Before undertaking this step, a decision needs to be made as to whether the gallbladder would be used for bypass if the tumour is not resected. However, the long-term results of choledochojejunostomy are better than those of cholecystojejunostomy. On the other hand, if the portal vein is occluded by the tumour and multiple venous collaterals have developed around the bile duct, the gallbladder may be the best option for the biliary bypass as long as the cystic duct is still patent and not too close to the tumour. Assuming that this rare situation does not exist, the gallbladder is removed in a standard fashion, and the bile duct is transected just above or below the cystic duct entrance but at least 2 cm from the tumour. This manoeuvre will expose the portal vein more fully.

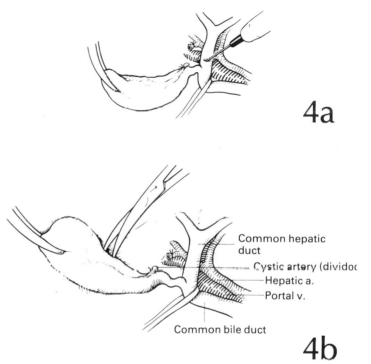

4a

Common hepatic duct
Cystic artery (divided)
Hepatic a.
Portal v.
Common bile duct

4b

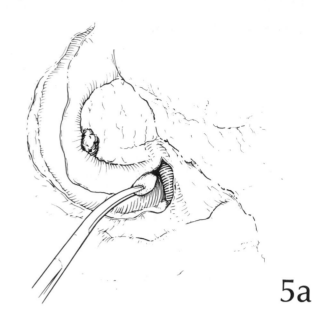

5a

Exposure of the superior mesenteric vein

5a–c To determine whether a tumour in the head, uncinate or neck of the pancreas is resectable, the superior mesenteric vein must also be exposed. To facilitate this manoeuvre, the transverse mesocolon is freed from the head and uncinate process, and the Kocher manoeuvre is extended to the third portion of the duodenum, thus exposing the right lateral edge of the superior mesenteric vein. Dissection of this vein is then carried up to the neck of the pancreas (*Illustration 5a*). Venous branches draining the transverse mesocolon and the head of the pancreas may need to be divided to continue tracing the superior mesenteric vein beneath the pancreatic neck. Dissection can then be continued between the superior mesenteric vein (below) and portal vein (above) and the neck of the pancreas. When this dissection is completed, fingers may be passed in this plane (*Illustrations 5b* and *5c*) to assess further the extent of the tumour. A judgement must be made at this point as to whether the tumour extends into the superior mesenteric or portal veins or into the superior mesenteric artery which lies to the left and somewhat behind (dorsal) the veins.

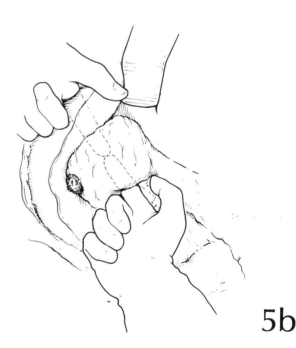

5b

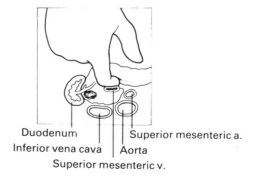

Duodenum

Inferior vena cava

Superior mesenteric v.

Superior mesenteric a.

Aorta

5c

Division of the duodenum

6 If the lesion is resectable, the next step is to divide the first portion of the duodenum. Multiple small vessels communicating between the first portion of the duodenum and the head of the pancreas have to be ligated before the duodenum can be divided. However, the right gastric artery, which usually extends from the common hepatic artery to the pyloric region, and associated nerves should be preserved. In addition, the first 2–3 cm of duodenum should be preserved, along with the pylorus. The pacemaker of the small intestine lies in this proximal segment of the duodenum, and preservation of the neurovascular supply should help with postoperative motility. Once adequate mobilization of the proximal duodenum has been completed, division with a GIA stapler is performed.

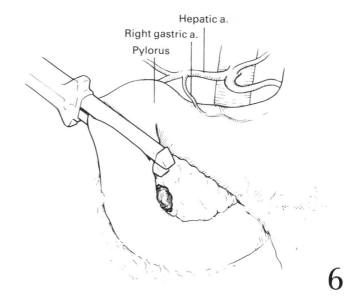

6

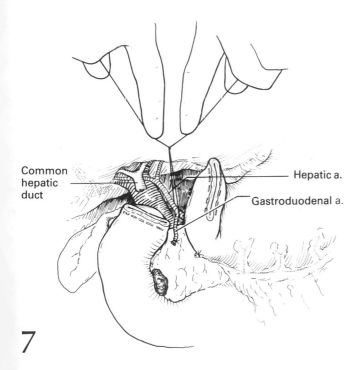

7

Division of the gastroduodenal artery

7 After the proximal duodenum has been divided, the gastroduodenal artery can be exposed more casily. A sufficient length of artery should be dissected to allow room for both ligation and suture ligation on the side leading from the hepatic artery. Care should be taken in this process not to interrupt flow through the hepatic artery. The gastroduodenal artery runs along the ventral surface of the neck of the pancreas and becomes the right gastroepiploic artery. This artery also needs to be ligated and divided to separate fully the pylorus from the specimen. If the patient has a replaced right hepatic artery extending from the superior mesenteric artery, this vessel usually runs ventral to the portal vein along its right side and dorsal to the common duct, also along its right side. Care should be taken to identify and preserve a replaced right hepatic artery which occurs in 15% of the population.

Division of the pancreatic neck

8 Despite division of the gastroduodenal and gastro-epiploic arteries, a considerable amount of blood continues to flow into the pancreatic neck through branches from the superior mesenteric artery. Larger vessels usually run along the cephalad and caudal borders of the pancreas at the neck, and placement of stay sutures along these borders of the pancreas reduces blood loss during division of the pancreatic neck. A vascular clamp applied to the specimen side will also minimize blood loss during this process. Protection of the portal vein with a finger or forceps is another wise move during the division of the pancreatic neck. Use of the cautery for the division also minimizes blood loss. If the tumour extends close to this margin, frozen section of the pancreatic neck should be performed at this point rather than when the entire specimen has been excised.

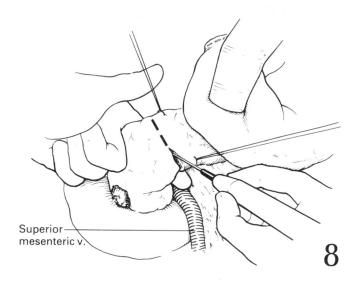

Superior mesenteric v.

8

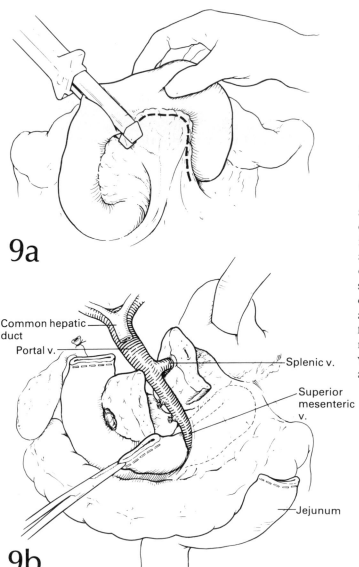

9a

Common hepatic duct

Portal v.

Splenic v.

Superior mesenteric v.

Jejunum

9b

Division of the jejunum

9a,b The ligament of Treitz is mobilized and the jejunum is then divided with a GIA stapler about 8–10 cm distal to the ligament. The mesentery is divided relatively close to the jejunum to avoid any injury to the superior mesenteric artery or vein. Usually, a double row of short vessels attaches the fourth portion of the duodenum to the uncinate process. Once these short vessels have been divided, the proximal jejunum can be passed behind the superior mesenteric artery and vein to the patient's right. This manoeuvre facilitates dissection of the uncinate process from the right and dorsal sides of the superior mesenteric vein, as well as from the right side of the superior mesenteric artery.

Dissection of the uncinate process

$10a,b$ At this point the only remaining attachments of the specimen are between the
uncinate process and the mesenteric vessels. Relatively
few venous branches drain from the uncinate process
into the superior mesenteric and portal veins. However,
these branches are relatively short and need to be
carefully ligated and suture ligated to avoid bleeding
from or narrowing of the superior mesenteric or portal
vein. In addition to these venous attachments, multiple
arterial branches extend from the superior mesenteric
artery into the uncinate process and these vessels
should be ligated close to the superior mesenteric
artery, especially if the tumour extends into the
uncinate process. During this dissection, care should be
taken to avoid injury to the superior mesenteric artery.
The chance of injuring the artery may actually be less if
it is identified and exposed in the process of dissection.

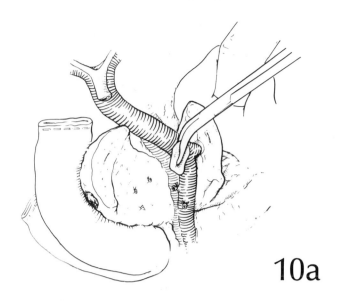

10a

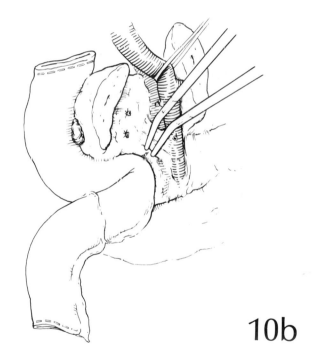

10b

Resected specimen

11a,b
The resected specimen consists of the gallbladder, the distal bile duct, the second, third and fourth portions of the duodenum, the proximal jejunum, and the head, neck and uncinate portions of the pancreas. When the resection has been performed for malignancy, frozen sections of the bile duct, duodenum and pancreatic neck and uncinate process are performed. If any of these margins, except the uncinate, are positive, further tissue may be removed in an effort to achieve a negative margin. In selected cases, however, resection of a segment of the portal or superior mesenteric vein may also be performed to achieve a negative margin. A primary anastomosis of the vein will normally suffice, but autologous vein is occasionally required to bridge the gap. Rarely, the coeliac axis is stenotic so that a significant proportion of the blood flow to the liver comes through collaterals in the pancreatic head. In this rare situation, an arterial bypass from the aorta or right renal artery to the hepatic artery or division of the arcuate ligament may need to be performed.

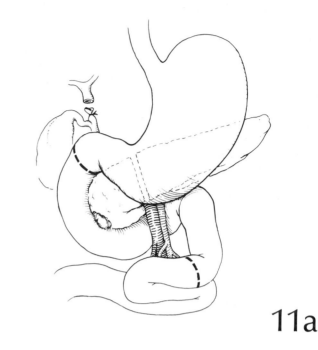

11a

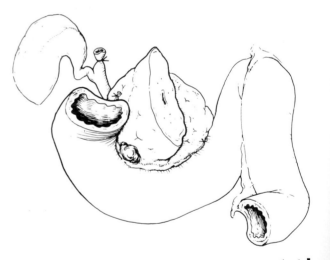

11b

Pancreatic anastomosis

12a–d A variety of methods exist to reanastomose the pancreas to the intestinal tract. Common options that are performed include an end-to-end (dunking) pancreaticojejunostomy (*Illustration 12a*), an end-to-side (mucosa-to-mucosa) pancreaticojejunostomy (*Illustration 12b*) or an end-to-side pancreaticogastrostomy (*Illustration 12c*). Any of these anastomoses may be stented with a short internal stent or with a longer stent which exits the jejunum and abdominal wall. If an end-to-side (mucosa-to-mucosa)

pancreaticojejunostomy is carried out, the outer layer is performed with 3/0 non-absorbable sutures which extend from the pancreatic capsule to the jejunal serosa (*Illustration 12d*). A 2–3 mm opening is made in the jejunum adjacent to the pancreatic duct, and an anastomosis is performed with 4/0 absorbable sutures. This anastomosis is usually stented with a short segment of paediatric feeding tube which is attached to the jejunum with a single 4/0 absorbable suture.

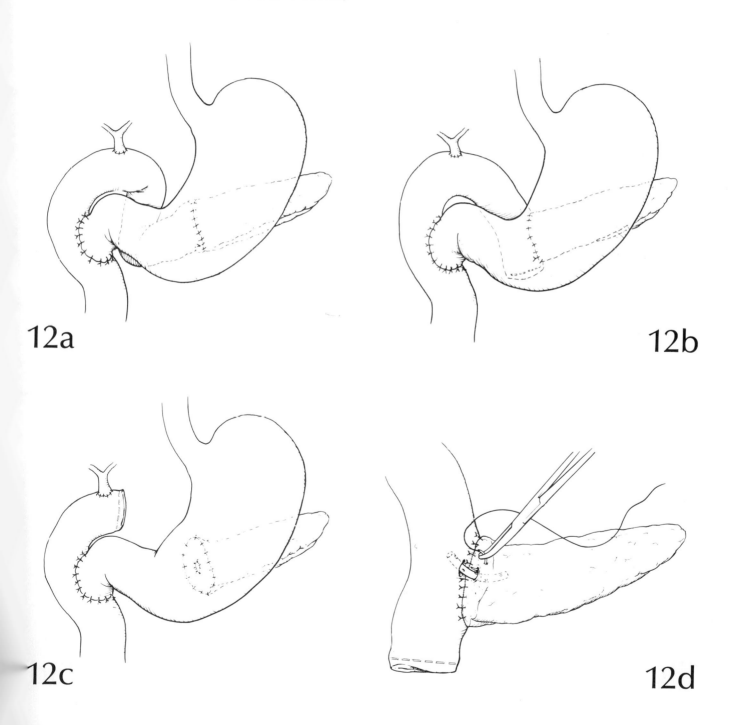

12a

12b

12c

12d

Hepaticojejunostomy

13a–d The hepaticojejunostomy usually lies only 6–8 cm distal to the pancreaticojejunostomy. The hepaticojejunostomy is performed in an end-to-side fashion and may be done in one or two layers. The anastomosis which is illustrated is two-layered with an outer layer of interrupted 4/0 non-absorbable sutures (*Illustration 13a*) and an inner layer of running 4/0 absorbable sutures (*Illustration 13b*). A T tube is placed through a separate stab incision in the common hepatic duct (*Illustration 13c*). The anterior row of sutures is also completed in two layers, and the jejunum is tacked to periportal tissues to take tension off the anastomosis (*Illustration 13d*). Fluorocholangiography is performed to assess proper positioning of the T tube and to check for leaks. The use of an operatively placed T tube or a preoperatively placed transhepatic stent is controversial. However, if a leak occurs at the biliary or the pancreatic anastomosis, external drainage may facilitate closure of the leak.

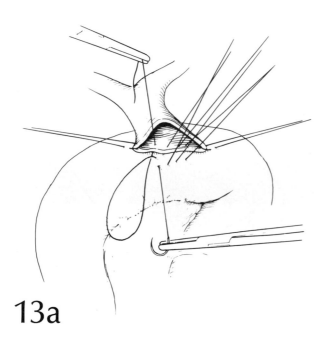

13a

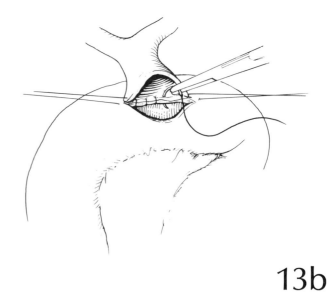

13b

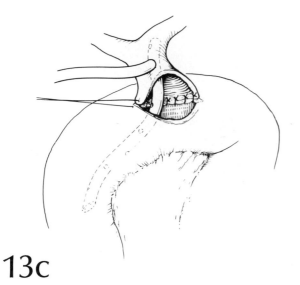

13c

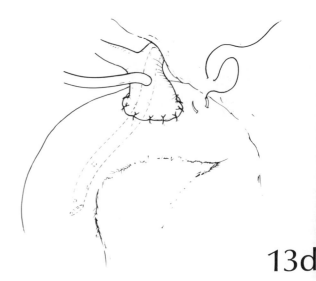

13d

Duodenojejunostomy

14a–d The third anastomosis is an end-to side duodenojejunostomy. This anastomosis is performed 15–20 cm distal to the hepaticojejunostomy. The duodenojejunostomy is performed in two layers. First, an outer layer of interrupted 3/0 non-absorbable sutures is placed (*Illustration 14a*). The staple line is removed from the duodenum, the blood supply is checked and an enterotomy is made in the jejunum (*Illustration 14b*). An inner layer of running 3/0 absorbable sutures is inserted (*Illustration 14c*) and the anastomosis is completed with an outer layer of interrupted 3/0 non-absorbable sutures (*Illustration 14d*).

This anastomosis is left just above the transverse mesocolon. However, the jejunum just below the anastomosis is tacked to the mesocolon to prevent internal herniation as well as obstruction. Two closed suction drains are inserted, one via the right flank and the other via the left upper quadrant. The right drain extends dorsal to the hepaticojejunostomy and ventral to the pancreaticojejunostomy. The left drain goes through the old ligament of Treitz area and lies behind (dorsal) the pancreaticojejunostomy. The T tube is brought out through a stab incision in the right upper quadrant. Both drains and the T tube are sutured to the skin, and the abdominal wall is closed in a standard fashion.

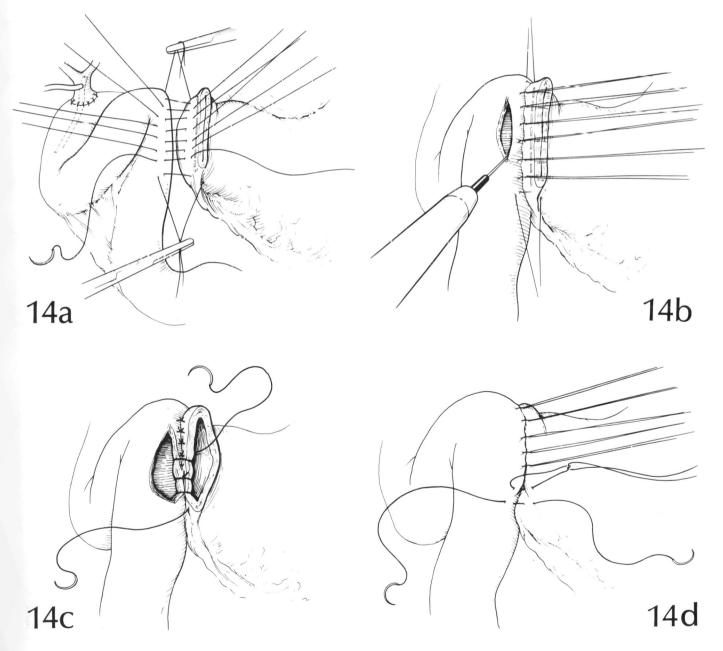

14a

14b

14c

14d

Postoperative care

Prophylactic antibiotics are normally stopped after 24 h. The routine use of octreotide to prevent a pancreatic anastomosis leak remains controversial. The nasogastric tube is left in until bowel function returns and drainage has diminished to less than 500 ml in 24 h. The incidence of delayed gastric emptying in the early postoperative period may be as high as 30–40% so the routine use of an intravenous prokinetic agent such as erythromycin has been recommended by some authorities. A pancreatic fistula may also occur in 5–15% of patients so the drainage fluid should be analysed for amylase on about the fifth postoperative day and again after oral intake has started. A T tube cholangiogram is performed on the fifth or sixth postoperative day. Prophylactic antibiotics directed at the organisms cultured from the bile are given before and for 24 h afterwards if no cholangitis occurs. If no bile or pancreatic leak is demonstrated and no cholangitis is experienced, the T tube is closed on the day after cholangiography. If a pancreatic or a bile leak is discovered, the T tube is left on drainage and a CT scan is performed. Any unusual fluid collections which do not communicate with an existing drain are percutaneously aspirated and drained.

In most circumstances in which a pancreatic leak is documented, the patient is kept on nil by mouth and total parenteral nutrition is begun. Re-exploration is usually not required unless bleeding develops. Oral intake is not begun until bowel function has returned, the stomach is properly emptying, and bile or pancreatic leaks have healed. Drains are not removed until the T tube has been closed, any fistulas are healed and the patient is eating. An unusual problem is drainage of very large amounts of ascites in the early postoperative period which requires urgent re-exploration to assess venous obstruction. On the other hand, if the ascites is chylous, an injury to a main lymphatic channel may have occurred, and this problem can usually be managed by stopping oral intake and beginnig parenteral nutrition. When the patient does begin eating, blood sugars and bowel movements are monitored. Most patients who do not have pancreatic endocrine or exocrine insufficiency before pancreaticoduodenectomy do not develop these problems after surgery, because more than half of the pancreas remains after the head of the gland has been resected.

Outcome

The mortality rate following pancreaticoduodenectomy has diminished significantly in recent years although morbidity remains high[1, 3–5]. In a recent series of 145 consecutive patients who underwent pancreaticoduodenectomy at The Johns Hopkins Hospital the hospital mortality was zero[3]. However, in this series, in which 81% of patients underwent a pylorus-preserving pancreaticoduodenectomy, the postoperative morbidity was 52%. The most common complication was delayed gastric emptying which occurred in 36% of the patients. Although some authorities have suggested that this problem is more common after pylorus-preserving pancreaticoduodenectomy, comparative data have not confirmed this contention[1]. Delayed gastric emptying is often caused by other intra-abdominal problems such as pancreatitis or a pancreatic fistula. When these other complications resolve, gastric emptying usually improves so that long-term problems with gastric stasis are unusual.

The next most common complication after pancreaticoduodenectomy is development of a pancreatic fistula[3–5]. In a recent randomized trial of pancreaticojejunostomy versus pancreaticogastrostomy performed at The Johns Hopkins Hospital the overall incidence of pancreatic fistula was 11%[5]. However, the incidence was the same regardless of the type of anastomosis employed. Pancreatic fistula can lead to intra-abdominal abscess, haemorrhage and death. However, careful monitoring of amylase levels in the drainage fluid resulting in early diagnosis, percutaneous drainage of intra-abdominal collections, and parenteral nutritional support have all diminished the severity of this complication. Total pancreatectomy, of course, avoids the problem of pancreatic fistula, but the overall morbidity is actually higher with total than with partial pancreaticoduodenectomy[1]. Moreover, with total pancreatectomy the diabetes mellitus can be quite brittle, and late problems with hepatic fibrosis have been reported.

In a collected series of 339 pylorus-preserving pancreaticoduodenectomies published in 1990, the hospital mortality was 4% which compared favourably with the 3% mortality reported in a collected series of standard Whipple procedures reported during the same time period[1]. During this period, the hospital mortality in collected series of regional and total pancreatectomies was 6% and 18%, respectively[1]. Since 1990 several large series of pylorus-preserving pancreaticoduodenectomies have been published with mortality rates of 0–2%.

Thus, pylorus-preserving pancreatiocduodenectomy can usually be performed with equal or greater safety than the other alternatives. On the other hand, controversy continues as to whether it provides the best chance for long-term survival in patients with cancer. Critics argue that the area resected is reduced and suggest that pylorus-preserving pancreaticoduodenectomy should not be performed for pancreatic cancer. However, advocates point out that the bile duct, uncinate process and pancreatic neck margins are usually closer to the tumour than the duodenal margin. Moreover, survival rates after the pylorus-preserving procedure have been the same or better than those with the classic Whipple procedure or with total pancreatectomy[1, 4]. Finally, the quality of survival can be better with pylorus-preserving pancreaticoduodenectomy than with either the classic Whipple procedure or with regional pancreatectomy[6].

References

1. Pitt HA. Curative treatment for pancreatic neoplasms: standard resection. *Surg Clin North Am* 1995; 75: 891–904.
2. Traverso LW, Longmire WP Jr. Preservation of the pylorus in pancreaticoduodenectomy. *Surg Gynecol Obstet* 1978; 146: 959–62.
3. Cameron JL, Pitt HA, Yeo CJ, Lillemoe KD, Kaufman HS, Coleman J. One hundred and forty-five consecutive pancreaticoduodenectomies without mortality. *Ann Surg* 1993; 217: 430–8.
4. Yeo CJ, Cameron JL, Lillemoe KD *et al*. Pancreaticoduodenectomy for cancer of the head of the pancreas: 201 patients. *Ann Surg* 1995; 221: 721–33.
5. Yeo CJ, Cameron JL, Maher MM *et al*. A prospective randomized trial of pancreaticogastrostomy versus pancreaticojejunostomy following pancreaticoduodenectomy. *Ann Surg* 1995; 222: 580–92.
6. Yasuda H, Takada T, Uchiyama K *et al*. Social function following pylorus-preserving pancreaticoduodenectomy for cancer of the head of the pancreas. *Asian J Surg* 1993; 16: 228–31.

Pancreatic cancer: palliative bypass

P. C. Bornman FRCS(Ed), MMed (Surg)
Professor of Surgery and Head of Surgical Gastroenterology, University of Cape Town and Groote Schuur Hospital, Cape Town, South Africa

J. E. J. Krige FRCS, FCS(SA)
Associate Professor, Department of Surgery, University of Cape Town and Groote Schuur Hospital, Cape Town, South Africa

Principles and justification

The complexity of palliative treatment of pancreatic carcinoma is often underestimated[1]. Most patients are elderly with comorbid diseases, and additional risk factors associated with obstructive jaundice such as renal failure, coagulation disorders and sepsis further compound management strategy. Palliative treatment should aim at minimizing hospital stay while improving and maintaining quality of life. Although there are no objective criteria to validate the benefits of relieving jaundice, patient morale and performance status are generally improved, particularly when pruritus is present. Duodenal obstruction is seldom a presenting symptom, but when present is usually an indication of advanced disease. The management of pain is often difficult, particularly during the terminal stages of the disease.

Non-operative stenting has provided an alternative option for biliary bypass[2,3]. Stenting is now the treatment of choice in high-risk or frail patients and in those with obvious advanced disease without duodenal obstruction. In elderly fit patients without overt metastatic disease, the choice between palliative bypass surgery and non-operative stenting will be largely determined by ease of access to centres with endoscopic and interventional radiological facilities and expertise in stenting. Surgically fit patients with locally advanced disease (who may survive longer) should undergo surgical bypass, as the initial advantage of stenting will be eroded by the subsequent need for stent replacement and the risk of duodenal obstruction.

Choice of operation

Despite careful preoperative evaluation, the final decision determining the choice of bypass is often made during laparotomy. Selection will depend on the presence of metastases, extent of the primary tumour, proximal bile duct infiltration and the degree of duodenal involvement. Other anatomical considerations such as previous biliary surgery (e.g. cholecystectomy), obesity and mobility of the small bowel mesentery also influence the choice of bypass.

Bypass surgery should be avoided when unexpected diffuse liver or peritoneal metastases, ascites and porta hepatis involvement by tumour are encountered. These patients should rather be referred for postoperative stenting unless a gastrojejunostomy is required for overt duodenal obstruction. The morbidity and mortality in this subgroup of patients is high and the bypass procedure often proves ineffective.

Biliary bypass

For biliary drainage the options are anastomosis of either the gallbladder or the bile duct to the jejunum or duodenum. External biliary drainage via a T tube is no longer acceptable and cholecystgastrostomy is of historic interest only.

Cholecystojejunostomy using a loop of proximal jejunum is the simplest method of palliative biliary bypass and has particular appeal in the high-risk patient. Only a small incision is required and the anastomosis is technically easy and safe. This bypass is now also performed laparoscopically.

In selecting the gallbladder for biliary bypass, the surgeon must ensure that the cystic duct is patent and that entry into the bile duct is not close to the upper limit of the tumour. A tense distended gallbladder does not necessarily indicate communication with an obstructed common bile duct, but may be caused by cystic duct obstruction. Accurate assessment of cystic duct compromise may be difficult to determine at operation even with careful dissection. It is also important to ensure that there is an adequate distance between the entry of the cystic duct and the level of obstruction. Cystic duct patency is best determined preoperatively by endoscopic or percutaneous transhepatic cholangiography, or intraoperatively by cholangiography via the gallbladder. It is generally accepted that 2–3 cm of clearance is required between the obstruction and the entry of the cystic duct to safeguard against recurrent biliary obstruction[4]. The indiscriminate use of the gallbladder may have been responsible for the poor results reported in some studies. The gallbladder should not be used when chronic cholecystitis and gallstones are present.

To avoid the development of cholangitis due to reflux of the bowel contents into the biliary system, either an enteroanastomosis or a Roux-en-Y jejunal loop has been recommended. There is, however, increasing evidence that this potential complication is overemphasized when used for short-term palliation. The Roux-en-Y jejunal loop is seldom used for gallbladder drainage as it adds a further anastomosis to the procedure. The Roux loop is preferable for bile duct drainage, particularly when a simultaneous duodenal bypass is contemplated. It is useful when technical difficulties due to a shortened small bowel mesentery (caused by obesity or tumour bulk) prevent the bowel from reaching the porta hepatis without tension. A choledochoduodenostomy may also overcome this problem, but later encroachment by tumour and the development of recurrent jaundice has limited its use.

Duodenal bypass

A gastrojejunostomy is clearly indicated in patients with clinically overt gastric outlet obstruction and in the symptomatic patient in whom there is evidence of duodenal infiltration or displacement by tumour on endoscopy, barium meal or at laparotomy. It must be emphasized that delayed gastric emptying may not only be due to a mechanical obstruction, but also occurs as a consequence of advanced disease. A gastrojejunostomy in this situation may not be effective. The role of a prophylactic gastrojejunostomy remains controversial, but a good case can be made when longer survival is anticipated as the risk of developing duodenal obstruction increases exponentially in patients who survive longer than 6 months[5].

The sequence of anastomoses when draining both the gallbladder and the stomach has never been standardized. The authors' support the rationale for doing the gastric bypass first using proximal jejunum as troublesome bile reflux is thus avoided. There is no need to add a vagotomy since the risk of subsequent stomal ulceration is negligible despite the biliary diversion.

Preoperative assessment and preparation

In the selection of palliative treatment, assessment of performance status, anaesthetic risk and tumour staging are important considerations in planning preoperative preparations and surgical strategy[6].

Associated medical conditions should be identified and treated and special attention given to those risk factors related to malignant biliary obstruction. Adequate rehydration, correction of haematocrit and initiating diuresis are important measures in preventing renal failure. Mannitol (500 ml of a 10% solution infused over 1–2 h) before or during surgery remains a useful diuretic when other measures fail to establish a diuresis. The administration of one or two doses of vitamin K usually corrects the deficient coagulation factors related to reduced absorption, but additional fresh frozen plasma may be required in patients with associated liver disease.

Antibiotics are the most effective means of combating the systemic effects of endotoxaemia and the increased susceptibility to sepsis in the jaundiced patient[7]. A combination of penicillin and an aminoglycoside is commonly used, but should be avoided in elderly patients and those with renal impairment. The use of a second generation cephalosporin fulfils the same need and has the advantage of being effective against staphylococci.

Several controlled trials evaluating preoperative biliary drainage have shown no reduction in postoperative morbidity and mortality and in some studies it has been associated with life-threatening complications such as haemorrhage and cholangitis[8]. Internal stenting avoids many of the disadvantages of external biliary drainage but its use has not gained widespread acceptance. The use of preoperative biliary drainage (preferably by internal stenting) is now restricted to selected cases with cholangitis or renal failure who do not respond to medical therapy.

Operation

Incision

1 A right subcostal incision is used in most patients because it provides easy access and good exposure of the operative field. The incision can readily be extended across the midline if required. A right transverse incision is preferable in obese patients and in those with hepatomegaly. A long midline incision extending from the xiphisternum to below the umbilicus can be used in patients with a narrow subcostal angle.

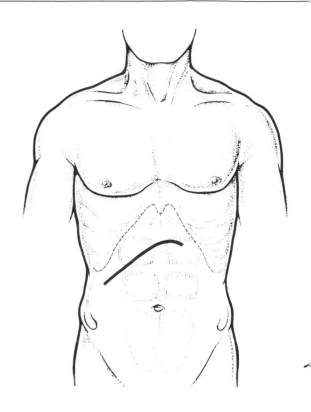

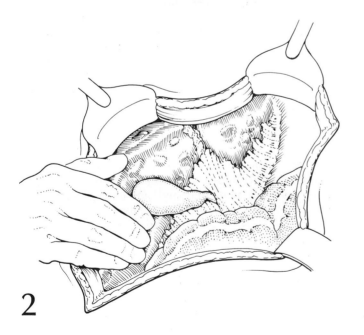

2

Exploration of the peritoneal cavity

2 A mechanical subcostal retractor facilitates exposure of the porta hepatis, especially if the bile duct is used for drainage. A systematic approach is used, first to exclude distant metastases, then regional nodal involvement and, finally, local tumour extension. Biopsies are taken of suspicious areas showing puckering, nodular implantation or fixation. Hepatic, omental serosal or peritoneal seedlings are usually immediately obvious and preclude resection. Special attention is paid to examination of the liver using bimanual palpation and, if available, intraoperative ultrasonography which may detect unsuspected deep-seated liver metastases. Portal vein involvement, invasion of the hepatic artery or superior mesenteric vessels, or extension of the tumour beyond the normal limits of pancreatic resection indicate non-resectability.

3 Extension of tumour from the neck of the pancreas or uncinate process along the superior mesenteric vessels into the base of the mesocolon is assessed by elevating the transverse colon and examining the mesocolon from below in the region of the ligament of Treitz. The base of the small bowel mesentery should also be examined for nodal involvement.

4 The gastrohepatic omentum is incised to allow inspection and palpation of the neck and body of the pancreas and to assess regional lymph nodes along the coeliac and hepatic arteries and in the porta hepatis (1). If nodal metastases or local tumour extension to surrounding structures is present, the tumour is incurable and a bypass is performed. If neither nodes nor extension are present, the lesser sac is exposed via the gastrocolic ligament which allows complete examination of the body and tail of the pancreas and the nodes along the splenic vessels and the splenic hilum (2). The opening is widened and the stomach retracted upwards using a malleable retractor or a Penrose drain placed around the stomach. This allows complete visualization of the neck, body and tail of the pancreas. The duodenum is Kocherized only if no distant or regional nodes are encountered and forms part of the assessment of resectability (3).

Preparation of the intestinal loop

The first loop of the jejunum is usually used to fashion the gastroenterostomy when this is necessary. The loop of jejunum distal to the stoma is next inspected either to fashion a Roux loop or, more simply, as an intact loop with or without an enteroanastomosis between afferent and efferent loops. The highest loop of the jejunum which reaches the right upper quadrant without tension is selected. An enteroanastomosis is made between the afferent and efferent loops approximately 20 cm from the apex of the loop.

The loop is next passed through an avascular window in the right transverse mesocolon so that it lies

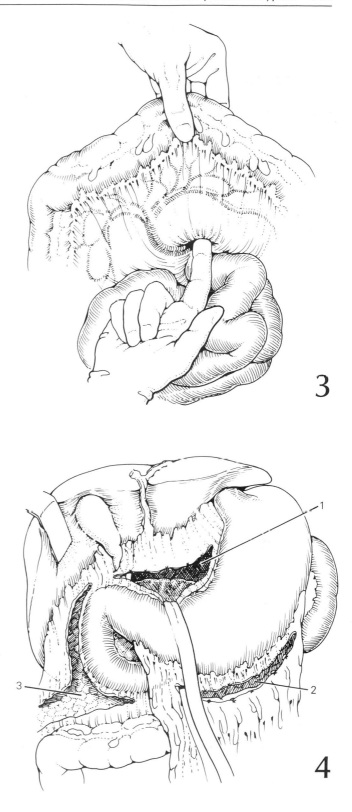

comfortably in the right subhepatic space. This retrocolic route facilitates exposure for the next phase because exposure and access is more difficult if the loop is brought in front of the colon, especially if a choledochojejunostomy is being performed.

CHOLECYSTOJEJUNOSTOMY

5 A suitable proximal jejunal loop which easily reaches the gallbladder is selected for an antecolic anastomosis. A retrocolic approach through the mesocolon of the hepatic flexure to the right of the middle colic vessels can be used if necessary. In the unusual situation where neither is possible, a Roux loop is used. A flexible approach is used when selecting the site of the gallbladder anastomosis. Either the fundus or the body of the gallbladder is suitable and the most prominent and accessible site is chosen. The gallbladder is first emptied using a trocar suction apparatus which allows it to be handled more easily than when grossly distended and avoids spillage of bile.

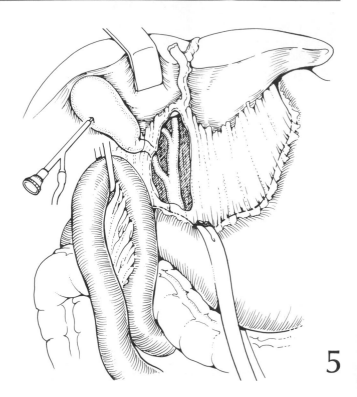

5

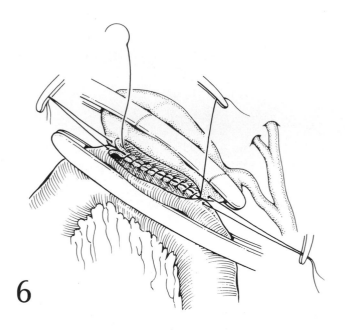

6

6 Non-crushing soft bowel clamps placed across the gallbladder and the small bowel are useful to avoid spillage. The jejunal loop and gallbladder are laid side-by-side and a continuous 3/0 monofilament suture is used to approximate the posterior walls. An incision is made in both the gallbladder and jejunum. The inner layer, incorporating the full thickness of the posterior wall of the gallbladder and the intestine, is anastomosed using a 3/0 continuous absorbable monofilament suture starting at one corner, and both the posterior and anterior inner layers are completed. A Connell stitch applied at each corner is useful to prevent mucosal pouting.

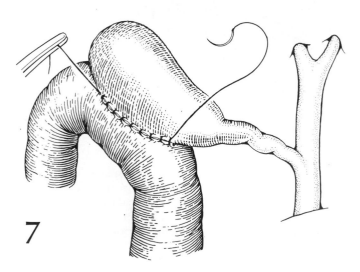

7

7 The anterior serosal surfaces are approximated using a continuous 3/0 suture. When the gallbladder wall is distended and thin, a two-layer anastomosis is preferred using 4/0 sutures and a thin needle to avoid bile leakage from the suture holes. For a thicker gallbladder wall a single-layer anastomosis is adequate.

CHOLEDOCHOJEJUNOSTOMY

8 The Roux loop is fashioned by transecting the jejunum approximately 15 cm beyond the ligament of Treitz. The proximal small bowel is held up and spread to transilluminate the mesentery and identify the vascular arcades so that the mesentery can be divided without compromising the blood supply. The authors divide only primary and secondary arcades before transecting the bowel. This usually provides sufficient length when the antimesenteric margin at the end of the loop is used for the biliary anastomosis. It is seldom necessary to divide the tertiary arcades and extend the division into the base of the mesentery. The bowel is transected between crushing clamps and the distal end of the Roux loop is secured by closure using two layers of an absorbable suture. Alternatively, staples can be used to divide the bowel and the end of the loop is closed by invagination using an absorbable suture.

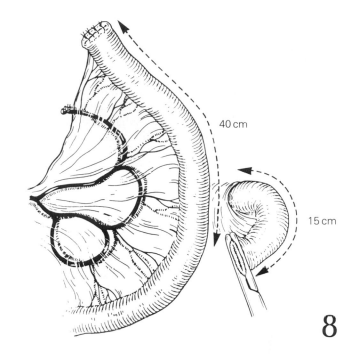

40 cm

15 cm

8

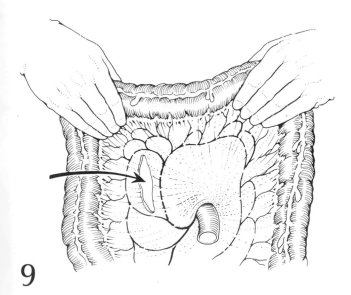

9

9 The transverse colon is retracted out of the wound and transilluminated to identify the middle colic vessels and their branches. An avascular site in the mesocolon which provides the shortest route to the porta hepatis is selected, usually to the right of the middle colic vessels. The mesocolon is opened with a scalpel or pair of scissors for a distance of about 8 cm to allow comfortable passage of the jejunal loop and accompanying mesentery.

10 The loop is manipulated through the gap in the mesocolon to a point where the end of the loop lies comfortably without tension adjacent to the porta hepatis at the site of the proposed biliary anastomosis.

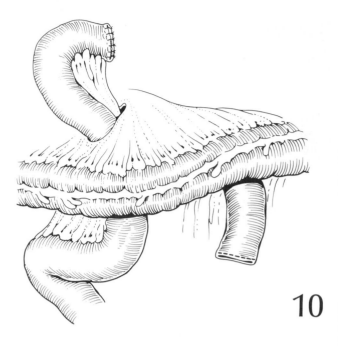

10

11 A cholecystectomy is not routinely performed. Removal of the gallbladder does, however, facilitate construction of the hepaticojejunostomy, especially if exposure is limited and a high anastomosis is required. In this situation dissection and removal of the gallbladder must be meticulous to avoid bleeding from the gallbladder bed. Emptying of the gallbladder before dissection may be useful when the gallbladder is grossly distended. The common bile duct is opened at least 2–3 cm above the macroscopic extent of the tumour. Two 5/0 stay sutures are placed at the site of the choledochotomy to support the duct and avoid injury to the posterior wall of the duct or adjacent structures during opening. The initial incision is made in the anterior wall with a no. 15 scalpel blade and the choledochotomy is enlarged to 3 cm using a pair of angled Pott's scissors. The decision whether to use interrupted or continuous sutures for the anastomosis is based on the size of the duct, the level of the anastomosis and the adequacy of exposure. A low anastomosis to a wide duct can be accomplished without difficulty using a continuous suture. For higher anastomoses, where exposure is less adequate, the technique for high bile duct reconstruction using interrupted sutures is recommended[9].

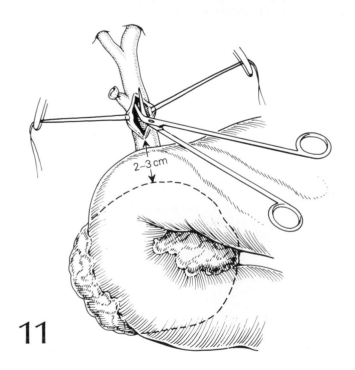

11

12 The selection of suture material and the size and diameter of the needle are governed by the thickness of the bile duct wall. When the wall of the bile duct is thin, 4/0 sutures, a thin needle and suture bites 2 mm apart and placed 2 mm from the edge are used. Particular care is taken to avoid undue traction on sutures placed in a thin-walled bile duct to prevent tearing of the duct wall. For ducts with thicker walls, 3/0 sutures, a larger needle and more generous bites can be used. A superior row of sutures which will constitute the anterior layer of the anastomosis is placed in the bile duct first before the posterior layer of sutures is inserted. The apex suture is placed first to mark the mid point of the anterior wall anastomosis. The sutures (absorbable monofilament) are now sequentially placed starting from the apex, working towards the two corner stay sutures. The needles are passed from the outside inwards to allow subsequent tying of the knots on the outside when the final sutures are placed through the anterior jejunal wall. This technique allows accurate and precise placement of the sutures and produces the best possible mucosa-to-mucosa approximation[9]. The needles on the anterior row of sutures are retained and each suture is clipped with a shod clamp and kept in sequential order on a clamp hanger. The row of upper sutures is lifted to elevate the anterior wall of the bile duct and facilitate exposure and placement of the posterior wall sutures. The end of the jejunal loop is positioned at a convenient distance below the inferior margin of the choledochotomy. A soft bowel clamp is applied across the jejunal loop 15 cm from the end after milking the contents back to avoid leakage and

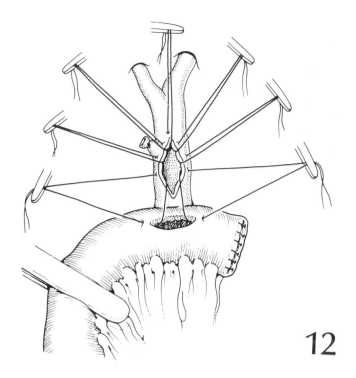

12

contamination of the operative field during the procedure. A linear incision is made into the antimesenteric margin of the jejunum near the closed end. The jejunal incision should be three-quarters the length of the biliary opening to avoid an ultimate discrepancy in size as the jejunal opening usually stretches with manipulation. Stay sutures are placed at each corner.

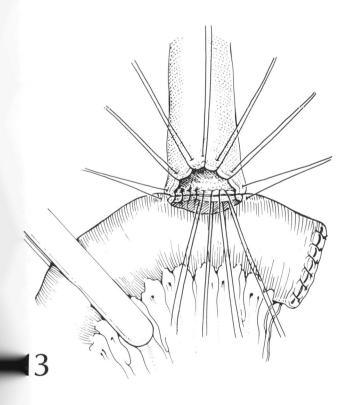

13

13 The posterior layer of sutures is placed starting from *within* the lumen of the bile duct, taking care that the full thickness of both the jejunal wall and the bile duct are incorporated in each suture to ensure accurate approximation and effective haemostasis. The needle is cut off each interrupted suture once placed. It is helpful to hold up the previously placed suture to allow close apposition of the two walls and accurate placement of the next stitch. The remainder of the posterior wall is completed with sutures placed every 3 mm. After all the sutures have been placed the jejunal limb is 'railroaded' upwards to lie in close proximity to the inferior margin of the choledochotomy. The posterior layer sutures are then tied serially. The tension applied on each knot is critical to ensure that each tie is snug and secure. The two corner stay sutures are held on shod clamps while the others are cut. The integrity of the posterior anastomosis should be assessed at this stage by inspecting the suture line from below by gently lifting and rotating the end of the loop upwards.

14 The technique of suture placement on the jejunal side is important. The needle is passed obliquely through the jejunal wall incorporating only 1 mm of mucosa from the cut edge and 3 mm of serosa. This prevents eversion and mucosal pouting and ensures a watertight closure.

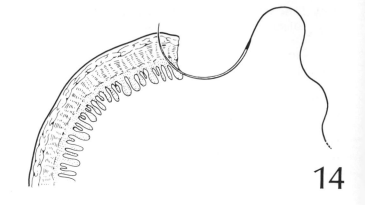

14

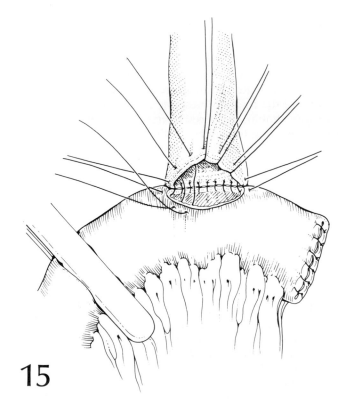

15

15 The previously placed anterior row of sutures is now used to complete the anastomosis by passing the needles from the inside outwards onto the anterior wall of the jejunum. The entire row is placed and the needles are cut from the sutures. The anterior layer of sutures is then serially tied, each knot being placed on the outside.

16 The enteroanastomosis between the end of the proximal jejunum and the side of the Roux loop 40 cm from the tip is fashioned below the transverse mesocolon. Before starting the anastomosis, particular attention is paid to ensure that the proximal small bowel mesentery is not twisted or rotated. Soft bowel clamps are applied to both the proximal jejunum and the Roux loop to avoid contamination of bowel content during the procedure. An incision is made on the antimesenteric margin of the Roux loop 40 cm from the end and a stay suture is inserted at each corner of the anastomosis. A double-armed 3/0 suture is inserted at the mid point of the posterior wall and tied. The posterior wall is completed using each of the sutures. The corner stay sutures are tied and each arm continued to fashion the anterior wall. The sutures are now tied at the point where they meet in the middle of the anterior layer.

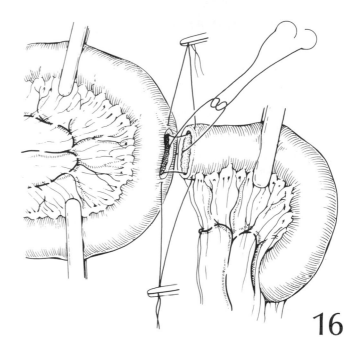

16

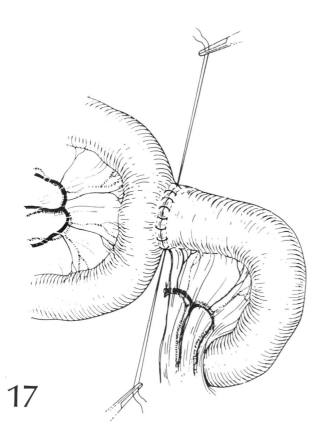

17

17 The ligated edges of the mesentery are examined to ensure that haemostasis is secure. The remaining defect in the transverse mesocolon adjacent to the jejunal loop is carefully closed using fine sutures and the divided surfaces of the mesentery are apposed to prevent internal herniation.

CHOLEDOCHODUODENOSTOMY

18 Before embarking on a choledochoduodenostomy, evaluation of the mobility of the duodenum and bile duct is essential to ensure absence of
tumour encroachment and tension-free approximation.
A Kocher incision with freeing of the lateral margin of
the duodenum may be required to achieve the
necessary mobility. The gallbladder is removed and the
choledochotomy performed between two 5/0 stay
sutures. A longitudinal incision is made in the post-
bulbar duodenum, the mid point of the incision being
centred on the choledochotomy. The duodenal incision
tends to stretch with manipulation and should therefore
always be slightly smaller than the biliary incision. A stay
suture is placed through each apex of the duodenotomy
to the mid point of each wall of the choledochal incision
(A). A similar stay suture is placed through the inferior
apex of the choledochotomy to the mid point of the
posterior wall of the duodenal incision (B). These three
stay sutures are tied to fashion the posterior wall of the
anastomosis. The anastomosis can be performed using
either a continuous suture beginning at the mid point of
the posterior wall or by using interrupted sutures.

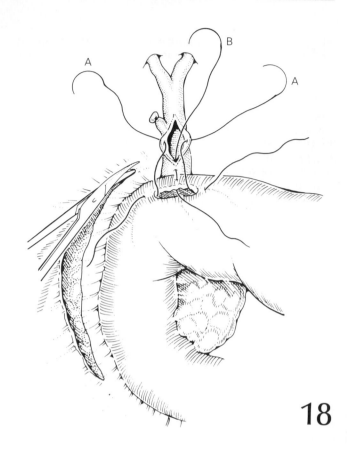

18

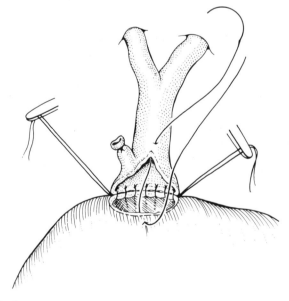

19

19 The posterior wall is completed by placing the
remainder of the interrupted 3/0 absorbable
monofilament sutures. The sutures are inserted so that
the knots are tied on the inside of the lumen. The
anterior wall is similarly constructed by placing a stay
suture from the mid point of the duodenum to the
superior apex of the choledochotomy.

20 Interrupted sutures are placed between the stay sutures to complete the anastomosis. The knots are tied on the outside. A 6-mm closed suction drain is placed in Morrison's pouch.

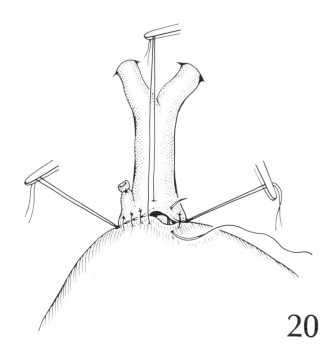

20

GASTROENTEROSTOMY

21 The gastroenterostomy can be performed by placing the jejunal loop either in an antecolic or a retrocolic position. The selection is often an arbitrary decision based on the extent of both local and regional tumour spread and anatomical factors including mobility of the small bowel mesentery and body habitus. It is important to place the gastroenterostomy in the antrum close to the greater curvature to avoid stomal malfunction. The site for the anastomosis on the anterior wall of the stomach is selected and marked by applying Babcock forceps. A loop of jejunum is then brought anterior to the colon for an isoperistaltic anastomosis. The loop is selected so that the afferent limb is short but not under any tension. An extra few centimetres of slack allows for any subsequent colonic distension without compromise behind the jejunal loop.

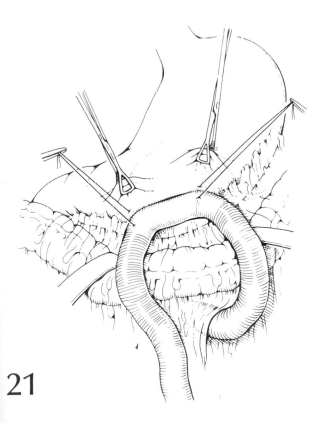

21

22 Corner sutures are first placed about 8 cm apart and the jejunum is attached to the stomach using a continuous row of 3/0 seromuscular sutures. This posterior row of sutures should be placed on the jejunum midway between the mesentery and the antimesenteric border. The opening in the stomach is made about 5 mm from the row of sutures, extending from one corner suture to the other, using cautery. If large submucosal vessels are encountered these are best secured by underrunning with 3/0 absorbable sutures. Fluid within the stomach is aspirated to avoid contamination during surgery. The opening in the jejunum is similarly made 5 mm from the previous suture line after applying a soft bowel clamp to prevent bowel content spillage. The jejunal opening should be slightly smaller than the gastric opening because the jejunal wall stretches and the opening gets larger during the performance of the anastomosis.

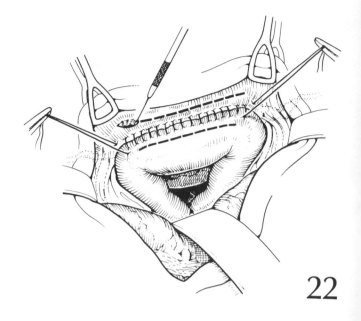

22

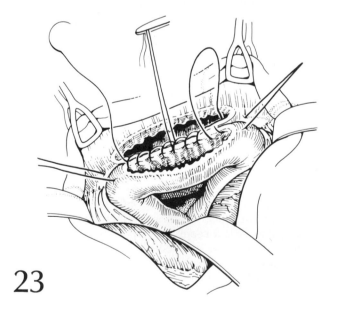

23

23 Next the posterior inner layer of sutures is placed. Continuous absorbable 3/0 sutures are used, beginning in the middle of the posterior wall and progressing laterally in both directions. These sutures are haemostatic and should encompass the full wall of both the stomach and jejunum. The suture is carried on to the anterior wall, bringing the edges of the stomach and jejunum together. This suture will form the inner layer of the anterior portion of the anastomosis. A Connell suture is useful and simplifies inversion of the mucosa when the corners of the anterior wall of the anastomosis are fashioned. Continuous 3/0 sutures are next inserted to complete the outer wall of the anterior portion of the gastroenterostomy.

24 The construction of a retrocolic gastrojejunostomy is similar to that of the antecolic
technique. The lesser sac is entered by dividing the
gastrocolic omentum and the posterior wall of the
stomach is exposed. The transverse colon is retracted
out of the wound and the transverse mesocolon
transilluminated to visualize the middle colic vessels
and its branches. An avascular portion of the mesocolon
is selected, usually to the left of the middle colic vessels,
and is opened for a distance of 8 cm.

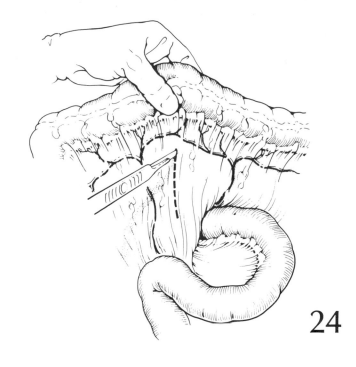

24

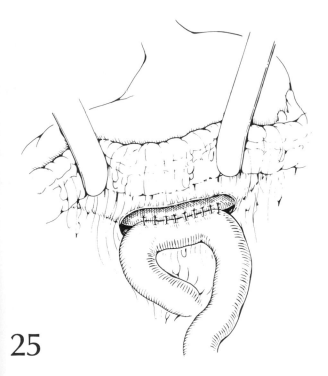

25

25 After completion of the anterior wall of the
gastroenterostomy the defect in the transverse
mesocolon is closed.

26 When a retrocolic Roux loop is used for biliary drainage, the same loop can be used for the gastric bypass. Passage through the transverse mesocolon should be near the hepatic flexure and to the right of the middle colic vessels. This route has the benefit of avoiding entry into the lesser sac and provides the shortest access to the porta hepatis. In addition, potential kinking of the loop is avoided by constructing the gastrojejunostomy first. The additional advantage of the gastric anastomosis above the biliary anastomosis is avoidance of troublesome bile reflux into the stomach.

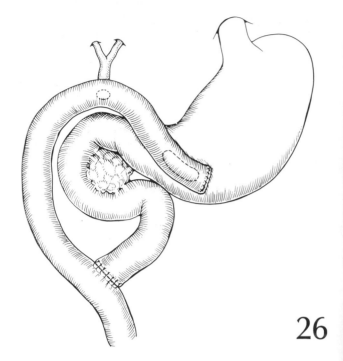

26

Postoperative care

Most patients can be managed in a general surgical ward during the postoperative period unless comorbid systemic illnesses require support in an intensive care unit. Fluid balance needs careful monitoring to avoid renal failure and perioperative antibiotic therapy should continue for 24 h unless other indications dictate longer treatment. The nasogastric tube can usually be removed after 2–3 days with return of bowel sounds, or when the nasogastric drainage is less than 500 ml over a 24 h period. Abdominal drains can be removed after 3–4 days unless the operation is complicated by a bile leak or bowel fistula.

Functional delayed gastric emptying is not infrequently encountered, particularly in patients with advanced disease who have undergone a gastroenterosotmy. Prokinetic drugs are usually unhelpful and some patients may require nasojejunal feeding or parenteral nutrition. Other complications include bleeding due to coagulopathy, renal failure as part of the hepatorenal syndrome, sepsis, and delayed healing with wound dehiscence and anastomotic leaks.

Reports on morbidity and mortality after palliative bypass operations remain distressingly high[10]. However, most complications can be avoided by careful selection of treatment options (including non-operative stenting), appropriate preoperative preparation and performance of operations by experienced surgeons.

References

1. Krige JE, Bornman PC, Terblanche J. Optimal palliation of pancreatic carcinoma. *S Afr Med J* 1992; 81: 238–40.

2. Bornman PC, Harries-Jones EP, Tobias R, Van Stiegmann G, Terblanche J. Prospective controlled trial of transhepatic biliary endoprosthesis versus bypass surgery for incurable carcinoma of head of pancreas. *Lancet* 1986; i: 69–71.

3. Smith AC, Dowsett JF, Russell RCG, Hatfield ARW, Cotton PB. Randomised trial of endoscopic stenting versus surgical bypass in malignant low bile duct obstruction. *Lancet* 1994; 344: 1655–60.

4. Singh SM, Reber HA. Surgical palliation for pancreatic cancer. *Surg Clin North Am* 1990; 63: 599–611.

5. Gudjonsson B. Cancer of the pancreas: 50 years of surgery. *Cancer* 1987; 60: 2284–303.

6. Bornman PC, Krige JEJ. Surgical palliation of pancreatic and periampullary tumours. In: Trede M, Carter DC, eds. *Surgery of the Pancreas*. Edinburgh: Churchill Livingstone, 1993: 497–513.

7. Keighley MR, Razay G, Fitzgerald MG. Influence of diabetes on mortality and morbidity following operations for obstructive jaundice. *Ann R Coll Surg Engl* 1984; 66: 49–51.

8. McPherson GA, Benjamin IS, Habib NA, Bowley NB, Blumgart LH. Percutaneous transhepatic drainage in obstructive jaundice: advantages and problems. *Br J Surg* 1982; 69: 261–4.

9. Voyles CR, Blumgart LH. A technique for the construction of high biliary-enteric anastomoses. *Surg Gynecol Obstet* 1982; 154: 885–7.

10. Schouten JT. Operative therapy for pancreatic carcinoma. *Am J Surg* 1986; 151: 626–30.

Illustrations by Gillian Lee and the late Robert Lane

Rectal biopsy

Robin K. S. Phillips MS, FRCS
Consultant Surgeon, St Mark's Hospital For Diseases of the Rectum and Colon and Homerton Hospital, London and Honorary Lecturer, St Bartholomew's Hospital Medical School, London, UK

Biopsy is a diagnostic procedure which, unless carried out correctly, may fail in its purpose. The biopsy may be mucosal, excisional, full-thickness, or taken from an abnormal structure. Each requires special care to achieve the best results.

Operations

MUCOSAL BIOPSY

1, 2 A simple mucosal biopsy is carried out for diseases which are primarily superficial, e.g. ulcerative, Crohn's and ischaemic colitis, amoebic disease, and solitary ulcer syndrome. No anaesthetic is required. The procedure is usually easy but may be difficult when the mucosa is very atrophic as in the chronic inactive phase of ulcerative colitis. A satisfactory result can be obtained with an 'Officer's' heavy biopsy forceps; the piece of mucosa is twisted off by rotating the instrument until the specimen comes away without traction. This reduces the possibility of bleeding from the biopsy site.

Sharp cutting forceps (including suction biopsy apparatus) should not be used unless the edges are sharpened regularly because, when blunt, bleeding may occur.

With flexible instruments there is also the opportunity for 'hot' biopsy. With this technique, the appropriate endoscopic biopsy forceps grasp the lesion, which is tented up. A coagulating diathermy current is then passed until the apex of the tented mucosa turns white, and the biopsy is taken. The technique is appropriate for sampling and destroying small polyps, but larger polyps require snare removal. Diathermy artefacts and the small risk of secondary haemorrhage make the use of the 'hot' procedure inappropriate for routine diagnostic biopsy.

Regardless of the method used, pathologists prefer a specimen that is not fixed 'curled-up' because the glandular structure becomes distorted. The biopsy should be pressed down, mucosa upwards, on a piece of ground glass, thick blotting paper or card before being placed in a fixative solution. It is probably wise to defer a barium enema examination for at least 1 week after a biopsy has been taken because of the small risk of intestinal perforation.

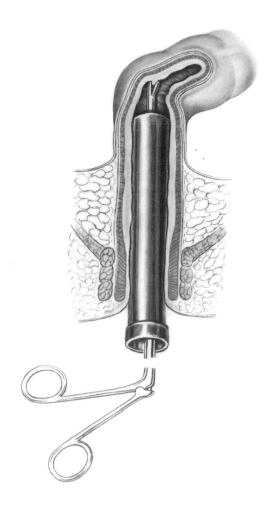

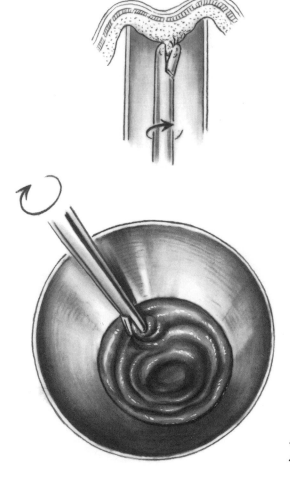

1

2

EXCISION BIOPSY

3 The forceps or snare is placed over the lesion or around its base and the whole structure is removed. In the case of a pedunculated lesion, the wire loop of the snare is passed over the polyp which is gently shaken until the wire lies around the stalk. The loop is tightened until it grips the stalk and then the instrument is retracted slightly so that minimal traction is exerted on the stalk. The diathermy current is passed using multiple very short bursts at 5-s intervals, tightening the wire slowly until the polyp is removed. *A long continuous current must never be used.*

If the pedicle bleeds, it should be touched with a fulgurating button using a coagulating current, or a swab of 1:1000 topical adrenaline may be applied.

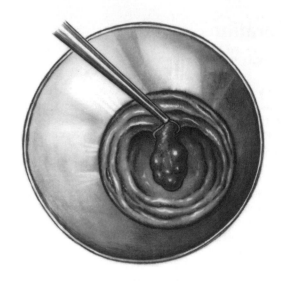

3

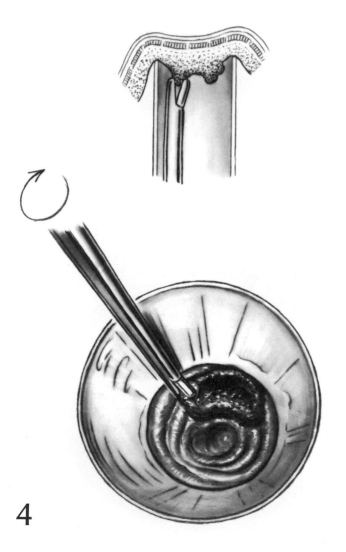

4

BIOPSY OF ABNORMAL STRUCTURES

When an abnormal structure such as a tumour is seen, two decisions must be made — whether it can be removed completely (excision biopsy) and, if not, from which area is a correct diagnosis (diagnostic biopsy) most likely to be obtained. All biopsies are liable to sampling error if only a part of the lesion is sampled. Thus, if a tumour is small or pedunculated, it should usually be removed totally either by twisting or by snaring using electrocoagulation. This can be done without an anaesthetic and the intestine does not normally require any special cleansing.

4 If the lesion is larger and not completely removable, the biopsy should be taken with Officer's forceps, from the edge where the mucosa alters its characteristics, e.g. the rolled everted edge of a malignant ulcer. If the lesion is within reach of the finger it may be reasonable to take the biopsy from the most indurated area. This is particularly necessary for patients with a villous adenoma, which is very soft when benign but becomes indurated when malignant, when it is recurrent, or after previous diathermy treatment.

It is very unwise and dangerous to make a blind 'grab' at a lesion, particularly when it is of uncertain nature, because bleeding and perforation may occur. If a whole polyp is removed, its stalk or base should be identified with a stitch because this is the area where tumour infiltration needs to be sought by the pathologist.

FULL-THICKNESS RECTAL BIOPSY

A full-thickness rectal biopsy may be required on some occasions to diagnose Hirschsprung's disease (aganglionosis) or some similar rare disorders with either hyperganglionosis or hypoganglionosis. In infants a full-thickness biopsy is usually unnecessary because the diagnosis of Hirschsprung's disease may be made: (1) by seeing abnormal nerve fibres in the submucosa of the mucosal biopsy; (2) by special staining techniques; (3) supported physiologically by an absent anorectal inhibitory reflex. In the adult in whom the diagnosis is suspected or if a megacolon is present, however, a full-thickness biopsy should be taken. These patients are usually very constipated and therefore it may be necessary to spend several days clearing the intestine. It is essential that the intestine should be clear before this diagnostic procedure is carried out to avoid dangerous extrarectal sepsis. A general anaesthetic is required.

Position of patient

The patient is placed either in the lithotomy or prone jack-knife position and an Eisenhammer or Parks' speculum is inserted. The biopsy is best taken from the left posterior quadrant. It must be from above the upper limit of the internal sphincter muscle, which is normally an aganglionic area. The anorectal ring is palpated to determine the upper limit of the sphincter complex.

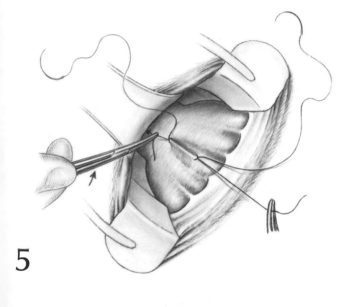

5

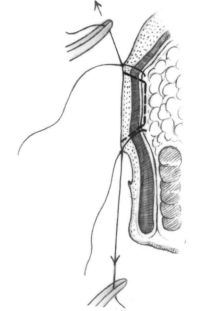

6

Incision

5, 6 Stay sutures of 2/0 absorbable material are placed through the thickness of the rectal wall 2–3 cm apart and tied. If they are correctly placed, incorporating muscle, a characteristic blanching occurs as they are secured. One end of the upper stitch is gripped in an artery forceps which is pushed forwards and upwards by an assistant. The lower stitch is pulled downwards and backwards by the operator. The other end of the upper suture with the needle attached is left in order to oversew the defect in one full-thickness layer when the piece of tissue has been removed. Thus, the purpose of the two stay sutures is to raise and control a full-thickness ridge of rectal wall and to facilitate removal of the tissue. Suction to remove blood may be helpful.

7 A transverse incision is made with scissors or with diathermy set on a coagulating current directly through the full thickness of the intestinal wall, just above the lower stay stitch. As soon as the muscle coat is seen, it should be grasped with Allis' forceps; the muscle layer should not be relinquished, otherwise it will retract and a mucosal biopsy can easily result.

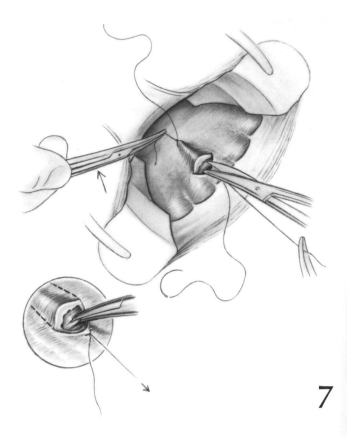

7

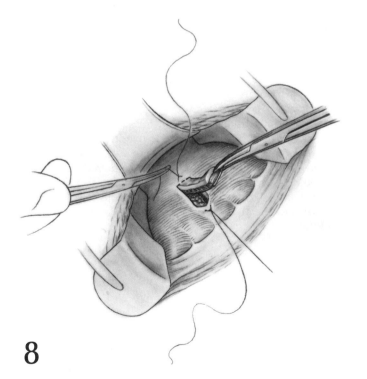

8

8 Parallel cuts 3 mm apart are made vertically up the rectum (longitudinally) to the upper stay suture and the specimen is removed.

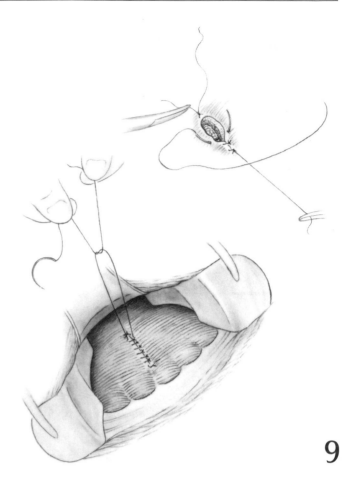

Wound closure

9 The defect is closed with interrupted 2/0 absorbable sutures taking all layers of the intestinal wall.

The retractor is closed slightly to see whether bleeding has been controlled. A further full-thickness stitch may be inserted if necessary and a piece of haemostatic gauze placed on the area.

9

Postoperative care and complications

No special treatment is needed after operation, but bulk stool softeners are preferred to oil-containing laxatives. No postrectal abscesses or fistulae have resulted from this procedure, nor has secondary haemorrhage occurred in the author's experience.

Sepsis prevention in colorectal surgery

Steven D. Wexner MD, FACS, FASCRS, FACG
Staff Colorectal Surgeon, Residency Program Director, Department of Colorectal Surgery, and Director of Anorectal Physiology Laboratory, Cleveland Clinic Florida, Fort Lauderdale, Florida, USA

David E. Beck MD, FACS, FASCRS
Staff Colorectal Surgeon, Department of Colon and Rectal Surgery, Oschner Clinic, New Orleans, Louisiana, USA

Operative technique is one of the most important factors that can limit morbidity and mortality rates in colorectal surgery. The measures described in this chapter complement but cannot replace good technique. Each surgeon uses multiple measures to obtain good results. Thus, the large number of factors involved has made it difficult to study the influence of each measure on the incidence of septic complications.

Biology of tissue contamination

Wound infections result from contamination with either skin or bowel flora, while intra-abdominal abscesses result from contamination with bowel contents. An adequate number of bacteria and a suitable environment must be present for an 'infection' to become established. A colony count of at least ten is usually required to produce infection in normal tissue. The presence of devitalized tissue, foreign bodies or haematoma reduces the number of bacteria required, re-emphasizing the importance of good surgical technique.

Skin flora contains predominantly Gram-positive cocci, whereas the intestine contains a mixture of bacteria (*Table 1*).

Patient factors are also important. The presence of a distant infection, such as within the urinary tract, significantly increases the incidence of postoperative sepsis. Patients with diabetes and other immunocompromised patients have well documented higher incidences of infections, probably caused by their reduced ability to suppress bacteria.

Bowel preparation

The major septic risk associated with a colonic resection is from colonic bacterial contamination. Preoperative preparation to 'clean' the bowel has become standard practice in colonic and rectal surgery, and consists of two components: mechanical cleansing and antibiotic preparation. A 'clean' colon reduces the incidence of infectious complications and anastomotic disruption, simplifies colonic surgery, and is certainly more aesthetically pleasing to the surgeon. The ideal mechanical bowel preparation would be safe, cost-effective, rapid, provide good cleansing, and cause minimal patient discomfort and inconvenience. Furthermore, it should be easy to administer, for both inpatient and outpatient usage. Several methods are available, but no method has yet fulfilled all these criteria.

Mechanical preparation options

Dietary restriction

This method is insufficient by itself to cleanse the colon adequately. However, 1–5 days of a clear liquid diet may be used as an adjunctive preparatory measure.

Cathartics

Cathartics stimulate bowel evacuation. Medications commonly used include castor oil, magnesium citrate, senna concentrate or bisacodyl. Regimens that employ these medications usually require 2–3 days to empty the colon of stool and are frequently combined with enemas and dietary restrictions. These agents have been associated with dehydration and electrolyte changes, and frequently cause abdominal cramps and anal irritation. In controlled trials using cathartics, adequate cleansing occurred in only 75% of patients. Some surgeons have reverted to the use of a phosphate soda preparation.

Enemas

Enemas (saline, soap suds, tap water) work by dilution or irritation. They are messy and uncomfortable for patients and the nursing staff, and rarely provide adequate cleansing when used alone. They may be helpful in patients with an obstructing lesion who should not be given any oral bowel preparation.

Oral lavage

Oral lavage methods, which usually require only 2–4 h, have been developed to reduce the time required for mechanical cleansing.

Three solutions have been described. The first is saline (1.5–2 l/h via a small 10-Fr nasogastric tube for 4–5 h), which has been associated with fluid and electrolyte disturbances and weight gain. It should not be used in patients with compromised renal or cardiovascular status and is rarely used in current clinical practice.

Mannitol is an osmotic agent which is not absorbed. It causes clinical dehydration and is metabolized by colonic bacteria, resulting in increased infection rates and combustible gas production. Because of these disadvantages and the risk of bowel gas explosions, mannitol should seldom be used.

Polyethylene glycol electrolyte gastrointestinal lavage (PEG lavage) is an isosmotic solution composed of polyethylene glycol 3350 and an electrolyte solution (sodium, 125 mmol/l; sulphate, 40 mmol/l; chloride, 35 mmol/l; bicarbonate, 20 mmol/l; and potassium, 10 mmol/l). In the USA, this solution is available commercially as Golytely and Colyte. It provides excellent cleansing in 90–100% of patients and is associated with neither fluid nor electrolyte problems. It has a mildly salty taste, is well tolerated by most patients, and clinical trials have demonstrated its superiority over other methods. A new solution, NuLytely, has an improved taste and, in controlled trials, appears to clean as well as other PEG lavage solutions.

Intraoperative lavage methods have been described for patients requiring emergency operations. Proponents of these techniques suggest that their use may allow the safe accomplishment of a primary anastomosis after resection.

The transrectal method involves placing a large Malecot or de Pezzar latex catheter (32–34 Fr) into the rectum via the anus. This allows irrigation of the left colon, which may be accomplished before or during the operation.

Although cumbersome, these latter two methods may adequately cleanse the colon, thus permitting a primary anastomosis in selected cases.

Antibiotic preparation options

Mechanical cleansing of the bowel reduces the amount of stool and bacteria, but does not alter the concentration of bacteria remaining in the colon. Use of appropriate prophylactic antibiotics in several prospective studies has reduced the incidence of infectious complications associated with colonic resections from 40–50% to approximately 5–10%. To be effective, the drugs must cover the spectrum of both Gram-negative and anaerobic bacteria adequately. Furthermore, they must be administered before bacterial contamination to provide adequate intraluminal and tissue levels. Finally, the duration of use must be short to reduce the development of resistant bacterial strains (less than 24–48 h).

Bowel flora

The colon contains a large number of bacteria. The species of bacteria and their mean stool concentrations are listed in *Table 1*. Bacteriological studies have demonstrated that there is a wide variation in the bacterial species between individuals, but that the flora of each person remains relatively stable over time.

Methods

Luminal antibiotics are inexpensive and effective. Overgrowth of resistant bacteria is avoided if these agents are used for less than 24 h. The systemic absorption of these agents is variable and there is controversy about the importance of luminal and tissue concentrations. These medications may cause gastrointestinal discomfort or diarrhoea. Appropriate agents are listed in *Table 2*. Product information should be consulted to confirm dosages.

Systemic (parenteral) antibiotics produce results equal to those produced by luminal medications if the appropriate drugs are used and if they are administered immediately before surgery. Adequate tissue levels must be present at the time of contamination. Appropriate agents and their recommended dosages are described in *Table 3*. Again the dosages should be confirmed before use.

Table 1   Colonic bacteria

Organism	Concentration in stool*
Anaerobic	
Gram-negative bacilli	
Bacteroides fragilis	10^9
Bacteroides spp.	10^8
Gram-positive cocci	10^7
Gram-positive bacilli	
Clostridia spp.	10^7
Aerobic	
Gram-negative bacilli	
Escherichia coli	10^8
Klebsiella spp.	10^6
Gram-positive cocci	
Streptococcus (*Enterococcus*)	
faecalis	10^6
Staphylococcus aureus	10^6

* Log counts/g stool

Table 2   Oral antibiotic agents

Medication	Bacterial cover*	Dosage
Erythromycin	Gram-positive, anaerobic	1 g
Neomycin	Gram-negative	1 g
Metronidazole	Anaerobic	500 mg

* An anti-aerobic agent must be combined with an anti-anaerobic agent. Acceptable combinations include erythromycin and neomycin or metronidazole and neomycin (see text)

Table 3   Parenteral antibiotic agents

Medication	Spectrum of cover	Dosage
Cefotetan	Gram-positive, Gram-negative, anaerobic	1 g (every 12 h)
Cefotaxime	Gram-positive, Gram-negative, anaerobic	1–2 g (every 8 h)
Cefoxitin	Gram-positive, Gram-negative, anaerobic	1–2 g (every 6 h)
Gentamicin	Gram-negative, aerobic	80 mg (every 8 h)
Clindamycin	Aerobic, anaerobic	150 mg (every 6 h)
Metronidazole	Anaerobic	500 mg (every 6 h)

Topical antibiotics can also be used at surgery. These have been found to be equivalent to other methods of prophylactic antibiotic administration in reducing infectious complications.

Combinations of antibiotic methods are difficult to justify because of the additional cost. When single methods have been compared with a combination of methods in prospective trials, there has been no statistical improvement unless the single method has an unusually large infection rate. However, despite the lack of consistent scientific support, the majority of surgeons utilize a combination of methods, usually oral and systemic agents together.

Recommendations

A 1-day preparation provides good cleansing and its short duration makes it cost effective.

Mechanical cleansing (PEG lavage preparation)

A clear liquid diet is started on the day before surgery. In the morning, PEG lavage is started: 240 ml orally every 10 min (1.5 l/h) until diarrhoea becomes clear and free of particulate matter.

Some surgeons also administer metoclopramide, 10 mg by mouth, 1 h before beginning PEG lavage as it may reduce nausea and bloating. Two bisacodyl tablets may also be administered after completing the PEG lavage to evacuate any remaining colonic fluid. Although clinically helpful in selected patients, these adjunctive medications have not demonstrated a significant improvement in controlled trials.

Antibiotics

One or more of the following regimens may be selected.

Oral antibiotics

Three doses of neomycin (1 g orally) and erythromycin (1 g orally) the day before surgery at 13.00, 14.00 and 23.00 hours. Metronidazole (1 g orally) may be substituted for the erythromycin.

Parenteral antibiotics

Any one of the following may be chosen.

1. Intravenous cefotetan, 1 g, on call to the operating room.

2. Intravenous cefoxitin, 1 g, on call to the operating room and every 6 h for three doses after surgery.
3. Intravenous cefotaxime, 2 g, and intravenous metronidazole, 1 g, on call to the operating room.

Topical

A first generation cephalosporin can be used, e.g. cefapirin sodium, 1 g/l of saline. The abdomen and wound should be irrigated at the end of the operation.

Intraoperative limitations of contamination

During surgery the important principles of adequate exposure, haemostasis and the correct operation performed in the proper manner remain extremely important. Bowel preparation as described above reduces but does not eliminate the potential for contamination. Additional measures are thought to be helpful but it has been difficult to document this in well controlled studies.

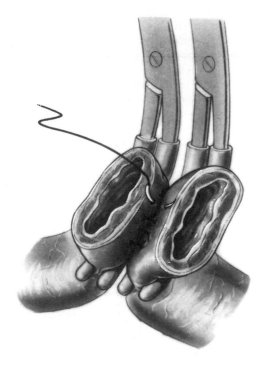

1

1 Traction sutures or atraumatic clamps can be used to keep the open ends of the bowel elevated. This in turn reduces the chances of intestinal contents spilling into the surgical field.

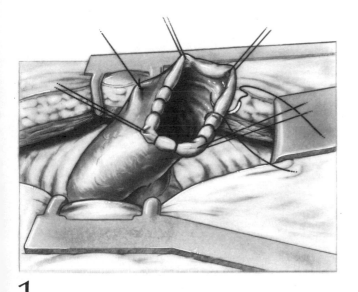

2

2 Atraumatic bowel clamps such as Glassman, Dennis or Satinsky clamps, or ties (umbilical tapes or Penrose drains) prevent retained intestinal contents from spilling into the open ends of the bowel and contaminating the abdominal cavity or wound. Swabbing the ends of the open bowel with povidone-iodine or an antibiotic solution may also aid in reducing infectious complications. Packing loops of bowel away from open ends of bowel and covering exposed loops with laparotomy pads or towels helps limit gross particulate contamination.

3 Sponges and plastic barrier drapes can be placed on the exposed wound edges: these probably help to prevent wound contamination. They have not, however, been proven statistically to reduce the incidence of wound infections.

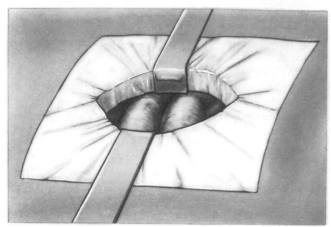

3

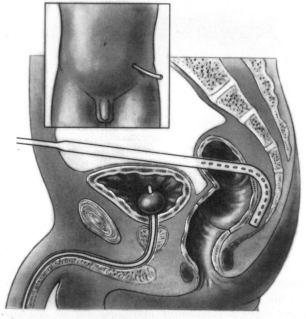

4

Drains

4 Multiple prospective studies have evaluated the use of abdominal drains. It is generally accepted that drains are ineffective in the abdominal cavity. However, the pelvis is different because it forms a rigid non-collapsible space that can store blood or peritoneal fluid. Both of these substances are excellent culture media for bacteria. Therefore, although placement of pelvic drains is reasonable, their use is not mandatory.

5   When suction drains are used they are generally removed on the second postoperative day. All studies have shown a reduced incidence of infection with closed suction drains when compared with Penrose drains.

Some authors have proposed irrigation of the pelvis to assist in evacuation of retained pelvic secretions and blood. However, a prospective controlled trial demonstrated no difference between suction sump drains with irrigation and those in which suction alone was employed.

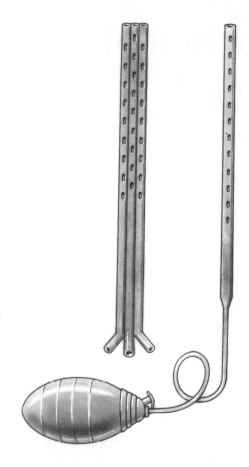

5

Wounds

Historically, the incidence of wound infection after colonic resection averaged 30–40%. These high incidences were associated with poor mechanical preparation. However, these studies were often uncontrolled and the antibiotics used would not have been considered effective by today's standards. Recent studies in which appropriate antibiotics were used have shown higher infection rates only in patients in whom inadequate cleansing was present. However, the difference frequently failed to reach statistical significance. Current postoperative wound infection rates are usually in the range below 5–10%.

Despite high residual colonic bacterial concentrations, an adequate bowel preparation generally permits primary skin reapposition. Packing the subcutaneous wound open with gauze is very effective in preventing superficial wound infections. This measure is appropriate in emergency operations on unprepared bowel in which gross faecal contamination is noted.

Further reading

Beck DE, DiPalma JA. A new oral lavage solution versus cathartics and enema method for preoperative colonic cleansing. *Arch Surg* 1991; 126: 552–5.

Condon RE. Intestinal antisepsis: rationale and results. *World J Surg* 1982; 6: 182–7.

Gorbach SL, Nahas L, Lerner PI, Weinstein L. Studies of intestinal microflora. *Gastroenterology* 1967; 53: 845–55.

Hares MM, Alexander-Williams J. The effect of bowel preparation on colonic surgery. *World J Surg* 1982; 6: 175–81.

Saadia R, Schein M. The place of intraoperative antegrade colonic irrigation in emergency left-sided colonic surgery. *Dis Colon Rectum* 1989; 32: 78–81.

Vernava AM III, Dean P. Preoperative and postoperative management. In: Beck DE, Wexner SD, eds. *Fundamentals of Anorectal Surgery.* New York: McGraw-Hill, 1992: 50–6.

Wilson SE, Sokol T. Antimicrobials in elective colon surgery. *Infect Surg* 1985; 10: 609–11.

Illustrations by Patrick Elliott

Anastomotic suturing techniques

Thomas T. Irvin PhD, ChM, FRCSEd
Consultant Surgeon, Royal Devon and Exeter Hospital (Wonford), Exeter, Devon, UK

History

The basic principles of intestinal suture were established more than 100 years ago by Travers, Lembert, Czerny and Halsted, and have since undergone little modification. However, these pioneers recognized the dangers of intestinal anastomosis. The breakdown or disruption of a suture line in the large intestine may result in peritonitis, faecal fistulation and serious or fatal septic complications. The factors that result in such complications are now well established, and it is apparent that safety in anastomosis of the intestine depends to a large extent on the technical expertise and judgement of the operating surgeon.

The development of stapling instruments for anastomosis of the intestine has added a new dimension to colorectal surgery. There is no difference in the healing properties of stapled or sutured anastomoses, but colorectal surgeons need to be familiar with both methods. Interestingly, it appears that techniques of hand suture have a longer learning curve than stapling methods[1].

Principles and justification

The factors that influence the healing of an anastomosis of the large intestine can be considered under two broad headings: surgeon-related variables and patient-related variables.

Surgeon-related variables

The multicentre Large Bowel Cancer Project co-ordinated from St Mary's Hospital, London[2], established that there was an enormous difference in the incidence of disruption of large bowel anastomoses in the hands of different surgeons, the incidence ranging from 0.5% to more than 30%. Such a wide variation could not be explained by differences in the patients undergoing surgery, and the results of this study imply that there are wide variations in the technical expertise and/or judgement of surgeons performing colonic and colo-rectal anastomoses.

The technical factors which may affect the outcome of anastomosis include: access and exposure, blood supply, suture technique, the use of drains and diversion of the faecal stream.

Access and exposure

Intestinal anastomoses will prove difficult if surgical access and exposure are unsatisfactory. This may result from inadequate anaesthesia, an inappropriate or inadequate incision, and imperfect illumination of the operative field. Poor access may also result from inadequate mobilization of the viscera, a problem which is especially likely to occur in operations involving a low rectal anastomosis.

The surgeon should never have to struggle with an anastomosis because of limited access. When difficulty is encountered, the problem should be carefully assessed and an attempt must be made to improve the exposure. If the difficulty seems insurmountable it is prudent to consider an alternative procedure which avoids an anastomosis or, if possible, to call upon a surgeon with greater experience of such surgery.

Blood supply

A good blood supply is vital to the healing of all wounds, and the preparation for an anastomosis must be meticulous to avoid disturbance of the blood supply to the cut edges of the bowel. The only absolute criterion of an adequate blood supply is the presence of free arterial bleeding from the cut edges of the gut. The absence of a visible or palpable arterial pulse is not necessarily of significance, but blanching or cyanosis of the edges of the bowel and the presence of a dark, venous type of bleeding are signs of an inadequate and thus an unacceptable blood supply.

Blood flow to an anastomosis may be compromised in several ways: undue tension on the suture line resulting from inadequate mobilization of the viscera; devascularization of the bowel during mobilization or preparation for the anastomosis; strangulation of the tissues by tightly knotted sutures; and the excessive use of diathermy coagulation to achieve haemostasis in the cut ends of the bowel.

Before starting an anastomosis the surgeon should ensure that the ends of the bowel can easily be apposed: if the bowel ends overlap it can be safely assumed that there will be no tension on the suture line. Haemostasis in the cut edges of the bowel may be achieved either by individual ligation of vessels or by the use of diathermy coagulation. The latter method has the disadvantage that it may result in a greater degree of tissue necrosis at the suture line, but it is certainly a less tedious technique than the ligation of vessels and, in practice, little tissue damage will result if diathermy is limited to controlling only major bleeding points. Minor oozing should be ignored, but significant arterial bleeding should be checked because these vessels retract within the tissues and produce unpleasant haematomas.

Some surgeons place non-crushing occlusion clamps across the bowel to avoid soiling of the operative field during intestinal anastomosis. However, it is important that these clamps are applied lightly and never across the mesentery of the intestine for fear of damaging the blood supply to the anastomosis.

Suture technique

Secure healing of an intestinal anastomosis is dependent on accurate apposition of the serosal or outer surfaces of the bowel, and this is achieved by the use of a suture technique which inverts the cut edges of the gut.

Most surgeons use an open method of intestinal anastomosis. 'Aseptic' or closed techniques of anastomosis achieved some popularity in the earlier part of this century because of the belief that the breakdown of anastomoses resulted from the bacterial contamination of the peritoneum which occurred during the construction of the open type of anastomosis. Several ingenious techniques of 'aseptic' anastomosis were devised, but they were not generally accompanied by a reduction in the incidence of anastomotic dehiscence. Some surgeons still use closed types of anastomosis for aesthetic reasons.

One aspect of the technique of intestinal suture which has remained the subject of controversy is the use of either one layer or two layers of sutures in an anastomosis. Probably a majority of surgeons now use a single layer of sutures on the grounds that it may cause less ischaemia, tissue necrosis or narrowing of the lumen than a two-layer method.

1a–d

The two-layer anastomosis (*Illustration 1a*) consists of an inner layer of sutures incorporating the full thickness of the bowel wall and an outer layer of sutures inserted through all layers except the mucosa. This second layer is frequently referrred to as a seromuscular stitch, but it should in fact include the collagenous submucosal layer of the bowel since more superficial sutures have a tendency to cut out. Single-layer techniques of suture are shown in *Illustrations 1b–d*. In *Illustration 1b* the suture is inserted from the mucosal aspect of the bowel through the full thickness of the bowel wall and inversion of the anastomosis results when the suture is tied. The Gambee stitch (*Illustration 1c*) is inserted through all layers of the bowel wall and is passed twice through the mucosa on each side of the anastomosis to secure mucosal inversion. The Gambee suture technique thus results in minimal inversion of the cut edges of the bowel. In *Illustration 1d* the suture is a submucosal stitch inserted from the serosal aspect of the bowel, as in the outer layer of a two-layer anastomosis. Matheson and Irving[3] have reported excellent results with this 'serosubmucosal suture' and other experts in colorectal surgery have now adopted this method.

The author uses a single-layer suture technique for colonic and colorectal anastomoses, and a two-layer method for anastomoses involving the caecum or terminal ileum.

Various absorbable and non-absorbable suture materials have been used for anastomosis of the intestine. Experimental studies have suggested that anastomoses made with absorbable sutures are weaker than those made with non-absorbable materials during the early phase of healing, but the difference is slight and probably has no clinical significance. It is usual for two-layer anastomoses to be made with absorbable sutures for the inner layer and non-absorbable sutures for the outer layer. Single-layer anastomoses are usually fashioned with non-absorbable materials.

Chromic catgut is the most popular absorbable suture material, and there is no convincing evidence that other materials such as polyglycolic acid, polyglactin, or polydioxanone are superior for intestinal suture. However, an increasing number of surgeons are using polyglactin (Vicryl) even in single-layer anastomoses.

Non-absorbable suture materials include silk, polypropylene and various synthetic polyesters. There are theoretical advantages to the use of monofilament non-absorbable suture materials (stainless steel wire, nylon or polypropylene) in that these materials provoke less tissue reaction than braided sutures, but these differences are slight and the monofilament sutures have inferior handling characteristics. The author prefers braided non-absorbable suture materials.

The size or gauge of the suture material used in anastomosis of the intestine is not standard, but 2/0 or 3/0 sutures are in common use in adult surgery. The use of ultrafine suture materials for adults is probably

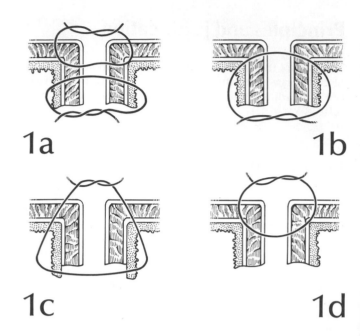

1a   **1b**   **1c**   **1d**

misguided because these sutures may cut through the bowel wall.

Use of drains

The use of peritoneal drains is regarded by some surgeons as a necessary feature of the management of anastomoses, particularly in surgery of the colon and rectum. Many protagonists of the use of drains claim that they safeguard the patient against anastomotic leakage by permitting the development of an enterocutaneous fistula when anastomotic dehiscence occurs rather than a diffusing faecal peritonitis. However, experimental studies have shown that foreign bodies, including drains, placed close to anastomoses actually increase the probability of anastomotic disruption. The value of drains is in removing any blood or serum which may collect in dead space, particularly after low anterior resection of the rectum when such collections may account for a significant incidence of 'late' dehiscence of the suture line.

The author uses small-calibre (Redivac) closed suction drains for the purpose of removing any blood or serum which may collect after operations involving significant dissection or mobilization of the viscera, and in operations complicated by significant faecal contamination. The drains are deliberately not placed in the vicinity of anastomoses and are removed after 48 h.

Faecal diversion

There has been considerable debate concerning the value of a temporary loop colostomy, caecostomy or loop ileostomy to protect anastomoses in the left colon or rectum. These procedures are usually reserved for 'high-risk' anastomoses such as a very low colorectal or coloanal anastomosis or an anastomosis made in the presence of unfavourable local conditions. There is no evidence that proximal faecal diversion prevents anastomotic dehiscence, but it does appear that the septic complications of dehiscence may be less serious when the faecal stream has been diverted.

It is therefore a matter of judgement as to when faecal diversion should be used to protect an anastomosis, and it is apparent from the literature and informal discussion with surgeons that there is considerable variation in the use of such methods. In the case of low colorectal anastomoses, some surgeons use intraoperative leakage tests as a guide to the need for a defunctioning colostomy. In such tests the rectum is distended with air and a colostomy is used if sites of visible leakage of air cannot be repaired. However, other surgeons have suggested that demonstration of an airtight anastomosis is no guarantee of uncomplicated postoperative healing.

In recent years, an intracolonic bypass procedure has been developed as an alternative to faecal diversion by colostomy or ileostomy for the protection of distal left-sided anastomoses in the large intestine[4]. A soft latex tube with a reinforced collar is sutured to the mucosa and submucosa of the bowel wall with absorbable sutures proximal to the anastomosis, thus creating a watertight seal and excluding the anastomosis from contact with the faecal content of the bowel. The device separates spontaneously from the bowel wall and is passed rectally after 2 weeks.

The author uses a loop transverse colostomy to protect the colorectal anastomosis in the following circumstances:

1. When the anastomosis is 6 cm or less from the anal verge.
2. When the anastomosis is close to the site of previous fistulation between the large intestine and the vagina or urinary bladder.
3. When the rectum has suffered irradiation injury.
4. When there are unusual technical difficulties with the anastomosis because of restricted access or obesity.
5. When a very large pelvic dead space exists following operations for extensive malignancies.

This protocol has resulted in complete freedom from life-threatening or fatal complications of anastomotic dehiscence in the author's unit during the past 15 years.

Some surgeons use a loop ileostomy in preference to a colostomy. However, it should be noted that closure of a loop ileostomy is technically more difficult than closure of a loop colostomy and the author would not recommend the use of a defunctioning loop ileostomy unless the surgeon is familiar with the technique of closure of this stoma.

The surgeon should avoid an anastomosis in the presence of established peritoneal sepsis and the bowel should be exteriorized as a colostomy or ileostomy.

Alimentary continuity can be re-established at a later date as an elective procedure.

Postoperative peritoneal sepsis and anastomotic complications may result when significant faecal contamination or soiling of the peritoneum occurs during surgery. In some cases, as in the surgery of advanced tumours of the large intestine, some degree of soiling may be unavoidable, but it should always be regarded as a serious complication. When gross faecal soiling occurs in conjunction with other local factors which may propagate peritoneal infection (residual tumour, extensive retroperitoneal dissection or traumatic injuries to other viscera), it is advisable to avoid an anastomosis and to exteriorize the bowel.

Patient-related variables

Bowel preparation

Faecal loading of the colon has an adverse effect on the healing of colonic or rectal anastomoses. The mechanical state of the bowel may determine the success or failure of anastomoses in the left colon or rectum, and is a major factor in the high incidence of dehiscence which follows primary anastomosis of the left colon in operations for acute obstruction.

In elective colonic surgery, thorough mechanical preparation of the bowel is an integral factor in the safe conduct of colonic and rectal anastomoses, but may be relatively ineffective when there is some degree of colonic obstruction. Dudley et al.[5] described an ingenious method of intraoperative colonic irrigation followed by primary anastomosis in cases complicated by obstruction. This method has found favour with other surgeons but the majority still prefer to avoid an anastomosis and exteriorize the bowel in the presence of gross large bowel obstruction. Alimentary continuity is re-established at a second operation. The author believes that there is a place for both methods. Intraoperative colonic lavage adds significantly to the operating time and may be inappropriate in operations on unfit patients.

Surprisingly, the bacterial content of the colon remains high despite mechanical preparation and it is customary to use antimicrobial agents to reduce the infectivity of the colonic contents. There is no convincing evidence that prophylactic antimicrobial therapy prevents anastomotic dehiscence, but it results in a reduction in the incidence of abdominal wound infection after intestinal surgery and the septic complications of anastomotic dehiscence may be less severe when the bowel is prepared with antibiotics. Most oral antibiotic regimens effective in 'sterilizing' the intestinal contents have the potential disadvantage that they may cause a clostridial pseudomembranous colitis, but the short-term use of systemic antibiotics is less likely to lead to this complication.

Systemic factors

The precise role of systemic abnormalities in the pathogenesis of anastomotic dehiscence has not been clearly defined, but it seems probable that such factors are of much less significance than the presence of local sepsis, colonic obstruction, or surgeon-related variables. The systemic factors which do appear to exert an unfavourable effect on anastomotic healing include advanced malignancy, malnutrition and colorectal operations resulting in excessive blood loss.

Severe malnutrition leads to reduced collagen synthesis and impaired healing of colonic anastomoses, and several factors may account for the relationship between excessive blood loss and the healing of anastomoses. Traumatic or bloody operations on the colon in experimental animals result in peritoneal sepsis and, as a consequence, an increased incidence of anastomotic dehiscence. This factor may partly account for the high incidence of anastomotic dehiscence in patients with advanced malignant disease since this seems to be largely a complication of extensive operations for the removal of fixed tumours. Moreoever, major intraoperative blood loss has disproportionately severe effects on the splanchnic circulation, and the resulting intestinal ischaemia may have adverse effects on colonic healing.

Preoperative

Preoperative assessment must take account of the general medical status or fitness of the patient as well as specific consideration of the intestinal disease and the appropriate method of surgical treatment. It should be noted that the majority of fatalities after surgery of the large intestine are due to complications of coexisting medical disease rather than to specific complications of surgery, and the risks are greatly increased in the elderly and in emergency operations. The surgeon is ultimately responsible for the safety of the patient, but the preoperative assessment is a joint exercise involving the anaesthetist and, on occasions, specialist physicians.

Preoperative investigations to determine the extent of the large bowel pathology will not be discussed here. The issues which do require discussion are: selection of the appropriate surgeon for the operation, informed consent, preparation of the large intestine, and perioperative antibiotic therapy.

Selection of surgeon

It is essential that the surgeon and anaesthetist have appropriate skills to treat the patient. This may seem an elementary point but the Confidential Enquiry into Perioperative Deaths[6] showed that surgeons and anaesthetists undertaking the treatment of patients who are seriously ill are sometimes lacking in appropriate skills or experience. It is the responsibility of the consultant in charge of the patient to ensure that the surgeon actually performing the operation has the appropriate experience.

Informed consent

Patients undergoing surgical operations in the UK remain less informed than their counterparts in the USA but this situation is changing. Department of Health guidelines suggest that patients must be informed of any substantial risk associated with the proposed treatment, and that they have the right to refuse certain types of treatment.

It is essential that the surgeon discusses with the patient the possibility of a stoma as part of the operative treatment, carefully explaining the reasons why such an arrangement might become necessary, and whether it is likely to be temporary or permanent. Some patients may not wish to have a stoma under any circumstances and the surgeon must be aware of this before embarking upon the operation.

Preparation of large intestine

Mechanical preparation

2 In the absence of partial or complete obstruction of the bowel, modern methods of mechanical preparation should ensure that the large intestine is virtually empty. These new methods achieve mechanical cleansing of the gut more rapidly than the traditional methods of purging or enema, and they involve the use of whole gut irrigation or powerful stimulant laxatives.

The original technique of whole gut irrigation involved the administration of 4 litres of normal saline by nasogastric tube every hour for a period of 3 h, but patient compliance was rather poor and there was some risk of salt and water absorption resulting in fluid overload in the elderly. The modern technique involves the administration of 3–4 litres of a polyethylene glycol electrolyte solution over a period of 3 h by oral ingestion or by nasogastric tube. The appearance of the colonic lumen through the colonoscope after whole gut irrigation is shown.

The most effective stimulant laxative is Picolax (sodium picosulphate and magnesium citrate). Two sachets are taken on the day before surgery, one in the morning and a second in the afternoon. This is the method used by the author.

Preoperative mechanical preparation should not be attempted if there is evidence of obstruction of the intestine, even if the obstruction is incomplete. The preparation will be ineffectual, unhelpful and potentially dangerous. In such circumstances, the surgeon must consider alternative strategies such as intraoperative colonic irrigation, resection of the obstructed bowel, the use of an intracolonic bypass tube or avoidance of a primary anastomosis.

Antimicrobial preparation

Various antibiotic regimens are used to reduce the infectivity of the gut content and to minimize the effects of faecal spillage during operations on the large intestine. Some surgeons limit the use of antibiotics to the perioperative period, while others also administer antimicrobial agents during preoperative mechanical preparation of the bowel.

The author gives patients oral metronidazole, 200 mg every 8 h, for 48 h before surgery.

Perioperative antibiotic therapy

It has been shown that perioperative use of intravenous broad-spectrum antibiotics results in a significant reduction in the incidence of abdominal wound sepsis in colorectal surgery. Such therapy may also reduce the risks of intra-abdominal septic complications, particularly in cases complicated by significant faecal soiling of

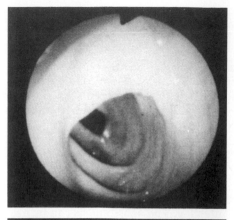

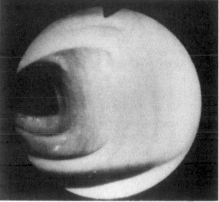

2

the peritoneum, and some surgeons use perioperative intravenous antibiotics in preference to preoperative oral medication. The antibiotics in most common use are second or third generation cephalosporins, and many surgeons combine these drugs with metronidazole because of its activity against *Bacteroides* spp.

The author uses the following regimen: cefuroxime, 1.5 g, is given by intravenous injection with induction of anaesthesia, and two further intravenous doses of 750 mg are given at intervals of 8 h. Metronidazole is not given routinely unless there is evidence of significant sepsis or faecal soiling at operation. In such cases, this drug is given in a dose of 500 mg every 6 h by intravenous infusion, and is continued together with cefuroxime for 3–5 days.

Anaesthesia

Nearly all abdominal operations on the large intestine are carried out under general anaesthesia with full muscle relaxation, although it is possible to carry out resections and anastomoses under spinal anaesthesia. Some significance has been attached to the use of parasympathomimetic drugs such as neostigmine in the reversal of muscle relaxants since the muscarinic effects on the large intestine might result in disruption of an anastomosis. The author is not convinced that such dangers exist in actual practice and has not encountered a case in which such complications ensued.

Operations

Anastomoses may be made end-to-end, end-to-side, side-to-end or side-to-side. In this section the indications for the use of the different types of anastomosis and the techniques of intestinal suture will be described.

END-TO-END ANASTOMOSIS

This method of anastomosis is applicable at any level in the large intestine. The anastomosis can be made either with a two-layer or a single-layer method of suture but the author, in common with many other surgeons, prefers the single-layer method for most colonic and colorectal anastomoses.

Single-layer method

Braided non-absorbable suture materials such as silk or a synthetic polyester are generally preferred, but some surgeons use an absorbable polyglactin (Vicryl) suture.

Methods of suture

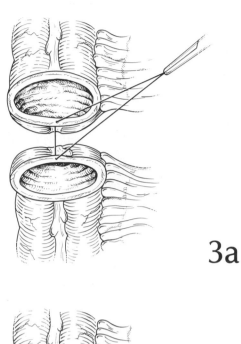

3a

3a–c Various suture techniques are used in single-layer anastomoses, and more than one technique may be used in an individual anastomosis. The suture may be a serosubmucosal stitch (*Illustration 3a*), a full thickness vertical stitch (*Illustration 3b*), or a horizontal mattress suture (*Illustration 3c*). Most anastomoses are made by the open method, but a closed technique of end-to-end anastomosis may be used if the colon is sufficiently mobile for the application of special occlusive clamps. Closed techniques of anastomosis were commonly used some 50 years ago when they were believed to be safer than open methods, but they are seldom used in modern surgical practice although they have considerable aesthetic value.

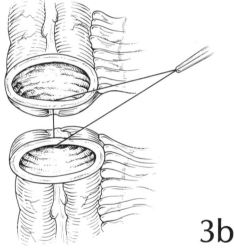

3b

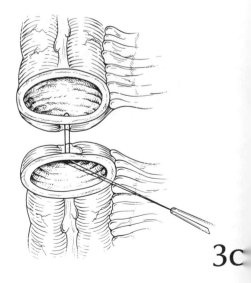

3c

Colonic anastomosis: serosubmucosal suture (open method)

4a–e Stay sutures are inserted at the mesenteric and antimesenteric borders of the intestine and at the midpoint of the posterior aspect of the anastomosis (*Illustration 4a*). The remaining sutures on the posterior aspect of the anastomosis are inserted at intervals not exceeding 5 mm (*Illustration 4b*) and the sutures are held in forceps until the layer is complete. The anterior layer is created in a similar fashion, beginning with a suture at the midpoint of the anastomosis (*Illustration 4c*). The sutures are held in forceps until the layer is completed (*Illustration 4d*), and secure inversion of the mucosa is achieved when they are tied (*Illustration 4e*).

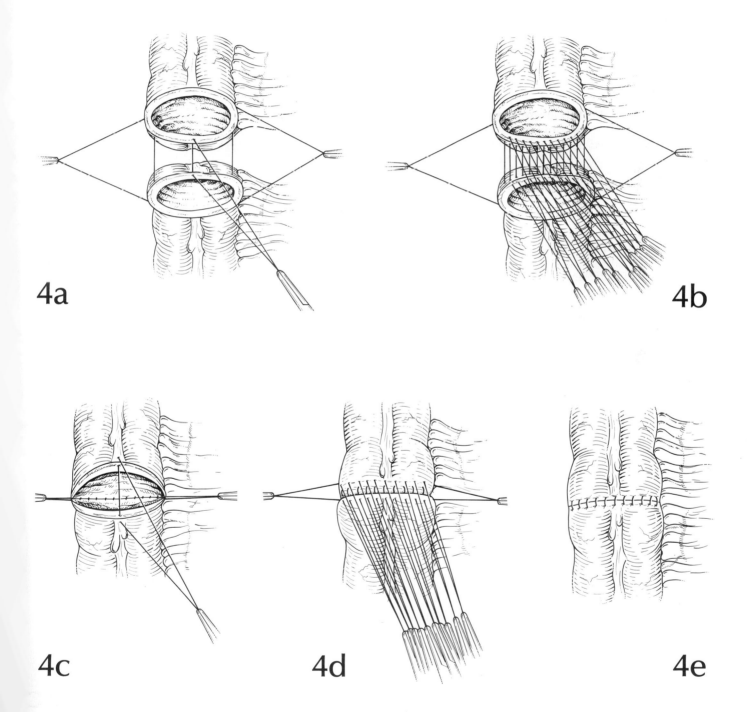

4a

4b

4c

4d

4e

Colonic anastomosis: serosubmucosal suture (closed method)

5a–c This method requires the use of Wangensteen's clamps and is applicable only when both ends of the bowel are sufficiently mobile and the access is sufficiently good to permit the use of these clamps. The technique thus has limited application and is mainly used in ileocolic anastomoses or anastomoses in the proximal colon; it is not suitable for colorectal anastomoses.

The ends of the bowel are held in the occlusive clamps and the posterior layer of serosubmucosal sutures is inserted in a similar fashion to an open anastomosis (*Illustration 5a*). The stitches should be inserted at least 5 mm from the edge of the clamp so that the clamps can be easily rotated, and each stitch must be sufficiently deep to incorporate the submucosal layer of the bowel wall. The sutures are tied after completion of the posterior layer. The clamps are then rotated and are held together with a double collar while the anterior layer of the anastomosis is completed (*Illustration 5b*). The stitches for the anterior layer can be placed closer to the occlusion clamps. The sutures of the completed anterior layer are held taut while the clamps are removed and are then tied, starting with the angle sutures at the mesenteric and antimesenteric borders.

An essential step on completion of the anastomosis is to separate the crushed ends of the bowel by firm pressure between finger and thumb (*Illustration 5c*). The surgeon must be absolutely certain that patency of the lumen has been established.

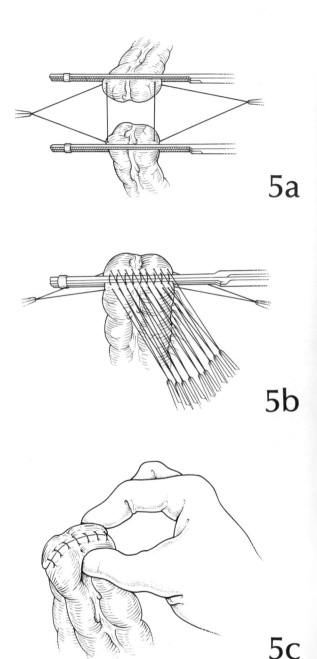

5a

5b

5c

Colorectal anastomosis: single-layer open technique

6a–g In the author's opinion, a single-layer suture technique is infinitely preferable to a two-layer method for colorectal anastomosis. Indeed, a two-layer technique is virtually impossible to use in the construction of very low colorectal anastomoses when access is limited.

A braided suture material such as silk is used, and the anastomosis begins with the insertion of three sutures through all layers of the bowel wall (*Illustration 6a*). The first two sutures are inserted at the mesenteric and antimesenteric borders of the intestine and a third suture is inserted at the midpoint between these sutures. The presence of this central stitch assists greatly in the subsequent insertion of equidistant sutures in the posterior aspect of the anastomosis. The posterior layer is completed with a series of through-and-through sutures incorporating all layers of the bowel wall, and the sutures are held in forceps until the layer is complete (*Illustration 6b*). The interval between each suture should be relatively small; otherwise there is a tendency for eversion of the mucosa to occur when the sutures are tied. Alternative suture methods may be used, such as a mattress technique (*Illustration 6c*) or a submucosal suture (*Illustration 6d*), but these sutures become more difficult in very low anastomoses. The author uses the method shown in *Illustrations 6a* and *6b*. The anterior layer of the anastomosis is made with a similar series of full thickness sutures knotted on the mucosa (*Illustration 6e*). A small gap in the suture line finally remains in the centre of the anterior layer, and this is closed with a submucosal suture inserted parallel to the edge of the suture line (*Illustration 6f*).

An alternative method of construction of the anterior layer is to use a series of vertical submucosal sutures as shown in *Illustration 4d* or horizontal mattress sutures (*Illustration 6g*).

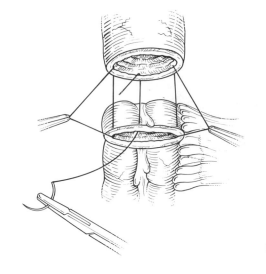

6a

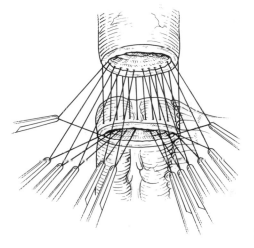

6b

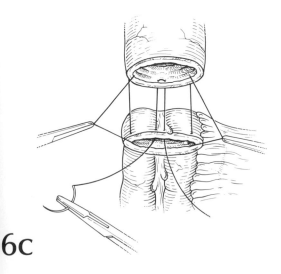

6c

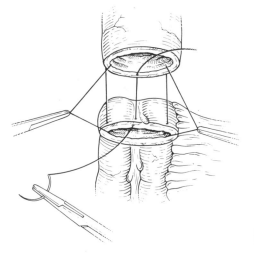

6d

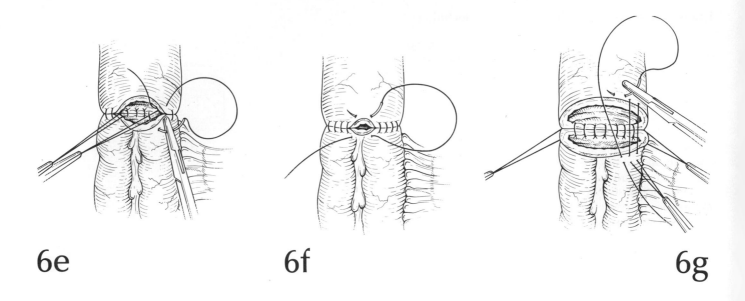

6e

6f

6g

Coloanorectal anastomosis

7a, b An end-to-end, overlapping, or sleeve-type anastomosis may be made between the colon and the upper part of the anal canal. In the Parks operation, the colon is pulled through a short rectal stump (after excision of the rectal mucosa) and anastomosed to the anal canal above the dentate line. A single-layer anastomosis is made with sutures which incorporate the anal mucosa, the internal sphincter muscle and the full thickness of the colonic wall (*Illustration 7a*). A bivalve anal speculum or retractor is required for this anastomosis, and the author uses a single layer of interrupted silk sutures, although absorbable sutures of chromic catgut or polyglactin may be equally satisfactory. Some surgeons insert a second layer of sutures through the outer edge of the rectal stump and the serosal layer of the colon (points A and A¹ of *Illustration 7b*), but the author finds this unnecessary and unusually difficult.

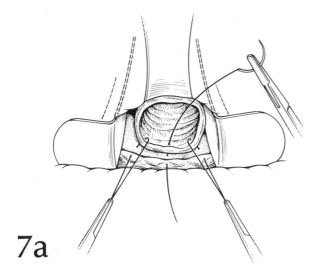

7a

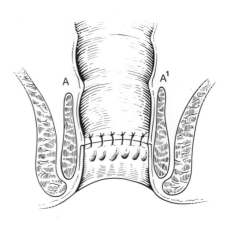

7b

Two-layer method

The author uses chromic catgut and non-absorbable sutures in these anastomoses, but some surgeons use polyglactin for all layers with excellent results.

Insertion of posterior outer layer of sutures

8a–c The divided ends of the bowel are held in crushing clamps and light occlusion clamps are applied across the bowel, care being taken to avoid the mesentery. The two-layer inverting anastomosis commences with the insertion of the outer layer of interrupted submucosal sutures on the posterior aspect of the anastomosis (*Illustrations 8a, b*). Non-absorbable sutures of silk or other braided material are used and they are inserted first at the mesenteric and antimesenteric borders of the intestine. The sutures are tied when this layer is complete and the crushing clamps can then be amputated (*Illustration 8c*), thus opening the bowel lumen.

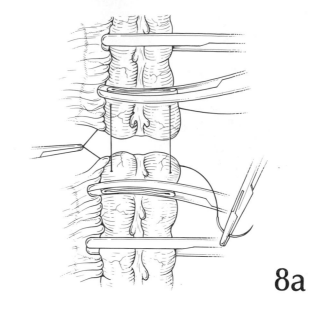

8a

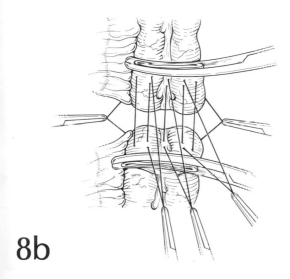

8b

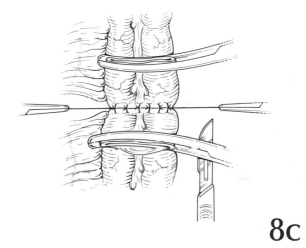

8c

Inner layer of sutures

9a–g A continuous chromic catgut suture which begins at the antimesenteric border is used for the inner layer of the anastomosis. The suture is inserted through all layers of the bowel wall and tied on the serosal aspect (*Illustration 9a*). A forceps is applied to the short end of the suture which will be used again on completion of this layer. A continuous over-and-over suture technique is used for the posterior aspect of the anastomosis, care being taken to include all coats of the bowel wall (*Illustration 9b*). The mesenteric corner of the anastomosis is securely invaginated by the use of the Connell suture technique (*Illustration 9c*) and inversion of the edges of the bowel is achieved when the suture is pulled taut (*Illustration 9d*). The anterior aspect of the inner layer of the anastomosis may be completed with an over-and-over suture technique, but a continuous Connell technique may be preferred (*Illustration 9e*). The mucosa and edges of the bowel on the antimesenteric aspect are invaginated as the last Connell stitch is pulled tight (*Illustration 9f*), and the suture is tied to its other end (*Illustration 9g*).

Some surgeons prefer to start the inner all-coats catgut layer in the midline posteriorly, using catgut with a needle at each end. This avoids knots at the weakest points – the mesenteric and antimesenteric borders.

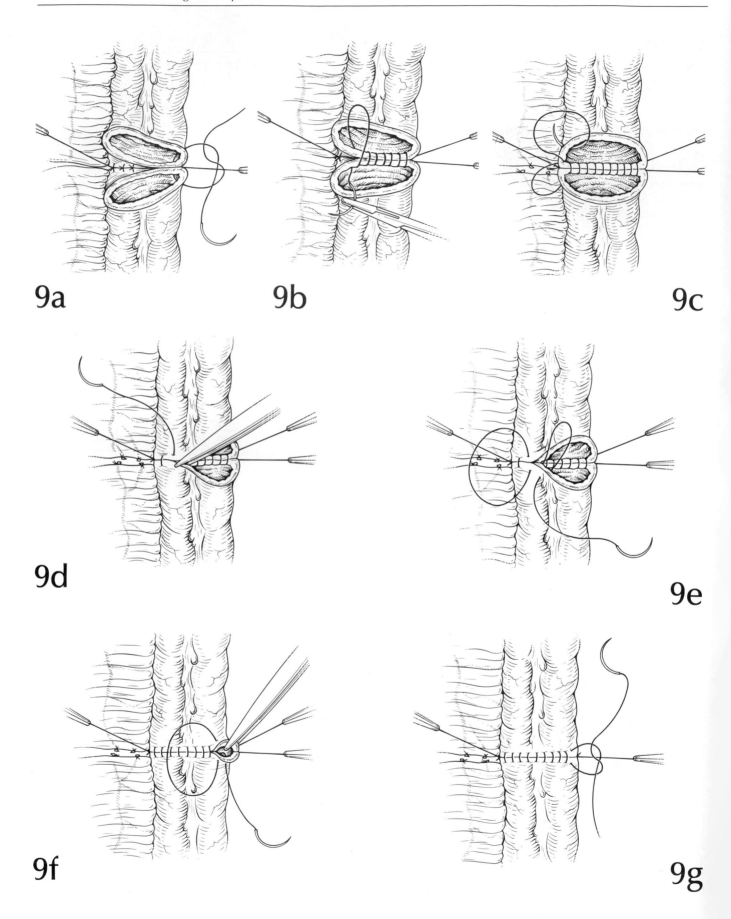

9a

9b

9c

9d

9e

9f

9g

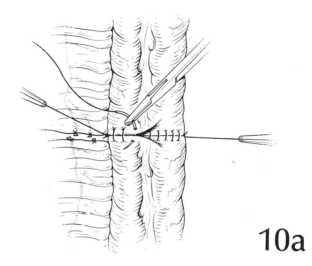

10a

Insertion of anterior outer layer of sutures

10a, b Interrupted non-absorbable submucosal sutures are then inserted on the anterior aspect of the bowel (*Illustration 10a*), and the anastomosis is completed (*Illustration 10b*).

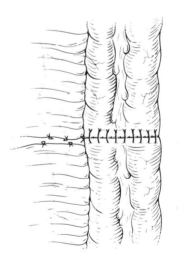

10b

Anastomosis starting with inner layer of sutures

11a–d Some surgeons prefer to begin the two-layer anastomosis with the insertion of the inner layer of catgut (*Illustrations 11a, b*). When this layer is complete, the outer layer of sutures is inserted on the anterior aspect of the anastomosis and the anastomosis is then rotated (*Illustration 11c*) so that the outer layer can be completed on the posterior aspect (*Illustration 11d*). This method is apt to prove unsatisfactory in obese subjects when the mesentery is laden with fat because, after completion of the inner layer, insertion of the outer layer of sutures on the posterior aspect of the anastomosis is difficult to achieve with precision when the mesenteric fat encroaches on the bowel wall.

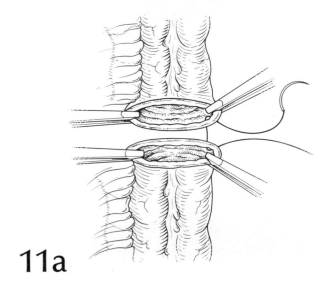

11a

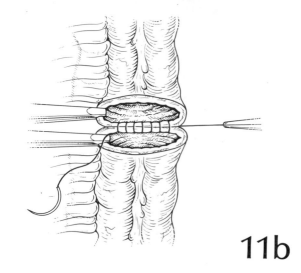

11b

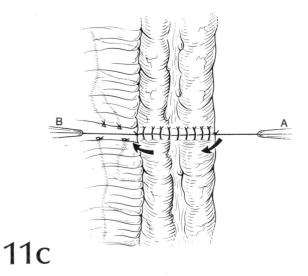

11c

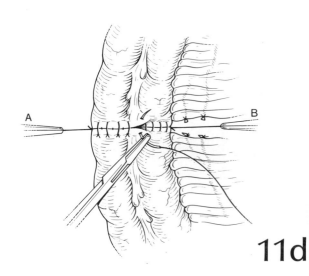

11d

Ileocolic anastomosis: correction for unequal ends of bowel

12a–d An end-to-end anastomosis is possible even when there is considerable disparity in the size of the two ends of bowel. This situation may arise in anastomosis of the ileum to the colon after right hemicolectomy or in operations for small bowel obstruction (*Illustration 12a*). The problem is solved by widening the orifice of the smaller lumen: the outer layer of submucosal sutures is inserted in an oblique fashion away from the cut edge of the bowel on the antimesenteric aspect in the end of the smaller calibre lumen (*Illustration 12b*), and the open end of the bowel is widened by cutting along the antimesenteric border (*Illustrations 12c, d*).

Most problems of disparity can be solved in this way, but some surgeons prefer to use an end-to-side technique of anastomosis in these circumstances.

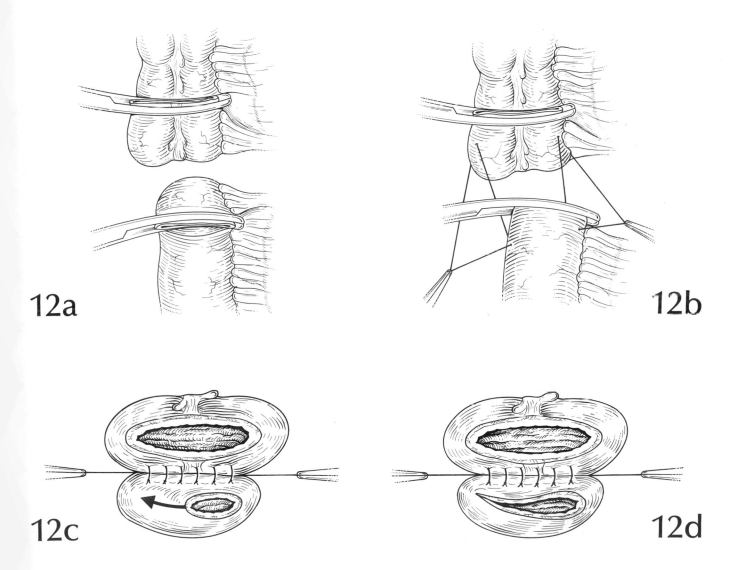

12a

12b

12c

12d

Colorectal anastomosis

It is the author's view that a two-layer suture technique has only limited application in colorectal anastomoses and that it is inappropriate for low colorectal anastomosis.

13a–d
A modified suture technique is used in a two-layer anastomosis in the extraperitoneal rectum. In a low colorectal anastomosis, where access may be restricted, it is often simpler to insert the outer layer of submucosal sutures parallel to the cut edge of the rectum as horizontal mattress sutures (*Illustrations 13a, b*). The use of this stitch in the extraperitoneal rectum is desirable also in that it is placed at right angles to the longitudinal muscle fibres, and there is less tendency for it to cut through the muscle tissue than a conventional vertical suture. The sutures are held in forceps until the outer layer is complete (*Illustration 13c*), and inversion of the suture line is achieved when these are tied (*Illustration 13d*).

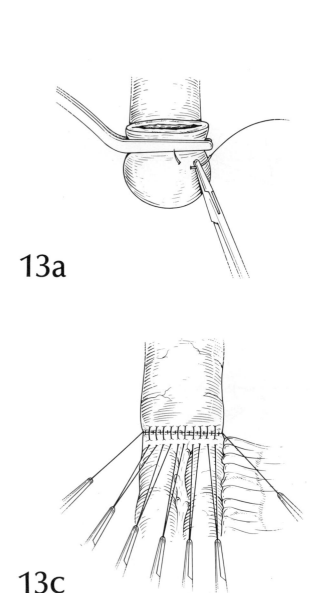

13a

13c

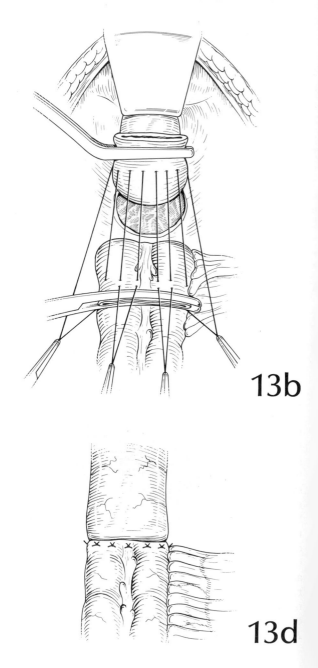

13b

13d

Caecorectal anastomosis

14 An end-to-end anastomosis may be made between the caecum and rectum after subtotal colectomy. A two-layer suture technique is used, but the author prefers a side-to-end reconstruction for this anastomosis, as shown in *Illustrations 17a–d*.

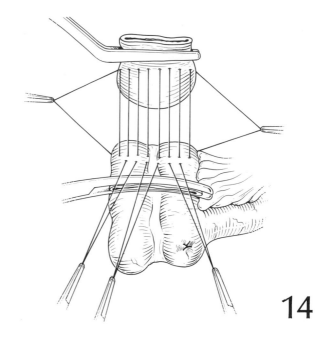

14

END-TO-SIDE AND SIDE-TO-END ANASTOMOSES

These methods are used less frequently than end-to-end anastomoses. The side-to-end method is used by some surgeons for caecorectal, ileorectal and colorectal anastomoses, and it appears to be the most common method for anastomosis of the ileum to the anal canal in the operation of restorative proctocolectomy. The end-to-side technique is favoured by some surgeons for ileocolic anastomosis, particularly when there is a significant disparity in the two ends of bowel.

Technique for closure of end of bowel

15a–h When an end-to-side or side-to-end anastomosis of the small or large intestine is performed, one end of the bowel must be closed. A two-layer inverting suture technique is used. The bowel is held in a crushing clamp, and a chromic catgut suture mounted on a straight needle is inserted through all layers of the bowel wall at the antimesenteric border (*Illustration 15a*). The suture is knotted, and the first layer starts as a continuous horizontal mattress suture (*Illustrations 15b, c*). The crushing clamp is removed as the suture is again knotted at the mesenteric border of the intestine. The suture is then returned towards the antimesenteric end as a continuous over-and-over stitch incorporating all layers of the bowel wall (*Illustrations 15d, e*) and is finally knotted at the antimesenteric end (*Illustration 15f*). Interrupted submucosal sutures of silk or other braided material are then inserted (*Illustration 15g*), and the end of the bowel is securely invaginated (*Illustration 15h*).

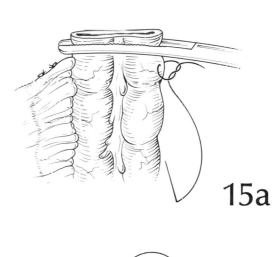

15a

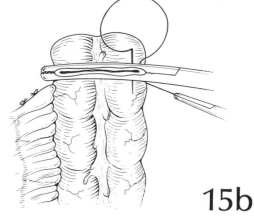

15b

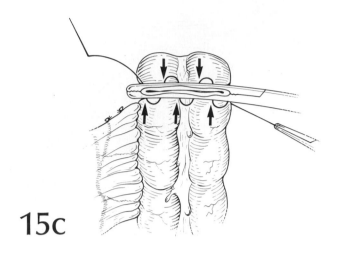

15c

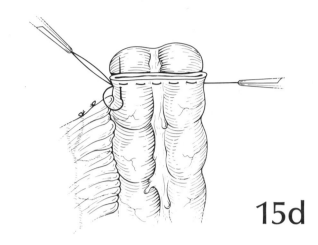

15d

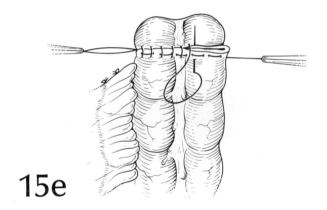

15e

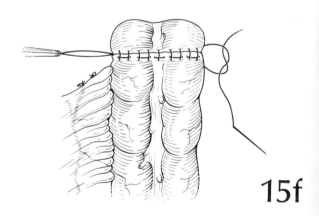

15f

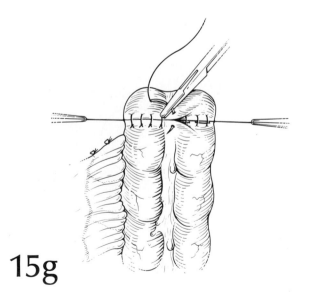

15g

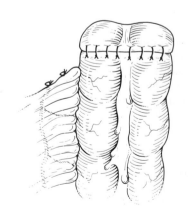

15h

Ileocolic and ileorectal/colorectal anastomoses

16a–d

In an end-to-side reconstruction after the operation of right hemicolectomy, the end of the colon is closed and the end of the ileum is anastomosed to the side of the colon using a standard two-layer inverting technique (*Illustrations 16a–c*).

In side-to-end colorectal anastomosis, the side of the colon is anastomosed to the end of the rectal stump (*Illustration 16d*). The author never uses this method in colorectal anastomosis but finds it useful in anastomosis of the caecum to the rectum and in anastomosis of the ileum to the rectum after the operation of subtotal colectomy if there is marked disparity in the size of the ileum and rectum.

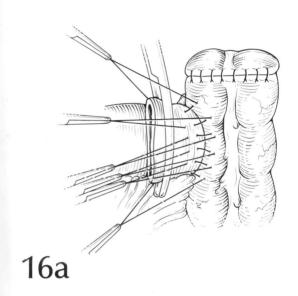

16a

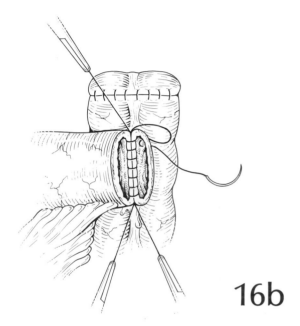

16b

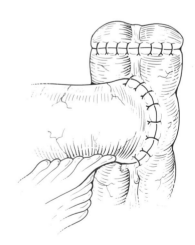

16c

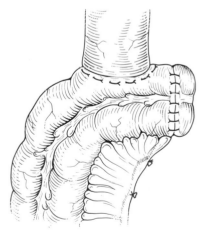

16d

Caecorectal anastomosis

17a–d In the method of anastomosis favoured by the author, the end of the caecum is closed (*Illustration 17a*) using the technique shown in *Illustrations 15a–h* and the side of the caecum is anastomosed to the cut end of the rectum. A two-layer suture technique is used, beginning with the insertion of an outer posterior row of silk submucosal mattress sutures (*Illustration 17b*). The inner layer of the anastomosis is made with a continuous chromic catgut suture incorporating all layers of the bowel wall (*Illustration 17c*) and the anastomosis is completed with an anterior layer of silk submucosal mattress sutures (*Illustration 17d*).

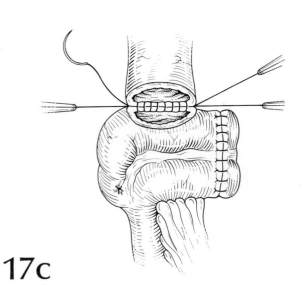

17a

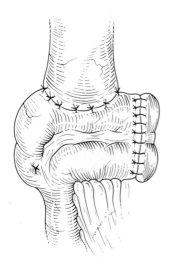

17b

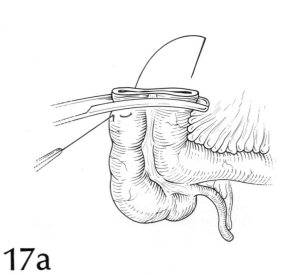

17c

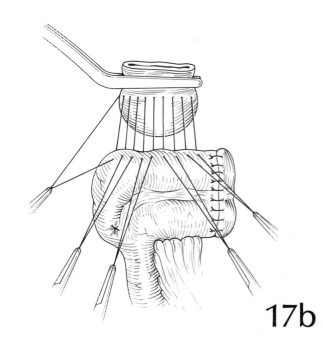

17d

Ileoanal pouch anastomosis

18 The most common method of anastomosis in the operation of restorative proctocolectomy involves suture of the side of the most dependent part of the ileal pouch to the lumen of the anal canal at or above the dentate line. A single-layer suture technique is favoured although some surgeons use a stapled anastomosis. It is customary and advisable to protect the anastomosis with a defunctioning loop ileostomy.

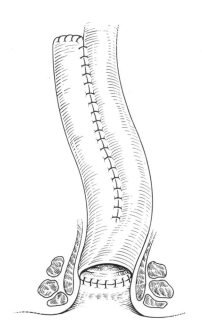

18

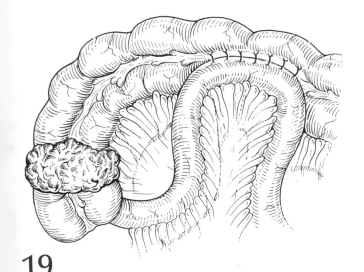

19

SIDE-TO-SIDE ANASTOMOSIS

19 The chief application of side-to-side anastomosis in the large intestine is in the relief of obstructions caused by irremovable neoplasms, particularly in the right colon. The ileum is anastomosed to the transverse colon beyond the site of obstruction using a two-layer suture technique.

A previous generation of surgeons frequently used side-to-side techniques of anastomosis in preference to the end-to-end method, but there is no evidence that the former method is safer and it may result in 'blind loop' problems associated with the closure of the two ends of bowel.

Postoperative care

Peritoneal drains are removed after 48 h, their purpose being to remove any collections of blood or serum during the early postoperative period.

Systemic antibiotics are usually limited to the perioperative period, but may be continued for 3–5 days when there is significant faecal soiling or bacterial contamination during surgery. Intravenous cefuroxime and metronidazole are used by the author.

A period of alimentary motor dysfunction inevitably follows anastomosis of the intestine and may or may not be apparent clinically. Nasogastric tubes are not required routinely but oral intake should be introduced cautiously. Early oral intake may result in abdominal distension and vomiting. In the author's practice, oral intake is restricted until the patient passes flatus, which usually occurs on about the fourth day.

Prolonged intolerance of oral intake, vomiting, fever or protracted ileus may indicate that anastomotic dehiscence has occurred. Gross disruption of an anastomosis is usually accompanied by evidence of peritonitis, fistulation or systemic signs of gross sepsis, but the signs may be less explicit in elderly subjects. A marked leucocytosis accompanying a non-specific general deterioration in the condition of the elderly patient should alert the surgeon to the possibility that anastomotic dehiscence has occurred.

Dehiscence is a complication which begins during the first few days after operation when the integrity and strength of the anastomosis are largely dependent on the sutures. Clinical features of dehiscence seldom arise *de novo* after the first postoperative week, although this may not be true for stapled anastomoses.

Anastomoses in the left colon or rectum may be examined radiologically on the 12th day using a water-soluble contrast medium such as Gastrografin. In most cases the study is of academic interest only, although small anastomotic leaks which are unassociated with clinical signs may be revealed. Occasionally, the study will confirm the clinical impression that a more serious degree of anastomotic disruption has occurred.

Ultrasonographic examination of the abdomen is helpful in the diagnosis of localized leaks, and perianastomotic abscesses may be drained percutaneously under ultrasonographic guidance. However, most abscesses associated with colorectal anastomoses will discharge spontaneously through the suture line. It may require considerable judgement on the part of the surgeon to determine when further surgery is indicated for the complications of anastomotic dehiscence.

Outcome

In expert hands, major resectional surgery of the large intestine is associated with a mortality rate of less than 5%, and most deaths are due to complications of coexisting medical disease rather than problems with the anastomosis. Fatalities due to disruption of the anastomosis are rarely encountered in the hands of skilled and experienced surgeons.

References

1. Friend PJ, Scott R, Everett WG, Scott IHK. Stapling or suturing for anastomoses of the left side of the large intestine. *Surg Gynecol Obstet* 1990; 171: 373–6.

2. Fielding LP, Stewart-Brown S, Blesovsky L, Kearney G. Anastomotic integrity after operations for large-bowel cancer: a multicentre study *BMJ* 1980; 281: 411–14.

3. Matheson NA, Irving AD. Single layer anastomosis after rectosigmoid resection. *Br J Surg* 1975; 62: 239–42.

4. Ravo B, Ger R. Temporary colostomy – an outmoded procedure? A report on the intracolonic bypass. *Dis Colon Rectum* 1985; 28: 904–7.

5. Dudley HAF, Radcliffe AG, McGeehan D. Intraoperative irrigation of the colon to permit primary anastomosis. *Br J Surg* 1980; 67: 80–1.

6. Buck N, Devlin HB, Lunn JN. *The Report of a Confidential Enquiry into Perioperative Deaths*. London: Nuffield Provincial Hospitals Trust, 1987.

Stapling in colorectal surgery

R. W. Beart Jr MD, FACS
Professor of Surgery, Mayo Clinic, Scottsdale, Arizona, USA

History

Surgeons continue to be interested in identifying the best way to create an intestinal anastomosis. In 1893, Nicholas pointed out that '... the ideal method of uniting intestinal wounds is yet to be devised'. Through the years, surgeons have devised numerous types of suture material; absorbable, non-absorbable, synthetic, non-synthetic, braided and monofilament, to create intestinal anastomoses. Mechanical stapling devices might be traced to the early work of Denans in Marseilles, whose work preceded the more famous Murphy Button by 66 years. In 1826, he invaginated intestinal ends over two silver rings, and then approximated the bowel with a special pair of forceps. Inversion was accomplished, and the entire circumferences of the serosal surfaces were opposed. Stapling devices were developed to overcome inadequacies with traditional suturing methods. Hultl produced a stapling instrument in 1911. It was cumbersome, weighed over 4.5 kg, and took hours to assemble. Petz designed an instrument, similar to Payr's crushing clamp, which placed a row of staples along both edges close to the stomach during gastrectomy. Between 1945 and 1950, a group of Russian engineers in Moscow, including Gudov and Androsov, developed methods to staple blood vessels together, prompted by the difficulties with traditional suture techniques experienced during World War II. Their developments continued up until 1970, and included many gastrointestinal stapling instruments[1].

Since that time, Ravitch and Steichen should be given the greatest credit for the proliferation of these instruments[2]. They initiated numerous publications outlining surgical techniques for the use of staplers to perform pneumonectomy, lobectomy, gastrectomy, end-to-end bowel anastomosis, and transection of multiple vessels. These instruments have now become commonplace and approximately 40% of intestinal anastomoses in the USA are created with these devices. It is appropriate to review the advantages of these instruments as well as the potential disadvantages that have been identified since the early 1970s.

When performing colonic surgery with staplers, there are four fundamental techniques which should be mastered: functional end-to-end anastomosis, end-to-side anastomosis, end-to-end anastomosis, and double/triple stapling methods.

Functional end-to-end anastomosis

1a, b In the functional end-to-end method, the bowel is mobilized completely, making sure that all tension has been relieved. The mesentery is dissected to the point where the bowel is to be transected. This can be achieved with a linear stapler which cuts as it divides and seals both ends of the bowel (*Illustration 1a*).

Alternatively, a clamp can be placed on the section to be removed and a stapling device placed across the end to be preserved (*Illustration 1b*). The stapler should be placed in the antimesenteric to mesenteric direction.

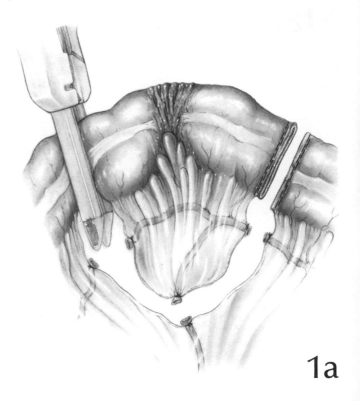

1a

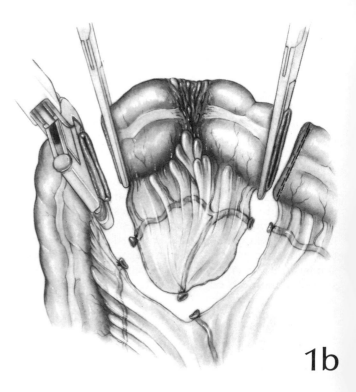

1b

2 The anastomosis is inspected on the inside of the bowel to look for bleeding points which may occasionally need to be ligated. The length of the anastomosis should not be less than 6 cm to provide an adequate lumen. If less than 6 cm, then a second linear staple cartridge should be used in the linear stapler.

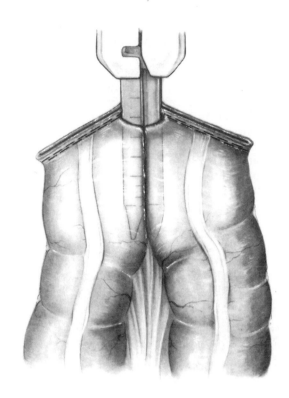

2

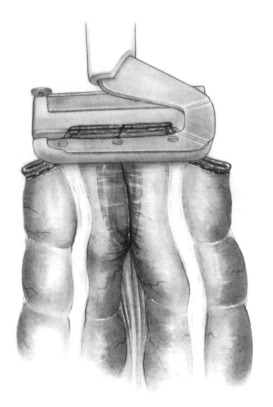

3

3 This leaves a defect at the site where the staplers were inserted, which can be closed with either a mechanical stapler or a traditional hand sewn technique. In either case, the closure should be from staple line to staple line, by distracting the two staple lines to form a triangular anastomotic defect. Two limbs of the triangle are the staple lines and the third limb is the closure of the defect. This creates a functional end-to-end anastomosis, which has been shown to heal well and function as well as an end-to-end anastomosis[3].

End-to-side anastomosis

4 An end-to-side anastomosis can be created as an alternative to the functional end-to-end anastomosis. The bowel is similarly mobilized and divided, but the ends of the remaining bowel are not sutured shut. Instead, a purse-string suture is placed around the end of the distal bowel (e.g. the transverse colon). After sizing the proximal bowel, the appropriate circular staple device is placed through the end of the proximal bowel (e.g. the terminal ileum) without the anvil.

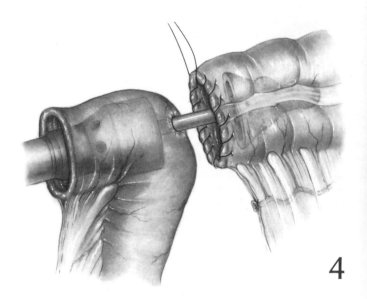

4

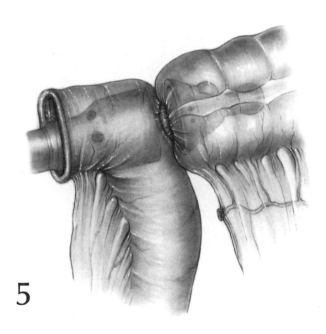

5

5 The circular stapler shaft is then extended through the antimesenteric side of the ileum and the anvil attached. The anvil is then placed into the end of the transverse colon and the purse-string tied around the shaft of the anvil, which is retracted into the stapling instrument.

6 An end-to-side anastomosis is created with a circular stapler, which is then withdrawn. The end of the ileum through which the stapler had been placed must then be closed with a linear stapler.

These two anastomotic techniques are used in similar situations. The functional end-to-end anastomosis requires four staple cartridges and is, therefore, somewhat more expensive than the end-to-side anastomosis. However, the end-to-side anastomosis has a short but real 'blind end', which theoretically may, at a future time, cause problems by the formation of a pulsion diverticulum. In both cases, the mesenteric defect can be closed. Neither anastomotic technique has been shown to be more secure or more rapid than traditional hand-sewn techniques. Therefore it becomes a matter of personal preference as to which technique a surgeon chooses to use.

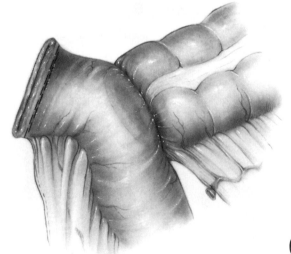

6

End-to-end anastomosis

The end-to-end anastomosis is most commonly created with the circular stapler. Typically, such an anastomosis will be created in the pelvis where the descending or sigmoid colon is being anastomosed to the rectum. With this technique, the patient must be placed in a modified lithotomy position so that access to the anus is possible. The bowel is resected to the point where the bowel is to be divided. Distally, a clamp is placed across the bowel at the proximal margin of transection, and the distal rectum is irrigated with water or cytotoxic agent to minimize the presence of any viable cancer cells.

7 A non-crushing bowel clamp can then be placed across the distal bowel, the bowel can be transected and a purse-string suture placed around the open rectum. Proximally, the bowel is transected and a purse-string suture needs to be placed, which can be done with a purse-string clamp. Automatic purse-string devices can be used both proximally and distally, but are quite expensive and probably offer minimal advantage.

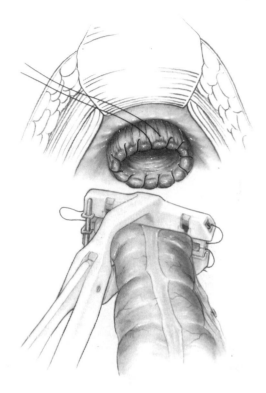

7

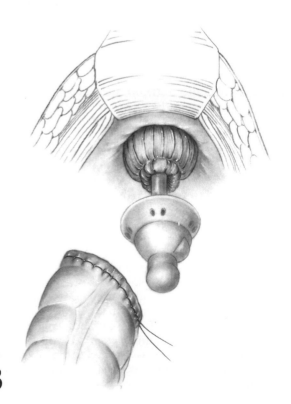

8

8 Once the purse-strings are placed, the circular stapler is inserted through the anus and advanced through the rectum. As it approaches the rectal purse-string, the assistant opens the stapling device, passing the anvil through the purse-string suture. The purse-string is then tightened around the shaft and the instrument is opened completely.

9   The proximal bowel is then placed over the anvil. Placing the bowel over the anvil can be difficult and, before doing this, the edge of the proximal bowel should be grasped with three narrow Allis' clamps, one-third of the circumference apart. The bowel can be dilated with ring forceps and glucagon can be given to relax the bowel. The Allis' forceps are then used to place the lumen over the posterior aspect of the anvil and, using blunt-tipped forceps, the anterior lip of the bowel is brought over the anvil anteriorly. The purse-string can then be tightened around the shaft of the anvil.

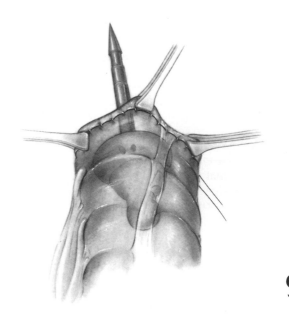

9

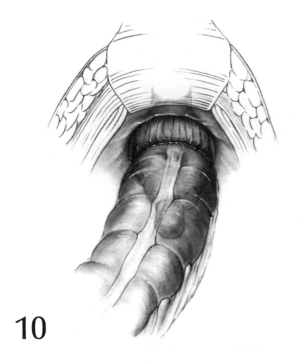

10

10   Under direct vision and making sure the bowel is not rotated, the anvil can then be tightened and the stapler can be fired. The stapler is then opened minimally and, using a rotating motion, is withdrawn from the anus. The operating surgeon, working the abdomen, should make an effort to place traction on the rectum to ease the stapler across the anastomosis because the anastomosis is smaller than the cartridge and removal of the stapler can be somewhat difficult.

At this point, the surgeon must ensure that the anastomosis is not under tension. This is done by making sure that the bowel is laying in the hollow of the sacrum. If there is any 'bow-stringing' across the hollow of the sacrum, the left colon and splenic flexure must be mobilized to remove any evidence of tension. The stapler rings should be inspected. They should be removed from the stapler carefully, maintaining their orientation, and the purse-string sutures should be cut so the rings can be opened fully. Unless the purse-string sutures are cut, small defects in the rings can be hidden. If a defect in the ring is identified, its location in the circumference of the bowel should be noted; this is made possible by having preserved its orientation. If the anastomosis cannot be adequately inspected, the rectum should be insufflated with air through the anus and the leak identified. If this can be repaired with sutures, diversion may be unnecessary. If a leak cannot be identified, or if there is any question about the integrity of the anastomosis, a diverting stoma is appropriate.

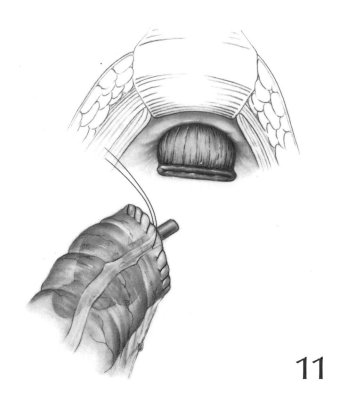

11

Double/triple stapling techniques

11 A double or triple staple technique is used in a similar situation to an end-to-end anastomosis. With these techniques, the bowel is similarly mobilized and the mesentery ligated and divided. The distal bowel is transected with a linear stapler.

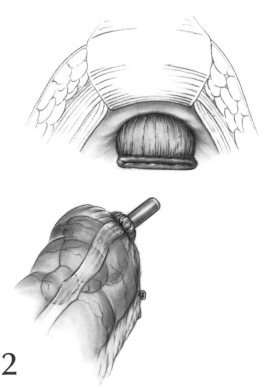

12

12 In the double stapling method, a purse-string suture is then placed in the proximal bowel after its division between clamps, and the detachable anvil inserted proximally with the purse-string suture being tied snugly onto the shaft of the anvil.

13a, b The circular stapler (without the anvil which has already been placed in the proximal bowel) is then passed through the anus and placed under some pressure against the rectal stump. The shaft of the instrument is then advanced and allowed to perforate the blind stump of the rectum adjacent to the staple line.

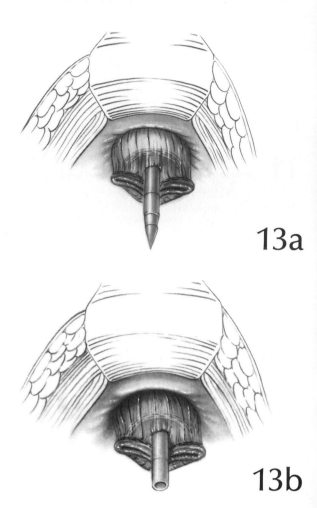

13a

13b

14 The anvil and the stapler are then reunited, making sure that the bowel is not rotated. The stapler is closed, fired and removed. However, it is vital to ensure that neither the vagina nor other pelvic structures are included in the anastomosis, and after the instrument is closed, all sides of the anastomosis must be carefully inspected before firing the apparatus.

It is desirable to ensure that the linear staple lines are not juxtaposed when this technique is used, and the bowel must not be under tension after the anastomosis has been completed.

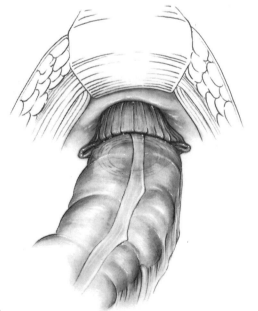

14

15 In the triple stapling technique, an enterotomy is made in the proximal bowel a few centimetres from its open end. The anvil is introduced, the colotomy closed with a purse-string suture, and the bowel is then transected distally.

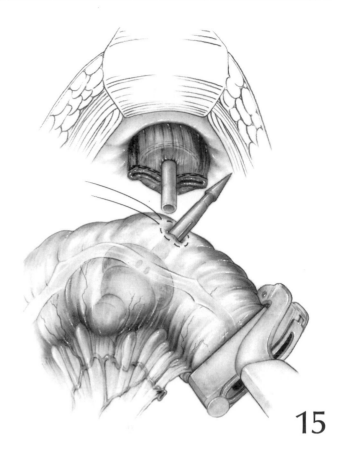

15

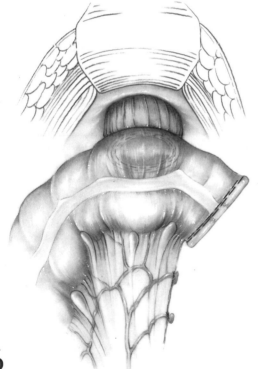

16

16 The anastomosis is completed as for the double stapling method described above.

Stapled pouch procedures

Stapling devices can be used to construct various types of ileoanal pouches with sutures or staples. The latter technique is less time consuming, although more expensive.

Advantages and disadvantages of staplers

Staplers have been proven to be an effective way of anastomosing the bowel. Traditional Halstedian techniques requiring inversion anastomosis have not been found to be necessary with staplers and an everted anastomosis is secure. It has not been shown that staplers save a significant amount of operative time for most anastomoses[3, 4]. For low-lying rectal anastomoses, it has been shown that perhaps as many as 15% of rectums will be preserved in situations where a traditional two-layered anastomosis cannot be performed[2]. Questions have been raised about whether or not metal is a promoter of carcinogenesis or may promote recurrence of cancer[5, 6]. However, the preponderance of recent data suggests that when the rectum is irrigated and margins of normal bowel are resected around cancers, local recurrences do not appear to be increased when compared with hand-sutured techniques[1, 5].

Stricturing has been noted with an increased frequency when the circular stapler is used. It is unclear whether this is a vascular problem or if there are other aetiologies. Most often, the stricture is a very thin web and can be easily dilated; it occurs in 30–40% of patients, but is functionally significant in only about 2%. It is also important to note that these staple lines are not haemostatic, and care must be taken to confirm that there are no bleeding vessels coming through the anastomosis. If this occurs, the bleeding point must be ligated. Staplers are clearly a more costly way to anastomose the bowel, and the prudent surgeon may choose not to staple anastomoses in all situations. However, these techniques are clearly advantageous in specific situations and should be part of the armamentarium of all general surgeons[7, 8].

References

1. Fraser I. An historical perspective on mechanical aids in intestinal anastomosis. *Surg Gynecol Obstet* 1982; 155: 566–74.

2. Ravitch MM, Ong TH, Gazzola L. A new, precise, and rapid technique of intestinal resection and anastomosis with staples. *Surg Gynecol Obstet* 1974; 139: 6–10.

3. Scher KS, Scott-Conner C, Jones CW, Leach M. A comparison of stapled and sutured anastomoses in colonic operations. *Surg Gynecol Obstet* 1982; 155: 489–93.

4. Beart RW, Kelly KA. Randomized prospective evaluation of the EEA stapler for colorectal anastomoses. *Am J Surg* 1981; 141: 143–7.

5. Gertsch P, Baer H, Kraft R, Maddern GJ, Altermatt HJ. Malignant cells are collected on circular staplers. *Dis Colon Rectum* 1992; 35: 238–41.

6. Phillips RKS, Cook HT. Effect of steel wire sutures on the incidence of chemically induced rodent colonic tumours. *Br J Surg* 1986; 73: 671–4.

7. Dziki A, Duncan M, Harmon J *et al*. Advantages of handsewn over stapled bowel anastomosis. *Dis Colon Rectum* 1991; 34: 442–8.

8. Heald RJ, Allen DR. Stapled ileo-anal anastomosis: a technique to avoid mucosal proctectomy in the ileal pouch operation. *Br J Surg* 1986; 73: 571–2.

9. Heald RJ. Towards fewer colostomies – the impact of circular stapling devices on the surgery of rectal cancer in a district hospital. *Br J Surg* 1980; 67: 198–200.

10. Hurst PA, Prout WG, Kelly JM, Bannister JJ, Walker RT. Local recurrence after low anterior resection using the staple gun. *Br J Surg* 1982; 69: 275–6.

Ilustrations by Richard Neave and the late Robert Lane

Surgical management of anastomotic leakage and intra-abdominal sepsis

Miles Irving MD, ChM, FRCS
Professor of Surgery and Consultant Surgeon, Hope Hospital, University of Manchester School of Medicine, Salford, UK

Sarah O'Dwyer MD, FRCS
Consultant Surgeon, The General and Queen Elizabeth Hospitals, Birmingham, UK

Principles and justification

Leakage from anastomosed bowel is almost always the result of bad judgement and/or poor technique at the time of construction. Leakage rates vary widely between surgeons and, although anastomotic leakage occurs even in the best of hands, very low rates can be attained and this must be the goal of all gastrointestinal surgeons.

Anastomotic failure occurs when the bowel is ischaemic, when it is inadequately mobilized (resulting in tension on the anastomosis), and when seromuscular apposition of the divided intestinal ends is inaccurate. Furthermore, the presence of severe malnutrition and intra-abdominal sepsis also compromise anastomotic healing and, therefore, when conditions for anastomotic healing are not ideal the surgeon should not hesitate to exteriorize the intestinal ends and reconstruct the intestine at a later date. It may be appropriate to protect a primary anastomosis by fashioning a proximal diverting stoma which can be closed when the anastomosis has healed. The role of intraluminal devices such as the Coloshield in protecting an anastomosis is unclear, and they have not gained wide acceptance. Should anastomotic leakage occur, prompt institution of the correct management will limit the risk of further major complications and death. The approach to this problem will depend upon the type of leakage and the general condition of the patient.

Anastomotic leaks can be categorized into four principal types:

1. Asymptomatic leaks.
2. Leaks associated with generalized peritonitis.
3. Leaks associated with localized infection or abscess formation.
4. Leaks associated with an enterocutaneous fistula.

Clinical presentation

Leakage associated with generalized peritonitis

Disruption of an anastomosis with leakage of enteric content can occur at any time after surgery but is most usual 2–5 days following the procedure. Bowel contents discharge into the abdominal cavity and the patient becomes tachycardic and shows signs of generalized peritonitis. In a short time peripheral circulatory failure develops, urine output falls and vital signs deteriorate. The degree of abdominal distension depends on the amount of gas leakage and may lead to a tense tympanitic abdomen with radiological evidence of pneumoperitoneum. The diagnosis of an anastomotic leak can be difficult, particularly in immunosuppressed and elderly patients where an intra-abdominal catastrophe can present as progressive postoperative confusion or deterioration in respiratory function. In most cases an experienced surgeon will be able to make a clinical diagnosis of anastomotic leakage, following which resuscitation and urgent laparotomy are required.

Leakage associated with abscess formation

An abscess should be suspected in a patient who fails to progress or where there is evidence of low-grade swinging pyrexia. Where there is a track to the surface erythema of the skin, swelling and tenderness indicate the site for drainage. Assessment of the pelvis by rectal examination may reveal a boggy swelling in the presacral space. A low pelvic abscess can be drained rectally or through the perineum. If such an abscess is associated with leakage from a colonic anastomosis, a defunctioning stoma may be necessary to prevent further pelvic abscess formation.

Leakage associated with an enterocutaneous fistula

In some cases of anastomotic leak, the surrounding inflammatory reaction is so marked that the leakage is confined and a generalized peritonitis does not occur. In these cases the patient develops pain and swelling in the area of leakage, which is associated with a raised temperature and constitutional disturbance. The remaining part of the abdomen remains soft although there may be a degree of intestinal obstruction, but normal bowel function may continue.

Eventually a fistula presents through the wound or drain site with the discharge of pus, gas and enteric content (singly or in combination), usually followed by relief of constitutional and obstructive symptoms.

Preoperative

Asymptomatic leakage

Small leaks from low rectal anastomoses are seen in a proportion of cases in which the integrity of the anastomosis is routinely checked postoperatively by radio-opaque enema. Similar small leaks almost certainly occur in anastomoses higher in the intestinal tract but these are rarely subject to such checks. Providing the leak is not associated with infection, as evidenced by persistent swinging pyrexia and signs of inflammation, and normal bowel function has returned, no intervention is required. The leak will heal spontaneously without complications.

Leakage associated with generalized peritonitis

The patient with generalized peritonitis requires aggressive intravenous fluid resuscitation using both crystalloid and colloid solutions and should be transferred to a high-dependency or intensive therapy unit before surgery if possible.

Measurement of central venous and pulmonary wedge pressures aids in the determination of the degree of circulatory failure and allows optimal fluid resuscitation with minimal cardiac overload. Arterial blood gases and acid–base status should be measured and mechanical ventilation may be necessary to reverse acidosis and to support pulmonary function. Blood cultures should be taken and intravenous antibiotics (such as metronidazole and cefuroxime) should be given immediately the diagnosis has been established. A urinary catheter is inserted at the outset of resuscitation and, wherever possible, surgery should be delayed until urinary flow is established. Pharmacological support (e.g. using dopamine and noradrenaline) may be required to bring about a satisfactory cardiac response and to maintain systemic vascular resistance. However, the presence of faecal peritonitis may prevent complete correction of circulatory failure before reoperation.

Leakage associated with abscess

Supplementary investigations (e.g. ultrasonography, computed tomography (CT) and indium-labelled leucocyte scanning) are useful in defining the anatomy and localizing occult collections of pus. In some cases, when there are strong clinical grounds for suspecting an abscess but radiological investigation has been inconclusive, laparotomy is justifiable.

Operations

Incision

Wherever practicable the previous incision should be reopened and extended as necessary to obtain adequate access. On opening the peritoneal cavity faecal fluid should be sucked out and a sample sent for urgent microbiological assessment.

MANAGEMENT OF LEAKS ASSOCIATED WITH GENERALIZED PERITONITIS

1 The soft fibrinous adhesions binding the abdominal contents together should be separated to release pockets of fluid that lie between the loops of intestine. This is best achieved by gentle digital dissection, gradually separating the tissues and following the bowel down to the site of the anastomosis. Every effort should be made to avoid perforating the intestine during this dissection.

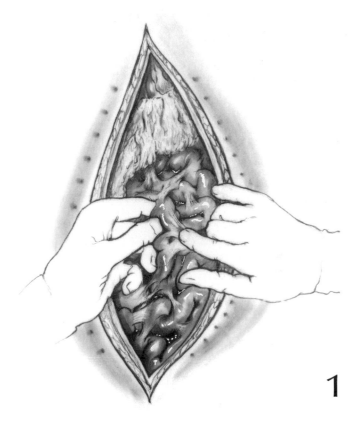

1

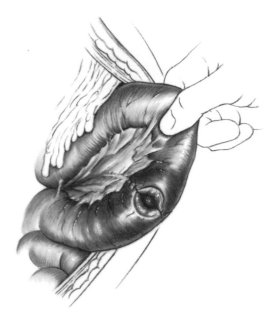

2

2 The leakage usually arises from a hole in one part of the anastomosis: only rarely will the whole anastomosis have come apart (although this may occur on exploration and mobilization). A small defect may be resutured, but this should not be performed in the great majority of patients. Similarly, taking down the anastomosis, resecting the area and then constructing a new anastomosis is dangerous because this second anastomosis, fashioned in the presence of generalized peritonitis, is also likely to leak. Even a loop stoma proximal to the disrupted bowel may be insufficient because there remains a length of 'loaded' bowel between the stoma and the point of leakage.

3 Once the site of leakage has been established the anastomosis is taken down and the ends separated. The abdominal cavity should be irrigated with copious quantities of saline at body temperature. Careful separation of loops of intestine and irrigation of paracolic, subdiaphragmatic and pelvic recesses must be continued until the irrigation fluid is no longer turbid or contains debris. Fibrinous exudates can be left as radical debridement has not been shown to be of value and may lead to blood loss and tissue damage.

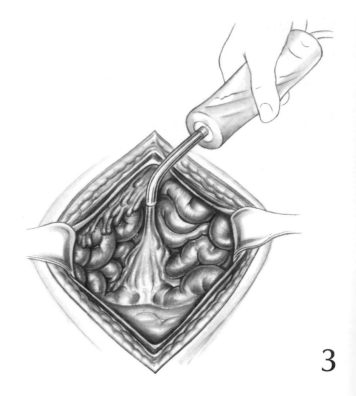

3

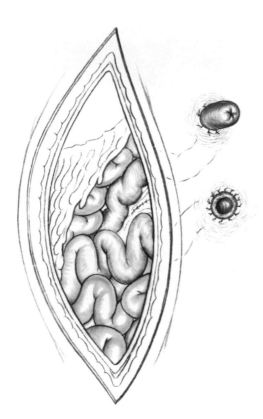

4

4 The intestinal ends must be separated and excised back to healthy tissue. Ideally, both ends should be brought to the surface through stab incisions away from the main wound and fixed with mucocutaneous sutures. It is important for the proximal stoma to be in a site where a bag can be applied successfully and this stoma should be constructed as a formal end ileostomy or colostomy. When the inflammatory reaction to generalized or prolonged peritonitis is severe, thickened mesentery and oedema of the intestinal wall may prevent eversion of the mucosa. In order to avoid a flush ileostomy, where possible about 5 cm of ileum should be brought out and tacked to the abdominal wall. Eversion can be performed under local anaesthesia a few days later.

5 Where there is only a short segment of bowel beyond the disrupted anastomosis (such as a rectal stump following an anterior resection), or where separation of the small bowel mesentery is difficult because of oedema, the stump or distal bowel should be closed in the manner of a Hartmann's operation and only the proximal limb brought out to the surface.

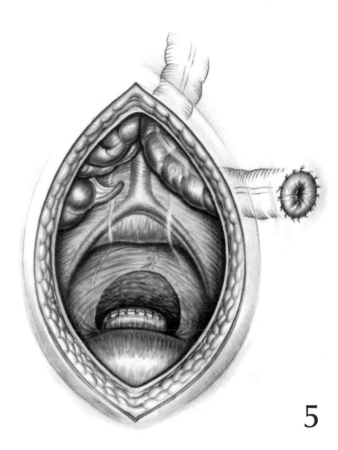

5

Wound closure

6a–c Following stoma formation the peritoneal cavity is washed with 1 litre of saline containing 1 g tetracycline. Sump suction drains are inserted into the right and left paracolic gutters positioned in the hepatorenal and rectovesical pouches, respectively. In the case of moderate peritoneal contamination it may be possible to close the deep layers of the abdominal wall with interrupted sutures of 1 polydioxanone, taking 1-cm bites of muscle and peritoneum on each side as a one-layer 'mass' closure. Tension sutures should not be used in closure of abdominal wounds. The skin and subcutaneous tissues are irrigated with tetracycline in saline lavage and primary closure is performed using monofilament sutures or metal clips. If there has been severe faecal contamination, the superficial layers can be left open and packed with gauze soaked in saline. The gauze pack is changed every 12 h until healthy granulation tissue is seen and the wound is clean. It may then be closed under local anaesthesia, usually some time after the fourth postoperative day.

In some cases of long-standing peritonitis it can be difficult to close the abdominal wall because oedema and inflammation render the intestine difficult to reduce into the abdominal cavity and because the abdominal wall is rigid. In such circumstances the authors recommend the use of relaxing incisions into the muscles of the abdominal wall at the lateral border of the anterior rectus sheath on either side of the midline wound.

In a very small number of cases, where contamination of the abdominal cavity is extremely severe or long-standing, or if there is a large intra-abdominal cavity unsuitable for treatment by tube drains alone, formal laparostomy may be necessary. Following thorough intra-abdominal toilet and siting of suction drains the abdomen or the abscess cavity is packed with saline-soaked gauze. In order to prevent coughing disturbing the packs, patients are ventilated for 24 h after laparostomy. The packs are changed 12–18 h after surgery and then twice daily, allowing absorption of purulent fluid into the packs and thereby preventing occult intracavity abscess formation.

Formation of granulation tissue, epithelialization and contraction of the wound occurs over 2–3 months and occasionally incisional hernia repair is required at a later date.

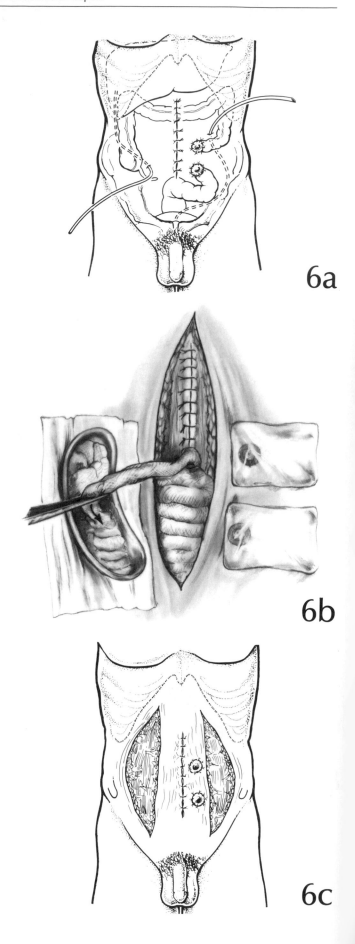

6a

6b

6c

MANAGEMENT OF LEAKS ASSOCIATED WITH ABSCESS FORMATION

7 Whenever a well-localized abscess is detected it should be drained by direct incision or, preferably, ultrasound- or CT-guided drainage. Following anatomical delineation of the abscess a drain is inserted and pus sent for microbiological culture. If preoperative scanning indicates evidence of loculation, further drains can be inserted to facilitate complete emptying of the cavities. If the abscess is chronic and has a thick wall, drains must be left *in situ* until repeat scanning indicates complete collapse of the cavity. Irrigation of the cavity may be necessary to remove any debris which collects as the abscess heals.

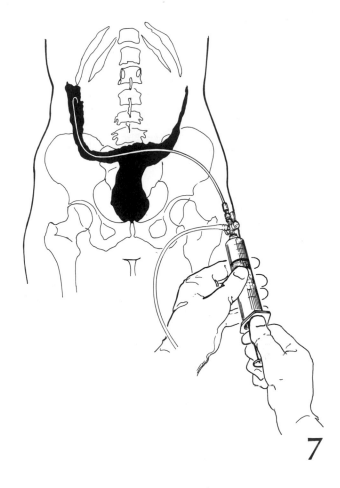

7

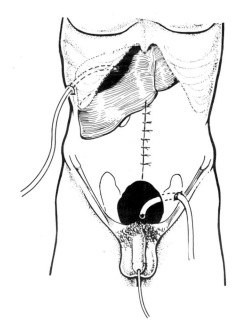

8

8 Abscesses which cannot be safely or adequately drained with the aid of scanning techniques require a formal surgical approach. In the case of an inadequately draining abscess with a track to the surface, this track can be used as a guide to the deeper cavity. In some cases laparotomy may be necessary to achieve satisfactory placement of large tube drains which should be positioned to allow drainage of debris and pus.

MANAGEMENT OF LEAKS ASSOCIATED WITH ENTEROCUTANEOUS FISTULA

With correct management 60–80% of enterocutaneous fistulae will heal with no operative intervention other than to drain abscesses. Five principles of management of such fistulae should be undertaken in the following sequence:

1. Fluid and electrolyte disturbances should be corrected.
2. The skin should be protected by application of stoma appliances.
3. Nutritional support should be started.
4. Focal sepsis should be detected and eliminated.
5. The anatomy of the fistula should be investigated and a decision made for conservative or surgical management.

Correction of fluid and electrolyte disturbances

9 A high output fistula, defined as one with a loss of over 500 ml in 24 h, can lead to rapid dehydration. Continuous replacement of the lost water and electrolytes is necessary until the loss ceases. During this time, application of a dependent drainage device may allow the patient to mobilize and minimizes the need for repetitive emptying of stoma bags.

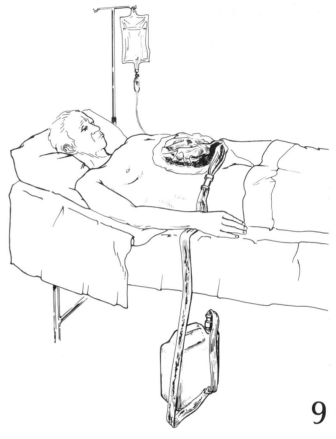

9

Protection of the skin around the fistula

10 The mouth of the fistula should be isolated with protective material such as Karaya or Stomahesive placed over the surrounding skin and a stoma bag fitted over this protective barrier.

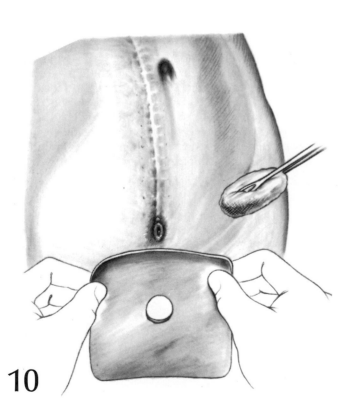

10

11 For confluent fistulae or those arising in large broken-down wounds it is important to prevent pooling of liquid bowel contents, and protection of the skin may necessitate introduction of suction catheters and the application of an extensive appliance on the abdominal wall.

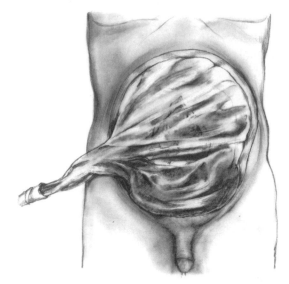

11

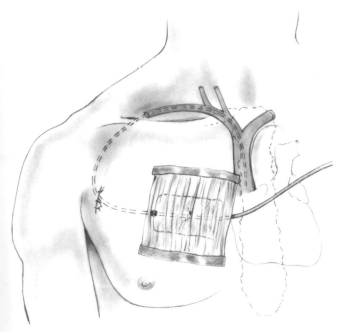

12

Nutritional support

12 Once fluid and electrolyte deficits have been corrected, parenteral nutrition should be commenced through a catheter positioned in a large vein, preferably with the tip in the superior vena cava. Tunnelling the feeding line so that it emerges on the anterior chest wall allows better access for the nursing staff, who should be trained in strict aseptic technique. By using dedicated feeding lines and trained staff exogenous line infection can be almost eliminated. Patients with terminal ileal or large bowel fistulae can usually be converted rapidly to enteral nutrition using a liquid low-residue formula. Peripheral intravenous feeding may be an alternative means of short-term adaptation to enteral feeding.

13 Patients with a high small intestinal fistula, a persistent high-output stoma or significant malnutrition will require parenteral nutrition until the fistula closes or reanastomosis of the bowel takes place. Using compact pumps it is possible to decrease the duration of feeding gradually so that the daily requirements are infused over 12 h during the evening and night. This allows the patient to exercise during the day when the feeding line is closed off using a heparin lock.

Detection and elimination of focal sepsis

The patient should be examined to establish whether sepsis is present, to determine the anatomy of the fistula and to ascertain whether there is obstruction distal to the fistula. Abscesses can be detected by a combination of clinical signs, CT, ultrasonography and isotope scanning and sinography. The anatomy of the fistula can be established by radio-opaque contrast studies and fistulography.

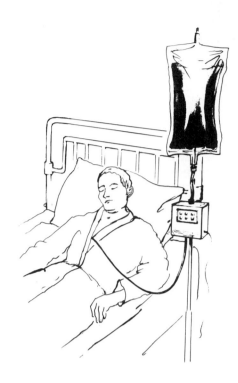

13

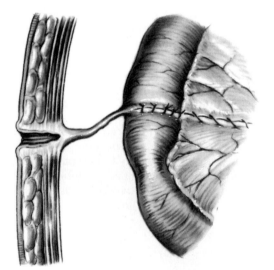

14

Continuing management of the fistula

14 If a fistula has a low output, and is shown on contrast study to be lateral and without distal obstruction then it will close with the management regimen outlined above, provided that there is no residual sepsis. Where there is a persistent track, fistuloscopy and insertion of tissue sealants can be helpful in occluding the track.

15a–d

If the bowel is completely disrupted (*Illustration 15a*), there is distal obstruction (*b*), an associated abscess (*c*), or muco-cutaneous continuity (*d*), the fistula will not close spontaneously. In these circumstances surgical operation is necessary and the type of surgery is dictated by the maturation of the fistula and the nutritional state of the patient. If, as a result of good nutritional management, the patient is well nourished (serum albumin >28 g/dl), and if sepsis has been eliminated, it is permissible to resect the fistula and reconstruct the anastomosis. If, however, the patient is anaemic, hypoalbuminaemic or septic, the bowel ends should be exteriorized as previously described. Reanastomosis can take place later when the patient is no longer septic and malnourished.

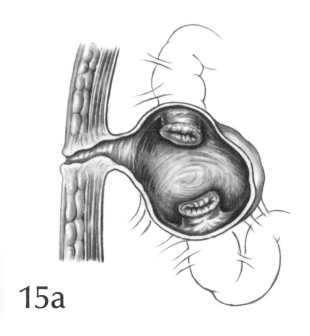

15a

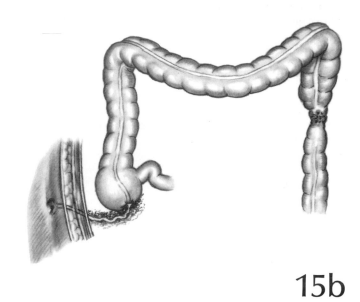

15b

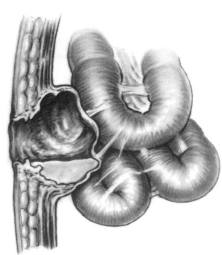

15c

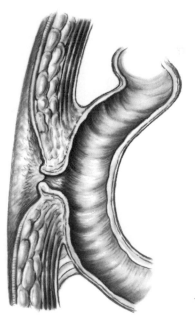

15d

Postoperative care

In the immediate postoperative period the patient may be haemodynamically unstable and is best managed in a high-dependency or intensive care area. Respiratory support may be required but prolonged mechanical ventilation is associated with increased complications and must be avoided wherever possible. Intravenous infusions should be continued until the stoma starts functioning, at which time oral intake can commence.

Postoperative antibiotics should be considered only if there has been gross contamination of the abdominal cavity or if there is recurrent septicaemia. Abscesses should be drained percutaneously following ultrasonographic or CT localization but surgical drainage may occasionally be necessary. Should the patient show evidence of ongoing sepsis a full infection screen is required and, if an infective focus cannot be identified or drained percutaneously, further laparotomy is necessary.

Restoration of intestinal continuity

Reanastomosis of the bowel should not be contemplated until all sepsis has subsided and the patient has regained lost weight. At the earliest this will be 3 months after all wounds have healed, but it may be better to leave the patient even longer, to allow intra-abdominal inflammation to subside and to make restoration technically easier. Early intervention increases the risk of bowel injury during division of adhesions and separation of bowel loops.

Interventional radiology in colorectal surgery

Henry W. Loose FRCR
Consultant Radiologist, Freeman Hospital, Newcastle-upon-Tyne, UK

Principles and justification

The development of new imaging methods, in particular the techniques of computed tomography (CT) and real time ultrasonography, has enabled precise localization of disease foci. The introduction of more refined fluoroscopic and angiographic equipment in parallel with the development of small-diameter catheters, guidewires and drainage tubes has rendered many abnormalities accessible for biopsy and drainage using guided percutaneous techniques.

The colon is readily examined by colonoscopy, but the paracolic tissues and other organs cannot be visualized, and severe haemorrhage may render colonoscopy ineffective. Angiography is often quicker and more precise, and embolization of the bleeding vessel through the arterial catheter may be a simple therapeutic measure, either as a definitive treatment or to enable resuscitation of the patient before surgical resection of the underlying pathological lesion.

Surgical relief of colonic obstruction is traditional and remains the treatment of choice, but a small proportion of patients can be treated using interventional radiological techniques, e.g. percutaneous caecostomy for relief of pseudo-obstruction, barium reduction of intussusception and balloon dilatation of colonic strictures.

Metastases from colonic carcinoma, particularly in the liver parenchyma, have on the whole defied successful therapy. Selective angiographic catheter placement and embolization or injection of cytotoxic agents have been shown to prevent tumour growth and are under active investigation.

Preoperative

Personnel

These techniques should be performed by radiologists who have specialized as full-time 'interventionalists'. It is important that the department offers adequate equipment, trained staff (both radiographic and nursing), as well as sufficient clinical experience to justify the substantial capital expenditure that is involved in maintaining a complete range of disposable equipment.

Anaesthesia

Local anaesthesia with mild sedation (diazepam, 10 mg intravenously) is usually sufficient for most procedures, and may be potentiated with pethidine hydrochloride, 25–50 mg intravenously if required. Some centres prefer oral diazepam in doses appropriate to the age of the patient and an intramuscular narcotic 1 h before the procedure.

Anxious patients benefit from Omnopon, 20 mg intramuscularly 30 min before the procedure. In a long procedure or in patients who require dilatation of a tract to a gauge larger than 8.5 Fr, a combination of midazolam hydrochloride, 5–10 mg intravenously with fentanyl citrate, 50–100 μg intravenously, is effective. All patients must be monitored with a visual display of pulse rate, blood pressure and oxygen saturation.

General anaesthesia is seldom required with the exception of children, and is contraindicated because the development of pain is a pertinent indication of ischaemia or overdilatation, which can only be appreciated if the patient is able to communicate with the operator.

Patient preparation

The appropriate puncture site, usually the femoral artery at the groin, should be shaved. Fluid by mouth should be encouraged because the incidence of depression of renal function secondary to the toxic effects of contrast medium rises significantly if fluid is withheld.

Diagnostic angiography causes little discomfort apart from a transient warmth and occasional feeling of micturition if the internal iliac vessels are filled.

Embolization of a solid organ, however, causes ischaemic pain that may require intravenous narcotics for 24–48 h after the procedure. An intravenous infusion should be *in situ* before embolization.

Extensive embolization may also cause a low-grade fever secondary to tissue destruction, nausea and a feeling of lassitude which has been termed 'postembolization syndrome'. These may require supportive therapy.

If angiography is to be performed for localization of the site of haemorrhage, additional personnel are required to monitor the vital signs and to maintain adequate fluid balance, blood volume and the airway, to enable the attention of the operating radiologist to be directed to the procedure.

Informed consent

The procedure should be discussed with the patient and informed consent obtained, preferably by the 'operating' radiologist. The radiologist should not proceed to intervene without full and complete discussion with other appropriate clinicians who are responsible for the care of the patient.

Equipment

Standard disposable catheters (5 Fr or 7 Fr) and wires (0.035 inch) in sterile packs are used. The 'sidewinder' shape facilitates entry into the coeliac and superior and inferior mesenteric vessels from a femoral approach, as the tip enters in a caudal direction after the catheter has been formed in the aortic arch.

Embolic materials

Autologous clotted blood is absorbed within 12 h and therefore is of little practical value. The most practical materials for vessel embolization are the absorbable haemostatic materials, such as surgical gelatin sponge (Gelfoam) cut into small fragments 0.25–1 mm in diameter. These are drawn into a syringe in 50% normal saline and 50% contrast medium and injected under fluoroscopy when the contrast medium is visible, which allows close monitoring of any change in flow pattern. Slow hand injection is required. As soon as the flow in the vessel is slowed, the catheter is withdrawn a few millimetres to ensure that the vessel is not obstructed, and contrast medium is injected to clear the catheter and repeated every 5 min. Further particles may be required if flow continues or a steel coil can be placed behind the surgical gelatin sponge to obstruct residual flow. Gelatin sponge is absorbed within a few days, but the clot will have consolidated at the point of haemorrhage. The coil causes permanent obstruction, but is soon bypassed by collateral flow.

Tumour embolization requires more permanent materials that are not absorbed such as polyvinyl alcohol (Ivalon), a plastic sponge that expands when wet. It is available ready packed and sterile as spheres or sheets which can be cut into fragments of appropriate size (150–590 μm) in the angiography room.

A most effective embolizing agent is absolute alcohol (70%), which is painful on injection but toxic to the endothelium and produces rapid permanent vessel closure. Alcohol can be used in end arteries, e.g. the hepatic or renal vessels, with distal catheter placement but it is inappropriate for embolization of intestine or other sites of dual arterial supply, such as the internal iliac vessel.

Steel coils or detachable balloons are used for occlusion of larger vessels and act in a fashion equivalent to surgical ligation. Coils are essentially short segments of wire (0.038 inch) with a circular memory. Dacron threads are tied around the wire and stimulate clot formation *in vivo*. Detachable balloons are used to close fistulae and the necks of aneurysms, but otherwise have little advantage over the coils and are more cumbersome to use. Liquid plastic polymers are used, but require extra skills and are outside the scope of this text.

If it is not possible to achieve good distal catheter placement, then embolization is unsafe. This can be overcome by the introduction of a coaxial 3-Fr catheter passed with a 0.025-inch steerable guidewire through the lumen of the diagnostic catheter and steered to a more peripheral position. Steel coils (0.025 inch) are available, and gelatin or polyvinyl alcohol sponges are made in a powder form (200 μm) for use through the small coaxial catheter.

An alternative to particulate embolization is the infusion of a vasoconstrictive drug through the arterial catheter, which may be left *in situ* for up to 24 h. Satisfactory persisting vasoconstriction is monitored by contrast injection every 2–4 h.

Operations

ANGIOGRAPHY

Acute colonic haemorrhage

Angiography is a quick and effective way to localize the site of lower gastrointestinal haemorrhage. It is important that the procedure is not delayed while resuscitation is carried out before the patient is sent to the radiology department, because gastrointestinal haemorrhage is often intermittent and the site will not be identified if the haemorrhage has ceased. Patient resuscitation can be performed during angiography if adequate skilled help is available. Emergency surgery in these patients carries a high mortality rate (20–50%), and accurate preoperative localization reduces this. Vasopressin infusion or transcatheter embolization may convert an emergency laparotomy into an elective resection.

A proctosigmoidoscopy should precede angiography to exclude a site of haemorrhage from the rectum or anal region. Acute lower gastrointestinal haemorrhage without haematemesis may be caused by bleeding below the oesophagogastric junction. Upper gastrointestinal endoscopy should precede angiography, but the occasional exception can be made if the haemorrhage is rapid. The three major abdominal vessels should be examined at angiography, and the site will be shown if the haemorrhage is greater than 0.5 ml/min.

Radionuclide studies have been disappointing except in those patients where haemorrhage is rapid, but may be helpful if angiography proves negative. Labelled red cells can be monitored over a 6-h period, although there is usually some free technetium released into the lumen of the gut which may lead to false positive identification of the site of blood loss.

The inferior mesenteric artery is injected first at a rate of 3 ml/s for 4 s as the distribution of the superior rectal artery can be obscured by a bladder that fills with excreted contrast medium; filming is continued for 12–16 s to include a full study of the venous phase.

The superior mesenteric artery is then injected at a rate of 8 ml/s for 5 s, and filming is performed for 16 s. Two separate injections may be required because the relatively small size of rapid sequence films may not be large enough to cover the distribution of the inferior and superior mesenteric arcades to include the splenic flexure.

The coeliac axis must always be examined (8 ml/s for 5 s) if the examination of the inferior mesenteric and superior mesenteric arteries proves negative.

Provocation angiography

The site of haemorrhage can be elusive and evade detection despite good quality angiography and

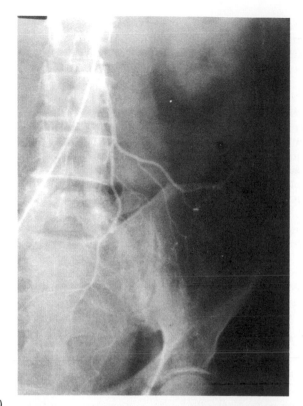

(a)

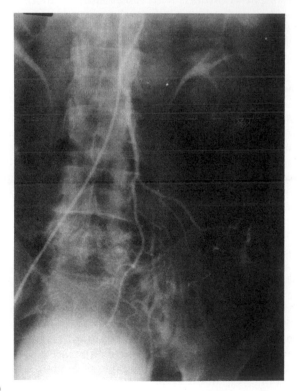

(b)

Figure 1   A 52-year-old man had had five large rectal bleeds in the previous 2 years, and a further bleed 24 h before angiography. (a) Initial angiography was normal. (b) Extravasation into sigmoid colon occurred after papaverine, 20 mg, and streptokinase, 5000 units for 4 h. Surgical resection then showed that the pathology was a bleeding diverticulum

radionuclide studies. The reasons are not clear, but intermittent vascular shutdown ('spasm') and clot formation when the systemic blood pressure is low contribute to negative angiographic findings.

Provocation angiography may be indicated. It is only performed with the full consent of the patient and his clinician. It is indicated in patients who have had repeated colonic bleeds requiring hospitalization and resuscitation and negative angiography, often on a number of occasions. It also may be indicated in those patients who require long-term anticoagulation, but who suffer repeated gastrointestinal bleeds without an identified cause.

The catheter is left in the artery that is thought to be the most likely supply vessel, i.e. inferior mesenteric or ileocolic vessel. A vasodilator is injected (papaverine, 20–30 mg or isosorbide dinitrate, 1–2 mg) and angiography is repeated. If this does not precipitate extravasation from the bleeding site, streptokinase, 5000 units/h for 4 h or tissue plasminogen activator, 0.5 mg/h is infused for 4–6 h and angiography is again repeated (see Figure 1a and b).

It must be emphasized that this procedure is only done with the full consent of the patient and full knowledge of a surgeon who may be required to perform emergency surgery if the resultant bleed cannot be controlled with vasopressin or embolization.

It is not effective or indicated in patients with chronic gastrointestinal bleeding or those that have not had an acute bleed in the previous 2–3 days.

EMBOLIZATION AND VASOPRESSIN

Vasopressin infusion is an effective method of controlling haemorrhage. It is not necessary to position the catheter highly selectively but it is left in the main trunk of the superior or inferior mesenteric artery. It is occasionally necessary to site the catheter in an aberrant middle colic artery which arises from the coeliac axis. It has been necessary to achieve more selective positioning in a few cases of postsurgical blood loss in the middle small intestine (anastomotic bleed) to achieve vasospasm.

Vasopressin, 100 units, is mixed with 500 ml of saline, (0.2 units/ml final strength) and then delivered at a rate of 30–60 ml/h. Angiography is repeated after 20 min, and if extravasation is still present the infusion rate is doubled to 60–120 ml/h or the concentration is doubled to 0.4 units/ml. If extravasation is still present after 20–30 min an alternative therapy should be undertaken. Further dose increases are unlikely to be of benefit. The infusion is continued for 24 h if good vasoconstriction is achieved.

Abdominal cramp is a sign of effective vasoconstriction, as vasopressin precipitates intestinal wall contraction which should subside after 20–30 min. If persistent, it is evidence of excessive vasoconstriction and the rate of infusion should be reduced.

The side effects of vasopressin are varied, but may be severe, particularly if manifest in the cardiovascular system (arrhythmias, severe hypertension, ischaemia of the legs). Development of intestinal ischaemia is rare, but recorded. Cerebral oedema may develop secondary to low serum sodium levels and all patients should remain on full monitoring and have regular electrolyte checks to avoid hyponatraemia. Local catheter complications (sepsis and haematoma) may also occur.

Transcatheter embolization of the intestine has been slow to be accepted because of the risks of resultant ischaemia. It is now, however, a real alternative, as the catheters can be removed and a long-term arterial infusion is avoided, thus minimizing patient discomfort. A definite end-point is also attained. It is a safe technique in the branches of the coeliac artery, but it is prudent for the catheter tip to be in a superselective situation.

There is evidence that selective embolization of the bleeding point in the intestine is a feasible therapy. It should only be performed when the catheter is superselective, which usually requires a coaxial system. Gelatin sponge plugs are used, though a single mini-coil may also be effective.

The incidence of symptomatic ischaemia is only 15% in published series, and fewer than 10% have required surgical intervention. Embolization may facilitate resuscitation of the patient and allow elective surgery to be undertaken. It can also be indicated in the patient in whom surgery is not feasible because of concomitant disease in other systems, for example severe cardiac or lung disease or irreversible clotting defects.

Acute haemorrhage (Figure 2a–d)

Acute haemorrhage at the site of a surgical anastomosis is effectively controlled by vasopressin. Severe blood loss from ischaemic colitis is also well controlled by vasopressin, but embolization is contraindicated.

The widespread use of sclerotherapy to control oesophageal varices has led to diversion of the portal venous blood to the superior and inferior mesenteric veins, and varices develop along postsurgical adhesions between intestine and parietes. They may present with lower gastrointestinal haemorrhage and can be controlled by vasopressin before surgical therapy or transhepatic portal vein embolization.

Angiodysplasia requires surgical resection, but acute blood loss can be controlled by vasopressin or embolization.

Tumours seldom present with acute blood loss and are normally diagnosed by other methods, but a small carcinoma in the caecum may be confused with angiodysplasia and may be overlooked at barium radiology or colonoscopy.

Vascular–enteric fistulae must always be considered when haemorrhage is severe particularly when a vascular graft is present. Colonic haemorrhage may

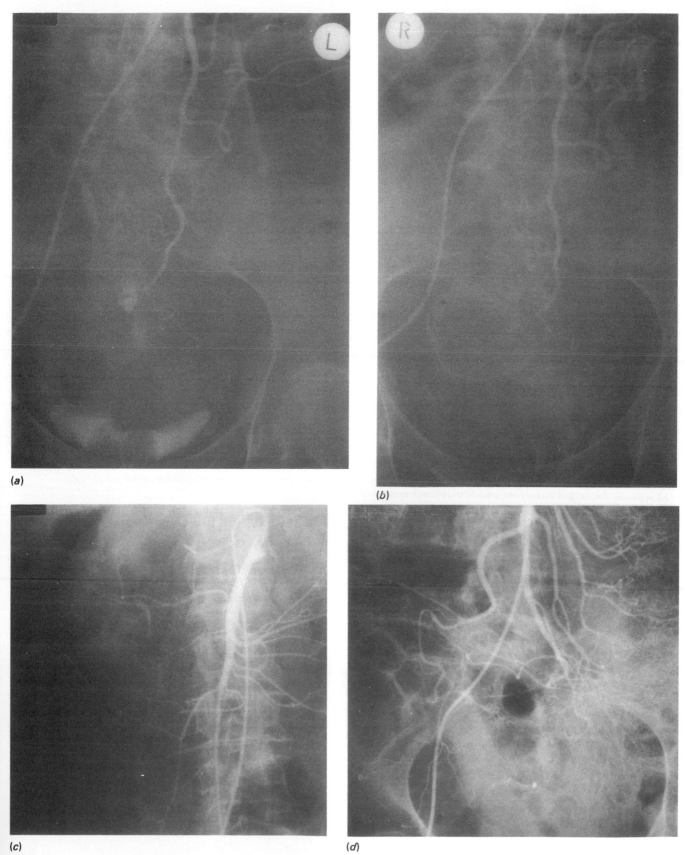

Figure 2   (a, b) In a woman aged 62 years, sigmoidoscopic biopsy showed a rectal carcinoma. Severe bleeding occurred, and angiography showed transection of the superior rectal artery. This was embolized with a surgical gelatin sponge plug and bleeding ceased. (c) In a man aged 72 years, injection of the superior mesenteric artery produced extravasation from a branch of the ileocolic artery, due to a bleeding diverticulum. (d) A woman aged 74 years suffered severe rectal bleeding. Injection of the superior mesenteric artery produced extravasation into the pelvic caecum. Surgical resection showed Dieulafoy's disease.

result if the iliac limb of a vascular graft erodes into the sigmoid or descending colon.

Haemorrhage after biopsy or polypectomy is usually simply managed by selective embolization.

Diverticular haemorrhage is usually more severe from the right colon than from the left and can be controlled with vasopressin, but embolization is quicker as a prelude to elective surgical resection.

Irresectable arteriovenous malformations of the rectum can be managed with repeated embolization.

Chronic colonic blood loss

Angiography is indicated in patients who have persistent anaemia with positive occult blood testing, and in whom other methods of investigation have failed to uncover the source of blood loss.

The three major intestinal vessels are examined as described in the previous section, but extravasation of contrast medium into the intestinal lumen will not be seen, the lesions being localized by their abnormal vascular pattern.

Leiomyomas and leiomyosarcomas are well defined, hypervascular and contain irregular tumour vessels. Carcinoids show a characteristic stellate distribution of the central vessels or may distort the root of the mesentery by an associated desmoplastic reaction.

Arteriovenous malformations may demonstrate large dilated tortuous feeding vessels, but these may be undetectable without good-quality venous phase films. A venous arteriovenous malformation can involve a long segment of the large intestine, and the arterial anatomy may be normal. The large number of tortuous, irregularly draining veins opacify poorly (up to 40 s after injection) and may fill after the normal venous drainage has cleared.

Angiodysplasia is regarded as an acquired condition and is predominantly seen in patients over 60 years old. The demonstration of early opacification of a draining vein alerts the angiographer to examine the antimesenteric border of that segment of intestine. Clusters of small arteries may be visible, but if very small an arterial abnormality may not always be detected. Most are detected in the right colon opposite the ileocaecal valve, but they may be found throughout both large and small intestine.

If angiography demonstrates an arteriovenous malformation or angiodysplastic lesion in the small intestine preoperative selective catheterization is indicated. Methylene blue, 1–2 ml, is injected through the catheter in the operating theatre to identify the appropriate small intestine segment. The specimen must be left intact and the artery injected to enable the pathologist to take sections of the appropriate area. A small angiodysplastic lesion or arteriovenous malformation will be missed if a strict protocol is not observed.

Meckel's diverticulum may be diagnosed by angiography if it is either distended with blood or associated with an elongated and straightened distal ileal branch of the superior mesenteric artery.

Carcinomas of the caecum, if small, may closely mimic the angiographic appearances of angiodysplasia, and the tumour vessels can be overlooked. Colonoscopic evaluation is advised in all patients, and angiodysplasia may be successfully treated with electrocoagulation or laser therapy at the same session.

EMBOLIZATION AND CYTOTOXIC THERAPY FOR HEPATIC METASTASES

The results of conventional treatment of hepatic metastases are poor; the response rate to 5-fluorouracil, for example, is less than 20%. A number of adjunctive therapies have been developed, including percutaneous injection of 70% alcohol, intermittent ischaemia and injection of radioactive agents. Embolization or chemo-embolization employing simultaneous cytotoxic drugs and particulate agents is being assessed.

Although there is a dual blood supply to the liver (portal vein, 75%; hepatic artery, 25%), liver tumours are predominantly supplied by the hepatic artery, which is accessible to percutaneous catheterization.

Iodized oil fluid injection angiography (*Figure 3a* and *b*)

Iodized oil fluid injection angiography has rendered smaller tumours visible, particularly if vascular, and is indicated if metastases have been identified in one liver lobe and resection is being considered. The technique involves direct infusion of 6–8 ml of iodized oil fluid (Lipiodol) into the main hepatic artery (peripheral to the gastroduodenal) with follow-up CT scan after 14 days. The iodized fluid oil is cleared from the liver parenchyma by the reticuloendothelial system, but persists in the abnormal circulation around the tumour where lymphatics are absent. It will demonstrate tumours of 2–3 mm in diameter. The effectiveness of cytotoxic agents depends on the degree of extraction and the level of concentration within the liver. It is attractive to assist the cytotoxic contact time by direct arterial injection attached to iodized oil fluid.

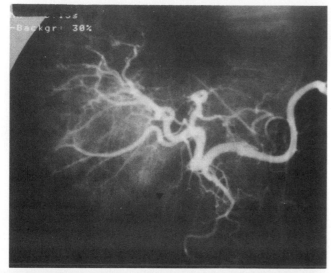

(a)

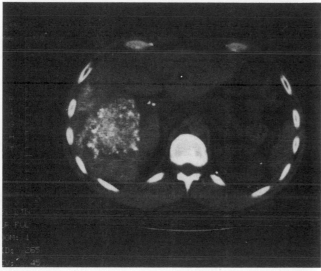

(b)

Figure 3   Iodized oil fluid injection angiography. (a) Coeliac axis injection shows a large vascular tumour in the right lobe of the liver (arrowed). (b) An injection of 6 ml into the hepatic artery followed by a CT scan after 10 days shows residual iodized oil fluid in the tumour in the right lobe, but the left lobe is clear of other metastases

Tumour embolization *(Figure 4a–d)*

The role of concurrent embolization is uncertain, but much evidence suggests that devascularization and consequent anoxia is an effective method to induce tumour necrosis. In the experience of the author, the more vascular the tumour, the greater the response to particulate embolization.

There is much uncertainty and dispute as to whether chemotherapy should be combined with particulate embolization. It is the author's practice to perform particulate embolization in all patients who undergo chemotherapeutic infusion of metastases. This is followed by repeat angiography, chemotherapy and further embolization each month for 3 months. A vascular tumour is embolized with permanent particulate material and steel coils, and follow-up angiography is devoted to embolization of recanalized and collateral vessels inclusive of the extrahepatic supply, such as the lumbar or intercostal, inferior phrenic or right colic vessels.

No patient who is motivated to undergo treatment should be excluded, but caution should be exercised if the portal vein is thrombosed. It is the author's policy not to proceed to particulate embolization of both right and left lobes if the portal vein is thrombosed, but single-lobe embolization has been undertaken without detectable complication.

An intravenous line must be in place before the procedure to facilitate administration of sedatives, antibiotics and analgesics as required. The procedure is covered by antibiotics for 5 days, which has reduced the incidence of hepatic abscess and sepsis to 2%.

Coeliac and superior mesenteric angiography are performed to evaluate the blood supply of the liver and establish the patency of the portal vein. Common anatomical variants include the right hepatic artery arising from the superior mesenteric artery (25%) and the left hepatic artery arising from the left gastric artery (5%).

A coaxial system of catheterization (2.2-Fr within 5 Fr) may be required, but it is usual to attain superselective positioning of the 5 Fr catheter using available guidewires. A small number of procedures require a brachial approach if a large liver distorts the angle of the origin of the coeliac artery.

The most effective form of chemoembolization is under assessment at different centres. It is possible to repeat percutaneous chemotherapy and therefore administer regular doses, usually on a monthly regimen. Iodized oil fluid is now given in the same syringe, which aids retention in the liver and around the tumour mass.

The author's regimen is a monthly treatment for 3 months. CT is carried out before embolization, at 3 months, 6 months and at 1 year. Repeat chemoembolization is performed at 6 months, at 1 year, 6-monthly to 3 years and then annually.

Absolute alcohol (70%), 2 ml, iodized oil fluid, 8 ml, and mitomycin C, 20 mg, are infused, followed by gelatin sponge powder. Polyvinyl alcohol replaces gelatin sponge at the third treatment. Starch microspheres of mitomycin, cisplatin, doxorubicin hydrochloride and 5-fluorouracil may be considered as alternative agents.

The assessment of the response may be difficult. Decrease in the size of the liver on palpation (75 cm), decrease of the tumour size on CT (50%), or decrease in serum carcinoembryonic antigen are commonly measured parameters.

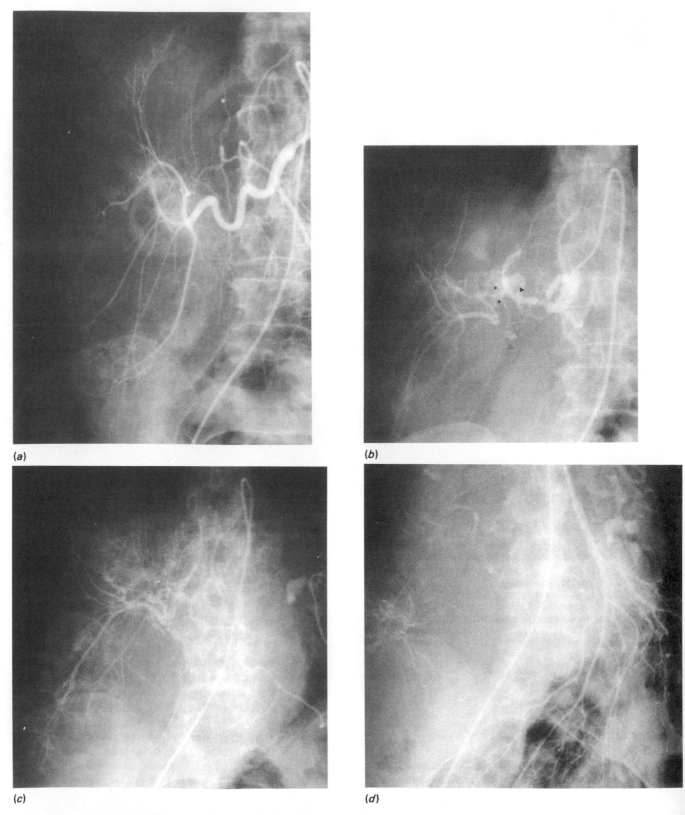

Figure 4   Particulate embolization for colonic metastasis. (a) Large vascular metastasis in right lobe; (b) 4 years after initial embolization, injection into the left hepatic artery (large arrowhead) shows cross-circulation into the right hepatic artery (small arrowheads). Note the residual tumour is much smaller but still perfused and the coil (open arrowhead) in the obstructed right hepatic artery stem; (c) and (d) the same, 4 years later. Multiple vascular metastases appear in the left lobe with enlargement of the original tumour. Injection of the superior mesenteric artery shows collateral supply from the right colic artery to the original tumour mass

Results

Comparison of the diameter of the mass underestimates the response, as there is a delay of 2–4 months before necrotic tumour is resorbed and metabolized. Clinical benefit may be evident without objective confirmation.

Assessment of the true benefit of chemoembolization for colonic metastases is not possible, as there are no controlled clinical trials. In the author's personal experience, particulate embolization with mitomycin and iodized oil fluid has a response rate greater than 50%, with clinical benefit in more than 70% of patients. The response is related to the vascularity of the tumour on angiography (the greater the vascularity the better the response to particulate embolization), the histological grade of the primary tumour and the time of diagnosis of metastases after the original surgical resection.

Percutaneous tumour injection of alcohol

Ultrasound-guided percutaneous injection of alcohol can be used as adjunctive therapy. It is indicated for metastases that are small in number (up to five) and small in diameter (2 cm), but may be used if a single tumour is large (4 cm). The volume of absolute alcohol injected is related to tumour size.

Early follow-up and assessment of response has been promising.

PERCUTANEOUS BIOPSY AND ABSCESS DRAINAGE

Percutaneous abscess drainage is now standard therapy, and laparotomy is very seldom performed.

Ultrasonic guidance is quick and effective, but occasionally lack of a 'window' due to overlying gas indicates other forms of imaging. It is important that the relevant images, whether fluoroscopic, ultrasonographic or computed tomographic are correlated before drainage is undertaken to avoid drainage of a necrotic tumour or asymptomatic haematoma.

Indications and imaging

It is not necessary to arrange for a surgical team to be on stand-by. An abscess can be drained even if there is enteric communication, if it is multilocular, or it is shielded by overlying structures.

It may be prudent to aspirate with a fine needle (22 Fr) and perform a Gram stain or cytology in a doubtful mass lesion before embarking on dilatation of a tract into the abscess cavity.

It may be necessary to insert more than one drainage tube in a large multilocular cavity or when the septa cannot be broken down by a catheter and wire combination.

Drainage is performed in the ultrasound suite and fluoroscopy is seldom required. If the cavity cannot be clearly visualized, it may be necessary to move the patient to the CT scanner and identify a suitable tract. Fluoroscopy is used at follow-up tubography to establish the presence (or absence) of an internal communication and to document healing of the cavity.

Percutaneous drainage is now routine for hepatic and renal retroperitoneal collections and peritoneal abscesses in subhepatic, subphrenic and paracolic spaces (see Figure 5a–c). The lesser sac and deep pelvic spaces (paravesicular and pararectal fossae) may require a CT scan as a diagnostic method to plan the safest and most suitable route of approach.

Technique and equipment

Several systems are used, and the choice is usually made on personal preference. The safest method is to guide a fine needle (20 Fr) into the cavity and insert a 0.18-inch diameter flexible-tip guidewire with a stiff shaft. The tract can then be dilated to 5 Fr with an angled dilator with an end hole and an additional side hole through which a larger diameter J-tip guidewire (0.35 inch) exits. The tract is then dilated to the required diameter before introduction of the drainage catheter.

'Pigtail' catheters, 8.5 Fr in diameter, are large enough to drain fluid collections and cysts, but thick pus, necrotic pancreatic abscesses and empyemas will require 14-Fr catheters with large side ports. Very occasionally, 20 Fr may be required. It is wise to utilize pigtail catheters with a locking device, usually a suture that fixes the pigtail into a loop in addition to skin sutures.

The cavity is irrigated and aspirated with saline at a low pressure to avoid sepsis. The radiologist should see the patient daily, and follow-up tubography under fluoroscopy is arranged for 48 h later. The tube is removed when the radiological criteria of closure of cavity and the clinical criteria of a normal leucocyte count, normalization of temperature and no drainage are met. The tube is only removed after discussion with the clinicians concerned. A simple abscess seldom requires drainage for more than 7 days.

Pericolic abscess drainage

Drainage of abscesses associated with local perforation of the colon, such as periappendicular or peridiverticular abscesses, or those associated with Crohn's disease, do not require percutaneous drainage if it is preferable to remove the abscess and the abnormal colonic segment at one surgical procedure. Drainage of a diverticular abscess, however, may permit a single elective surgical resection and anastomosis instead of a two-stage surgical procedure. Furthermore there is debate as to whether the appendix requires removal

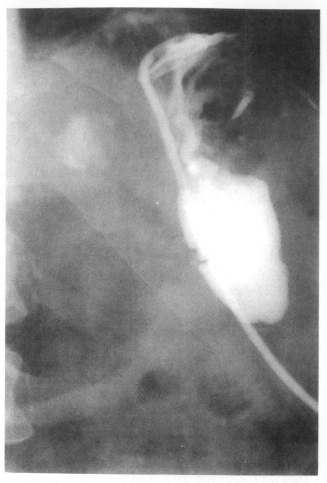

(a)

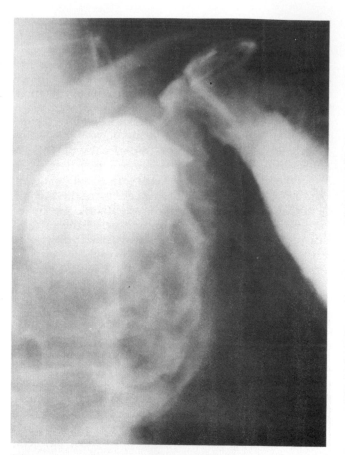

(b)

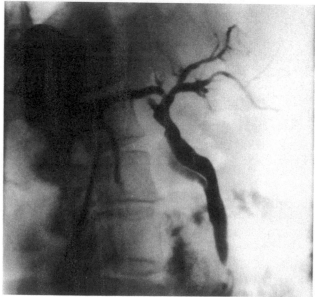

(c)

after drainage of an appendicular abscess and Crohn's disease abscesses may be drained without resort to surgical resection if no enteric communication is present.

Pericolic abscesses are best drained under CT guidance as they are intimately related to the intestine. In the pelvis drainage may be achieved by direct rectal or vaginal puncture and tract dilatation using the same techniques if imaging demonstrates intimate contact.

Diverticular and appendiceal abscesses often require a longer period of drainage (2 weeks) if an enteric connection is present. Successful drainage and closure of fistulae is achieved in more than 90% of cases.

Haematomas may be simply aspirated, but if they contain clot and fibrous tissue they may not drain. No haematoma should be formally drained unless it is painful or is causing obstruction, to avoid introduction of secondary infection.

DILATATION OF STRICTURES

Benign anastomotic strictures of the rectum and sigmoid colon are easy to catheterize using 'arterial'

Figure 5   (a) Drainage of an abscess with enteric connections. (b) Drainage of a left subphrenic abscess after a perforated sigmoid diverticulum, showing communication with the gastric fundus. Spontaneous closure occurred after 4 weeks of catheter drainage. (c) Drainage of a hepatic abscess (secondary to diverticulitis). Spontaneous rupture to right bile duct occurred. Spontaneous closure occurred after 3.5 weeks of catheter drainage

techniques and equipment. More proximal strictures are best approached by colonoscopy.

Dilatation of these strictures is possible with balloon catheters that inflate to 2–3 cm in diameter. Prolonged expansion is required, but the inflation pressure is usually insufficient to eliminate the narrowed segment. It is a procedure that is at best temporary and the symptoms and the stricture usually recur within 1 month. Repeated dilatations may be undertaken.

PERCUTANEOUS CAECOSTOMY (*Figure 6a–c*)

Obstruction of the colon is treated by surgical means, but percutaneous caecostomy may be indicated in those patients who are unfit for anaesthesia or in the frail, elderly patient with pseudo-obstruction.

The technique is identical to that for drainage of an abscess. Percutaneous enteric drainage kits are available for introduction of gastrostomy tubes, but these are not normally required for drainage of a large dilated caecum.

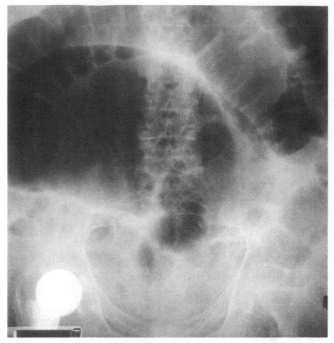

(a)

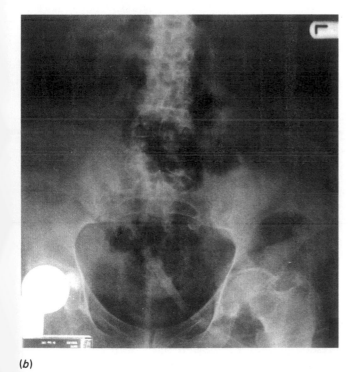

(b)

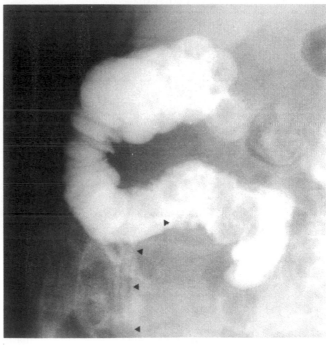

(c)

Figure 6   A women aged 91 years suffered repeated episodes of pseudo-obstruction of the sigmoid colon. (a) Gross dilatation of the caecum and colon to the sigmoid colon region. (b) At 24 h after percutaneous caecostomy, resolution of the dilated colon was demonstrated. (c) Injection of contrast through a balloon catheter 24 h after insertion. (With acknowledgement to Dr L Murthy, Freeman Hospital).

Illustrations by Peter Cox

Proctoscopy and sigmoidoscopy

J. D. Hardcastle MA, MChir, FRCS, FRCP
Professor of Surgery, University Hospital, Queen's Medical Centre, Nottingham, UK

Principles and justification

Indications

Proctoscopy is used to inspect the region of the anorectal ring and anal canal. The diagnosis and treatment of haemorrhoids (injection or banding) and other minor anal problems can be carried out through a proctoscope of adequate size.

Sigmoidoscopy is part of the routine examination of patients complaining of symptoms suggestive of rectal or colonic disease. It is indicated in all patients with rectal bleeding or a change of bowel habit. It should be performed before barium enema examination. Flexible sigmoidoscopy may also be indicated to confirm any biopsy lesions seen on barium enema examination and in the follow-up of patients who have had previous rectal or left colonic resection for colorectal cancer. In patients with rectal bleeding over the age of 50 years, flexible sigmoidoscopy should be performed to exclude polypoid lesions in the distal colon.

Contraindications

Anal stenosis or an acute anal fissure rendering proctoscopy painful are contraindications. These will be detected by preliminary digital examination of the anal canal.

A severe degree of anal stenosis may make it difficult to pass a rigid or flexible sigmoidoscope. When this is present, it is usually possible to dilate the stricture sufficiently to pass either a small-calibre rigid sigmoidoscope or a flexible fibreoptic sigmoidoscope. The incidence of perforation with flexible sigmoidoscopy is very low, but the examination should terminate if the patient complains of severe discomfort, and particular care should be taken in patients with acute inflammatory bowel disease.

Preoperative

No special preparation is required for proctoscopy.

Bowel preparation and medication for sigmoidoscopy

Rigid sigmoidoscopy can be performed without bowel preparation, but in many patients faeces present in the rectum will obscure the view and possibly limit the distance to which the sigmoidoscope can be passed. Examination without bowel preparation has the advantage that it enables the contents of the upper rectum to be inspected. For flexible sigmoidoscopy, a single phosphate enema provides adequate bowel preparation in the majority of patients, a second enema being only very occasionally necessary.

Sigmoidoscopy may be carried out in the outpatient department. After explanation, the patient undresses, puts on a gown and is given a phosphate enema. The patient should not be examined for at least 30 min, preferably after the bowels have been opened twice. This results in adequate clearance of the left side of the colon. Neither sedation nor analgesia is required, and antispasmodics have been shown to be of no help. The procedure should be terminated if severe pain is experienced.

In patients with artificial joints and valvular heart disease, prophylactic antibiotics should be given, as transient bacteraemia has been reported.

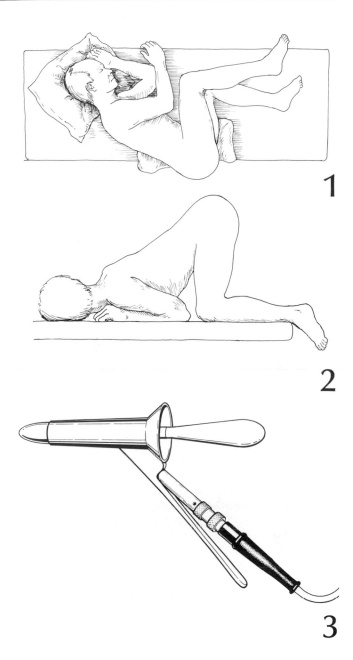

Operations

PROCTOSCOPY

Position of patient

1,2 The left lateral position as described for sigmoidoscopy is satisfactory; however, the knee–elbow position is sometimes preferred and can most conveniently be achieved by the use of a purpose-built tilting examination couch.

Instruments

3 Proctoscopes of many different sizes and types are available. The simple tubular proctoscope illustrated is useful for routine proctoscopy. Satisfactory disposable instruments are available. A 20-cm (8-inch) pair of non-toothed dissecting forceps is essential for cleaning the rectum with soft cotton-wool swabs. A fibreoptic light source is preferred because of its greater reliability and intensity of light.

Insertion and examination

The lubricated proctoscope with the obturator in place is passed with firm pressure into the anal canal in a direction toward the umbilicus. As the instrument is felt to enter the rectum, it is directed more posteriorly and passed to the full extent. The obturator is withdrawn and the light adjusted. The proctoscope is held steady in the rectum with the left hand, leaving the right hand free for carrying out necessary manipulations such as swabbing away any excess mucus, and for injection of haemorrhoids. The lower rectum is inspected by gentle rotation of the instrument so that the whole circumference of the wall can be seen; as the instrument is slowly withdrawn the mucosa becomes darker as it enters the upper anal canal and the mucous membrane closes over the end of the instrument. Haemorrhoids, if present, may prolapse into the proctoscope, especially if the patient is asked to strain. The lower end of the anal canal should be inspected for evidence of fissure. If it is decided to pass the instrument again it should be withdrawn completely and the obturator replaced.

RIGID SIGMOIDOSCOPY

Instruments

4 A number of instruments is available. The most useful for diagnostic purposes is the 25-cm Lloyd-Davies sigmoidoscope (internal diameter, 19 mm), which is available in lengths of 30 cm and 20 cm and is particularly useful if polypectomy is to be performed. Instruments with a distal circumferential light source are available with attachments, making it possible to perform polypectomy and other manipulations while maintaining inflation of the rectum. An insulated distal end of the instrument is advisable when performing polypectomy in order to avoid accidental burning of the rectal mucosa. A plastic disposable instrument is also available, which is satisfactory for routine diagnostic work.

Cup biopsy and grasping forceps are necessary together with a supply of soft cotton-wool swabs, so that fluid can be removed from the rectum. A long suction tube is particularly helpful in patients with fluid rectal contents.

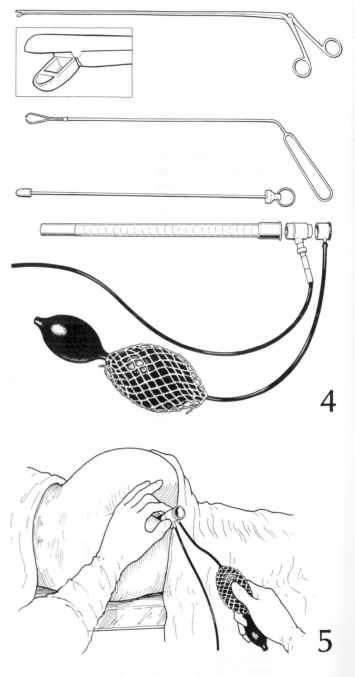

4

5

Insertion

5 Patients should be warned that during the course of sigmoidoscopy they will experience a desire to defaecate. After lubrication of the anal canal during digital examination of the rectum, the instrument is inserted pointing towards the umbilicus with the obturator in place, care being taken not to damage the anterior rectal wall. When the instrument is felt to enter the lower rectum, it is directed posteriorly and the obturator removed. The rectum is then gently inflated with air to allow the sigmoidoscope to be advanced through the lumen. Further passage may require depression and anterior movement at the proximal end of the instrument in order to find the intestinal lumen. Discomfort may be experienced as the instrument is passed into the lower sigmoid colon.

Unless the lumen of the sigmoid colon is clearly seen, the sigmoid colon has not been entered; the instrument can only be advanced by further stretching of the upper rectum. Inspection of the whole mucosa can be achieved by rotating the instrument during removal, taking care not to miss lesions hidden behind the mucosal rectal valves or rectal folds. Throughout the whole of the examination, the instrument is held in the left hand while the right hand holds the inflation bellows and bulb, which can be gently squeezed between the thumb and index finger to control the degree of inflation. The instrument should be passed with the minimum degree of inflation as this is one of the main factors causing discomfort and may make negotiation of the rectosigmoid angle more difficult.

Biopsy of neoplasms

The sigmoidoscope is manipulated so that the lesion is at the end of the instrument. The glass window is then removed, and although this causes deflation of the rectum, if the sigmoidoscope has been correctly positioned the lesion remains within view. Biopsies can then be taken under vision and should never be performed blindly. Excess bleeding at the site can be controlled by pressure from a cotton-wool swab or occasionally 1:1000 topical adrenaline. An instrument that allows a biopsy to be taken while maintaining inflation of the rectum may, at times, prove valuable.

Polypectomy

6 Polyps with a stalk can be removed with a diathermy snare technique. The polyp is grasped by polyp-holding forceps which have previously been passed through the loop of the diathermy snare. The snare is then passed over the polyp, care being taken not to take an excess of normal mucosa into the snare by excessive traction on the forceps; if this is done there is a danger of perforation of the intestine. Closure of the snare during application of diathermy will slowly coagulate the stalk of the polyp which can then be removed by the holding forceps.

Instruments that have facilities for polypectomy while maintaining inflation of the rectum are in some cases easier to use, as this makes more accurate placement of the snare possible without the use of polyp-holding forceps. After polypectomy the patient should be re-examined to make sure that the intestine has not been perforated and to inspect the coagulated area for bleeding; if necessary, the area can be coagulated with the small ball electrode.

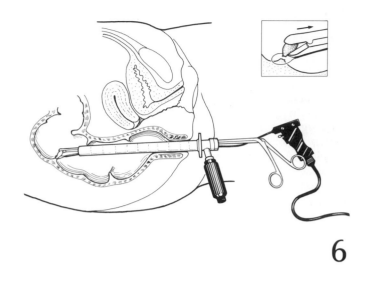

6

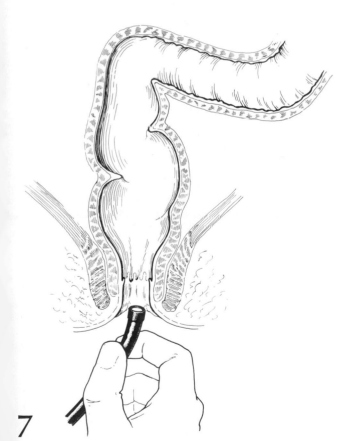

7

FIBREOPTIC SIGMOIDOSCOPY

Insertion

Patients should be placed on a couch or bed, initially in the left lateral position. A rectal examination should be performed to exclude a low anal or rectal lesion and to slightly stretch and lubricate the anal canal. Local anaesthetic gel is helpful if the digital examination is painful.

7 The tip of the sigmoidoscope should be well lubricated and inserted 'sideways' with slight finger pressure for a distance of 4–5 cm.

Initial inspection usually reveals a red blur as the tip of the instrument is against the rectal mucosa; the rectum should be gently inflated and the instrument withdrawn slightly, adjusting the flexible end until the lumen is in sight. The focus control should be adjusted and any residual fluid or faeces sucked out. The sigmoidoscope may then be advanced along the lumen of the rectum to the rectosigmoid junction.

Negotiation of the rectosigmoid junction

8 An attempt should be made to pass around this corner under direct vision with minimal insufflation of air, by angling the tip of the instrument at about 15 cm. In patients with an acute angulation of the rectosigmoid region, it may not be possible to keep the lumen in sight. In this case the tip of the instrument should be gently advanced across the mucosa but without causing it to blanch. If, as the instrument is inserted, movement across the mucosa is not seen the sigmoidoscope should be withdrawn until the lumen comes into view again and a further attempt made to advance the instrument, angulating the tip in the direction of the lumen. It may help to twist the shaft of the sigmoidoscope during the manoeuvre to bring the tip into the correct position rather than to use the instrument control. If the tip becomes fully deflected the instrument will not advance further and it will again form a loop. Care must be taken to insufflate only small volumes of air to prevent an increase in the acuteness of the rectosigmoid angle and discomfort for the patient.

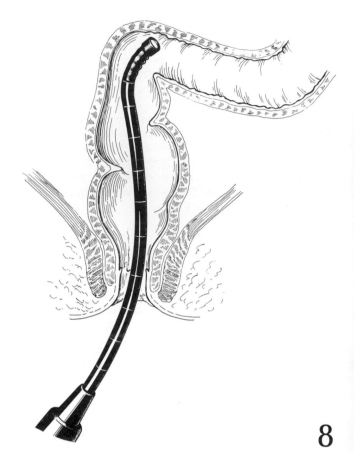

8

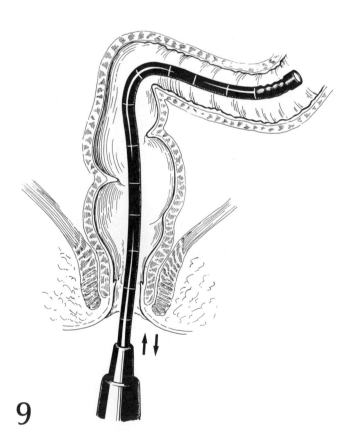

9

Negotiation of the sigmoid colon

9 By a combination of manipulation of the tip of the sigmoidoscope and twisting of the shaft, it is possible to reach the sigmoid colon in most patients. If a large loop forms, this can be reduced by withdrawing the instrument and at the same time rotating the shaft in a clockwise direction. This results in a straightening of the sigmoid colon and allows further advancement. If the tip does not advance rapidly along the sigmoid colon, short advancement and withdrawal movements of the shaft will cause the sigmoid colon to 'concertina' over the instrument.

More complicated procedures such as the 'alpha' manoeuvre (as described in the chapter on pp. 590–601), should be reserved for the experienced colonoscopist and are seldom necessary with flexible sigmoidoscopy.

Many patients experience discomfort as the sigmoid colon is negotiated, and this can be eased by the patient or assistant pressing on the abdomen at the site of discomfort. Alteration of the patient's position to prone may assist the angulation of the sigmoid colon, particularly if a mobile tumour is present.

In patients who have had an anterior resection or sigmoid colectomy, the sigmoidoscope can be passed more rapidly through to the descending colon.

Full insertion and withdrawal

Occasionally, the instrument tip may reach the splenic flexure with a characteristic view of the triangular transverse colon. In the majority, however, insertion is only possible to the descending colon and, furthermore, only part of the lumen is usually visualized in this direction. The main examination of the colon should be undertaken under slow instrument withdrawal, keeping the lumen *in view all the way*. If the instrument has a ratchet tip control, this should be used to prevent rapid passage around acute angles and for careful examination of the sigmoid colon. Biopsy or removal of samples for cytology of a lesion should be done during withdrawal – the lesion may be cleaned by injecting water down the irrigation channel. Polypectomy can also be performed, and the technique for this is described in the chapter on pp. 590–601.

During withdrawal of the instrument, as much air as possible should be aspirated in order to increase the patient's comfort.

Care and disinfection of flexible sigmoidoscopes

An assistant or nurse should be trained in the care, cleaning and disinfection of the equipment according to the manufacturer's instructions.

Immediately after use, instruments should be washed in fresh detergent solution, any adherent debris brushed away, and fresh detergent flushed through all hollow components. Instruments should then be cleaned in an ultrasonic cleaner, rinsed in tap water and disinfected with 2% alkaline glutaraldehyde. Some disinfectants give rise to skin reactions, and staff should be aware of the danger and wear gloves. Adequate ventilation should be provided in the area where glutaraldehyde is used for disinfection.

Postoperative care

No special postoperative observation is necessary after routine sigmoidoscopy. If the patient has had a snare polypectomy performed, however, a warning should be given that bleeding may occur after the operation and if this is excessive, medical aid should be sought. Barium enemas should not be given for several days after a biopsy because of the risk of extravasation of barium.

Colonoscopy and polypectomy

Christopher B. Williams FRCP
Consultant Physician, St Mark's Hospital for Diseases of the Rectum and Colon, St Bartholomew's Hospital and King Edward VII Hospital for Officers, and Honorary Consultant Physician, The Hospital for Sick Children, London, UK

Principles and justification

Indications

After clinical assessment, proctosigmoidoscopy or flexible sigmoidoscopy, and sometimes barium enema, colonoscopy is indicated when the clinical problem has not been resolved, when radiology demonstrates a possible or definite lesion requiring removal or biopsy, and when there has been bleeding or anaemia. Colonoscopy should replace diagnostic laparotomy for most patients with suspected disease of the colon or terminal ileum. Examination through a stoma is technically relatively easy and is usually preferable to contrast studies, which are often difficult to perform and interpret. Therapeutic possibilities include laser photocoagulation, sclerotherapy and stricture dilatation. Colonic snare polypectomy is the procedure of choice for removal of almost all colonic polyps.

Contraindications and complications

There are few contraindications to colonoscopy, but there are occasional serious complications (1 in 2500 perforation rate, 1 in 10 000 mortality rate) so that the procedure should not be undertaken or vigorously pursued without good clinical reasons. Colonoscopy can provoke cardiac arrhythmias and should not be undertaken after recent myocardial infarction. Bowel perforation can occur and colonoscopy is, therefore, contraindicated or should only be performed with great caution and expertise in any form of acute colonic disease where perforation is likely (e.g. very severe acute ulcerative colitis, Crohn's disease and ischaemic colitis). It is similarly contraindicated in the acute phase of diverticulitis.

Chronic severe diverticular disease or a colonic stricture may make the examination difficult and more likely to weaken the instrument, but the results of successful examination may avoid surgery. Postoperative adhesions (e.g. after hysterectomy) may make the colon fixed and result in a traumatic insertion. Use of a small diameter paediatric instrument (colonoscope or gastroscope) may help in all these conditions.

Preoperative

Bowel preparation

For limited colonoscopy (flexible sigmoidoscopy) a 100-ml phosphate enema without dietary preparation should give an adequate view except in patients with stricturing or diverticular disease. Otherwise bowel preparation for colonoscopy must be rigorous and the reasons for this should be explained to patients to obtain their full cooperation. Iron tablets and constipating agents are stopped 4–5 days before the examination but other medications are continued.

In purge regimens a clear liquid diet is started 24 h before colonoscopy and an aperient (senna or bisacodyl) is given on the afternoon or evening before examination. A further dose of high-volume aperient (magnesium citrate) or large-volume cleansing enemas are given on the day of colonoscopy. Nasal tube lavage using warmed isotonic electrolyte solution infused at a rate of 2–3 l/h for 3 h will produce a perfectly clean colon without enemas. Oral lavage involves drinking 3–4 litres of balanced electrolyte–polyethylene glycol solution over 2–3 h and is a highly effective preparation for those who can tolerate the volume and salty taste.

There is a risk that an explosive gas mixture will form after preparation with mannitol or other carbohydrate-based agents; these should not be used before polypectomy unless the risk is eliminated by the use of carbon dioxide insufflation. The use of carbon dioxide has the added advantage of leaving the patient less distended at the end of the procedure when compared with air insufflation.

Medication

Premedication is unnecessary before colonoscopy except in highly nervous patients or children. If a gentle endoscopic technique is used, sedation during the procedure may also be unnecessary, especially in confident and motivated patients or those known to be easy to examine – such as after resection of the sigmoid colon. Intravenous diazepam, 5–10 mg, or midazolam, 2–5 mg, combined with pethidine, 25–50 mg, makes the procedure easily tolerated by the patient (half dosage for elderly patients). Benzodiazepines alone contribute amnesia but are only weakly analgesic. Additional doses of pethidine can be given when necessary and can be completely reversed by intravenous or intramuscular naloxone. Antispasmodics are not routinely used by all endoscopists but if there is spasm intravenous hyoscine butylbromide, 40 mg, or glucagon, 0.1 mg, will help accurate examination on withdrawal of the instrument, or during insertion if there is severe diverticular disease.

General anaesthesia is generally contraindicated because pain supplies the only warning that the bowel or mesentery is being overstretched.

Choice of instrument

Shorter (130–140 cm) colonoscopes may have slight mechanical advantages over longer (165–185 cm) instruments in use and maintenance but, except in expert hands, will not always reach the caecum, especially if radiography shows a redundant bowel. Thinner and more flexible paediatric instruments are available and should be used both for children and when there is stricturing or fixation of the bowel causing problems with standard instruments.

Sterilization of the instrument requires rigorous measures, including perfusion of all channels and parts with glutaraldehyde solution or gas sterilization with ethylene oxide, particularly after examination of patients with mycobacterial infection or before those with immunodepression.

Is radiographic control needed?

Most examinations do not require radiographic screening control and most colonoscopists never use it. In the learning phase and for the less experienced, however, the extra information given can be invaluable, sometimes making difficult procedures quicker, safer and less traumatic. It will also help to localize obstructing lesions found unexpectedly at colonoscopy.

Technique

Position of patient

Most endoscopists start with the patient in the left lateral position and it is often possible to complete the examination without a change. If there are mechanical difficulties at any stage of the procedure, however, a change to the prone or supine position may alter the position of the bowel and make examination easier. The prone position helps to compress loops and also to reach the last few centimetres to the caecal pole; the supine position has the advantage of allowing palpation and visualization of the light transilluminating the abdomen. The right lateral position improves visualization of a fluid-filled descending colon and also greatly facilitates passage around the splenic flexure.

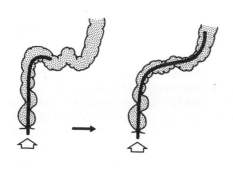

1

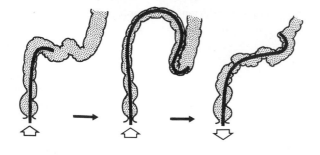

2

Insertion and passage through the rectosigmoid

1 The colonoscope tip and perianal region are lubricated, a digital examination of the rectum performed and the instrument is gently inserted. Initially there is no view because the tip is against the wall of the rectum and the instrument is withdrawn to disimpact it before a view can be obtained by insufflating air, angling the tip and rotating the instrument shaft as necessary.

In passing the many bends of the rectosigmoid the object is to distend or stretch the bowel as little as possible to keep it short, ideally passing almost straight into the descending colon. This is easier to suggest than to achieve, but is the ideal and is made more likely by observing the following points:

1. As little air as possible should be insufflated while keeping some view.
2. The bowel lumen should be followed accurately.
3. If the view is poor, even for a few seconds, the instrument should be withdrawn slightly and the direction reassessed.
4. Blind pushing should be avoided, although on acute bends this may be necessary for a few seconds, providing the general direction is certain.
5. If the tip will not angle round a bend the surgeon should try 'corkscrewing' by pulling back and twisting the shaft clockwise or anticlockwise.
6. The instrument should be pulled back repeatedly after passing any major bend and before starting each inward push. This straightens the colonoscope and shortens the colon, making insertion easier and more comfortable.

Sigmoid 'N loop': hook and twist manoeuvre

2 The most common situation on reaching the junction of the sigmoid and descending colon, in spite of all care, is for there to be an 'N loop', bowing up the sigmoid and resulting in a tip angulation which makes direct passage into the descending colon difficult or impossible. If the tip can be coaxed a short way round the bend, thus looking into the descending colon, it will be 'hooked' retroperitoneally so that the instrument can be withdrawn 20–30 cm to reduce and straighten out the loop. Because of the normal spiral configuration of the sigmoid loop, putting a strong (usually clockwise) twisting force (torque) on to the shaft of the colonoscope while it is withdrawn will help in straightening out this loop and keeping the tip in the descending colon. Occasionally, where the sigmoid colon is long or unusually mobile, an anticlockwise twist may work better because atypical looping can result when the descending colon is not fixed retroperitoneally in its usual left paravertebral position.

Sigmoid 'alpha loop'

3 Sometimes, especially in patients with a redundant colon, a loop is obviously forming but the tip none the less runs inwards without discomfort to the patient. This suggests that a spiral 'alpha' loop is forming (easily confirmed when fluoroscopy is used). If an alpha loop is suspected, the colonoscope should be pushed in as far as is comfortable for the patient, preferably to the splenic flexure, which uses about 90 cm of the instrument.

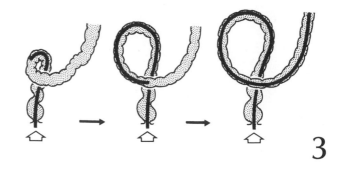

3

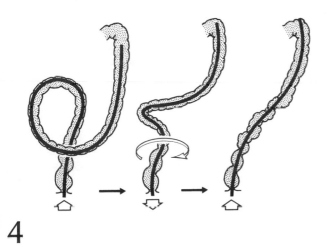

4

Straightening out loops

4 Having reached the upper descending colon or splenic flexure, a sigmoid loop should normally be removed, because loops create friction in the control wires, cause stress in the instrument and may hurt the patient. To remove the loop, the colonoscope shaft should be withdrawn firmly until the tip begins to slide or resistance to withdrawal is felt, usually at 45–50 cm insertion depth. When pulling back, the application of a clockwise twist often helps to prevent the tip of the colonoscope from slipping back prematurely.

Keeping straight or stiffening the sigmoid colon

5 Once the colonoscope is straightened, with its tip in the descending colon and the sigmoid colon convoluted and shortened, some care may be needed to prevent the sigmoid loop reforming. Continued clockwise (occasionally anticlockwise) twist on the shaft helps to keep it straight during insertion. Shaft insertion without tip movement (loss of 1:1 relationship) indicates relooping and the instrument is immediately pulled back again. Having an assistant push firmly in the left iliac fossa resists the tendency of the sigmoid loop to rise up from the pelvis.

In a few patients with a very redundant colon in whom unavoidable sigmoid looping occurs (but total colonoscopy is indicated), a 'stiffening' or overtube may be needed. This is a plastic tube which is placed in position over the colonoscope, lubricated with jelly and passed over the *straightened* instrument to stop it from flexing. Insertion of a stiffener is ideally carried out under radiographic control with to-and-fro rotary movement used to avoid catching redundant mucosa. A softer low-friction 'split' overtube is available which can be positioned over the endoscope after insertion (and taped over the split) which avoids having to withdraw the colonoscope and does not need fluoroscopy.

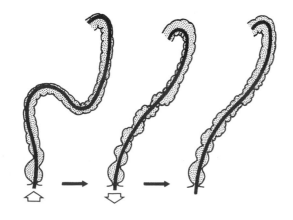

5

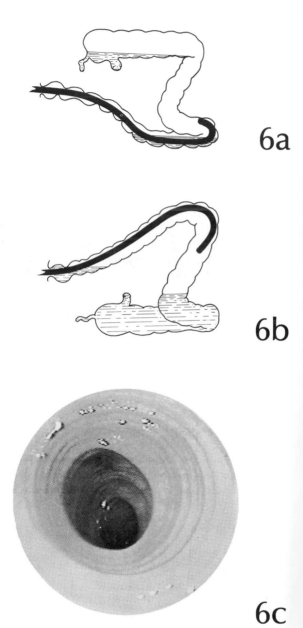

6a

6b

6c

Position and the splenic flexure

6a–c In the left lateral position the descending colon is deflated and filled with fluid. Changing the patient to the right lateral position not only improves the view in the descending colon (particularly important if there is blood or residual fluid), but also causes the transverse colon to flop down and open out the splenic flexure, making this point much easier to pass.

The instrument shaft should be pulled back and straightened out to 50 cm before tackling the splenic flexure or transverse colon; failure to do this accounts for most cases where the proximal colon is described as being difficult to pass. To prevent the sigmoid loop reforming, excessive tip angulation should be avoided, hand pressure by the assistant should be used over the left iliac fossa and a gentle clockwise twisting force maintained on the shaft while pushing gently inwards. Too rapid or aggressive pushing merely loops up the sigmoid.

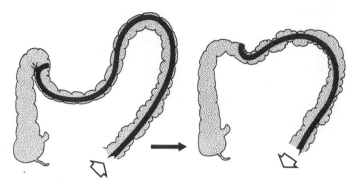

7a

Redundant transverse colon

7a–c The transverse colon may push down into a deep loop that makes it difficult and painful to reach the hepatic flexure. If this happens the correct procedure is to withdraw the instrument 30–50 cm to shorten the transverse loop; this withdrawal may need to be repeated several times, the tip advancing a few centimetres each time until the loop straightens. Deflation also helps to shorten the hepatic flexure, making it easier to reach and to pass. If the right lateral position has been used to pass the splenic flexure, the patient is changed back to the normal left lateral position when the proximal transverse colon is reached, thus facilitating insertion up to and around the hepatic flexure.

Difficulty in the transverse colon is often due to recurrent looping in the sigmoid colon, and continued abdominal pressure in the left iliac fossa may be more effective than trying to affect the transverse colon with pressure in the upper abdomen or left hypochondrium.

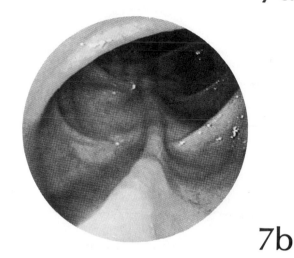

7b

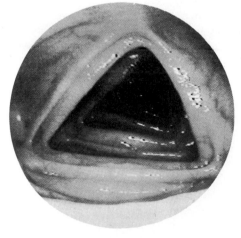

7c

Passing the hepatic flexure

8 Having reached and deflated the hepatic flexure, and then angled around it into the ascending colon, the transverse colon loop may remain, making it difficult to pass the rest of the instrument into the ascending colon. Paradoxically, by withdrawing the colonoscope forcibly 30–50 cm, so straightening out the transverse loop, it becomes easier to pass it onwards.

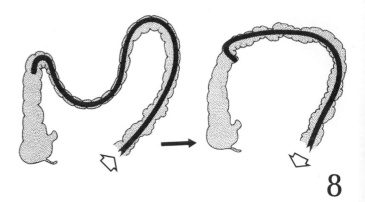

8

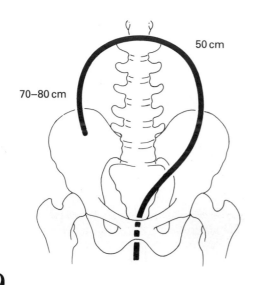

9

9 The hepatic flexure is a 180° hairpin bend and major angulation may be required, even though the view is imperfect. A combination of both control knobs and recurrent minor aspirations should be used to reduce the size of the flexure as far as possible to angle progressively around the hepatic flexure while simultaneously maintaining a limited mucosal view by pulling back if necessary. As soon as the ascending colon is seen it is deflated and shortened by aspiration and, while steering carefully to avoid further haustral folds, the colonoscope should spontaneously descend towards the caecum.

Reaching the caecum

If there is difficulty in reaching the caecal pole, changing the patient's position to prone or supine may be helpful. Excessive push pressure usually only loops up the sigmoid colon.

10 The colonoscope is known to have reached the caecum when the bulge and slit opening of the ileocaecal valve is seen or, 5 cm beyond this, the appendix orifice is identified at the junction of the taeniae coli. If these anatomical features are not obvious, and experience is sometimes needed to be sure, there is a danger of mistaking the hepatic flexure for the caecum. Transillumination should be visible in the right iliac fossa if the room is darkened and the instrument light is bright enough or a palpating finger can be seen indenting the bowel wall through the colonoscope.

The fully straightened colonoscope at the caecal pole is 70–80 cm from the anus, then during withdrawal the splenic flexure is at 50 cm and descending colon at 40 cm. However, during insertion and in cases where the caecum has not been reached, because loops invariably form, these distance rules do not apply and localization may be impossible without radiographic control, although transillumination and palpation may give some indication.

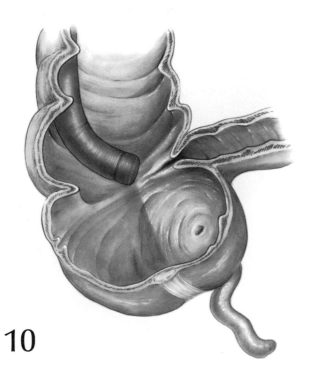

10

Entering the terminal ileum

11 The ileum joins the caecum through the variably shaped bulging or slit-like ileocaecal 'valve' on the first prominent haustral fold about 5 cm back from the caecal pole.

Deflation can help to locate the valve opening by making it bulge or bubble, but some valves may only be obvious after retroverting the instrument tip in the caecal pole to visualize a slit on the underside of the ileocaecal fold.

To enter the ileum the valve must first be identified, then the instrument straightened to 70–80 cm for maximum manoeuvrability. Ideally the valve should be placed at the top or bottom of the view for ease of entry using tip angulation with the up/down control. The caecum should be deflated slightly to make the region more supple, the tip angled towards the lower lip of the valve and (as seems appropriate) either pushed in or pulled back slowly so that the tip slips into the enveloping lips of the valve, with a 'red out'. Finally, the valve should be opened up by insufflation and passed into the ileum, which appears granular due to the villous surface seen in air (under water the villi show their characteristic frond-like configuration).

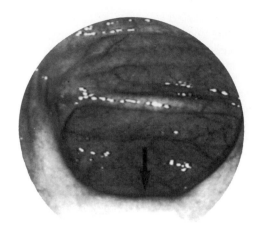

11

Examination

To some extent the colon is seen during insertion of the instrument but more active examination is normally undertaken during withdrawal of the colonoscope. Fastidious care is necessary to see behind folds, especially when the bowel has been convoluted by straightening the instrument.

Usually it is best for the endoscopist to control the instrument using a one-handed technique during withdrawal, even if an assistant has helped with insertion. Very active manoeuvring of the controls, with corkscrewing rotation and to-and-fro movements of the shaft, may be necessary to avoid blind spots. Examination of the bowel on withdrawal may sometimes take as long as insertion of the instrument.

Postoperative care

In most cases no particular care is needed after colonoscopy apart from a few minutes of rest and some food and drink. If sedation has been used the patient must be warned not to drive a vehicle for 24 h. When the patient appears and feels well he or she can be safely discharged, preferably with an escort. Most examinations are performed on a day-care basis.

POLYPECTOMY

Safety

The principle behind colonoscopic polypectomy is to prevent bleeding by adequate electrocoagulation of vessels before transection, because the endoscopist operates 'single handed' without the surgeon's ability to use artery forceps or ligature should bleeding occur. On the other hand, avoidance of excessive heat damage is also essential to prevent necrosis of the colon wall, which can occur as a secondary phenomenon even when there has been little visible whitening at the time. This is the reason for a 'postpolypectomy syndrome' of peritoneal pain and fever, and also of secondary or 'delayed' haemorrhage due to damaged submucosal arterioles exposed by ulceration. Judgement is required as to the amount of current required – 'not too little; not too much'. Most experts use coagulating current alone with a relatively low power setting, relying on passage of time (usually 5–15 s) and applying progressive mechanical tightening of the snare during current application to cause first heating and whitening locally and then slow transection below the polyp tissue.

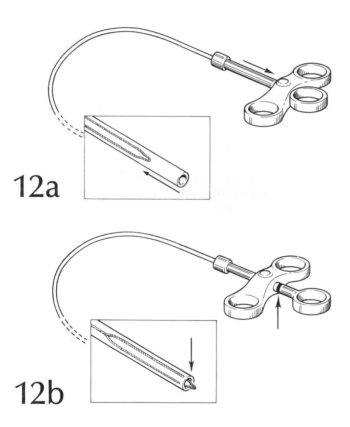

12a

12b

Adjusting the polypectomy snare

12a, b For efficient electrocoagulation it is fundamental to 'neck' the stalk tissue to cause local current concentration, because heating increases as the square of current concentration and as the cube of snare loop tightening. Adjustment of the snare before the procedure is a necessary preliminary. The handle/wire assembly should be examined on a bench to ensure that it has an easy action with good 'feel', full opening and full closing. When completely closed (*Illustration 12a*) the tip of the wire should retract at least 15 mm, and preferably 20 mm, into the outer plastic sheath, to allow for inevitable crumpling of the sheath during forcible closure around a polyp stalk. Full closure is necessary for adequate necking and subsequent transection of a large stalk, which will greatly decrease the risk. Another invaluable safety measure (*Illustration 12b*) is to make an indelible mark on the snare handle at the point corresponding to the closure of the snare tip to the end of the plastic sheath. This mark on the handle indicates the correct snare closure point to the assistant, avoiding unintended mechanical 'cheese-wiring' through a small polyp, but also gives a measurable advance warning if the snare has entrapped the polyp head or if the stalk is unexpectedly large.

Small polyps

13 Polyps up to 5 mm in diameter are common but, because of their small size, can be disproportionately awkward to catch with the snare and troublesome to retrieve or aspirate for histology. Use of electrically insulated 'hot biopsy' forceps is an effective compromise, allowing electrocoagulation of the tented-up basal tissues of the small polyp while usually obtaining an adequate biopsy of the sample, which is protected from current flow within the jaws of the forceps. For safety, only the apex of the polyp is grasped and tented up towards the lumen by angling or twisting the instrument and pulling back the forceps slightly. Current is applied for only 2 s or less to cause localized electrocoagulation limited to the vasculature in the pseudopedicle – the 'Mount Fuji' effect of whitening at the apex of the small 'mountain' of pulled-up tissue.

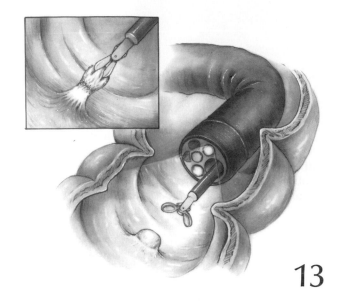

13

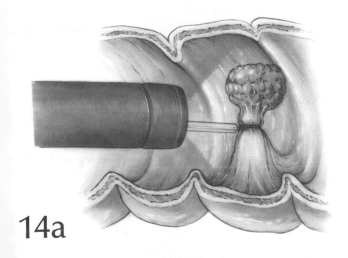

14a

Stalked polyps

14a, b The snare is manoeuvred over the polyp head and on to the upper part of the stalk, preferably leaving a short margin of normal tissue below the head for identification by the histopathologist. The snare loop is closed gently, correct closure of the handle to the previously made mark (*see* above) is checked and then the stalk is moved around for better visualization and to ensure that the colon wall has not been entrapped by the loop. Finally, continuous low-power coagulating current is applied, initially with quite gentle squeeze pressure on the handle but, as soon as visible swelling or whitening indicates local electrocoagulation, the squeeze is increased to sever the head. If any bleeding occurs (other than back-bleeding from the polyp head), the snare is quickly opened and the basal part of the stalk regrasped for a few minutes, with or without gentle extra electrocoagulation.

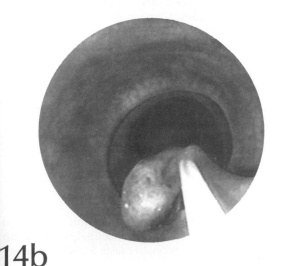

14b

Broad-stalked polyps

15 Semipedunculated polyps with bases or stalks over 1 cm in diameter present a problem in achieving sufficient depth of electrocoagulation to occlude all vessels in the feeding plexus. Basal injection with 1:10 000 adrenaline solution, 1–5 ml, with a long flexible sclerotherapy needle, can be used either before snaring or as an emergency measure should bleeding occur. Longer thick stalks can be preinjected in their mid-portion with 1 ml of a sclerosant–adrenaline mixture to ensure long-term effect, providing there is room to snare above the injection point which swells significantly.

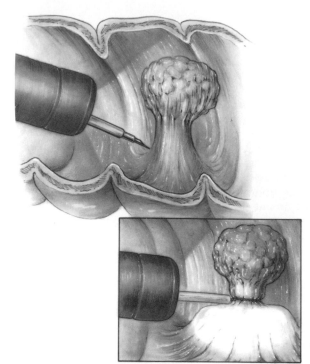

15

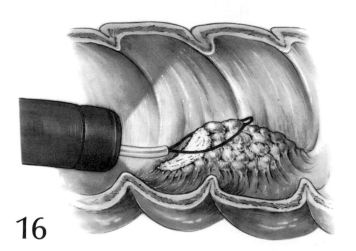

16

Large or sessile polyps (piecemeal removal)

16 Polyps over 2–3 cm in diameter without a compressible stalk are hazardous to snare in a single portion because the higher power current and longer application time required risk transmural heating and perforation. If such heating occurs, an unsedated patient will usually report immediate peritoneal pain which is an early warning to abandon the procedure (unless deflation suggests that the pain is actually due to distension of the colon). Piecemeal removal of larger sessile polyps (in up to 20–30 smaller portions, and in repeated sessions if necessary) keeps control of the procedure and provides a reasonable degree of safety, but allows removal of nearly any polyp if the patient can tolerate the long procedure time(s) involved. Snaring with the colonoscope tip in retroversion may be needed to entrap any part of a sessile polyp which is invisible on the proximal side of an acute haustral fold. Because some of these polyps will prove to be malignant, and surgery therefore possibly indicated, it is often wise to obtain initial histology by partial (80–90%) removal before repeating the procedure and removing the more risky basal parts of the polyp. Very fully informed patient consent of the risks involved are clearly essential before undertaking a hazardous polypectomy.

Making a nearby 1-ml tattoo injection of a 1:10 dilution of sterilized Indian ink facilitates follow-up examinations. The mark probably lasts for life, certainly for many years.

Retrieving polyps

The normal way to retrieve a snared polyp for histological examination is to catch the head with the polypectomy snare and pull it back with the endoscope. For very large polyps the patient may need to squat and then strain to relax the anal sphincter for successful final delivery. Multiple larger polyps may require multiple reinsertions of the endoscope for individual snare retrieval (an overtube can be used). Alternatively, 500–600 ml of tap water are syringe-injected through the instrument channel above the snared polyps or polyp fragments with additional air insufflation, and a disposable enema given after withdrawing the endoscope to stimulate spontaneous evacuation into a pan from whence they can be retrieved.

Follow-up

Judgement is necessary about the correct interval for follow-up. Some polypectomy sites heal completely within 2–3 weeks and are thereafter impossible to identify accurately. Thus, a malignant polyp site should be checked and tattooed within this time. On the other hand, a longer period is desirable to allow resolution of tissue damage before checking for regrowth of benign tissue after removal of benign sessile polyps.

Polyps can be missed at colonoscopy and it is sometimes justifiable to perform a check examination within a year. High-risk patients with multiple adenomas or malignancy need initial checks at 1–2 years but in many other patients examination at 3-yearly or even longer intervals is probably adequate.

Further reading

Cotton PB, Williams CB. *Practical Gastrointestinal Endoscopy*, 3rd edn. Oxford: Blackwell Scientific Publications, 1990.

Laparoscopic-assisted appendicectomy

Robert W. Bailey MD
Division Head, General Surgery, Greater Baltimore Medical Centre, Baltimore, Maryland, USA

Karl A. Zucker MD, FACS
Professor of Surgery, University of New Mexico School of Medicine, Albuquerque, New Mexico, USA

History

The recent introduction of laparoscopic cholecystectomy has had an enormous impact on the practice of general surgery. The advantages of this innovative procedure have been documented in several recent series[1,2]. Substantial reductions in the length of hospital stay, recovery period, postoperative discomfort and health care costs have led to its rapid acceptance. The first description of a laparoscopic incidental appendicectomy was in 1983 by Semm in Germany[3]. In 1987, Schrieber reported the first laparoscopic experience in a group of women with acute appendicitis[4]. He demonstrated the safety and efficacy of this approach in a clinical situation that is usually encountered by general surgeons. Several medical centres have subsequently adopted laparoscopy as the primary technique for the diagnosis and treatment of acute appendicitis.

Pier *et al.* recently published their experience with 625 consecutive laparoscopic appendicectomies[5]. Only 14% were histologically normal, and fewer than 2% of the patients required the procedure to be converted to an open laparotomy (most of these were in the first 50 cases). The operative morbidity rate was minimal, with only one case of appendiceal stump leakage and two patients developing intra-abdominal abscesses requiring interval laparotomy. They reported an operative time of less than 30 min and a wound infection rate below 2%[5]. Valla *et al.* have also shown the benefits of laparoscopic appendicectomy in a group of 465 paediatric patients with ages ranging from 3 to 16 years[6]. These and other reports have demonstrated that the appendix can be safely removed under laparoscopic guidance in the majority of patients, including those with extensive inflammation or atypical anatomy.

Principles and justification

Indications

A recent review of the literature suggests a possible role for incidental appendicectomy in patients between the ages of 10 and 30 years[7], but the indications are less clear for those of 30–50 years of age, and no benefit is apparent in those older than 50 years. As the risk of mortality from future acute appendicitis is so small and the benefits of a prophylactic appendicectomy are unconvincing, incidental appendicectomy, either under laparoscopic guidance or by open laparotomy, is not commonly performed at most institutions.

An appendicectomy performed solely as an incidental procedure, e.g. during elective gallbladder surgery, must be differentiated from the removal of a normal appendix during exploration for presumed appendicitis. Reasons offered for removal of a normal appendix following explorations for presumed acute appendicitis include: (1) the assumption by surgeons that any patient with a right lower quadrant incision has had their appendix removed; (2) to avoid future diagnostic confusion in any patient who may suffer from repeated episodes of lower abdominal pain, i.e. inflammatory bowel disease or gynaecological disorders; (3) failure to accurately determine the presence or absence of early acute appendicitis by gross inspection only; and (4) avoiding the risk of another anaesthetic in the future.

Although a conventional right lower quadrant incision is not made during laparoscopic appendicectomy, the growing popularity of this procedure may also result in possible confusion regarding the presence of an appendix. The remaining indications for removal of a normal appendix would apply regardless of the surgical approach. Because most surgeons agree with removal of a non-inflamed appendix during an open procedure, the authors' bias has been to recommend removal of a normal-appearing appendix during laparoscopic exploration for presumed appendicitis unless contraindicated by other intra-abdominal findings.

Contraindications

Absolute contraindications to attempting laparoscopic appendicectomy are few. Patients presenting with evidence of advanced intestinal obstruction, generalized peritonitis, or uncorrectable bleeding disorders should primarily undergo an open procedure. Although laparoscopic removal of the appendix may be technically possible in such circumstances, the operative time can be greatly increased.

Relative contraindications would include: previous lower abdominal surgery; evidence of localized abscess formation, i.e. a mass on palpation; suspicion of malignancy; or pregnancy. Whether such cases should be attempted will depend mostly on the capabilities of the surgeon. With increased exposure and operative experience, even the most difficult case can be successfully approached under laparoscopic guidance.

Potential advantages of laparoscopic appendicectomy

It is anticipated that many of the same advantages as with laparoscopic cholecystectomy will also be realized with laparoscopic appendicectomy.

Laparoscopic appendicectomy allows a more thorough exploration of the abdominal cavity than would be possible through a small right lower quadrant incision. This is particularly important in those patients presenting with evidence of lower abdominal peritonitis who appear to have a normal appendix. It also allows definitive treatment of other abdominal or pelvic pathology, as deemed appropriate by the operative findings. Conversion to a midline laparotomy may be avoided if the entire abdomen can be examined under laparoscopic guidance.

Laparoscopic appendicectomy shortens hospitalization and recovery periods[8,9]. Patients are generally able to leave the hospital 24 h after uncomplicated laparoscopic appendicectomy. Most are able to return to their normal activity within 2–3 days. Postoperative discomfort is also diminished. Although the pain following open appendicectomy is usually moderate to minimal, patients often complain of noticeable discomfort for 1–2 weeks and require oral narcotic analgesics. Almost no postoperative pain is experienced after laparoscopic appendicectomy.

Finally, the incidence of postoperative wound complications is reduced. Contamination of the wound is assumed following removal of a severely inflamed or perforated appendix through a traditional right lower quadrant or midline incision. During laparoscopic surgery the appendix can be removed without coming into direct contact with the fascia or subcutaneous tissues. In addition, the smaller less traumatic trocar puncture sites appear to diminish the incidence of wound complications such as abscess, cellulitis, dehiscence and necrotizing fasciitis[5].

Potential disadvantages of laparoscopic appendicectomy

The appendiceal stump may be difficult to mobilize and secure. Until recently, atraumatic intestinal clamps, angled forceps and curved scissors have not been available for laparoscopic surgery. In the past, methods of ligating the appendix were limited to pretied ligatures of plain or chromic catgut. Many surgeons were hesitant to rely on such sutures to close an appendiceal stump, particularly with inflamed tissues and a contaminated field. Recent refinements of laparoscopic suturing techniques and the development of endoscopic intestinal stapling devices have made closure of the appendiceal stump a simple manoeuvre.

Operative time can be expected to be increased during a surgeon's early attempts at any new laparoscopic procedure. Current reports from centres with extensive experience with this technique indicate that the length of a laparoscopic appendicectomy is comparable to the traditional method[5,6,8,9].

In some patients, atypical anatomy, extensive inflammation, dense adhesions, or abscess may necessitate abandoning the laparoscopic approach in favour of an open laparotomy. This will increase the length of the operation and may result in confusion if the patient believes that the need for conversion was the result of an intraoperative complication. Fortunately, the need to convert to an open technique is uncommon with increasing experience[5,6]. Patients should always be informed that any laparoscopic procedure may need to be converted to an open laparotomy and that this decision usually represents sound surgical judgement to minimize operative risk.

Preoperative

Preoperative evaluation and preparation for patients undergoing laparoscopic appendicectomy is nearly identical to that for patients undergoing traditional surgery. The basic guidelines for the safe performance of a laparoscopic procedure, e.g. stomach and bladder decompression, should be adhered to strictly. All other adjuvant measures, e.g. preoperative antibiotics, should be administered as for open appendicectomy.

Anaesthesia

Most therapeutic laparoscopic procedures require general anaesthesia. Regional anaesthesia, however, has been successfully employed on occasion for laparoscopic cholecystectomy[1]. With further refinement of operative and anaesthetic techniques, such options may become more readily acceptable in the future. Specific details concerning the use of anaesthesia during laparoscopic surgery have been previously published[10].

Operating room arrangement

1 The endoscopic imaging equipment, instrument table and energy devices, i.e. lasers and electrosurgery units, must be arranged to permit the surgical team to work comfortably in the lower abdomen. The video monitors should be placed near the foot of the table in clear view of the entire surgical team. Similarly, the insufflator should be positioned so that the surgeon can monitor the intra-abdominal pressure throughout the procedure. A basic laparotomy instrument set should be immediately available in the operating room.

The patient is positioned supine on the operating room table with both arms tucked-in at the side. If the arms are abducted they may hinder the ability of the surgical team to work in the lower abdomen and pelvis. The surgeon stands on the left side of the patient with the assistant standing directly opposite.

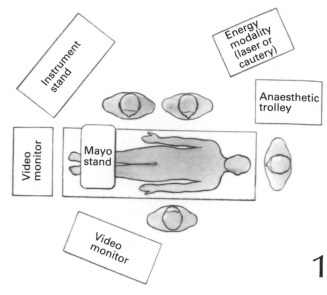

1

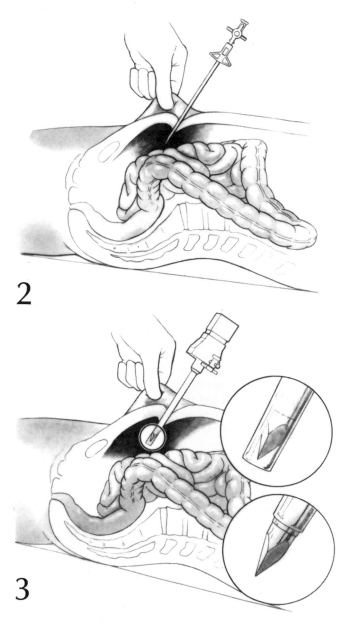

2

3

Operation

Establishment of a pneumoperitoneum

A pneumoperitoneum is established using currently accepted techniques (as described in the chapter on pp. 161–176). The patient is placed in a 10–20° head-down (Trendelenburg) position, and a 1.0–1.5-cm incision is made within the infraumbilical folds of the umbilicus.

2 A specially designed insufflation (Verres) needle is inserted into the abdominal cavity, and its position is confirmed by aspirating with an attached syringe and monitoring the insufflation pressure through the needle.

3 The peritoneal cavity is distended with carbon dioxide until a pressure of 12–15 mmHg is achieved. The needle is withdrawn and a 10-mm or 11-mm laparoscopic trocar and cannula are inserted through the same incision and into the distended abdomen.

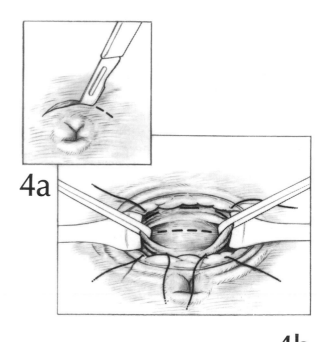

4a

4b

$4a–c$ An alternative method of establishing the pneumoperitoneum is the open or Hasson technique[11]. A larger (approximately 2–3-cm) periumbilical incision is made, and the peritoneal cavity is entered under direct vision. A specially designed laparoscopic cannula with a blunt tip is guided into the abdomen and a purse-string suture closes the fascial opening around the sheath to create an airtight seal.

Diagnostic laparoscopy

A complete survey of the abdominal cavity is performed using a forward-viewing or side-viewing laparoscope introduced through the umbilical cannula. An angled telescope offers greater versatility in cases where the appendix is hidden from view, such as with a retrocaecal location. The diagnosis is confirmed, the extent and severity of the inflammatory process is determined, and the feasibility of a laparoscopic approach is assessed.

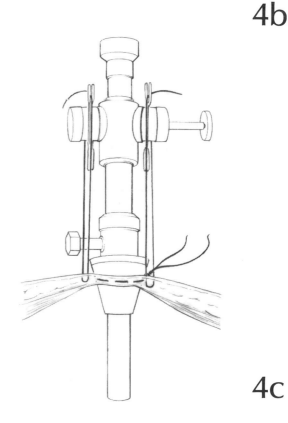

4c

Accessory cannula placement

5 Insertion of additional trocars and cannulae is performed under direct laparoscopic vision. The locations of the epigastric vessels are identified and care is taken to avoid injury to them. Two accessory sheaths are often sufficient to complete the operative procedure; however, additional cannulae may be necessary to retract surrounding tissues. The two accessory sheaths are usually placed in the right anterior axillary line (at a site parallel or just cephalad to the umbilicus) and in the midline just above the pubic symphysis. In more complex cases with severe inflammation or atypical anatomy (i.e. retrocaecal appendix) a fourth cannula is often usefully inserted in the right upper quadrant of the abdomen.

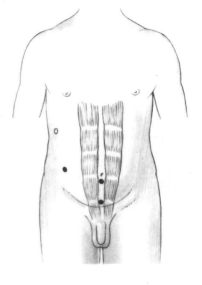

5

The sizes of cannulae used will depend on the technique and instrumentation employed. The most commonly used cannulae are available in diameters ranging from 5 mm to 12 mm. The authors generally use 10-mm sheaths so that a wide range of instruments, such as fan retractors and bowel-grasping forceps, can be introduced. The automatic intestinal stapler (Endo-GIA) requires a 12-mm cannula, and if its use is anticipated an appropriately sized sheath should be placed above the pubic symphysis. The additional trauma to the abdominal wall is negligible when using these larger devices, and difficulties are avoided that can occur when the surgeon is unable to introduce an instrument because an existing cannula is too small.

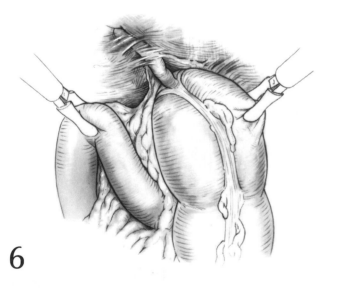

6

Identification and mobilization of the appendix and caecum

6 Following visual inspection of the abdominal cavity, the right colon and caecum are identified. The taeniae coli can be traced towards the caecum and appendix. Atraumatic bowel-grasping forceps are used to elevate the caecum and terminal ileum into the operative field.

7 Curved dissecting, i.e. Metzenbaum-like, scissors may be used to free the lateral and inferior peritoneal attachments of the appendix and/or the right colon. These scissors may be connected to an electrosurgery generator to deliver a monopolar current and facilitate haemostasis. Low-power settings (generally less than 30 W) and short bursts of energy should be used to avoid injury to surrounding structures. Alternatively, a free-beam or contact-tip laser device may be used for dissection in this area[12]. The appendix is identified and mobilized into the operative field.

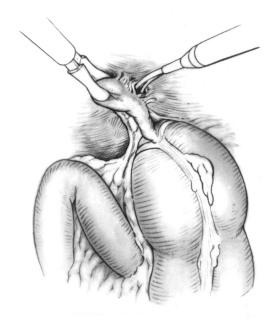

7

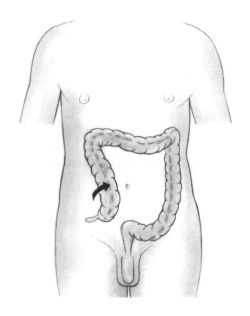

8

8 If the appendix is behind the caecum or deep in the pelvis, the ascending colon must be freed from its peritoneal attachments in order to retract it cephalad and towards the midline. This manoeuvre generally requires additional instruments and a fourth cannula is placed in the upper right abdomen.

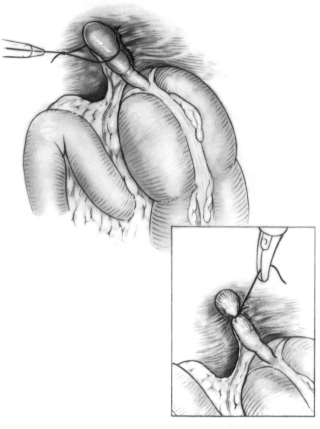

9 Once mobilized, the appendix is grasped at its tip with atraumatic forceps. If the appendix proves difficult to hold due to extensive inflammation or necrosis, a pretied laparoscopic ligature may be used to encircle the tip of the appendix. This suture may then be used as a point of retraction.

9

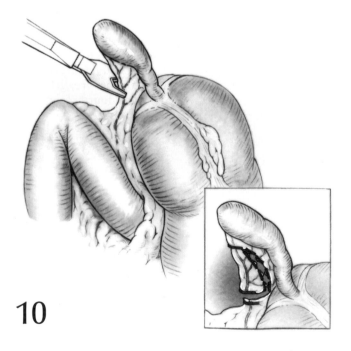

10

Dissection of the mesoappendix

The blood supply to the appendix may be divided in either a retrograde or an antegrade manner. Confusion exists, however, as to the distinction between a retrograde and an antegrade dissection. To avoid any such confusion, the subsequent narrative will refer to an antegrade dissection as that which originates at the junction with the caecum.

10 In the absence of significant inflammation, the appendiceal artery may be readily isolated at the base of the appendix with an angled dissecting forceps and controlled with either surgical clips or direct suture ligation.

The remaining mesoappendix is then divided between clips or with monopolar or bipolar electrocautery.

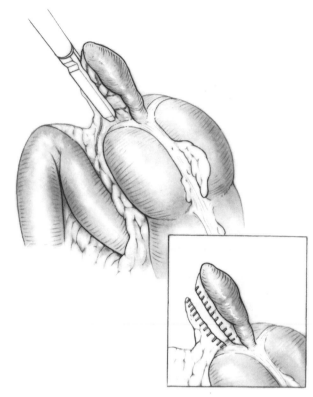

11a

11a, b
Alternatively, the entire mesoappendix may be ligated and divided with an automatic stapling device using a vascular cartridge.

If the base of the appendix cannot be readily identified, then the blood supply can be sequentially ligated beginning at the tip of the appendix (retrograde dissection). The dissection should be continued until the base of the appendix and its junction with the caecum is freed from any adhesions or peritoneal attachments.

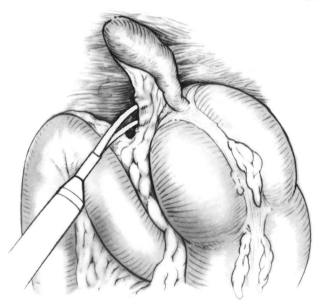

11b

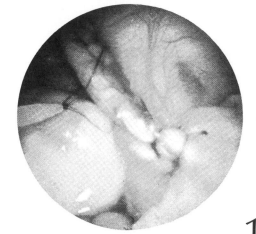

12a

Ligation and division of the appendix

12a, b Previously, the most common method of securing the appendix involved the use of pretied laparoscopic ligature made of 0 chromic catgut or synthetic suture. Two ligatures are placed near the junction with the caecum and a third placed on the proximal portion of the inflamed appendix. The appendix is divided, leaving the two ligatures on the caecum intact. The appendix may be sharply divided with a scissors, using monopolar or bipolar electrical current, or with laser energy. Many surgeons prefer to use an electrosurgery instrument in order to 'sterilize' the exposed mucosa. Extreme care must be taken to avoid burning the caecum, particularly when using monopolar current. This can lead to subsequent necrosis, sloughing of tissue and caecal fistula.

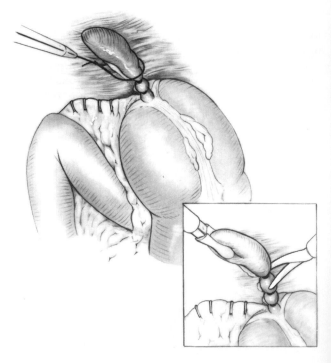

12b

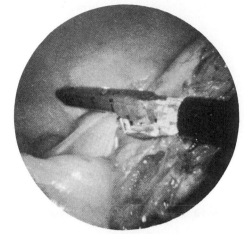

13a–c An alternative method uses an intestinal stapling device, which is fired across the base of the appendix, simultaneously dividing it between several rows of staples.

13a

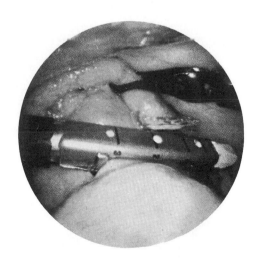

13b

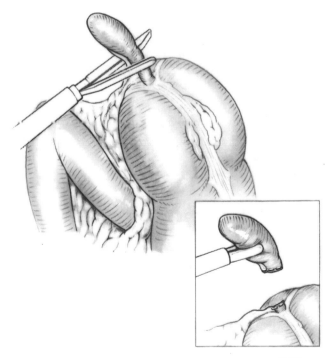

13c

14a–d With either of the above techniques, the base of the appendix remains everted. If desired, the apendiceal stump may be inverted or invaginated into the wall of the caecum with a purse-string or Z-type suture; however, few laparo-scopic surgeons have found this necessary. Recently, a large prospective trial involving traditional open surgery has shown no advantage with inverting the base of the appendix[13].

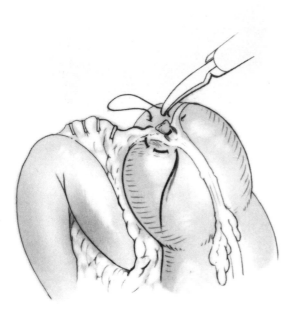

14a

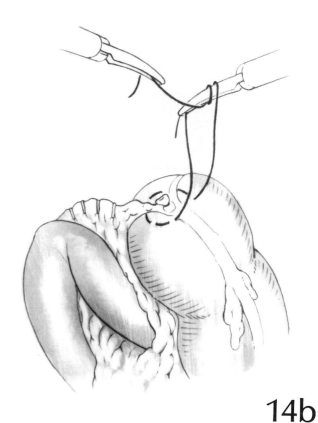

14b

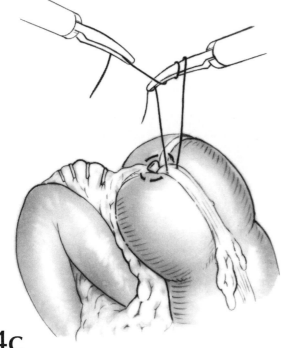

14c

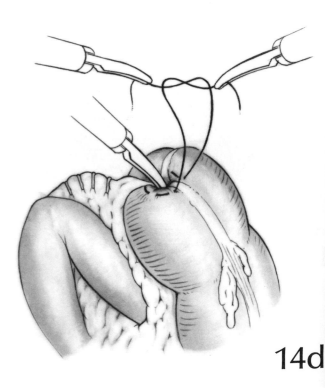

14d

Extraction of the appendix

15a, b An attempt should be made to remove the appendix and any other contaminated material without coming into contact with the anterior abdominal wall. This has been shown to almost eliminate the risk of postoperative wound infections[5,6]. If the appendix is not too enlarged, it can be first withdrawn into one of the 10-mm or larger accessory cannulae and then the entire sheath (with the enclosed specimen) removed from the peritoneal cavity.

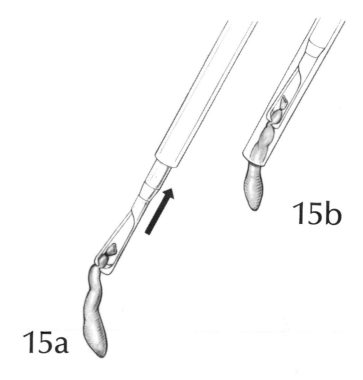

15b

15a

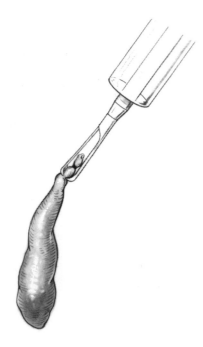

16 If the appendix will not easily pass through a 10-mm or 12-mm cannula, a 20-mm appendiceal extractor sheath can be exchanged for one of the sheaths already positioned (preferably at the umbilicus). The larger diameter of this conduit will permit the extraction of most appendices.

16

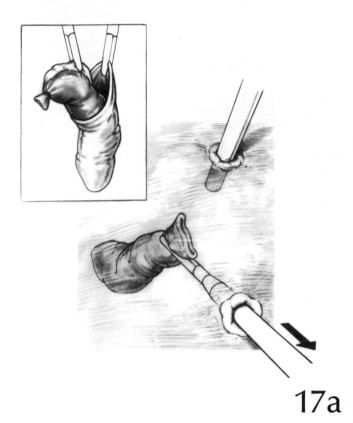

17a

17a, b Another popular method involves placing a sterile condom (or the finger of a large surgical glove) into the abdomen and placing the appendix within this reservoir. The appendix is then removed through one of the cannulae or through an enlarged fascial opening without coming into contact with the abdominal wall. This technique is particularly useful for removing a necrotic or fragmented appendix. Commercially available 'bags' are also available which have incorporated a number of useful improvements.

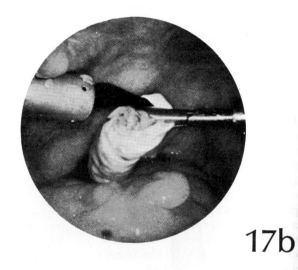

17b

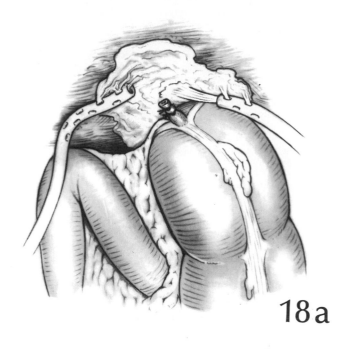

Irrigation and drain placement

18a, b Once the appendix has been detached, the lower abdomen and pelvis are irrigated with large quantities of saline. Contaminated material and debris are removed with a pool-tip aspiration cannula or atraumatic forceps. The operative field is inspected for adequate haemostasis and the appendiceal stump re-examined to ensure proper closure.

Closed suction drainage catheters may be used in cases of localized abscess formation. The drains are trimmed to the desired length and placed into the abdomen through one of the larger laparoscopic cannulae. The drainage catheter is then held in place with a pair of forceps, and the external tip is brought out through one of the accessory cannulae. The entire sheath is then removed with the catheter and the drain is secured to the skin.

18a

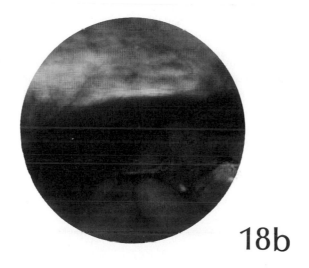

18b

Postoperative care

Postoperative care is similar to that following open appendicectomy. Patients undergoing laparoscopic surgery, however, generally experience a more rapid return of bowel function and earlier ambulation and discharge from hospital[8,9]. The severity of the underlying inflammatory process, however, will continue to exert a major influence on the postoperative course of the patient. Antibiotics, analgesics and intravenous fluids are administered as are clinically necessary. The larger umbilical fascial defect should be closed with one or more synthetic sutures. The smaller accessory puncture sites generally do not require fascial closure. If a large (i.e. 12-mm) cannula has been used at one of these locations or if the fascial opening has been enlarged to extract the specimen, it should be closed in a similar fashion. The skin is approximated with either sutures or staples. Wound problems should be few with the avoidance of abdominal wall contamination.

Outcome

Experience with laparoscopic appendicectomy is growing. Current reports indicate that laparoscopic appendicectomy is indicated for all but a few patients, provides definitive treatment of the underlying disease process, and can be performed with an acceptable incidence of operative morbidity and mortality. Recently published prospective randomized clinical studies comparing conventional appendicectomy with the laparoscopic method have demonstrated a shortened hospital stay and more rapid return to normal activity with the laparoscopic approach[8,9]. Laparoscopy has the additional advantage of allowing examination of the entire abdominal cavity, and in many cases can be used to manage other disorders which may have mimicked acute appendicitis. It has yet to be demonstrated whether laparoscopic appendicectomy will decrease the incidence of long-term complications, such as pelvic adhesions or small intestinal obstruction.

References

1. Bailey RW, Zucker KA, Flowers JL, Scovil WA, Graham SM, Imbembo AL. Laparoscopic cholecystectomy: experience with 375 consecutive patients. *Ann Surg* 1991; 214: 531–41.

2. Spaw AT, Reddick EJ, Olsen DO. Laparoscopic laser cholecystectomy: analysis of 500 procedures. *Surg Laparosc Endosc* 1991; 1: 2–7.

3. Semm K. Endoscopic appendectomy. *Endoscopy* 1983; 15: 59–64.

4. Schreiber JH. Early experience with laparoscopic appendectomy in women. *Surg Endosc* 1987; 1: 211–16.

5. Pier A, Gotz F, Bacher C. Laparoscopic appendectomy in 625 cases: from innovation to routine. *Surg Laparosc Endosc* 1991; 1: 8–13.

6. Valla JS, Limonne B, Valla V *et al*. Laparoscopic appendectomy in children: report of 465 cases. *Surg Laparosc Endosc* 1991; 1: 166–72.

7. Fisher KS, Ross DS. Guidelines for therapeutic decision in incidental appendectomy. *Surg Gynecol Obstet* 1990; 171: 95–8.

8. McAnena OJ, Austin O, O'Connell PR, Hederman WP, Gorey TF, Fitzpatrick J. Laparoscopic *versus* open appendicectomy: a prospective evaluation. *Br J Surg* 1992; 79: 818–20.

9. Attwood SEA, Hill ADK, Murphy PG, Thornton J, Stephens RB. A prospective randomized trial of laparoscopic *versus* open appendectomy. *Surgery* 1992; 112: 497–501.

10. Hasnain JU, Matjasko MJ. Practical anesthesia for laparoscopic procedures. In: Zucker KA, ed. *Surgical Laparoscopy*. St Louis: Quality Medical Publishing, 1991: 77–86.

11. Fitzgibbons RJ, Salerno GM, Filipi CJ. Open laparoscopy. In: Zucker KA, ed. *Surgical Laparoscopy*. St Louis: Quality Medical Publishing, 1991: 87–97.

12. Saye WB, Rives DA, Cochran EB. Laparoscopic appendectomy: three years' experience. *Surg Laparosc Endosc* 1991; 2: 109–15.

13. Engstrom L, Fenyo G. Appendicectomy: assessment of stump invagination versus simple ligation: a prospective, randomized trial. *Br J Surg* 1985; 72: 971–2.

Illustrations by Jenny Halstead and Susan Hales

Open appendicectomy

Graham L. Newstead FRACS, FRCS, FACS
Senior Lecturer in Surgery, University of New South Wales and Associate Director, Division of Surgery, Prince of Wales and Prince Henry Hospitals, Sydney, New South Wales, Australia

Principles and justification

Differential diagnosis

The contradiction of appendicitis is that the classic history of central abdominal colic becoming constant right iliac fossa pain may occasionally be due to other pathology, yet acute appendicitis may present with a variety of subtle differences both in symptoms and signs. Any patient in whom appendicitis is suspected, however, should undergo appendicectomy, which may be preceded by laparoscopy. The suspicion of mesenteric adenitis should delay surgery only if signs are minimal and hospitalization allows continuous reassessment. This is particularly important in children, as progression to peritonitis may be rapid. Possible gynaecological pathology may warrant pelvic ultrasonography, consideration of laparoscopy and exclusion of pregnancy.

Recurrent mild right iliac fossa pain, not uncommon in children, should be treated by exclusion of other causes before consideration of interval appendicectomy, indicated in selected patients. A faecolith may be present within the lumen despite normal histology, yet its implication is uncertain.

Incidental appendicectomy for a normal appendix should be undertaken only in special circumstances. Appendicectomy to facilitate appendicostomy may be used for intraoperative colonic lavage in the presence of obstruction.

Masked diagnosis

Retrocaecal appendicitis may be more severe than apparent on palpation, due to the dilated caecum acting as a buffer between the inflamed appendix and the anterior abdominal wall.

Appendicitis in a long rectocaecal appendix or with a caecum situated high in the right hypochondrium may mimic acute cholecystitis. A long intrapelvic appendix may present as a pelvic abscess and be confused with tubo-ovarian pathology in women.

Particular care must be taken in assessing elderly and immunocompromised patients, in whom the clinical signs of appendicitis may be masked, as may the diagnosis.

Special situations

The presence of a mass does not preclude appendicectomy, as it may indicate a phlegmon and not an abscess. A chronic mass requires consideration of such factors as the patient's age and associated history. In the absence of acute signs, initial assessment of the caecum and terminal ileum by colonoscopy or radiology may be most appropriate. Appendicectomy during pregnancy is safest during the second trimester. If surgery is necessary, discussion with the patient's obstetrician and employment of a gentle surgical technique will usually avoid miscarriage or early onset of labour. At all times, early operation is preferable and safest.

Preoperative

An intravenous infusion should be commenced and a preoperative dose of broad-spectrum antibiotic is administered to all patients to cover aerobic and anaerobic organisms; it should be continued if there is significant peritonitis. A nasogastric tube should be inserted to empty the stomach in those patients experiencing excessive vomiting or who have definite peritonitis. The abdomen should be shaved (if required) in order to facilitate extension of an incision in the right iliac fossa or to accommodate a midline incision if needed. Informed consent should be obtained and advice given to the patient regarding prevention of deep vein thrombosis and postoperative deep breathing exercises. Consideration should be given to the use of subcutaneous calcium heparin and antiembolism stockings in adults, particularly if there is a history of previous deep vein thrombosis. An indwelling urinary catheter should be inserted in patients with peritonitis; all others should be encouraged to void before surgery.

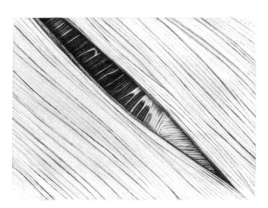

1

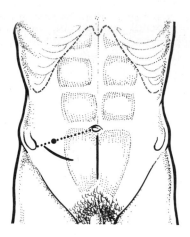

2

Anaesthesia

A fasting time of 4 h is preferred. After premedication, the patient is transferred to the operating theatre where general anaesthesia is induced and maintained with muscle relaxation and endotracheal intubation.

Operation

Position of patient

The patient is placed in the supine position. Calf compressors or muscle stimulators, if available, are used in adults and an adhesive diathermy pad applied to the thigh.

Preparation of abdomen

The entire abdomen is prepared with suitable antiseptic to allow extension or change of incision if required. The right lower quadrant is square draped to also allow access to the midline and the right flank above the anterior iliac crest.

Incision

1   The point of maximal tenderness elicited before anaesthesia should be compared with palpation of the abdomen following anaesthesia; muscle relaxation may facilitate palpation of a mass. These factors and concern for cosmesis will determine the area over which the incision should be centred. McBurney's point, being at the junction of the lateral third and medial two-thirds of a line passing from the antero-superior iliac spine to the umbilicus, is the classic surface marking for the base of the appendix, but the preferred incision may be somewhat transverse, keeping to the skin creases, initially to a maximum of 5 cm, but allowing lateral extension above the iliac crest if required.

A midline incision in patients with peritonitis and/or an indefinite diagnosis of appendicitis provides satisfactory exposure.

Splitting the aponeurosis of the external oblique muscle

2   The skin is incised, and the subcutaneous fatty and membranous layers of the superficial fascia are divided. The superficial circumflex and superficial epigastric veins may require ligation. The skin and fat are retracted, and a small incision is made in the lateral aspect of the fibres of the external oblique aponeurosis. A pair of scissors with the jaws opened a little is then pushed in the direction of the fibres, downwards and medially to their insertion into the anterior surface of the rectus sheath.

Splitting the internal oblique and transversus abdominis muscles

3 The fleshy muscle fibres of the internal oblique pass upwards and medially to insert into the anterior aspect of the lateral edge of the rectus sheath. An incision is made in the line of the most medial fibres, which are split by blunt dissection to separate them. At this point some small intermuscular vessels may be encountered which can be secured by diathermy. The tip of the forceps is angled laterally to split the deeper transverse fibres of the transversus abdominis muscle, which insert into the lateral edge of the rectus sheath. These muscle fibres are similarly split. The wound retractors are replaced to include these muscle layers.

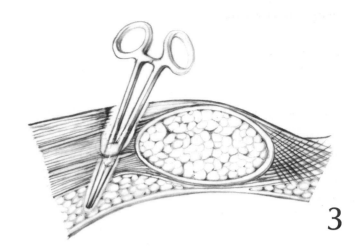

3

Opening the peritoneum

4 The extraperitoneal fat covering the peritoneum is gently cleared by blunt dissection and the peritoneum is grasped with an artery forceps. The tissue held by the forceps is inspected to ensure that no intestine has been trapped, and a second forceps is applied and further inspection made. The peritoneum between the two forceps is incised along the line of the skin incision for a small distance to allow inspection of the peritoneal cavity, again to ensure that no intestine has been inadvertently included. The incision is extended with scissors, the retractors are placed into the peritoneal cavity and the wound edges are elevated. A sample of any turbid fluid present is collected in a syringe and the air evacuated before it is placed in the container so that culture for both aerobic and anaerobic organisms may be undertaken. If there is a small amount of thick material, a little saline may be instilled to allow aspiration of a satisfactory sample.

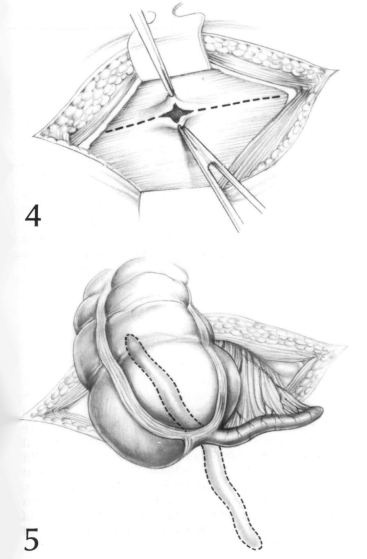

4

5

Identification of the appendix

5 If a taenia coli is immediately visible, it may be traced by index finger to the inferior pole of the caecum. The appendix may be immediately palpable and lie free, or it may lie behind the terminal ileum, pass down into the pelvis, or more commonly, pass superiorly behind the caecum.

Exploration of the peritoneal cavity

6 If the appendix is found to be normal, the index finger should be passed into the pelvis, particularly in women to examine the right fallopian tube and ovary. With wound retraction it may be possible to place a Babcock's tissue forceps on the round ligament to enable visual inspection. In smaller patients, the left fallopian tube and ovary may be digitally assessed. A gauze swab on a sponge-holding forceps should be used to exclude free blood or pus within the pelvis. The terminal ileum should be delivered, inspected and returned segment by segment until the distal 60 cm of ileum have been assessed to exclude ileal disease and a Meckel's diverticulum. The mesentery should also be checked for lymphadenopathy.

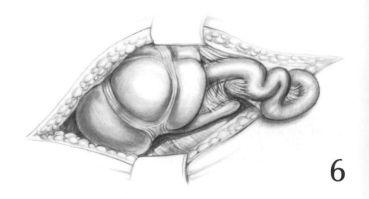

6

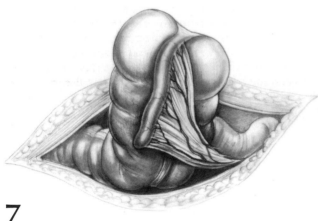

7

Delivery of the appendix

7 Retraction of the wound edges and easy palpation of the appendix may allow the application of Babcock's forceps to deliver the appendix into the wound, but perforation of an inflamed or gangrenous appendix must be avoided. If the appendix lies in the retrocaecal position, the caecum is grasped with non-toothed forceps and gently drawn inferiorly and then rocked up into the wound. This process can be gently repeated until the appendix base is visible. Scissors or diathermy may be used to divide any vascular adhesions covering the lateral aspect of the appendix as it lies adherent to the posterior aspect of the caecum. Retrograde appendicectomy may be required, necessitating lateral extension of the incision. Retrograde appendicectomy with medial extension of the incision may be required for a long fixed pelvic appendix (*see* later under '*Special circumstances*').

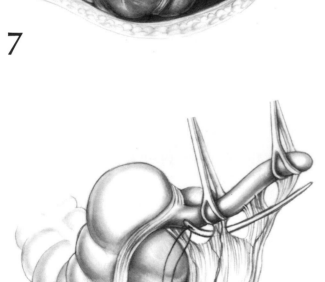

8

Division of the mesoappendix

8 The appendix is displayed between one pair of Babcock's forceps applied gently towards the tip and another near the base. Small windows are developed at the junction of the mesentery with the appendix using blunt forceps. The resultant pedicles containing the branches of the appendiceal vessels are ligated and divided. If the mesentery is thick, oedematous, or short, stitch ties may be required.

9 The appendiceal artery arises from a posterior branch of the ileocolic artery. It may be retrieved by inspecting behind the ileocaecal valve. The peritoneal fold beneath the caecum may need division to provide adequate mobilization if exposure is difficult. If the vessel is still unsecured, the wound incision may be extended medially or laterally as appropriate.

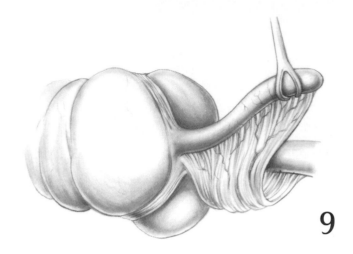

9

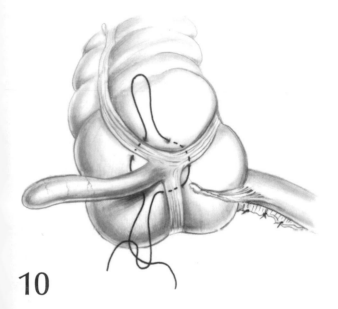

10

Insertion of purse-string suture

10 If invagination of the appendix stump is preferred, a circumferential purse-string suture is placed 1 cm away from the base of the appendix, gathering small seromuscular bites of caecal wall and ensuring that the line of the now divided mesenteric attachment is not picked up, thus avoiding a small recurrent branch of the appendiceal artery. The purse-string is left loose.

No purse-string suture is required if invagination is not intended.

Clamping, ligation, division and invagination of the appendix stump

11 The appendix is held somewhat vertically and crushed just above its base. A 0 chromic catgut tie is used to ligate the appendix base at this mark. The artery forceps is then applied to crush the appendix 5 mm above the ligature. A gauze swab is laid along the index finger and the appendix held along the index finger on the gauze by the thumb. An artery forceps is applied to the edge of the appendix between the ligature and the crushing forceps. The appendix is divided between the ligature and the crushing artery forceps. It is delivered to a dish, with the gauze swab and the crushing forceps, as 'unsterile'. The small remaining amount of mucosa visible outside the basal ligature may be scraped with a scalpel blade onto a further gauze swab, also placed into the waiting dish.

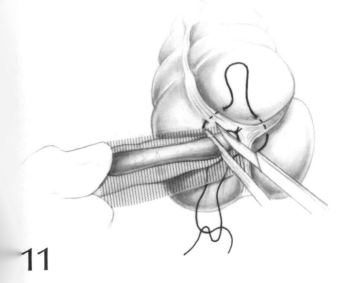

11

12 A decision to bury the appendix base requires that it be invaginated into the caecum and the purse-string suture is gently tightened and tied. If invagination is incomplete a further seromuscular bite to fully invaginate the stump may be obtained.

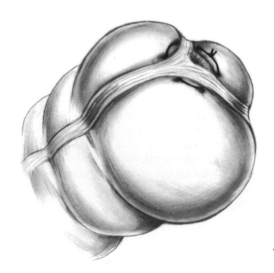

12

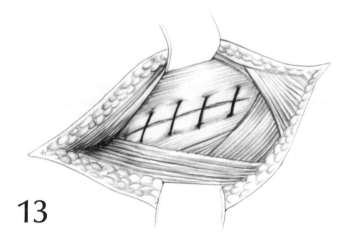

13

Wound closure

13 Warm normal saline should be poured into the right iliac fossa and pelvis and aspirated until the return is clear. Wound retractors are placed deep to the muscles and outside the peritoneum. Small artery forceps are placed at either end of the peritoneal incision and in the middle of its upper and lower edges. A continuous absorbable suture is inserted, ensuring at all times that intestine is not accidentally caught by the needle. An intraperitoneal drain should only be required if there is significant oozing or if a chronic abscess cavity has been opened.

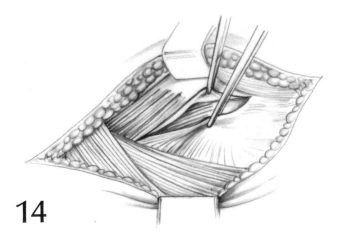

14

14 Further saline lavage is applied to the wound before muscle closure. The external oblique aponeurosis is retracted and interrupted absorbable sutures are used to loosely approximate the split layers of the transversus abdominis and internal oblique muscles without tension to avoid ischaemia, picking up the fascia of the internal oblique muscle rather than the muscle bundles.

15 A continuous absorbable suture is used to close the external oblique muscle, preferably burying the knot in thin patients. The membranous layer of subcutaneous tissue is approximated with interrupted absorbable sutures and the skin closed with interrupted or subcuticular sutures.

When significant pus has been encountered, it may be considered preferable to employ delayed wound closure, despite adequate intraperitoneal lavage. In such circumstances, interrupted absorbable sutures should be used in the muscular and aponeurotic layers. Loose approximating sutures are placed through the skin and subcutaneous layers for later tying.

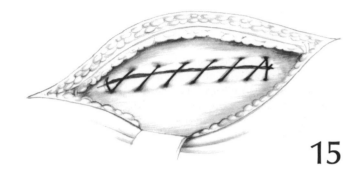

15

Special circumstances

Medial wound extension

16 By incising the lateral edge of the rectus sheath in the medial corner of the wound, the rectus muscle is exposed so that it can be further retracted medially. Care must be taken to avoid damaging the inferior epigastric vessels, which pass posterior to the rectus muscle. In the presence of peritonitis, the potential for infection in the rectus sheath space must be considered.

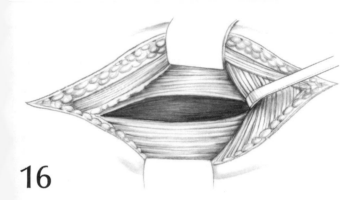

16

Lateral wound extension

17 This is necessary to deal with a high retrocaecal or subhepatic appendix. The skin incision should be extended above the iliac crest towards the lateral abdomen and flank. The muscle layers may be further split laterally, but fibres of the internal oblique and the transversus abdominis muscles may need to be divided to gain optimum exposure.

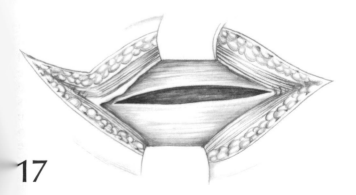

17

Retrograde appendicectomy

18 Having exposed the base of the appendix at its junction with the caecum, an artery forceps is passed through the mesentery and the appendix base is clamped, ligated, divided and invaginated with a purse-string suture in the manner described above. The mesoappendix is then secured from the base of the appendix towards its tip by serial clamping, division and ligation. At each stage the caecum is gently pushed superiorly within the abdominal cavity to give exposure to the portion of mesoappendix being ligated.

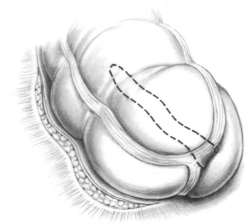

18

19 When it is necessary to extend the incision laterally for this purpose, incising the lateral peritoneum in the right paracolic gutter will allow the caecum and ascending colon to be gently pushed medially, thus exposing more of the elongated appendix.

19

Appendiceal tumour

20 If the appendix contains a tumour less than 2 cm in diameter, near the tip and apparently confined to the appendix, appendicectomy should include as much mesoappendix as possible. Most of these tumours will be carcinoid tumours. If the tumour is greater than 2 cm in diameter, it should also be managed initially by appendicectomy, the need for subsequent right hemicolectomy being determined by the microscopic features characteristic of carcinoid tumours and adenocarcinomas.

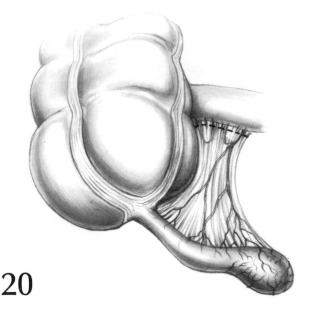

20

Mass in the right iliac fossa

21 After incising the peritoneum, the caecum and appendix are inspected to ascertain the underlying pathology. If omentum is adherent it may be gently separated, thus delineating the aetiology. The terminal ileum should be inspected for evidence of inflammation, and obvious evidence of local tumour extension should be excluded. Extension of the incision may allow a more definitive assessment. If the appearance of the appendiceal inflammation suggests Crohn's disease that does not involve the caecum, the appendix may be removed, in which case care must be taken to ensure seromuscular apposition of the uninvolved caecum adjacent to the base of the divided appendix. If Crohn's appendicitis does involve the adjacent caecum, a modified right hemicolectomy may be required.

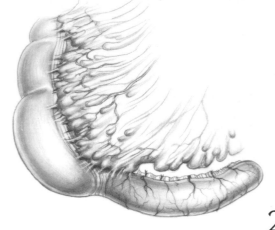

21

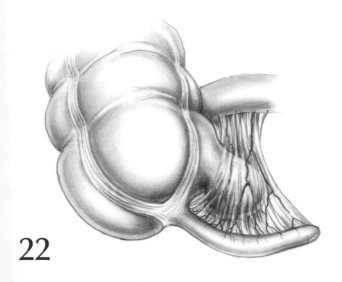

22

22 Localized diverticulitis of the caecum may occur, and if this can be confirmed by careful inspection, a decision on whether to close without resection or to carry out a segmental resection can be made. If the mass precludes a definitive diagnosis, it is reasonable to proceed as if dealing with a caecal tumour.

23 Tumours of the caecum may cause acute appendicitis. The caecum should be palpated carefully, and if an associated mucosal mass lesion is present, the wound may need to be closed and a midline incision made to allow an immediate right hemicolectomy to be undertaken.

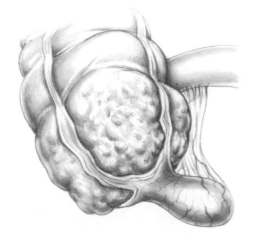

23

Postoperative care

After reversal of muscle relaxation and extubation, the patient is transferred to the recovery room and kept under routine observation until awake and stable. Suitable analgesia and antiemetics are prescribed. Intravenous infusion is continued until abdominal progress is satisfactory, and oral fluids are then introduced. Intravenous antibiotics are continued if peritonitis was present. Sutures remain for 1 week, but may be removed after 3 days and replaced by adhesive strips if desired.

Complications

Wound infection

After 24 h the wound dressing may be removed to allow frequent inspection. Minor cellulitis may be treated with appropriate antibiotics. Localized tenderness with fever may be treated by removal of a suture and probing to release accumulated pus.

Peritoneal abscess and septicaemia

This is relatively uncommon. Increasing abdominal or pelvic pain with diarrhoea after 1 week associated with fever may indicate the necessity for antibiotics after blood cultures have been taken. Other causes should be excluded. Computed tomography with needle aspiration of a collection may be considered.

Intestinal fistula

Conservative treatment is appropriate, and a small intestinal series, barium enema and perhaps colonoscopy may eventually be required, before consideration of re-exploration.

Further reading

Bak M, Asschenfeldt P. Adenocarcinoid of the vermiform appendix. A clinicopathologic study of 20 cases. *Dis Colon Rectum* 1988; 31: 605–12.

Cerame MA. A 25 year review of adenocarcinoma of the appendix, a frequently perforating carcinoma. *Dis Colon Rectum* 1988; 31: 145–50.

Engstrom L, Fenyo G. Appendicectomy: assessment of stump invagination versus simple ligation: a prospective, randomised trial. *Br J Surg* 1985; 72: 971–2.

Lewin J, Fenyo G, Engstrom L. Treatment of appendiceal abscess. *Acta Chir Scand* 1988; 154: 123–5.

Ruiz V, Unger SW, Morgan J, Wallack MK. Crohn's disease of the appendix. *Surgery* 1990; 107: 113–17.

Illustrations by Gillian Lee and Kathleen I. Jung

Ileostomy

John R. Oakley FRACS
Staff Surgeon and Head, Section of Enterostomal Therapy, Department of Colorectal Surgery, The Cleveland Clinic Foundation, Cleveland, Ohio, USA

Victor W. Fazio FRACS, FACS
Chairman, Department of Colorectal Surgery, The Cleveland Clinic Foundation, Cleveland, Ohio, USA

Principles and justification

Indications

The three types of ileostomy (end ileostomy, loop ileostomy and loop-end ileostomy) have differing indications.

End ileostomy

An end ileostomy is constructed under many varied circumstances:

1. At the completion of abdominal colectomy or after proctocolectomy performed for inflammatory bowel disease.
2. In patients with familial adenomatous polyposis in whom abdominal colectomy and ileorectal anastomosis is contraindicated because of rectal carcinoma, where a 'sea' of rectal polyps would make the future control of polyps difficult, or where restorative ileal pouch–anal anastomosis is not considered advisable or is not desired by the patient.
3. In the rare circumstances where multiple synchronous carcinomas are present in the large bowel.
4. A 'temporary' end ileostomy is sometimes constructed after ileal or ileocaecal resection for perforating Crohn's disease, ileocaecal trauma, obstructing right colonic lesions, or after complex fistula surgery. Subsequent removal of the ileostomy and reanastomosis of the bowel may be carried out.
5. Rarely in inflammatory bowel disease to allow the patient's general condition to improve before elective colectomy, but this is seldom advised.
6. When constructing an ileal conduit for urinary diversion.

Loop ileostomy

A loop ileostomy may be used to provide diversion (usually temporary) in the following conditions:

1. Above an ileal pouch–anal anastomosis for mucosal ulcerative colitis or familial polyposis.
2. Above an ileorectal anastomosis for inflammatory bowel disease.
3. Above a continent ileal reservoir.
4. Above enterocutaneous fistulae, before or after surgical resection.
5. Proximal to colorectal or coloanal anastomoses when a loop colostomy is judged to be technically difficult or undesirable.
6. In certain cases of ileocaecoappendiceal sepsis (such as perforating Crohn's disease).
7. To complement colonic decompression in certain cases of toxic megacolon.
8. Proximal to any distal bowel anastomosis where the anastomosis is tenuous because of radiation effects or malnutrition, or where it lies in proximity to a septic inflammatory 'nest'.
9. For certain cases of severe perianal Crohn's disease where proctocolectomy is not acceptable to the patient.

The advantage of a loop ileostomy is that the mesenteric vessels are not divided in its construction, so that ischaemia is virtually impossible. The major disadvantage is that the amount of ileal protrusion above the skin level is limited and with passage of time is more prone to recession than an end stoma.

Loop-end ileostomy

A loop-end ileostomy may be used as a primary procedure for the definitive stoma in patients with ileal urinary conduits or in obese patients with a thick abdominal wall where it would be difficult to maintain sufficient blood supply to allow the end of a divided bowel to reach beyond the skin level. Occasionally, a previous loop ileostomy may be converted to a loop-end stoma by transection and closure of the efferent limb of the ileum just inside the peritoneal cavity. In these patients, the mesenteric defect is not obliterated unless a loop-end ileostomy is constructed during a primary procedure.

Preoperative

The preoperative preparation required largely depends upon the underlying condition for which the ileostomy is planned. The surgeon, stoma nurse and sometimes also a trained lay ostomy visitor, should discuss the implications of surgery with the patient and his or her family, providing reassurance and encouragement. Most patients will benefit from reading pertinent literature available from local or national stoma associations.

Siting the stoma

1, 2 Rehabilitation of the patient begins before the operation, with selection of the optimal stoma site. It is preferable to mark a stoma site first with the patient seated, when any crease or fold of skin will become more prominent, and then to check the position with the patient supine.

The following rules apply:

1. Use the summit or apex of the infraumbilical fat mound.
2. The mark should be in the middle of, or at least within the surface marking of, the rectus abdominis muscle.
3. The mark should be at least 4 cm from the planned incision line.
4. The stoma site and the adjacent skin should be away from creases, scars, the umbilicus, any prominences and anticipated future incisions. Using a commercially available standard size template facilitates correct placement.
5. A site where the skin has been injured, e.g. from a skin graft, burn, or radiotherapy, must be avoided.

At the selected site a vertical line is marked downwards from the umbilicus, and a horizontal line is marked outwards from the lower border of the umbilicus.

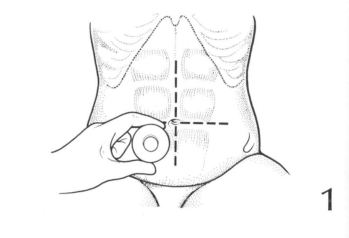

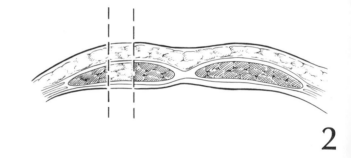

Marking the stoma

3 Once the position of the faceplate is determined with the patient seated, the patient is asked to lie down while the faceplate is held in position. An indelible mark is then made by placing a drop of India ink or methylene blue over the stoma site; a needle prick produces a tattoo which cannot be washed away during preoperative bathing or when preparing the abdominal wall with antiseptic solution.

Anaesthesia

General anaesthesia with relaxants and endotracheal intubation is used. Peroperative intravenous broad-spectrum antibiotics are given. A nasogastric tube is inserted after induction of anaesthesia and the bladder is catheterized if a bowel resection is contemplated.

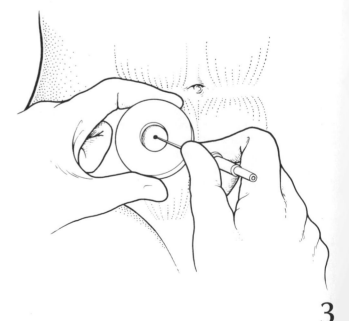

Operation

END ILEOSTOMY

Position of patient

A supine or modified lithotomy-Trendelenburg position is used, depending on whether a combined abdomino-perineal proctectomy is to be part of the procedure.

Incision

The incision is made in the midline, skirting just to the left side of the umbilicus. If colectomy is planned, the incision is carried to the upper epigastrium to a point where the surgeon judges that the splenic flexure can be safely mobilized. Because of the possibility of future stoma revision and relocation (especially when operating for Crohn's disease), a midline incision is very much preferred over a paramedian approach so that the sites for possible future stomas are left intact.

Division of the terminal ileum

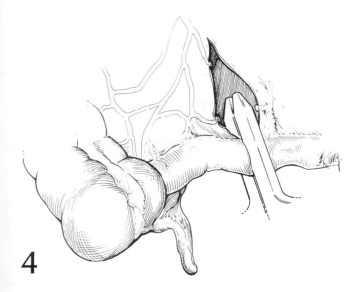

4 In the absence of ileal disease, the ileum is transected 7–10 cm from the ileocaecal valve unless a later ileal pouch–anal anastomosis is contemplated, in which case the terminal ileal division should be 1–2 cm proximal to the ileocaecal valve. To minimize contamination in the course of later delivery of the end of the ileum through the abdominal wall, a linear stapling instrument should be used.

Ileostomy aperture

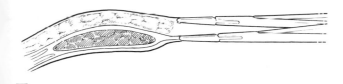

5 The cut edge of the linea alba and the dermis at the level of the stoma site are then grasped with Kocher (or similar) clamps and retracted medially.

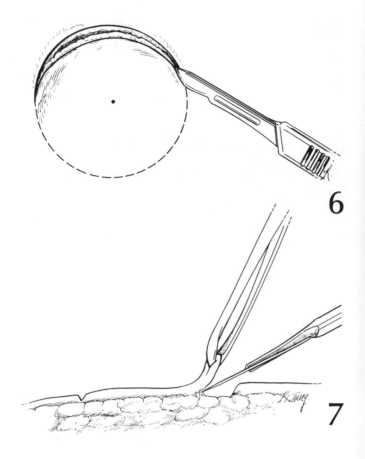

6,7 A circumferential incision, 2–2.5 cm in diameter, is made around the previously marked stoma site. No trephine is made; only the skin disc is excised. The subcutaneous fat is preserved to minimize the chances of a dead space and accumulation of a parastomal seroma or abscess, and to add support to the stoma as it traverses the subcutaneous tissues. The sagittal view (*Illustration 7*) shows excision of the skin disc and preservation of the fat.

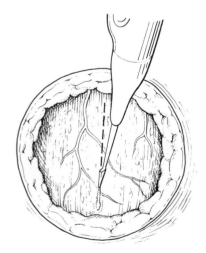

8 A vertical incision is made through the subcutaneous tissue. Any bleeding from the skin edge, which is usually minor, should be left to stop spontaneously, as coagulation could severely traumatize the skin and cause mucocutaneous separation.

9 An abdominal pack, or a sponge, is then placed within the peritoneal cavity behind the rectus muscle while the surgeon maintains medial traction on the wound edge to ensure that the rectus muscle does not slip laterally during the course of fashioning the ileostomy aperture. This manoeuvre is facilitated by the operator's hand pushing upwards from inside the abdomen over the area of the ileostomy aperture.

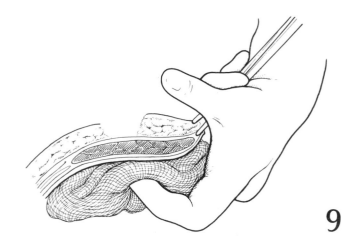

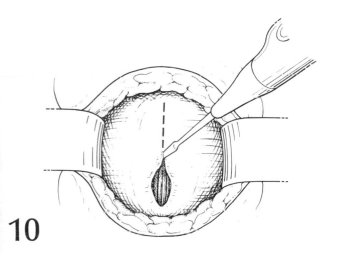

10 Scarpa's layer of fascia is incised and short right-angle retractors are positioned medially and laterally to display the anterior rectus sheath. The cutting cautery incises the sheath for 3–3.5 cm in a vertical direction; lateral cruciate incisions are not necessary.

11 An artery forceps is inserted perpendicularly down to the posterior sheath and the jaws gently opened in the horizontal plane, minimizing the risk of injury to the inferior epigastric vessels. Before the instrument is withdrawn, medial and lateral retractors are placed to prevent the vertical fibres of the muscle springing back and making identification of the site of rectus split difficult. A muscle splitting, rather than a muscle cutting, procedure is used to minimize the risk of postoperative hernia or prolapse of the ileostomy.

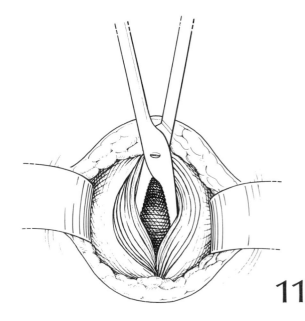

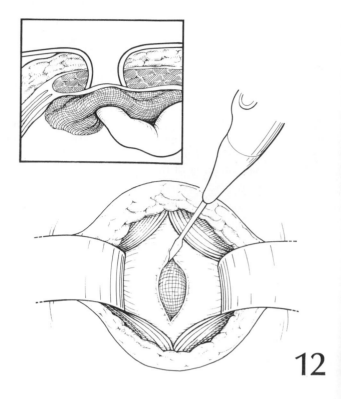

12 With an assistant maintaining lateral and medial retraction of the rectus muscle and exposing the posterior rectus sheath, and the surgeon pushing upwards from inside the abdomen, the posterior rectus sheath and peritoneum are divided in the vertical plane, cutting directly on to the sponge, which protects the operator's left hand.

13 The aperture size is tested: for the surgeon who uses size 7 or 8 gloves, the optimal size corresponds to a snug two-finger aperture such that the distal interphalangeal joint of the middle finger and the pulp of the index finger can be seen. If the aperture is too large, prolapse or parastomal hernia may occur; if too narrow it may become obstructed.

14 Manipulation of the aperture may cause bleeding from the rectus muscle or tributaries of the inferior epigastric vessels. A large pair of Kelly forceps may be passed through the aperture and used as a retractor to check for any bleeding.

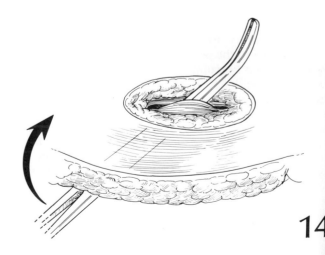

Fashioning the stoma

15 The terminal ileum is prepared for drawing through the aperture by dividing the mesentery 0.5–1.0 cm from the bowel wall so as to preserve a vascular arcade close to the bowel. This reduces the bulk of the mesentery and straightens the terminal ileum. Sufficient length of bowel should be prepared to pass through the thickness of the abdominal wall and to protrude 5–6 cm beyond the level of the skin. It is wise to suture ligate the divided vessels to ensure that the ligatures are not dislodged when passing the bowel through the stoma. Arterial bleeding from the distal mesenteric attachment confirms a good blood supply to the stoma.

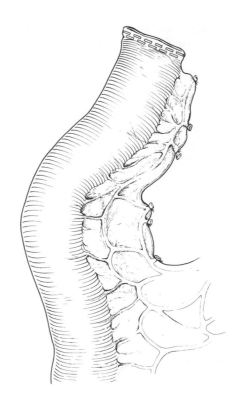

15

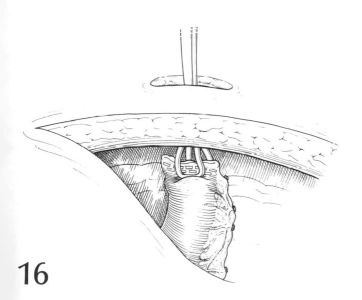

16

16 A Babcock clamp is passed through the stoma aperture, grasping the prepared ileum and drawing it gently through the abdominal wall so that the ileal mesentery lies in a cephalad direction to facilitate later obliteration of the mesenteric defect. A 6-cm length of exteriorized ileum is optimal.

17 Although some surgeons prefer to obliterate the mesenteric defect by suturing the cut end of the mesentery to the lateral abdominal wall, or by fashioning an extraperitoneal ileostomy, these techniques can be time consuming and technically difficult. The authors' preference, after completion of the colectomy, is to suture the cut edge of the mesentery to the anterior abdominal wall. This is achieved using interrupted or continuous 2/0 chromic catgut (or other absorbable material) sutures, starting at the mesenteric attachment to the bowel and suturing the free edge of the mesentery to the back of the abdominal wall approximately 2.5 cm lateral to the wound edge. At the cephalad end the suture is continued to the free lower edge of the falciform ligament. Residual transverse mesocolon or redundant lesser omentum may be included in the stitch. Care must be taken not to injure significant vessels in the free edge of the mesentery.

Stabilizing sutures of 3/0 chromic catgut, or absorbable sutures of 3/0 chromic catgut or Vicryl are usually placed between the seromuscular layer of the ileum and the peritoneum around the internal aperture. These sutures may be omitted in patients with Crohn's disease because they increase the risk of fistula formation, but if they are inserted carefully without taking deep bites into the bowel, the risk is reduced and they probably add another safeguard against ileal prolapse.

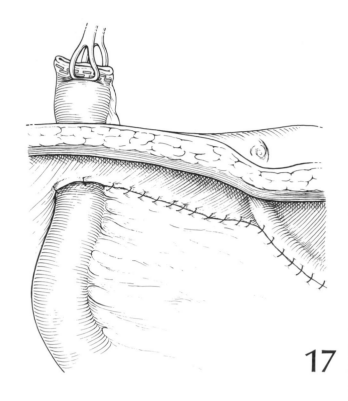

17

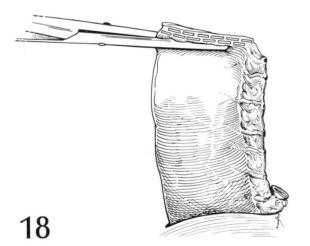

18

Maturing the ileostomy

18 The end of the ileostomy is opened after the main incision has been closed and is isolated with drapes to minimize bacterial wound contamination. Arterial or 'nuisance' bleeding from the cut end of the bowel is a sign of bowel viability.

19 One of the problems that confronts the surgeon and the stoma therapist is the late occurrence of a gully or 'moat' at the mucocutaneous junction of the stoma, which tends to occur as the patient gains weight, notwithstanding the initial satisfactory placement of the stoma. To minimize this effect, the skin edge can be everted by placing radial sutures of 3/0 catgut between the bowel wall and the subcutaneous fat. The seromuscular bowel stitch is placed about 1 cm above the skin level and is sutured to the most superficial part of the subcutaneous fat, bringing the suture out at the fat–epidermis junction. As the suture is tied a slight concertina effect is produced, which reduces any tendency for formation of a parastomal gully.

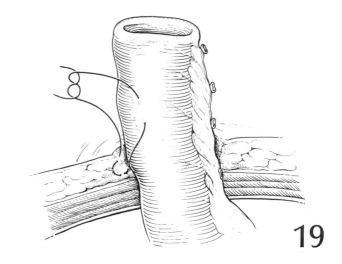

19

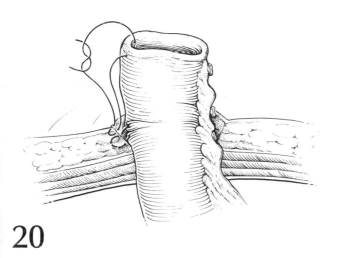

20

20 Radial sutures of 3/0 chromic catgut are placed at the four compass points of the stoma, through full-thickness bowel edge and sutured to the subcuticular skin. They should be placed vertically rather than tangentially or horizontally through the subcuticular skin, because minor degrees of vascular compromise here may cause separation of the mucosa and serositis of the exposed ileum. The sutures should not go through the external skin because of the risk of ileal mucosal island implantation, which may cause early separation of the stoma appliance.

21a, b Four additional sutures are then placed between the four compass-point sutures and the sutures are tied down, everting the stoma.

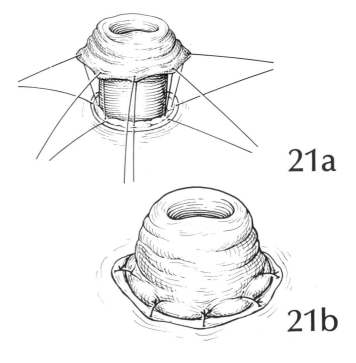

21a

21b

22 The maturing sutures may alternatively be inserted through full-thickness bowel edge and through the seromuscular layer of the bowel wall at skin level before passing through the subcuticular skin. This produces a three-point suture which helps to keep the stoma everted, especially in the patient with flabby subcutaneous tissue where there is little support for the stoma. This type of suture is best avoided in patients with Crohn's disease because of the risk of development of skin-level fistulae.

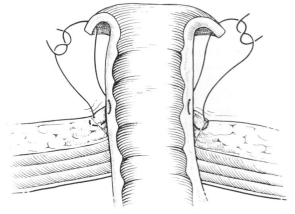

22

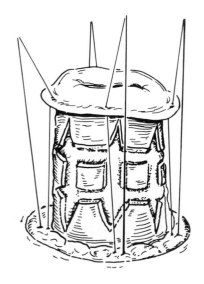

23

23 An alternative method of constructing the end ileostomy is to add a two-directional myotomy to the spout. This minimizes the risk of stoma recession and is appropriate for short stomas or in patients with a thick abdominal wall.

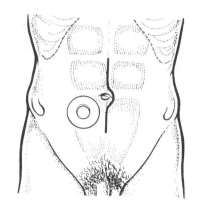

24

LOOP ILEOSTOMY

24 A midline incision is used. Positioning is as for an end ileostomy.

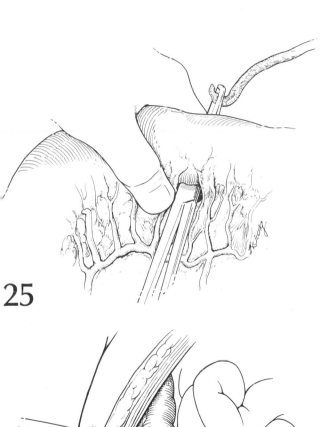

25

26

25, 26 When a loop ileostomy is being placed proximal to an anastomosis or for diversion above distal small bowel pathology, it should be created 15–20 cm proximally, depending on the thickness of the abdominal wall. The distance above an intact ileocaecal valve may be reduced to 10–15 cm. At the apex of the loop selected, a tape is brought through a small window made in the small bowel mesentery, to act as a retractor. It is important to be able to differentiate the proximal from the distal site of the loop, because as the loop is brought through the abdominal wall aperture, it may rotate and not be recognized. Therefore, each site should be tagged, adjacent to the apex of the loop, with sutures of different material, colour or length.

27a–e

The ileostomy loop is brought through the abdominal wall aperture using curved forceps to grasp the ends of the tape, and checking the orientation of the loop so that the proximal end is cephalad and the distal end caudad. An ileostomy rod is placed under the loop. Possible injury to the mesenteric vessels can be minimized by placing a Kocher clamp on one end of the tape and making several twists in the tape. As the tape is pulled through the mesentery, detorsion or rifling of the Kocher clamp will lessen the risk of damage by the clamp. The rod is grasped by one of its eyelets and gently brought through the mesentery to support the loop.

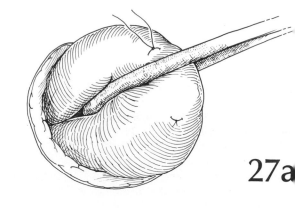

27a

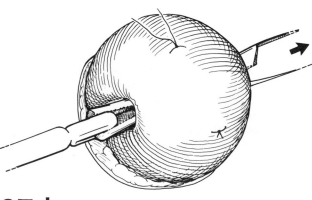

27b

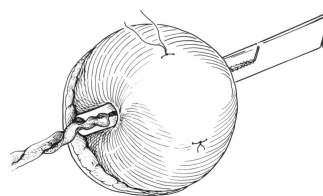

27c

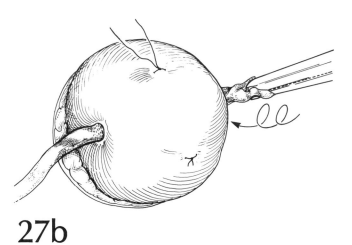

27d

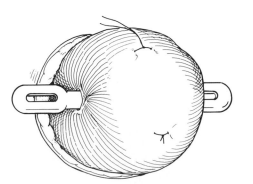

27e

28 The abdomen is closed and the main incision isolated from the ileostomy with drapes. The identifying tags may now be removed. An incision is made in the loop on its caudad and distal side across 80% of its circumference approximately 0.5 cm above, and parallel to, the skin. If the incision is flush with the skin, mucus may escape from the recessive limb and cause a faulty seal with the appliance.

Bleeding may occur as the enterotomy is extended towards the mesenteric edges, and the incision should stop about 5 mm short of the mesentery on both sides. A useful technique to minimize bleeding is to make an initial seromuscular incision with scissors, allowing the submucosa to pout out. Selective light electrocoagulation of the visible submucosal vessels can then be performed before completing the enterotomy.

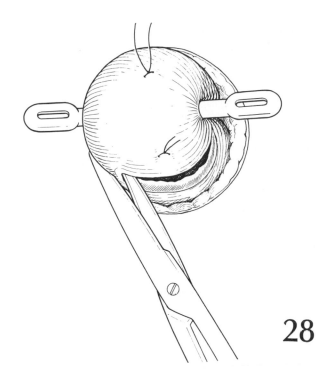

28

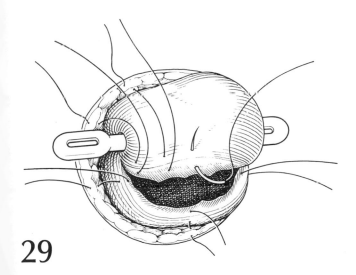

29

29 Sutures of 3/0 chromic catgut are then placed, for both loops, through full-thickness bowel edge and then through the subcuticular layer of skin. The sutures are tagged and not tied down until all have been inserted because it is difficult to place them with accuracy next to the rod. On the caudad, or lower, side three sutures are usually sufficient; one adjacent to the rod on each side and one centrally placed. Five sutures are usually needed on the cephalad side.

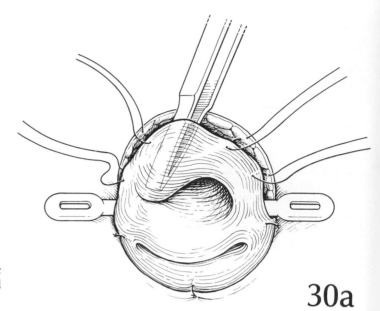

30a

30a, b The caudad sutures are tied before the cephalad part of the bowel is everted with the help of the blunt end of a pair of tissue forceps.

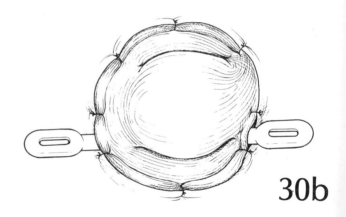

30b

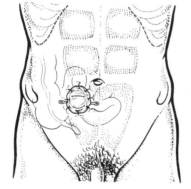

31

31 The completed loop ileostomy in the distal small bowel to divert the faecal stream from the colon is shown.

LOOP-END ILEOSTOMY

This may be performed at the time of colectomy or by conversion of a loop ileostomy to a loop-end ileostomy. In the latter instance, the distal limb is transected and oversewn just inside the peritoneal cavity. The following illustrations show the technique for construction of the loop-end stoma at the time of colectomy.

32, 33 The line of transection of the ileum is chosen close to the ileocaecal valve using hand sutures or a linear stapling device. A moist tape is placed around the ileum, passing through a small mesenteric window 7–10 cm above the transected bowel after judging the amount of small bowel that will be needed to traverse the thickness of the abdominal wall. The closed distal end should lie just within the peritoneal cavity.

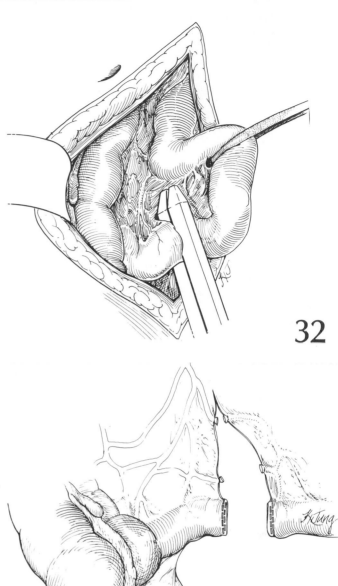

32

33

34 The abdominal wall aperture is made in the same way as for conventional ileostomy and the loop drawn through, after marking the proximal and distal ends with differing sutures as with loop ileostomy. The mesenteric defect is to be obliterated, and the functional end lies caudad and the non-functional end cephalad. This allows the cut edge of the small bowel mesentery to be aligned easily with the anterior abdominal wall.

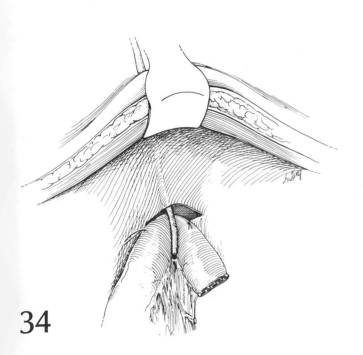

34

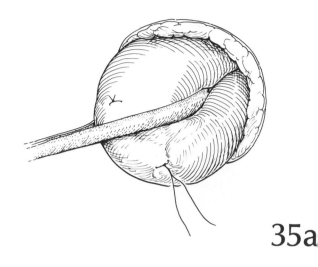

35a, b Using the tape, the loop is drawn through the abdominal wall aperture until 2–3 cm protrude beyond the skin. The tape is replaced by a short plastic ileostomy rod. Stabilizing sutures of 3/0 chromic catgut may then be placed between the seromuscular layer of the loop and the subcutaneous fat to facilitate further eversion of the skin, but this manoeuvre is optional.

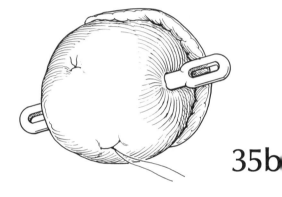

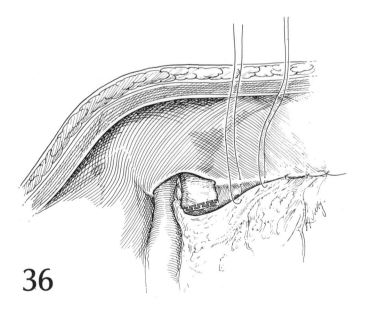

36 The mesentery of the small bowel is sutured to the anterior abdominal wall 2–3 cm lateral to the main incision using interrupted or continuous absorbable sutures. The suture line is carried cephalad up to and on to the free edge of the falciform ligament and caudad to the internal aspect of the abdominal wall aperture. Seromuscular sutures may also be placed between the limbs of the loop and the peritoneum of the ileostomy aperture.

37 An enterotomy is made on the cephalad side of the loop across 80% of the circumference of the ileum, about 0.5 cm above skin level.

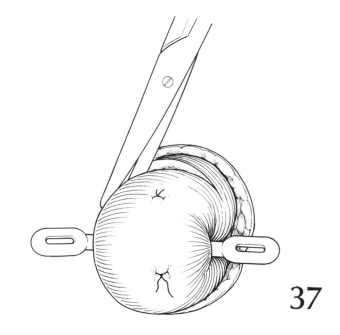

37

38a–c Sutures of 3/0 chromic catgut are placed through the full thickness of the cut edge of the ileum and sutured to the subcuticular layer of skin: three sutures are usually required on the defunctioned side and five on the functional side. The sutures should be placed so that the rod remains slightly eccentric and closer to the defunctioned side. As described for loop ileostomy, the sutures are not tied until all have been inserted. The blunt end of a pair of tissue forceps aids eversion.

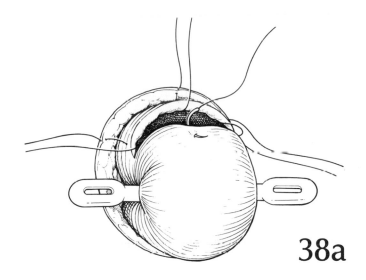

38a

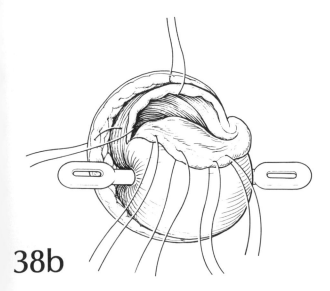

38b

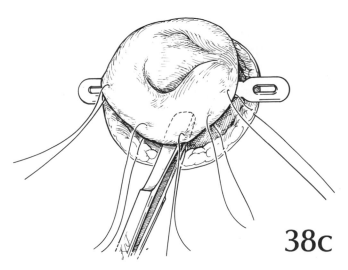

38c

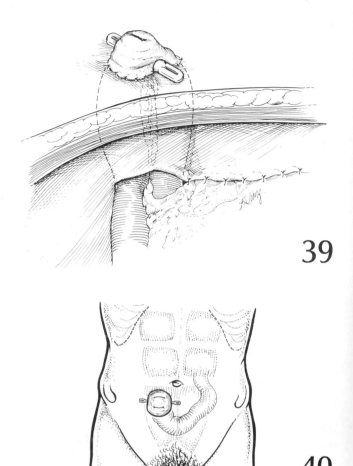

39, 40 The main incision is closed before breaching the ileal lumen, as for other types of ileostomy construction, but for clarity the completed stoma is shown with the incision unclosed.

Note

In cases of extreme obesity, the fashioning of an ileostomy, even a loop ileostomy, may be extraordinarily difficult. In such cases a generous (8–10 cm) incision is made in the peritoneum and posterior rectus sheath of the internal aperture so that the bowel can be brought through the abdominal wall easily. However, before delivering the bowel through the aperture, sutures of 1 Prolene are placed on both sides of the extended incision and left untied. After the bowel has been delivered to a length that satisfies the surgeon, these sutures may be tied, partly closing the defect; the surgeon should watch for any ischaemic effects on the bowel produced by these ties. This manoeuvre will help to reduce the possibility of formation of a parastomal hernia.

Postoperative care

Early management

A skin barrier is applied to the stoma in the operating room, the most suitable being a large karaya disc which can be applied over the ileostomy rod in the case of a loop or loop-end stoma. An open-ended transparent pouch with adhesive backing is attached to the skin barrier using hypoallergenic paper tape to secure the periphery of the pouch to the skin. The clear pouch allows easy inspection of the stoma in the postoperative period, with special attention being paid to stoma colour, skin separation and oedema. Two-piece pouches are available, the extra length of which rests in the bed next to the patient so that the weight of the contents does not cause separation of the pouch from the skin. One-piece units are also available, which have the advantage that they can be used by personnel who are less skilled in stoma management.

Approximately 3–5 days after surgery, the patient is instructed in the care of the stoma. Until that time the stoma therapist or nurse checks the pouch daily. Usually 3 or 4 days of careful instruction are required before the patient can confidently assemble and apply the pouch to the stoma.

Ileostomy equipment

The essential components are a *skin barrier* to which a *pouch* is attached. One-piece and two-piece appliances are available, the latter having detachable and disposable pouches. The barrier protects the skin and encourages irritated, denuded, and eroded skin to epithelialize. The most common barriers are karaya (which is available as a wafer, ring, paste, or powder) and gelatin–pectin based products (wafers, rings, powder, or paste) such as Stomahesive and Hollihesive. The skin barrier may be supplied with the opening precut to various sizes, or the patient may need to cut it to an appropriate size and shape. Almost all modern stoma equipment is disposable.

Many combinations of one-piece and two-piece systems, drainable and non-drainable pouches, precut and uncut skin barriers are available. Most appliances are self-adhesive, in some an in-built convexity of the skin barrier is useful to adhere to the skin around a recessive stoma or one located on a 'flabby' abdominal wall. Various skin sealants (gels, sprays, wipes, and liquids) are available as added protection to the surrounding skin.

Application of the pouch

The skin is prepared with a fat solvent such as non-medicated soap. The stoma diameter is measured, using calipers or a commercially available template, to obtain the correct aperture size, which should be slightly larger than the base of the stoma. The patient will need to cut the aperture to the appropriate size unless a precut barrier or faceplate is to be used. A gelatin–pectin based or karaya ring or a rim of paste may be added to the barrier, with or without a convex insert, in order to obtain a better seal around the base of the stoma. The faceplate is then placed centrally over the stoma and attached to the skin and secured with the in-built adhesive tape or by a 'picture frame' of microporous tape. It is advisable to protect the skin with a sealant before applying the tape. In a one-piece system the pouch will be supplied attached to the appliance, but in a two-piece system the pouch should be applied at this stage. A pouch cover made of cotton is useful in hot weather and for patients with vinyl sensitivity.

Home-going equipment

By the time of discharge from hospital most patients will be fitted with a 'permanent' appliance. The type selected will depend on the configuration of the stoma, the surrounding skin and the abdominal wall, and also on the patient's personal preference, type of employment and lifestyle. An experienced stomal therapist should fit the patient with the most appropriate form of pouch. Some trial and error may be necessary and a large order for equipment should not be placed until the time of the postoperative visit, several weeks after surgery.

Follow-up

The patient is seen in the outpatient clinic approximately 6 weeks after surgery when it is necessary to remeasure the stoma diameter because shrinkage has usually occurred. The patient's skin is checked, any problems are discussed, and further encouragement is given.

Complications

Mucosal slough

Slough of mucosa results from ischaemia or excessive tension, and if minor requires no treatment. Slough of part of the everted muscle as well, or mucocutaneous separation, may leave exposed serosa of the non-everted part of the ileostomy, delaying the maturation of the stoma.

Degrees of pseudo-obstruction may be encountered, and late stenosis at the skin level (Bishop's collar deformity) may be seen if the defect is significant. Early surgery and revision are not indicated except for the obviously necrotic stoma or where there is wide circumferential separation or ischaemia at the mucocutaneous junction.

High output

In the early postoperative period a watery green effluent may be noted. Caution should be exercised in interpreting this as a sign of return of normal bowel function: it may indicate pseudo-obstruction or ileus, which may be recognized by finding mucous clumps or strands which are grey-white in appearance. Oral intake should be withheld until a thicker brown effluent is noted.

After the patient resumes normal eating and drinking, the effluent may remain high in volume: codeine, diphenoxylate, loperamide, tincture of laudanum, or combinations of these may be used to reduce the output to 700–1000 ml/day. Psyllium seed derivatives sometimes help to thicken the stool.

Parastomal irritation

There are many causes of parastomal irritation, including a poor seal, candidiasis, parastomal ulceration, allergy to the pouch material or adhesive tape, folliculitis, trauma to the skin from frequent pouch changes, pressure ulcers, psoriasis and eczema. Most of these problems can be resolved by very careful stoma management, and the involvement of a stoma therapist is invaluable.

Ileostomy fistula

This may occur early as a result of suturing the bowel wall to the rectus fascia (as opposed to the peritoneum or subcutaneous fat), or late secondary to faceplate trauma or recurrent disease, particularly Crohn's disease. If it is symptomatic, surgical revision is required, but often the fistula opening is adjacent to the mucocutaneous junction and the fistula can be incorporated into the pouching system.

Paraileostomy ulceration

When extensive paraileostomy ulceration occurs requiring debridement which leaves a large raw area, a non-seal and non-adhesive appliance may temporarily be required to allow healing. A non-adherent dressing is applied over the ulcer and the pouch held in position by a belt, with the dressing being changed two or three times a day until the ulcer is small enough to allow a conventional pouch to be applied.

Ileostomy obstruction

Bowel obstruction after ileostomy may occur at any time because of adhesions, volvulus, or entrapment of the bowel in the fascial closure. Food bolus obstruction is also seen after this operation: ingestion of poorly digested food (string vegetables, corn, popcorn, peanuts, fruit skins) may produce a picture of bowel obstruction, especially in the first 3 months after surgery. Predisposing causes such as low-grade or partial obstruction by adhesions or recurrent Crohn's disease may exist.

Bolus obstruction should be treated conservatively; irrigation of the ileostomy by gentle lavage with 50–100 ml saline introduced through a small catheter, repeated at intervals until an adequate return is seen. The bolus should then break up and this is recognized by the presence of vegetable fibre in the returned irrigation fluids.

Ileostomy recession

Recession of the ileostomy may be treated by good stomal therapy techniques, particularly the employment of various degrees of convexity, either built in or added to the appliance. If this treatment is unsuccessful, stoma revision (usually without laparotomy) may be required (*see* chapter on pp. 668–682).

Ileostomy prolapse and hernia

Fixation of the mesentery and limiting the abdominal wall aperture will usually prevent prolapse. Prolapse may sometimes be managed by local revision of the ileostomy but relocation is often required. A small paraileostomy hernia beside a stoma where the bowel has been brought through the belly of the rectus muscle and the abdominal wall defect may be repaired and the ileostomy revised without relocation. However, if the hernia defect is large, or if it occurs with a stoma located outside the rectus muscle, local revision is unlikely to be successful and relocation is almost always required (*see* chapter on pp. 668–682).

Ileostomy closure

Timing of closure

Oedema and friability of the tissues, which occur early after ileostomy construction and persist for several weeks, increase the complications associated with closure. The operation should be deferred for at least 2 months, and preferably 3 months, after stoma construction.

Preoperative preparation

Before a loop ileostomy is closed, the integrity of any distal anastomoses or suture lines should be assessed in the distal bowel and distal obstruction or disease ruled out. This is usually achieved by standard endoscopy and by water-soluble contrast radiology.

Formal bowel preparation for ileostomy closure is not usually necessary, but administration of clear liquids for 12–24 h before surgery and preoperative enemas (to empty any residual colonic segment) are usually advisable. Broad-spectrum antibiotics are administered peroperatively.

Anaesthesia and positioning

General anaesthesia, with muscle relaxation to facilitate mobilization of the stoma from the abdominal wall and subsequent closure of the defect, is indicated. Surgery is usually performed with the patient supine, or in the modified lithotomy (Lloyd-Davies) position if other surgery is to be performed at the same time.

Incision

41 A circumferential incision is made adjacent to the mucocutaneous junction, leaving a sliver of skin 1–2 mm wide attached to the bowel. Taking any additional skin results in an unnecessarily large defect with prolonged healing time and greater potential for distortion and puckering. It is not normally necessary to make transverse or vertical extensions of the circular incision, although the surgeon should not hesitate to do so later if there is any difficulty in mobilizing the stoma.

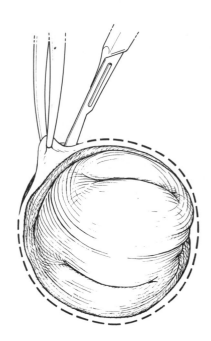

41

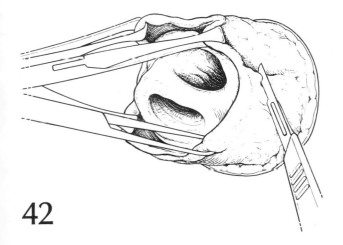

42

Mobilization of ileostomy from abdominal wall

42 The small rim of skin attached to the bowel is grasped by four Allis forceps and the subcutaneous tissue is freed from the serosal surface of the bowel by sharp dissection using a size 15 scalpel blade

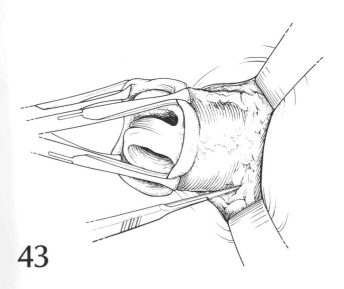

43

43 Gentle retraction with small right-angle retractors and countertraction on the bowel forceps facilitates the dissection, which should proceed around the circumference of the bowel, gradually deepening the dissection. It is necessary continually to move the retractors and to use deeper bladed retractors as the dissection passes deep to the anterior rectus sheath and to the fibres of the rectus muscle. Scalpel dissection with adequate retraction and appropriate countertraction will usually allow mobilization to the peritoneal level, but occasionally fine scissor dissection may also be necessary.

44 Once the peritoneal cavity is entered, an index finger can be placed deep to the posterior sheath, and the filmy adhesions attaching the bowel to the back of the abdominal wall can be broken down by gentle sweeping of the index finger around the circumference of the internal opening, combined if necessary with some sharp dissection under direct vision. The bowel, mesentery and any attached omentum must be freed from the abdominal wall for a distance of 2–3 cm from the internal opening.

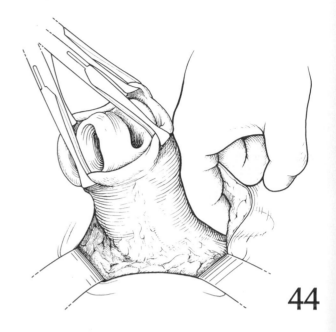

44

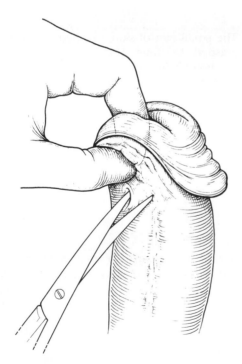

45

Preparation of the bowel for closure

45 The edges of the bowel which had been everted for the ileostomy construction are returned to their normal configuration by dividing the adhesions between the everted and adjacent segments of bowel wall. This is best achieved by scissor dissection against an index finger inserted into the functional end of the bowel, while gentle traction is applied to the rim of skin attached to the edge of the bowel.

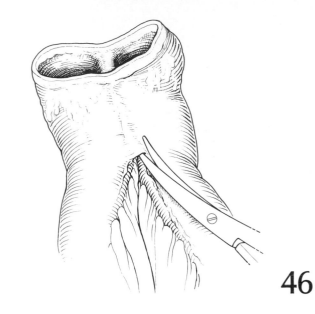

46

46, 47 After mobilization from the abdominal wall, the loops of bowel proximal and distal to the stoma will lie almost parallel to one another, with filmy adhesions maintaining this relationship. These adhesions need to be divided to straighten out the bowel and to prevent postoperative angulation and potential obstruction at the point of closure.

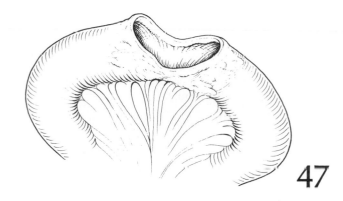

47

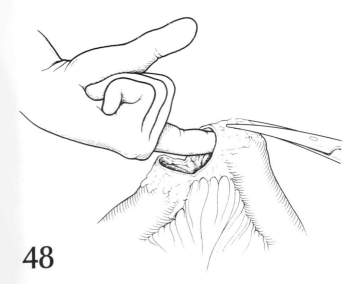

48

48 Any residual subcutaneous fatty tissue or fibrous scar is then excised from the bowel serosa.

49 The attached sliver of skin is trimmed from the bowel edges, leaving a soft, pliable, and freely bleeding bowel edge. It is important to excise all areas of fibrosis and scarring; these areas can often be located by feel more easily than by sight.

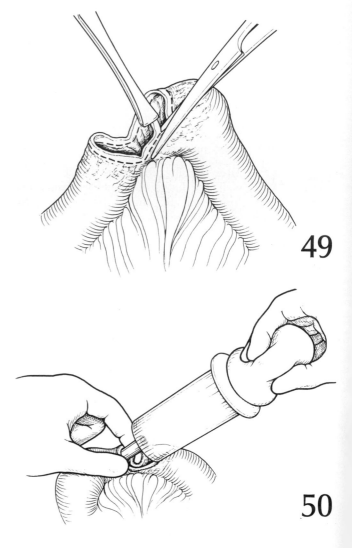

49

50 It is expedient to test each limb of the bowel for an unrecognized enterotomy by the instillation of a weak solution of coloured antiseptic such as povidone-iodine (Betadine).

50

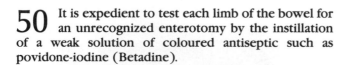

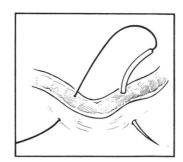

Closure of the bowel defect

51 The defect in the bowel is closed transversely with interrupted absorbable sutures of 3/0 Vicryl or 3/0 chromic catgut. The sutures are inserted through the seromuscular tissues and pass through the groove between the muscle and the submucosa of the bowel, rather than being full thickness. This assures accurate approximation of bowel layers and helps to maintain an inverted suture line.

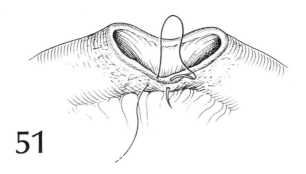

51

52 The initial two stitches are placed at the mesenteric ends of the defect, tied, and tagged to produce gentle lateral retraction. An antimesenteric stitch is then placed halfway between the two lateral stitches, and if there is discrepancy in the length of bowel on either side, intervening 'halfway' sutures can be placed to facilitate accurate bowel closure. These sutures are temporarily left untied and tagged with a small artery clamp.

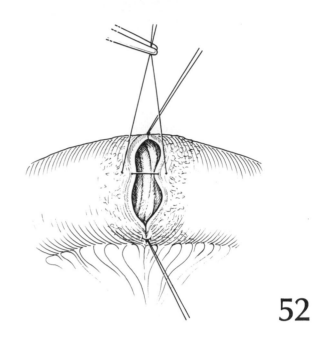

52

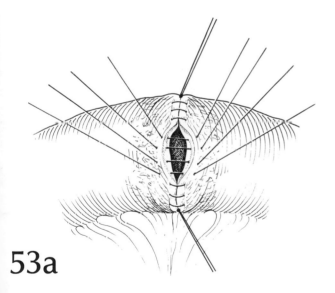

53a

53a, b Sutures are placed and tied from each end; the central four or five are placed and left untied until all have been inserted.

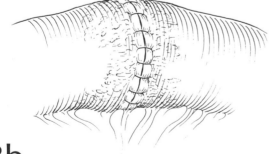

53b

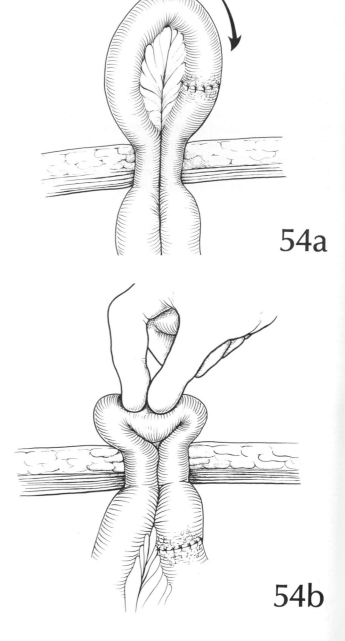

54a, b The closed bowel is irrigated with saline before being replaced into the abdominal cavity, which is best achieved by first replacing the bowel containing the suture line. Careful handling of the sutured bowel and gradual 'milking' of the remaining bowel back into the abdominal cavity using gentle finger compression prevents disruption of the suture line.

Closure of the abdominal defect

55 The defect in the abdominal musculature is closed parallel to the rectus muscle fibres by three or four full thickness sutures of strong absorbable material such as 1 Vicryl, with the knots placed deep to the posterior rectus sheath.

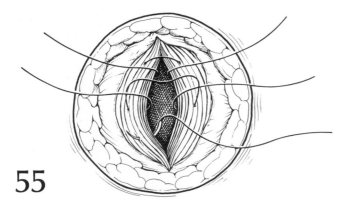

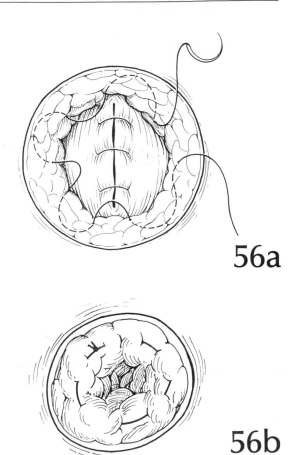

56a

56b

56a, b
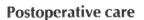
The depth of the subcutaneous wound is reduced by placing a purse-string suture of 2/0 chromic catgut approximately half-way between the fascia and the skin, but tied loosely so as not to distort or pucker the wound. Any residual defect is loosely packed with petrolatum (Vaseline) gauze and heals by secondary intention within several weeks. This produces a small, flat, undistorted scar which can be used again for a stoma site if necessary. Any attempts to primarily close the circular skin defect result in a puckered scar and are not recommended.

Postoperative care

The patient is maintained with postoperative fluids, and oral intake is restricted until bowel function resumes. Nasogastric suction is employed for about 24 h but is not continued routinely unless there are excessive amounts of aspirant. Peroperative antibiotics are not usually continued beyond the first 24 h.

The petrolatum (Vaseline) gauze packing is removed after 3 days, and a non-adherent dressing is applied and changed as necessary until the wound heals. The patient is advised to take a low-residue diet for 6–8 weeks to reduce the chance of a bolus obstruction at the ileostomy closure site where oedema persists for several weeks. Normal diet can be recommended after 8 weeks.

Acknowledgements

Illustrations 2, 3, 5, 8–12, 15–17, 19–22, 24, 26, 28–31, 37, 38, 40–56 have been drawn from roughs prepared by Joseph A. Pangrace at The Cleveland Clinic Foundation.

Tube caecostomy

Robin K. S. Phillips MS, FRCS
Consultant Surgeon, St Mark's Hospital for Diseases of the Rectum and Colon and Homerton Hospital, London, and Honorary Lecturer, St Bartholomew's Hospital Medical School, London, UK

James P. S. Thomson DM, MS, FRCS
Consultant Surgeon and Clinical Director, St Mark's Hospital for Diseases of the Rectum and Colon, London, Honorary Consultant Surgeon, St Mary's Hospital, London, Honorary Lecturer in Surgery, Medical College of St Bartholomew's Hospital, London, Civil Consultant in Surgery, Royal Air Force and Civilian Consultant in Colorectal Surgery, Royal Navy, UK

Principles and justification

Indications

Tube caecostomy procedures are now very uncommon, but can be used to achieve distal bowel gaseous decompression. However, this method does not divert the faecal stream and requires a considerable amount of nursing care to maintain its patency. After on-table colonic irrigation (*see* chapter on pp. 397–416), it is sometimes tempting to leave the irrigating catheter *in situ*, both to decompress the colon and to permit antegrade radiological examination of an anastomosis. However, the quality of such films is poor, and complications have been reported by leaving the tube *in situ*.

Caecostomy may be useful in the management of pseudo-obstruction but other techniques, such as colonoscopic decompression, are now available. Where there is impending caecal rupture, tube caecostomy cannot be relied upon as there may already be full-thickness necrosis of the bowel wall, thus mandating bowel resection.

Preoperative

Caecostomy is usually performed concomitant with another procedure and thus the preparation of the patient will be for the other procedure. When, however, it is used in a patient with a large bowel obstruction, the same efforts to optimize the patient's condition should be taken as for a more extensive procedure.

Anaesthesia

The operation can be performed under local or general anaesthesia depending on the condition of the patient.

Operation

Principles of technique

A large-bore balloon catheter, such as a 30-Fr Foley catheter, is inserted and secured in the caecum with its distal end directed towards the hepatic flexure. The caecum is in turn sutured to the anterior abdominal wall.

It is usual to remove the appendix, as it is theoretically possible for its lumen to be obstructed by the tube. Where the caecum is mobile the removed appendix stump may be a suitable site for the tube, but it is usual to place the tube in the anterior caecal wall to simplify the placement of sutures between the caecum and the anterior abdominal wall.

Caecostomy by mucocutaneous suture should not be undertaken, as the effluent is essentially ileal and without a suitable spout, skin excoriation will develop rapidly. Furthermore, formal closure as opposed to tube removal would then become necessary.

Incision

1 When a tube caecostomy is constructed in association with a colonic anastomosis, a stab incision is made in the right iliac fossa. If caecostomy alone is performed, a small oblique incision some 6 cm in length is made over the caecum.

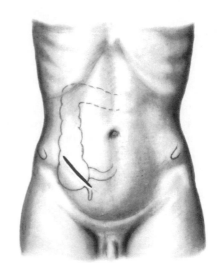

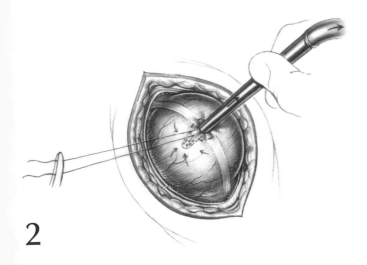

Opening the caecum

2 A purse-string 2/0 suture of soluble material is placed in the caecum at the site of the anterior taenia. If the caecum is grossly distended it may help first to aspirate the gas by puncturing the caecum with a large-bore needle attached to the suction tubing, thus allowing some of the tension to be relieved. This will allow a soft bowel clamp to be placed across a portion of the caecum so that when the caecum is opened and the Foley catheter is introduced there will be no spillage.

Insertion of caecostomy tube

3a, b The Foley catheter is introduced with the drainage end occluded to avoid spillage. The balloon is inflated and the purse-string pulled up against the tube and knotted. The soft bowel clamp can then be removed and suction applied to the Foley catheter if more decompression is required. It may be necessary to place a second purse-string suture at this stage to ensure a watertight fit.

Appendicectomy can then be performed.

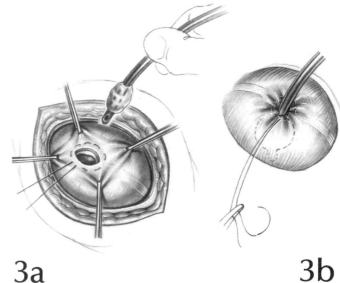

Securing caecum to anterior abdominal wall

4 Four 2/0 sutures of the same material are inserted one after another between the seromuscular layer of the caecum and the anterior abdominal wall. It helps if they are clipped but not tied until all four have been inserted.

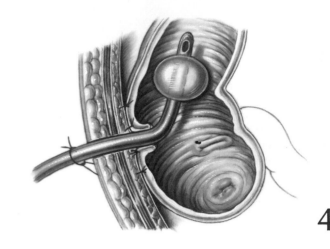

4

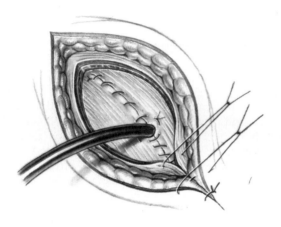

5

Wound closure

5 If an incision in the right iliac fossa has been made, then it should be closed.

Securing tube to anterior abdominal wall

6 The tube is secured primarily by a suture to the anterior abdominal wall. Undue pulling up of the Foley balloon catheter should be avoided as this may cause some ischaemic necrosis of the caecal wall against the anterior abdominal wall. The catheter is then secured to the abdominal wall with adhesive tape and attached to a urine drainage bag to create a closed system.

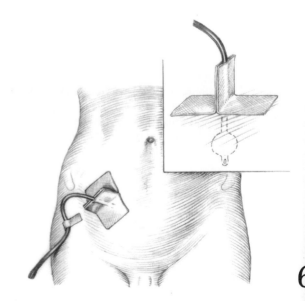

6

Postoperative care

Care of tube

After the first 36 h, the caecostomy tube is washed through every 6 h with 100 ml of physiological saline warmed to body temperature. At least the same volume should then be siphoned from the system. There is a theoretical risk of water intoxication if plain water is used, particularly if larger volumes are employed.

Removal of tube

A fistula between the caecum and anterior abdominal wall should be well established by the seventh postoperative day, depending on the nutritional state of the patient. The securing stitch on the abdominal wall should be removed and the balloon deflated. The catheter can be left to fall free spontaneously, which it usually does by the ninth day. Provided there is no distal obstruction in the bowel, the opening will close. Only very rarely is a formal closure required.

Laxatives

Mineral laxatives may increase faecal fluid, thereby keeping the fistula open; they should therefore be avoided.

Illustrations by Gillian Lee and the late Robert Lane

Colostomy

Robin K. S. Phillips MS, FRCS
Consultant Surgeon, St Mark's Hospital for Diseases of the Rectum and Colon and Homerton Hospital,
London, and Honorary Lecturer, St Bartholomew's Hospital Medical School, London, UK

James P. S. Thomson DM, MS, FRCS
Consultant Surgeon and Clinical Director, St Mark's Hospital for Diseases of the Rectum and Colon, London,
Honorary Consultant Surgeon, St Mary's Hospital, London, Honorary Lecturer in Surgery, Medical College of
St Bartholomew's Hospital, London, Civil Consultant in Surgery, Royal Air Force and Civilian Consultant in
Colorectal Surgery, Royal Navy, UK

Principles and justification

Types of operation and indications

A colostomy diverts faecal flow onto the anterior abdominal wall and may be either temporary or permanent. A temporary stoma is sometimes used in a staged operation in the management of malignant large intestinal obstruction or with certain anal operations. A permanent colostomy is performed in association with operations to excise the rectum and sometimes for patients with idiopathic faecal incontinence.

The four main types of colostomy are:

1. Loop colostomy.
2. Double-barrelled colostomy.
3. Divided colostomy (Devine).
4. Terminal colostomy.

Loop colostomy

This is the most usually formed temporary colostomy. Its site depends on the reason for its construction and may be either in the transverse or in the sigmoid colon. In principle, a loop of colon is brought to the surface, secured by mucocutaneous suture and held in place by a rod until it becomes adherent (usually 5–8 days) when the rod can be removed.

Loop stomas are now less commonly constructed in cases of obstruction or complicated diverticular disease than in the past, as more surgeons embark on immediate intestinal resection in the treatment of these conditions. Thus, the majority of loop stomas are used to defunction

a distal anastomosis, but may be used with certain anal operations (some high anal fistulae or anal sphincter repair, particularly in cases of Crohn's disease).

The advantages of a transverse loop colostomy include its ease of construction and ease of closure. The disadvantages are: its site in the right upper quadrant (though there is nothing to prevent the surgeon from mobilizing the hepatic flexure so that the stoma can be sited in the more convenient right iliac fossa); its tendency to prolapse; and the vulnerability of the marginal artery during closure (and hence of the distal colonic blood supply if the inferior mesenteric artery has previously been ligated at its origin). Because of these disadvantages, some surgeons prefer to construct a loop ileostomy to defunction the distal intestine (as described in the chapter on pp. 627–653).

Double-barrelled colostomy

This is the type of colostomy used in the Paul–Mikulicz operation. A 'spur' is constructed between the two antimesenteric limbs of the colostomy, which can subsequently be divided using a linear cutting stapler. In theory the colostomy should then close spontaneously, but it is usual for a formal closure to be necessary. The operation is becoming obsolete, although it could be used in an unfit patient with a volvulus after resection of the sigmoid colon.

Divided colostomy

This colostomy is constructed in the usual way but with a tongue of skin separating the two limbs of the stoma. Because it is as easy to close the distal limb subcutaneously, and because a conventional loop stoma provides satisfactory bowel defunctioning, a divided colostomy has little place in current surgical practice.

Terminal colostomy

This end stoma is usually constructed in association with operations to excise the rectum (as described in the chapter on pp. 766–781) or Hartmann's operation (as described in the chapter on pp. 798–806). It may be necessary, however, in cases of irremediable faecal incontinence, when the operation can be performed without a laparotomy solely through a trephine incision, taking great care not to inadvertently close the proximal colon and secure the distal limb! The colostomy is formed from the sigmoid colon which is brought out through an incision in the left abdominal wall.

Closure of loop colostomy

A temporary loop colostomy is closed when there is no longer a need to defunction the distal intestine. If a colostomy has been constructed to cover a healing anastomosis, then it is essential that total healing of the anastomosis has occurred before undertaking the colostomy closure. This may partly be assessed endoscopically, when the bowel can also be seen to be healthy and not cyanosed or oedematous, but it is important to perform contrast radiology in addition because tracks may be overlooked with the endoscope. Anteroposterior and lateral films should be taken. Colostomy closure is easiest if undertaken at least 2 months after the original operation, and is most difficult if undertaken in the first month.

Preoperative

Bowel preparation

When circumstances allow, a full bowel preparation is preferable. Many of the conditions, however, for which a loop stoma is constructed are 'urgent' or 'emergency' in nature, which precludes bowel preparation. Perioperative systemic antibiotics are given against aerobic and anaerobic organisms.

Before colostomy closure, the proximal intestine should be prepared in the usual way, but taking into account that there is less intestine to empty. If the distal intestine contains any barium it must be washed out because the barium may solidify and cause intraluminal obstruction. Otherwise, distal loop washouts are unnecessary. The perioperative antibiotic regimen favoured by the surgeon for colonic surgery should be used.

Anaesthesia

General anaesthesia is preferred because traction on the mesentery causes pain and nausea. It is possible, however, to perform these operations under local or regional anaesthesia. Colostomy closure is best performed under general anaesthesia.

Operations

LOOP COLOSTOMY

Incision

1 The sites of incision for a transverse colostomy and a left iliac fossa sigmoid colostomy are shown in *Illustration 1*. The ideal siting for a transverse colostomy is in the right iliac fossa, but the hepatic flexure must be mobilized in order to achieve this. If a transverse colostomy is to be performed, for example, as the first stage of a staged colonic resection, then the incision (usually 6 cm) must be in the right upper abdomen, midway between the umbilicus and the costal margin, and placed over the rectus abdominis muscle but extending just lateral to its lateral margin.

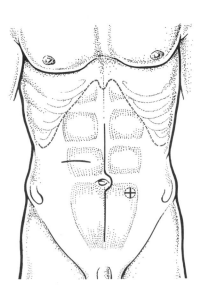

1

2 The incision is deepened through the anterior rectus sheath. The rectus abdominis may either be divided or split in the line of its fibres, and then the abdomen is opened.

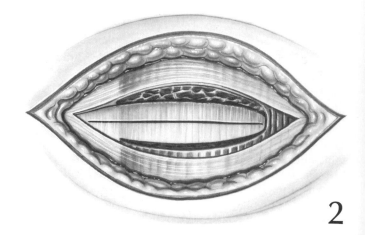

2

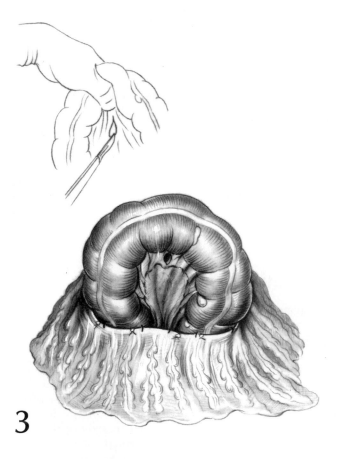

3

Preparation of the colon

3 A transverse colostomy may be prepared either by making a window in the omentum or by lifting the free edge of the omentum upwards and dissecting the intact omentum from its largely avascular attachment to the colon. A nylon tape is passed through the mesentery in order to draw the colon up to the surface where the tape is substituted with a plastic rod.

Opening the colostomy

4 The colon may be opened longitudinally or transversely. A transverse incision damages fewer of the encircling vessels in the colonic wall, is easier to secure and probably easier to close.

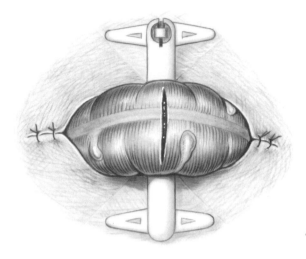

4

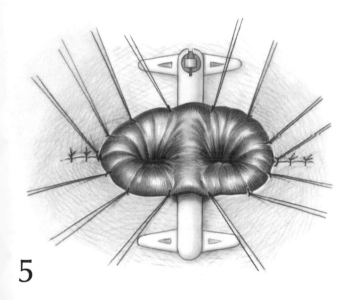

5

Mucocutaneous suture

5 Once open, the colostomy is sutured to the skin with interrupted sutures of 2/0 or 3/0 absorbable material mounted on a taper-cut needle, which penetrate the entire thickness of the intestinal wall but which pass through the subcuticular layer of the skin. The wound is cleaned and a stoma appliance is fitted immediately.

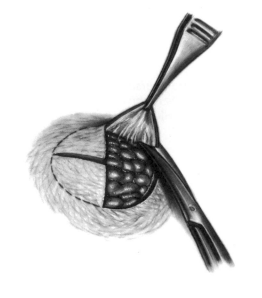

6a

TERMINAL COLOSTOMY

Incision

6a, b The exact site should be marked before the operation to ensure that an appliance will fit satisfactorily away from the umbilicus and the anterior superior iliac spine. A disc of skin approximately 2 cm in diameter is excised. This can be done most accurately using a cruciate incision and excising the four pieces of skin to complete the circle. The alternative of picking up a piece of skin and slicing it off with a knife results in a wound that is oval rather than round and which has edges that in places are only a partial thickness depth. When a laparotomy is also to be performed, a more satisfactory trephine incision is obtained when it is made before the main laparotomy incision.

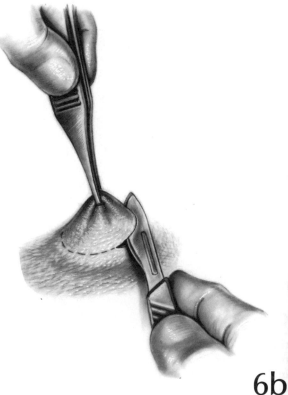

6b

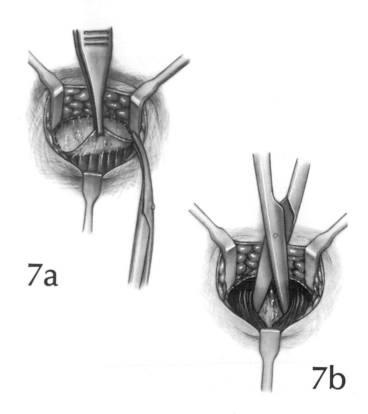

7a, b A cylinder of superficial fascia is removed, taking care to obtain good haemostasis. The dissection through the abdominal wall is aided by three equidistantly placed Langenbeck's or phrenic retractors. A disc of anterior rectus sheath is next removed, the rectus muscle is split, and the abdomen is carefully entered.

7a

7b

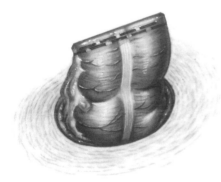

8

Delivery of colon through abdominal wall

8 The colon is delivered through the anterior abdominal wall. If it remains totally intraperitoneal, it is desirable for the space between the mesocolon and the abdominal wall (the lateral space) to be closed using non-absorbable sutures. This prevents the possible complication of internal herniation of the small intestine. Alternatively, the colon may be brought to the surface extraperitoneally.

Mucocutaneous suture

9 Before the main abdominal incision is closed, it is important to ensure, by adequate mobilization of the colon, that there will be no tension on the mucocutaneous suture line. Once the main abdominal incision has been sutured and dressed, the clamp on the distal colon is removed and a mucocutaneous suture is performed with 3/0 absorbable sutures placed into the dermal layer and through the muscularis serosal layers, avoiding mucosal penetration.

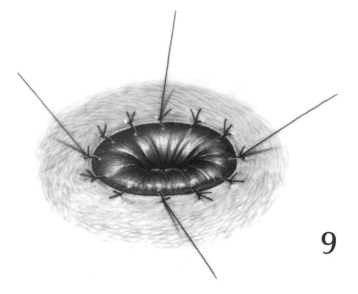

9

CLOSURE OF LOOP COLOSTOMY

A loop colostomy may be closed using one of two techniques:

1. Simple closure: after mobilization of the colon the opening is sutured (half-anastomosis).
2. Excision of the colostomy and anastomosis: the site of the colostomy is excised and the continuity of the colon is restored by end-to-end anastomosis.

In both these instances, the operation is conducted so that the colon is returned to within the peritoneal cavity. So-called extraperitoneal closure of the colostomy is seldom performed and is unsatisfactory because inadequate mobilization has been performed and the anastomosis is almost always under tension.

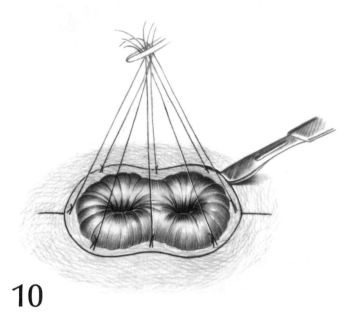

10

Mobilization of the colostomy

10 Between four and eight strong silk sutures are placed around the mucocutaneous junction of the colostomy allowing good control of the colon during mobilization. The incision is made around the edge of the colostomy taking a small fringe of skin approximately 2 mm wide. If necessary, the incision may be enlarged at either end of the colostomy in the transverse plane.

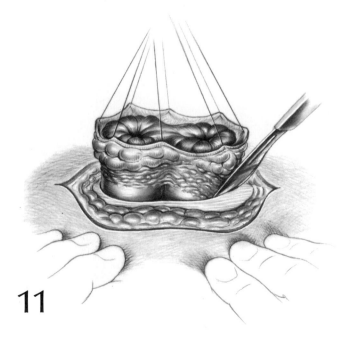

11

11 With traction applied to the colostomy using the stay sutures, the tissues of the anterior wall are freed from the colon. Great care must be exercised to remain in the correct plane and avoid damage to the colon. There is usually little blood loss during this procedure. If haemorrhage does occur, this suggests the surgeon is in the wrong plane.

Removal of the skin edge and unrolling of the colostomy edge

12 The rind of skin is removed and the edge of the colostomy is unrolled. Palpation of the proposed anastomotic edge between finger and thumb confirms when the unrolling is complete, and the colon is then ready for closure.

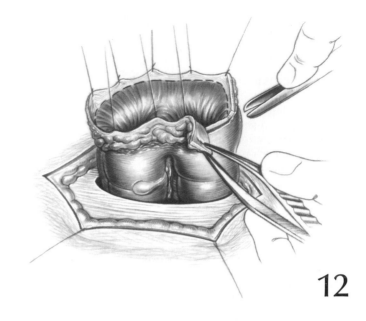

12

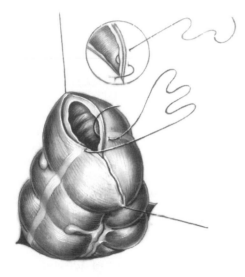

13a

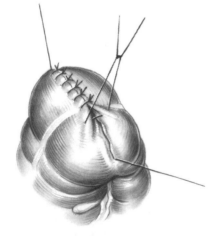

13b

Simple closure of the colon

13a, b This may be achieved in any way with which the surgeon is familiar (as described in the chapter on pp. 528–550): two-layer (usually a continuous inner absorbable suture and an outer interrupted non-absorbable layer); one-layer (usually an interrupted serosubmucosal stitch of either absorbable or non-absorbable material); or with the stapler (usually a functional end-to-end anastomosis; described in the chapter on pp. 551–560).

Wound closure

14 A single layer of strong monofilament absorbable or non-absorbable sutures is inserted into all layers, taking large bites on either side of the wound. After all sutures have been placed they are then tied so that the edges of the abdominal wall are closely, but not tightly, approximated. The skin wound is closed, and if haemostasis is in any way in doubt a wound drain is employed.

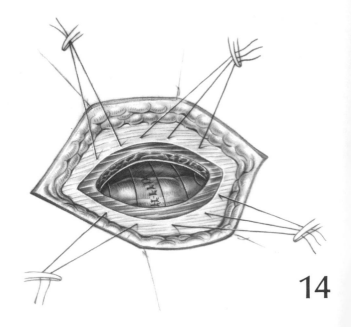

14

Postoperative

General management

The general care of the patient will be largely determined by the indication for performing the colostomy. It is wise to maintain intravenous fluids until the patient has at least passed flatus.

It is important to check the viability of the intestine in the early postoperative period and also to make sure that it has not retracted.

It is unusual for the patient to require a nasogastric tube after colostomy closure. Intravenous fluids are maintained until flatus is passed and then a diet is gradually reintroduced.

Care of the colostomy

It is usual to fit an appliance as soon as the colostomy has been constructed. As the effluent from a transverse loop colostomy may be somewhat liquid, codeine phosphate, loperamide, or other constipating agents may be useful.

With a terminal colostomy, particularly in a younger and motivated patient, there is much to recommend colostomy irrigation for long-term management, after the patient has completely recovered from surgery.

Complications of colostomy

Delayed complications are described in the chapter on pp. 292–306.

Loss of viability

This will occur early in the postoperative course if the blood supply to the colostomy has been compromised.

It necessitates reconstruction of the colostomy with viable colon. On occasion, however, only the last 1–2 cm of mucosa are ischaemic. As this will heal without intervention, it pays to examine the terminal few centimetres of the intestine endoscopically before deciding on revision.

Separation of the colostomy

This is usually the result of tension at the mucocutaneous junction, and if this occurs circumferentially the colostomy will need to be re-established. Partial separation may also be caused by tension or infection. It will usually heal spontaneously provided that less than half the circumference is involved.

Infection

Although surgery is performed in a potentially septic field, it is very rare for sepsis to complicate the construction of a colostomy. This does occasionally happen, however, with surrounding cellulitis, and there may be some separation of the edge of the colostomy. A haematoma surrounding the colostomy may be a predisposing factor, which emphasizes the importance of good haemostasis in the colostomy wound. Provided that there is adequate drainage, the colostomy will heal but subsequent scarring might lead to some stenosis at the mucocutaneous junction.

Complications of colostomy closure

Wound infection

This is usually avoided if perioperative antibiotics have been employed and there has been no wound haematoma.

Wound hernia

Hernias do occur in these wounds, and occasionally they are complicated by strangulation.

Breakdown of the colonic suture line

This either results in a faecal fistula, which usually closes spontaneously, or peritonitis, which will require the colostomy to be re-established

Distal anastomosis abscess

If the colostomy is closed before satisfactory healing of the anastomosis has occurred, an abscess may develop at this site. This may also necessitate re-establishment of the colostomy. If the proper indications for performing colostomy closure have been observed, however, this complication should not occur.

Illustrations by Peter Cox

Complications of ileostomy and colostomy

Hasse Jiborn MD, PhD
Associate Professor, Department of Surgery, Malmö General Hospital, University of Lund, Malmö, Sweden

Göran R. Ekelund MD, PhD
Associate Professor and Chairman, Department of Surgery, Malmö General Hospital, University of Lund, Malmö, Sweden

General technical considerations

Surgery for stoma complications requires an atraumatic technique to avoid damaging the intestinal wall so that it can be used for reconstruction; accidental perforation might result in fistula formation. The skin around the stoma should be incised with a knife or diathermy (preferably with a needle tip) and the stoma mobilized using careful dissection by needle tip diathermy or by a fine pair of scissors; mobilization is best achieved when tissues are under some tension. For good results even these 'minor' operations should be performed only when adequate assistance is available.

1 To get good access for this 'keyhole' surgery appropriate retractors should be used, such as the Löfberg's type which was originally developed for surgery of the thyroid gland.

If the stoma site is going to be reused and the original size is appropriate, the skin should be incised immediately (about 1 mm) outside the mucocutaneous junction in order not to create too large a skin opening. If additional incisions are needed for access, care must be taken to obtain perfect alignment of the subcutaneous tissue and the skin to produce a smooth scar, which is essential for safe function of the appliance.

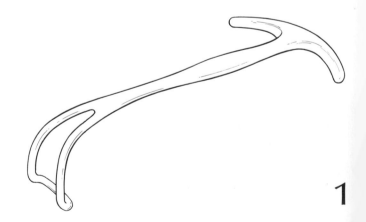

1

Suture material

The following suture materials are recommended:

Peritoneum and intestinal wall: 3/0 synthetic absorbable braided (e.g. Dexon, Vicryl) or monofilament (e.g. Maxon, PDS).

Fascia closure: 2/0 synthetic absorbable monofilament (e.g. Maxon, PDS) or braided (e.g. Dexon, Vicryl).

Mucocutaneous suture: 4/0 non-absorbable monofilament (e.g. Novafil, Prolene, Ethilon) or 3/0 synthetic absorbable braided (e.g. Dexon, Vicryl).

Skin suture: 3/0 non-absorbable monofilament.

Absorbable monofilaments may be preferred to braided sutures for parastomal hernia repair because they are less likely to maintain infection and they retain their strength longer than braided sutures. Non-absorbable suture material should be used only for deep sutures to secure any mesh grafts in repair of parastomal hernia.

Complications of ileostomy

Ileostomy complications are common. Most can be managed by experienced stoma care, but 30–40% require surgical revision[1,2]. The most frequent complications are obstruction, recession and prolapse; less common are parastomal hernias, fistulae, ulcerations and granulomas.

Obstruction

Obstruction may be caused by stenosis developing at skin and/or fascial levels. A food bolus is often the immediate cause of overt obstruction and this is usually managed by irrigation with 100 ml warm saline through a Foley catheter gently introduced into the stoma.

Intra-abdominal adhesion is another cause of obstruction. Recurrent disease must be considered in patients with Crohn's disease.

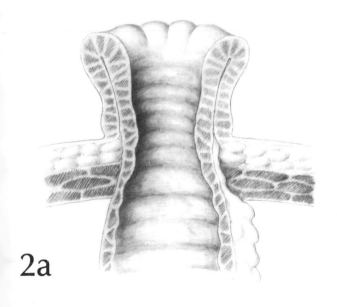

2a

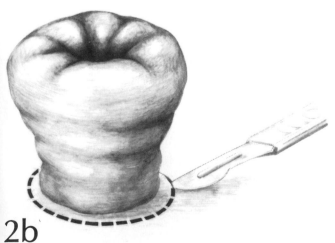

2b

Stenosis

Stenosis of the stoma can be managed by local repair.

2a, b The skin is incised around the stoma immediately outside the strictured zone; this should create a 2–3-cm wide (two-finger wide) opening in the skin. Care should be taken not to create a larger opening.

3a, b

The stoma is straightened, mobilized in the subcutaneous plane and the eversion reduced. The distal part of the ileum with the stricturing scar tissue is then excised.

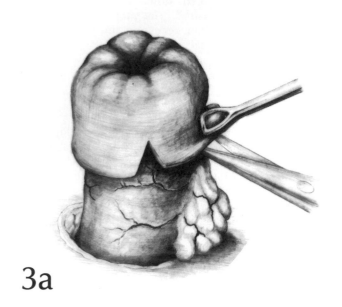

3a

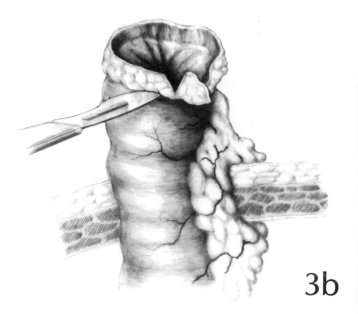

3b

4a, b

The stoma is explored with a finger for any additional stricture at the fascial plane; if such a stricture is discovered, dissection is continued beyond the fascia. Part of the junction between ileum and fascia is opened and the fascia incised to create an adequate opening (not too large because of the risk of herniation).

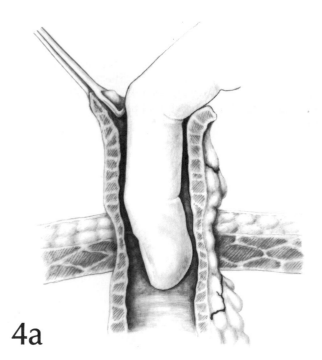

4a

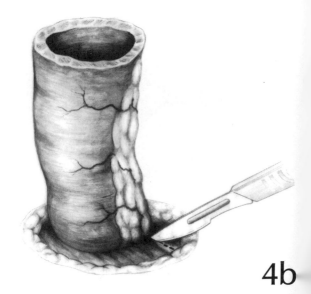

4b

5 The ileum is again everted and sutured to the skin with 4/0 non-absorbable monofilament: skin to seromuscular in the proximal limb at the skin plane; full thickness for the end of the ileum. The surgeon should be careful not to penetrate the bowel wall with the *seromuscular* bite because of the risk of fistula formation.

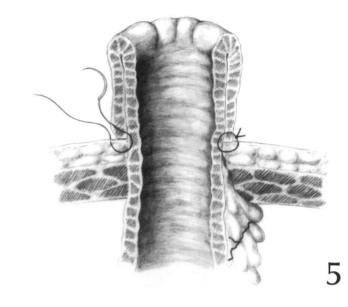

5

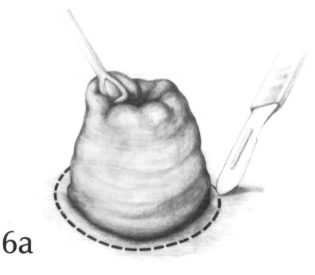

6a

Recession

Recession results from either too large an abdominal opening or inadequate fixation of the ileum at the fascial plane. Recession often occurs at night when the patient is lying down and may result in leakage because of impaired fitting of the appliance.

Local repair of stoma

6a, b The stoma is detached at the muco-cutaneous junction, straightened, the eversion reduced and mobilized down into the peritoneal cavity to gain extra length.

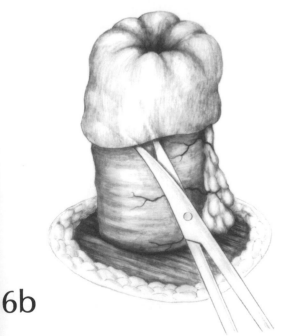

6b

7a, b The stoma is sutured to the peritoneum circumferentially with interrupted 3/0 absorbable sutures with seromuscular bites. If the opening in the fascia is too large, one or two interrupted sutures are placed in the aponeurosis to obtain an appropriate narrowing using 2/0 absorbable monofilament or braided sutures. The length of the ileum projecting outside the skin level should be 6–8 cm (if too long, the excess should be resected).

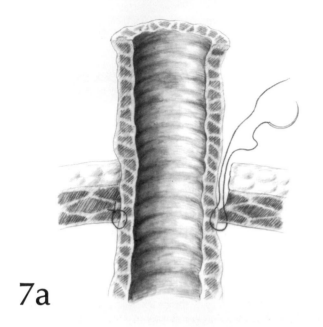

7a

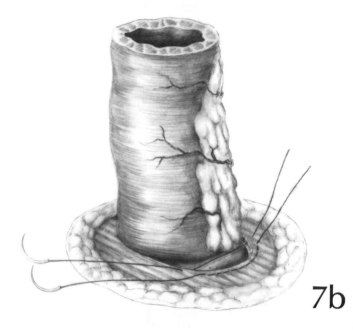

7b

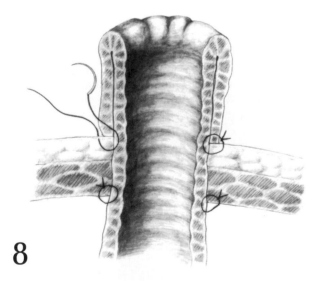

8

8 The ileum is everted and the mucocutaneous junction is re-established.

9a, b Too large a skin opening may be reduced by the Mercedes manoeuvre[3]. Two or three triangular skin excisions (with acute angles and the bases placed centrally) are made around the stoma and closed by non-absorbable monofilament sutures.

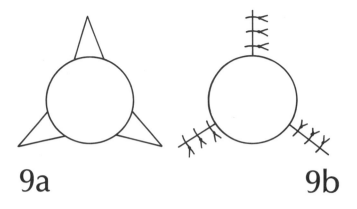

9a

9b

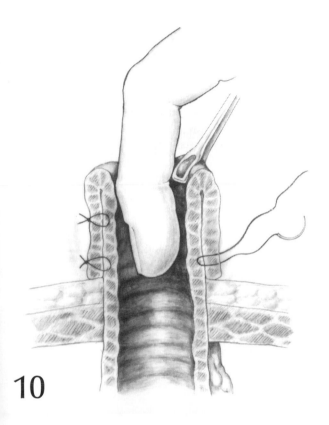

10

Local fixation of stoma with repair

Local fixation can often be achieved without detachment of the stoma.

10 The stoma is everted by grasping it with a pair of Babcock's forceps introduced into the stoma. The index finger is inserted into the stoma and interrupted 3/0 absorbable sutures are placed through the full thickness of the outer intestinal wall and the seromuscular layer of the inner wall, guided by the index finger to avoid penetration of mucosa in the inner layer and to lessen the risk of fistula formation.

11 Another method of fixation is to use the GIA stapler *without* the blade instead of sutures. The retracted ileostomy is pulled out to a length of about 4 cm by inserting three pairs of Babcock's forceps 120° apart, one at the mesenteric region. The GIA stapler *without* the blade is placed towards the mucocutaneous junction between the forceps and fired. Three parallel rows of staples are created. Care should be taken to avoid placing the instrument over the mesentery since this may cause necrosis of the ileostomy. The stoma, even with correct placement of staples, is unsightly for about 6 weeks but gradually returns to a more normal appearance[4].

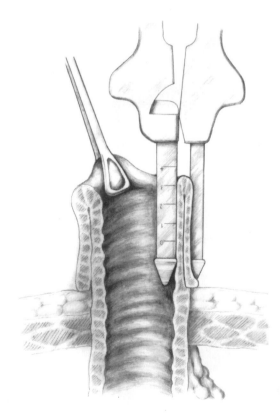

11

Retraction

Retraction (or fixed recession) is often caused by insufficient intestine being used for the construction of the stoma. By dissecting the stoma to the peritoneal level, sufficient intestinal length can often be mobilized to reconstruct the stoma with adequate length (2–4 cm). For operative technique, *see* section on Recession, page 671.

Recurrent Crohn's disease should be suspected when retraction develops and if this is in fact the case the problem should be managed accordingly, usually by radiological examination, endoscopy followed by laparotomy, resection and construction of a new stoma.

Prolapse

12a–c The same operative technique can be used as described for recession, i.e. reduction of the eversion and mobilization of the stoma to the fascial plane. The base of the stoma is secured to the peritoneum (fascia) by interrupted seromuscular sutures, after which the abundant ileum is resected. The stoma is reconstructed with mucocutaneous sutures.

If the mesentery has been completely detached and an excessive length of ileum can be pulled out of the stoma site, laparotomy may sometimes be necessary to reattach it to the peritoneum using interrupted absorbable sutures. The stoma should then be reconstructed (*see* chapter on pp. 627–653).

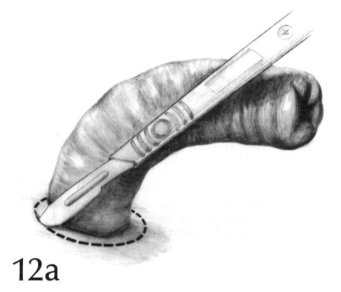

12a

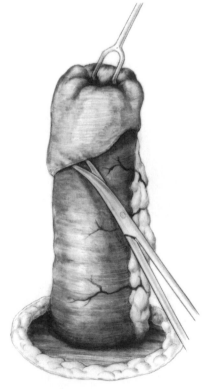

12b

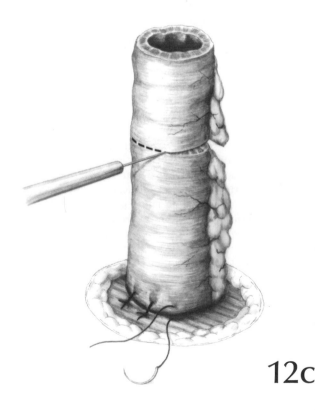

12c

Excessive length of stoma

A stoma which is too long is usually caused by misjudgement at the time of construction. The ileum should be detached at the mucocutaneous junction, eversion of the stoma reduced, amputated to the appropriate length, and resutured mucocutaneously (*see* section on Prolapse, page 674).

Parastomal hernia

Parastomal hernia is relatively rare in connection with ileostomy.

Local repair

13a, b The stoma is detached from the mucocutaneous junction and the ileum is mobilized to the fascial level. If access is necessary, a transverse 'help' incision may be made in the skin and subcutaneous tissue.

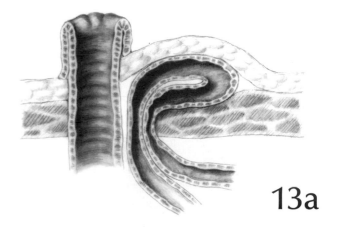

13a

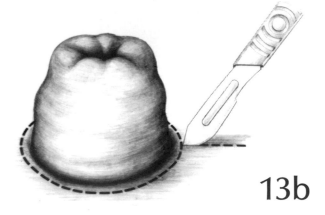

13b

14a–c The hernial sac is dissected free and excised. The aponeurosal defect is closed by interrupted 2/0 absorbable sutures through all layers, including the peritoneum, leaving an adequate opening for the ileostomy. This should be checked by the index finger in the stoma. The stoma is refashioned (*see* section on Recession, page 671). If a 'help' incision has been performed this is closed with interrupted subcutaneous sutures and skin sutures. Care must be taken to create a smooth scar.

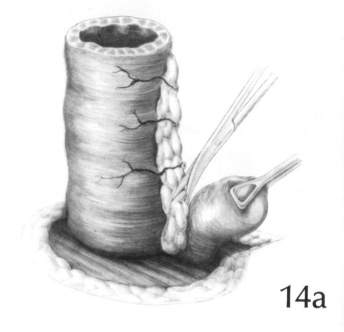

14a

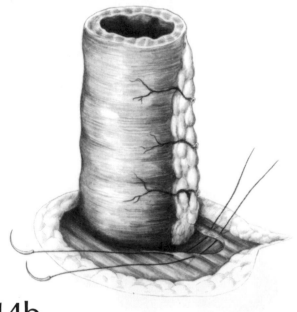

14b

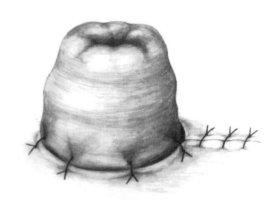

14c

Resiting of the stoma

In case of hernial recurrence the stoma may be resited by laparotomy. Before bringing the patient to surgery it must be ensured that the new stoma site has been selected appropriately (usually in the opposite lower quadrant), if possible with the aid of a stoma care nurse, and has been marked.

The stoma is detached at the mucocutaneous junction and dissected free down to the peritoneum. The stoma is dissected and closed at the end by staples or a running suture. Laparotomy is performed through a low midline incision (usually through the old incisional scar), the distal ileum and mesentery are detached and mobilized to fit the new stomal position.

Parastomal fistula

Fistulae may occur from trauma caused by pressure of the appliance flange and are thus located at skin level. Deeper fistulae usually arise from non-absorbable sutures having been placed too deep or too firmly in the bowel wall, and these fistulae usually originate at the fascial level. Recurrent disease must always be considered in patients with Crohn's disease and managed accordingly.

Preoperative assessment

The fistulous tract is assessed by a probe to search for the inner opening but probing must be performed with great care to avoid making false openings. Fistulography, enterography and ileoscopy are of value in locating fistulae and in the search for recurrent Crohn's disease.

Operative technique

Fistulae at the skin level may heal spontaneously after appliance correction.

Deeper fistulae require laparotomy, ileal resection and stomal reconstruction. If peristomal tissues in the bowel wall are not destroyed by the fistula and there is no gross infection, the stoma may be reconstructed at the original site, otherwise the stoma must be resited.

Ulceration

Peristomal ulceration is often due to recurrent Crohn's disease. If ulcerations are not accompanied by local recurrence in the ileum requiring resection, they usually heal if overhanging skin is excised and the ulcer is thoroughly curetted.

Granuloma

Granulomas in the stoma base are often caused by mechanical pressure by the appliance, which should be corrected if possible. Excision and cauterization are usually followed by recurrence. Granulomas may be an indication of fistula, which should be treated accordingly.

Complications of colostomy

Complications are also common with colostomies and have been reported in up to 50% of patients. Colostomy complications may occur early in the postoperative course (such as stomal necrosis) or may develop many years after operation (such as paracolostomy hernia[5]).

Necrosis

If necrosis of the stoma occurs, it appears early after operation. The disturbed mesenteric circulation, which is the cause of stomal necrosis, may be the result of too extensive mesenteric dissection, stretching of the colon in order to reach the abdominal wall or, sometimes, entrapment of the mesentery in the abdominal wall opening. Stoma necrosis is most common in obese patients and after emergency surgery with bowel distension.

15 Necrosis results in mucocutaneous separation of part of, or the entire, circumference of the stoma. The extent of mucosal necrosis is often not obvious but must be discovered. It can be judged using a glass test tube inserted gently into the stoma, illuminated with a torch. The mucosa is visible through the test tube and its condition can be judged[6]. If only partial and superficial necrosis is observed (well distal to the fascial plane) conservative treatment with repeated observations may be employed. If deep necrosis or total separation and retraction of the stoma has occurred, laparotomy with further mobilization of the colon must be performed and a new stoma established.

Stricture and retraction

Partial necrosis and mucocutaneous separation, if managed conservatively, often results in stricture formation and stomal retraction. A stricture and retraction of a colostomy should be managed surgically similar to that described for ileostomy complications.

Prolapse

Prolapse is most common in loop transverse colostomies and less common with end colostomies.

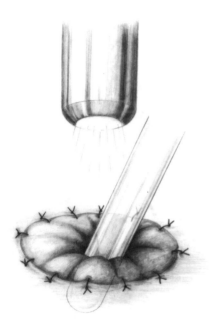

15

Loop transverse colostomy

Construction of a loop transverse colostomy should be avoided because of its significant complications and problems of management. Other methods should be considered, such as primary resection with or without a covering loop ileostomy (*see* chapter on pp. 727–745).

If, however, the prolapse of a loop transverse colostomy presents, conservative treatment can be used if the stoma is temporary and early further surgery considered. If the stoma is to be permanent, the transverse colostomy may be divided and transformed into a terminal end colostomy and a distal mucocutaneous fistula.

16a, b The stoma is detached at the mucocutaneous junction and mobilized to the peritoneum. The colon is transected at the stoma region and the distal part of the mesentery divided to allow separation of the two bowel ends. Any redundant colon is resected. The distal end is brought out as a mucocutaneous fistula via a separate stab incision to the left of the midline and secured to the skin by mucocutaneous sutures using 4/0 non-absorbable monofilament.

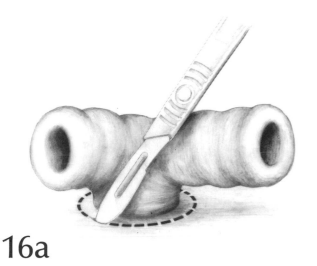

16a

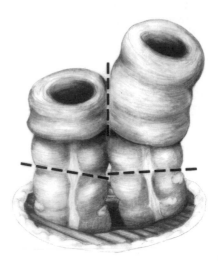

16b

17a, b The proximal terminal colon is secured to the peritoneum by interrupted 3/0 absorbable sutures with seromuscular bites in the colon. If the fascia opening is too large it can be narrowed by one or two interrupted 2/0 absorbable sutures. The stoma is reconstructed by mucocutaneous sutures.

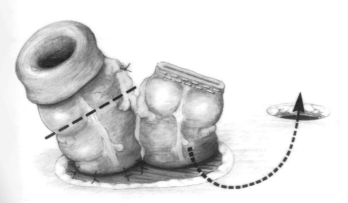

17a

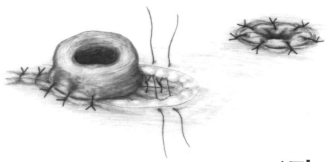

17b

End colostomy: local repair

18a–d
A similar procedure as for ileal prolapse is employed. The stoma is detached at the mucocutaneous junction and dissected to the peritoneal cavity.

The redundant colon is pulled out. The mesentery and the colon are secured to the peritoneum by interrupted 3/0 absorbable sutures. The excess colon is resected 1–2 cm above the skin level and sutured to the skin.

End colostomy: resiting of stoma

If the prolapse is recurrent or is combined with a hernia, laparotomy and resiting of the stoma must be considered. The same technique as has been described for resiting of an ileostomy may be employed (page 677).

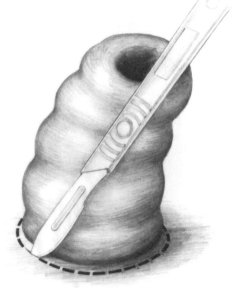

18a

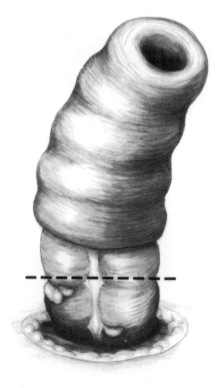

18b

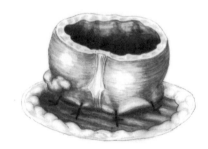

18c

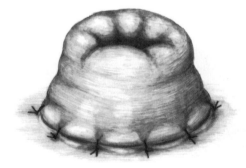

18d

Parastomal hernia

Some degree of parastomal hernia is common with end colostomies. Most should be managed conservatively with special care of appliances and girdles, because they are harmless to the patient, and the results of surgery are disappointing, with a high incidence of recurrence.

If the hernia is very discomforting (for example, it interferes with the wearing of an applicance, with irrigation of the colon, or causes unacceptable cosmetic problems), surgical correction must be considered. Symptoms are often aggravated if the hernia is combined with other complications such as stenosis or prolapse. Bowel strangulation may occur in a parastomal hernia but is rare and requires urgent surgery.

Two surgical options are available, local repair (with or without support of a synthetic mesh) and resiting of the stoma with closure of the abdominal defect at the original stoma site. Resiting of the stoma is often advocated, because local repair is accompanied by a high recurrence rate.

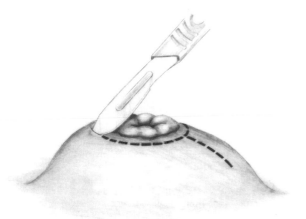

19

Local repair

19 The skin is incised circumstomally about 1 mm outside the mucocutaneous junction and then the stoma is dissected down to the fascia.

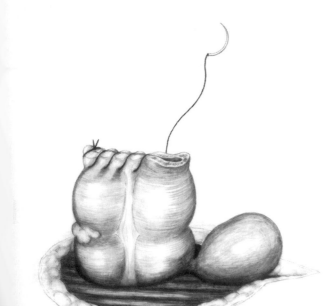

20

20 The stoma is closed by a running suture (e.g. non-absorbable monofilament). The hernia is identified and dissected to the peritoneal plane. A lateral transverse skin incision is often needed to expose the area.

21 The hernial sac is excised and the edges of peritoneum grasped with clamps. The stoma is now secured to the peritoneum by interrupted 3/0 absorbable sutures with seromuscular bites. The aponeurosal defect is closed by interrupted sutures through all layers, including peritoneum, using 2/0 absorbable monofilament leaving an adequate opening for the stoma. The transverse 'help' incision is closed by interrupted absorbable sutures in the subcutaneous layer and non-absorbable monofilament skin sutures (care must be taken to create a smooth scar). The distal margin of the stoma is resected and the mucocutaneous junction is restored (*see* section on Prolapse, page 674).

If necessary the aponeurosis may be reinforced by a sheet of synthetic mesh (e.g. Marlex, Gore-tex) sutured to the fascia with interrupted non-absorbable monofilament sutures. A more extensive method, raising a large skin flap and reinforcing the entire aponeurosal area surrounding the stoma, is described by Leslie[7].

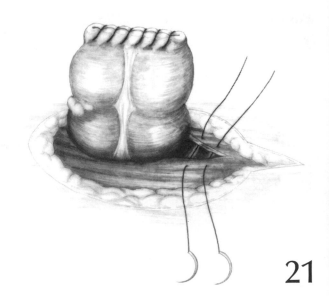

21

Resiting of stoma

The stoma and hernia are mobilized as above. Laparotomy is performed through a midline incision. The stoma is completely disconnected from its original site. The abdominal defect at the original stoma site is repaired in a routine fashion (the peritoneum is closed by a continuous 2/0 absorbable suture, the fascia by interrupted 2/0 absorbable sutures and the subcutaneous tissue and skin are left for secondary healing). The colon is mobilized to fit the new stoma site, the location of which must be carefully chosen before surgery. For details of the stoma construction, *see* chapter on pp. 658–667.

References

1. Carlstedt A, Fasth S, Hultén L, Nordgren S, Palselius I. Long-term ileostomy complications in patients with ulcerative colitis and Crohn's disease. *Int J Colorectal Dis* 1987; 2: 22–5.

2. Weaver RM, Alexander-Williams J, Keighley MRB. Indications and outcome of reoperation for ileostomy complications in inflammatory bowel disease. *Int J Colorectal Dis* 1988; 3: 38–42.

3. Todd IP. Mechanical complications of ileostomy. *Clin Gastroenterol* 1982; 11: 268–73.

4. Winslet MC, Alexander-Williams J, Keighley MRB. Ileostomy revision with a GIA stapler under intravenous sedation. *Br J Surg* 1990; 77: 647.

5. Allen-Mersh TG, Thomson JPS. Surgical treatment of colostomy complications. *Br J Surg* 1988; 75: 416–18.

6. Ekelund G, Hagenfeldt I. Postoperative control of newly established enterostomas. *Coloproctology* 1980; 2: 404–5.

7. Leslie D. The parastomal hernia. *Surg Clin North Am* 1984; 64: 407–15.

Resection of the small intestine for inflammatory bowel disease

Olle Bernell MD
General Surgeon, Department of Surgery, Huddinge University Hospital, Huddinge, Sweden

Göran Hellers MD, PhD
Chairman, Department of Surgery, Huddinge University Hospital, Huddinge, Sweden

Principles and justification

In most cases, small intestinal resection is an emergency procedure that is carried out in patients with intestinal obstruction, or less commonly, in patients with a vascular catastrophe or to remove a tumour. In such cases, neither the indications for, nor the technique of, intestinal resection pose any substantial problems. It is usually quite simple to identify the correct level for intestinal resection and to create a 'routine' end-to-end anastomosis (as described in the chapter on pp. 528–550).

In contrast, in patients with inflammatory bowel disease, the problems are different. The fate of the anastomosis is affected by the indications and the timing of surgery, and it is also more difficult to decide on the correct level for the resection.

In managing the intestinal lesion in Crohn's disease, it is therefore important to consider both the strategy and the tactics of the surgical approach. The most important strategic decision for an individual patient is to decide how soon into a period of medical therapy surgery might be undertaken. Surgery might be advised early in the natural history before serious complications arise in patients who are not doing well on medical therapy, e.g. those who require high doses or chronic use of steroids. In contrast, the surgical approach might be very conservative with surgery postponed until complications arise.

Once surgery is undertaken, the length of intestine affected by Crohn's disease, and therefore the amount to be resected, will have an impact on the likelihood of postoperative short bowel syndrome. Furthermore, the surgical plan must recognize that it is likely that patients with Crohn's disease will require a series of operations during the overall natural history of the condition. Thus, considerable clinical judgement is required to decide on the length of intestine to be resected in an individual patient.

From the tactical point of view, the timing of surgery and the preoperative and perioperative management of each operative procedure must be considered carefully. The aim here is to achieve safe anastomotic healing and to reduce the risk of immediate and late surgical complications.

Indications

Surgery for small intestinal Crohn's disease is performed either to achieve remission or to alleviate the symptoms of obstruction and/or septic complications. Surgery to achieve remission is carried out in patients who have active disease and in whom the symptoms cannot be controlled by medical treatment. Such patients are often malnourished and have a low serum albumin concentration because of the protein-losing enteropathy caused by the inflammatory process. These patients are often febrile (from local perforation and abscess formation) and have enteroenteric or enterocutaneous fistulae or extraintestinal manifestations of Crohn's disease, e.g. arthritis, ankylosing spondylitis or pyoderma gangrenosum. In addition, some patients may have small intestinal bacterial overgrowth caused by chronic intestinal obstruction, as well as intermittent colicky abdominal pain associated with this problem.

Preoperative

In patients with very active disease, it is often wise to postpone surgery for a few days to correct fluid and electrolyte imbalance. It is also advantageous to try to control the activity of the intestinal inflammation with short-term, perioperative, high-dose steroids. Small intestinal bacterial overgrowth should, if possible, be eliminated by nasoenteric intubation of the upper small intestine and direct administration of antibiotics. These antibiotics can be given both enterally and systemically using agents active against aerobes and anaerobic bacteria (as described in the chapter on pp. 522–527). Formal bowel preparation is advisable if there is a risk of fistulae into the large intestine or if there may be Crohn's disease of the large intestine which will require removal. In the absence of these possibilities, mechanical bowel preparation is unnecessary, and a few days on a liquid diet is sufficient. Perioperative steroid cover to prevent steroid crisis and subcutaneous mini-dose heparin to mitigate the risks of deep venous thrombosis and thromboembolic problems should be given.

Anaesthesia

Patients should be operated on under general anaesthesia supplemented by muscle relaxants. Continuous epidural block can be used for postoperative pain relief.

Operation

Extent of resection

Over the past two decades, there has been a major discussion about the possible benefits of extensive compared with conservative intestinal resection in Crohn's disease, and also about the use of frozen sections at the margins of resection to help to determine the extent of resection. It is now clear that extensive resection does not reduce the risk of recurrent inflammatory bowel disease in the residual small intestine. In addition, frozen sections have not been shown to be of value in deciding on the extent of resection, because in macroscopically normal intestine, which can be used for anastomosis, there are often histological features of Crohn's disease.

Thus, the selection of the site for intestinal resection rests with the judgement of the individual surgeon. It is recognized that surgeons should be 'conservative' in the amount of intestine resected because of the risk of recurrent disease requiring further resection, and also because some proximal intestinal thickening is secondary to obstruction rather than the ulcerative process *per se*.

Surgeons are advised to carry out a very limited resection and then immediately to open the specimen. If there is no major mucosal disease close to the resection margin, an anastomosis can be fashioned even if one or both ends of the remaining intestine is thickened. On the other hand, if the mucosal surface is severely ulcerated, an additional section of intestine can be removed.

In patients without obstructive disease, the intestinal wall is often much less oedematous, and the resection can be performed very close to the obvious Crohn's lesion. There is no reason to carry out a wedge resection of the mesentery associated with the intestine to be resected. The mesentery should simply be trimmed so that it can be easily closed.

Incision

In patients with inflammatory bowel disease, a midline incision should always be used, despite the greater risk of postoperative hernia formation, so that sites for stomas are not compromised. Exposure is greatly facilitated by extending the incision at least 5 cm above the umbilicus.

Suture material

One layer of interrupted absorbable sutures is sufficient, because it has been repeatedly shown that non-absorbable sutures do not offer any advantages and their persistence might be associated with fistula formation. The author's preference is 3/0 polyglactin (Vicryl).

Technique

1 After exploratory laparotomy, a pair of crushing clamps is used for each transection. The gut is 'shaved off' the crushing clamp on the healthy side of the intestine. The clamp should be narrow and firm, so that only 2–3 mm of gut is crushed within the jaws of the clamp. In Crohn's disease, the significantly diseased part of the small intestine most often has fat wrapping around the serosal aspect of the gut. The clamp should be placed across the intestine at a point where there is minimal fat wrapping, so that the ulcerated part of the intestine is excised.

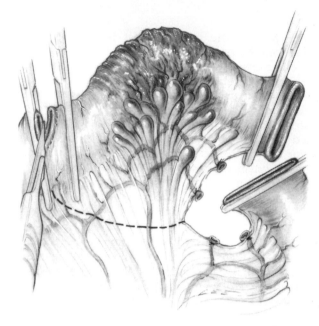

1

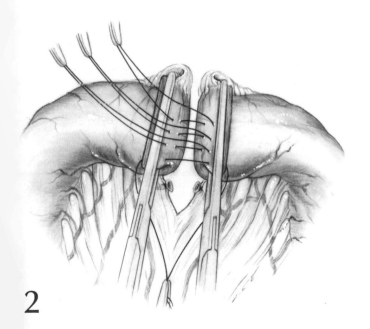

2

2 The crushing clamps are left *in situ* and a row of interrupted sutures is placed to fashion the posterior anastomosis. Once this row of sutures has been completed, they are tied serially and divided. The 'end' sutures are tied but are maintained as 'stay' sutures.

3 The part of the intestine that is closest to the anastomosis on both sides of the clamps is gently squeezed empty and a soft clamp is placed about 5 cm from the anastomotic site on each side. The area for the anastomosis is surrounded by warm, moist packs from the remaining part of the abdominal contents. The crushing clamps are removed and the intestinal lumen is opened on both sides. The inside of both ends of the intestine can be inspected. It is unnecessary to trim the 2–3 mm of crushed intestine because this zone provides haemostasis. If any bleeding points occur, they can be managed with diathermy.

If no linear ulcers are seen on either side, a second (anterior) row of interrupted sutures is placed. The sutures should be inserted about 3 mm from each other and placed through the serosa and muscle, taking in the submucosal plane but without penetrating mucosa. These sutures are then tied serially to complete the anastomosis.

The mesenteric defect is closed with a few interrupted absorbable sutures, making sure that there is no impairment of the blood supply to the intestine.

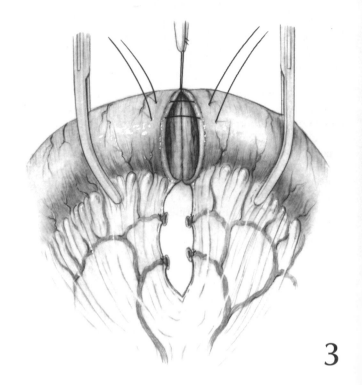

3

4 The soft bowel clamps are removed, and confirmation of an anastomotic lumen is obtained by gently palpating the anastomosis with the thumb and the index finger, making sure not to stretch or disrupt the suture line.

After completing the anastomosis, the area is washed with warmed physiological saline. The packs are removed, and the abdominal contents are again irrigated with significant volumes of warmed physiological saline. The abdomen is closed in the conventional manner. Drains are not necessary unless there is a chronic abscess cavity (an 'inflammatory nest') that requires drainage.

In patients with the unusual complication of free perforation from Crohn's disease with intra-abdominal sepsis, it is wise to consider construction of an end ileostomy and mucous fistula at completion of the resection. The intestine can be reconstructed at a later date when the patient has completely recovered (as described in the chapter on pp. 627–653).

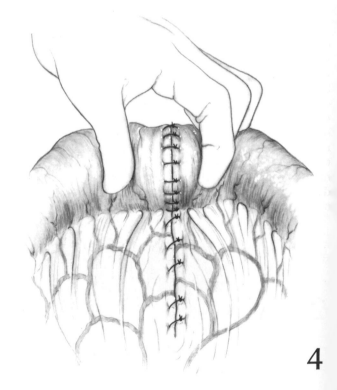

4

Postoperative care

The nasogastric tube is maintained until the patient is fully awake and then withdrawn as soon as possible. The patient is immediately mobilized. The postoperative feeding regimen is as follows. On the first day, 300 ml of liquid is a normal allowance; on the second day, the patient can usually take 500–1000 ml liquid by mouth; on the third day, it is usually not necessary to maintain the intravenous infusion, and a full liquid diet is usually tolerated; on the fourth day, the patient can usually eat normal, solid food.

Illustrations by Gillian Lee Illustrations and the late Robert Lane

Conventional colectomy

D. A. Rothenberger MD
Clinical Professor of Surgery and Chief, Division of Colon and Rectal Surgery, University of Minnesota Medical School, Minneapolis, Minnesota, USA

Principles and justification

Colon resections are performed for a wide variety of conditions including neoplasms (both benign and malignant), inflammatory bowel diseases, and other benign conditions such as colonic haemorrhage, procidentia or megacolon. Although the indication for colectomy will alter some of the technical details, the operative principles underlying the conduct of colon resections are well established. This chapter outlines these general principles and highlights some of the major alterations in technique designed to accommodate the specific demands of common variables such as malignancy, obstruction, inflammation and infection.

Preoperative

Patient status

Colectomy has become a safe operative procedure but remains a major undertaking with significant potential for morbidity. The surgeon must assess each patient for reversible risk factors such as anaemia, dehydration, electrolyte imbalance and malnutrition. Medical diseases such as diabetes, hypertension and cardiopulmonary problems should be optimally controlled. A detailed history of any pre-existing gastrointestinal dysfunction, especially of problems such as dumping syndrome, diarrhoea, irritable bowel symptoms or anal incontinence, must be obtained because such information may alter the extent of colectomy and the decision to perform a restorative anastomosis.

Disease status

Complete evaluation to determine the extent and nature of the primary colonic disease and to exclude other pathology is essential to proper planning of a colectomy. Several commonly encountered clinical problems deserve special consideration.

Carcinoma

The surgeon should anticipate potential problems which could affect resection of the primary lesion. For instance, a bulky, palpable lesion of the right colon may have invaded the duodenum or involve the ureter. Computed tomography might clarify the situation and facilitate planning of the operation. Before performing a colectomy for carcinoma, one must exclude synchronous lesions, preferably by colonoscopy examination or with an air contrast barium enema and proctoscopy. A search for distant metastases is worthwhile if the information would alter the operative approach. For instance, one may decide not to operate for a non-obstructing colonic cancer if there are extensive pulmonary metastases.

Obstruction

Colonic obstruction alters the usual preoperative assessment. The upper tract is decompressed with a nasogastric tube and the colon is evaluated with a water-soluble contrast enema to determine the extent, site, nature and degree of the obstruction. If the obstruction is partial and there is no evidence of impending perforation, the distal colon and rectum are cleansed with gentle enemas. Often, a limited oral bowel preparation becomes feasible and one can thus convert an emergency situation into a semielective operation in prepared bowel (as described in the chapter on pp. 727–745).

Inflammatory bowel disease

The surgeon must determine whether proctectomy should accompany colectomy for Crohn's disease or ulcerative colitis. Rectal function may be safely preserved by performing an ileorectal anastomosis if anal sphincter function is adequate, the rectum is compliant, the risk of neoplasm is not excessive, and the rectal disease is not severe.

Infection

Sepsis may dominate the clinical course of many patients with colonic pathology. Diffuse peritonitis obviously requires immediate laparotomy, but localized peritonitis secondary to a confined perforation and a walled-off abscess can often be controlled non-operatively by percutaneous drainage, guided by computed tomography or ultrasonography, and use of broad-spectrum antibiotics. Sepsis associated with colovesical, colouterine, colovaginal or colocutaneous fistulae often clears quickly after institution of systemic antibiotics. The goal is to convert an emergency situation to an elective operation on a prepared bowel as described in the chapters on pp. 699–716 and 717–726.

Genitourinary tract assessment

An intravenous pyelogram is not indicated routinely before a colectomy, but if the surgeon has reason to suspect retroperitoneal or genitourinary tract involvement, assessment of the ureters is indicated. This is probably best accomplished by a computed tomographic scan performed with intravenous contrast. If a retroperitoneal, periureteric or pelvic mass or inflammation is anticipated, ureteric stents placed via cystoscopy just before colectomy can be invaluable to avoid inadvertent injury to the ureters.

Stoma planning

The surgeon should anticipate those cases in which there is likely to be a need for a stoma, either temporary or permanent, and provide the patient with information regarding this possibility before the operation. Enterostomal therapy consultation before surgery is invaluable to select and mark a site on the abdomen for a stoma.

Bowel preparation

The majority of colectomies are performed electively and thus a complete bowel preparation is usually feasible. Standard bowel preparation may be conducted over a 24-h period and (in most instances) on an outpatient basis, allowing the patient to be admitted on the morning of surgery. The patient drinks only clear liquids for 24 h and consumes 4 litres of polyethylene glycol solution over 2–4 h in the afternoon the day before surgery. A sodium phosphate enema is given 2 h before surgery. Two doses of metronidazole and neomycin sulphate are given the day before surgery after the lavage preparation, and an intravenous second-generation cephalosporin is administered within 1 h before the incision is made. If patients anticipate they could not tolerate a large-volume oral lavage preparation, alternatives such as an oral sodium phosphate preparation or traditional cathartics and enemas can be substituted.

A nasogastric tube is usually placed to empty the stomach but is generally removed at the completion of the operation unless there was evidence of partial obstruction. For distal colonic lesions, the rectum is irrigated with sterile water through a proctoscope.

Anaesthesia

An epidural catheter for narcotic infusion is often used to supplement a general anaesthetic and to provide initial postoperative analgesia for 48–72 h. Once a general anaesthesia is induced, a Foley urethral catheter is inserted into the bladder.

Definition of terms

1 A variety of terms are used to describe different types of colectomy. These terms are somewhat misleading since they refer primarily to the portion of the colon resected and not precisely to the extent of mesentery or omentum resected with the colon. The mesenteric clearance technique dictates the extent of colonic resection. In general, a proximal mesenteric ligation will eliminate the blood supply to a greater length of colon and require a more extensive 'colectomy'. The mesenteric clearance technique used in a given instance is determined by the nature of the primary pathology (malignant *versus* benign), the intent of the resection (curative *versus* palliative), the precise location of the primary pathology, and the condition of the mesentery (thin and soft *versus* thickened and indurated). In general, the curative resection of a colonic malignancy is best accomplished by performing a radical mesenteric clearance with proximal vessel ligation and concomitant resection of overlying omentum. Resection of a benign process does not require wide mesenteric resection and the omentum can be preserved if desired.

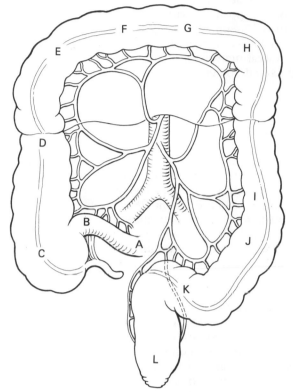

1

A → C	:	Ileocaecectomy
±A + B → D	:	Ascending colectomy
±A + B → F	:	Right hemicolectomy
±A + B → G	:	Extended right hemicolectomy
±E + F → G ± H	:	Transverse colectomy
G → I	:	Left hemicolectomy
F → I	:	Extended left hemicolectomy
J + K	:	Sigmoid colectomy
±A + B → J	:	Subtotal colectomy
±A + B → K	:	Total colectomy
±A + B → L	:	Total proctocolectomy

Operation

Position of patient

For most colectomies, the patient is placed in a modified lithotomy position with the legs supported by Allen stirrups. Pneumatic compression stockings are used routinely to minimize the risk of thromboembolism and peripheral neuropathy. The supine position is used for right-sided colectomies.

Incision

2   The choice of incision varies widely depending on the particular circumstances of each case.

Knowledge of the underlying pathology, extent of disease, level of the splenic flexure, physical appearance of the patient, previous surgical incisions, and availability of qualified assistants all influence the surgeon's decision. If in doubt, a midline incision is used because it can be extended to expose any area within the abdomen. The midline incision is preferred for patients with inflammatory bowel disease because such patients may require frequent reoperations and may eventually need a stoma. The surgeon usually stands opposite the segment of intestine to be resected, i.e. on the left side of a patient undergoing a right colectomy and vice versa. A first assistant stands across from the surgeon and, when appropriate, a second assistant stands between the legs of the patient who is in a modified lithotomy position. Self-retaining abdominal retractors facilitate exposure and fibreoptic headlights clearly illuminate the operative field, enhancing the safety and ease of the operation.

Exploration

After the incision has been made, the presence of ascites or peritoneal contamination is noted. The surgeon should confirm the preoperative diagnosis and determine resectability of the primary pathology. The uninvolved small and large intestine is assessed to determine the adequacy of the bowel preparation and the presence or absence of obstruction, inflammation, oedema or other factors that might alter the decision to perform a primary anastomosis. All viscera accessible to the surgeon are examined in a standard sequence. Conditions such as an aortic aneurysm, ovarian mass, gallstones or liver metastases may require a change in the operative plan.

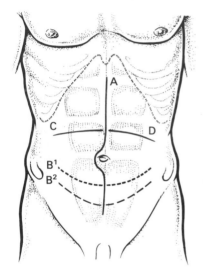

2

A. Midline: versatile
B. Transverse infraumbilical (high and low): primarily for pelvic exposure; if placed near level of umbilicus (B^1), useful for sigmoid colectomy and total colectomy
C. Right trans-supraumbilical: for right colectomy
D. Left trans-supraumbilical: for left colectomy
C + D: used for subtotal colectomy, extended left and right colectomy

Extent of resection

After laparotomy and complete exploration, the surgeon can finalize plans for resection based on knowledge of the patient's primary and secondary pathology.

3 It is useful to think in anatomical terms based on knowledge of colon mesenteric anatomy. For instance, if the goal is to perform a curative resection of a caecal cancer, the planned resection should encompass its field of lymphatic spread. This will require proximal ligation of the ileocolic vessels, including the terminal ileal and right colic vessels and usually the right branch of the middle colic artery. Thus, approximately 15 cm of terminal ileum, the ascending colon, and the right transverse colon to the middle colic artery will be resected. On the other hand, if a cancer of the hepatic flexure is to be resected, the ileocolic and right colic vessels will be resected together with the entire middle colic artery. Thus, less terminal ileum will be removed because the distal ileal vessels will be left intact, but more transverse colon will be resected to ensure removal of the lymphatic bed of the primary lesion along the middle colic vessels. Cancers of the splenic flexure and proximal descending colon may theoretically spread to the lymphatics near the middle colic or the inferior mesenteric arteries. A radical resection with proximal ligation of these two major vessels at their origin would require resection of most of the transverse, descending and sigmoid colon. This would make restoration of continuity difficult. A better alternative, because it does not appear to compromise cancer curability and it eases the technical difficulty of doing a primary anastomosis, is to ligate the left branch of the middle colic artery near its origin from the main trunk, and the left colic artery near its origin from the inferior mesenteric artery. Thus, the right transverse colon and the sigmoid colon can be preserved and a relatively easy colocolic anastomosis achieved.

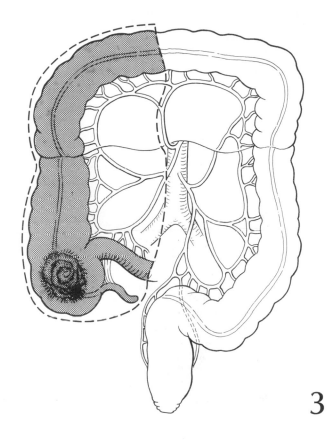

3

Mobilization

The first step is to mobilize the bowel that is to be resected by dividing its peritoneal attachments. The extent of the planned resection determines the type and extent of mobilization of the colon that is necessary. The goals of mobilization are: (1) to expose the mesenteric vessels which need division and ligation; (2) to keep retroperitoneal and other adjacent structures away from the field of resection; and (3) to free sufficient lengths of intestine proximally and distally to allow a tension-free, well vascularized anastomosis to be performed. Thus, for an isolated sigmoid resection, one often has to mobilize the entire left colon including the splenic flexure to conduct a colorectal anastomosis. In general, for a descending colon lesion, it is best to begin by mobilizing the sigmoid colon, then the descending colon, and finally the left transverse colon. After resection of the descending colon and its mesocolon, a tension-free colocolic anastomosis is performed. Similarly, if an isolated segment of transverse colon is to be resected, it is usually necessary to mobilize both the splenic and hepatic flexures. Usually a mid-transverse colonic resection is incorporated into an extended right, an extended left, or a subtotal or total colectomy. For the last procedures, the author finds it most convenient to begin with mobilization of the entire left colon followed by mobilization of the right side, meeting near the midline in the lesser sac.

Right colectomies

4 The caecum and terminal ileum are gently re-tracted anteromedially by the surgeon's right hand to expose the lateral and inferior peritoneal attachments. Electrocautery with a blade tip is used to incise through the posterior peritoneum, taking care not to penetrate the mesentery. The surgeon's left index finger is inserted into this plane and easily directed upwards towards the hepatic flexure.

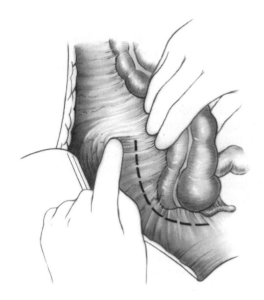

4

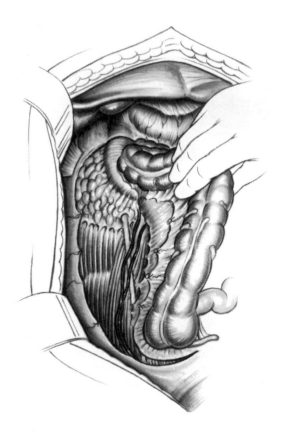

5

5 The assistant incises the exposed, thinned out peritoneum overlying the surgeon's finger with electrocautery. The terminal ileum, caecum including the appendix, and the distal ascending colon is thus mobilized.

6 The underlying right ureter and gonadal vessels are kept posteriorly in the retroperitoneum. By applying gentle anterior retraction on the mobilized right colon the surgeon exposes the duodenum, which is left unharmed in the retroperitoneum by dividing any remaining tissue tethering the colon to the retroperitoneum. Excessive anterior retraction of the colon at the level of the hepatic flexure may result in a tear of one of the fragile veins located in the base of the mesentery near the duodenum. If such a vein is noted to be under tension during the mobilization procedure, it is best to suture ligate and divide it before a troublesome tear occurs. If a tear occurs, packing is used to control the bleeding and to prevent a large haematoma from forming in the base of the mesentery. The packing is slowly removed to reveal the torn vessel, which is suture ligated.

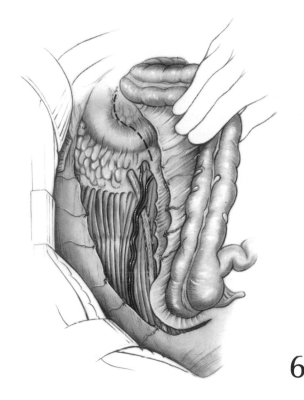

6

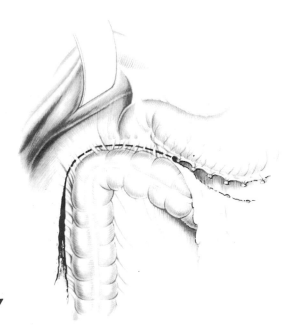

7

7 Adhesions to the gallbladder are divided under direct view. If the omentum is to be resected with the transverse colon, it is divided between clamps with preservation of the gastroepiploic vessels along the greater curvature of the stomach. If the omentum is to be preserved, it is retracted upwards over the stomach, and the relatively avascular attachments between the colon and omentum are divided with electrocautery.

Left colectomies

8 Mobilizations of the sigmoid, descending and left transverse colon are considered together. The sigmoid colon is retracted anteromedially by the surgeon's left hand to expose the lateral peritoneal attachments. Electrocautery dissection along the white line of Toldt is instituted.

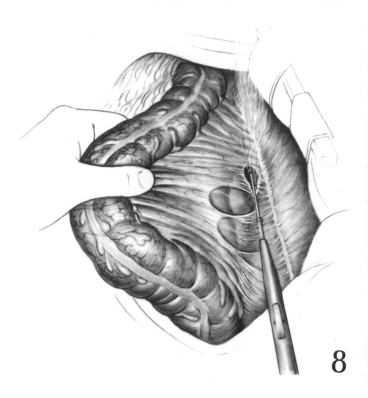

8

9 The full thickness of the peritoneum is incised but the mesentery itself is not entered. The gonadal vessels and left ureter are gently displaced posteriorly using a stick sponge. The surgeon's right hand is inserted into the plane posterior to the descending colon and used to separate the colon from the retroperitoneal structures. It is important to get into the proper plane of dissection. If too deep, troublesome retroperitoneal bleeding occurs and, if too superficial, the colon will remain fixed to the retroperitoneum. By rolling the right hand out from under the descending colon, the right lateral peritoneal attachments are exposed for division by the assistant positioned between the patient's legs.

It is important not to pull down on the descending colon because this can result in a splenic injury. Instead, the thrust of the dissection is upwards towards the splenic flexure. The surgeon's left hand retracts the now mobilized sigmoid and distal descending colon anteromedially, allowing its mesentery to serve as a fan-like retractor, keeping the small intestine from interfering with the remaining lateral mobilization. At this time, the splenic flexure is visualized, and any peritoneal bands to the spleen or splenic–omental adhesions are divided under direct view by electrocautery. Once that is accomplished, the left transverse colon is gently retracted inferiorly towards the left lower quadrant by an assistant. The surgeon's right hand in the plane posterior to the descending colon is gently passed up to the splenic flexure. By rolling the right hand, the remaining lateral peritoneal attachments are exposed for division by the assistant.

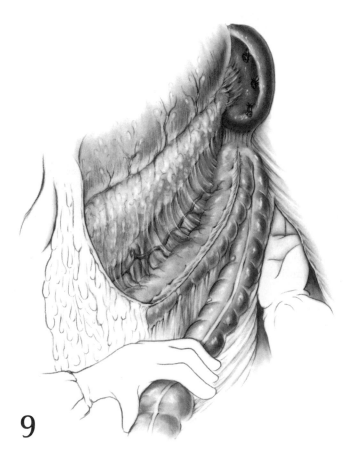

9

10 At this point, it is important to stay adjacent to the superolateral margin of the colon. The splenocolic ligament is often quite thick and may be best divided between clamps and secured with ties. Omental adhesions may overlie this area and must be clamped and divided initially to expose the deeper attachments. As these attachments are divided, the left colon is held up in a fan-like manoeuvre to enhance exposure of the retroperitoneum. As the splenocolic ligament is divided, the lesser sac is entered and the dissection continues medially. The omentum is handled as noted earlier. If the splenic flexure is difficult to expose, it is sometimes helpful to enter the lesser sac in the midline before completing division of the splenocolic ligament. Thus one can work at the most difficult point of dissection from two sides: along the left transverse colon from within the lesser sac, and along the descending colon in the retroperitoneum.

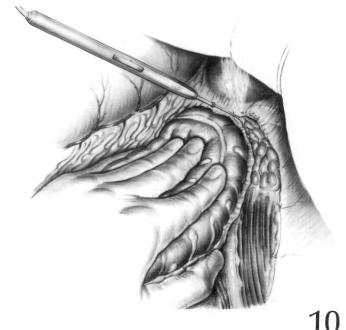

10

Division of mesentery and resection

11 The mobilized colon is retracted so that its mesentery can be exposed and transilluminated. The primary vessels such as the ileocolic, middle colic and inferior mesenteric or their major tributaries are exposed by incising the overlying peritoneum. These major vessels are triply clamped, divided and doubly tied on the proximal end. For cancers, a proximal ligation is standard.

If mobilization was properly performed, this step should be quite safe because the ureters, gonadal vessels, duodenum and other retroperitoneal structures should be out of the field of mesenteric vessel ligation. For benign conditions, ligation is performed where 'comfortable', without risking proximal mesenteric dissection. Once the major vessels are divided, the mesentery supplying the intestine at the sites of the proposed anastomosis is assessed, divided between clamps, and ligated. Inflammatory conditions such as Crohn's disease may thicken the mesentery, making division in the standard fashion quite hazardous. Suture ligation and small bites of tissue can overcome this problem. A short distance of only 1 cm or less is cleared along the mesenteric surface of the intestine to allow accurate suture placement without compromising the vascularity of the anastomosis. The mesenteric flow at the proposed anastomotic sites should be pulsatile. The blood supply to the splenic flexure area is variable and may be tenuous, especially in elderly patients, after ligation of the middle colic artery or the inferior mesenteric artery. If there is doubt about the adequacy of the blood supply, the left colon should be resected.

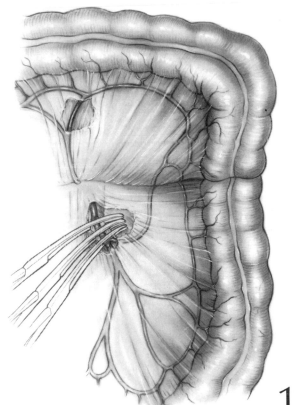

11

If a hand-sewn anastomosis is planned, non-crushing clamps are placed across the intestine at the sites for division, with two crushing clamps being placed in parallel on the 'specimen side' of the non-crushing clamps. The intestine is resected and is sent to the pathology department for review of the adequacy of resection.

Mesenteric closure

12 Mobilization should allow the two ends of intestine to come together without tension. After alignment, the mesocolon is closed with a continuous polyglycolic acid suture from its base near the proximal ligation point to within 5 cm of the site of anastomosis. This is best accomplished at this stage since the base of the mesocolon defect is most easily exposed before the anastomosis is created. Care is taken not to damage any vessels along the cut edges of the mesocolon which might diminish blood flow to the anastomosis. The remaining 5-cm gap in the mesentery is closed after completion of the anastomosis.

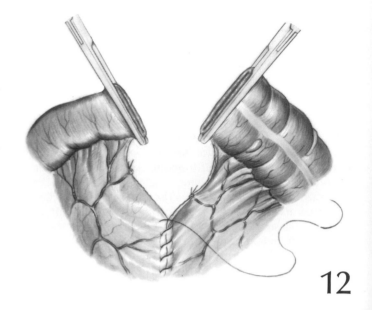

12

Anastomosis

Ideally, a primary anastomosis is performed following a colectomy. The surgeon's sound judgement is essential to assure success. Factors that must be considered include the patient's overall status, the condition of the peritoneal cavity, the condition of the intestine and completeness of its preparation, and the assurance that the necessary technical demands of an anastomosis, i.e. vascularity, lack of tension, and accurate approximation, can be met. We generally prefer a semiclosed, hand-sutured, minimally inverting technique approximating the intestine in an end-to-end fashion (as described in the chapter on pp. 528–550).

13 The site of anastomosis is isolated from the surrounding field with laparotomy pads. The bowel clamps are held parallel, approximately 3 cm apart, by the assistant, who directs the tips towards the surgeon's dominant hand.

The clamps are rotated through 90° to expose the posterior wall, and interrupted 4/0 seromuscular sutures are placed at approximately 1-cm intervals. The sutures at the mesenteric and antimesenteric sides are left untied and tagged.

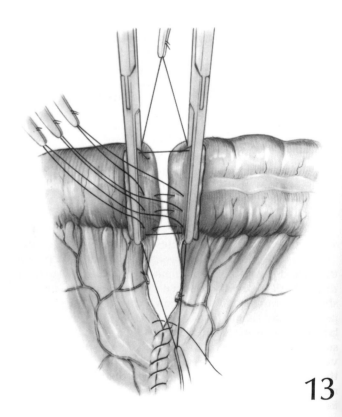

13

14 The other sutures are serially tied and trimmed as the assistant holds the parallel Dennis clamps together. The Dennis clamps are rotated through 180°, thus exposing the anterior wall. A series of 4/0 seromuscular sutures are placed about 1 cm apart and the ends tagged. Occlusion of the intestine 3–4 cm from the ends is achieved by gentle digital compression or by a shod non-crushing clamp gently applied across the intestinal lumen only.

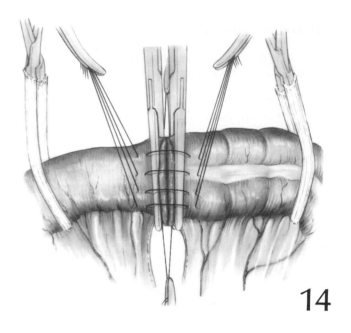

14

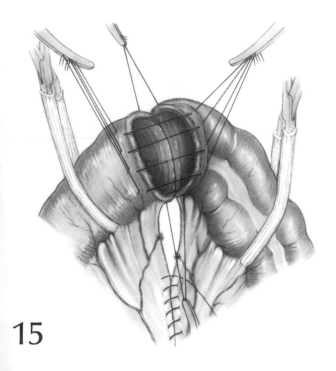

15

15 The non-crushing clamps are removed from first one cut end of intestine and then the other. While the tagged sutures are held up to open the intestinal lumen, an assistant is ready to use suction if any stool begins to leak from the cut end.

16 After ensuring that none of the sutures have inadvertently picked up the opposite wall and that there are no major arterial 'pumpers', the surgeon ties all suture pairs. Proximal occluding pressure or shod clamps are removed. The anastomosis is completed by placing 4/0 interrupted, full-thickness sutures between each of the previously placed sutures. The surgeon must be certain that the anastomosis is well vascularized, widely patent, under no tension, and that the technique was not compromised in any way. The mesocolic suture is completed up to the wall of the intestine.

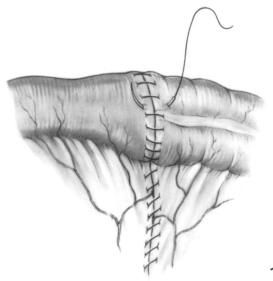

16

Alternative anastomotic techniques

Unique problems demand flexibility on the part of the surgeon, and other anastomotic techniques may be preferred.

Size discrepancy

Major size discrepancy in the two limbs of intestine does not usually pose a problem if the technique described above is used. The technique of continually halving the distance to guide suture placement on each end of cut intestine can be used to easily accommodate a major size discrepancy. An acceptable alternative anastomotic technique is a side-to-side functional end-to-end stapled anastomosis (as described in the chapter on pp. 551–560). A total abdominal colectomy and ileorectal anastomosis may involve two limbs of intestine with major size discrepancy. If the rectum is large and the ileum small, the author's preferred approach is to use a double-staple technique (as described in the chapter on pp. 551–560).

Distal anastomosis

Most colonic anastomoses are easily accessible and lend themselves to suturing. If a distal anastomosis to the upper or middle third of the rectum is required after a segmental or total colectomy, the circular stapled end-to-end anastomosis may be easier (as described in the chapter on pp. 551–560).

Oedematous bowel

Obstruction often results in oedematous bowel which can be hazardous to approximate because sutures or staples may pull out. A two-layer technique or reinforcement of a stapled anastomosis may be preferable in such situations. Alternatively, the oedema may preclude a safe primary anastomosis, and a colostomy or ileostomy may be necessary as a first step (as described in the chapter on pp. 727–745).

Wound closure

After achieving haemostasis, the abdomen is irrigated, fluid is suctioned, and the fascia is closed, usually with a running, heavy, slowly absorbable monofilament suture. The subcutaneous tissue is irrigated, and in most instances the skin is approximated by subcuticular sutures or skin staples.

Postoperative care

Nasogastric aspiration is maintained after the operation if there was evidence of obstruction, but otherwise it is not used unless the patient develops nausea, distension or vomiting. Clear liquids are begun when the patient has a soft abdomen with normal bowel sounds and expels flatus and/or stool without nausea, vomiting or distension. If tolerated, the diet is advanced to a normal intake over the next 2 days. Intravenous fluids are maintained until the patient is taking sufficient fluids orally. The urinary catheter is normally discontinued between the second and fourth day after surgery. If there is evidence of infection or sepsis without an obvious aetiology, the surgeon must suspect a leaked anastomosis (as described in the chapter on pp. 561–572). Patients have generally recovered sufficiently to be discharged 6–8 days after surgery.

Illustrations by Gillian Oliver and the late Robert Lane

Elective surgery for sigmoid diverticular disease

Mark Killingback FRCS, FRCSEd, FRACS
Sydney Adventist Hospital, Sydney, Australia

Principles and justification

Patients may have significant clinical problems attributable to diverticular disease caused by functional colonic muscle abnormalities without local inflammation of the colon being present. This concept has led to a better understanding of the indications for surgical treatment. Furthermore, there may be a discrepancy between the clinical and radiological assessments in these patients – a barium enema may underestimate or exaggerate the apparent significance of the diverticular disease.

In recent years there has been a better appreciation of the response of symptoms to dietary manipulation. The effect of increasing food residue with a high fibre diet has greatly reduced the number of patients requiring surgery for 'failed medical treatment'.

Indications

Caution must be exercised in attributing abdominal and intestinal symptoms to diverticular disease, particularly in those patients whose principal complaint is chronic abdominal pain. Irritable bowel syndrome may be indistinguishable from the symptoms of non-inflammatory functional chronic diverticular disease. The author does not believe that there is any pathological relationship between these two conditions.

Prophylactic resection of sigmoid diverticular disease is not justified in the early stage of the disease in an attempt to prevent complications, such as perforation and fistula formation. Their development is largely unpredictable and is often the first manifestation of the disease. If symptoms have become refractory, however, surgery is indicated because the inflammatory focus has become irreversible and will cause progressive fibrosis of the wall of the colon, the mesentery and the pericolic tissues with or without a concomitant abscess.

Most elective resections are performed for complicated disease such as chronic phlegmonous diverticulitis, chronic pericolic or pelvic abscess and fistulae. Some of these patients will present for a second-stage elective procedure after a previous laparotomy for acute diverticulitis, drainage of an abscess, or frank peritonitis.

Despite conservative management with a high-residue diet and unprocessed bran, persistent symptoms may warrant elective surgery. In this group, patients with irritable bowel syndrome should be diagnosed and excluded.

Repeated attacks of acute diverticulitis of significance may occur with evidence of peritoneal irritation, fever and systemic effects. Such attacks usually settle with antibiotic therapy in a few days, but often leave a focus for subsequent attacks. Such an episode which subsides slowly and leaves a focus of tenderness, with or without a mass on palpation, is better managed by resection in an otherwise fit patient. If the attack is less severe in an elderly patient with accompanying medical problems, it may be preferable to observe the patient for a period and advise surgery on the basis of future episodes.

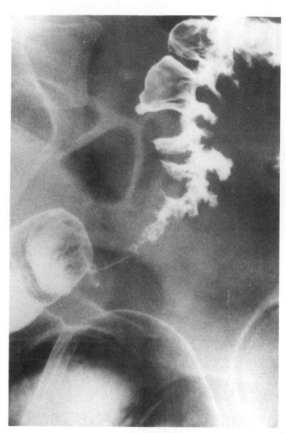

1a

1a, b A persistent inflammatory mass for more than 4–6 weeks is an indication for resection in the fit patient. Invariably it will be associated with a stricture on radiography (*see Illustration 1a*), and this in turn will raise the possibility that a carcinoma is present. Although the inflammatory stricture usually shows mucosal continuity (*see Illustration 1b*) indicating its benign nature, the radiograph can appear indistinguishable from a carcinoma.

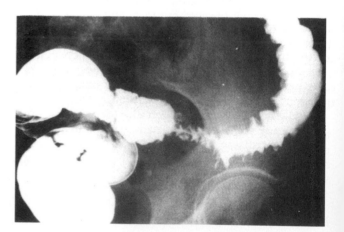

1b

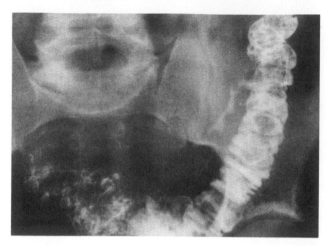

2 A barium enema may show extravasation beyond the wall of the colon, indicating localized perforation. There may or may not be an associated stricture, and it is likely that there is an associated inflammatory mass. While this situation may be tolerated in the unfit patient without symptoms, the colon is best resected.

2

Flexible sigmoidoscopy or colonoscopy can differentiate some but not all of these lesions, because stenosis, fibrosis and angulation of the colon may impede the passage of the endoscope. Computed tomography (CT) can be very helpful in acute diverticulitis by demonstrating a related abdominal or pelvic abscess. Its value in patients with chronic or intermittent symptoms, however, is yet to be demonstrated.

Colovesical and colocutaneous fistulae are common and may complicate sigmoid diverticulitis. Less common fistulae are colovaginal, coloenteric and colofallopian, but diverticular disease can form a fistula into any organ and many bizarre fistulae have been described. Such fistulae are usually an absolute indication for surgery, but in frail patients without evidence of an active abscess or ascending renal tract infection (colovesical fistula), the compromise for conservative treatment may be acceptable.

Resection is usually indicated as a secondary procedure if emergency surgery for acute diverticulitis with peritonitis has previously been carried out. Such patients may have an associated fistula, and a proximal stoma may be present. Patients in whom a Hartmann operation has been performed as an emergency will need careful assessment to see if further resection of proximal and/or distal residual disease is needed before an anastomosis is carried out.

Interval elective surgery is indicated very occasionally between recurrent episodes of profuse colonic bleeding. While most bleeding of this type is due to vascular dysplasia (most often from the right colon), bleeding from diverticula may be demonstrated by angiography and histology. If colonoscopy, scintigraphy, or angiography has demonstrated a bleeding site, a segmental resection can be performed. If the episodes of bleeding recur significantly without localization, colectomy and ileorectal anastomosis should be considered as an elective treatment.

Preoperative

Preparation for the patient with diverticular disease is the same as for any major colorectal operation and will include a full blood count, blood biochemistry, chest radiography and electrocardiography. Intravenous pyelography is not mandatory before sigmoid resection for uncomplicated disease, but is important if complications are evidenced by the presence of a palpable mass or radiological stricture, which may be close to the left ureter on the pelvic brim and left wall of the pelvis. It may also reveal an incidental urinary tract abnormality, such as ureteric duplication, deviation of the ureter, non-functioning of one kidney, or obstruction of the ureter by the inflammatory disease in the pelvis.

Mechanical bowel preparation is carried out the day before surgery by the oral administration of 3 litres of polyethylene glycol preparation over a 2-h period. Usually with this preparation no additional aperients or enemas are administered. During the intraoperative and early postoperative period, prophylatic broad-spectrum antibiotics are given parenterally.

Ureteric catheterization

In patients in whom a large pelvic inflammatory mass is evident on rectal examination, considerable extraperitoneal pelvic fibrosis is likely. In such patients, the introduction of ureteric catheters before operation is most helpful. The author has employed ureteric catheters in 9% of patients resected.

Operation

Position of patient

The Lloyd-Davies position (modified lithotomy-Trendelenburg position) with Lloyd-Davies stirrups is preferred. This allows better retraction by the second assistant standing between the patient's legs, vaginal examination which may assist in a difficult anterior dissection (particularly after a hysterectomy) and is necessary for the use of the intraluminal stapling instrument, which is the author's preferred method of anastomosis.

Incision and laparotomy

A midline incision is made from the pubic symphysis to as far above the umbilicus as necessary to gain wide exposure. A thorough laparotomy is performed to assess the diverticular disease, its complications and any other intra-abdominal pathology.

In assessing the diverticular disease, the possibility of carcinoma must be considered. If there is doubt about such a diagnosis, the problem is usually diverticular disease. Any attachment of the diverticular disease to adjacent organs should be noted. The extent of the diverticular disease along the colon proximally must be assessed, as well as any abnormal muscular thickening. A similar examination of the rectosigmoid and upper rectum is important to assess possible inflammatory disease and associated muscle changes with diverticula.

Despite preoperative investigations and careful intraoperative assessment, real doubt may exist that the disease is benign. In this situation a careful examination of a preoperative barium enema may show mucosal continuity along the stricture, indicating that the disease is not malignant. While flexible sigmoidoscopy may not have been useful before operation, its use during the operation, assisted by the abdominal surgeon, may confirm a diagnosis.

If carcinoma cannot be excluded, then the surgeon will need to perform an appropriate cancer operation, resecting adherent organs *en bloc*. Although resecting a segment of bladder wall *en bloc* for diverticulitis (mistaken for carcinoma) may be surgically acceptable, further extension of radical pelvic surgery is not. In such a circumstance, it is preferable to dissect between the bladder and the sigmoid pathology, and extend the operation as appropriate if examination of the lumen of the resected sigmoid has revealed carcinoma. Distending the bladder with saline may lift the pathological segment out of the pelvis and facilitate this part of the operation.

Mobilizing the sigmoid and descending colon

3 After placement of a plastic ring wound protector in the abdominal wound, incision of the parasigmoid peritoneum along the line of the mesenteric and parietal fusion will expose the gonadal vessels and lower part of the ureter. Careful identification of the mesenteric layer of the left colon will ensure the correct anatomical plane.

Gentle digital dissection medially and upwards is used to displace the colon mesentery forwards, and the gonadal vessels, left ureter and perinephric fascia posteriorly. Troublesome bleeding may occur if large ovarian veins are not manipulated with care. This dissection should stop at the mid-point of the left kidney, as further manipulation may cause a traction injury to the splenic capsule which is not under vision during this manoeuvre.

With the upper sigmoid and lower descending colon retracted to the right, further identification of the course of the left ureter to the pelvic brim is made. The inferior mesenteric artery and vein are clearly identified from this left aspect, distinctly enveloped in fascia. Dissecting across the aorta immediately behind these structures will prevent damage to the preaortic nerve plexus, and when followed distally will lead to the correct anatomical plane for presacral dissection.

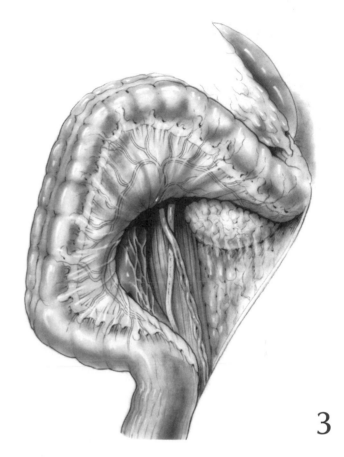

3

Specific difficulties in resecting sigmoid diverticulitis

The apex of the sigmoid colon is often fixed into the pelvis by adhesion to a deep chronic pelvic abscess, and until this is mobilized adequate dissection of the sigmoid colon is not possible. This pelvic dissection can often be achieved by careful 'pinching off' manoeuvres. In other instances, however, sharp scalpel dissection (too tough for scissors) or diathermy is required to cut through the very hard fibrosis that may join the sigmoid colon to the parietal peritoneum or pelvic structures. It is in this circumstance that ureteric catheters, which can be palpated, are most helpful.

4 If the sigmoid colon cannot be mobilized from the pelvis as the first step in the operation, then exposure of the left ureter will be difficult. Dissection in this area, and then to the left pelvic brim, will be facilitated by transecting the colon as an early step in the operation and lifting the sigmoid colon forward to expose the left posterior abdominal wall and the pelvic brim. This latter area can be a potentially hazardous dissection, with thick fibrosis obscuring the left ureter and left common iliac vessels. In such a circumstance, the sigmoid can be mobilized from this site by dissecting the adherent sigmoid in its intramural plane, thus avoiding damage to vital structures.

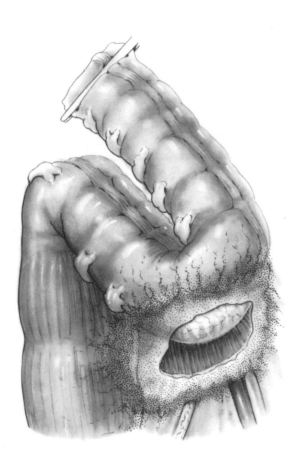

4

Splenic flexure mobilization

In most resections for diverticulitis, mobilization of the splenic flexure will be necessary. Up to this point in the operation, care is taken to avoid traction on the left aspect of the greater omentum and the splenic flexure of the colon to avoid capsule injuries to the spleen.

Mobilization of the splenic flexure is best performed by the surgeon operating from the right side of the table with the first assistant standing between the patient's legs, which maximizes his view and ability to assist. A second assistant on the left side of the table retracts the wound and the left costal margin. It is for this part of the operation that the incision in the upper part of the wound should be adequate.

5 The first three steps in mobilization are: (1) release of omental adhesions to the anterior border of the spleen; (2) release of omental adhesions to the left paracolic gutter at the level of the lower pole of the spleen; and (3) division of the peritoneum between the colon and the lower border of the spleen. This peritoneum is over the upper pole of the left kidney, and the incision is continued laterally to complete the incision of the left paracolic gutter.

These three manoeuvres release the spleen and will effectively prevent traction injuries to the splenic capsule.

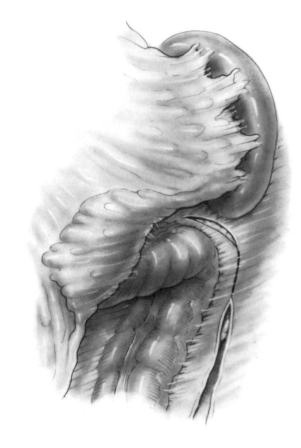

5

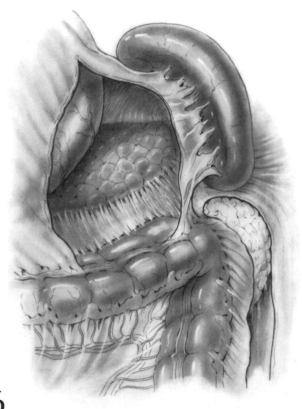

6

6 With the greater omentum retracted upwards and to the right, the lesser sac can be exposed by incising above the left transverse colon and/or opening the left lateral limit of the lesser sac, which is a short distance proximal to the splenic flexure.

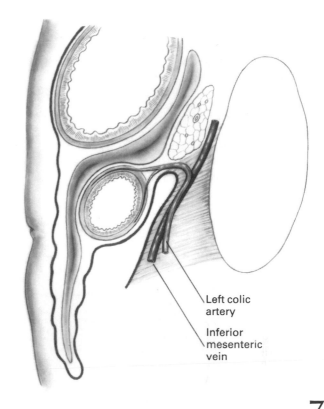

Left colic artery

Inferior mesenteric vein

7

7, 8 With the structures on the posterior wall of the lesser sac exposed, further mobilization (if required) can be achieved by dividing the anterior layer of the transverse mesocolon, which will allow the left colic vessels adjacent to it and the peritoneum posterior to these vessels to be dissected from the left perinephric fascia. Care must be taken medially of the inferior mesenteric vein, if it is to be preserved. The splenic flexure will now be fully mobilized.

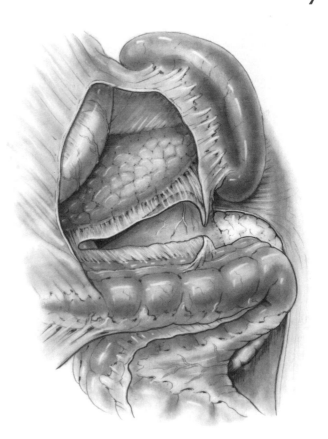

8

9 If necessary, division of the inferior mesenteric vein below the duodenum will give further length to the left colon by allowing the course of the left colic artery to 'unwind', which is thus preserved as an additional source of circulation to the left colon.

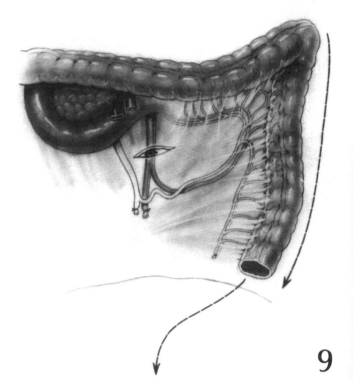

9

Selecting the proximal level of resection

In deciding the proximal extent of resection, several aspects are important. Obviously, active chronic infection in the colon and mesentery must be included. Muscle thickening, which may be proximal to the sigmoid colon, is best removed, and it is preferable to remove colon that contains many diverticula.

10 In the fit patient it may be reasonable to include the descending colon and distal transverse colon in order to remove extensive diverticulosis. More proximal excision of the colon requiring division of the middle colic vessels is not recommended.

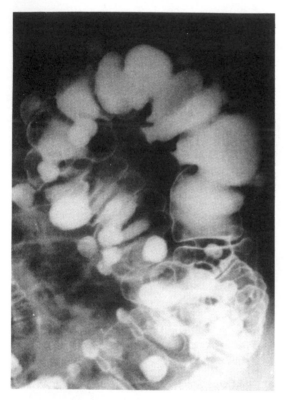

10

11 It may be difficult to detect diverticula if there is much pericolic fat. By 'milking' gas and fluid into the segment in question, the luminal pressure will increase and expand the colon, causing occult diverticula to 'balloon' and be revealed. Although one or two diverticula can be inverted at or near the anastomosis if unavoidable, it is preferable to use normal colon free of diverticula.

In the author's series, the level of proximal resection was near the sigmoid descending junction in 60% of patients, and at varying levels to the distal transverse colon in the remaining 40%.

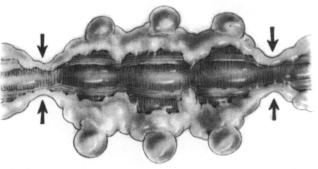

11

Vascular preparation of the colonic mesentery

12 If the proximal level of resection is in the vicinity of the sigmoid—descending colon junction, the left colic artery should be preserved, and the inferior mesenteric vein and artery ligated below the origin from that artery. This ligation is similar to cancer surgery, as there is no advantage in ligating branches and tributaries of the sigmoid vessels closer to the intestinal wall. If more proximal colon is to be removed, then both the inferior mesenteric artery and vein will be divided.

The marginal vessels of the descending colon run close to and parallel to the colon, but in the proximal sigmoid colon these vessels are often further from the intestine and lie in a looped formation, making them more vulnerable to inadvertent surgical interruption.

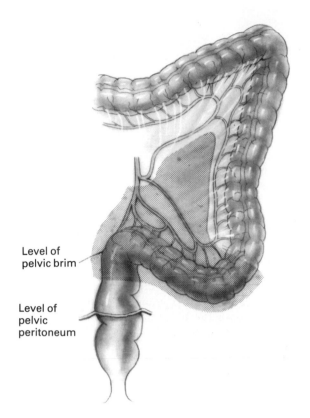

Level of
pelvic brim

Level of
pelvic
peritoneum

12

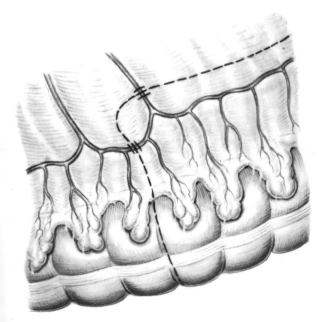

13

13 Division of the marginal vessels should be more distal than the level of the colon transection ('overshoot') to provide a safe margin to avoid damage to the vasa breva and vasa longa, which are related to the area for anastomosis. The marginal artery flow should be tested by allowing it to bleed. If flow is poor, and more proximal resection is inadvisable, this may be an indication for a proximal stoma.

Stapled anastomosis in diverticular disease

14 The author's preference is to use circular stapling wherever possible after resecting diverticular disease. The results are satisfactory, but not all patients are suitable, and approximately 5% of patients are best managed with a sutured anastomosis. These are patients with chronic pelvic floor fibrosis, which restricts the safe use of the stapler, patients who exhibit persistent spasm of the upper one-third of the rectum even under anaesthesia, and patients whose left colon is markedly contracted after a period of defunctioning by a proximal stoma.

The stapling technique is a good discipline for the surgeon, because both the proximal and distal ends of intestine must be normal, supple and free of inflammatory changes or muscle thickening for the technique to be satisfactory.

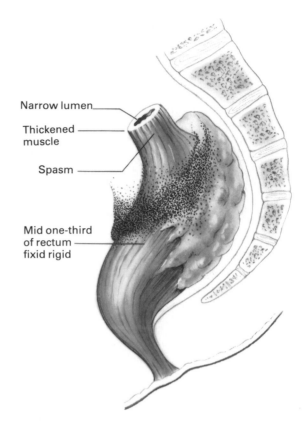

Narrow lumen
Thickened muscle
Spasm
Mid one-third of rectum fixid rigid

14

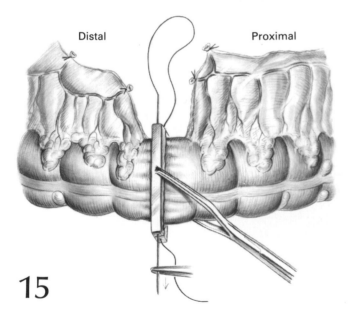

Distal   Proximal

15

Preparation of the colon

Minimal excision of terminal branches of the vasa breva and vasa longa should occur to secure a bare segment of colon for anastomosis. For convenience, one or two obtrusive appendices epiploicae can be excised (preserving the vasa within the base of the appendix).

15 A 1.5-cm segment of colon can be cleared to facilitate the application of an occlusive bowel clamp, and immediately proximal to it a purse-string clamp that is used in all cases to insert a purse-string suture. This clamp should leave no more than 1.0 cm of 'bare' colon between it and the proximal pericolic fat and vessels. A double-ended 0 polypropylene (Prolene) round-bodied malleable needle (3.5 metric) is passed through the purse-string clamp, and the colon is divided between the clamps.

16 Before dividing the colon, a nylon tape is tied around it (being careful not to include the marginal vessels) 10 cm proximal to the area for anastomosis. The edges of the colon are held in a pair of Babcock's forceps and a segment is thoroughly irrigated with water to remove all faecal debris.

If the colon is poorly prepared or loaded with faeces, intraoperative colonic lavage should be performed via the caecum or ileum to cleanse it completely.

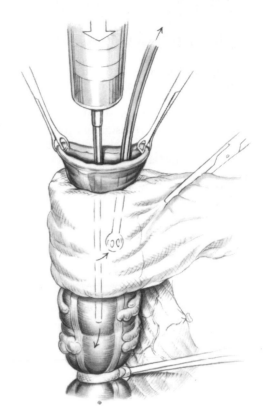

16

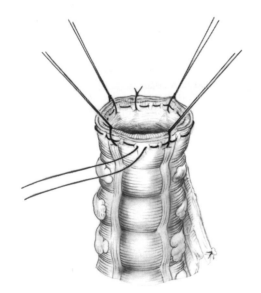

17

17 Four stay sutures are then placed on the margin of the divided colon. Two of these should pass through the antimesenteric taenia. A fifth short suture is used to 'trap' the mesenteric taenia. These five sutures include the purse-string suture to reinforce its function, and the stay sutures facilitate the insertion of the anvil into the colon.

Selecting the distal level of resection

The distal level of excision is also determined by the site of inflammation in the wall and mesentery of the intestine. It is important to remove distal diverticula that may be obscured in the pericolic and perirectal fat just above or below the rectosigmoid junction. Careful examination of the barium enema radiograph may also help to localize the distal limit of diverticula formation. The longitudinal muscle coat is usually thickened in the rectosigmoid region and sometimes in the upper rectum, and it is preferable to remove this abnormality. Therefore, the distal level of dissection is usually below the promontory of the sacrum through the upper third of the rectum.

18 Unusually, extensive diverticular disease may affect the upper one-third of the rectum.

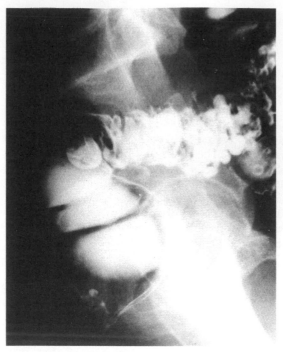

18

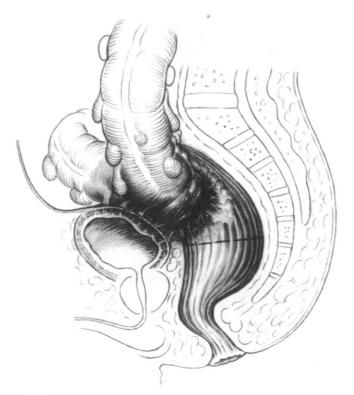

19 Secondary involvement of the upper one-third of the rectum is important in determining the distal level of transection. If a pelvic abscess involves the rectovaginal or rectovesical pouch but leaves the upper part of the rectum unaffected, the level of transection can be through healthy intestine in the upper one-third of the rectum. If this part of the rectum is abnormal due to contiguous inflammation, the transection level must be far enough distal to be through healthy rectal wall. In some cases this will mean an extraperitoneal level, and very occasionally through the lower one-third of the rectum.

19

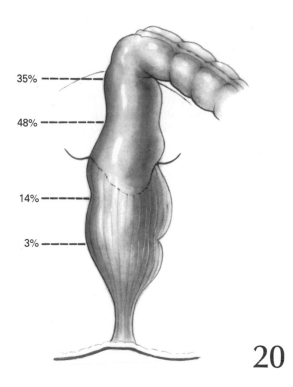

20 The levels of distal resection of 172 consecutive cases are shown.

20

Preparation of the rectum

With the usual level of transection in the upper one-third of the rectum, the presacral space is dissected, but not completely to the tip of the coccyx. The peritoneum lateral to the rectum is usually incised and a variable division of lateral ligaments of the rectum performed. At the selected level the mesorectum is divided transversely between artery forceps. The left forefinger and thumb are used to feel the wall of the rectum and 'pinch' the mesentery safely away from the intestine to allow safe application of the forceps. As this posterolateral clearing of the rectum occurs, the released rectal wall stretches to reveal at least 2 cm of 'bare' rectum suitable for anastomosis.

21 A right-angled rectal clamp is applied to the proximal part of the bare rectal wall (from right to left). The rectum is thoroughly irrigated through the anus with a rectal catheter through a proctoscope. The water is delivered by hand pump or large syringe to allow meticulous cleansing of all faecal debris, which is vital to the technique of circular stapling through the anus.

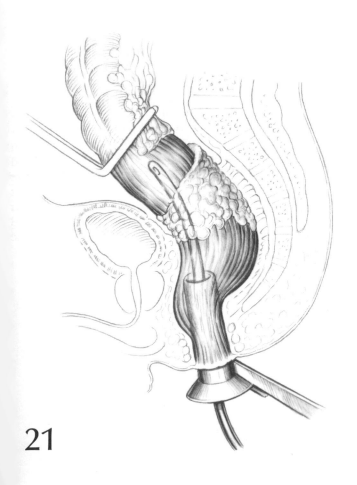

21

22 The purse-string clamp is applied right to left and used in 99% of patients to insert the purse-string in the wall of the rectum.

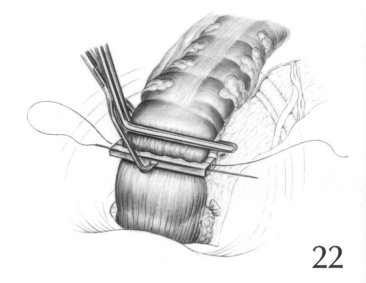

22

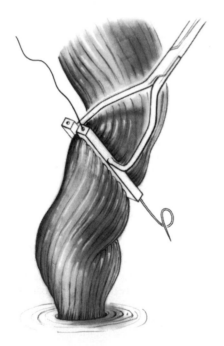

23

23 This manoeuvre is more difficult if the transection level is extraperitoneal, but it is achieved by rotating the rectum anticlockwise and angling the right side of the clamp upwards. Bending the soft needle as it emerges from the clamp on the left side overcomes any further difficulty.

The rectum is divided 3–4 mm above the purse-string clamp, and the specimen is removed. Before the purse-string clamp is removed, a Foss–Eisenberg non-crushing right-angled clamp is placed to control the rectum and stop bleeding from the cut edge. At least eight silk stay sutures are inserted and tied to trap the purse-string suture, to improve its function and to assist in control of the rectal stump.

Specific recommendations on stapling technique

Not all the details of the technique of circular stapling are described here, but certain important points are emphasized, of which some are specifically important in treating diverticular disease. For example, spare anvil heads in various sizes should be available to test the diameter of the colon so that the appropriate stapler will be selected, and hyoscine butylbromide, 20 mg given at least 5 min before the insertion of the stapler, is effective in overcoming spasm in the colon and rectum. The diameter of the stapler is not related to postoperative narrowing of the anastomosis, and there is no need to 'stretch' the intestine excessively to fit a larger size of stapler. In addition, the perineal operator should examine the anal canal and gently dilate it if there is stenosis sufficient to obstruct the stapler.

24 The abdominal operator should insert the right forefinger into the cleansed rectal stump to guide the stapler through a tight anal canal and to prevent any sudden thrust against the rectal wall.

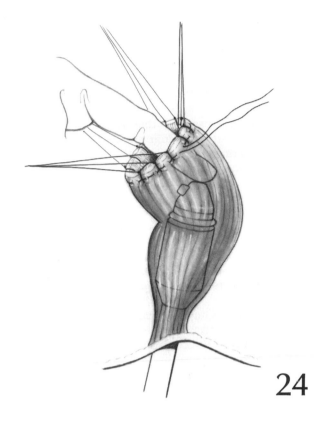

24

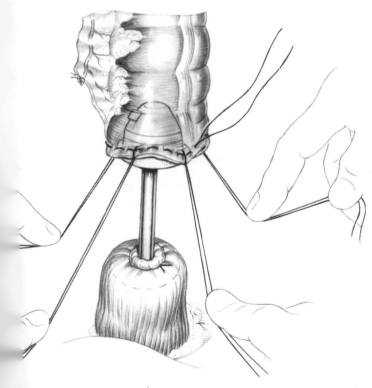

25

25 The detachable anvil head has greatly facilitated safe insertion into the colon, but if not available then the technique shown is recommended, using the stay sutures to 'see-saw' the colon gently over the anvil.

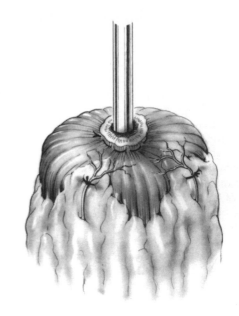

26 Significant arteries that lie over the edge of the anvil or the cartridge should be underrun with a 3/0 polyglactin suture, as they may cause significant postoperative bleeding or haematomas in the anastomosis.

It is specifically important in diverticular disease that, in the final stages of approximation of the cartridge or anvil, two or three pauses in the compression are necessary to allow the fluid to be squeezed from the compressed muscle; muscle damage may otherwise occur and the taenia may evert and escape the line of the staples.

The author has no experience with or enthusiasm for using the 'stab' technique in the closed rectal stump after a Hartmann resection and prefers to dissect out the rectum to obtain healthy and supple rectal wall for anastomosis.

26

Colovesical fistula

The management of a colovesical fistula is principally that of the diseased colon with all its implications. The fistula in the bladder wall is usually not a difficult technical problem and may not be identifiable. The operation is usually performed in the chronic phase of diverticulitis, and a preliminary colostomy followed by a second-stage resection is usually unnecessary. Blunt digital dissection will usually separate the colon from the bladder and if a small defect is noted in the vault of the bladder (usual site) it may, in some instances, be closed with a single layer of 2/0 polyglactin suture. On rare occasions a larger defect in the bladder wall is present with fibrotic margins, and in these circumstances excision of the defect in the wall of the bladder is preferable with a two-layer closure: the inner (mucosal) layer with continuous 2/0 plain catgut and an outer (mucosal) layer with interrupted 2/0 polyglactin sutures. It is important to separate the bladder repair from the colorectal anastomosis, particularly in the presence of chronic residual pelvic granulation tissue which could subsequently suppurate. If omentum is available, it can be placed between the intestinal anastomosis and the bladder. The use of the prolonged pelvic drainage technique (*see Table 1*) will prevent the sequence of sepsis—anastomotic defect and possible anastomotic—vesical fistula.

The indications for a complementary proximal stoma are those referred to when resecting diverticulitis and are not specifically related to the problem of the colovesical fistula (*see* below).

The bladder is drained with a urethral catheter, during which time urinary drainage is checked to ensure blockage of the catheter does not go undetected. It is in this circumstance that use of the new smaller suprapubic catheters may be preferable to drainage with a urethral catheter. Whichever method is used, the bladder should be drained for 10 days.

Drains

Anastomotic drains, as such, are not used. Presacral drains, in a fully dissected presacral space, remain of unproven value, even though they are often used in the belief that they may prevent secondary pelvic sepsis, which may damage the anastomosis. Presacral drains are certainly useful if optimal haemostasis in the pelvis is difficult to achieve.

27 Prolonged drainage at the site of a chronic abscess (the inflammatory 'nest' of Turnbull) is important. It is indicated if the parietal walls/floor of the abscess cannot be excised (even though the granulation tissue may be cleaned by curettage). This focus, if not controlled by drainage, will form a secondary abscess and damage the anastomosis. It may also take a long period to resolve. The principle is to convert the infected site to the dimension of the drain with carefully balanced, continuous irrigation—suction until a well established channel exists around the drains. The regimen is shown in *Table 1*.

Table 1   Prolonged pelvic drainage

Day	Irrigation with saline via 12-Fr Nelaton catheter*	Suction via a 20-Fr Ventrol sump drain†
1	6 l/24 h	−80 mmHg
2–10	1 l/24 h	−80 mmHg
11	Remove	Remove

*Indoplast Pty Ltd, Sydney, Australia; †Mallinckrodt, Athlone, Ireland.

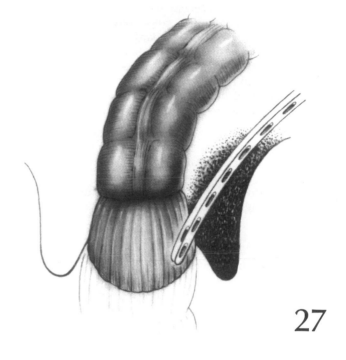

27

28 On day 11 the two drains are replaced with one Nelaton catheter which is used for the sinogram. This usually shows the optimum size of track, which signifies that the previously infected pelvic space has been 'neutralized'. The drain can be gradually removed over the next 5 days. This technique has enabled anastomoses to be performed in the presence of a chronic pelvic abscess and has practically eliminated the Hartmann operation as an elective procedure.

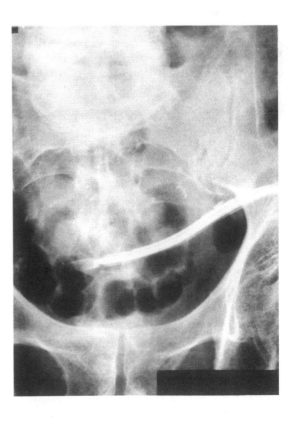

28

Indications for a proximal stoma

If the above criteria are used to select the proximal and distal ends of intestine for anastomosis, the use of a proximal stoma at the time of operation will be minimal. Currently, the author uses a proximal stoma in fewer than 10% of cases. In recent years, preference for a loop ileostomy instead of a loop colostomy has developed in association with higher standards of stomal management. In the event of a long-term stoma being necessary, the loop ileostomy is associated with a lower incidence of prolapse and hernia.

The following indications may each, or in combination, be reasons for performing a proximal stoma:

1. Technical problems with the anastomosis, such as muscle separation, tearing or haematomas, or demonstrated leaks that cannot be overcome satisfactorily by supporting sutures.
2. Poor blood supply to the colon or rectum despite all care having been taken with vascular preparation.
3. Thickened and oedematous wall as a result of pre-existing large intestinal obstruction.
4. Residual inflammatory changes in the rectum near the anastomosis which may not be resectable for some reason.
5. A combination of factors such as poor general health, prolonged and complex operation, and significant blood loss.

Postoperative care

Intravenous therapy usually continues for 7 days. Nasogastric intubation and aspiration are not used routinely, but they are used promptly if indicated by intense nausea, hiccoughs, abdominal distension, or vomiting. This approach is used in 30–40% of patients. Oral feeding is usually not commenced until the seventh day. The urethral catheter is removed on the fourth day. If a loop ileostomy is present, the plastic rod under the loop is removed on the tenth day.

As part of an ongoing study on anastomotic healing, the author routinely has the anastomosis assessed by a limited Gastrografin enema 10–12 days after surgery. A small catheter must be used, and no pressure can be generated in the rectum during the injection of contrast material as anastomotic disruption might occur. Specific instruction must be agreed by the radiologist for this investigation or, alternatively, the surgeon or surgical assistant should conduct the test. Although not necessarily recommended as routine postoperative monitoring it is wise to carry out at least this investigation before an operation to close a proximal stoma.

Complications

Postoperative complications are those that might follow any resection of the left colon and rectum. Secondary sepsis related to the chronic infected focus may occur if prolonged drainage is mismanaged. If a septic focus does occur, it may be possible to drain it by a CT-guided catheter, but in some instances it will still take a long time to resolve.

Outcome

Since the strict insistence on the use of a normal rectal segment for the anastomosis to avoid any inflammatory change in the intestinal wall, the author's anastomotic leakage rate has beome insignificant. On occasion, the upper rectum at the sacral promontory becomes involved in the inflammatory process because of contiguous inflammation in the sigmoid colon, and under these circumstances the extraperitoneal middle one-third of the rectal segment or below may be required for the anastomosis. In 109 consecutive stapled anastomoses for elective resections of diverticular disease, two (1.8%) minor leaks have occurred, which have only been detected on routine postoperative contrast radiography.

Illustrations by Gillian Lee and Paul Richardson

Colonic surgery for acute conditions: perforated diverticular disease

J. M. Sackier MB, FRCS
Associate Professor of Surgery, University of California, San Diego, California, USA

History

Colonic diverticula are acquired pulsion herniations consisting of mucosa and submucosa which occur at the small openings for nutrient vessel entry most commonly found on the antimesenteric border of the bowel[1]. The most frequent site for occurrence is the sigmoid colon but, in reducing order of frequency, they are also found in the descending, transverse and ascending colon.

Occasionally a giant diverticulum may be found alongside the sigmoid colon, but this is rare. The disease is extremely common and is found in approximately 10% of adults in the western world by the age of 40 years and in 65% by 80 years of age. Most diverticulosis is asymptomatic and acute perforations may be the first presentation.

Classification

The choice of treatment largely depends upon the extent of the disease at the time of presentation. The classification proposed by Hinchey and colleagues[2] is of value.

1a–d

Stage 1:   a pericolic abscess confined by the mesentery.

Stage 2:   a pelvic abscess caused by local perforation of a pericolic abscess.

Stage 3:   peritonitis resulting from rupture of a pericolic or pelvic abscess into the general peritoneal cavity. There is no communication between the lumen of the bowel and the abscess cavity because of obliteration of the neck of the diverticulum by the inflammatory process. This is also known as acute noncommunicating diverticulitis.

Stage 4:   faecal peritonitis resulting from free perforation of the diverticulum. This usually develops rapidly and is also known as acute communicating diverticulitis.

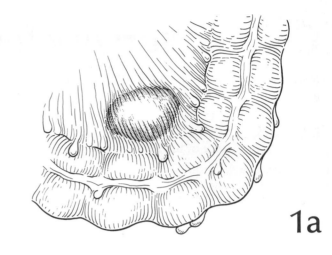

1a

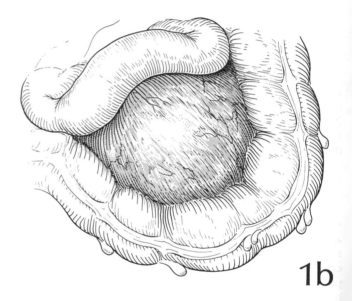

1b

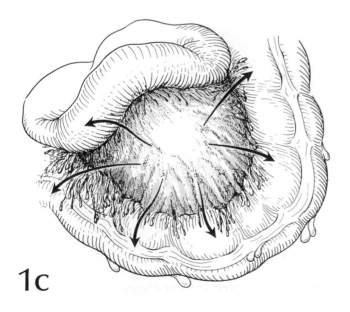

1c

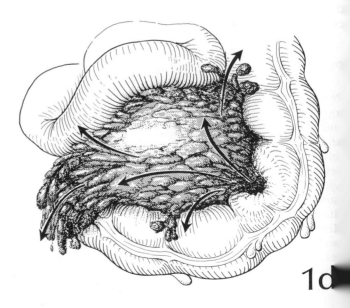

1d

Preoperative

Assessment

Patients who present with acute diverticular disease should be admitted to hospital for resuscitation, conservative treatment and the establishment of a more specific diagnosis.

Initial investigations should include a full blood count, and assessment of the function of the kidneys, heart and lungs. If cardiac disease is present, it may be necessary, if the patient is in an unstable haemodynamic state, to use a Swan-Ganz catheter to help manage cardiopulmonary function. Radiographic films of the chest and abdomen (erect and supine) are required. The most accurate test to stage the disease is the abdominal computed tomography (CT) scan, which can differentiate a bowel phlegmon, local abscess and free perforation.

Barium enema should be avoided because of the risk of perforation, producing a barium peritonitis which may be life-threatening. If a contrast study is thought necessary, a water-soluble medium should be used. Endoscopy is usually unhelpful because it is difficult to negotiate a tortuous and inflamed sigmoid colon. However, it may be of some value to see an unbreached mucosa which can help to differentiate acute perforated diverticulitis from a perforated carcinoma.

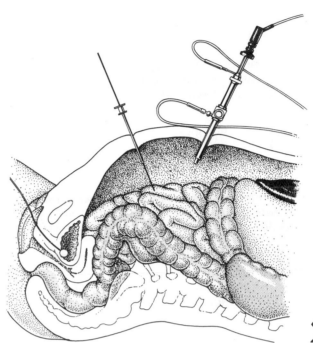

2

2 Occasionally it may be difficult to reach a firm preoperative diagnosis, especially in the elderly or rotund patient. In this circumstance, diagnostic laparoscopy may be useful. If free pus or faeces is seen, then the patient requires immediate laparotomy. Patients who have a localized peridiverticulitis can avoid open surgery. A unilocular abscess can be drained under direct vision as an alternative to drainage under CT control.

Preparation

Preoperative resuscitation and treatment are instituted together in the form of intravenous fluids, antibiotics and no oral intake. Nasogastric intubation is usually unnecessary and merely adds to the patient's discomfort. If, at the time of CT scan a localized abscess with defined walls is identified, it may be treated initially with percutaneous drainage under radiological guidance. This may avoid an emergency operation, although a high percentage of patients will require later elective resection. Although many of these patients are moderately sick, some (particularly the elderly) may need vigorous resuscitation and cardiopulmonary support aided by a Swan-Ganz catheter. Occasionally, perforated diverticulitis may present with fasciitis of the

abdominal wall or the thigh. This complication may be associated with a gas-forming organism and is an indication for early surgery and wide debridement of the area. Occasionally, further early surgery is required for excision of the fasciitis. More usually, and apart from the obvious free perforation or ruptured pericolic abscess, the indication for surgery is failure to improve on maximum medical therapy 24–48 h after admission to hospital.

Anaesthesia

General anaesthesia with endotracheal intubation is required. Regional spinal anaesthesia adds unnecessarily to the time taken for the surgery but can be used.

Position of patient

The patient is positioned supine on the operating table with the legs in stirrups. This position distributes the assistants around the operating table and provides access to the perineum to irrigate the rectum, to use an end-to-end stapling machine, and occasionally to allow for a cystoscopy to place ureteric stents. The abdomen and perineum are prepared and draped.

Selection of operative procedure

The choice of surgical procedure will depend not only on the extent of disease, but on the experience of the surgeon, the clinical condition of the patient before and during the operation, and the severity of coexisting disease. For instance, the surgeon confident and skilled in techniques of primary anastomosis may choose to perform a Hartmann's procedure in a patient who becomes unstable during surgery or for patients who are on steroids because of the high incidence of anastomotic breakdown under these circumstances.

3a–f The full spectrum of surgical choices is as follows.

1. Proximal diverting colostomy and placement of drains (*Illustration 3a*).
2. Bowel exteriorization (von Mikulicz operation, *Illustration 3b*) – of historical interest only.
3. Resection with colostomy and mucous fistula (*Illustration 3c*).
4. Resection with colostomy and Hartmann's pouch (*Illustration 3d*).
5. Resection and primary anastomosis with or without proximal defunctioning stoma (*Illustrations 3e, f*).

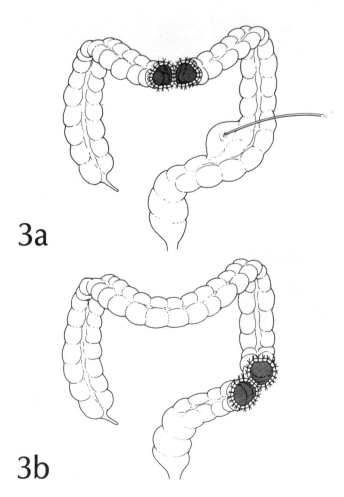

3a

3b

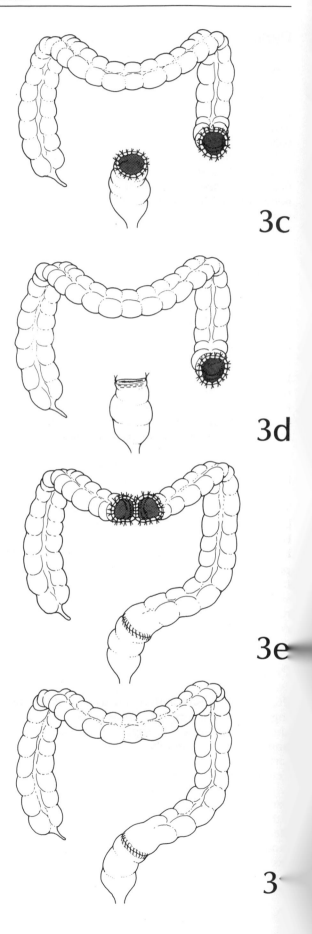

3c

3d

3e

3

Proximal diverting colostomy and placement of drains

At one time this was standard therapy for the treatment of perforated diverticular disease which was supplemented with local suture plication if a hole was seen in the intestinal wall. However, over the past 20 years it has become accepted that this is inadequate therapy because stool located between the site of the stoma and the intestinal perforation will frequently continue to emerge into the peritoneal cavity resulting in an expected high mortality rate. However if, at the time of abdominal exploration, an acute phlegmonous diverticulitis is found *without* free perforation or abscess formation, local irrigation of the inflamed area (with or without local drains and with or without a defunctioning proximal loop stoma) has been reported to be associated with a good outcome. Under adverse conditions, an inexperienced surgeon might treat free perforation of the intestine with vigorous intraperitoneal irrigation, proximal stoma and local perforation closure using an absorbable synthetic suture material buttressed with omentum. Such a procedure should be seen as a temporary measure until such time as the patient can be transferred for more definitive therapy or the availability of a more experienced surgeon. Preferably, a fully trained surgeon should proceed to one of the excisional techniques described below for the treatment of perforated diverticular disease.

Resection with colostomy and mucous fistula

This procedure results in the removal of the diseased bowel but gives the patient two stomas to manage. The benefit of a mucous fistula is that bowel reconstruction is somewhat easier than after a Hartmann procedure.

Resection with Hartmann's pouch

When there is an insufficient length of distal colon to bring to the abdominal wall, the bowel may be closed as a Hartmann's pouch with either sutures or staples. The stump should then be secured to the sacral promontory with non-absorbable sutures to prevent it from descending into the pelvis and to facilitate subsequent bowel reconstruction. The second operation to reconstruct the bowel is often a difficult procedure because of small intestine adhesions in the pelvis which obscure the Hartmann's pouch. These adhesions tend to resolve with time; therefore a 16–20-week waiting period is recommended before the second operation. The commonly experienced difficulties with intestinal reconstruction after the Hartmann procedure and its associated morbidity and mortality rates should be borne in mind when contemplating the optimum procedure for each individual patient.

Resection with primary anastomosis

Resection of the diseased bowel to include the rectosigmoid junction followed by immediate bowel anastomosis is a controversial recommendation. The belief that an anastomosis in the presence of peritonitis may lead to a higher incidence of anastomotic failure has dissuaded many surgeons from performing this procedure. However, experience has shown that the overall morbidity and mortality rates from 'staged' procedures are as high or even higher than from a carefully planned and executed single-stage operation. Furthermore, if the surgeon is unsure about the security of the anastomosis, a proximal stoma (loop colostomy or loop ileostomy) is an additional safeguard which is relatively simple to reverse at a later date. Two developments have made the operative approach safer: first, 'on-table' orthograde colonic lavage[3,4], and second, the intraluminal bypass tube[5] (Coloshield).

Operations

COLOSTOMY WITH DRAINAGE

A lower midline incision is made and the diagnosis of a localized abscess is confirmed. If frank peritonitis or faecal soiling is found, bowel resection is then the preferred treatment.

4 The abscess is usually located in the mesentery or between the mesentery and lateral abdominal wall. Gentle blunt dissection with the operating finger placed in a gauze swab, working downwards from the abdominal wall, will allow the cavity to be entered. Soft Penrose drains should be placed and brought out laterally with as straight a tract as possible to facilitate drainage.

The adjacent small bowel may adhere to the mass and should be gently separated away, taking care not to injure the serosa of the bowel.

In placing the colostomy (*see* chapter on pp. 658–667) the surgeon should remember that the greater the distance from the distal limb to the perforation, the more faecal material can leak; however, placing the colostomy close to the perforation may render subsequent resection difficult.

On rare occasions it may be considered safer to close a perforation with interrupted, absorbable synthetic sutures as a temporary measure. Great care is necessary because the tissues are friable and the perforation may be enlarged, which would then mandate intestinal resection.

RESECTION WITH COLOSTOMY AND MUCOUS FISTULA

A lower midline incision is made and extended above the umbilicus as required. The patient is placed in a head-down position and rotated towards the right so that the small intestine drops away from the operative field. Once the small intestine has been carefully dissected free of the mass, it is placed in warm moist packs. The sigmoid colon is gently manually retracted towards the midline to expose the fascial layer of Toldt, which is incised, taking great care to note the gonadal vessels and ureter, which may be palpated and visualized as it lies over the iliac vessels.

The colon should be palpated above until normal bowel is felt. To prevent further faecal soiling, a soft clamp should be placed across the bowel at this point; this will form the proximal line of resection.

The distal dissection should be carried down towards the peritoneal reflection beyond the diseased bowel at the top of the rectum.

If there is any concern about the presence of malignant disease, a cancer operation should be performed. The distal margin is defined and clamps are

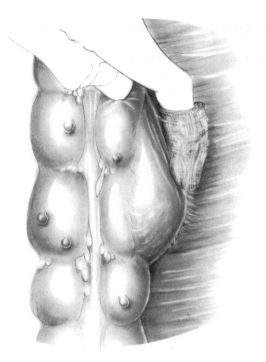

4

placed at the resection margin in the upper rectum. The vessels may be secured and divided close to the intestine when the surgeon is certain that a malignancy is not present. However, in practice this is difficult because the mesentery tends to be oedematous and thickened and it is usually technically easier to locate and divide the vessels towards the base of the mesentery.

It will usually be necessary to mobilize the splenic flexure to provide sufficient length to fashion an anastomosis without tension, but great care should be taken to avoid splenic injury. The intestine may be divided using the GIA stapling device and this renders it easier to draw the proximal colon through the circular incision for the colostomy.

Once the specimen has been resected, the abdomen should be copiously lavaged and the site of the colostomy in the abdominal wall should be chosen. Ideally this should be along a line joining the anterior superior iliac spine with the umbilicus, but the state of the patient's abdomen and previous scars and skin creases may dictate otherwise (*see* chapter on pp. 658–667).

The closed distal intestine is brought out of the lower end of the wound and secured to the skin. The abdomen is then closed in layers. Once the main wound has been covered, the colostomy is sutured with interrupted mucocutaneous sutures of chromic catgut.

If there is gross peritoneal soiling, a delayed primary closure of the skin may be used by inserting a series of interrupted, loosely tied sutures to the skin and interposing this with a ribbon gauze soaked with povidone-iodine. The ribbon gauze is changed twice daily by the nursing staff. If the wound is clean at 3 days the pack may be removed and the sutures tightened.

HARTMANN'S PROCEDURE

5 The operation is carried out as described in the previous section; however, if the distal bowel is too short to be brought out as a mucous fistula, the upper rectum may be closed as a Hartmann's pouch with a transverse stapling device or by suture. The pouch should then be secured to the sacral promontory with two large silk sutures to prevent the upper rectum from falling into the pelvis, becoming kinked (which may result in a small closed loop bowel obstruction), and to facilitate finding the rectal stump at a subsequent operation. It is unnecessary to place drains into the pelvis.

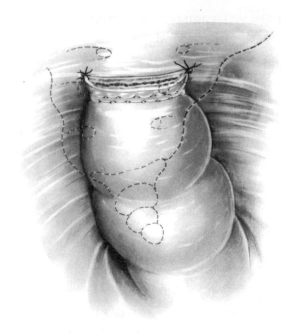

5

RESECTION WITH PRIMARY ANASTOMOSIS AND PROXIMAL COLOSTOMY

During this operation it is necessary to locate healthy intestine with minimally thickened muscle, and splenic flexure mobilization is usually required to achieve this objective. However, splenic flexure mobilization should not be attempted in the unstable patient or by the inexperienced surgeon.

6 The anastomotic technique should be the surgeon's preference. The author uses an interrupted single layer of inverting sutures with absorbable synthetic material (2/0 polygycolic acid). The usual tenets of colonic anastomosis must be strictly adhered to: there must be no anastomotic tension (by mobilization of the splenic flexure); a good blood supply (pulsatile bleeding) should be present; and careful attention must be paid to the technical details of suture placement (*see* chapter on pp. 528–550). It is useful in this circumstance to place the sutures in guy-rope fashion and run them down in groups once the posterior layer has been completed.

If the pelvis is narrow, the surgeon may choose to use a stapled anastomosis, but the ends of the intestine tend to be sufficiently thickened that concern for staple penetration through the intestinal wall may be justified.

A right-sided proximal transverse colostomy is then raised, which should be reversed at about 6 weeks after operation once a contrast study demonstrates anastomotic integrity. The use of drains should be avoided.

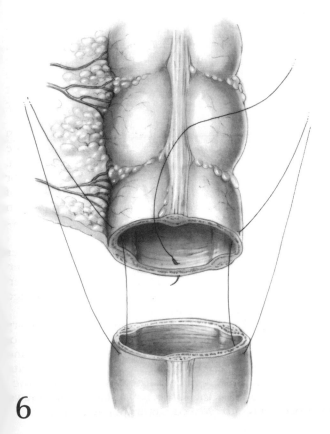

6

RESECTION WITH PRIMARY ANASTOMOSIS WITH NO COLOSTOMY

As mentioned earlier, this is a challenging procedure for an experienced surgeon. Two recent developments may improve success: first, on-table colonic lavage (*see* chapter on pp. 727–745) and second, the intracolonic bypass tube.

Intracolonic bypass tube

This device has been demonstrated experimentally to be of value in reducing faecal soiling of the anastomosis and is associated with improved anastomotic healing. It has been used in colonic perforation[6] as an adjunct to primary anastomosis to avoid the need for a proximal defunctioning stoma.

7a, b After the diseased bowel has been removed, it is necessary to evert a cuff of approximately 4 cm of proximal colon. This is easier when there has been an element of obstruction which leads to proximal colonic dilatation. Four intraluminal stay sutures of silk are placed, and a gentle traction eversion is achieved. Babcock forceps may also be placed on the edge of the intestine and a section of proximal colon induced through this lip. If the intestine is very contracted, Hegar dilators can be used to widen it. The author has not found the administration of glucagon to be of value.

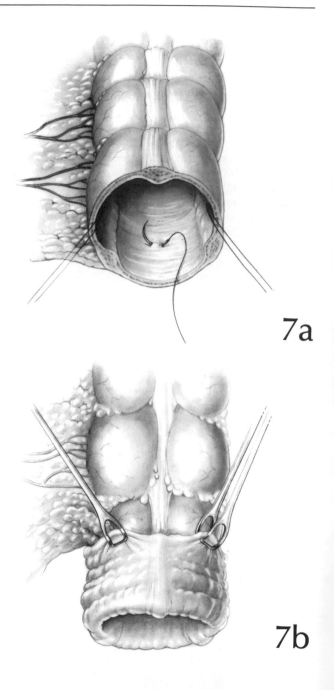

7a

7b

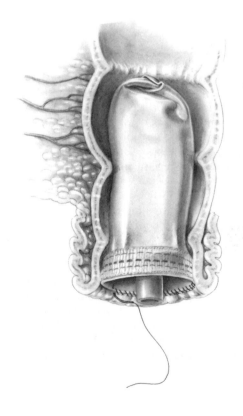

8

8 An appropriately sized intracolonic bypass tube is selected, always trying to use the largest available but without forcing the device into position. The tube is folded in parachute fashion and may be lubricated to ease insertion. If the intestine is very contracted, it is preferable to open the bypass tube so that the proximal polyester reinforcing band can be apposed directly to the inside of the lumen of the proximal bowel. The tube should be sutured to the proximal colon with a locking, running stitch of 2/0 polyglycolic acid, being sure to pick up mucosa and submucosa. There is a very definite feel to incorporating this latter bowel layer and some experience is required to recognize this sensation.

9 Once the tubocolonic anastomosis has been completed, it should be checked by trying to insert a pair of mosquito forceps in between the tube and the colon to look for gaps. If present, they should be closed with interrupted polyglycolic acid sutures.

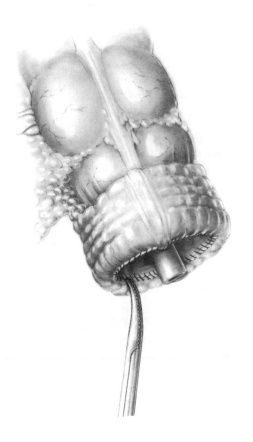

9

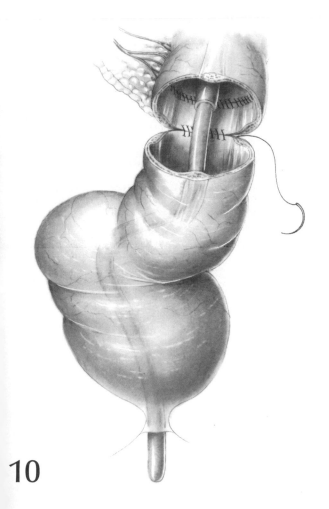

10

10 The everted cuff should now be returned to its previous position and the serosa of the colon checked for perforation of the tubocolonic anastomotic line. If present, a serosal horizontal mattress suture should be placed.

For a sutured anastomosis, the rectal probe is now attached to the intraluminal bypass tube; this is a useful 'handle' to lift up the intestine. The author prefers a single layer of interrupted inverting polyglycolic acid sutures and these are now placed. The rectal probe is then passed distally and retrieved at the anus by an unscrubbed assistant.

The tube can be unravelled at this juncture, but the author prefers to leave it in position because of the risk of perforating the tube with the anterior sutures.

The anterior layer of colorectal anastomotic sutures is now placed.

Traction on the rectal probe will lead the intraluminal bypass tube to unravel and come to lie across the anastomosis while providing for luminal continuity.

If the assistant gently pulls on the rectal probe, the surgeon will be able to feel the tubocolonic anastomosis and ensure that it is patent.

11 Once the mesenteric defect, peritoneal cavity and abdomen have been closed, the surgeon's attention should be directed to the perineum. Gentle traction should be placed on the tube and it should then be incised. A finger should be placed inside the lumen of the tube to ensure that the latex surfaces are not adherent so that faeces may pass. The tube may now be fully cut across and will then retract and come to lie within the rectal ampulla.

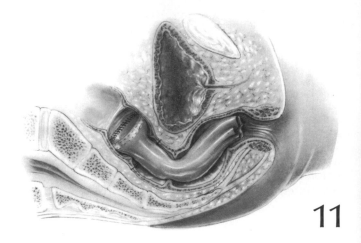

11

Postoperative care

Antibiotics should continue and be adjusted as indicated by the sensitivity of intraoperative cultures. Intravenous fluids should be administered according to metabolic need. The patient should ideally spend the first 24 h in the intensive care unit, as elderly patients are at great risk from the complications of septicaemia. A nasogastric tube is usually necessary and will have been placed during operation. The urinary catheter may be discontinued when the patient has achieved fluid balance and is alert enough to urinate. When the ileus resolves, the nasogastric tube may be spigotted and residual volumes taken. When these decrease, the nasogastric tube is removed, oral fluids are commenced and the patient can progress to a normal diet. For the patient with a colostomy, nursing care should be supplemented with psychological support.

References

1. Painter NS, Burkitt DP. Diverticular disease of the colon: a deficiency disease of Western civilization. *BMJ* 1971; 2: 450–4.

2. Hinchey EJ, Schaal PGH, Richards GK. Treatment of perforated diverticular disease of the colon. *Adv Surg* 1978; 12: 85–109.

3. Munro A, Steele RJC, Logie JRC. Technique for intra-operative colonic irrigation. *Br J Surg* 1987; 74: 1039–40.

4. Radcliffe AG, Dudley HAF. Intraoperative antegrade irrigation of the large intestine. *Surg Gynecol Obstet* 1983; 156: 721–3.

5. Ravo B. Colorectal anastomotic healing and intracolonic bypass procedure. *Surg Clin North Am* 1988; 68: 1267–94.

6. Ravo B, Mishrick A, Addei K, Gastrini G, Pappalardo G, Gross E. The treatment of perforated diverticulitis by one-stage intracolonic bypass procedure. *Surgery* 1987; 102: 771–6.

Illustrations by Gillian Lee

Colonic surgery for acute conditions: obstruction

L. P. Fielding MB, FRCS, FACS
Chief of Surgery, St Mary's Hospital, Waterbury, Connecticut, Clinical Professor of Surgery, Yale University School of Medicine, Connecticut, USA and Visiting Clinical Scientist, St Mary's Hospital, London, UK

Principles and justification

Large bowel obstruction is a relatively common complication of lesions in the colon and rectum, usually caused by a primary tumour. The discussion in this chapter will be centred on this aetiology, although the principles of mangement can be applied to any other cause of large gut obstruction. The two specific disease processes of toxic megacolon and volvulus are discussed in other chapters (*see* pp. 750–765). One of the problems about discussing the relative merits of different methods of treatment of intestinal obstruction is that there is no clear definition of the condition. It seems reasonable, therefore, to divide the subject into three subsections: (1) bowel stenosis resulting in faecal loading but without obstruction to intestinal gas; (2) complete obstruction to the onward flow of faecal matter, fluid and gas, but without major systemic upset; and (3) the addition of major systemic metabolic problems, usually caused by longstanding obstruction with or without bowel perforation.

The implications for therapy of these three subsets of large bowel obstruction will be discussed at the relevant points during the chapter. In a survey[1] which reviewed the clinical practice of 84 surgeons, it was clear that there was a spectrum of methods employed to treat these conditions. However, the overall figures indicated that immediate tumour resection (with or without bowel reconstruction) was practised more frequently at all sites than the method of bowel decompression followed at a later date, by tumour resection (staged resection): right colon 96%; splenic flexure 75%; left colon 55%. Over the last 10 years the trend towards immediate resection, even for left-sided obstructing colonic tumours, appears to have increased. Thus, at each site primary tumour excision will be described first and a staged procedure will be described as an alternative method of treatment.

Preoperative

General assessment of patient on admission

1   The severity of clinical illness suffered by patients with intestinal obstruction is very variable, ranging from the patient with colicky abdominal pain alone to a severely ill person with gross systemic and metabolic derangement associated with multiorgan failure. It is worthwhile, therefore, to review systematically all principal body systems, obtain baseline information on each and be prepared to monitor the function of all. In particular, in haemodynamically unstable patients, a Swan–Ganz catheter is necessary to assess cardiac function and provide fluid resuscitation to establish maximal cardiac output without central overload. Pulmonary and renal function need to be reviewed and supported. This will generate a large volume of information which should be integrated by an experienced surgeon and the most ill patients should be placed in the critical care unit. It seems that the key to good results is the presence and active participation of a senior and interested surgeon at *all* stages of management.

Anaesthesia

It is usual for these patients to have general inhalation anaesthesia with muscle relaxants and positive pressure ventilation. Some anaesthetists will include as part of their technique an epidural or spinal anaesthetic, which will reduce the need for muscle relaxant drugs and their reversal. The latter techniques improve the operative field, reduce blood loss and assist with immediate postoperative pain control.

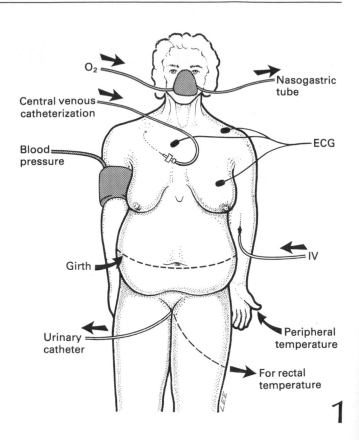

1

Operations

Position of patient

2   It is useful to place the patient in the lithotomy-Trendelenburg position with Allen stirrups, which allows an approach to be made to the anal canal during surgery and places a second surgical assistant in a position to be of greater help than when the patient is in the simple supine position (*see Illustration 3* on page 48). However, this operative set-up does have its disadvantages in that it is somewhat more difficult for the instrument nurse to see the operative field (and therefore to assist the surgeon), and the anaesthetist will need to make special arrangements to maintain access to the patient's head and shoulders.

The essential features of the position are that there should be a small sandbag under the sacrum, which should be sited at the end of the table proper (the bottom leaf of the table should be removed), and that the legs are in the stirrups, which are also level with the end of the table. This allows the legs to be raised, but the hip joint is abducted then flexed to a *minimal* degree. A large neurosurgical type of overtable is placed above the head end of the operating area. Once this position has been achieved, the patient is catheterized, placed in 15° head-down tilt, cleansed and draped.

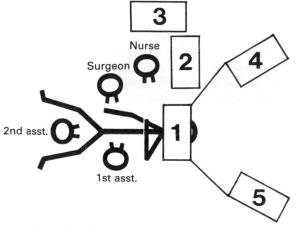

1, overhead table; 2, instrument trolley; 3, instrument trolley; 4, anaesthetic machine; 5, anaesthetic table

2

Abdominal incision

3 Assuming that the object of therapy is to carry out a primary tumour resection, a long midline incision skirting the umbilicus is made at the very start of the procedure. The incision should extend from the pubic skin crease to two-thirds of the way between the umbilicus and xiphisternum. In patients with gross intestinal obstruction and obesity, a full length pubis to xiphisternum incision should be carried out.

Some surgeons may disagree with an immediate tumour resection and wish to fashion a so-called 'decompressive loop transverse colostomy', in which case a modest-sized left paramedian incision or a midline incision is carried out to preserve the upper right quadrant for the stoma.

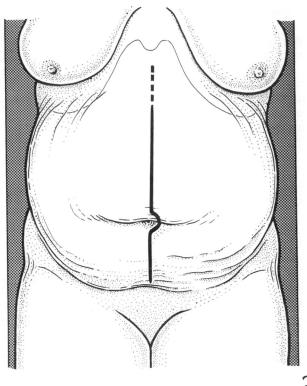

3

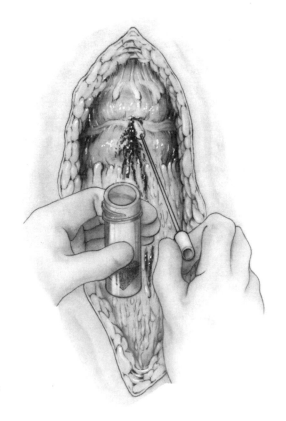

4

Bacteriology

4 Once the abdomen is opened there is always some free fluid present, some of which should be placed in a sterile screw-capped pot and sent for aerobic and anaerobic culture.

Bowel decompression

Once the abdomen has been opened, irrespective of the site of the obstructing lesion, the next procedure is to deflate the distended bowel, which will allow greater access to the abdominal cavity and reduce the risk of intestinal perforation. The caecum is inspected to make sure a perforation has neither taken place nor is imminent. Assuming that the caecum is undamaged three techniques are described that can be used singly or in combination.

Needle aspiration

5   A 14-gauge intravenous needle is attached to the sucker system and passed obliquely through a taenia coli into the lumen of the transverse colon. Care is taken to keep the tip of the needle within the luminal gas rather than the fluid content because if the needle touches fluid faeces it immediately becomes blocked. Gas can be transferred from the remainder of the bowel to the transverse colon by applying pressure in both flanks simultaneously.

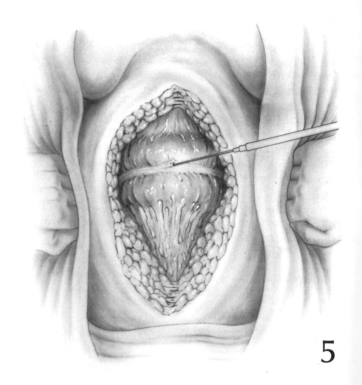

5

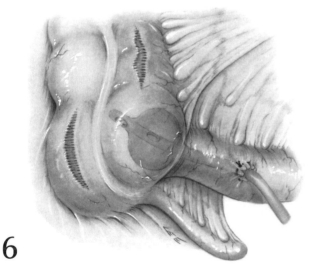

6

Foley catheter decompression

6   It is frequently found that simple needle aspiration alone is not adequate to decompress the right side of the colon. This can be achieved by passing a large Foley catheter through a purse-string placed in the distal ileum, through the ileocaecal valve and then on into the colon. Gentle intermittent suction on the catheter will eventually allow considerable quantities of liquid faeces to be aspirated, thus decompressing the bowel

An alternative site of access to the bowel for the Foley catheter is the appendix stump. However, this site may be more prone to leakage.

Small bowel decompression

7 In patients with an incompetent ileocaecal valve (or as a secondary phenomenon to adherence to a tumour) the small bowel itself is frequently found to be distended. If this occurs in the distal small bowel, fluid may be 'milked' into the caecum and then aspirated through the Foley catheter (*see Illustration 6*). When the upper part of the small intestine is affected, gas and fluid may be 'stripped' back through the pylorus into the stomach and then aspirated through a large nasogastric tube.

It must be noted at this point that if a segment of small bowel is attached to the primary tumour or if a lymph node with secondary tumour is present the small bowel must *not* be 'peeled-off' but must be resected *en bloc* with the tumour and then the bowel reconstructed. This is a basic concept in surgery for tumours and if it is not observed the surgeon can expect to find a cluster of intraperitoneal secondary deposits occurring 9–18 months after tumour resection. Once the bowel has been decompressed, a full laparotomy is possible.

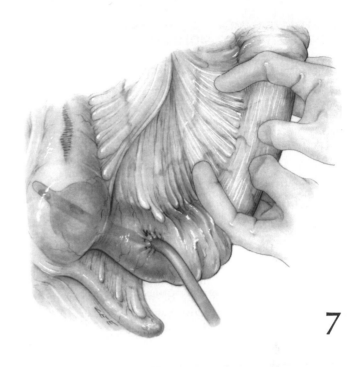

7

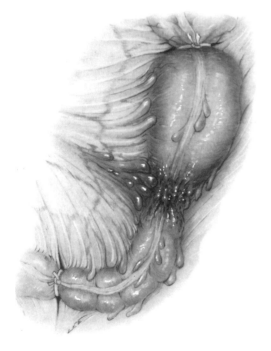

8

Laparotomy findings

8 First, the nature of the obstructing lesion should be sought and, if it is a tumour, some assessment of its mobility should be made gently at this stage of the operation. Sites of secondary spread to the peritoneum or liver are sought and then a systematic laparotomy is carried out.

Assuming that the tumour is considered removable, tapes are tied around the bowel both proximal and distal to the obstructing tumour to prevent intraluminal spread of malignant cells. The remaining small and large bowel are packed away into the abdominal cavity or may be exteriorized into a plastic bag.

Once the large and small bowel have been completely decompressed, resective surgery can continue as for the elective case.

IMMEDIATE TUMOUR RESECTION FOR OBSTRUCTING LEFT-SIDED COLONIC LESIONS

The mobilization of a left-sided tumour may be divided into six basic phases:

Phase 1: division of arterial supply and venous drainage and visualization of the left ureter.
Phase 2: mobilization of the left colon.
Phase 3: mobilization of the splenic flexure.
Phase 4: complete distal mobilization.
Phase 5: division of the bowel.
Phase 6: consideration of immediate anastomosis.

Phase 1: securing vascular supply

Depending on the bulk of the transverse colon and small bowel, it may be possible to pack these organs into the upper abdomen, or it may be necessary to place the small bowel in a plastic bag which can then be exteriorized on the abdominal wall.

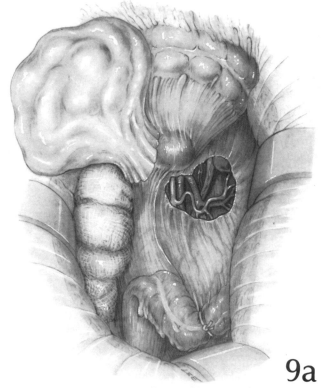

9a, b The aorta is displayed below the fourth part of the duodenum and, assuming that a radical resection is possible, the inferior mesenteric artery is divided at its origin from the aorta (for distal lesions, this vessel may be divided just distal to the ascending branch of the left colic). The mobilization of this part of the mesentery requires the control of small arteries and veins by electrocoagulation.

The dissection then moves 1.5–2 cm left and laterally where the inferior mesenteric vein is found running due 'north' to join the splenic vessel. This structure is divided according to the level of division of its sister artery.

9a

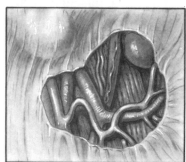

9b

10 As the mesentery is mobilized and lifted forward, the central portion of the left ureter must be identified and protected. The dissection is then carried laterally in front of the plane containing the ureter, continuing the mobilization of the bowel mesentery. The mesentery is divided at the site of bowel division. There should be at least 5 cm of normal-looking bowel between the tumour and the resection margins. There is usually more at the proximal resection site because this site is determined by the colour of the bowel after the required vessels have been divided – at least 5 cm must be removed proximal to the site at which the bowel colour changes from pink to blue.

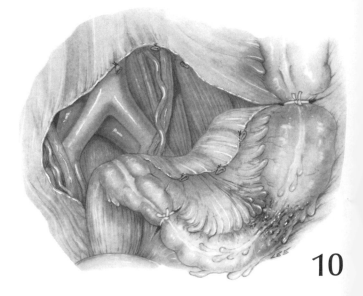

10

Phase 2: mobilization of the tumour

11 The colon is then lifted forward and to the patient's right; and the congenital adhesion of the sigmoid colon is divided revealing the ureter and iliac vessels. The peritoneum overlying the left paracolic gutter is similarly divided. There is usually a tendency for the gonadal vessels to be taken forward on to the specimen. If these structures are well away from any tumour and are not fixed or tethered, they may be swept posteriorly and preserved. If the tumour is at the rectosigmoid junction or in the upper rectum itself, the rectum will require mobilization (*see* chapter on pp. 766–781).

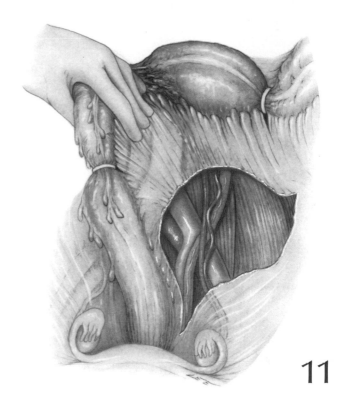

11

Phase 3: mobilization of the splenic flexure

In almost all radical left-sided resections it is necessary to mobilize the splenic flexure and this procedure is carried out in three separate stages. The surgeon should stand to the patient's right.

Posterior dissection

12 Having started to divide the peritoneal reflexion in the left paracolic gutter, the surgeon carries this incision in the peritoneum upwards towards the spleen. The colon itself is pulled across to the patient's right and with blunt dissection the mesentery to the colon is separated from perirenal fat. At this stage of the procedure it is very easy to go too far posteriorly and lift the kidney forward. This must be avoided because it leads into the wrong plane and also opens up, unnecessarily, a false plane.

12

13 Once the correct plane is achieved this tissue line is developed by blunt finger and gauze dissection until the surgeon's hand comes to lie behind the splenic flexure.

No attempt is made at this time to pull the colon down towards the pelvis because this may rupture small adhesions on the spleen itself.

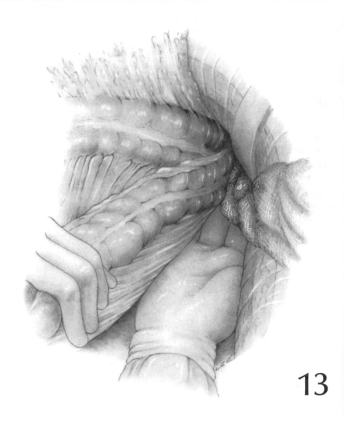

13

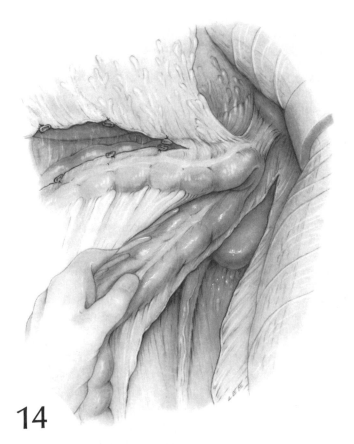

14

Anterior dissection: mobilization of the great omentum

14 If the lesion is distal the omentum may be dissected free from the 'bloodless plane' of the colon, gradually working towards the apex of the splenic flexure. Here again the transverse colon should not be pulled forcibly towards the midline for fear of splenic damage.

15 For more proximal lesions, when the left part of the omentum needs to be taken *en bloc* in a specimen, the great omentum is mobilized from the stomach by dividing the short vessels leading from the epiploic arch to the greater curve. When the short vessels from the splenic hilum are encountered, the left gastroepiploic vessel is divided and the dissection directed to the apex of the splenic flexure.

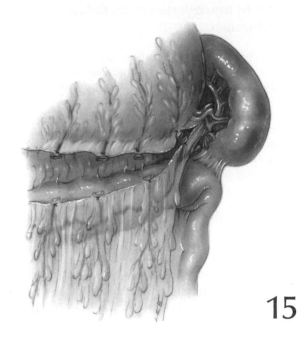

15

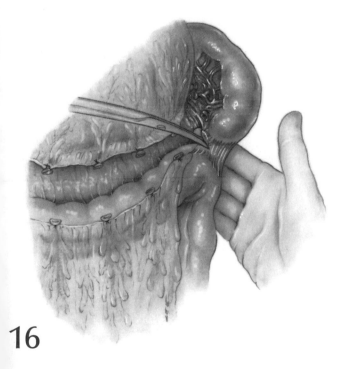

16

Release of splenic flexure

16 Having established the posterior and anterior parts of the dissection, the operator's right hand is placed behind the splenic flexure and, using long dissecting scissors with the left hand, the remaining attachment of the splenic flexure to the spleen is divided under direct vision. Sometimes vessels at this point need to be formally ligated.

For tumours near the splenic flexure, when direct invasion of the spleen or the tail of the pancreas may have occurred, the dissection follows the line between the left gastroepiploic vessels and the stomach but continues up, dividing the short gastric vessels. The peritoneum around the spleen is divided, mobilizing this structure, which can then be brought down with the tail of the pancreas to be taken *en bloc* with the resected specimen. The splenic vessels are divided. The pancreas is divided by traversing the gland with a knife and three structures will then need to be ligated separately – the superior and inferior pancreatic vessels and the pancreatic duct. It is usually possible then to suture the tail of the pancreas by interrupted sutures to complete its closure.

Phases 4 and 5

The mobilization of the distal colon is then completed to a point at least 5 cm distal to the tumour. The proximal and distal points of bowel transection are now ready to be divided before discarding the specimen.

Phase 6: immediate *versus* delayed anastomosis

At this point in the operation the surgeon must decide either to prepare for an immediate anastomosis or to delay this procedure to a second operation. If the patient is relatively fit, if the bowel is judged to be suitable to take sutures securely and if the surgeon is confident of achieving primary anastomotic union, the anastomosis is performed. If not, the anastomosis is delayed. The techniques involved in these two procedures will be discussed in turn.

'On-table' orthograde bowel lavage[2]

Before an anastomosis can be constructed safely the proximal bowel needs to be mechanically empty, which can be achieved by 'on-table' bowel lavage. A Foley catheter is inserted into the distal ileum as described for bowel decompression (*see Illustration 6*).

17, 18   A long length of presterilized anaesthetic scavenging tubing is attached very firmly, with a watertight fit, to a 10-cm long metal connector, which is inserted into the bowel, having discarded the specimen some 8 cm distal to the site of the eventual anastomosis. Packs need to be placed carefully around the area to catch any spillage and three tissue-holding (Babcock) forceps are placed on the edge of the bowel to aid the introduction of the anaesthetic tubing. Once the metal connector is in place, two strong nylon tapes are secured around the bowel, tying the colon to the metal tube.

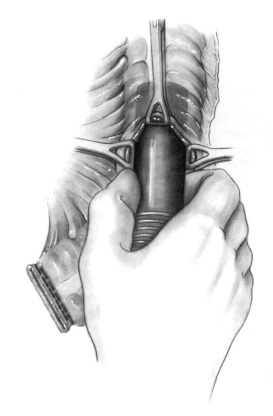

17

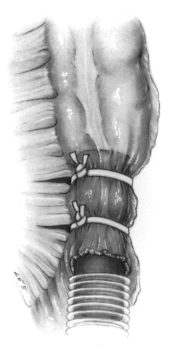

18

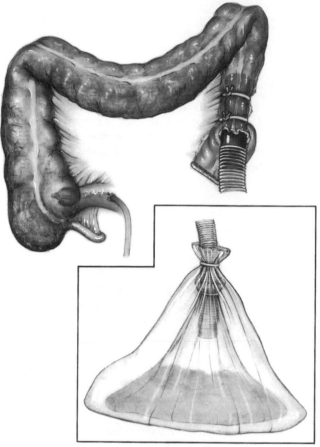

19 The distal end of the anaesthetic tubing is placed over the table and into two plastic bags, one inside the other, and tied on to the tubing to form a closed system. Physiological saline or Hartmann's solution, which must be warmed to body temperature to avoid cooling the patient, is then instilled into the proximal colon through the Foley catheter.

19

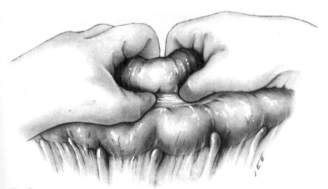

20 While this fluid is progressing through the colon, any faecal matter is broken down by finger pressure into pellets of not more than half the diameter of the anaesthetic scavenging tubing.

20

21a, b Blockage of the tubing by faeces will eventually cause extreme technical difficulty and result in faecal contamination of the peritoneal cavity. The irrigant fluid is helped around the colon by intermittent pressure on the ascending and transverse and (possibly) descending colon, so that no segment becomes over-distended.

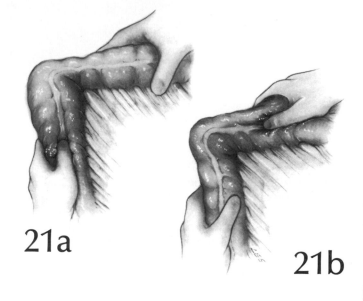

21a

21b

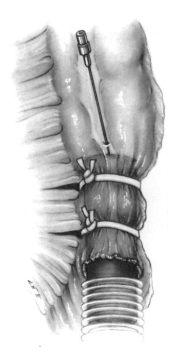

22

22 As fluid flows down the anaesthetic tubing, a negative pressure is produced, sucking the colon into the tubing. This can be avoided by placing a large intravenous hypodermic needle, which acts as a vent, through the proximal colon.

23 The procedure is continued until all faecal residue has been manipulated out of the colon and the effluent is running clear.

The distal (usually somewhat damaged) colon is then discarded, along with the anaesthetic tubing, at the site of anastomosis.

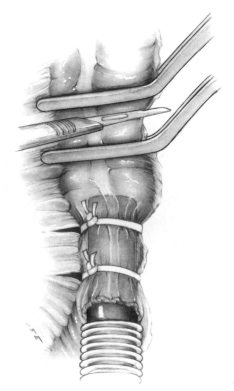

23

Cleansing of the distal segment

24 A proctoscope is passed into the anal canal and through it a large calibre (28 Fr) Foley catheter is inserted. Through the catheter physiological saline is introduced to wash the rectum and low sigmoid colon below the occluding clamp. At the end of this procedure the irrigant fluid is changed to mercury perchloride 1:500, which will prevent seeding of any residual malignant cells at the anastomotic site.

A second crushing clamp is placed distal to the first and the intervening short segment of colon is discarded. The anastomosis then proceeds and the author uses an open technique of one-layer, interrupted, musculosubmucosal sutures, 3–4 mm apart (*see* chapter on pp. 766–781). After the anastomosis, this area and the whole peritoneal cavity are extensively lavaged with warmed physiological saline containing tetracycline (1 g/l). If the anastomosis is below the peritoneal reflexion suction drains are placed anteriorly and posteriorly. These are removed on the second day postoperatively. The author does not use drains after an intra-abdominal anastomosis.

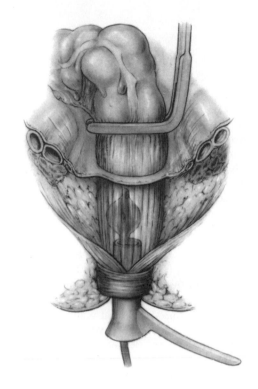

24

Techniques for delayed anastomosis

If the conditions to consider a primary anastomosis do not apply, the proximal colon should be brought out as an end-colostomy using the techniques described in the chapter on pp. 798–806. One modification of this technique which has been found useful after adequate bowel decompression is to bring the bowel out through the abdominal wall leaving the bowel closed for some 2–3 days to allow the bowel to adhere to its surroundings before being contaminated by faeces.

If the distal end of the bowel is not long enough to reach the anterior abdominal wall the rectum is irrigated as described above. The second crushing clamp is placed across the bowel after this irrigation and the intervening short segment of gut is gradually excised at the same time that the rectal stump is oversewn using the 'cut and stitch' method to prevent any rectal contents spilling into the pelvis. Alternatively, the rectal stump may be stapled closed with a TA 55 stapler.

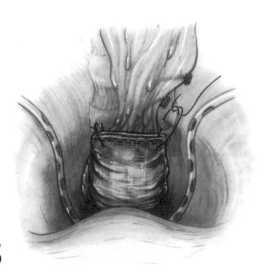

25 In order to avoid the rectum falling into the pelvis and becoming kinked, the apex of the rectal stump is sutured to the presacral fascia. This will assist in a subsequent operation if reconstruction is undertaken (*see* chapter on pp. 798–806).

Two suction drains are placed into the pelvis and removed when no further serosanguineous fluid is obtained.

25

26a, b If the distal bowel is long enough to reach the anterior abdominal wall, the distal bowel may be divided between crushing clamps of the Zachery–Cope design – the distal crushing element is not removed from the bowel, which is brought out through the lower end of the laparotomy incision. Sufficient length of bowel needs to be left so that a gauze dressing may be placed underneath this crushing clamp to raise it above the closed abdominal wound surface by about 2–3 cm.

The length of 'proud' bowel may be excised once it has become fixed into the wound (8–10 days) thus forming an open mucous fistula. The rectum itself should not be mobilized in order to make adequate length to bring to the abdominal wall as this opens up planes in the pelvis which may give rise to troublesome, and occasionally severe, pelvic sepsis. If there is not adequate length, it is better to close the distal bowel as a Hartmann's procedure (*see* above).

Before closing the abdomen, any site of tumour attachment or any possible peritoneal or liver secondary tumours should be biopsied so that adequate tumour staging can be obtained in consultation with the histopathologist.

An alternative method of handling the distal bowel is to divide it using the GIA machine, leaving sufficient length for the bowel to rest easily 0.5–1.0 cm above the abdominal wall skin once closed. At the end of the closing sequence, the bowel is *not* opened but sutured to the skin. Depending on the patient's further management, the site may remain closed, be opened as a stoma or, if there are no plans to reconstruct the bowel and if there is no distal obstruction in the rectum, the bowel above the level of the skin can be trimmed under local anaesthesia and a simple running absorbable suture used to close the stoma. Eventually the skin will heal over the area, leaving the closed bowel end in the subcutaneous tissue where it can be opened with ease should the need arise.

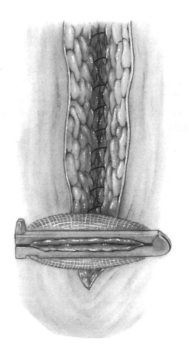

26a

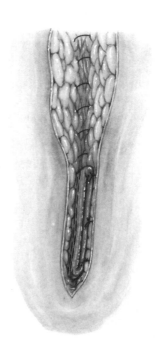

26b

Closing sequence

After all these procedures, extensive lavage is carried out with warmed physiological saline containing tetracycline 1 g/l to remove blood and debris, to prevent possible contamination of faecal matter and also to reduce the *concentration* of organisms within the abdominal cavity and on the wound. All these patients run the risk of intra-abdominal complications of sepsis or adhesive obstruction and therefore it is important to have the most efficient technique of gastric decompression. For this reason the author performs a gastrostomy in all these patients, except those who have been on long-term steroids.

27a, b Abdominal wall closure is achieved with a mass suture technique, using a continuous 1 polydioxanone suture; each bite should be 1 cm from the incision line and each loop of the suture placed 1 cm apart. In the obese patient, care should be taken to include as little fat as possible because the tension in the suture line will rapidly diminish as the fat gives way.

Deep tension sutures should never be used. If there is any significant tension on the abdominal wall because of bowel distension or increased oedema of the bowel caused by the resuscitation fluids, forcing the bowel closed merely increases intra-abdominal tension and reduces the vascular supply to the gut. Furthermore, the increased tension in the abdominal wall may give rise to disruption or a serious fasciitis with tissue breakdown.

To avoid closing the abdominal wall under great tension, a mesh insert should be sutured in place to the fascia to maintain the gut *in situ*. One edge of the mesh is trimmed in a curve to fit the abdominal wall opening. The edge itself is then folded over so that there is a double layer of mesh being attached to the fascial edge. Once the first side of the mesh is in place, the abdominal wall is placed into a position where the second edge of the mesh can be trimmed, and once sutured will lie as 'snug' fit, but without tension.

When the patient's general condition has improved and the abdomen has become soft and less distended, the mesh may be divided in the midline, the omentum and bowel beneath gently lifted away from it. The mesh is then sutured, taking 2-cm bites of mesh on either side of the midline to gradually approximate the fascial edges. With a large mesh insert, this may need to be performed more than once. Subsequently, under general anaesthesia the mesh is removed and a routine mass closure of the fascial layer carried out. Although this process of mesh insert and 'graduated removal' appears laborious, it is important to remember that gut blood flow and venous return must not be compromised in these already very ill patients.

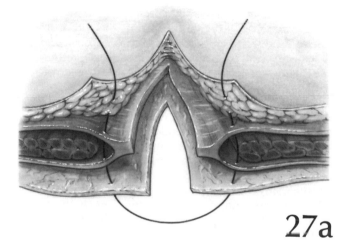

27a

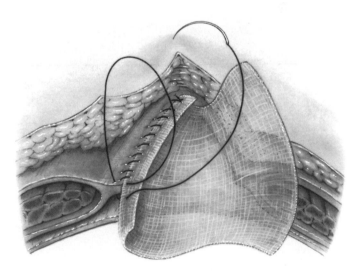

27b

28 Finally, after a further irrigation, the skin and subcutaneous tissues are lightly packed with dry gauze in preparation for delayed primary closure 48–72 h later.

Protection of anastomosis after immediate bowel reconstruction

This is a controversial subject in elective surgery and more so in patients undergoing immediate tumour resection and anastomosis in the face of bowel obstruction. The author's preference is to decide before starting the anastomosis whether undue difficulty will be encountered. If difficulty is likely, the author prefers not to proceed to anastomosis, but to construct an end colostomy and to either close the distal rectum as a Hartmann's procedure or to bring it out as a mucous fistula. The occurrence of a clinically significant anastomotic leak, especially in these patients (who are frequently elderly and ill) is, in the author's view a greater risk than that associated with the second operation when the patient has fully recovered. Furthermore, some patients may wish not to undergo a second procedure, having successfully survived the first.

Some surgeons advocate anastomotic 'protection' in all potentially compromised anastomoses (in the setting of obstruction, after irradiation, and even after ultra-low

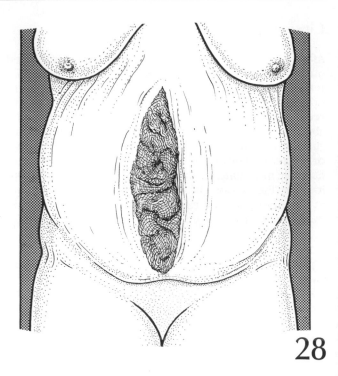

28

anterior resection of the rectum), by loop ileostomy (*see* pp. 627–653), transverse loop colostomy (*see* pp. 658–667). or the insertion of a Coloshield apparatus. The author has not used an anastomosis-protecting stoma or Coloshield in the setting of obstruction but recognizes that this represents a reasonable approach to anastomotic protection.

IMMEDIATE TUMOUR RESECTION FOR OBSTRUCTING RIGHT COLONIC LESIONS

The principles of management for these lesions are the same as those for obstructing left-sided tumours, but the detailed anatomy is different.

Securing vascular supply

29 The mesentery to the distal part of the small bowel is spread out towards the patient's right iliac fossa, so that the vascular supply may be studied.

Nylon tapes are passed around the small bowel and large bowel proximal and distal to the lesion to occlude the lumen. The ileocolic, right colic (and for transverse colon tumours the middle colic) vessels are divided at their origins.

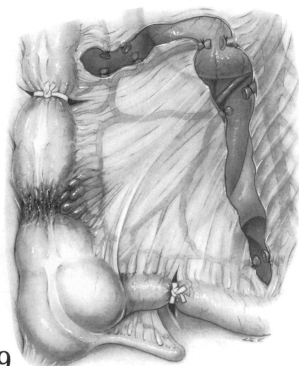

29

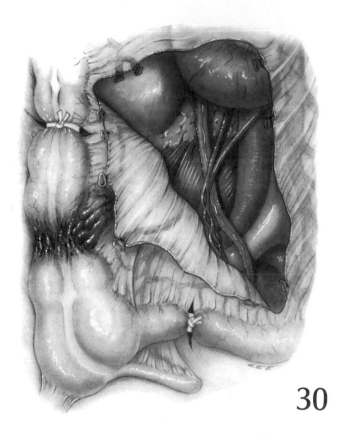

30 The dissection is then taken to the deep side of the mesentery supplying the bowel which is lifted forward, and the ureter, vena cava and aorta are identified.

30

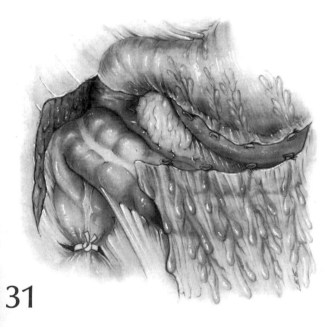

31

31 The hepatic flexure is then mobilized: either the greater omentum is dissected free in the 'bloodless plane' or, for lesions near the hepatic flexure, the omentum is mobilized between the right gastroepiploic vessels and the greater curve of the stomach. In the latter case the dissection is taken down over the inferior part of the first and second parts of the duodenum, dividing the right gastroepiploic vessel at its origin. The dissection is then taken laterally, dividing the top end of the peritoneum overlying the right paracolic gutter. The plane of the dissection at this point is the duodenum and great care must be taken not to damage this structure.

32 Before these two dissections are joined, it is useful to return to the pelvic brim and divide the peritoneum demonstrating the ureter and iliac vessels. Once these structures have been identified, the peritoneum under the caecum is mobilized and the remaining portion of the right paracolic gutter is mobilized.

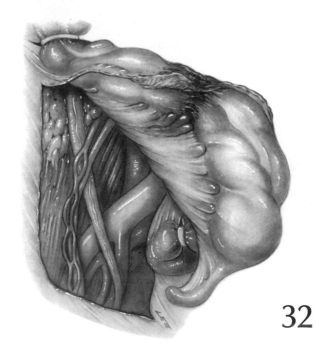

32

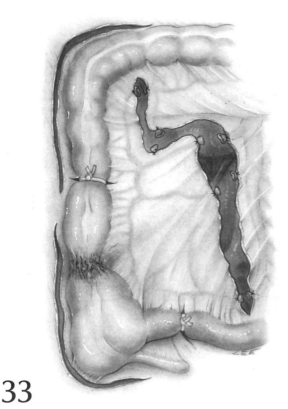

33

33 The parts of the dissection are then joined by lifting the tumour forward: the medial part, where the principal vessels have been ligated; the superior part, bordered by the duodenum; the inferior part, in which the ureter and iliac vessels have been identified; and the lateral part of the paracolic gutter.

As the tumour is lifted forward, the gonadal vessels tend to adhere to the underside of the dissection. They may frequently be left *in situ*, being mobilized by blunt dissection; however, if adherent to the tumour, they are divided.

Finally, the proximal small bowel and distal colon are divided between crushing clamps.

Immediate *versus* delayed anastomosis

It is usual for an immediate anastomosis to be carried out but if there is 'peritonitis' of the bowel surface or the bowel wall itself is very friable, the bowel ends should be brought out. However, in most patients a very carefully performed end-to-end anastomosis can be constructed.

If there is heavy distal colonic faecal loading, a retrograde on-table gut irrigation may be carried out, using a similar technique to that described above.

Closing sequence

The procedures are the same as those described above: lavage with warmed physiological saline containing tetracycline 1 g/l; no drains; gastrostomy; mass closure of abdominal wall; delayed primary closure of skin and subcutaneous tissues.

All these patients should, at the end of the procedure, continue to have positive pressure ventilation and be managed, where possible, in an intensive therapy unit. There is strong evidence that even short periods of hypotension or hypoxia will prejudice the long-term outcome, and the risks of respiratory/cardiac failure will be mitigated by accepting this advice on every occasion. Furthermore, an intensive therapy unit gives an opportunity for careful measurement of urinary output, good pain control, adequate physiotherapy and detailed clinical observation by staff experienced in the care of the seriously ill.

EXTENDED RIGHT HEMICOLECTOMY

For obstructing lesions of the distal part of the transverse colon, splenic flexure and proximal descending colon, an extended right hemicolectomy is a useful procedure. The anatomical dissection will be a combination of the techniques described above and will allow, in most patients, immediate anastomosis.

DELAYED RESECTION POLICY (STAGED RESECTION)

Some surgeons remain of the opinion that immediate tumour resection for left-sided obstructing lesions is not to be undertaken and that a 'defunctioning' transverse colostomy should be carried out as the only primary procedure. The author does not advocate this method.

PAUL–MIKULICZ OPERATION: DOUBLE-BARRELLED COLOSTOMY

Some surgeons, after a radical resection, have brought the ends of the colon out through a single opening in the abdominal wall, so that a full laparotomy to reconstruct bowel continuity may be avoided. If this procedure is carried out, the bowel ends can be mobilized, trimmed, sutured or stapled and returned to the abdominal cavity without further bowel mobiliza-

tion. However, the operation is difficult to get 'just right' and perhaps the safest procedure is a simple end colostomy and mucous fistula, as described above. One of the dangers of the Paul–Mikulicz procedure is that the small bowel is always at risk by attachment to the underside of the two limbs of the colostomy; because of the local nature of the mobilization, this adherence of small bowel may not be appreciated and fistula formation may occur. The author does not favour the use of this procedure.

MANAGEMENT OF FIXED TUMOUR

If the tumour is found to be fixed or adherent to vital structures, no attempt should be made to resect it at the first operation. In particular, surgeons should refrain from trying to develop a plane of cleavage directly between the tumour and the attached organ. Under these circumstances, the following sequence is suggested:

1. For right-sided lesions, an ileocolonic anastomosis is fashioned to establish an internal bypass. For more distal lesions, a transverse colostomy is necessary.
2. Before undertaking the bypass or transverse colostomy, decompression of the bowel should be undertaken using the techniques described above. Before an ileocolonic anastomosis, the segment of the small bowel to be used should be chosen as the site for Foley catheter decompression; for more distal lesions, the site of the transverse colostomy is used for needle decompression.
3. Radiopaque 'clips' are placed around the tumour area (it may be possible to irradiate the lesion and render it operable).
4. Closing sequence as described above.

Once the patient has recovered from the acute illness and after the consideration of radiotherapy, the patient should undergo a second laparotomy by an experienced colorectal surgeon in an attempt to excise the primary tumour.

References

1. Fielding LP, Stuart-Brown S, Blesovsky L. Large bowel obstruction caused by cancer: a prospective study. *BMJ* 1979; ii: 515–17.

2. Dudley HAF, Radcliffe AG, McGeehan D. Intraoperative irrigation of the colon to permit primary anastomosis. *Br J Surg* 1980; 67: 80–1.

Colonic surgery for acute conditions: massive haemorrhage

E. L. Bokey MS, FRACS
University of Sydney, Department of Colon and Rectal Surgery, Concord Hospital, Concord, New South Wales, Australia

P. H. Chapuis DS, FRACS
University of Sydney, Department of Colon and Rectal Surgery, Concord Hospital, Concord, New South Wales, Australia

Principles and justification

The most common causes of massive haemorrhage of the large intestine are angiodysplasia and diverticulosis of the colon. Other causes include inflammatory bowel disease (notably Crohn's disease), ischaemic colitis, and radiation injury to the colon. Haemangiomas, leiomyomas, lipomas and colonic varices are rare causes, and secondary haemorrhage after endoscopic polypectomy may occur very occasionally. The presence of telangiectasias on the lips and buccal mucosa suggests the Osler–Rendu–Weber syndrome (hereditary haemorrhagic telangiectasia) as the cause for bleeding. Some patients with angiodysplasia are more likely to bleed if they have associated aortic valve disease[1].

Preoperative

Initial assessment

Most patients with massive haemorrhage ideally should be cared for in a high-dependency area and their management is largely influenced by the rate of bleeding. Initial resuscitation is often necessary before an accurate history can be obtained or a complete physical examination performed. Resuscitation includes the insertion of an adequate peripheral line, a urinary catheter and a nasogastric tube and preferably a central venous line. A careful history, including details of drug usage, may provide a clue to the source of haemorrhage, but often the history and physical examination are not helpful.

If the patient's condition improves and the bleeding stops spontaneously there is time to select appropriate investigations. However, should bleeding persist, urgent investigations become necessary. Early upper endoscopy may exclude gastric and duodenal lesions. Proctoscopy to exclude bleeding haemorrhoids is useful and simple to perform. Sigmoidoscopy (preferably with a flexible instrument) may identify distal pathology.

Colonoscopy

1 Emergency colonoscopy is possible at the time of bleeding, but must be carried out by an experienced endoscopist. Generally, it is best performed once the patient is stabilized and following an adequate bowel preparation. Excessive air insufflation should be avoided as this will efface the mucosa and collapse small arteriovenous malformations. Typically, angiodysplasias seen at colonoscopy are multiple, bright red in colour with a central vessel and a peripheral flare. They occur throughout the colon but are usually found in the right side.

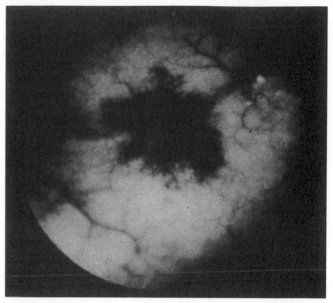

1

Angiography

2 Selective angiography is sometimes helpful, but its success is proportional to the rate of bleeding and the experience of the radiologist. Diagnostic features of angiodysplasia include a vascular blush, early draining vein, and large submucosal veins. Extravasation of contrast material into the lumen confirms the bleeding site. If an active site is identified, selective injection of vasopressin may be successful as an interim measure to stop bleeding. Occasionally, if the bleeding site has not been identified, the catheter may be left *in situ* for further emergency angiographic studies should bleeding recommence.

The illustration shows the late arterial phase with the catheter in the superior mesenteric artery, from which the right hepatic artery is arising. There is moderate extravasation of contrast into the bowel lumen from the right colic artery, adjacent to the pyelogram. Also note gallstone near 'R' marker.

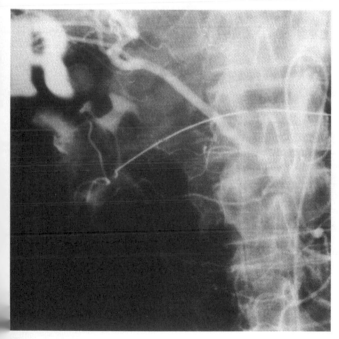

2

Nuclear scanning

Nuclear scanning generally lacks the accuracy of angiography. This investigation may take up to 4 h to complete and is recommended only in a relatively stable patient. Occasionally, a technetium-labelled sulphur colloid scan will demonstrate the bleeding site, if bleeding is occurring at the time of injection, usually at the same rate as that required for angiography (minimum 1 ml/min). A ^{99m}Tc scan may demonstrate bleeding from ectopic gastric mucosa in a Meckel's diverticulum.

Endoscopic management

Coagulation

If diagnosed, angiodysplasia may be treated successfully by endoscopic coagulation. Hot biopsy forceps or laser may be used, according to personal preference. Coagulation using the hot biopsy forceps requires a setting of 2–3 V. The mucosa is touched or lightly grasped by the forceps and the current is applied until blanching occurs. Treatment for lesions larger than 5 mm diameter should begin around the periphery of the lesion and be directed to its centre. It is advisable not to overdistend the colon to avoid perforation.

Laser

Coagulation with a neodymium yttrium aluminium garnet (NdYAG) laser can be performed using a similar technique with the laser enabled at a power setting adjusted to deliver 40 W for 0.5 s at a working distance of 1 cm. This low setting is chosen to avoid perforation of the thin-walled right colon. At the completion of colonoscopy, the colon must be deflated to avoid delayed perforation.

Operation

The details of surgical treatment depend on whether the cause and source of haemorrhage have been identified and whether the operation is urgent or elective.

Whenever possible the patient should be counselled by a stomal therapist, and all patients (even those who are bleeding profusely) should be sited for an ileostomy and sigmoid colostomy.

Unknown source of haemorrhage

The procedure of choice is total colectomy with ileostomy, rectal mucous fistula or oversewing of rectal stump.

Patients are catheterized and placed in stirrups. A long midline incision is made. A full laparotomy is performed (with careful palpation of the small bowel); this usually confirms blood in the colon but rarely discloses the cause. Blood in the small intestine may be present when the source of bleeding is in the colon. Arteriovenous malformations cannot be identified by inspection or by palpation. The presence of diverticula does not imply that they are the cause of haemorrhage. It is best to avoid intraoperative endoscopic manoeuvres. They are time consuming, potentially hazardous, and rarely helpful.

If the patient's condition permits, an immediate ileorectal anastomosis may be performed.

Known source of haemorrhage

The procedure will depend on the cause and site of the haemorrhage.

If angiodysplasia has been identified in the right colon, then right hemicolectomy with immediate ileotransverse anastomosis is performed.

In the rare event that a sigmoid diverticulum in the left colon has been identified as the source of bleeding, a Hartmann's procedure is advised.

Profuse bleeding is rare in patients with inflammatory bowel disease. Where it occurs it is usually associated with Crohn's disease. When bleeding becomes life-threatening despite intensive medical treatment, emergency total colectomy with ileostomy and rectal mucous fistula may become necessary. It is important to ensure that the rectum can be exteriorized without tension. It should not be oversewn or stapled and returned to the pelvis as these patients are at significant risk of anastomotic disruption. On very rare occasions, if the rectum as well as the rest of the colon is bleeding profusely, an emergency proctocolectomy may be necessary.

The surgical specimen

3 The cause of bleeding is often not identified before or during surgery, because angiodysplasias are difficult to see with the naked eye. Arterial injection of barium into the resected specimen may help the pathologist to confirm the diagnosis[2].

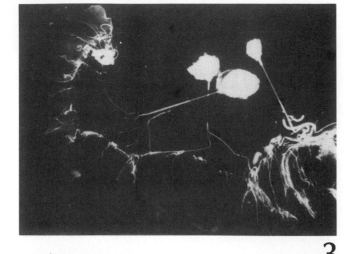

3

4 Examination of the open specimen after barium injection will show areas of barium pooling in the mucosa and will direct the pathologist as to where tissue should be sampled for sectioning.

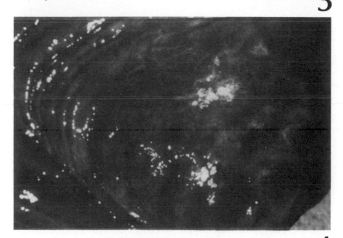

4

5 Histological examination will show barium-filled vascular spaces in the mucosa, continuous with ectatic submucosal vessels typical of angiodysplasia[3].

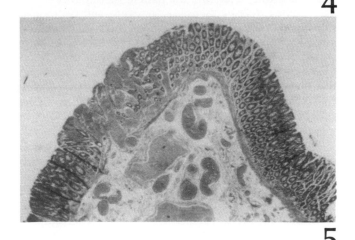

Acknowledgements

Illustration 2 is reproduced by courtesy of Dr G. R. Faithful.

5

References

1. Price AB. Angiodysplasia of the colon. *Int J Colorectal Dis* 1986; 1: 121–8.

2. Alfidi RJ, Caldwell D, Riaz T *et al*. Recognition and angio-surgical detection of arteriovenous malformations of the bowel. *Ann Surg* 1971; 174: 573–82.

3. Hayward PG, Bokey EL, Chapuis PH, Kneale KL, Faithful GR. The use of barium injection studies to confirm the diagnosis of colonic angiodysplasia. *Coloproctology* 1984; 6: 156–7.

Illustrations by Angela Christie

Colonic surgery for acute conditions: volvulus of the colon

David N. Armstrong MD, FRCSEd
Clinical Instructor, Department of Surgery, Yale University School of Medicine, New Haven, Connecticut, USA

G. H. Ballantyne MD, FACS, FASCRS
Associate Professor of Surgery, Department of Surgery, Yale University School of Medicine, New Haven, Connecticut, USA

History

Torsions of the colon have plagued mankind throughout history. The Greeks called this condition 'ileus', the Romans 'volvulus'. The natural history of sigmoid volvulus was detailed in the Papyrus Ebers from dynastic Egypt – the twist of colon either 'rotted in the belly' or it untwisted and the patient rapidly recovered. Asclepiades defines 'ileus' as 'a severe and prolonged twisting of the intestine'. The method of treatment advocated by Hippocrates suggests that he was treating sigmoid volvulus. He advised insertion of a ten-digit long (about 22 cm) suppository into the rectum, and this manoeuvre often relieved the obstruction. Indeed, this technique heralded the modern derotation of sigmoid volvulus with a rigid sigmoidoscope 25 cm in length.

Treatment of all forms of intestinal obstruction remained primarily non-operative until late in the 19th century. Although Praxogaras, in ancient Greece, had advocated 'making an incision in the pubic region, then cutting open the rectum, removing the excrement, and sewing up the rectum and abdomen', few physicians had entrusted their patients to surgeons for these heroic measures. Occasional descriptions of operative treatment of intestinal obstruction crept into the surgical literature after the Renaissance. In 1692, for example, Nuck reported the successful reduction of a volvulus by 'gastrostomy'.

Satisfactory techniques for enteric suturing and anaesthesia did not evolve until the 19th century. Successful operative treatment of colonic obstruction and sigmoid volvulus became more common in the 1880s. Atherton reported the first successful operative detorsion of a sigmoid volvulus in Boston in 1883. Treves, in his monograph on intestinal obstruction published in 1884, recommended colectomy when a gangrenous colon was encountered. In 1889, Senn sought to apply the principles advocated by Travers for the treatment of obstruction. He advised enterotomy for decompression of the intestine proximal to the volvulus. Because of the high likelihood of recurrence, Senn also suggested 'shortening of the mesentery' of the sigmoid colon (sigmoidopexy). Thus, by the close of the 1890s, operative treatment of sigmoid volvulus rapidly became, for many, the standard therapy.

Operative detorsion or obstructive resection of the Paul–Mikulicz type remained the recommended treatment of colonic volvulus for the first half of the 20th century. In the second half, however, primary therapy of sigmoid volvulus has returned to non-operative techniques. In 1859, Gay had observed during an autopsy of a patient who had died from a sigmoid volvulus that 'with a tube, per rectum, the bowel could be relieved of its contents; and then, by rolling the body over, the bowel (would) right itself'. This form of therapy, of course, brings to mind the ten-digit suppository used by Hippocrates for decompression of patients with volvulus. Unfortunately, the value of non-operative decompression of sigmoid volvulus with a rigid sigmoidoscope and rectal tube was not widely recognized until 1947, when Bruusgaard reported his results in the treatment of 168 episodes of sigmoid volvulus. His data demonstrated that whenever possible, patients with sigmoid volvulus should undergo non-operative techniques for decompression and derotation of the twisted sigmoid colon.

Caecal volvulus occurs less commonly than sigmoid volvulus. Classical physicians were silent on this condition. In 1646, Fabricius Hildanus described the autopsy of a young boy who had succumbed to a caecal volvulus and Treves accumulated only five cases of caecal volvulus. The first major treatise on caecal volvulus was published in 1900 by Von Manteuffel and the first major series in English in 1905 by Smith and Perry. Throughout the 20th century, three different operations have been advocated for this condition: caecopexy, caecostomy and right hemicolectomy. Because of the great success of non-operative decompression for the treatment of sigmoid volvulus, similar attempts have been made for the non-operative reduction of caecal volvulus but with intermittent success.

In English-speaking countries, sigmoid rather than caecal volvulus is more commonly encountered. Non-operative decompression and derotation of a sigmoid volvulus followed by elective sigmoid resection has become the standard therapy. In contrast, caecal volvulus generally requires urgent operative treatment after resuscitation.

Principles and justification

Aetiology

Large intestinal volvulus accounts for 3–5% of large intestinal obstruction in Western populations, and for over 50% of obstruction in the 'volvulus belt' of Africa and the Middle East.

Volvulus of the sigmoid colon occurs in the presence of three conditions:

1. Elongation of the sigmoid colon.
2. Narrowing of the base of the sigmoid mesocolon (mesosigmoiditis).
3. A torque force applied to the sigmoid colon.

In the West, the sigmoid colon elongates as a result of neurological disease, laxative abuse, or chronic constipation, most often seen in occupants of chronic care facilities. The base of the sigmoid mesocolon becomes foreshortened as the scar tissue generated by the chronic mesosigmoiditis contracts. This occurs because of repeated episodes of torsion.

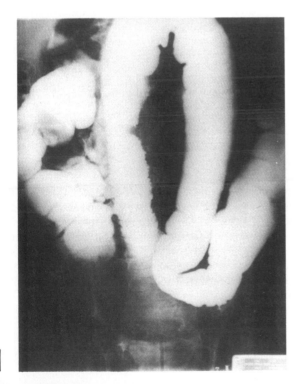

1 Barium enemas in these patients reveal the close apposition of the descending colon–sigmoid colon junction to the rectosigmoid junction. As a result, the narrow base acts as a fulcrum, about which the sigmoid colon twists.

In African and Middle Eastern societies, a high-fibre diet results in an overloaded sigmoid colon whose weight provides the rotational force to initiate torsion. A shift in the relative positions of the intra-abdominal organs, as seen in pregnancy or tumours, may also precipitate an episode of sigmoid volvulus.

1
Barium enema showing close apposition of descending colon junction and rectosigmoid junction in a patient who has had recurrent episodes of sigmoid volvulus.

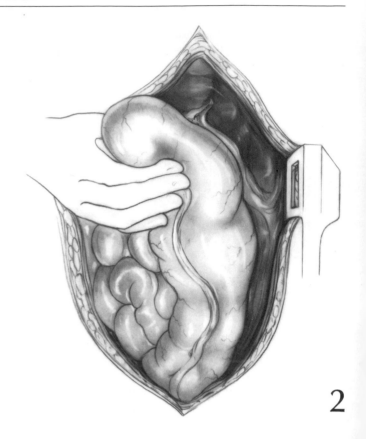

2 Caecal volvulus occurs in patients with incomplete peritoneal fixation of the caecum. In a series of post mortems in the USA, the caecum retains a complete mesenterium ileocolicum commune without any retroperitoneal fixation in about 11% of patients. Axial torsion of the caecum can produce a caecal volvulus when the right colon retains this degree of mobility.

In another 25% of patients, the ascending colon is fixed to the retroperitoneum, but the caecum remains unattached. In these patients the caecum can fold anteriorly, producing a caecal bascule. Thus, the caecum of about one-third of the American population has sufficient mobility that it can twist and generate a caecal volvulus.

Indications

Large intestinal volvulus is a life-threatening condition. Non-operative reduction of the volvulus provides excellent initial therapy for the majority of patients with sigmoid volvulus and an occasional patient with caecal volvulus. Unfortunately, following non-operative reduction, there is a high probability of recurrence with a high concomitant mortality. Consequently, almost all patients in whom a colonic volvulus is discovered should undergo definitive operative treatment during the same hospitalization.

Choice of operation

Sigmoid volvulus

When non-operative reduction of sigmoid volvulus is achieved, the patient can receive a standard mechanical and antibiotic bowel preparation. This allows construction of a primary anastomosis after resection of the twisted segment. When non-operative detorsion can not be achieved, the patient must undergo emergency sigmoid resection. Under these circumstances, a temporary stoma may be required. Simple sigmoidopexy is followed by too high a recurrence rate to be recommended.

Caecal volvulus

Non-operative derotation of a caecal volvulus is seldom achieved. As a result, almost all patients afflicted by caecal volvulus require emergency surgical intervention after a rapid period of resuscitation and stabilization. Necessarily, the patients undergo operation without a bowel preparation. Excellent results have been reported after three operations: caecopexy, caecostomy and right hemicolectomy.

Caecopexy

Caecopexy prevents future torsion of the right colon by fixation of the ascending colon to the abdominal wall near the right gutter. The major advantage of this procedure is that the colon is not opened, and thus no contamination of the abdominal cavity occurs. The great disadvantage of the procedure, however, is that decompression is not achieved and the right colon remains distended. Hence, closure of the abdomen is difficult. In addition, large quantities of 'toxins' remain within the colon, and bacterial translocation may continue to plague the patient in the postoperative period.

Caecostomy

In this operation, the caecum is intubated with a large catheter, decompressed and drained of its faecal contents. In addition, the right colon is secured in place both by sutures, as in caecopexy, and by the caecostomy tube. Consequently, the right colon is decompressed and drained. Recurrence rates of caecal volvulus after caecostomy are very low. None the less, the greatest disadvantage of a caecostomy is the risk of contamination of the abdomen during decompression of the caecum and placement of the catheter. In addition, abdominal wall infections can occur around the caecostomy site. This may lead to separation of the caecum from the abdominal wall and drainage of caecal contents into the free abdominal cavity. Finally, persistent drainage through the caecocutaneous fistula requires prolonged wound care and lengthens the period of disability after operation.

Right hemicolectomy

Right hemicolectomy offers a definitive treatment for caecal volvulus and avoids the problems of caecopexy and caecostomy. Resection of the right colon eliminates any chance of recurrence of caecal volvulus. Transection of the ileum and transverse colon with stapling instruments, which simultaneously seal both the specimen side and the patient's side of the intestine eradicates any significant abdominal contamination. The obstructed segment and its contents of 'toxins' are removed, and the risk of persistent sepsis is minimized. As the distended segment is removed, closure of the abdominal wound is also facilitated. In most patients a primary anastomosis can be safely constructed.

Preoperative

Clinical presentation

The average age of patients with volvulus is 60–66 years. Caecal volvulus occurs more commonly in patients who have undergone operations that partially or completely mobilize the right colon. Sigmoid volvulus is more commonly reported in blacks than other ethnic groups and more commonly in men than in women. Patients generally have a sedentary lifestyle and may be inhabitants of chronic care facilities, such as nursing homes or psychiatric hospitals. Many report a prolonged history of constipation.

Patients develop the signs and symptoms of colonic obstruction with abdominal distension, abdominal pain and obstipation evolved over 3–5 days. Some become nauseated or begin to vomit. Physical examination typically reveals abdominal distension, increased tympany and perhaps some abdominal tenderness. On digital examination, the rectal vault is often empty.

Diagnosis

3–5 The characteristic appearance of a caecal or sigmoid volvulus on a plain abdominal radiograph will confirm the diagnosis in the majority of patients. The distended intestine assumes two characteristic silhouettes in caecal volvulus: the appearance of a 'coffee bean' in axial torsion of the caecum and ascending colon and a solitary inverted tear-drop in caecal bascule. In sigmoid volvulus, the colon often appears like a 'bent inner tube'.

In doubtful cases, a limited Gastrografin enema will reveal the characteristic 'bird's beak' appearance of the apex of the sigmoid volvulus in the proximal rectum. During rigid or flexible sigmoidoscopy, spiralling folds of mucosa at the rectosigmoid junction establish the diagnosis.

Occasionally the sigmoid volvulus spontaneously derotates before the diagnosis is documented by abdominal radiography. Under these circumstances, colonoscopy can often confirm that the sigmoid colon was recently twisted. Colonoscopic examination in these patients reveals discrete segments of inflammation at the rectosigmoid junction and at the descending colon–sigmoid junction. Each segment of inflammation is about 5 cm in length and is characterized by loss of the vascular markings, thickening of the intestinal wall, erythema and sometimes granularity or friability. These findings strongly support the diagnosis.

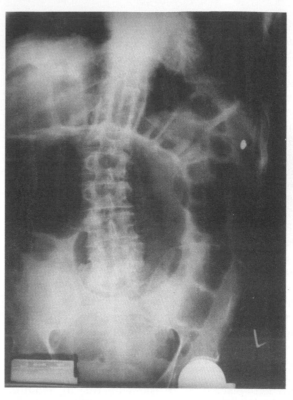

3

Abdominal radiograph of caecal volvulus produced by axial torsion of the caecum and ascending colon showing 'coffee bean' appearance of obstructed right colon.

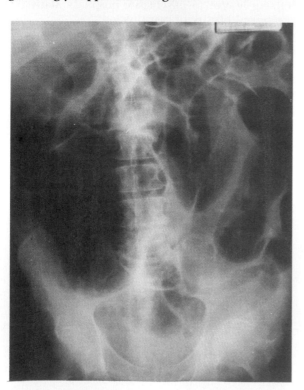

4

Abdominal radiograph of caecal volvulus produced by a caecal bascule showing 'inverted tear-drop' appearance of obstructed caecum.

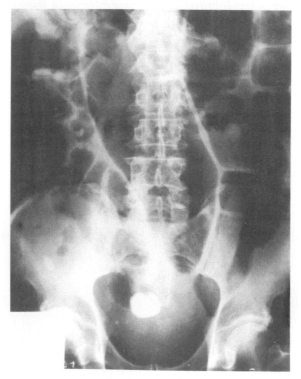

5

Abdominal radiograph of sigmoid volvulus showing 'bent inner tube' appearance of obstructed sigmoid colon.

Resuscitation

The first priority is resuscitation of the patient, although these patients generally appear reasonably stable. Colonic obstruction carries a very high mortality rate, however, because it precipitates large volume shifts and often generates cardiovascular complications because of endotoxin and bacterial translocation.

All patients are admitted to a surgical intensive therapy unit. Oxygen saturation is monitored by pulse oximetry. Pulse, blood pressure and central venous pressure are continuously monitored. A Swan–Ganz catheter is required when the patient has significant associated cardiac disease. The patient is laid in the left lateral position to improve venous return, which may be compromised as a result of massive abdominal distension. Oxygen is given because splinting of the diaphragm impedes respiratory efforts and results in shunting of blood through the pulmonary circulation. A Foley catheter is inserted to help assess fluid balance. All patients should be intubated with a nasogastric tube because of the high mortality rate from aspiration of gastric contents. Parenteral antibiotics to cover aerobic and anaerobic organisms must be given to all patients to treat potential sepsis and as prophylaxis against inadvertent perforation during sigmoidoscopic intubation.

The rate of fluid resuscitation is determined by the success of non-operative attempts at derotation of the volvulus. If an emergency operation proves necessary, the patient is rapidly resuscitated over a 4–8-h period with a balanced electrolyte solution. If the volvulus is successfully reduced, the patient is rehydrated more cautiously over a 48-h period.

Non-operative decompression and derotation of sigmoid volvulus

The patient is placed in the left lateral position. A 25-cm rigid sigmoidoscope is advanced into the rectum under direct vision. Air insufflation is not generally required. Spiralling folds of rectal mucosa are traversed at the rectosigmoid junction. Intubation of the obstructed loop of sigmoid colon is heralded by the almost explosive propulsion of gas and liquid stool through the sigmoidoscope. The tip of a well-lubricated no. 32 rubber rectal tube is pushed gently into the sigmoid colon through the sigmoidoscope. This serves to maintain decompression of the sigmoid colon during the few days before elective resection of the sigmoid colon.

On occasion, initial attempts at detorsion of the volvulus are unsuccessful. The patient is placed in the knee–elbow position; this may allow the colon to fall away and open up the angle of the volvulus. The temptation to push a narrow, rigid probe into the apex should be resisted, as this may perforate the already compromised intestinal wall. If visibility is poor, the end of the sigmoidoscope is placed directly on the twist at the rectosigmoid junction. Without moving the sigmoidoscope, the tube is pushed up the sigmoidoscope, so that the tip lies at the apex. Undue force should never be used, nor attempts to poke blindly. There will be no doubt when decompression has been achieved. A polythene-lined bucket should be on hand to avoid unnecessary spillage from the sudden, forceful rush of gas and liquid stool.

In some patients the rigid sigmoidoscope is not long enough to reach into the obstructed segment of sigmoid colon, but a flexible sigmoidoscope or colonoscope can be advanced into the twisted segment. There is no sudden rush of gas and fluid, as the endoscope works with a closed system. The obstructed sigmoid colon is slowly decompressed with suction. The flexible instruments are not as effective for drainage of the faecal contents of the sigmoid colon because of the narrow calibre of the suction channel. None the less, decompression of the sigmoid colon with flexible instruments will generally result in detorsion of the volvulus.

Successful non-operative reduction of volvulus

Sigmoidoscopic decompression is successful in over 90% of patients in whom the sigmoid colon remains viable at the time of presentation. When successful, decompression should be confirmed radiologically, and the rectal tube taped securely to the buttocks. The patient is stabilized and assessed for surgery, undergoes a standard mechanical and antibiotic bowel preparation, and elective surgery is scheduled 5–7 days later.

Unsuccessful non-operative reduction of volvulus

When endoscopic attempts at detorsion of the volvulus fail, the patient should receive operative therapy immediately following adequate resuscitation because the sigmoid colon is strangulated and usually necrotic.

Operations for sigmoid volvulus

Position of patient

For operations to correct sigmoid volvulus, the patient is placed in the Lloyd-Davies position.

Incision

A lower abdominal midline incision extending to the umbilicus allows adequate exposure for correction of sigmoid volvulus. Care must be taken when entering the peritoneum not to inadvertently cut the distended colon.

COLOPEXY

Several techniques of colopexy have been described. The simplest involves suturing the sigmoid colon to the lateral abdominal wall using interrupted sutures. More elaborate methods include enclosing the sigmoid in a lateral retroperitoneal 'pouch', plicating the mesentery (mesenteropexy), Gore-tex banding of the sigmoid colon to the abdominal wall, and sigmoid colostomy. All of these techniques have recurrence rates similar to those in unoperated patients and, furthermore, are often more time-consuming than a simple resection.

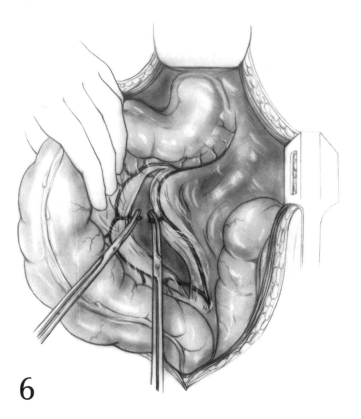

6

RESECTION: SIGMOID COLECTOMY

Sigmoid resection provides the simplest approach and has the lowest rate of recurrence. The small intestine is packed into the right upper quadrant with warm, moist packs. The sigmoid colon is mobilized on its primitive mesentery by dividing the 'white line' laterally. As a result of repeated torsions, the mesocolon is foreshortened and the peritoneal reflection shifted laterally. This often facilitates the dissection. The left ureter is identified and preserved.

Extent of resection

6 As a result of foreshortening of the mesentery, the peritoneal reflection of the rectum and the descending colon are brought into close proximity. Recurrence rates are lowest after simple resection of the omega loop of the sigmoid colon. More extensive resection is unnecessary. The inferior mesenteric artery is preserved, as this is a benign disease process, and this will ensure an adequate blood supply to the proximal rectum. The sigmoid branches are divided near their origin on the inferior mesenteric vessels. The remaining mesentery is divided between clamps and tied with 3/0 silk. The sites of transection are chosen to allow a well-perfused, tension-free anastomosis.

Side-to-side (functional end-to-end) colorectal anastomosis

7a, b The intestinal wall is not cleared of mesenteric tissue. The descending colon is transected near its junction with the sigmoid colon with a GIA 60 stapler. This closes both the descending colon and the specimen with double rows of titanium staples. Even in unprepared colon, faecal soiling seldom occurs. The rectum is divided just distally to the rectosigmoid junction, also with a GIA 60 stapler. The distal descending colon and the proximal rectum are usually contiguous because of scarring of the mesentery from chronic mesosigmoiditis.

The antimesenteric sides of the rectum and descending colon are aligned with two silk sutures. One is placed 1 cm from the end of the two staple lines near the mesentery. The second suture is placed 6 cm from the staple lines. The corners of the two staple lines are excised with curved Mayo scissors. A third GIA 60 stapler is introduced through the two colotomies. The third staple line should run along the taenia on the descending colon. After firing the stapler, the staple line is inspected for haemostasis. The edges of the remaining enterotomy are approximated with four Allis' clamps. The silk suture near the enterotomy is removed. The previous staple lines at the end of the rectum and descending colon can be aligned so that they either form an X or one continuous everted closure. The enterotomy is closed using a TA 55 stapler with 3.5-mm staples. A third silk suture is placed in the 'crotch' at the end of the third GIA staple line.

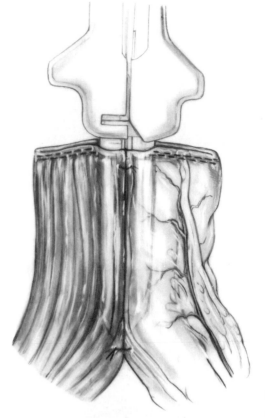

7a

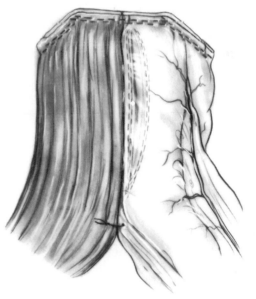

7b

End-to-end colorectal anastomosis (double stapling technique)

8 The points of resection are identified at the descending colon–sigmoid colon junction and the rectosigmoid junction. The proximal rectum is divided with the GIA 60 stapler. In some patients it may be necessary to use the Roticulator-55 stapling device to close the rectum, because the shape of the pelvis does not allow access with the more bulky GIA device. The specimen side of the rectum is secured with a right-angled bowel clamp, such as a Foss–Pemberton clamp. The intestine is divided and the specimen removed.

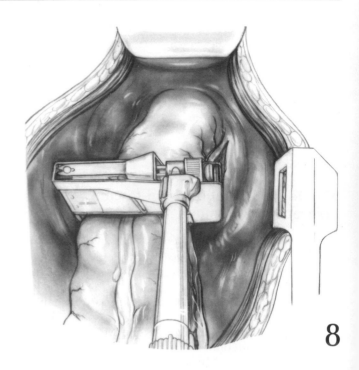

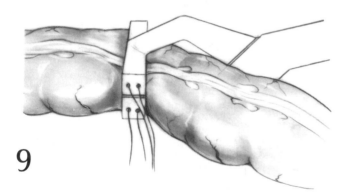

9 Mesenteric attachments and epiploic fat tags are cleared from 2.5 cm of intestinal wall. An automatic purse-string device is applied at the distal limit of the cleared colonic wall. A crushing bowel clamp is placed across the specimen side of the intestine near the purse-string. The intestine is divided with a scalpel or pair of heavy scissors. The purse-string device is left attached to the intestine and acts as a clamp until the specimen is removed. The wound is inspected for haemostasis.

10 The purse-string device on the descending colon is opened. The edges of the colon are grasped with three Babcock's clamps. The colon is usually dilated from the recent obstruction and does not require dilatation. The diameter of the colon is measured with sizers. Whenever possible, the 31-mm Premium CEEA should be used. When necessary, the descending colon can be dilated with the surgeon's thumb, or alternatively by slow distension with water in a Foley catheter with a 30-ml balloon. The anvil shaft assembly of the Premium CEEA is detached from the central rod and positioned within the descending colon. The purse-string is tightly tied within the groove on the shaft.

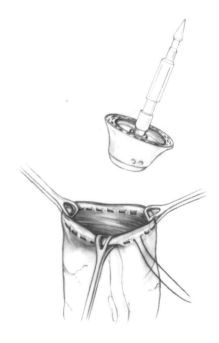

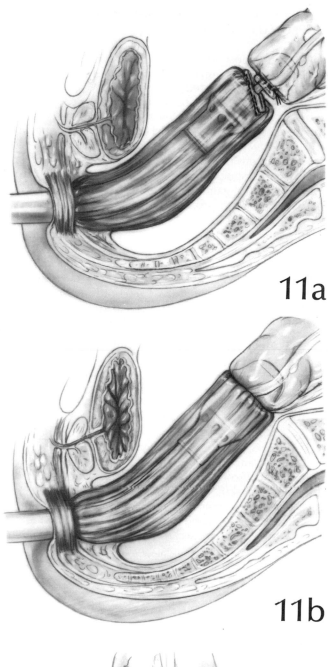

11a–c The anus is dilated to admit four fingers. The trocar is positioned in the centre rod of the Premium CEEA and withdrawn below the level of the staples. The head of the stapler is introduced into the rectum and advanced to the stapled closure of the proximal rectum. The trocar is advanced through the centre of the staple line by turning the wing nut at the base of the stapler. Once the tip of the trocar becomes visible, scissors are used to open the overlying intestinal wall. This facilitates passage of the trocar and prevents tearing of the rectum.

The centre rod is advanced until its orange neck is visible. The trocar is removed. The shaft of the anvil is inserted into the centre rod. The wing nut is turned until the green area becomes visible in the tissue thickness gauge. The stapler is fired. One Lembert suture of 3/0 silk is placed anteriorly on the staple line. This is used to provide counter traction as the stapler is withdrawn. The anvil is opened three and a half turns, twisted left and right and removed. The 'doughnuts' of tissue should be complete circles.

A rigid sigmoidoscope is introduced into the rectum and the staple line is inspected for haemostasis. The pelvis is filled with water. The rectum is insufflated until air escapes through the anus around the sigmoidoscope. The anastomosis should be air-tight; no air bubbles should float to the surface of the water in the pelvis.

Wound closure

The fascia is closed with a continuous monofilament suture (1 polydioxanone). The skin edges are approximated with a continuous subcuticular absorbable suture (4/0 coated polyglycolic acid). A sterile dressing is applied to the wound.

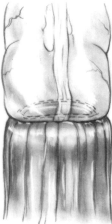

FAILED NON-OPERATIVE REDUCTION OR SUSPECTED ISCHAEMIC GUT

Failed sigmoidoscopic reduction or the presence of local peritonitis require urgent operative reduction and resection of the twisted sigmoid loop. A low midline incision is mandatory to provide the necessary exposure of an often enormously dilated sigmoid loop. Where possible, the surgeon should not untwist the colon because this manoeuvre may 'release' the contained stagnant venous blood into the circulation, which might cause septic shock. Similarly, the obstructed succus entericus would gain access to an absorptive surface in the intestine, both proximal and distal to the volvulus, with a similar outcome. Therefore, the colon should be clamped in the twisted position, and the mesentery clamped to occlude the vessels. Once control has been obtained, the colon can then be untwisted and removed.

The sigmoid colon generally twists anticlockwise, the caecum clockwise. When the base of the mesocolon is inspected, the direction in which to reduce it will be obvious. Several options for resection are available:

1. Paul–Mikulicz exteriorization and resection.
2. Hartmann's procedure.
3. Resection and primary anastomosis.

Paul–Mikulicz resection

The abdomen is entered through a lateral flank incision and the strangulated segment of sigmoid colon is exteriorized through the incision. The sigmoid loop is amputated at skin level distal to crushing clamps. A double-barrelled colostomy is fashioned using interrupted all-coats intestine to subdermal sutures and a few interrupted sutures are placed between the two adjacent limbs of the colostomy. This procedure is of largely historical interest.

Hartmann's procedure

Colorectal anastomoses constructed when the patient has not received a mechanical and antibiotic bowel preparation carry a high risk of leakage. Perforation of the sigmoid colon and significant peritoneal soiling also increase the risk of primary anastomosis. The incision, mobilization and resection of the sigmoid colon are the same as described above. Additional mobilization of the descending colon may be required, so that its divided end will reach the anterior abdominal wall. When the colon is unprepared, transection of the gut with a GIA 60 stapler minimizes the risk of spillage of stool. The apex of the rectal pouch is sutured to the sacral promontory with two or three non-absorbable sutures. This prevents retraction and allows easy identification of the pouch when the time comes for closure of the colostomy (as described in the chapter on pp. 798–806).

Resection and primary anastomosis

In selected patients with colonic obstruction, primary anastomoses have been constructed with a satisfactory outcome and with low leakage rates. Absence of peritoneal soiling and viable intestinal ends are prerequisites. Intraoperative cleansing of the colon is required (as described in chapter on pp. 727–745). The procedure is as described for sigmoid colectomy.

Operations for caecal volvulus

Position of patient

The patient is placed in a supine position. Access to the anus is not required.

Incision

The abdomen is entered through a midline incision for caecal volvulus. It should extend from the mid-epigastrium to below the umbilicus. Other incisions are possible but may interfere with the positioning of a stoma if a primary anastomosis proves unwise.

CAECOPEXY

12 The volvulus is derotated. Interrupted sero-muscular sutures of 3/0 silk are placed along the antimesenteric border of the ascending colon. These are used to secure the right colon to the abdominal wall near the right gutter. Low rates of recurrence of volvulus after this simple technique have been reported, but additional fixation of the ascending colon with an elevated flap of parietal peritoneum or polyvinyl alcohol sponge has been advocated.

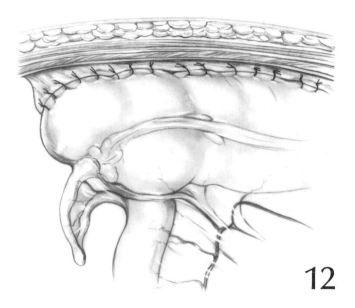

CAECOSTOMY

The caecal volvulus is untwisted. A colotomy is made through the anterior taenia coli of the caecum. The caecum and ascending colon are decompressed and drained of as much faecal material as possible with a large-core suction catheter. Irrigation of the caecum with warmed saline may be necessary to obtain satisfactory drainage of the right colon. Alternatively, the appendix can be excised and the caecum cannulated through the appendiceal orifice.

13 Two concentric purse-string sutures of a strong non-absorbable suture, such as 2/0 silk, are placed around the colotomy. The caecum is intubated with the largest available Mallincrot or Foley catheter. The catheter is secured in place with the purse-string sutures.

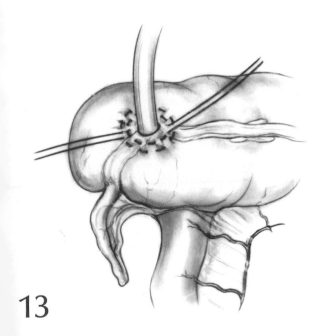

14 Interrupted seromuscular sutures of 3/0 silk are used to secure the antimesenteric border of the right colon within the right gutter, as with a caecopexy. A small stab wound is made approximately at McBurney's point in the right lower quadrant. A curved clamp is passed through the abdominal wall and used to withdraw the end of the catheter through the stab incision. Interrupted seromuscular sutures of 3/0 silk placed around the catheter seal the caecum to the anterior abdominal wall. Two heavy sutures, such as 1 silk, bind the catheter to the skin and prevent migration of the catheter.

After closure of the abdominal incision, a bulky dressing is placed around the catheter. This dressing maintains the first few centimetres of the catheter in a position perpendicular to the abdominal wall, which prevents kinking at the level of the fascia. The catheter is placed on continuous suction.

After the operation, the caecostomy catheter requires frequent attention. It must be cautiously irrigated with water several times a day. Abdominal radiographs should be obtained to confirm continued satisfactory decompression of the caecum. The catheter is removed approximately 3 weeks after the operation. In the majority of patients, the caecocutaneous fistula will spontaneously close. Occasionally, operative closure is required.

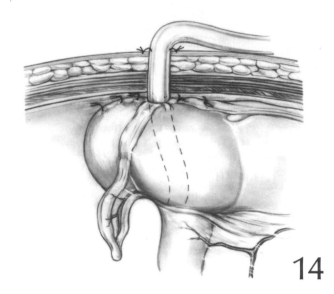

14

RESECTION: RIGHT HEMICOLECTOMY

Mobilization of the caecum is facilitated by the presence of a long mesentery. The retroperitoneal attachment of the caecum is opened near the common iliac vessels and the ureter is identified. A hand is passed palm-up behind the ascending colon and anterior to the ureter up to the hilum of the kidney. With the ascending colon retracted anteriorly, the lateral attachments of the colon are incised up to the hepatic flexure. The attachments of the mesocolon to the duodenum are sharply divided. The right colon is mobilized medially to the vena cava and the mesentery of the terminal ileum is freed of its retroperitoneal fixation. This allows sufficient mobility for the terminal ileum to be rotated up to the transverse colon for the anastomosis.

The lesser sac is entered through the avascular plane between the omentum and transverse colon. The omentum is freed from the proximal half of the transverse colon and preserved. The remaining points of fixation of the hepatic flexure are divided with cautery.

15 The right colon is elevated. The terminal ileum is divided with a GIA 60 stapler near the end of the ligament of Treves. The ileal arcades in the mesentery are divided between curved clamps. The ileocolic, right colic and right branch of the middle colic vessels are identified and divided near their origin and doubly ligated with 2/0 silk sutures.

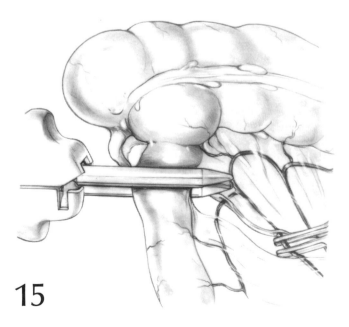

15

16 The transverse colon is divided with a GIA 60 or GIA 80 stapler near the preserved arcades of the left branch of the middle colic artery. The remaining mesentery near the chosen points of resection are divided between clamps and tied with 3/0 silk sutures. The specimen is held off the field and opened to ensure that no unsuspected neoplasms are found near the margins of resection.

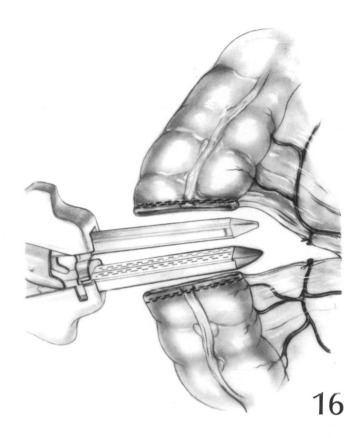

16

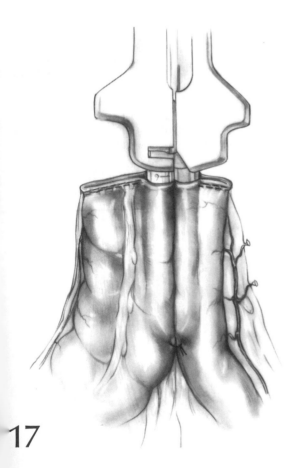

17

Side-to-side (functional end-to-end) ileocolic anastomosis

17 If the operation has proceeded smoothly without significant contamination of the abdomen with faecal material, a primary anastomosis can be constructed. The caudad surface of the transverse colon and the cephalad surface of the terminal ileum are approximated and fixed with two sutures of 3/0 silk. The mesentery of the terminal ileum is inspected to ensure that it is not twisted. The corners of the two staple lines are opened with a pair of heavy Mayo scissors. A large-bore suction catheter is passed into both the transverse colon and terminal ileum. The anastomosis is constructed along the antimesenteric border of the transverse colon with a GIA 60 stapler and the staple line inspected for haemostasis.

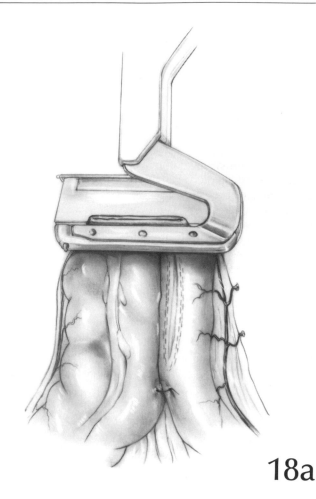

18a

18a, b The silk suture near the enterotomy is removed. Four Allis' clamps are used to approximate the intestinal wall of the remaining enterotomy. This is closed with a TA 55 stapler using 4.8-mm staples. A 3/0 silk suture is placed in the 'crotch' of the anastomosis and the abdomen is liberally irrigated with warmed saline.

BROOKE ILEOSTOMY

If the caecum has ruptured or there is gross spillage of stool into the abdominal cavity, a primary anastomosis should not be constructed. An end (Brooke) ileostomy and mucous fistula are fashioned (as described in the chapter on pp. 627–653). The closed end of the transverse colon is tacked to the cephalad end of the incision. It is not opened. The abdominal incision is closed, and the wound protected. The stapled closure of the terminal ileum is excised with a pair of curved Mayo scissors and the stoma constructed.

Closure

The fascia is closed with a continuous monofilament suture (1 polydioxanone). The wound is irrigated with an antibiotic-containing solution and the skin edges are left open. The wound is packed with gauze soaked in povidone-iodine. The skin wound can be closed 3–4 days after operation with Steri-strips.

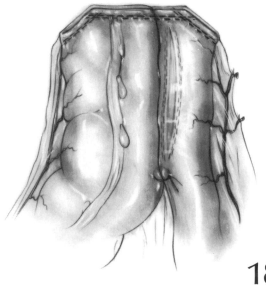

18b

Postoperative care

The management of patients after operation for large intestinal volvulus is the same as after resection of the colon for other diseases. The patient receives one additional dose of antibiotics after surgery. The nasogastric tube is removed on the first day after operation and the Foley catheter is removed when the patient is ambulatory. The patient begins eating when postoperative ileus resolves and is observed for signs and symptoms of abdominal sepsis and wound infection. If an intra-abdominal abscess is suspected, computed tomography of the abdomen with both intravenous and oral contrast media is performed. Abdominal abscesses can often be treated with percutaneous drainage.

Preliminary assessment of the integrity of a stapled anastomosis can be made on the basis of a plain abdominal radiograph. The staples of an intact anastomosis will form one of several different continuous patterns depending on the type of stapling technique that was used. A break in the continuity of the staple line strongly suggests anastomotic dehiscence. If an anastomotic leak is suspected, a Gastrografin enema is given to confirm its presence. Clinically significant dehiscence of the anastomosis is generally treated by removing it and constructing an ileostomy or colostomy. If no complications evolve during the postoperative course, the patient is discharged 7–10 days after operation.

Outcome

The results of treatment for large intestinal volvulus are largely determined by the condition of the twisted segment of colon at the time of operation. When the colon is viable, hospital mortality rates below 10% can be achieved in patients with either sigmoid or caecal volvulus. Unfortunately, the mortality rate of necrotic sigmoid colon is extremely high. Thus, early treatment either by non-operative or operative means is the primary determinant of outcome.

Caecopexy is followed by a 5–10% recurrence rate of volvulus. Recurrence after caecostomy is rare. Right colectomy obviously precludes recurrence. None the less, hospital mortality rates for patients afflicted with caecal volvulus are primarily determined by the condition of the intestine at the time of operation; mortality rates of 12% have been reported for patients with viable intestine at the time of operation and 32% for those with a necrotic right colon. As Lord Moynihan stated in 1905: 'Anything over a 10% mortality is the mortality of delay.'

Further reading

Ballantyne GH. Review of sigmoid volvulus: history and results of treatment. *Dis Colon Rectum* 1982; 25: 494–501.

Ballantyne GH. Review of sigmoid volvulus: clinical patterns and pathogenesis. *Dis Colon Rectum* 1982; 25: 823–30.

Ballantyne GH. The meaning of ileus: its changing definition over three millenia. *Am J Surg* 1984; 148: 252–6.

Ballantyne GH, Brander MD, Beart RW Jnr, Ilstrup DM. Volvulus of the colon: incidence and mortality. *Ann Surg* 1985; 202: 83–92.

Burke JB, Ballantyne GH. Cecal volvulus: low mortality at a city hospital. *Dis Colon Rectum* 1984; 27: 737–40.

Anterior resection of the rectum

R. J. Heald MA, MChir, FRCS, FRCSEd
Consultant Surgeon, Colorectal Research Unit, Basingstoke District Hospital, Basingstoke, Hampshire, UK

Prepared with the advice and collaboration of the former author of this chapter:

J. C. Goligher FRCS
Emeritus Professor of Surgery, University of Leeds, Leeds, UK

History

Until 20 years ago, anterior resection of the rectum, although a well established procedure, was considered appropriate for only the 30–50% of patients in whom the tumour was in the upper part of the rectum: it is now the accepted operation for 80–90% of all patients with rectal cancer. However, some of the lower lesions so treated impose special difficulties and carry a greater risk of complications.

Three important changes in surgical technique have led to the increased usage of this operation: (1) the recognition that a margin of clearance of 2.0 cm of apparently uninvolved intestinal wall beyond the palpable distal edge of the growth (or possibly less) is adequate, instead of the 5-cm margin previously considered necessary; (2) the availability of stapling devices that enable a colorectal anastomosis to be constructed with good results as low as the top of the anal canal; and (3) the appreciation that a thorough dissection and complete mobilization of the rectum and the cancer by the abdominal operator is necessary before deciding whether a sphincter-saving resection is possible.

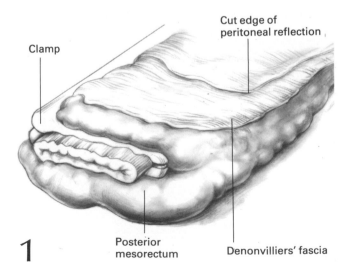

Clamp

Cut edge of peritoneal reflection

Posterior mesorectum

Denonvilliers' fascia

1

1 Good results can be attained by rectal mobilization in which the avascular plane between the visceral and parietal structures is identified under direct vision as a delicate filamentous latticework of areolar tissue. This encapsulation of the rectum and its mesorectum within a surgically definable plane provides one of the finest opportunities in surgery for a clear monobloc resection of a cancer-bearing organ and its principal field of direct, lymphatic and vascular spread. The precise development of the plane in the depths of the pelvis does, however, present special difficulties, and failure to excise this monobloc of tissue completely may explain the considerable differences in the incidence of local tumour recurrence recorded by different surgeons[1, 2].

Principles and justification

Several procedures are appropriate, depending on the circumstances. Each should be considered carefully.

Abdominoperineal excision (*see* also pp. 782–797)

This procedure is appropriate only for carcinomas that invade the anal sphincter or for those tumours which, after full mobilization in the visceroparietal plane, are so close to the sphincter that a clamp cannot be placed safely below the palpable edge of the tumour with an adequate margin of clearance. Thus, an abdominoperineal excision is more frequently necessary in an obese man with a narrow pelvis than in a woman. It may also be preferred to a very low anterior resection when anal sphincter tone and function are impaired, although some surgeons may prefer to undertake a Hartmann's procedure (*see* chapter on pp. 798–806) in this situation.

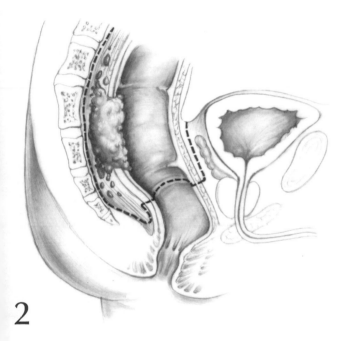

2

Low anterior resection with total mesorectal excision

2 The authors believe that the complete mesorectum should be removed as part of the proper clearance of all mid and low rectal tumours[3]. After full mobilization, the distal 'tail' of the mesorectum may be trimmed posteriorly and removed with the specimen to leave a 3–4-cm reservoir of rectal muscle tube above the anal canal. The precise site of the tumour will determine the length of distal rectum that can remain. The anastomosis (for which most surgeons will find the stapled technique easier) may thus lie up to 5 cm from the dentate line.

Usually, mobilization of the splenic flexure will be necessary to achieve an adequate length of colon for an anastomosis at this level. In addition, the large cavity created in the pelvis must be 'filled' with viable tissue and effectively drained with suction for the first 48 h after surgery. The large size of this cavity and the small size of the rectal reservoir distal to the anastomosis are important factors contributing to the risk of anastomotic leakage (*see* also chapter on pp. 561–572).

Many surgeons regard temporary defunctioning of the anastomosis by a proximal loop transverse colostomy or loop ileostomy as a wise precaution in these cases of very low anastomosis.

High anterior resection and mesorectal division

3 In this procedure the mesorectum is transected 5 cm below the tumour and the anastomosis is constructed in the middle third of the rectum, giving a rectal stump 8–10 cm long above the dentate line. Thus the size of the cavity remaining in the pelvis is smaller, and the higher and relatively easier anastomosis can be made manually or stapled according to the surgeon's preference. It is appropriate for patients with tumours above the peritoneal reflection in whom mobilization achieves sufficient length for the mesorectum to be divided 5 cm below the lower edge of the cancer. Full mobilization of the splenic flexure is usually unnecessary, suction drainage can often be omitted, and defunctioning is almost never required. The procedure is less of an undertaking than a low anterior resection with complete mesorectal excision and is associated with a much lesser incidence of anastomotic dehiscence and other complications.

Surgeons vary in the frequency with which they use high anterior resection. One of the authors (RJH) feels it appropriate in only about 15% of true rectal cancers because of the fear of local tumour recurrence arising from lymphatic and other satellite deposits of growth in the mesorectal tissues which are not excised. High anterior resection is used rather more frequently by JCG, particularly in patients whose rectal lesions lie 10 cm (or more) above the anal verge when measured at the preoperative sigmoidoscopy.

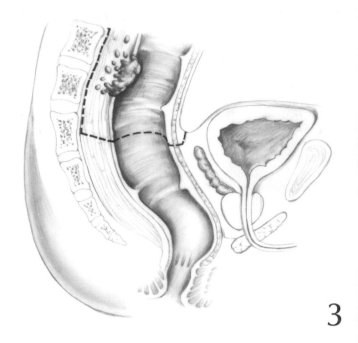

3

Abdominoanal, abdominosacral and abdominotransanal resections

These operations were popular with some surgeons when anterior resection was confined to growths of the upper rectum. The development of low anterior resection techniques and the advent of staplers have made these methods less useful alternatives.

Extended Hartmann procedure

The extent and technique of excision of tissue in this operation is identical to that of a low anterior resection, but no anastomosis is performed. Instead the patient is left with an iliac colostomy, an intact anal canal, and a small (open or closed) distal rectal stump, extending just above the pelvic floor (*see* chapter on pp. 798–806). It is appropriate for patients in whom an anastomosis is undesirable or likely to be unduly risky, a colostomy is acceptable, and in whom the tumour can be mobilized sufficiently for the bowel to be divided below it with an adequate margin of clearance. It may be particularly applicable if irremovable extensions of growth in the pelvis make local recurrence inevitable, or if the reason for avoiding an anastomosis is a patulous anal sphincter.

Local excision

This is appropriate for small mobile cancers in the lower half of the rectum that have not invaded the muscle coat of the intestinal wall, particularly those so close to the anal sphincter that only an abdominoperineal excision would provide adequate clearance. The indication is considerably strengthened if the patient is deemed to be an especially poor risk for abdominoperineal excision.

Preoperative

Clinical assessment

Frail patients may be judged unsuitable for the major surgery involved, and thus assessment of the general and cardiopulmonary condition of the patient is of great importance. Cardiac function tests may be useful, and assessment of peripheral vascular supply to the legs is always necessary because acute (and possibly fatal) postoperative leg ischaemia can occur when visceral collaterals, which have maintained a tenuous arterial supply to the legs, are interrupted by surgery[4].

The quality of the anal sphincter and its tone on rectal examination are also important: a patient prone to leakage or incontinence with a patulous sphincter would be unsuitable for very low colorectal or coloanal anastomosis. Previous intestinal resections and/or coexisting gastrointestinal disease causing diarrhoea or urgency might also influence the decision as to the most appropriate operation. The patient's own desire to avoid a stoma needs to be balanced against any of these relative contraindications.

Biopsy

A biopsy to confirm the diagnosis is essential before proceeding to surgery of this magnitude. However, the presence of a high-grade (poorly differentiated) tumour is no longer regarded as a contraindication to the performance of a sphincter-conserving operation.

Imaging

Both computed tomography (CT) and ultrasonography have enabled identification of local tumour spread and nodal metastasis. Substantial extrarectal spread more than 5 mm in diameter, or obvious nodal spread, apparent on a CT scan may also provide a guide towards the use of full-dose preoperative radiotherapy. Improved CT, ultrasonography and magnetic resonance imaging techniques will give the surgeon more precise information concerning the extent of tumour spread.

An intravenous pyelogram is of value with lesions which are close to the ureter (e.g. rectosigmoid, sigmoid and caecal tumours) and in the few large fixed rectal tumours which occupy the whole pelvis. However, it has little relevance to the routine mid-rectal carcinoma because the ureter is anterior to such lesions.

The entire large intestine should be examined using either double-contrast radiology or colonoscopy to exclude the presence of synchronous tumours (which occur in 3.5–4.0% of cases) and polyps. When the obstructive nature of the primary rectal tumour makes this impossible, careful palpation at operation should be combined with colonoscopy during the first 6–12 months after surgery to establish that the patient has a truly 'clear colon'.

Examination under anaesthesia

Patients should be examined rectally under general anaesthesia, and bimanual abdominovaginal examination in a woman should always be performed. In selected cases, cystoscopy may be necessary for bladder inspection and to insert ureteric stents. The assessment of tumour mobility and the extent of invasion of local structures will help the selection of locally advanced tumours for preoperative radiotherapy. Assuming that the surgeon decides to proceed with an operation, a urethral catheter is then inserted.

Bowel preparation

An empty large intestine is desirable, and can be achieved satisfactorily by combining clear fluids by mouth for 48 h before surgery with oral laxatives. During surgery, if more than minimal residual faeces are found in the colon, an on-table lavage can be performed (*see* chapter on pp. 727–745). Systemic antibacterial agents, including those effective against anaerobes (such as metronidazole) are commenced 1–2 h before surgery and administered every 6 h thereafter for 24 h.

Operations

LOW ANTERIOR RESECTION WITH TOTAL MESORECTAL EXCISION

Position of patient

The lithotomy-Trendelenburg position is used which ensures a choice of operation in the light of the operative findings (sphincter-saving resection or abdominoperineal excision). In the event of a restorative resection, this position permits the anal insertion of a staple gun. The patient is kept horizontal during the initial abdominal phase of the operation and only tilted 15–20° head down when the pelvic dissection commences.

Good lighting of the operative field is extremely important. It can be obtained by readjusting the readily moved and focused operating room lights to meet the needs of different phases of the dissection, a headlight (which some surgeons find rather irksome) and by incorporating lights into retractors.

Incision and abdominal exploration

4 The best access to the abdomen and pelvis is provided by a long vertical median or left paramedian incision extending from the pubic symphysis to well above the umbilicus. In obese male patients, anything short of an incision from the pubic symphysis to the xiphoid is unlikely to be satisfactory. Some surgeons advocate a long transverse incision, but in the authors' experience this is less satisfactory for the pelvic dissection than a conventional vertical approach.

The next step is a thorough exploration of the abdominal cavity to determine the presence of any extensions of the growth, special attention being directed to the liver, the greater omentum and peritoneal surfaces, the small intestine, the entire large intestine, and finally the rectum and the primary lesion itself. If no contraindication to excision is found, a self-retaining retractor is inserted. Loops of small intestine must be displaced away from the intended dissection in the left lower abdomen by enclosing it in a plastic bag which is then placed to the patient's right in front of the abdominal wall, into the right upper peritoneal compartment, or by packing the individual coils of intestine into the right upper compartment with a 20-cm wide roll of gauze, tightly rolled and held in place by an assistant's hand or a Finnochetto retractor.

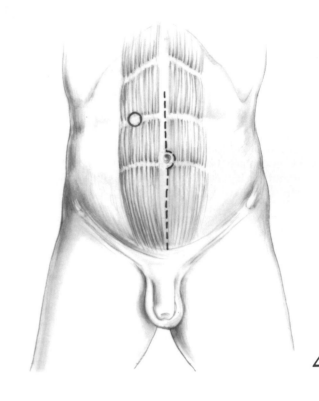

4

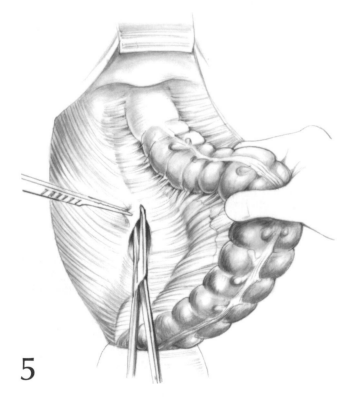

5

Initial incision of the visceral peritoneum

5 This will generally begin to the left or to the right of the pelvic brim. The left side is customary, the white lines of congenital adhesions between the left leaf of the mesosigmoid and the posterior parietal peritoneum providing a convenient starting point. It is important to gain access to the avascular plane between the mesentery and the surrounding parietal structures: a valuable clue to this is the mobility of the tissues which can be readily seen through the transparent peritoneum. A perfectly avascular plane can be developed in front of the bifurcation of the presacral nerve as it crosses the aortic bifurcation.

The process of lifting forward the superior rectal vessels and mesorectum is thus initiated. If a perfect avascular plane is not readily found to the left of the mesocolon, the operator should make a corresponding incision on the right side where vision and lighting are often better. The orientation provided by this plane is important for the satisfactory dissection of the more distal parts of the dissection.

6 Further dissection is divided into three stages.

1. Extension of the peritoneal cut around the left side of the splenic flexure, fully mobilizing the left colon and exposing the termination of the inferior mesenteric vein.
2. Extension of the right cut to encircle and facilitate the ligation of the inferior mesenteric artery and vein.
3. Extension of both planes downwards into the pelvis around the fully mobilized mesorectum, rectum, and the cancer.

The order in which these procedures are performed will vary according to circumstances: for example mobilization of the splenic flexure is not needed if an abdominoperineal excision becomes necessary, if the tumour can be resected with mesorectal division and a relatively high anastomosis, or if a trial dissection leads to the decision to refer the patient for radiotherapy; in some low cases an exceptionally long and well vascularized sigmoid may be safely used for the anastomosis. In all these situations the early mobilization of the splenic flexure would be inappropriate.

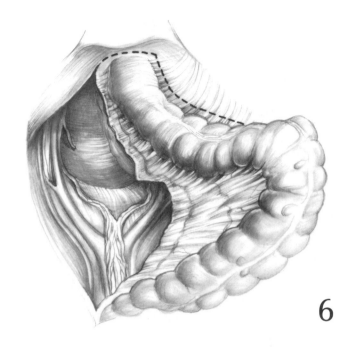

6

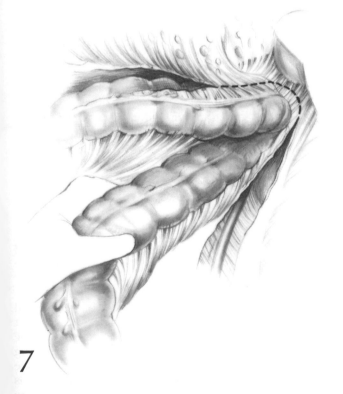

7

Mobilization of the splenic flexure

7 The wound is retracted superolaterally to the left while the peritoneum is divided and the subperitoneal fascia divided as a separate layer. The gonadal vessels, the ureter and the autonomic nerve plexuses are carefully preserved. The omentum is lifted forwards and upwards and the colon dissected from its posterior leaf and down from the adhesions to the hilar region and lower pole of the spleen. If the correct planes are followed, it will become apparent that the entire blood supply of the omentum comes from the gastric leaves so that the mobilization of the left colon should be virtually bloodless. Various adhesions can, however, make this part of the operation tedious. Once near the midline, the omentum becomes so mobile that later it can be brought down into the pelvis to wrap around the anastomosis.

Ligation and division of the inferior mesenteric vessels

8 In most cases the inferior mesenteric artery will be ligated and divided about 2 cm from the aorta in order to preserve those autonomic nerves which split around its origin. Some distance away, above and to the left, the inferior mesenteric vein disappears behind the lower border of the pancreas to the left of the duodenojejunal flexure. For a low anastomosis, the vein is best divided here because this gives the greatest amount of mobility to the splenic flexure so that the colon can lie easily in the bottom of the pelvis. In approximately 10% of patients a substantial branch from the superior mesenteric artery lies near the inferior mesenteric vein and supplies the descending colon. Judgement is required to determine if this vessel should be preserved or if it must be divided to provide sufficient intestine to reach the pelvic floor.

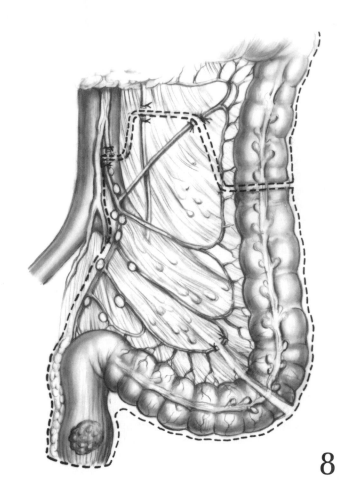

8

Mobilization of the mesorectum, rectum and cancer

This is the most important stage of the operation. The surgeon must develop a mental picture of the exact position of the tumour and its local spread based on the initial investigation and the preoperative assessment. To cut across or to leave satellites of tumour in the pelvis is to expose the patient to a very high risk of local recurrence.

Many surgeons prefer to divide the colon at this stage to facilitate the posterior and lateral dissections. The GIA stapler is ideal for this, but the colonic end will need to be revised and washed out later before the anastomosis is undertaken.

Posterior dissection

9 The avascular areolar tissue plane which surrounds the mesorectum must now be identified. The posterior surface of the mesorectum is similar to a bilobed lipoma. As the rectum is lifted gently forwards from the bifurcation of the presacral nerves, the areolar plane is opened under direct vision by sharp dissection and is extended downwards around the curve of the sacrum in the midline, past the coccyx, and forwards in front of the anococcygeal raphe. A St Mark's retractor (with integral illumination) greatly helps this process, particularly during the distal parts of the dissection which require the mesorectum to be drawn forwards so that the lowest part of the dissection can be seen.

Lateral dissections

10 The lateral attachments are mobilized by extending the plane of dissection forwards from the posterior midline around the side walls of the pelvis. It is important to appreciate that the inferior hypogastric plexuses curve forwards tangentially around the surface of the mesorectum in close proximity to it. The slender nervi erigentes (on which erection depends) lie more posteriorly in the same plane as the presacral nerves, which should be seen and preserved, although it is all too easy to 'tent-up' the nerves and cut them.

The nervi erigentes curve forwards from the sacral foramina; they converge like a fan to join the presacral nerves and form the neurovascular bundles of Walsh[5]. Thus the nerves lie at the outer edges of Denonvilliers' fascia and are in great danger at 10 o'clock and 2 o'clock in the anterolateral position just behind the lateral edges of the seminal vesicles. More distally they curve forwards out of danger.

As the dissection moves deeper into the pelvis, one or two middle rectal vessels may be divided: occasionally one is of sufficient size to demand diathermy or ligation after occlusion by carefully placed slender curved artery forceps. If the areolar plane surrounding the mesorectum has been faithfully followed, it is unlikely that there will be enough lateral pedicle to divide between clamps as has often been recommended.

If bleeding is encountered, a small adrenaline-soaked swab should be placed on to the bleeding point and attention moved to another part of the dissection. Any bleeding will be more easily controlled after the tumour has been removed.

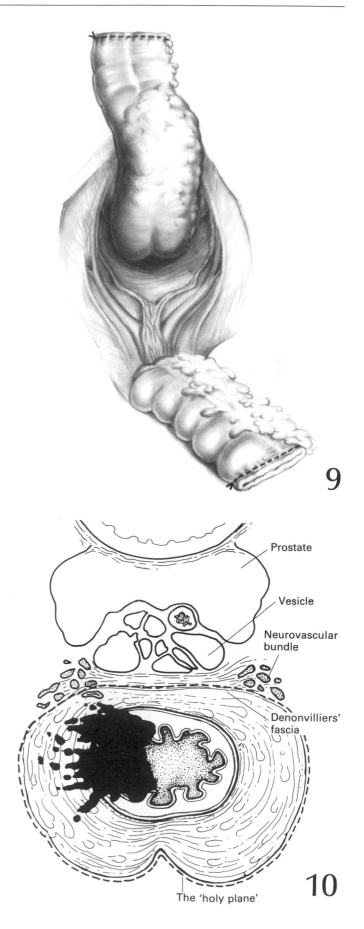

9

Prostate

Vesicle

Neurovascular bundle

Denonvilliers' fascia

The 'holy plane'

10

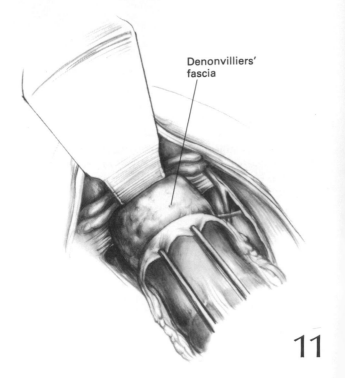

Denonvilliers' fascia

11

Anterior dissection

11, 12 In the male, a transverse incision is made through the peritoneum anterior to the peritoneal reflection in the pelvis, to descend straight to the superior aspect of the seminal vesicles. In drawing the tumour upwards it is important not to pull directly on the intestinal wall and tumour for fear of rupturing the tumour, and increasing the risk of local recurrence by malignant cell spillage. After the peritoneum at the rectovesical pouch has been divided, the posterior cut edge of the peritoneum should be grasped by long haemostats and gentle upward traction applied. This manoeuvre lessens the chance of the tumour being pulled apart.

A swab is laid on the anterior surface of the rectum, and the plane of dissection downwards immediately in front of Denonvilliers' fascia may now be developed, with great care, in the midline. Even greater care is required as this plane is extended laterally to meet the lateral dissection, because it is at the outer edge of Denonvilliers' fascia that the autonomic nerve fibres converge to form the neurovascular bundles that control both potency and bladder function. Denonvilliers' fascia marks the anterior limit of the dissection plane and the anterior surface of the 'tumour package'. It lies like a bib in front of the anterior mesorectum behind the vesicles, and below it fuses with the posterior fascia of the prostate. Therefore the fascia must be divided with scissors to 'cone-down' onto the anterior wall of the lowest few centimetres of the rectum, but this should not occur until well beyond the lower edge of the cancer.

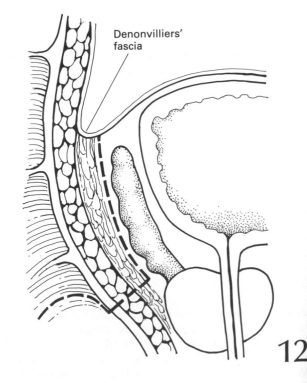

Denonvilliers' fascia

12

13 In the female, anterior dissection is generally straightforward provided that the uterus is lifted well forward. A common difficulty is to find a clean avascular plane behind the cervix and posterior fornix without encountering bleeding from the venous plexus. The peritoneal reflection itself may adhere to the posterior fornix; in this case (and the cancer permitting), the anterior peritoneal cut may be placed at the level of the posterior fornix to enter the dry plane just behind the posterior vaginal wall. Denonvilliers' fascia, often less well developed than in the male, is excised as the anterior surface of the specimen.

Anterolateral dissections

The joining of the anterior and lateral dissection planes is critical in the preservation of the pelvic autonomic nerves. It is particularly important in the male, but placement of the cuts requires careful judgement in both sexes. The anterior plane in the midline is clear of the nerves while the front of the lateral plane is marked by the presacral nerves and neurovascular bundles which have already been identified. The peritoneal and subperitoneal cuts are 'coned' medially to preserve these bundles as they curve inwards, and the lateral mesorectal edge is developed forwards to Denonvilliers' fascia and the circle is thus completed

Extended resections in special cases

Adherent adjacent organs should be excised *en bloc* with the primary tumour without splitting open a malignant adhesion. Although about half the adhesions to a cancerous segment are not caused by tumour invasion, it is safer to resect attached organs rather than to peel them away.

Uterus and vagina

It is practical to enter the vaginal vault at this stage and to excise a segment of vaginal wall with the cancer if the tumour is tethered or fixed at this point. However, if the cancer is large or fixed it is wise to clear all the anterior tissue medial to the nerves and the ureters and to perform a hysterectomy with excision of the vaginal vault and posterior vaginal wall before completing the anterior resection. If there is a large vaginal defect which cannot be closed, a low colorectal anastomosis should be wrapped around with the mobilized omentum and a loop stoma should be fashioned to defunction

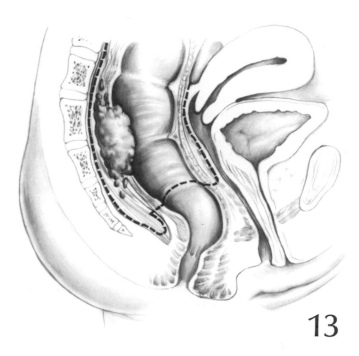

13

the anastomosis. These patients should not have sexual intercourse for several months after the operation until the area has healed.

Seminal vesicles

If these are very close to the tumour, the plane anterior to the seminal vesicles may be safely entered, allowing their excision *en bloc* with the rectum, carefully preserving the ureters. The neurovascular bundles will be in particular danger in such a dissection.

Prostate

It is occasionally appropriate, although difficult, to cut away an adherent part of the prostate or, when the prostate is greatly enlarged, to precede the rectal excision with a prostatectomy. The authors have encountered cases where transvesical or retropubic prostatectomy was necessary simply for access. The modern nerve-preserving 'radical prostatectomy' may be used as a part of extended *en bloc* anterior resection in a very small number of selected patients. The operation requires that the neurovascular bundles are carefully dissected distally, dividing the vessels emerging from them, ligating the troublesome penile dorsal venous complex, and removing the whole prostate with its capsule[5]. The distal prostatic urethra must be carefully divided above the triangular ligament.

Ureters

The ureters may be involved in rectosigmoid or colonic cancer but are seldom in danger in dissection for mid or low rectal cancer. However, it is always safe to divide the tissues anterior to the ureteric tunnels in both sexes because they pass in front of the nerve plexuses and are crossed only by the vasa, which may be sacrificed. If one ureter is invaded or obstructed, the adherent portion should be resected. Depending on the size of the resulting defect and height of the ureteric resection, it may be possible to effect a scalloped end-to-end anastomosis of the ureter or to implant the proximal end into the bladder or the opposite ureter[6]. The authors favour ureteroureterostomy as the most useful option and a pigtail stent across the interureteric anastomosis is a desirable safety measure if urological back-up is not readily available.

Bladder

The bladder may be involved in high (intraperitoneal) rectal cancers and the segment can be resected as a disc followed by reconstruction. The management of a mid-rectal tumour with anterior invasion of the bladder base is more difficult: it may be best approached by opening the bladder, catheterizing the ureters and resecting the bladder base at the point of adherence. A course of preoperative irradiation may facilitate such an operation. If firm attachment to the base of the bladder is encountered, the surgeon may be advised to close the abdomen without a resection, arrange a full course of radiotherapy, and then carry out a full laparotomy 8–12 weeks later, when conditions for curative resection may be more favourable.

Inferior hypogastric nerve plexuses and presacral nerves

Much of this chapter has emphasized the exploration of the plane within these nerves so that they may be preserved. If, however, a large tumour is invading the area, these must be resected with the cancer and the prevascular plane outside the nerves along the aorta and major vessels developed (a 'peri-adventitial strip'). If only one side is affected, the nerves on the other side may be preserved. There may, particularly in a female patient, be no serious functional consequences to nerve section, but stripping away of nerves not involved by the cancer is unnecessary.

Internal iliac nodes and the pelvic side wall

There is a wide variation in the reported incidence of internal iliac node involvement. Some surgeons regard lateral lymph node clearance as an essential part of radical surgery[7], but most limit extended resections to cases where there is either direct invasion and fixation of the region of the internal iliac vessels or a palpable or visible abnormal node within the chain concerned. If the tumour is found on preoperative evaluation to be bulky or fixed, a full course of preoperative irradiation will improve local cancer control and avoid the morbidity of extended lateral pelvic wall clearance. However, in the presence of direct invasion surgery may be modified to include ligation of the anterior division of the internal iliac artery and vein, and clearance of the pelvic side wall in the plane lateral to these vessels. Venous bleeding may be troublesome and this step should not be undertaken lightly. The nerve plexuses on the relevant side will be sacrificed; therefore they should be carefully preserved on the other side if possible.

Synchronous primary tumours

Arguments have been advanced for subtotal colectomy and ileorectal anastomosis for multiple cancers, and occasionally proctocolectomy with an ileal pouch and ileoanal anastomosis may be justified. However, ultra-low resection is more likely to be followed by good functional results when proximal large intestine is preserved. There is no evidence that a synchronous tumour may not be treated as effectively by a separate conventional resection without sacrificing the entire large bowel. This approach is preferred when the rectal cancer necessitates a low or ultra-low anastomosis. However, the remaining parts of the large intestine will need to be reviewed at regular intervals.

Liver metastases

This has become a highly specialized subject and is fully covered in the chapter on pp. 573–584. Small superficial and accessible deposits should be excised with a margin of normal liver of at least 1 cm whenever possible. However, the surgeon should be certain that there are no other metastases before undertaking synchronous resection of liver metastases. Intraoperative ultrasonography is used to determine the full status of the liver with regard to metastasis: when more deeply seated deposits are detected, it is better to complete the rectal excision and to document the full extent of the disease. In the postoperative period, CT scanning may give a clear picture of the extent of hepatic involvement, possibly avoiding fruitless re-exploration. Liver metastases should not normally be biopsied as implantation may occur.

Anastomosis

The most challenging part of the operation is now complete and the specimen is attached to the pelvic floor by a clean tube of anorectal muscle. The objectives remaining are to produce a perfect low anastomosis and to avoid implanting malignant cells into the soft tissue of the pelvis or the anastomosis itself.

14 The last remnants of the mesorectal 'tail' are drawn upwards with a swab and trimmed off the back of the rectum to create a clean muscle tube. The operator must carefully judge the position of the lower edge of the tumour. The intestinal wall is compressed with a finger and thumb distal to the tumour, and a right-angled clamp is placed below these with a 'safe' margin of intestinal wall between. Most rectal cancers may safely be given a clearance of 2 cm or less. Microscopic mural spread beyond the palpable lower edge is very rare and the compromise of mural margins does not appear to be a significant cause of local recurrence[8].

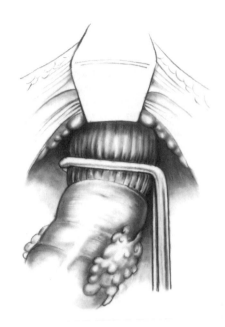

14

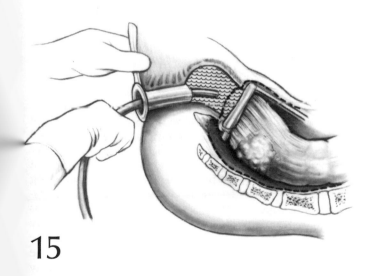

15

15 A proctoscope is introduced anally and fluid is delivered by a 50-ml syringe or through a catheter. Plain water is more cytocidal than saline; aqueous cetrimide or povidone-iodine solutions are probably best for this purpose.

Once the intraluminal washout is complete, and with the pelvis itself still awash with aqueous cetrimide, the anorectum is divided, preferably with a pair of large Goligher scissors. A few millimetres of intestinal wall should be left beyond the clamp so that it does not slip off. Upward traction must be applied only to the clamp; traction on the intestine itself may pull the cut edges through the clamp, with consequent spillage of malignant cells.

It may be difficult to achieve complete haemostasis, particularly in a long, narrow male pelvis. The middle rectal arteries themselves seldom bleed significantly and may usually be left until the pelvic side wall can be more readily inspected after the tumour has been removed. Gentle diathermy or a few ligatures are generally all that is required, although haemostatic gauze with local pressure may be helpful if a wide area of pelvic wall persists in oozing. Excessive use of diathermy may damage the hypogastric plexuses and should be avoided.

16 Insertion of the distal purse-string suture is important for a good stapled anastomosis. Upward pressure in the perineum is essential to bring the rectal stump into view. The principal operator's left hand should be inserted through the anus, or an assistant should apply direct pressure on a large swab. Countertraction with a St Mark's or wide-lipped pelvic retractor draws the bladder and vesicles forwards away from the anorectum which is thus made accessible for the suture. A 0 nylon or polypropylene (Prolene) suture (2/0 is rather easily broken) is mounted on a small half-circle atraumatic needle. A simple over-and-over continuous suture is appropriate, taking bites 5 mm from the cut edge of bowel and 5 mm apart.

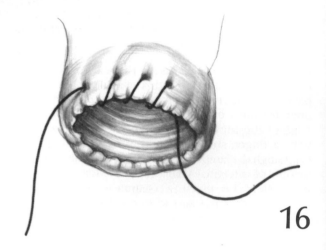

16

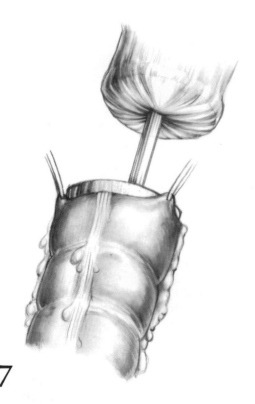

17

17 A pulsatile blood supply is essential so that the marginal artery is divided at a more distal point than the bowel itself. Usually, after full splenic flexure mobilization and double high ligations, the wide, well vascularized bowel which was formerly in the region of the spleen will be ready to lie comfortably in the sacral hollow without tension. However, great care is necessary in planning good vascular divisions that will preserve both adequate length and excellent blood supply for the crucial colonic component of the anastomosis. The proximal purse-string suture generally poses no problem and is performed with a simple over-and-over continuous stitch with 0 polypropylene.

The colonic end should be sucked out and washed clean with a cytocidal solution before being prepared for the anastomosis. This can be accomplished through the open bowel end using a 50-ml syringe and the sucker. The colonic end is eased over the anvil with the aid of three Babcock forceps. The intestinal wall drawn down onto the shaft should be cleaned of any mesenteric fat that may otherwise become interposed between the inverted opposed rims of colon and rectum. There is little good, and some harm, however, in cutting back the mesentery beyond the exact outer point of the inverted rim.

18 If the anvil has been disconnected from the body of the stapler, the introduction of the latter into the anus must be aided with lubricant and the assistant's fingers. The abdominal operator may pass a finger down through the lumen from above to meet the stapler, ease aside the mucosa and facilitate its upward passage. With the spindle fully advanced the lower purse-string suture is tightened and the upward-facing disc of rectal wall cleaned of any excess mesenteric fat.

The two halves of the stapler are now fixed together and the instrument is closed, taking great care not to catch adjacent structures such as vaginal wall or vesicles. When the gap is just within the recommendations (i.e. the widest permissible to avoid crushing the inturned rims), the gun is fired.

To remove the stapler, the gap between the shaft and the anvil must be opened while the gun is tilted, rotated and gently manipulated down through the anastomosis. The perineum may be steadied by the abdominal operator's left hand and the fingers used to help ease the instrument through the anal canal.

19 The purse-string sutures and a complete ring of intestinal end should be identified from both the rectal and the colonic sides in order to check the gun rings. Cutting and withdrawing the purse-string will avoid errors with a very slender ring. The anastomosis may be further checked by filling the pelvis with water and injecting air into the rectum through the anus.

20 If anastomotic integrity is in doubt it is common practice to add reinforcing sutures, and formation of a defunctioning loop stoma is wise in such a case. Only the distal (anorectal) ring should be sent for histology to confirm that tumour has not spread distally.

A double-stapling technique has many advocates, although it has not been proved superior to the use of a single-stapling approach. The TA55 or RL60 staplers may be used to divide the rectum about 5 cm from the dentate line or the TA35 or RL30 may be used to divide the anorectum in a very low anastomosis. To accommodate the thickness of the intestinal wall, the longer staple length is required. These staplers must be used only after the right-angled clamp has been applied and cytocidal washout completed. This means that the double-stapling method is inappropriate in the case of a very low-lying tumour because there is not enough room to place both the occlusive right-angled clamp and the stapler below the tumour. The technique does, however, save time if there is sufficient length of rectal stump to apply the stapler and clamp simultaneously.

With an ultra-low anastomosis, a J pouch may be created in the end of the proximal colon and stapled to the anus.

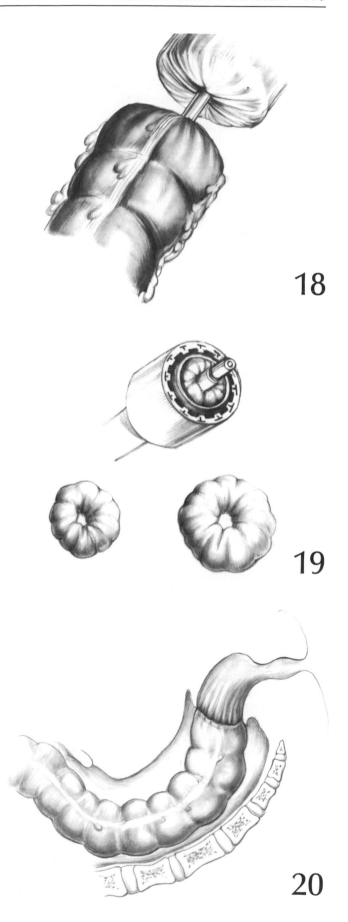

18

19

20

Defunctioning stomas

The question of whether to defunction a low or ultra-low anastomosis with a stoma remains controversial. With few exceptions, anastomotic leakage is reported in 10–15% of patients with anastomoses below 5 cm. The authors have adopted a cautious approach to intestinal defunction in such cases and use a loop right transverse colostomy. This stoma must be placed well to the right in the transverse colon because damage to the blood supply of the left transverse colon would be disastrous. We prefer to avoid a defunctioning ileostomy in the belief that episodes of band obstruction are more likely to occur after formation of a distal ileal stoma and its subsequent closure than after a loop transverse colostomy, which is performed entirely in the supracolic compartment. The stoma is closed 6–8 weeks after surgery, after a water-soluble contrast study has shown satisfactory healing of the colorectal anastomosis.

HIGH ANTERIOR RESECTION AND MESORECTAL DIVISION

Tumours above the peritoneal reflection, with a sigmoidoscopic height of about 10–15 cm from the anal verge, would not usually be considered by most surgeons to require an operation of the magnitude of a low anterior resection with total mesorectal excision. Treatment in these cases is by high anterior resection of the rectum, the initial stages of which are identical to those described for low resection except that mobilization of the splenic flexure may not be necessary.

After posterior mobilization of the rectum and the upper part of the lateral dissection have been performed, the tumour is lifted well out of the pelvis so that the mesorectum may be divided 5 cm below the lower edge of the cancer to ensure that any tumorous lymphatic invasion close to the primary lesion is removed. The superior rectal vessels are clamped and ligated, and the rectal wall is carefully cleaned and clamped as previously described.

The wall is then divided immediately below the clamp. Normally there is no problem in bringing down the upper sigmoid or descending colon for either a stapled anastomosis, using the technique described for low anterior resection (*see* also chapter on pp. 551–560), or manually inserted sutures. Anastomoses at this level should not require defunctioning and, because the pelvic cavity is largely filled by the remaining rectum and mesorectum, there is usually no need for suction drainage.

Postoperative management

Pelvic drains

Sump drains require continuous suction by extrinsic pumps. Interruption of suction during the transfer of the patient from the operating room to the ward may allow blood clots to form and block the air channel. Therefore, the authors prefer to use two medium-sized suction drains which are connected to the operating room pump as soon as they are inserted and to a closed suction bottle as soon as the abdominal closure is commenced. The suction bottle can be transported with the patient to the ward without further attention.

Anastomotic leakage

The large cavity created by rectal and mesorectal excision does not readily drain despite suction, and may become the site of an infected presacral haematoma which can become a presacral abscess. In the second or third week after surgery, this abscess may discharge through or near the anastomosis into the bowel lumen and may occasionally require further opening of the abscess into the rectum to give adequate drainage. The closer the anastomosis is to the anus, the greater the risk of a chronic abscess and possible anastomotic failure.

Anastomotic leakage of a different kind may sometimes occur during an apparently good recovery[9]. This problem may be caused by 'faecal extrusion': peristalsis driving the faeces downwards against a closed sphincter and forcing faecal material through the anastomosis into the pelvic tissues, leading to pelvic sepsis and septicaemia. Thus, despite the apparent initiation of normal bowel function, such patients sometimes become unwell, develop abdominal pain and peritonitis or simply deteriorate in a way that leads to suspicions of pulmonary embolus or cardiac event. In such patients an urgent radio-opaque enema should be undertaken to identify the leakage as the cause of septicaemia.

Anastomotic leakage is managed as in the chapter on pp. 750–765.

Loop stoma

Once the patient has progressed satisfactorily and the likelihood of anastomotic leakage is small, the supporting bar under the loop stoma can be removed, usually 10–14 days after surgery. If there are signs of an anastomotic leakage, then the supporting bar should be retained for a few extra days. About 4–5 weeks after surgery, a water-soluble contrast enema is carried out as a prelude to closure of the colostomy to make sure that the anastomosis is intact. If a leak is observed, the stoma should be left in place for a further few weeks and the contrast study repeated.

Anastomotic stricture

All low stapled anastomoses may be readily palpated during follow-up visits. A narrowing to 1–2 cm is very common in the early months and gentle dilatation may be appropriate at the time of colostomy closure, and occasionally in the ensuing months. Persistent symptomatic stricture is rare unless there has been colonic ischaemia, inadequate colonic length or gross pelvic sepsis. It cannot be overemphasized that the colon proximal to a low anastomosis must lie without tension in the hollow of the sacrum to avoid ischaemic complications. Very occasionally, reoperation may be required to achieve sufficient length of colon.

Postoperative anorectal function

If the sphincters were effective before surgery, it is rare for incontinence or stool seepage to be a problem with even the lowest anastomosis. Urgency and frequency of defaecation (the 'absent reservoir' syndrome) improves gradually over the initial 12–18 months. Very occasionally, reversion to a permanent colostomy may be requested by the patient and should be considered if symptoms are severe.

Local recurrence

This chapter is dedicated to techniques designed to prevent the dismal complication of local tumour recurrence, which is seldom amenable to curative treatment. If pelvic recurrence occurs, the patient should be considered for a full course of irradiation therapy, and further surgery can be contemplated 8–12 weeks after the end of this treatment. A repeat anterior resection may, very occasionally, be possible, or an abdominoperineal resection or a pelvic exenteration may be indicated.

Adjuvant therapy

Most surgeons believe that full-dose radiotherapy confers some benefit in selected cases, particularly for the locally advanced bulky lesion. Preoperative radiotherapy has the advantage that much of the fully irradiated tissue is removed by subsequent surgery. This treatment also has the theoretical attraction that it may shrink the tumour sufficiently to render the surgical dissection planes less likely to be transgressed by viable cancer cells. The role of chemotherapy is somewhat more controversial, although its use is undoubtedly on the increase.

References

1. Philips RKS, Hittinger R, Blesovsky L, Fry JS, Fielding LP. Local recurrence after curative surgery for large bowel cancer. The overall picture. *Br J Surg* 1985; 71: 12–16.

2. Hermanek P, Friedl P. Locoregional recurrence in rectal carcinoma. Experience from a German multicentre study (SGCRC). *Abstr Acta Chirurg Austr* 1991; (Suppl. 93): 9–10.

3. Heald RJ, Husband EM, Ryall RDH. The mesorectum in rectal cancer surgery – the clue to pelvic recurrence? *Br J Surg* 1982; 69: 613–16.

4. Ward AS, Heald RJ. Leg ischaemia complicating colorectal surgery. (In press).

5. Walsh PC, Schlegel PN. Radical pelvic surgery with preservation of sexual function. *Ann Surg* 1988, 208: 391–400.

6. Cranston D. Ureteroureterostomy. In: Whitfield HN, ed. *Operative Surgery: Genitourinary Surgery*, 5th edn, Volume 1, Oxford: Butterworth-Heinemann, 1993: 180–2.

7. Hojo K, Sawada T, Moriya Y. An analysis of survival and voiding, sexual function after wide iliopelvic lymphadenectomy in patients with carcinoma of the rectum, compared with conventional lymphadenectomy. *Dis Colon Rectum* 1989; 32: 128–33.

8. Karanjia ND, Schache DJ, North WRS, Heald RJ. 'Close shave' in anterior resection. *Br J Surg* 1990; 77: 510–12.

9. Karanjia ND, Corder AP, Holdsworth PJ, Heald RJ. Risk of peritonitis and fatal septicaemia and the need to defunction the low anastomosis. *Br J Surg* 1991; 78: 196–8.

Illustrations by Francis E. Steckel

Abdominoperineal excision of rectum

John J. Murray MD
Staff Surgeon, Department of Colon and Rectal Surgery, Lahey Clinic Medical Center, Burlington, Massachusetts, USA

Malcolm C. Veidenheimer MD
Vice-Chairman, Department of Surgery and Chief of the Division of General Surgery, HCI International Medical Centre, Clydebank, UK

Principles and justification

Indications

Abdominoperineal resection for the treatment of patients with distal rectal carcinoma remains the standard against which all other options of treatment must be compared. As described by Miles in 1908, the operation involves abdominal exploration with ligation and division of the proximal lymphovascular pedicle and mobilization of the rectum. The perineal dissection permits subsequent removal of the rectum. Although the two phases of the operation can be performed as sequential steps that involve repositioning the patient from the supine to the lateral decubitus position, the operation is most commonly performed as a synchronous combined procedure with two teams operating simultaneously when the lesion has been judged to be resectable. Although small carcinomas in the distal rectum may be treated with curative intent by local measures such as electrocoagulation or full-thickness excision, abdominoperineal excision is the customary treatment for most tumours involving the distal third of the rectum and for selected bulky tumours of the mid-rectum. Abdominoperineal excision of the rectum is also performed for inflammatory bowel disease. When undertaken for this diagnosis, the abdominal dissection differs from the technique described in this chapter so that the autonomic innervation to the bladder and sexual organs is preserved. The perineal dissection in patients with inflammatory bowel disease can be confined to the intersphincteric plane to reduce the size of the perineal wound.

Preoperative

Preoperative preparation begins with endoscopic and digital examination of the rectum to assess the size and location of the tumour. For carcinomas located in the anterior quadrant of the distal rectum, this evaluation includes an assessment for possible involvement of the prostate and bladder in men and the rectovaginal septum in women. A full course of preoperative radiation therapy may facilitate subsequent abdominoperineal excision of large tumours or tumours that appear fixed because of extension to other pelvic structures. Computed tomography, magnetic resonance imaging and transrectal ultrasonography may further delineate the extent of the pelvic tumour, but this information is unlikely to alter the plan of treatment. A definitive assessment regarding the resectability of a rectal carcinoma can only be made at laparotomy.

All patients require mechanical cleansing of the colon before operation. A lavage preparation using a balanced electrolyte solution with polyethylene glycol is employed in this department at present. Patients receive oral antibiotics before operation to reduce bacterial colonization of the large intestine. Parenteral antibiotics are provided during the operative period. Patients are seen before operation by an enterostomal nurse who begins instruction in stomal care. The enterostomal nurse also selects the most appropriate site on the abdominal wall for the colostomy. Prophylactic measures to reduce the risk of deep vein thrombophlebitis are mandatory in patients undergoing abdominoperineal excision of the rectum.

Operation

Position of patient

1 The patient is placed in the lithotomy Trendelenburg position with a pad beneath the sacrum to provide simultaneous access to the abdomen and perineum. The legs are positioned in stirrups that provide support to the knees and feet while avoiding compression of the peroneal nerve. A Foley catheter is inserted into the bladder using sterile technique. We have not found the routine use of ureteric catheters to be helpful. Their use is restricted to patients who have previously undergone extensive pelvic surgery or who have received radiation to the pelvis. A 2/0 purse-string suture of silk is used to occlude the anal orifice.

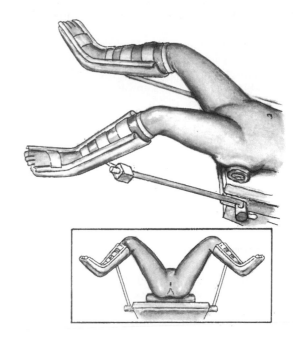

1

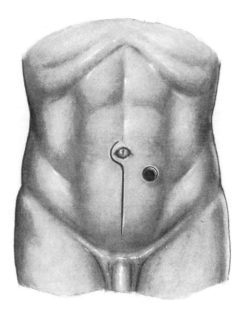

2

Incision

2 A midline incision extending cephalad from the superior margin of the pubic symphysis and passing to the right of the umbilicus provides access to the abdominal cavity without encroaching on potential sites for placement of the abdominal stoma. The colostomy should be situated over the body of the rectus muscle to reduce the risk of paracolostomy herniation. The site should be chosen to avoid deformities of the abdominal wall and bony contours. Most commonly, the best site for the stoma is in the left lower quadrant at the apex of the infraumbilical skin fold. In this location the stoma is easy for the patient to see, enabling correct placement of the colostomy appliance.

Technique

3 The extent of colonic resection necessary to accomplish abdominoperineal excision of the rectum is determined by the blood supply to the rectum and the level at which the proximal vascular pedicle is ligated. The left colic and superior rectal arteries, as well as a variable number of sigmoid branches, originate from the inferior mesenteric artery. The middle rectal arteries are derived from the internal iliac arteries and pass across the superior aspect of the levator ani muscles. The inferior rectal arteries originate from the pudendal arteries and have anterior and posterior branches that pass through the ischiorectal fossae. Ligation of the superior rectal trunk adjacent to the bifurcation of the aorta preserves the left colic artery. This approach improves perfusion to the proximal sigmoid colon and permits the apex of the sigmoid loop to serve as the site for proximal transection of the colon. Ligation of the inferior mesenteric artery at its origin from the aorta to encompass the para-aortic lymphatic tissue in the operative specimen has not been demonstrated to improve the chance for cure after abdominoperineal excision of the rectum. High ligation of the vascular pedicle impairs the blood supply to the proximal sigmoid colon, however, and usually requires more extensive resection of the colon.

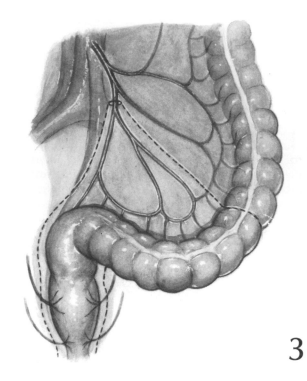

3

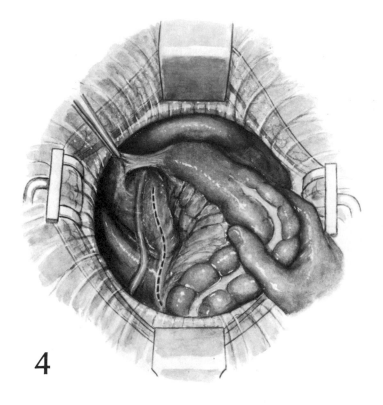

4

4 After exploration of the abdomen to assess the full extent of the tumour, a plastic drape is placed around the margins of the wound to minimize contamination of the skin. Exposure is maintained with a self-retaining retractor. Congenital adhesions in the left paracolic gutter are divided to begin mobilization of the sigmoid and rectosigmoid colon.

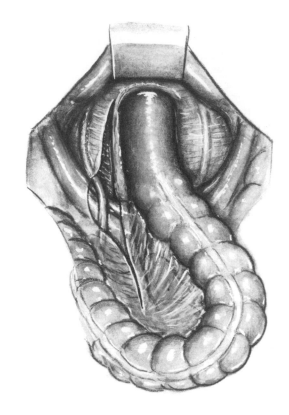

5 The peritoneum along the base of the rectosigmoid mesentery in the left gutter is incised with scissors. The incision is extended proximally across the sigmoid mesentery to the planned site for transection of the colon. The incision is carried distally across the brim of the pelvis and extends to the base of the bladder. During the course of this dissection, the left ureter is identified and protected.

5

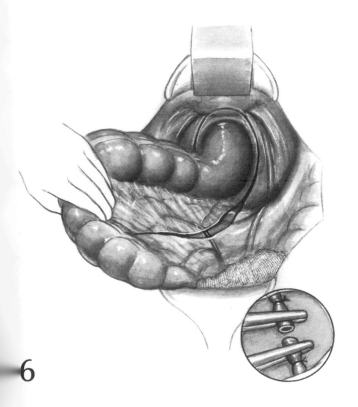

6 The sigmoid colon is retracted to the left. In a similar fashion, the peritoneum on the right side of the sigmoid mesentery is incised. The incision begins adjacent to the planned site for proximal transection of the colon. The dissection proceeds across the sigmoid mesentery to a point adjacent to the aortic bifurcation. From this point, the incision is extended along the root of the rectosigmoid mesentery and across the pelvis to the base of the bladder. The peritoneal incisions are joined across the base of the bladder just above the floor of the rectovesical pouch. Before the peritoneum is incised, the right ureter can usually be identified as it crosses the brim of the pelvis. The branches of the inferior mesenteric vessels are isolated, divided between clamps and ligated.

6

7 After the vascular pedicle has been divided, the remaining sigmoid mesentery is dissected from the posterior abdominal wall with scissors. Dissection progresses in a caudad direction, exposing the sacral promontory. While maintaining anterior traction on the rectosigmoid, the presacral space is entered by inserting dissecting scissors into the loose areolar tissue just anterior to the sacral promontory.

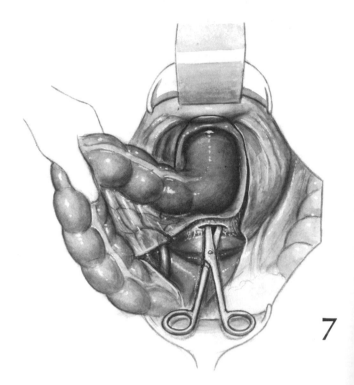

7

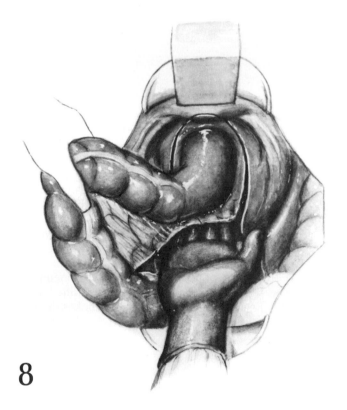

8

8 When the plane of dissection has been demonstrated, the right hand is inserted, and the rest of the presacral dissection is accomplished by blunt finger dissection and gentle anterior displacement of the rectum.

9 Blunt dissection in the presacral space is carried distally to the level of the tip of the coccyx, which can be appreciated on the back of the middle finger. Care is taken to ensure that the dissection is performed in a plane anterior to the presacral fascia to avoid injury to the presacral venous plexus. As the dissecting hand is swept laterally in the presacral space, the lateral attachments proximal to the lateral ligaments are thinned. These proximal lateral attachments are avascular and can be divided with sharp dissection.

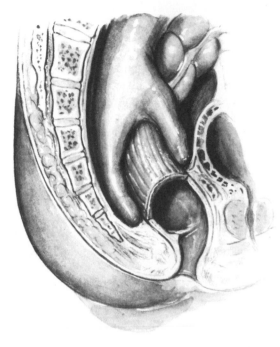

9

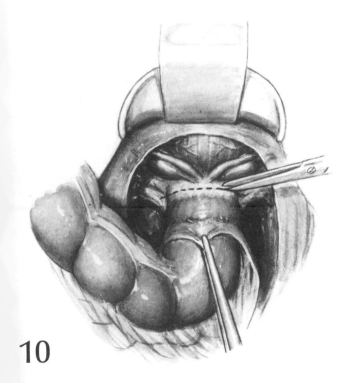

10

10 The anterior dissection, aided by retraction on the posterior edge of the peritoneal incision, is now carried to a deeper plane. The posterior wall of the bladder and the seminal vesicles are demonstrated by a combination of sharp and blunt dissection. Denonvilliers' fascia is exposed and incised by sharp dissection. In women, the anterior dissection commences at the base of the pouch of Douglas and exposes the cervix and the posterior fornix of the vagina.

11 Incision of Denonvilliers' fascia exposes the longitudinal muscle of the rectal wall. While countertraction on the rectum is maintained, the bladder and prostate are swept away from the anterior rectal wall by blunt finger dissection. Dissection in this plane is carried distally until the indwelling Foley catheter can be palpated within the membranous urethra when the examining finger is pressed against the undersurface of the pubic symphysis. In women, the posterior vaginal wall is swept from the rectum by finger dissection. This dissection should be carried into the distal third of the rectovaginal septum.

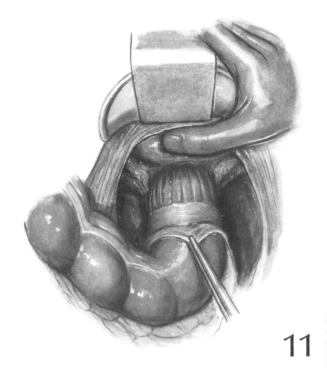

11

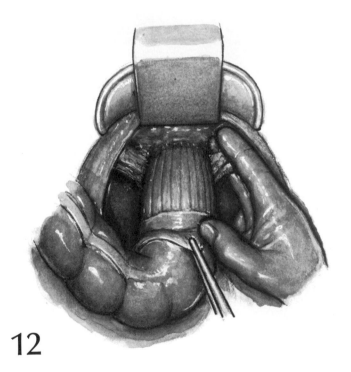

12

12 Lateral mobilization of the rectum is completed. The lateral ligaments may contain branches of the middle rectal vessels. While the rectum is displaced to the opposite side of the pelvis, the lateral ligament is thinned by placing the index finger in the anterior plane of the rectal mobilization and the middle finger in the posterior plane. The fingers are moved back and forth to thin the intervening band of tissue.

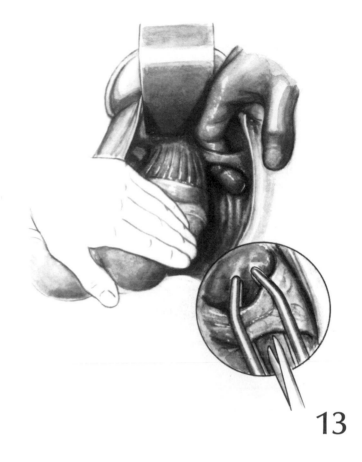

13

13 By means of a corkscrew movement of the index finger passed along the lateral border of the rectum, the lateral ligament on each side of the rectum is hooked on the finger, clamped and divided. Division of the lateral ligaments should be accomplished as close to the pelvic side wall as possible to encompass adjacent lymphatic tissue in the operative specimen. After division of the lateral ligaments, abdominal mobilization of the rectum is completed.

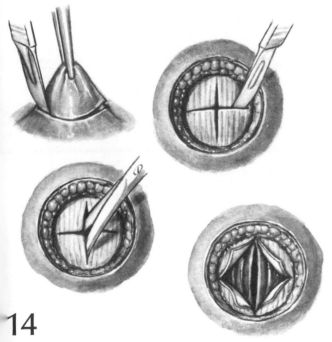

14

14 While midline traction on the lower abdominal wall is maintained by means of a Kocher clamp, the previously marked skin site for the colostomy is grasped in a Kocher clamp. A circle of skin approximating the diameter of the colon is excised. In obese patients, a plug of subcutaneous tissue and fat is removed with the overlying circle of skin. A cruciate incision is made in the exposed anterior sheath of the rectus muscle. The fibres of the rectus abdominis muscle are split using Mayo scissors and the peritoneum is incised. The defect in the abdominal wall should be of sufficient size to accommodate two fingerbreadths.

15 The colon is divided with a linear intestinal stapling instrument. The proximal end of the colon is drawn through the defect in the abdominal wall using Babcock clamps.

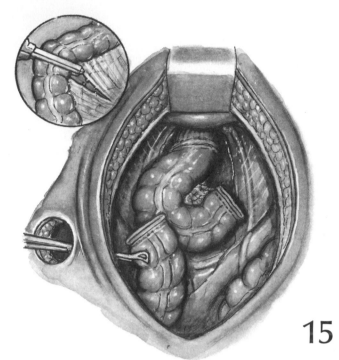

15

16 After the surgical specimen has been removed, the pelvic cavity is irrigated. The peritoneum along the pelvic side walls is mobilized to a degree that will permit closure with a continuous suture of absorbable material. Alternatively, the pelvic peritoneum can be left unapproximated. In this instance, closed suction drainage catheters are placed in the depths of the pelvis and brought through abdominal stab wounds.

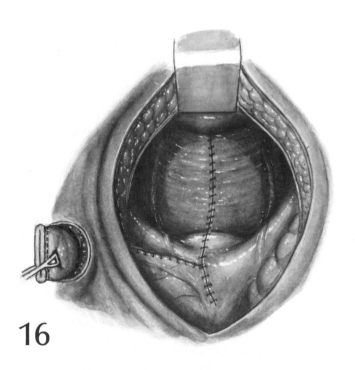

16

17 Adjuvant radiation therapy to reduce the risk of local recurrence of the tumour has become standard practice in the management of patients with advanced carcinoma of the rectum. Operative measures to exclude the small intestine from the pelvis may reduce the risk of radiation injury. A pedicled flap of omentum based on the left gastroepiploic vessels can be used to obliterate the pelvic dead space and displace the small intestine. The omentum is dissected from the transverse colon, permitting entry into the lesser peritoneal sac. The right half of the omentum is separated from the greater curvature of the stomach. Care is taken to preserve the gastroepiploic vessels as well as the omental blood supply arising from the left gastroepiploic artery.

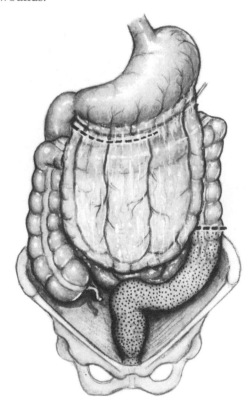

17

18 The pedicle of omentum is brought lateral to the afferent limb of the colostomy in the left paracolic gutter to fill the pelvic cavity and displace the small intestine.

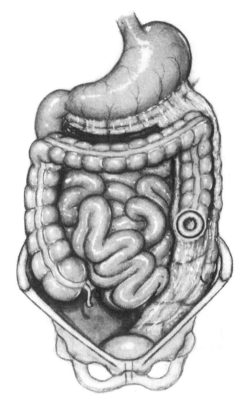

18

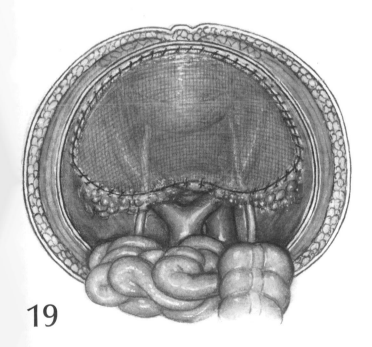

19

19 If the omentum is attenuated or unavailable, absorbable polyglycolic acid mesh can be used to create a temporary intestinal sling that will exclude the small intestine from the radiation portals during the period of treatment. The sling is anchored to the posterior abdominal wall below the aortic bifurcation with two 2/0 polyglycolic acid sutures. The sutures are run laterally in opposite directions, with care taken to avoid the ureters and iliac vessels. The sutures are continued across the lateral paracolic gutters and along the posterior aspect of the anterior abdominal wall.

20 Fixation of the mesh to the abdominal wall advances in a cephalad direction as the sutures are run from the posterior abdominal wall to the anterior abdominal wall. The sutures are approximated in the anterior midline above the level of the umbilicus as the midline fascial incision is closed. Closed suction catheters are placed in the pelvis below the sling to evacuate any fluid collections.

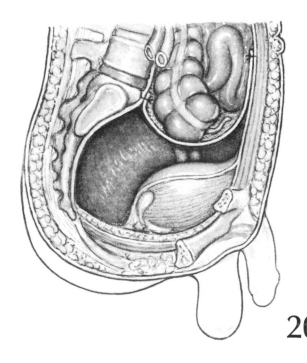

20

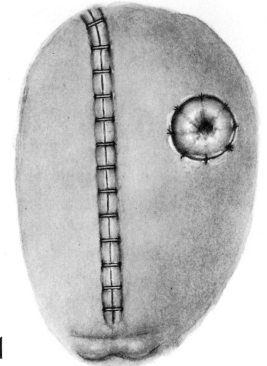

21

21 Copious irrigation of the wound before closure of the skin diminishes the incidence of wound infection. The colostomy is completed by immediate mucocutaneous anastomosis using sutures of 4/0 chromic catgut. A disposable colostomy appliance is secured to the abdominal wall in the operating room.

22 When abdominoperineal excision of the rectum is to be performed synchronously by two operating teams, the perineal dissection is started when the resectability of the lesion has been confirmed by the abdominal surgeon. When two operating teams are not available, the abdominal dissection is performed first and the perineal excision of the specimen performed after the colostomy has been fashioned and the abdominal incision has been closed. A rectangular or elliptical incision is outlined using electrocautery. The anterior margin of the dissection overlies the deep transverse perineal muscle. The incision extends posteriorly to the tip of the coccyx. To provide countertraction, the edges of the skin are grasped with Lahey double-hook clamps and the perianal skin is grasped with Kocher clamps.

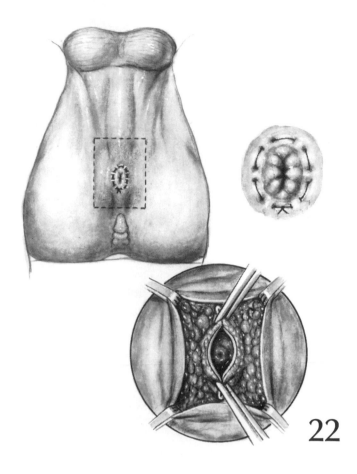

22

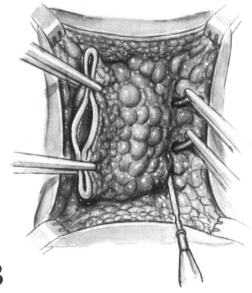

23

23 The dissection begins laterally. The perianal fat is divided with electrocautery or blunt scissors, providing entry to the ischiorectal fossa. The anterior and posterior branches of the inferior rectal arteries are isolated, divided and ligated.

24 A self-retaining retractor facilitates exposure in the ischiorectal fossa. The anterior dissection is deepened along a plane at the posterior border of the deep transverse perineal muscle.

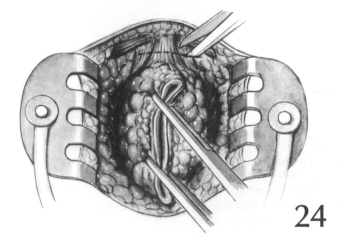

24

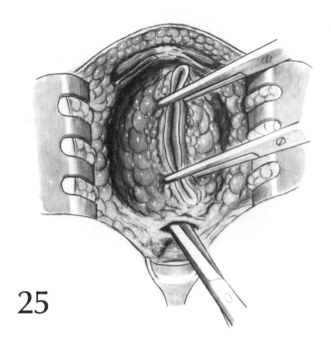

25

25 The anococcygeal ligament is divided by scissors dissection. The presacral pelvic space is entered along a plane anterior to the tip of the coccyx by dividing the levator muscles in the posterior midline. The perineal surgeon is guided by the fingers of the abdominal surgeon, which have been placed in the presacral space. The point of the scissors should be directed anteriorly, aiming at the umbilicus, to avoid inadvertent stripping of the presacral fascia. At this juncture, the abdominal and perineal dissections meet. The rectum and anus will be free in the midline posteriorly.

26 An index finger inserted through the precoccygeal incision is swept across the superior aspect of the levator muscles on each side of the pelvis, and the muscles are divided with scissors or electrocautery. The levator muscles should be divided as close to the pelvic side wall as possible to include a liberal portion of muscle and perirectal fat with the operative specimen. Dissection through the levator muscles is usually avascular.

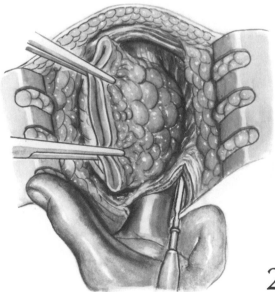

26

27 The abdominal surgeon passes the rectum through the open posterolateral perineal wound. After careful palpation to avoid injury to the urethra, the remaining attachments of the rectum to the recto-urethral muscle are divided.

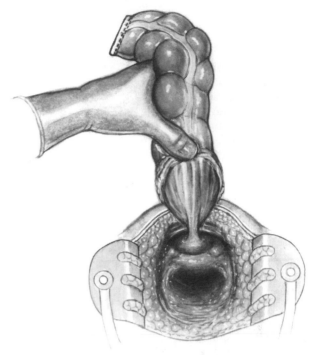

27

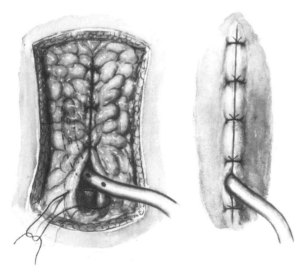

28

28 The perineal wound is copiously irrigated. When the pelvic peritoneum has been closed, a sump suction drain is placed into the pelvic cavity and brought through the posterior aspect of the perineal wound. When the pelvic cavity is to be drained from above, no drains are necessary in the perineal field. No attempt is made to approximate the levator muscles. The ischiorectal fat and subcutaneous tissues are approximated in two layers with interrupted sutures of 2/0 absorbable material. The skin incision is closed with interrupted sutures of nylon.

29 Because of the proximity of the rectum and vagina, and the presence of lymphatic channels within the rectovaginal septum, excision of carcinoma involving the anterior or lateral quadrants of the distal rectum in women should include posterior vaginectomy to ensure adequate clearance of the tumour and to reduce the potential for local recurrence.

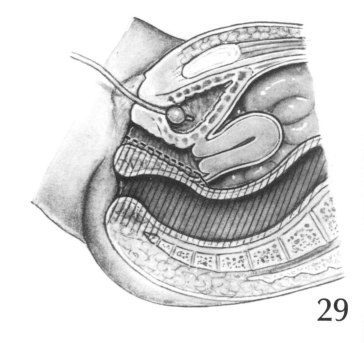

29

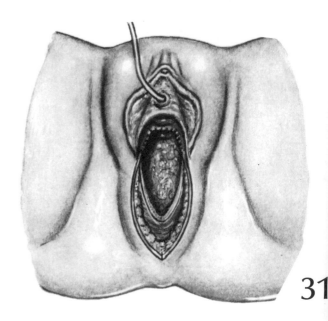

30

30 When the perineal dissection is started in women, the lateral margins of the perianal incision are carried anteriorly to the posterolateral aspects of the labia. After the levator muscles are divided and the specimen is delivered posteriorly, the incisions at the base of the labia are extended proximally as full-thickness incisions along the lateral walls of the vagina. A full-thickness transverse incision across the posterior fornix completes the dissection, and the specimen is removed.

31 Reconstruction of the vagina is unnecessary. Bleeding from the transected vaginal wall is controlled with electrocautery or with a continuous running suture of absorbable material. The ischiorectal fat and subcutaneous tissues are approximated in two layers with interrupted absorbable sutures.

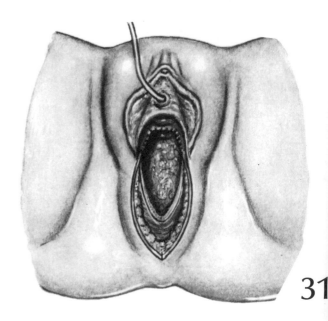

31

32 Closure of the skin incision is carried anteriorly to the base of the labia to reconstruct the posterior fourchette. The vaginal orifice should accommodate three fingerbreadths. A soft suction catheter is placed through the defect in the posterior vaginal wall to drain the pelvic cavity.

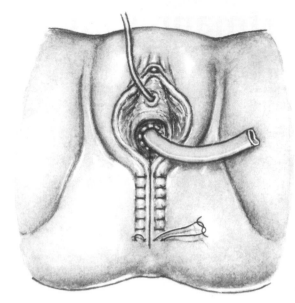

32

Postoperative care

Routine postoperative nasogastric decompression is unnecessary. Ambulation with assistance starts on the first postoperative day. Intake is restricted to intravenous fluids until spontaneous passage of flatus through the colostomy occurs. At this time, a liquid diet is prescribed. The diet is subsequently advanced to an unrestricted diet over the ensuing 24–48 h. When suction catheters are used in the perineal wound, they are removed on the fourth postoperative day. Subsequent care of the perineal wound requires sitz baths and irrigation of the perineal sinus with normal saline solution three times a day. These measures are unnecessary when drains have not been placed in the perineal wound. In this instance, abdominal drains are removed when their daily output has decreased to 20 ml

or less. The Foley urethral catheter is left indwelling for 5–7 days after abdominoperineal resection. For patients with symptomatic prostatic enlargement, transurethral resection of the prostate may be necessary after abdominoperineal resection because of compromised bladder function after excision of the rectum. Before discharge from the hospital, patients are instructed in the specifics of managing the stoma, including the option of irrigation of the colostomy.

Acknowledgements

The illustrations in this chapter are reprinted with kind permission of the Lahey Clinic.

Hartmann's operation

Pascal Frileux MD
Professor of Surgery, Hôpital Laennec, Paris, France

Anne Berger MD
Consultant Surgeon, Hôpital Laennec, Paris, France

History

1 In 1923 Henri Hartmann[1] described an operation which is now defined as a resection of the sigmoid colon with construction of a terminal colostomy and closure of the rectal stump. A variable length of rectum may also be resected. The indication was initially cancer of the upper or middle third of the rectum, at a time when anterior resection had not been developed. Today Hartmann's operation is usually performed as an emergency procedure to treat the complications of various colorectal diseases.

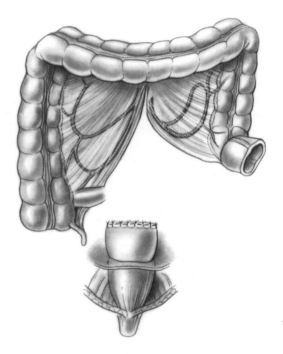

1

Principles and justification

Indications and contraindications

Hartmann's operation is indicated when it is necessary to perform an emergency resection of the sigmoid and/or rectum, when it is unsafe to perform a primary anastomosis, and when it is impossible to raise a mucous fistula owing to an insufficient length of bowel distal to the resection. The advantage of Hartmann's operation over simple diversion is that resection of the lesion is carried out at the primary stage.

Benign diseases

Hartmann's operation represents the 'gold standard' in patients with perforated diverticulitis with generalized peritonitis. There is, however, now a tendency towards primary anastomosis in selected cases[2].

Hartmann's operation is indicated in patients with ischaemic colitis requiring resection when the sigmoid colon is involved[3].

Acute colitis, in the form of toxic megacolon or fulminant colitis, may require an emergency colectomy but it is generally agreed that primary coloproctectomy should be avoided in this situation, and total abdominal colectomy is favoured. Some choose to close the rectal stump, while others (including the authors) prefer a sigmoid mucous fistula to avoid the possible complications caused by leakage from the suture line in the rectum. If Hartmann's procedure is selected, it is necessary to place a tube in the rectal remnant to drain the secretions produced by the inflamed mucosa.

Other indications include: trauma with extensive destruction of the sigmoid or rectum, including iatrogenic perforation; volvulus of the sigmoid colon (*see* chapter on pp. 750–765) with peritonitis and necrosis of the sigmoid colon; and postoperative sepsis after anterior resection in cases where the anastomosis cannot be conserved because of necrosis of the bowel or major disruption of the anastomosis[4].

Malignant diseases

While there was a place for Hartmann's operation in 1921 in the elective therapy of rectal cancer, this is no longer the case because re-establishment of continuity is often not carried out and the patient is left with a permanent colostomy. Malignant obstruction is now better treated by reconstruction after resection. The main indications for Hartmann's operation are in poor risk patients and in some palliative cases associated with perforation of a rectal carcinoma[5].

Operation

The following description applies to cases of perforated diverticulitis.

Position of patient

The patient is placed in the lithotomy position with stirrups.

Incision

2 While some surgeons favour a left paramedian incision, most perform a midline incision from the pubis to midway between the umbilicus and xiphoid. The edges of the incision are protected with surgical drapes.

The peritoneal fluid is first sampled for bacterial analysis and is then aspirated. Full exploration of the peritoneal cavity is undertaken to identify the primary lesion and occasional associated diseases. In cases of perforated diverticulitis, the origin of the peritonitis is easily recognized.

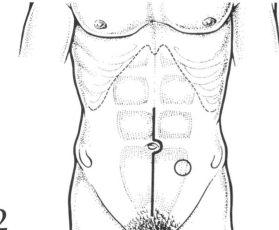

2

Resection

3   The vessels in the mesocolon are ligated close to the colon, as in any benign disease. The first step is to mobilize the colon, starting from the descending colon where inflammation is minimal. The ureter is identified and the mobilization proceeds distally, using either sharp or blunt dissection according to the type of the inflammatory lesions. There is usually an easy plane of dissection between the sigmoid and the posterior elements (ureter and gonadal vessels), but adhesions may be dense at the level of the pelvic brim. The vessels and mesentery are ligated and divided.

The site of proximal division of the colon varies with the extent of the inflammation; usually it is the limit between the descending and sigmoid colon. A GIA stapler or crushing clamps are used to divide the colon to avoid contamination.

The site of distal division is usually at the level of the sacral promontory because: gross inflammatory lesions rarely extend beyond this point, and if this is the case, they are confined to the mesocolon and do not involve the bowel itself; a sigmoid resection extending down onto the rectum, at the level of the peritoneal reflection, would make the re-establishment of continuity significantly more difficult.

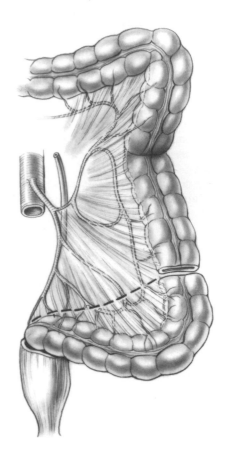

3

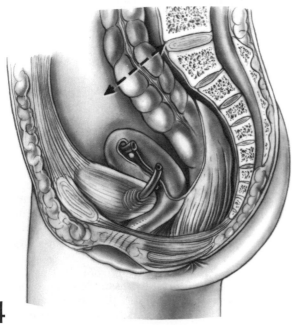

4

4   After the posterior aspect of the rectum at the level of the sacral promontory has been cleared, the rectum is closed using a TA 55 stapler. A clamp is placed above the staple line and the rectum is divided. A suture line over the staples is not necessary, but the rectal stump may be sutured to the sacral promontory to keep it from folding over into the pelvis.

Peritoneal lavage

In the case of peritonitis, thorough peritoneal lavage using saline is indicated to remove fibrinous exudate and pus.

Construction of left iliac colostomy

A separate incision is made in the left iliac fossa at a point equidistant from the anterior iliac spine and the umbilicus. A circle of skin 3 cm in diameter is excised, followed by a cross-shaped incision in the fascia and peritoneal layer. The passage for the colostomy should admit two fingers. If possible, the site of the colostomy should be chosen before the operation, but in emergencies this is not always possible. This colostomy is temporary; therefore, it is not necessary to make a subperitoneal tunnel as for a permanent colostomy (*see* chapter on pp. 782–797). The colon must be well vascularized and brought out without traction; this may require mobilization of the descending colon. The colostomy remains clamped until the abdominal wall has been closed.

Drainage

5 The main postoperative complication of Hartmann's operation is leakage from the rectal suture line. To minimize the consequences of a leak, effective drainage of the pelvis is necessary. The use of tubes, corrugated drains or Penrose drains has been suggested[6], but capillary drainage as described by Mikulicz[7] is used in this department. Large gauze packing is placed in the pouch of Douglas and is exteriorized through the inferior end of the midline incision. The Mikulicz packing is left in place for 12 days and removed under mild analgesia[7]. In addition to efficient drainage, we believe that this technique provides good healing of the peritoneum in the pelvis, thus facilitating reoperation for restoration of continuity.

In the case of generalized peritonitis, some surgeons advocate drainage of the right subphrenic, left subphrenic and subhepatic spaces.

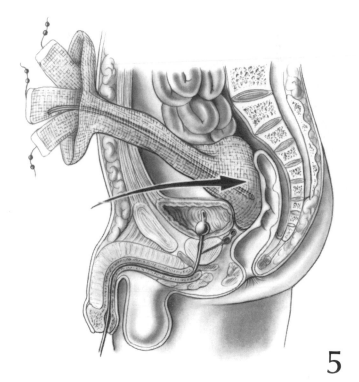

5

Closure of the abdominal wall

A conventional technique may suffice, but if the patient is old or fragile or there are factors which might lead to abdominal dehiscence in the postoperative period, it is recommended that polyglactin (Vicryl) or polyglycolic acid (Dexon) mesh is placed beneath the abdominal wall.

Evacuation and drainage of the rectum

Gentle dilatation of the anus followed by evacuation and irrigation of the rectal contents is a useful precaution.

Postoperative care

Some patients will require monitoring in an intensive care unit for the management of cardiopulmonary problems. Otherwise, routine postoperative care is required, including inspection of the colostomy and drains. The Mikulicz packing is irrigated from the seventh day to facilitate its removal. Rectal examination can help the diagnosis of pelvic sepsis and sometimes allows the evacuation of a purulent collection.

Outcome

Complications

The incidence of complications is high, approximately 30%, because of the presence of coexistent morbid conditions in elderly, malnourished and septic patients with urinary and pulmonary problems being common.

Sepsis and wound disruption

This occurs in about 25% of patients and in as many as 60% after emergency surgery. Intra-abdominal abscesses requiring percutaneous or surgical drainage occur in 5% of patients[6].

Colostomy complications

These types of complications should be rare, but necrosis may occur: if this is extensive, reoperation may be required[8]; if limited to 1–2 cm of the more distal gut, conservative treatment will suffice. Necrosis is particularly frequent in cases of ischaemic colitis. Most peristomal abscesses can be managed conservatively in the absence of stomal necrosis.

Rectal stump leakage

This occurs in approximately 10% of patients, but results of studies have ranged from zero[9] to 30%[10]. When the pelvis has been drained by a Mikulicz pack, leakage is signalled by a persistent discharge of pus and leakage of water-soluble contrast media seen during diagnostic radiography. Effective drainage may be required to prevent progressive pelvic sepsis and this can usually be achieved through the rectal stump.

Haemorrhage and retention of pus

This may occur in the rectal stump in acute colitis[11]. Conservative treatment with irrigation and packing may be ineffective and emergency proctectomy may very occasionally be required.

Small bowel obstruction

Small bowel obstruction may occur in the early postoperative period because of inflammatory adhe-sions or recurrent foci sepsis. Guidelines for management are the same as after any major abdominal operation.

Mortality rate

The mortality rate after Hartmann's operation is about 11%, but ranges from 4% to 30%. The mortality rate increases after emergency surgery and in malignant disease. However, most recent series report a lower mortality rate of about 3% for this operation[6].

RESTORATION OF CONTINUITY

The overall rate of restoration of 66%[12] is greater in cases of diverticular disease than in those of cancer, and is increasing with the use of circular staplers[9]. Because the mortality rate of this second procedure is low (0–5%), it is justifiable to propose bowel reconstruction in all cases. However, careful preoperative evaluation is necessary and the timing of surgery is important.

Preoperative

Assessment

Colonoscopy should be carried out to detect neoplasia, diverticular disease or other focal abnormalities in the proximal colon. The rectal stump should be assessed by digital examination and radiography to detect any leak from the suture line and to evaluate the length, volume and compliance of the remaining rectum. Endoscopy and biopsies may be useful, especially in cases of inflammatory bowel disease. Ultrasonography, computed tomography scanning, chest radiography and tumour marker assessment may be useful in patients with malignant disease to detect metastasis, which greatly reduces the indications for further surgery.

The time taken to re-establish bowel continuity is of great importance and depends on the nature of the initial disease and the severity of infection at the time of the first operation. In patients with malignant disease, the delay should be approximately 6 months[3]. In cases of diverticular disease when the procedure is performed in the absence of diffuse sepsis, the delay for reoperation can be quite short (3 months), while delay of 4–12 months is recommended if diffuse sepsis has occurred[13].

Approximately 10% of patients refuse reoperation. These patients are usually elderly and have become used to their colostomy and fear the pain and complications of further surgery. Others have severe or multiple comorbid conditions or an advanced stage of neoplasia, and should be spared the risk of an additional procedure.

Preparation

Bowel preparation is the same as for any colonic surgery. Rectal contents are evacuated and irrigations of the rectal stump are carried out. In 'easy' cases (long rectal stump with normal rectal wall), a conventional colorectal anastomosis may be considered; however, in more 'difficult' cases (short rectal stump or prior operations on the pelvis), the surgeon must be prepared to use either a circular stapler or special techniques, such as the pull-through operations.

Operation

The 'easy' case

The patient is placed in the lithotomy position (*see* page 48). A long midline incision is made, reaching the xiphoid process to give good exposure to the splenic flexure. The operation starts with the dissection of adhesions and a complete exploration of the abdominal cavity. The rectal stump is identified on the sacral promontory where it may be found to be tightly adherent to loops of small bowel, to the uterus in women, and to the posterior aspect of the bladder in men. The aim is to free these adhesions without damage and then find the presacral space so that the limits of the rectal remnant can be identified. This may be difficult because the top of the rectal stump can be adherent posteriorly and the ureters may be pulled towards the midline by the pelvic inflammation. It is useful to localize the ureters before proceeding to dissection of the rectum, and some surgeons pass ureteral catheters at the start of the operation. The dissection may be facilitated by using a sigmoidoscope or inflating the rectum through a Foley catheter to find the apex of the

rectum[14]. Others use a large calibre bougie or Hegar dilator. The presacral space is opened and the dissection proceeds downwards posteriorly and laterally. Once a sufficient length of rectum is mobilized (2–3 cm), the level for bowel section is selected where the rectum is supple and large.

The colostomy is dissected from the abdominal wall using instruments which will be discarded because they become contaminated. The left colon and splenic flexure are mobilized, and the end is resected, taking care to prepare a healthy segment of bowel which can reach the level of anastomosis without tension. The anastomosis is then performed as described in the chapters on pp. 528–550 and 551–560. Thorough haemostasis of the operative field and irrigation of the peritoneal cavity terminate the procedure.

The 'difficult' case

Sutured anastomosis

If there has been a leak from the rectal suture line, the top of the rectal stump, including the site of leakage, must be resected, whatever the technique of anastomosis. In the presence of a short rectal stump, the top being below the peritoneal reflection, the operation is often difficult and should be undertaken by a highly experienced surgeon. Despite the use of a sigmoidoscope or a Hegar dilator, localization of the rectal stump is difficult because the bladder (in men) or the uterus/vagina (in women) may be adherent posteriorly to the sacrum, burying the rectal stump. It may only be possible to find a small passage to the rectum from above. If access to the rectum is found posteriorly, then a retrorectal pull-through is indicated (Duhamel operation), provided that the superior part of the rectal stump has not been injured.

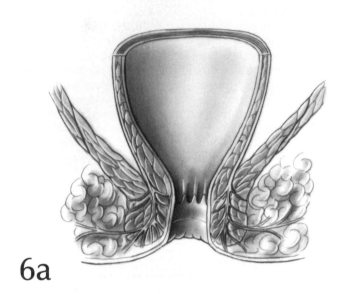

6a

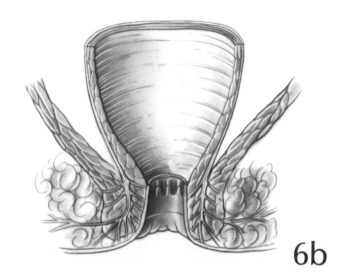

6b

6a–c If the rectal stump is really very short, or has sustained injury during mobilization, it is possible to carry out a mucosal proctectomy from below and to fashion a coloanal anastomosis, which results in a combination of a Soave and Parks operation.

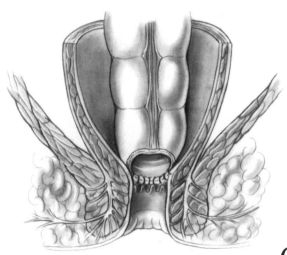

6c

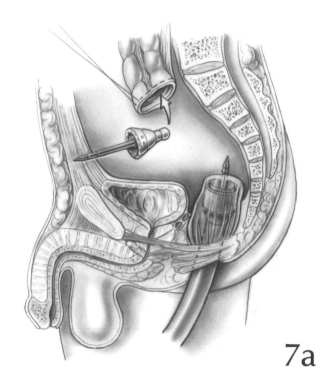

7a

Stapled anastomosis

7a, b The circular stapler is well adapted to this operation[15]; the instrument with the central stem alone is passed through the anus and perforates the rectal stump after minimal dissection, either at the top or at the anterior aspect. However, dissection should be sufficient to avoid taking another organ (bladder, ureter or vagina) between the shaft and the anvil. If the top of the rectum needs to be resected, a double-stapling technique may be used (*see* chapter on pp. 551–560).

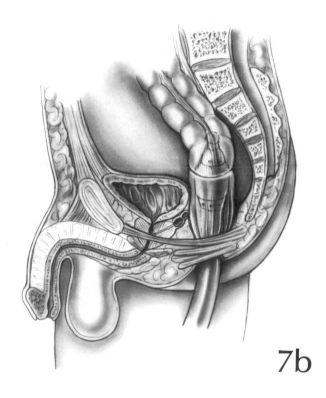

7b

Restoration of continuity in inflammatory bowel disease

The technique in this case is either ileorectostomy (*see* chapter on pp. 687–698) or ileoanal pouch anastomosis, depending on the specific diagnosis: Crohn's disease or mucosal ulcerative colitis.

Postoperative care

When a protective colostomy has been constructed, it should be closed 2 months later after digital and radiological examination of the anastomosis. Anastomotic stenosis is a late complication, and is more prevalent with the use of a small diameter staple machine and after pelvic sepsis associated with anastomotic leakage.

Outcome

The mortality rate is low, ranging from 0% to 5% and complications include wound sepsis, anastomotic leakage and urinary problems.

In conclusion while the indications for Hartmann's operation have changed since 1923, it remains a useful technique in emergency colorectal surgery. It is a safe operation, provided that pelvic drainage is efficient. Restoration of continuity is reasonably easy if the rectal stump is long enough; otherwise it may be challenging.

References

1. Hartmann H. Nouveau procédé d'ablation des cancers de la partie terminale du colon pelvien. *Congrès Français de Chirurgie* 1923; 30: 22–41.

2. Hackford AW, Schoetz DJ, Coller JA, Veidenheimer MC. Surgical management of complicated diverticulitis. The Lahey Clinic experience, 1967 to 1982. *Dis Colon Rectum* 1985; 28: 317–21.

3. Gallot D, Jauffret B, Goujard F, Deslandes M, Sezeur A, Malafosse M. L'intervention de Hartmann. Etude rétrospective de 86 cas. *Ann Chir* 1992; 46: 491–6.

4. Frileux P, Quilichini MA, Cugnenc PH, Parc R, Levy E, Loygue J. Péritonites post opératoires d'origine colique. A propos de 155 cas. *Ann Chir* 1985; 39: 649–59.

5. Doci R, Audisio R, Bozzetti F, Gennari L. Actual role of Hartmann's resection in elective surgical treatment for carcinoma of rectum and sigmoid colon. *Surg Gynecol Obstet* 1986; 163: 49–53.

6. Bell GA, Panton ON. Hartmann resection for perforated sigmoid diverticulitis. A retrospective study of the Vancouver General Hospital experience. *Dis Colon Rectum* 1984; 27: 253–6.

7. Orsoni JL, Mongredien PH, Anfroy JP, Charleux H. Le drainage selon Mikulicz dans les abdomens infectés. Etude critique, technique et résultats à propos de 93 malades. *Chirurgie* 1982; 108: 234–42.

8. Schein M, Decker G. The Hartmann procedure. Extended indications in severe intra-abdominal infection. *Dis Colon Rectum* 1988; 31: 126–9.

9. Cuilleret J, Espalieu PH, Balique JG, Berger JL, Youvarliakis P, Charret P. La place actuelle de l'opération de Hartmann: à propos de 50 cas. *J Chir* 1983; 120: 173–8.

10. Hulkko OA, Laitinen ST, Haukipuro KA, Stahlberg MJ, Juvonen TS, Kairaluoma MI. The Hartmann procedure for the treatment of colorectal emergencies. *Acta Chir Scand* 1986; 152: 531–5.

11. Ona FV, Boger JN. Rectal bleeding due to diversion colitis. *Am J Gastroenterol* 1985; 80: 40–1.

12. Haas PA, Haas GP. A critical evaluation of the Hartmann's procedure. *Am Surg* 1988; 54: 380–5.

13. Lubbers EJ, De Boer HM. Inherent complications of Hartmann's operation. *Surg Gynecol Obstet* 1982; 155: 717–21.

14. Gervin AS, Fisher RP. Identification of the rectal pouch of Hartmann. *Surg Gynecol Obstet* 1987; 164: 176–8.

15. Ramirez OM, Hernandez-Pombo J, Marupidi SR. New technique for anastomosis of the intestine after the Hartmann's procedure with the end-to-end anastomosis stapler. *Surg Gynecol Obstet* 1983; 156: 367–8.

Anorectal conditions: introductory comment

James P. S. Thomson DM, MS, FRCS
Consultant Surgeon and Clinical Director, St Mark's Hospital for Diseases of the Rectum and Colon, London, Honorary Consultant Surgeon, St Mary's Hospital, London, Honorary Lecturer in Surgery, The Medical College of St Bartholomew's Hospital, London, Civil Consultant in Surgery, Royal Air Force and Civilian Consultant in Colorectal Surgery, Royal Navy

In the practice of coloproctology, many patients who require treatment will have one of the troublesome anal conditions described in this section of the volume. Although surgery is often indicated, it is essential to be certain that a patient requires operative treatment because even the simplest procedure may result in complications and conservative measures are often effective. A critical review of symptoms, particularly in regard to type, location and severity, and an assessment of whether these symptoms 'match' the physical findings, is of paramount importance.

It is important that anorectal operations are not undertaken by those inexperienced in the field because there is a need for a high level of specialist training to prevent complications and to achieve the best results. In addition, adequate training will allow more procedures to be performed on a short stay or even on an outpatient basis.

Before embarking on planning the treatment of the anal disorder itself it is, of course, mandatory to exclude disease in the more proximal rectum and colon. Sometimes this has a bearing on the planning of the management of the anal problem, e.g. Crohn's disease; sometimes the symptoms may be similar, e.g. anorectal bleeding and a serious diagnosis may be potentially overlooked, and sometimes a separate asymptomatic pathology may be detected.

Although most operations will be performed under general anaesthesia, it is possible to use regional techniques (spinal or caudal blocks) or local infiltrative anaesthesia. The instruments required for anorectal surgery are generally unsophisticated, although specifically designed anal retractors are very helpful. A laser may be used to replace a scalpel or scissors, but the evidence does not suggest that this technique confers any particular advantage and it involves a large capital investment.

Haemorrhoids

Haemorrhoids may present with a variety of symptoms of which bleeding and prolapse are the most common. Discomfort and pain may also occur as the result of simple engorgement of the external plexus at defaecation or when complications such as thrombosis or fissure occur. Other symptoms include mucous discharge and its derived pruritus.

The majority of patients who present with symptomatic haemorrhoids (bleeding, pain, prolapse) will have normal bowel function, but a few may have severe constipation leading to straining at defaecation. These patients will need advice about bowel regulation and in severe cases will need to be investigated by colonic transit time, pelvic floor and anal canal studies. For the 'common' type of symptoms, dietary advice, bulking agents, injection sclerotherapy or infrared coagulation or banding are adequate treatment. However, those symptoms related to an external haemorrhoidal component will almost certainly not respond to these measures and will require operative treatment, as will those patients who have failed to respond to first-line 'office procedures'. Whether an open or closed operative technique is adopted depends on training and surgeon preference. Both methods when well done give excellent results. However, it is essential to remember two important details: secondary haemorrhoids require attention if symptomatic recurrence is to be avoided, and all the fibres of the internal sphincter must be identified and preserved to avoid postoperative problems with continence.

In the rare patient in whom there are long-standing circumferential haemorrhoids or prolapse, circumferential anoplasty (modified Whitehead haemorrhoidectomy) is regaining some popularity but care must be exercised to avoid any loss of the epithelium distal to the line of the anal valves. This anoderm must be relocated back up into the anal canal so that mucosa does not present at the anus which would result in mucous leakage ('wet anus'). The same caution must be observed for the Délorme procedure for the treatment of mucosal prolapse.

Complications of haemorrhoids such as acutely presenting haemorrhoidal thrombosis are usually managed non-operatively, although a more aggressive approach for immediate surgery has its advocates. A 'perianal haematoma' may be simply evacuated but postoperative haemorrhage may occur if the lesion is inadequately dressed with gauze and recurrence is common. An increasing number of surgeons therefore advocate immediate local resection for perianal haematomata.

Sepsis

Some of the most difficult problems for surgical treatment in the anorectum are those caused by local sepsis. The fundamental principle of operative treatment is to eradicate the sepsis while preserving full anal function. However, these two objectives are sometimes in conflict when a fistula tract crosses the sphincter mechanism and this dichotomy helps to explain the variety of techniques employed to classify and to treat fistulous disease.

While it can be presumed that most patients who have anorectal sepsis have non-specific infection (probably arising in the anal intermuscular glands), other associated pathology must be sought and excluded (e.g. Crohn's disease, intrapelvic sepsis, and occasionally pilonidal disease, infected dermoid cyst, hidradenitis suppurativa and, more recently, a resurgence of tuberculosis). Initially an abscess should be managed by simple drainage. The pus should be cultured because the presence of gut organisms is strongly indicative of an underlying fistula, but the growth of staphylococci eliminates this aetiology. Once the sepsis with its associated hyperaemia and swelling has settled a second assessment, preferably under anaesthesia, is carried out to seek possible associated pathology as described.

Although this plan provides a very general framework for management, fistula surgery has been bedevilled by difficulties with terminology. The seminal account by Parks et al.[1] has been of great value in helping us to change our emphasis for the definition of a 'low' and 'high' fistula from a simple anatomical statement of the site of the internal fistula opening in the anorectum to the use of terms to describe the functional relationship of the fistulous tract to the puborectalis component of the external anal sphincter (high fistulae being above the puborectalis and low fistulae being through or below the puborectalis muscle or superficial to the external sphincter). Most fistulae (perhaps 85%) are quite simple to treat because the fistulous tract is either subcutaneous (a bridged fissure) or intersphincteric (lying between the internal and external sphincters involving only the lower part of the external sphincter muscle itself). It should be noted that the internal opening of subcutaneous (submucous) fistula might lie at an anatomically 'high' level in the anal canal above the anorectal ring. However, because all the fistulous tract (sepsis) lies on the luminal side of the external sphincter mechanism, the lesion can be laid open without any loss of anal function. By contrast, the fistulae which traverse the sphincter mechanism (transsphincteric) can be substantially more difficult to treat and test the surgeon's skills. The 'low' variety are trans-sphincteric and pass through or below the puborectalis sling; the rare 'high' suprasphincteric variety have an internal opening above the puborectalis sling. In these fistulae it is therefore the course of the tract rather than the anatomical site of the internal opening which determines the nomenclature and this accounts for the alternative treatments which are well described in this section of the book.

Postoperative care of the wounds in these patients cannot be overvalued; pocketing, exuberant granulation tissue, mucosal bridging and the ingrowth of hair must be avoided by regular wound examination and hair shaving. If, despite these measures, there is a failure of wound closure and consolidation, other undiagnosed disorders should again be sought.

Pilonidal disease

Both pilonidal cysts and sinuses can be difficult to eradicate and a simple approach is recommended: laying open the sepsis, leaving the base *in situ*, and allowing it to heal with great attention to shaving local hair until the wound has healed and consolidated, which may take several months.

Rectovaginal fistula

Perhaps more accurately termed 'anovulval' or 'anovaginal' in most instances, it is often the result of childbirth injury rather than sepsis and is frequently associated with sphincter damage. Preoperative assessment of sphincter function by physiological testing and endoanal ultrasonography may therefore be of value. The excellent descriptions for operative treatment which follow should lead to successful management.

Ulceration

Anal fissure is the second most common condition seen in a rectal clinic and is by far the most common cause of anal ulceration. Other aetiologies include Crohn's disease, primary chancre, herpetic ulceration (often associated with HIV infection) and anal tumours. Many patients with the common 'idiopathic' variety of fissure are well treated by dietary change and stool bulking agents, although for recurrent or persistent fissures lateral sphincterotomy is undoubtedly the operative treatment of choice. In addition, it is usually advisable to excise a sentinal skin tag, hypertrophied anal papilla (anal polyp) and any overhanging tissue edges around the fissure.

Anal dilatation is advanced as an alternative to lateral sphincterotomy but there is no need to 'stretch' the whole of the internal sphincter, external sphincter and puborectalis sling which may result in compromised anal function. Even with lateral sphincterotomy, soiling may occur after defaecation as a result of the creation of a 'funnel-shaped' anal canal. Simple wiping with a damp cotton wool pledget to remove residual mucus and faeces will effectively help this problem and the accompanying pruritus ani.

Anal stenosis

This condition is quite uncommon and may have an inflammatory or structural aetiology. Local fungal and sometimes bacteriological infection may be difficult to treat and a dermatological opinion may be helpful. Anal stenosis because of structural damage following inappropriate surgery may be treated conservatively with a well lubricated anal dilator but may also require re-epithelialization procedures.

Condylomata acuminata

Anal and perianal warts caused by human papilloma virus, frequently associated with homosexuality, are a reminder that sexually transmitted disorders affect the anal region and may coexist with the more usual anal disorders. Inappropriate surgical treatment of anal warts may lead to excessive pain, scarring, and even anal stenosis. Although the treatment described is simple, effective and safe, careful postoperative follow-up is needed because further wart formation may occur.

Anal cancer

Malignant tumours of the anal canal are of many different histological types and are now managed by a multidisciplinary team of a surgeon, oncologist and radiotherapist. Nevertheless, surgery is important for localized disease and in the early diagnosis of these lesions.

The chapters which follow in this section of the book cover the field of anal canal disorders and will guide the surgeon well to perform careful and effective surgery.

References

1. Parks AG, Gordon PH, Hardcastle JD. A classification of fistula-in-ano. *Br J Surg* 1976; 63: 1–12.

Evacuation and excision of perianal haematoma

T. G. Allen-Mersh MD, FRCS
Consultant Surgeon, Westminster Hospital, London, UK

C. V. Mann MA, MCh, FRCS
Consulting Surgeon, The Royal London Hospital and St Mark's Hospital for Diseases of the Rectum and Colon, London, UK

Principles and justification

A perianal haematoma usually develops suddenly as a result of occlusion and swelling of one of the haemorrhoidal veins at the anal verge. The distended vein produces a tender swelling in which thrombosis rapidly develops. The natural history of the condition is of an acutely painful swelling which persists for several days and then slowly subsides as the clot is organized leaving an external anal skin tag. Occasionally, the haematoma causes pressure necrosis of the overlying skin, and the thrombus is extruded spontaneously. Although the lesion is usually solitary, occasionally multiple thromboses occur.

Indications

The usual course for the condition is spontaneous resolution, therefore there are no absolute indications for surgical intervention. The later the patient presents, the stronger the case for conservative management.

The principal advantage of surgical intervention is that it provides immediate relief of pain because the lesion is eliminated. Therefore, if the patient is seen early (within 48 h of onset), operative treatment is usually advised. Surgery is also indicated if an abscess develops to prevent the development of a subcutaneous fistula. The size of the thrombosed vein may also indicate the need for surgery, because a very large haematoma will subside to leave a large skin tag which may then be a source of pruritus and perianal soiling. Multiple lesions usually require surgical intervention.

Contraindications

The main hazard is an acute thrombosed haemorrhoid as a complication of a blood dyscrasia in acute leukaemia or polycythaemia.

Preoperative

No special preparation is required.

Anaesthesia

The operation is performed under local anaesthesia (lignocaine hydrochloride 1% with adrenaline 1:200 000). In the more nervous patient, however, where there is no contraindication, general anaesthesia may be preferred.

Operation

Position of patient

The left lateral (Sims) position with the pelvis raised on a sandbag is ideal. In an obese patient, the upper buttock may need to be strapped or held back by an assistant.

Under general anaesthesia the lithotomy or prone jack-knife position can be used.

Injection of local anaesthetic

1 The skin is gently cleansed with aqueous chlorhexidine gluconate 1:2000 solution. The finest needle should be used for the local anaesthetic injection, and the infiltration should include the skin around the area. Infiltration into the thrombus is usually not helpful and may result in premature leakage or bursting of the thrombosed area.

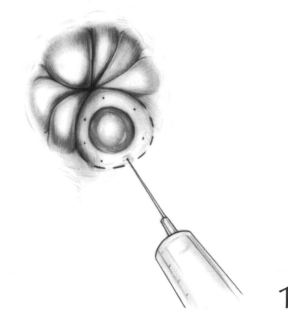

Evacuation of the haematoma

2 A short incision 1–2 cm long is made on the surface of the thrombosed haemorrhoid. The clot can then be removed with forceps as it is usually fairly solid. The redundant skin forming the sac around the clot is excised with fine scissors or a small scalpel.

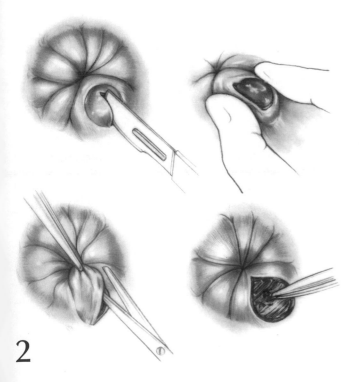

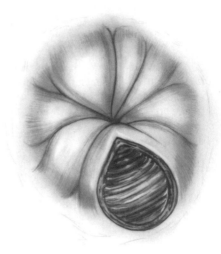

3 After the lesion has been removed the cavity should be gently curetted to ensure that all clot has been removed. The raw area between the anal mucosa and perianal skin is left open to drain, but as the edges tend to fall together naturally, it closes spontaneously within a few days. Excision of surplus skin and mucosa at the time of removal of the thrombus reduces the likelihood of anal tag formation.

Postoperative care

The wound is dressed with an absorbable cellulose mesh dressing, which is simply tucked over the raw area and covered with an external pad. A stool bulking and softening agent (sterculia granules 10 ml twice daily) is prescribed for 2 weeks to ensure the passage of a soft stool while the perianal area is tender. The patient is advised to take frequent warm (sitz) baths to soothe and cleanse the operation site. It is particularly helpful if this is done after each defaecation to ensure that the anal area is kept as clean as possible.

Healing of the wound takes 5–7 days. The patient will usually be relieved by excision of the tender thrombosed area, but should be warned that some pain will return once the local anaesthetic applied for the operation has worn off. It is advisable to prescribe an oral analgesic for 2–3 days.

Complications

Infection and abscess formation

If the clot is incompletely evacuated, the wound may become infected, producing cellulitis and persisting pain. In this event, attention should be given to ensuring that adequate drainage of the wound has been achieved by further trimming of the wound edges if necessary or evacuation of any retained clot. If this is required, it is usually better done under general anaesthesia when optimal conditions are more easily achieved. Antibiotics are not usually necessary.

If an abscess develops, it should be treated in the same way as a perianal abscess by incision or deroofing

under general anaesthesia. The pus should be cultured, and if *Escherichia coli* is detected, the patient should be examined to exclude the possibility of an anal fistula.

Skin tag

This will only form if evacuation, as opposed to excision, of the thrombosed haemorrhoid has been performed. If a large skin tag does form either after conservative management or inadequate excision, it can be excised under local anaesthesia.

Fistula

If large loose folds of skin remain after evacuation of the haematoma, superficial cross-healing of the wound edges can occur, leaving a subcutaneous fistula track. If this should happen, the fistula track should be laid open and the edges trimmed back so that proper healing of the wound from the base can occur.

Further reading

Bailey H. *Bailey and Love's Short Practice of Surgery*. 18th edn. London: HK Lewis, 1981: 1093 pp.

Goligher JC. *Surgery of the Anus, Rectum and Colon*. 5th edn. London: Baillière Tindall, 1984: 143 pp.

Management of uncomplicated internal haemorrhoids

Hak-Su Goh BSc, FRCS
Senior Consultant and Head, Department of Colorectal Surgery, Singapore General Hospital, Singapore

Principles and justification

Uncomplicated internal haemorrhoids do not bear pain-sensitive mucosa from or below the dentate line. They are enlarged and displaced anal cushions, which are first-degree, second-degree and small third-degree haemorrhoids and present with bleeding, perianal pruritus, or prolapse. They can be readily treated on an outpatient basis, by injection, banding, infrared coagulation, or a combination of these methods. Injection acts by stimulating submucosal fibrosis, which shrinks and anchors the anal cushions to their normal positions. Banding removes excessive internal haemorrhoidal tissues by strangulation. Infrared coagulation causes thrombosis of feeding vessels and induces haemorrhoidal involution. These techniques are all effective in treating internal haemorrhoids, but each has advantages in specific circumstances.

Management of haemorrhoids should include careful proctosigmoidoscopy to exclude inflammatory bowel disease, polyps, or carcinoma of the rectum. It is also important to alleviate factors that could aggravate or cause recurrence of haemorrhoids, such as prolonged and excessive straining at stool and chronic constipation. Apart from advice on a healthy diet of fresh fruits and vegetables, management should include a course of bulk laxative.

Infrared coagulation is a new method of treating internal haemorrhoids that is gaining widespread use. It acts by the generation of infrared light that penetrates tissue and instantly converts to heat to coagulate the tissue. When applied to the base of a haemorrhoid, the mucosa and blood vessels in the submucosa are coagulated and sealed to the muscularis. This reduces blood flow to the haemorrhoid, causing it to involute.

Indications

Injection is effective in controlling bleeding, particularly when the haemorrhoids are not bulky (first-degree and small second-degree haemorrhoids). It is useful in recurrent bleeding following haemorrhoidectomy and can be used to supplement banding. Smaller primary, as well as accessory, haemorrhoids can be injected after the larger ones have been banded. Sometimes this method is helpful for pruritus, but it is usually ineffective for bulky or prolapsing haemorrhoids.

Banding serves as the 'gold-standard' for the treatment of uncomplicated internal haemorrhoids. It is particularly effective for bulky and prolapsing haemorrhoids (second-degree and third-degree haemorrhoids).

Infrared coagulation is effective in bleeding haemorrhoids. It is useful in hepatitis B or human immunodeficiency virus (HIV)-positive patients, as it does not cause bleeding or tissue sloughing. It is particularly useful in patients who are receiving anticoagulants, who are immunocompromised, or who are pregnant. Like injection, it is not very effective for prolapse.

Contraindications

Injection should not be used in the presence of thrombosis or sepsis, active inflammatory bowel disease, or in bleeding associated with immunodeficiency disorders, such as acute leukaemia. While injection can be repeated, the interval should not be within 3 weeks because of the risk of causing injection ulcers which can bleed profusely. Injection is best avoided during pregnancy.

Banding should not be used for external haemorrhoids. All contraindications for injection also apply to banding.

Preoperative

No special preparation or anaesthesia is needed for injection of haemorrhoids. Occasionally, a simple enema (Fleet) can be administered when the rectum is loaded with soft faeces.

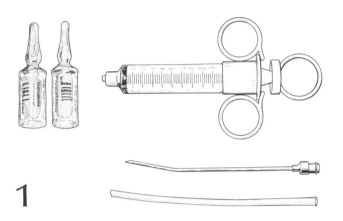

1

Operations

Position of patient

For injection, banding, or infrared coagulation of haemorrhoids, patients can be placed in either the left lateral (Sims) position or the semi-inverted (jack-knife) position on a proctological table.

INJECTION OF HAEMORRHOIDS

Instruments

1 With increasing awareness of hepatitis B and HIV infections, a 10-ml disposable plastic syringe with a three-finger grip and a long angulated needle has replaced the traditional Gabriel glass syringe. The sclerosant used is 5% phenol in vegetable oil (almond). A wide-bore plastic 'straw' facilitates drawing of the oily sclerosant into the syringe. A pair of long forceps and small pieces of gauze should be kept handy for wiping mucosal surfaces or for applying pressure if there is bleeding during injection. A lighted proctoscope provides a steady, bright illumination.

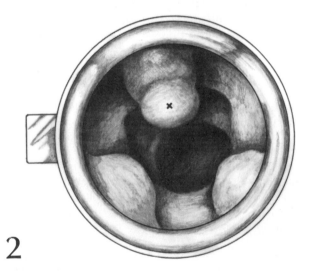

2

Injection

2 Injection is at the base of the haemorrhoids and into the submucosal plane. All the haemorrhoids can be injected in one session, and 3 ml of sclerosant is used for each site. It is best to start with the lowest haemorrhoid, so that if bleeding or leakage occurs, the remainder will not be completely obscured.

Precautions

3 Injection should be painless. If there is pain, the needle has been placed too near the dentate line and should be withdrawn and placed higher up the anal canal. If there is resistance, the injection is in the wrong plane, particularly if there is blanching of the mucosa. It indicates that the injection is in the mucosa and can cause ulceration with the risk of bleeding. The needle should be advanced into a deeper plane. When bleeding occurs on withdrawal of the needle, it is easily stopped by pressure. If bleeding does not stop with pressure, the area should be ligated with a rubber band.

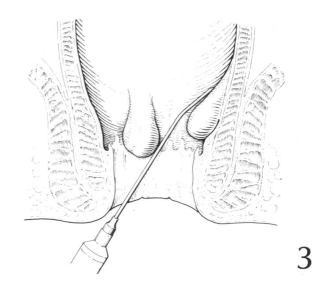

3

BANDING OF HAEMORRHOIDS

Instruments

4 Many versions of haemorrhoid ligators are available. They all have the same basic design, with a drum to trap haemorrhoidal tissue and a triggering mechanism to fire rubber bands. The instrument with the simplest design is often the most reliable. Two rubber bands are loaded onto the drum. Haemorrhoids can either be grasped with a long angulated forceps or a suction device. Grasping forceps are simple and reliable and are more widely used. A lighted proctoscope is preferred, and an assistant is needed to hold the proctoscope in place for the operator to grasp and fire at the same time.

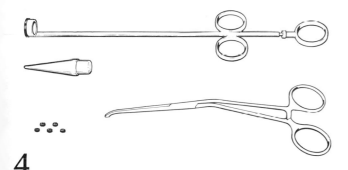

4

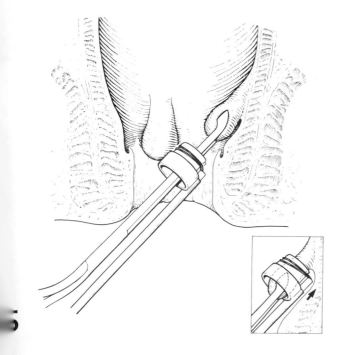

Banding

5 With the proctoscope in place and the haemorrhoid to be banded clearly visualized, the haemorrhoid is grasped with the forceps and drawn through the drum of the ligator. The patient should not feel any pain when the haemorrhoid is grasped. The ligator is then pushed to the base of the haemorrhoid and fired. Again, there should be no pain, although the patient may feel an urge to defaecate. Banding should start with the biggest haemorrhoid, and all of them may be banded in one session provided there is no discomfort. Otherwise, one or two haemorrhoids are banded first and the remainder 4–6 weeks later.

Precautions

6 Bands should not be placed too near the dentate line because they can catch sensitive mucosa or induce thrombosis of overlying external haemorrhoid and cause severe swelling and pain. When banding small haemorrhoids, a small volume of sclerosant or 0.5% bupivacaine hydrochloride with 1:100 000 adrenaline can be injected into the ligated mass to make it more tense and encourage sloughing.

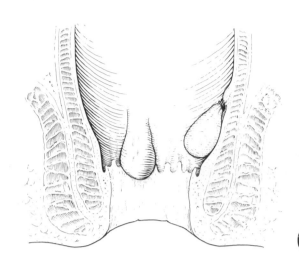

6

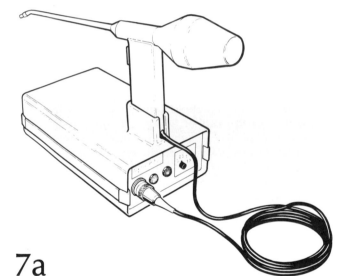

7a

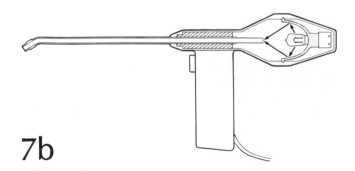

7b

INFRARED COAGULATION

Instruments

7a, b The infrared coagulator has a 15-V tungsten–halogen lamp as the infrared energy source. The light is reflected by a 24-carat gold-plated surface and carried through a quartz glass light-guide to a sapphire contact tip. The temperature at the tip reaches 100°C. The heat generated causes tissue coagulation, and the depth of coagulation is determined by the time of exposure. The automatic timer range is from 0.5 to 3.0 s, giving a coagulation depth range of 0.5–2.5 mm. The working setting is between 1.0 and 1.5 s to give a depth of 1 mm.

Coagulation

8a, b The instrument is switched on and the timer set at 1.0–1.5 s. With the haemorrhoids clearly visualized through a proctoscope, the tip of the coagulator is placed in firm contact with the base of the haemorrhoid using light pressure. The tip should not be embedded in the tissue. The instrument is then fired to the end of each automatically timed setting. A circular whitish eschar will appear on the mucosa after each exposure; three to five exposures are made in a semicircle around the base of the haemorrhoid, allowing a gap of a few millimetres between each. The tip of the coagulator should be wiped with damp gauze, after each exposure if necessary, to remove debris which may smoulder and carbonize, thereby damaging the tip.

Precautions

As each infrared exposure is so easy to execute, it is important to place the tip of the instrument accurately to avoid misfiring, thereby causing pain.

Postoperative care

No specific care is required following injection, but constipation should be treated. Patients can resume normal activities after injection. Some patients may feel faint and light-headed immediately after injection, but this is transient, lasting only 5–10 min. A short rest is all that is required.

Complications

Too much sclerosant or injection into the mucosa can cause injection ulcers, which may bleed profusely. An emergency under-running suture of the bleeding vessels may be required to stop the bleeding.

Extrarectal injection can give rise to pain and fever, or haematuria and prostatitis, if it is into the prostate. These complications may require intravenous antibiotics.

Mild tenesmoid discomfort is often felt following banding, and this is relieved with a non-steroidal anti-inflammatory drug, such as ketoprofen. A bulk laxative should be given to treat constipation and minimize the risk of prolapse due to straining.

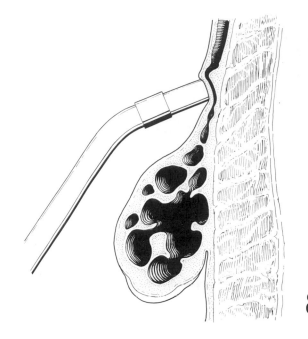

8a

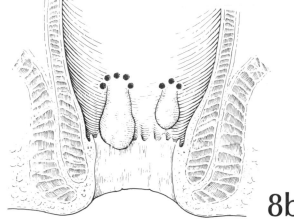

8b

When bands are placed too low or when they induce oedema and thrombosis, severe pain results. This is first treated conservatively with strong analgesics and sitz baths. If pain persists, the rubber bands should be removed under general anaesthesia.

At 7–10 days after banding the haemorrhoids slough off. In 1–2% of cases secondary haemorrhage, severe enough to require hospital admission, requires an under-running suture to control the bleeding. This is best carried out under general anaesthesia.

Very occasionally, banding of haemorrhoids can give rise to severe systemic sepsis, particularly in immuno-compromised patients. Immediate intravenous antibiotics and desloughing are required to control the sepsis.

Though not common, bleeding and pain can occur within 24 h of infrared coagulation. The bleeding is mild and stops spontaneously, while pain is easily controlled with simple analgesics.

Open haemorrhoidectomy (St Mark's ligation/excision method)

T. G. Allen-Mersh MD, FRCS
Consultant Surgeon, Westminster Hospital, London, UK

C. V. Mann MA, MCh, FRCS
Consulting Surgeon, The Royal London Hospital and St Mark's Hospital for Diseases of the Rectum and Colon, London, UK

Principles and justification

Indications

Surgical treatment offers the best chance of permanent cure of haemorrhoids because no other method approaches the precision and certainty of an expertly performed operative haemorrhoidectomy. The principal indication for operative haemorrhoidectomy is large, third-degree haemorrhoids. However, second-degree haemorrhoids associated with skin tags are frequently best treated by this method as it ensures that skin tags are removed. Where other treatments, such as banding or phenol injection, have failed to relieve symptoms of haemorrhoids, operation can still cure the patient.

Occasionally, persistent bleeding from haemorrhoids can result in severe anaemia. Where bleeding from another site in the gastrointestinal tract has been excluded, operative treatment results in more rapid control than treatment by non-operative methods.

The open method combines removal of the haemorrhoidal cushions and adjacent skin tags with excellent drainage of the contaminated wound. Complications are rare and symptom relief is achieved in most cases. The main drawback of operative haemorrhoidectomy is pain during the first postoperative week; this will be discussed later.

Contraindications

All operations on the anal area are best avoided in patients with inflammatory bowel diseases such as Crohn's disease or ulcerative colitis. Patients with active pulmonary or intestinal tuberculosis should not undergo operation since tuberculous infection of the anal wounds may occur.

Patients with asymptomatic HIV disease may undergo haemorrhoidectomy, but in the more advanced stages of HIV disease (CDC group 4) wound healing is impaired and elective anal surgery should be kept to an absolute minimum. These patients may have symptoms from inflamed and ulcerated anal mucosa associated with enlarged haemorrhoids. The temptation to 'tidy' the anus by surgical excision of haemorrhoids should be resisted.

If possible, gross obesity should be reduced and skin sepsis, e.g. fungal infection, should be treated before surgery. Haemorrhoids frequently become troublesome during pregnancy and operative haemorrhoidectomy is best avoided until after delivery. Future pregnancies may cause new haemorrhoids to develop and patients should be warned of this.

Rarely, patients with portal hypertension may develop large haemorrhoids associated with portosystemic shunting. Haemorrhoidectomy in this situation can result in considerable bleeding and is probably better avoided.

Acute prolapse and thrombosis of haemorrhoids (strangulated piles) can be operated on if the patient is seen early after the onset of the complication at a time when generalized anal oedema has not yet developed. In addition to excision of the thrombosed haemorrhoid, other non-thrombosed haemorrhoids can be excised provided adequate skin bridges are preserved. Once there is obvious cellulitis of the anal margin or if there is so much oedema that adequate skin bridges cannot be preserved, it is safer not to embark on open haemorrhoidectomy.

Old age is not a contraindication to surgical treatment providing that a safe anaesthetic can be given, e.g. by a caudal method. However, an irregular bowel habit, especially constipation, should be corrected before surgery because the patient who fails to pass a regular formed stool after operation or who uses purgatives to liquefy the motions may develop faecal impaction or anal stenosis.

Haemorrhoids, however painful or disabling, are harmless. Treatment should never introduce a significant element of risk to the patient.

Preoperative

All patients who complain of bleeding from the anus should undergo rectoscopy at least to the rectosigmoid junction (20 cm from the anal verge) to confirm that a rectal source of bleeding, such as a carcinoma, is not present. Where there is darker bleeding or any suggestion of a change in bowel habit, the patient should undergo barium enema or colonoscopy. Haemorrhoidectomy should not be performed until any concurrent disease in the colon or rectum has been treated.

Other than the usual preparation to ensure that the patient is fit for anaesthetic, very little specific anorectal preparation is required for haemorrhoidectomy. The patient is admitted on the evening before or early on the morning of operation and is given a disposable phosphate enema to clear the left colon and the rectum of stool. The enema must be given at least 2 h before surgery, otherwise the enema fluid may remain within the rectum and will flow into the anal canal at the time of surgery.

Anaesthesia

Most patients are very nervous at the prospect of a haemorrhoidectomy and premedication is important in preparation for the anaesthetic.

General anaesthesia is supplemented by local anaesthetic administered by the surgeon (1% solution of lignocaine with adrenaline 1:200 000).

In elderly or unfit patients, a caudal block can be used; some surgeons employ the caudal or epidural method routinely to supplement general anaesthetic to provide excellent analgesia and relaxation of the anal sphincter. However, in the hands of the less experienced operator, the total relaxation of the internal sphincter which results from caudal anaesthesia makes internal sphincter identification more difficult, with an increased risk of internal sphincter injury.

Operation

Position of patient

The patient is placed in the full lithotomy position with the buttocks lifted over the edge of the table. Some surgeons prefer to carry out the procedure with the patient prone and the table split in a jack-knife position. Both positions are satisfactory and the choice depends on the surgeon's preference. In the conscious patient, who is being operated on under local anaesthesia, the left lateral position can be less embarrassing and uncomfortable. In these circumstances the left lateral Sims position with the buttocks raised on a sandbag offers reasonable exposure, especially if the upper buttock is firmly retracted by strapping. If the patient has cardiac or respiratory insufficiency, this position is better tolerated than full lithotomy because there is neither embarrassment of diaphragmatic action nor gross postural effects on venous return to the heart, so that the cardiac output remains stable.

Once the patient has been positioned, perianal hair can be shaved using a scalpel blade before the skin is prepared and towels applied.

Injection of local anaesthesia

1 When the patient has been anaesthetized and is in the lithotomy position, the perianal skin is prepared with a mild antiseptic solution (cetrimide 1% or aqueous chlorhexidine gluconate 1:2000). The anal canal is carefully cleaned with cotton wool pledgets soaked in cetrimide until all faecal particles have been removed.

Local anaesthetic solution is then injected sub-cutaneously into each haemorrhoidal mass. An injection of 2–3 ml at each site is sufficient to ensure a dry field; excessive injection distorts the operative field, making it more difficult to estimate what is to be removed and the size of the skin bridges which are to remain. Infiltration should extend beneath the mucocutaneous junction and the lining of the lower part of the anal canal, but need not include the upper half of the anal cushion.

Further local anaesthetic solution (3–5 ml) is injected into each ischiorectal fossa just to the medial side of the ischial tuberosity to block the inferior haemorrhoidal branches of the pudendal nerve. A 5-cm no. 20 needle can be passed from a central posterior puncture forwards and laterally until it strikes the periosteum of the ischial tuberosity 2.5 cm above its lowest point. The needle is then withdrawn 1–2 mm and the infiltration carried out, having ensured by aspiration that a vein has not been entered. This partial pudendal nerve block relaxes the external anal sphincter and provides useful postoperative analgesia.

It is advisable to wait for 3–5 min after local infiltration to allow the full haemostatic and anaesthetic effects to develop.

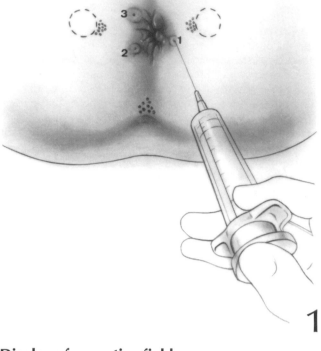

1

Display of operative field

If anal sphincter tone is increased, a gentle two-finger dilatation of the sphincter is performed to allow the anal canal to be opened. If the sphincter is of normal tone or atonic as a result of the nerve block, this step is unnecessary and may be damaging. Elderly patients should never have the sphincter dilated.

2 Dunhill forceps are placed on the perianal skin just outside the mucocutaneous junction opposite each primary haemorrhoidal cushion (left lateral, right anterior and right posterior; 3, 7 and 11 o'clock). Skin tags should be included in the area of perianal skin to be removed. Gentle traction on the forceps then brings each haemorrhoidal mass into view.

At this stage a careful note is made of the areas of skin and mucosa (skin bridges) which should remain between each area from which the haemorrhoidal cushions are to be dissected. It is usual to leave a skin bridge between each excised haemorrhoidal cushion and these should be greater than 1 cm wide to avoid a significant risk of postoperative anal stenosis.

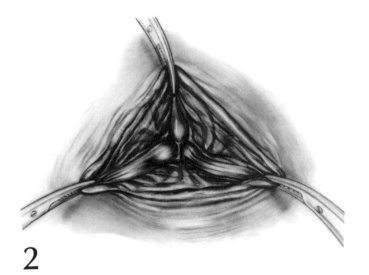

2

Triangle of exposure

3 As the internal haemorrhoids are pulled down, a second pair of Dunhill forceps is placed on the main bulk of each haemorrhoidal mass; further traction exposes the pedicles of the haemorrhoids and produces the so-called 'triangle of exposure' which is caused by the stretching of pink columnar cell mucosa between the apices of each taut pedicle. When the second pair of Dunhill forceps is clipped to each haemorrhoid, care must be taken not to include the internal sphincter muscle by taking too deep a bite. Intervening small haemorrhoids may be taken with separate forceps and approximated to the nearest primary forceps so that they are included with the main haemorrhoid in the subsequent section.

Once the triangle of exposure has been achieved the haemorrhoids are ready to be dissected and removed. It is a mistake to carry the pedicle dissection higher than this exposure allows because there is a risk of narrowing the upper anal canal if too much mucosa is gathered at the anorectal junction, and the excision of large amounts of anal epithelium will result in reduced anal sensation.

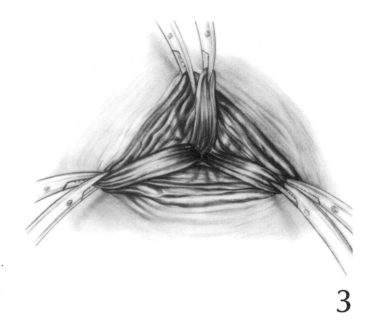

3

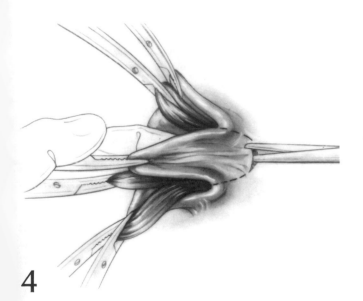

4

Start of dissection

4 The haemorrhoids are dissected in turn. For a right-handed surgeon it is convenient to start with the left lateral haemorrhoid, the others being temporarily held out of the way with slight traction by the assistant. The two forceps are held in linear fashion in the palm of the left hand, with the left forefinger in the anal canal on the pedicle of the haemorrhoid pressing lightly outwards to stretch the pedicle gently over the pulp of the finger. The blades of a pair of blunt-nosed scissors are placed alternately at each edge of the base, as seen from its cutaneous aspect, and the tissues divided towards the median plane until the incisions meet. The subcutaneous space superficial to the lowest (white) fibres of the internal sphincter and deep to the external (red) sphincter muscle is then exposed and can be opened up.

Further dissection

5 Dissection is continued in a coronal plane superficially at first, but almost at once this is changed to medial to the internal sphincter muscle and is directed towards the pedicle of the haemorrhoids in the submucosal plane. The borders of the dissection taper towards the base of the haemorrhoids and upward mobilization is not continued more than is necessary to allow easy control of the pedicle as previously defined by the triangle of exposure.

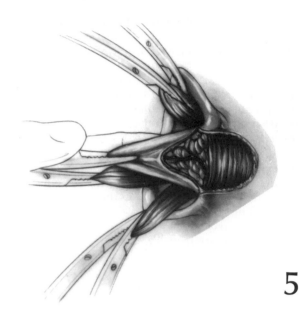

5

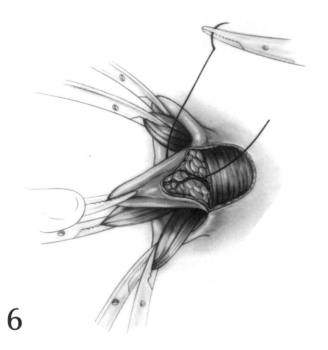

6

Ligation of pedicle

6 As the pedicle is exposed by dissection, traction on the haemorrhoid should be eased. Once the haemorrhoid has been defined, the pedicle is suture-ligated with a slow dissolving suture material (e.g. 2/0 Vicryl) with the knots tied on the luminal aspect. It is not necessary to use very strong material for the pedicle ligation; a large knot of non-absorbable material can excite a foreign body reaction and even cause a fistula.

Once the pedicle has been secured and traction on the pedicle released to check that vessels have been safely controlled by the ligature, the pedicle is cut through, leaving a good cuff. The ends of the ligatures are left long so that the pedicle can easily be identified and recovered to control persistent oozing. The pedicle is then allowed to retract to its normal position in the upper anal canal.

Procedure for remaining haemorrhoids

7 The other haemorrhoids are removed in a similar fashion. The right anterior haemorrhoid is usually the smallest and easiest to deal with, and is frequently left until last because, when the patient is in the lithotomy position, bleeding from the front of the anal canal may obscure subsequent dissection posteriorly. If the patient is prone, the sequence should be reversed. Intact bridges between perianal skin and anal mucosa must be preserved between each dissection site, and should be not less than 1 cm wide.

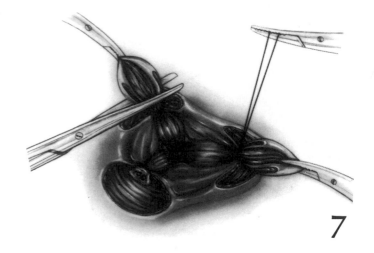

7

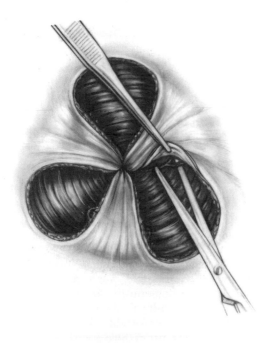

8

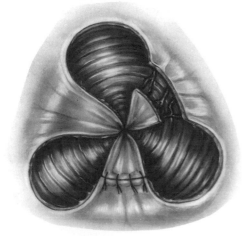

9

'Filleting' of skin bridges

8, 9 If large external veins are seen beneath the residual bridges, they can be removed by dissection beneath the margins of the bridges from each side ('filleting') or by dividing the bridges, removing the underlying veins, and then sewing the bridges back in place with fine catgut. When the divided skin bridges are being reconstituted, the rectal mucosa must not be dragged down to the anal verge, because mucus seepage from the anus would result. It may be necessary to remove a short segment of the rectal mucosa which forms the upper part of the skin bridge so that when the cut edges are sewn together the squamous epithelium is taken up into the anal canal.

Trimming of wounds

10 After all the pedicles have retracted into the upper anal canal, the mucosal defects are critically inspected for persistent bleeding and for redundant flaps of mucosa or perianal skin. Any redundant tags of skin are removed, and puckering of the skin bridges can be reduced by anchoring sutures of slowly dissolving 3/0 suture material. Haemostasis of any small bleeding points, either from the mucosal edges or from the raw area of the mucosal wounds, is controlled by light application of diathermy or by ligation with 3/0 Vicryl sutures. Occasionally, in the presence of diffuse bleeding, the application of a swab soaked in adrenaline solution (1:1000) is preferred to excessive diathermy.

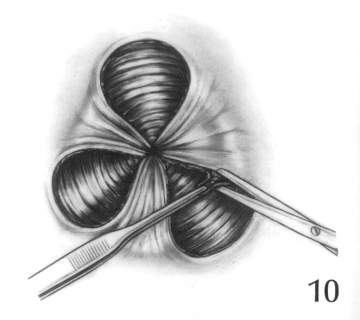

10

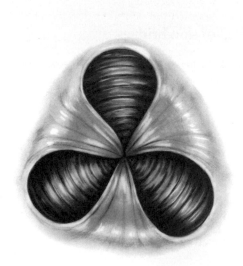

11

Final appearance and dressing

11 The final appearance of the operated area should resemble a clover leaf and the wounds should be completely dry before a dressing is applied. Dressings are a matter of personal choice, except that greasy or oily materials should be avoided as they prevent proper drainage of serosanguineous exudate from the raw anal mucosal defects. Dressings such as cellulose mesh which dissolve spontaneously can be lightly tucked in over each raw area. Bulky anal packs should be avoided because they are uncomfortable. The wound should be dry at the end of the procedure and there should be no need for anal tamponade. In occasional cases, where packing is thought to be justified because of difficulty with haemostasis, the use of gelatin sponge is useful because it provides some initial tamponade and haemostasis but decomposes quite quickly. This avoids the risk of hurting the patient which occurs when a non-absorbable pack is removed from the anal canal.

A thick pad of cotton wool is then laid over the perineum and held in place by either a T bandage or Tenafix pants.

Postoperative care and complications

The dressings remain undisturbed for 24 h. They are then removed and the patient is allowed to soak the area in a warm bath. A clean pad is applied and held in place with the T bandage or Tenafix pants. The patient is started on a combination of magnesium hydroxide and liquid paraffin (Mil-Par) and Normacol (fibre) granules, both 10 ml twice daily. On this regimen, the majority of patients will have a bowel action by the third postoperative day. The patient should be encouraged to have a bath after each bowel action and clean external dressings are then reapplied. Once the patient has had a satisfactory bowel action, Mil-Par can be discontinued, but Normacol granules are continued for the first 6 weeks to ensure a soft bulky stool while the anal canal is healing.

There is some controversy about routine digital examination after haemorrhoidectomy. However, there is a risk of faecal impaction and a gentle digital examination of the anal canal and lower rectum on the fifth postoperative day is recommended. If impaction is present, a disposable sodium dihydrogen phosphate enema is given. If an impaction is not identified until a later stage, when there may be complete blockage with liquid overflow, it may even require disimpaction under anaesthesia.

Pain control may be difficult after haemorrhoidectomy, being most severe on about the third postoperative day when the first bowel action occurs. Initial pain control can be achieved with routine postoperative analgesia and a caudal block at the time of operation. Strong oral or intramuscular analgesics, including opiates, are often necessary, with a sedative (e.g. diazepam) helping to overcome the anxiety of defaecation. Other methods, such as internal sphincterotomy at the time of haemorrhoidectomy and the application of topical anaesthetic cream have been tried but do not provide any significant reduction in pain. The use of diathermy or a laser beam for haemorrhoid dissection has been claimed to reduce postoperative pain.

However, in these authors' experience, while there may be slight differences in postoperative pain using these methods, the problem of pain-induced inhibition of defaecation is not overcome. Epidural anaesthesia provides good pain control, but this approach cannot be justified because of the complications and practical difficulties of the technique.

While there are no definite contraindications to day-case haemorrhoidectomy, this can only be recommended where the patient has suitable home conditions and the medical service has made appropriate arrangements for home supervision.

In the first 24 h after operation bleeding may occur from small vessels which appeared not to be bleeding at operation because of spasm or because a ligature becomes loose. Bleeding can occur later because of stool disturbing a ligated pedicle, excessive straining in a nervous patient, or necrosis of the ligated pedicle. It is important to recognize that bleeding after haemorrhoidectomy can be life-threatening. The volume of blood passed is an unreliable guide to the extent of bleeding, because in the presence of a continent sphincter the majority of the blood may pass up into the colon. When a fall in blood pressure or rise in pulse rate occurs, re-examination of the anal canal and identification of the bleeding point is required.

A digital examination should be carried out 1 month after operation to ensure that an anal stenosis is not developing. At this stage the wounds should be granulating well but will not be fully healed. There may be some slight persisting serosanguineous discharge from the healing wounds which necessitates a small pad. During the second postoperative month the wounds should heal completely and a pad should be unnecessary after 2 months. Occasionally, one of the wounds can persist as an anal fissure with continuing pain and discharge. If this problem persists, an internal anal sphincterotomy is indicated.

Management of acute anorectal sepsis

R. H. Grace FRCS
Consultant Surgeon, The Royal and New Cross Hospitals, Wolverhampton, UK

Principles and justification

Anorectal sepsis is a common minor surgical emergency; unfortunately it is often poorly managed and has a recurrence rate of 25–48%[1–3], resulting in discomfort, the need for further surgery, increased time lost from work, and damage to the anal sphincter.

Aetiology

1 Anorectal sepsis begins as an intermuscular abscess secondary to infection of an anal gland[4–8]. Extension of this downwards between the internal and external sphincters or through the lowermost fibres of the external sphincter produces a perianal abscess; extension through the external sphincter complex into the ischiorectal fossa produces an ischiorectal abscess; extension upwards or medially into the submucosal plane produces a high intermuscular or submucosal abscess. The track from the anal canal to the intermuscular abscess to the abscess cavity constitutes a fistula but not all anorectal abscesses are associated with such a fistula. Recent microbiological studies[9, 10] have shown that, although an abscess from which an intestinal organism has been cultured is likely to be associated with a fistula, those from which a skin organism is cultured (mainly *Staphylococcus aureus* or skin-derived *Bacteroides*) are not.

Indications

The diagnosis of anorectal sepsis is usually obvious: the patient complains of a painful lump by the anal canal and the severity of pain is such that the history is short. Examination reveals perianal swelling, usually associated with erythema of the overlying skin with local tenderness to palpation. There is, however, a small group of patients in whom the diagnosis may be delayed. This group complains of pain but there is no obvious swelling and no erythema; rectal examination is very uncomfortable. The unwary surgeon or general practitioner may ignore the patient's symptoms, or may consider the possibility of a fissure, but may miss the true diagnosis of submucosal sepsis. Any patient who complains of persistent anal pain of short duration in whom no fissure is visible should undergo an examination under anaesthesia as an emergency to identify the cause of the symptoms, which will frequently be found to be a submucosal abscess.

Any rationale for the initial treatment of anorectal sepsis on presentation must assume that a fistula is present because microbiology is not available; a past history of sepsis at the same site is strong evidence that a fistula is present.

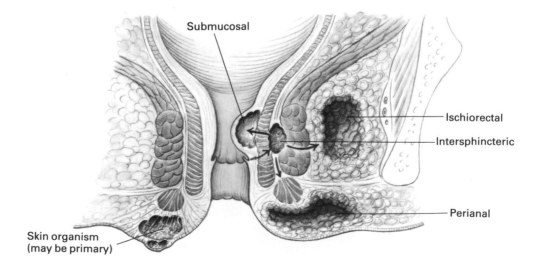

Submucosal

Ischiorectal

Intersphincteric

Perianal

Skin organism (may be primary)

1

Surgical management

The correct management of anorectal sepsis is governed by aetiology and should relieve the immediate symptoms, prevent recurrent sepsis and minimize healing time and thereby time lost from work.

Three drainage procedures have traditionally been described: incision and drainage; saucerization; incision and drainage with primary suture.

Incision and drainage

2a, b Linear incision over the point of maximal tenderness or induration releases the pus; a small drain may be left *in situ*, or the wound may be lightly packed with a dilute hypochlorite dressing. This technique will relieve the immediate symptoms and minimize healing time but will do nothing to prevent recurrent sepsis if a fistula is present.

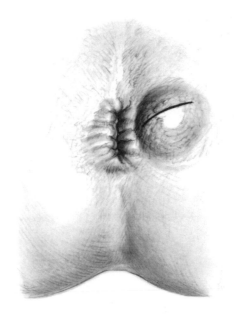

2a

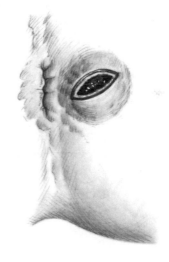

2b

Saucerization

3 A cruciate incision is made over the point of maximal tenderness or induration, followed by excision of the triangles of skin to allow 'good drainage'. If a fistula is present this technique will relieve the immediate symptoms but does not prevent recurrent sepsis and, with a large wound, is associated with a prolonged healing time.

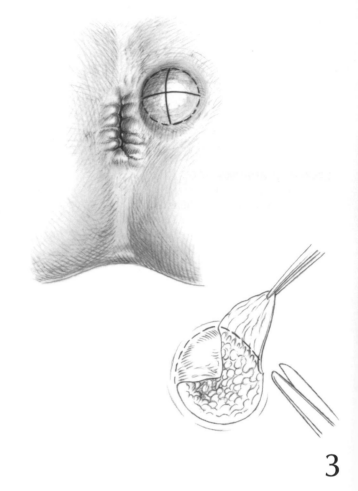

3

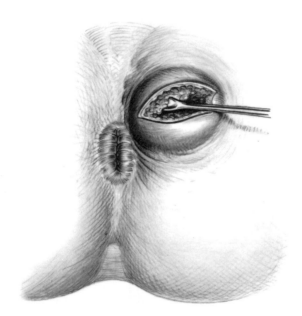

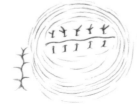

4

Incision and primary suture

4 A linear incision is made over the point of maximal tenderness or induration; the abscess cavity is curetted, and the wound sutured to obliterate this cavity. This technique, under antibiotic cover, will relieve the immediate symptoms and minimize healing time but will not prevent recurrent sepsis if an underlying fistula is present.

These three procedures all ignore the possibility of a fistula. Logical management requires the surgeon not only to drain the abscess but also to look for a fistula and treat it appropriately.

Operation

The management described in this chapter is simple, logical, and takes note of the anatomy and microbiology, recognizing that at the time of presentation no bacteriological data are available.

First examination under anaesthesia

5 The patient is examined under general anaesthesia in either the lithotomy or the jack-knife position. Visual examination and then careful palpation define the extent of induration and determine whether the abscess is perianal or ischiorectal; a large area of erythema does not necessarily indicate ischiorectal sepsis.

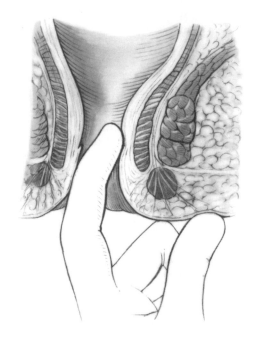

5

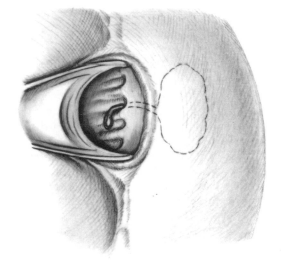

6

6 The anal canal is then inspected using a Sims or Eisenhammer speculum. The surgeon should look for pus draining into the anal canal through an internal opening at the dentate line. Gentle pressure on the abscess from the outside may help to identify the internal opening by the appearance of pus at the dentate line.

Incision and drainage

7a, b The abscess is drained through a linear incision, the cavity is curetted and the pus sent for microbiological examination. The incision may be radial (*Illustration 7a*) or circumanal (*Illustration 7b*): the radial incision may damage the underlying sphincter musculature.

The line of incision should reflect the direction of any potential fistula track: a perianal abscess will probably be associated with a low fistula track running directly towards the anal canal, which indicates a radial incision; an ischiorectal abscess may be associated with a 'high' fistula running posteriorly, or sometimes anteriorly, and a circumanal incision is preferred.

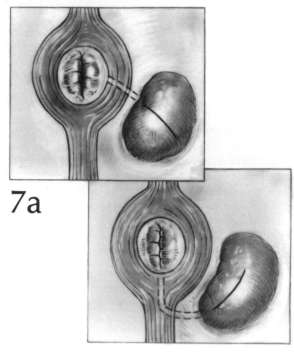

7a

7b

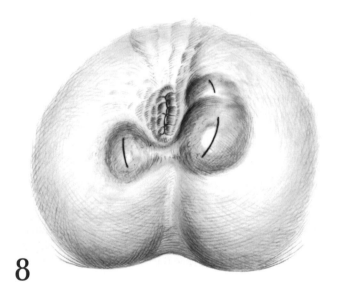

8

8 Anorectal sepsis may present with bilateral abscesses where the cavities connect in the midline and are usually associated with a fistula. Drainage of the abscess cavity will require at least one incision on either side and, depending on the extent of the sepsis, may require further incisions anteriorly or posteriorly. Most bilateral abscesses are associated with a posterior fistula.

9 In acute sepsis the relationship of the fistula track to the sphincter muscle may be difficult to establish. This is a particular problem anteriorly where the sphincter is more difficult to define because of oedema and induration. If the internal opening has been defined by the observation of pus in the anal canal it may be further defined using a hooked Lockhart-Mummery probe placed into the internal opening at the dentate line. A finger in the abscess cavity will help to identify the tip of the probe. If no pus has been observed in the anal canal, a fistula probe may be used to explore the abscess cavity and its relationship to the anal canal and the sphincter. However, all these manoeuvres should be performed with extreme caution because over-enthusiastic probing may produce a false track. When there is no obvious internal opening it is safer to await microbiology and perform a second examination under anaesthesia after the acute episode has settled.

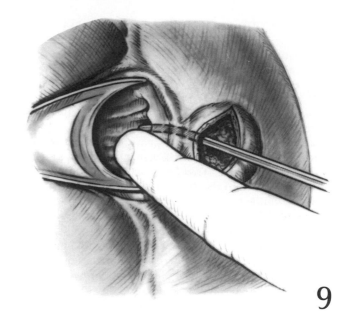

9

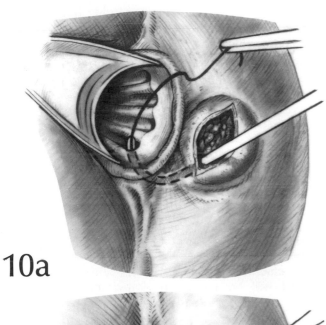

10a

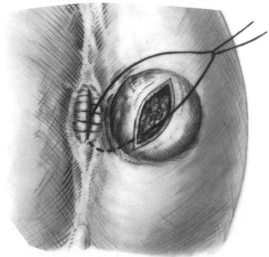

10b

10a, b If a fistula track has been defined its management depends upon the relationship of the track to the sphincter complex but oedema may make this difficult. A low fistula is easily laid open as described in the chapter on pp. 834–847. However, more complex anatomy is best managed initially by the use of a seton suture. An atraumatic 0 nylon suture on a large curved needle may be placed by guiding the needle along the groove in the Lockhart-Mummery probe; this may be done twice before tying the suture. The relationship of the seton suture to the sphincter may be further assessed at a subsequent examination under anaesthesia when the acute episode has settled.

Alternative management of the fistula is to leave its track unmarked until a second examination, when it can be treated (*see* chapter on pp. 834–847).

Microbiology

If no fistula is found at the first examination, further management depends upon the microbiology. Culture of intestinal organisms requires a second examination under anaesthesia 7–10 days later; growth of a skin organism means that no second examination under anaesthesia is required[9, 10].

Second examination under anaesthesia

If a fistula is found but not laid open at the initial examination under anaesthesia, it is defined again and then either laid open or managed with a seton suture.

If no fistula was found at the first examination, the incision is extended to give a good view of the abscess cavity which is then curetted. The fistula track will be marked by granulation tissue projecting from the fistula track into the cavity; this will remain even after the area has been curetted. The Lockhart-Mummery probe is gently passed into the track and if the fistula is low the track should be laid open and the wound edges trimmed. The management of a high fistula depends upon the extent of the external sphincter which lies below the fistula track. If a significant amount of the sphincter needs to be divided, treatment should include initial use of a seton suture. If the fistula track cannot be demonstrated, no further action should be taken.

Postoperative care

Analgesia will be required, but the patient with an abscess or abscess and fistula will rarely experience as much pain as a patient who has undergone haemorrhoidectomy.

Following first examination under anaesthesia, if no fistula is found, the abscess cavity should be packed as necessary for haemostasis with dilute hypochlorite solution in the dressing, which will be removed on the following day. The patient should be discharged home with instructions on wound management (*see* below).

Normal bowel action should be encouraged by the third or fourth postoperative day. A high-fibre diet combined with mild laxatives will ensure that there is little problem.

Wound management

The patient should bathe at least twice a day and after the bowels have been opened. The wound is irrigated with dilute hypochlorite (Milton) (1:40) solution and dressed with a flat dressing soaked in dilute hypochlorite which is tucked into the wound; the wound should not be packed and ribbon gauze should never be used. The anal dressing should be held in place with close-fitting elastic underwear which holds the dressing comfortably in place.

The passage of an anal dilator twice a day from the third postoperative day ensures that the smaller, low anal fistula wounds heal without 'bridging'. The larger, high fistula wounds do not require an anal dilator, but a further examination under anaesthesia may be required 2 weeks later to ensure that no bridging has taken place

and that the wound is healing satisfactorily. If pus is present at the later examination, there may be an unresolved problem which requires further evaluation.

Antibiotics

With adequate surgical drainage of the abscess there is no place for antibiotics in postoperative management except in cases with fulminating gangrene, tuberculosis, or in immunosuppressed patients.

Special situations

There are four special situations in which management may need to be modified.

Crohn's disease

The management of anorectal sepsis in Crohn's disease is part of the overall management of the disease and certain principles should be clearly understood:

1. Perianal sepsis is always associated with a fistula.
2. Large anal wounds do not heal well.
3. Management should be aimed primarily at relieving symptoms but with very conservative surgery.
4. There is a high incidence of recurrent sepsis if treatment does not include opening of the fistula.
5. A course of metronidazole and co-trimoxazole may be indicated.
6. Medical management may include steroids or azathioprine.

Abscess plus low fistula

Management may include laying open a fistula as the wound will be small, but simple drainage may be preferred.

Abscess with high fistula

The fistula should be laid open only with extreme caution because a large wound may be very slow to heal, or may never heal. A seton suture may be used in this situation for long-term drainage.

Abscess with multiple fistulae

The management almost certainly consists of drainage of the abscess; if sepsis continues, however, it may eventually be necessary to excise the rectum.

Tuberculous infections

This possibility should be considered in populations in whom tuberculosis is endogenous. Surgical management of the acute abscess should be on the principles already discussed because the results of bacteriological culture will not be available for at least 6 weeks. If tuberculous infection is suspected, a special request for suitable culture should be made. If it is positive, the patient will require anti-tuberculous therapy. The patient usually has evidence of tuberculosis elsewhere.

Fulminating anorectal sepsis

These infections are rare, may not be clostridial in origin[11,12] but are associated with definite mortality and considerable morbidity rates. Surgery must be radical, aiming to excise *all* the necrotic tissue until the edges are clean and bleeding; further procedures must be carried out if the first procedure is not sufficiently radical and if there is evidence of spreading cellulitis. These are the only patients with anorectal sepsis who require broad-spectrum antibiotics, taking account of microbiology when it becomes available. There may be a place for hyperbaric oxygen if there are gas-forming organisms, but the need for this has not been well defined. Control of diabetes is not usually difficult but is important.

Hydradenitis suppurativa

Hydradenitis suppurativa is a chronic low-grade sepsis of the skin which is probably associated with an abnormality of the apocrine gland system. The patient presents with multiple areas of discharge which connect by superficial subcutaneous sinus tracks. The areas most affected are the perianal skin, the perineum, the scrotum and the axillae; the nape of the neck and the face are less often involved. Men are more often affected than women. When the perineum and scrotum are involved, the condition may be very extensive and the patient may be a social outcast because of the associated offensive odour.

The microbiology of hydradenitis suppurativa has not been extensively studied but the organisms most frequently cultured are anaerobic Gram-positive cocci and the asaccharolytic group of *Bacteroides*[13].

The diagnosis is usually obvious with the classic areas of discharge with oedematous skin between external openings of the sinus tracks; the skin between these openings may be prominent and raised into thickened scarred folds. The alternating sepsis and healing causes scarring and contraction which may be a problem, particularly in the axillae with limitation of shoulder movements.

Surgical management of the perianal, perineal, and scrotal disease depends upon the extent and severity of the involvement. The oedematous folds of skin may need to be excised, but conservative surgery with preservation of skin can produce very good results. The surgical wounds in these areas heal rapidly, which is surprising in the light of the extent of the sepsis.

There is often epithelialization of some sinus tracks which should be laid open using the Lockhart-Mummery fistula probes; there is often a honeycomb of such sinuses. When they have all been laid open and curetted, the skin edges should be excised using sharp fistula scissors, preserving as much normal skin as possible.

The surgeon should accept the idea of conservative staged procedures if the involvement is extensive. The more radical procedure of wide excision of the affected skin and grafting is rarely required. There is no need for antibiotic cover.

References

1. Buchan R, Grace RH. Ano-rectal suppuration: the results of treatment and factors influencing recurrence rate. *Br J Surg* 1973; 60: 537–40.

2. Vasilevsky C, Gordon PH. The incidence of recurrent abscess or fistula-in-ano following ano-rectal suppuration. *Dis Colon Rectum* 1984; 27: 126–30.

3. Schouten WR, Van Vroonhoven TJ. Treatment of ano-rectal abscess with or without primary fistulectomy. *Dis Colon Rectum* 1991; 34: 60–3.

4. Nesselrod JP. In: Christopher F, ed. *A Textbook of Surgery*. 5th edn. Philadelphia: Saunders, 1949: 1092–114.

5. Eisenhammer S. The internal anal sphincter and the ano-rectal abscess. *Surg Gynecol Obstet* 1956; 103: 501–6.

6. Eisenhammer S. A new approach to the ano-rectal fistulous abscess based on the high intermuscular lesion. *Surg Gynecol Obstet* 1958; 106: 595–9.

7. Eisenhammer S. The ano-rectal and ano-vulval fistulous abscess. *Surg Gynecol Obstet* 1961; 113: 519–20.

8. Parks AG. Pathogenesis and treatment of fistula-in-ano. *BMJ* 1961; i: 463–9.

9. Grace RH, Harper IA, Thompson RG. Anorectal sepsis: microbiology in relation to fistula-in-ano. *Br J Surg* 1982; 69: 401–3.

10. Eykyn SJ, Grace RH. The relevance of microbiology in the management of ano-rectal sepsis. *Ann R Coll Surg Engl* 1986; 68: 237–9.

11. Ledingham IMcA, Tehrani MA. Diagnosis, clinical course and treatment of acute dermal gangrene. *Br J Surg* 1975; 62: 364–72.

12. Brightmore T. Perianal gas-producing infection of non-clostridial origin. *Br J Surg* 1972; 59: 109–16.

13. Eykyn SJ, Phillips I. Miscellaneous anaerobic infections. In: Finegold SM, George WL, eds. *Anaerobic Infections in Humans*, Volume 26. San Diego: Academic Press, 1989: 567–89.

Low anal fistula

P. R. Hawley MS, FRCS
Senior Consultant Surgeon, St Mark's Hospital for Diseases of the Rectum and Colon and Consultant Surgeon, King Edward VII Hospital, London, UK

Principles and justification

A fistula is an abnormal communication between any two epithelial-lined surfaces. An anal fistula is one in which there is an opening between the anal canal and the perianal skin. Most fistulae arise from abscesses originating in the anal glands. Anatomical studies show that there are between six and ten of these glands situated around the anal circumference, each discharging through a duct into an anal crypt, sometimes with two entering the same crypt; some crypts have no glands entering them. In at least half the cases, the glands penetrate the internal sphincter and extend into the longitudinal fibres, but not beyond them, into the external sphincter complex. Histologically, they are lined by stratified mucus-secreting columnar epithelium, but occasionally part may be lined by squamous epithelium. Cystic dilatation and infection of these glands is always situated deep to the internal sphincter muscle. Thus, the anal glands may be regarded as diverticula of the anal canal and, like diverticula in any part of the alimentary tract, are subject to stasis and secondary infection. Ducts that pass through the internal sphincter will not be able to discharge their contents so readily into the anal canal, for the muscle tone will tend to compress the lumen of the duct.

An anal fistula is virtually a sign of disease in the anal gland. This explains why there is no detectable opening into the anal canal in 30% of cases. While anal glands are distributed evenly around the circumference of the anal canal, 60% of all fistulae arise in the midline posteriorly, probably because this is the site of anal fissure, inflammation and fibrosis resulting in stasis and infection of the posterior gland. Another 20% of fistulae arise in the midline anteriorly, and the remaining 20% are distributed around the rest of the anal canal.

There are other aetiological factors. Tuberculosis, which used to be a common cause of anal fistulae, is now responsible for less than 1%. Anal fistulae are common in inflammatory bowel disease, particularly in Crohn's disease. Foreign bodies, usually from the ingestion of pieces of bone or fragments of wood, may result in a persistent fistula until these are removed. Commonly, a fistula is preceded by an abscess, and if an abscess in this region of the body is recurrent, it is almost certain that a fistula exists even if the tract cannot be identified. A neglected fistula will result in recurrent abscesses and progressive inflammation over many years. Malignancy very seldom occurs in a chronic fistula unless it is a 'congenital fistula', which is a minor degree of reduplication. Such fistulae are usually lined by rectal mucosa in their upper parts, with islands of squamous epithelium in the lower or external aspect of the fistula, and may not communicate with the anal canal. Not uncommonly malignant change occurs in these fistulae, resulting in a mucus-secreting adenocarcinoma, usually of low-grade malignancy.

A low fistula is one in which the tract can be laid open without division of the puborectalis muscle, thus preserving continence; 95% of all anorectal fistulae are low fistulae. Complex high fistulae are often iatrogenic, from injudicious probing of a low fistula with an upward extension in the intersphincteric or trans-sphincteric space. Approximately 60% of all anorectal fistulae are intersphincteric, even if their external opening is a considerable distance from the anal verge. They may cross the lower fibres of the external sphincter, but are still essentially intersphincteric. Trans-sphincteric fistulae occur in 30% of patients; a few in addition will have an upward supralevator extension that requires drainage.

Anatomy and classification of fistulae

Anatomy

1 The essential anatomy of the anal region is shown in *Illustration 1*. It should be noted that the ischiorectal fossa is a pyramidal space, the apex of which is above the anorectal ring. The anorectal ring marks the junction of rectum and anal canal and is formed by the puborectalis fibres of the levator ani muscle passing around the intestine and blending with the external sphincter. Complete incontinence results if all the anal sphincters, including the anorectal ring, are divided; section of muscle below this level may lead to some impairment of control or mucus leakage, depending on the amount of muscle divided.

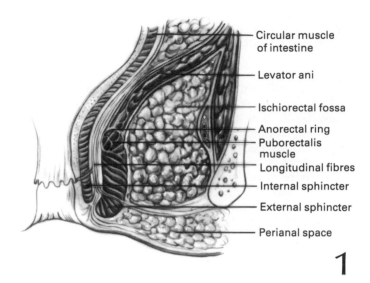

Circular muscle of intestine
Levator ani
Ischiorectal fossa
Anorectal ring
Puborectalis muscle
Longitudinal fibres
Internal sphincter
External sphincter
Perianal space

1

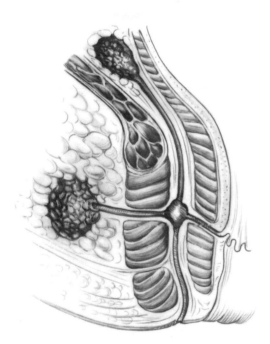

2

Classification of fistulae

2 Almost all anal fistulae result from infection of anal glands situated in the intersphincteric plane. An abscess in the anal gland leads to an abscess cavity in the intersphincteric space. From this focus infection may track laterally, medially, upwards or downwards, before or after tracking circumferentially.

[These illustrations represent the fistulae in two dimensions, but it must be remembered that in reality most are three-dimensional.]

3 About 60% of all fistulae are intersphincteric, usually passing downwards in the intersphincteric space to form a perianal abscess. When this discharges, a fistula results. The external opening is not usually close to the anus in the intersphincteric groove, but tracks laterally along the longitudinal fibres, and the external opening is 2–3 cm or more from the anal verge.

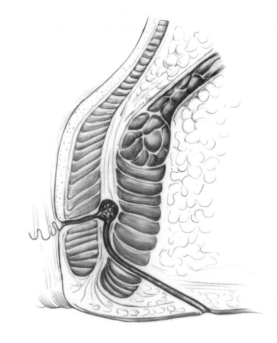

3

4 Pus may track upwards from the infected anal gland, remaining in the intersphincteric plane but pushing its way above the anorectal ring to cause a swelling and induration above the anorectal ring. This type of abscess often extends circumferentially and sometimes occurs without any downward extension, so that there is no external opening of the fistula. The abscess may break back into the anal canal by tracking medially, which gives a secondary opening, usually at a higher level than the primary opening, which is nearly always at the level of the dentate line.

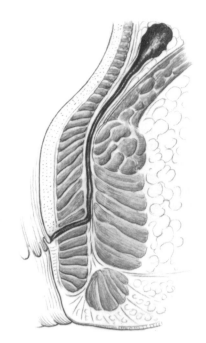

4

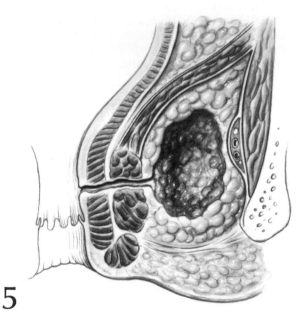

5

5 Pus from the infected anal gland may penetrate laterally through the external sphincter muscle to infect the ischiorectal fossa. This will result in an ischiorectal abscess, which will usually drain downwards through the investing fascia and the perianal fat to exit through the skin, resulting in a fistula that is termed a trans-sphincteric fistula. A difficulty arises because the site of penetration through the external sphincter muscle is often not at the same site as the tract penetrating through the internal sphincter. The fistula first tracks upwards in the intersphincteric plane and then breaks through the external sphincter at a higher level and sometimes through the puborectalis muscle. Uncommonly, the lateral extension will be above the puborectalis muscle, resulting in a true high fistula. The term 'high' trans-sphincteric fistula is the term given by some to this type of trans-sphincteric fistula, when the outward extension passes through the upper part of the external sphincter muscle. It is, however, by definition a low fistula.

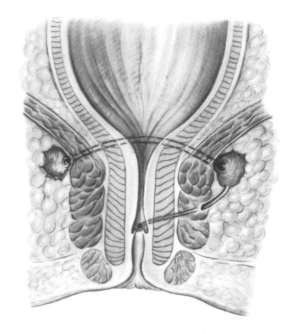

6 Infection of the intersphincteric plane or ischiorectal fossa may track around circumferentially, and the fistula between the crypt and the intersphincteric plane, which usually lies in the midline posteriorly, may not be the site of penetration through the external sphincter. The trans-sphincteric part of the fistula may penetrate more laterally and also at a higher level. The ischiorectal abscesses themselves may track around circumferentially, resulting in a so-called horseshoe fistula. These trans-sphincteric fistulae and abscesses are normally limited above by the levator muscles, but may push them up on one side, suggesting a supralevator origin.

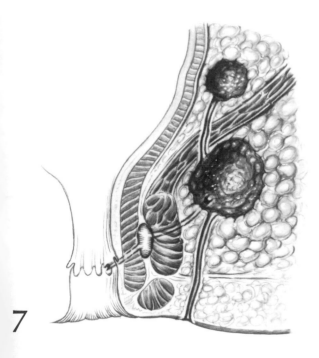

7 Very occasionally, the tract may spread upwards through the levator muscle and, even more uncommonly, into the rectum above the anorectal ring. Many of these high fistulae are probably iatrogenic in nature, but can occur with foreign bodies. A supralevator abscess associated with an ischiorectal abscess must be adequately drained, but if the puborectalis muscle is intact, the fistula can be dealt with as a low fistula. A supralevator hole in the rectum will need to be closed, possibly with a covering colostomy, but the primary cause must be dealt with first.

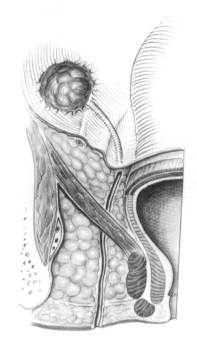

8

8, 9 Very uncommonly, a fistula arises from a supralevator origin and passes directly through the pelvic floor, either intersphincterically or through the levator, to open onto the perineal skin. These fistulae are termed extrasphincteric, and do not arise from anal gland disease. The origin is from pelvic inflammatory disease, such as diverticular disease, Crohn's disease, appendix abscess, pelvic abscess, or pyosalpinx. It may arise from a pelvic fracture penetrating the intestine. In these circumstances, the primary cause is dealt with and the fistulous tract simply curetted out, and left to heal.

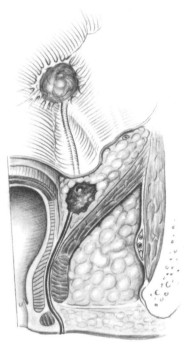

9

Principles of operative treatment

The object of treatment of a fistula is to eradicate the septic focus and permanently eliminate the fistula tract, this being accomplished with minimal disruption to the sphincter complex. Treatment of more difficult fistulae usually results in a compromise between complete cure of the fistula and complete continence. Some surgeons take the view that it is essential to cure the septic process that causes the patient's symptoms, and that this may only be accomplished with minor degrees of sphincter impairment, such as difficulty in controlling flatus or watery stool during an attack of diarrhoea. Other surgeons will take the view that the sphincter complex must not be disrupted in any way, often resulting in a persistent fistula or even recurrent attacks of abscess formation.

There are three methods of treating a low anal fistula, depending on the preference of the surgeon. The fistula may be laid open, it may be treated with an encircling ligature known as a seton, or the sepsis may be eliminated and the origin repaired by an advancement flap. All three of these methods are used in the treatment of low anal fistulae and will be described.

The instruments that are required include a malleable probe, a set of Lockhart-Mummery probe directors and a set of lachrymal probes, as many of the tracts are narrow and fibrosed and larger probes will not pass through them. It is useful if the lachrymal probes and one of the probe directors have an eye for the passage of a seton. A pair of fistula scissors (Miltex) and an Eisenhammer retractor should be available.

Preoperative

A recurrent discharging sinus or abscess in the perineum normally indicates that a fistula is present, and this will not heal until surgery is undertaken. The patient is carefully examined including sigmoidoscopy and proctoscopy. If it is thought that the fistula may be caused by Crohn's disease, a rectal biopsy and investigations of the gastrointestinal tract should be carried out before considering whether the fistula should be treated surgically.

Preparation

The rectum should be emptied by a disposable enema or suppositories.

Anaesthesia

General anaesthesia is necessary for all except the most superficial fistulae. Full relaxation should be avoided as there should be sufficient tone in the sphincter muscles to enable the operator to palpate the external sphincter and puborectalis muscle.

Position of patient

The patient should be in the lithotomy position with the buttocks well down over the edge of the table. Alternatively, the prone jack-knife position may be used and can be helpful for the high anterior fistula.

Operative examination

The perianal region is shaved, and before starting the operation the whole area should be carefully palpated. The index finger should feel around the anus externally, identifying the intersphincteric groove and recognizing induration, whether radial or circumferential. With the index finger within the anus, the location of any induration should be identified, in which quadrants, and whether above or below the puborectalis. An internal opening may be palpable. It must be remembered that most fistulae open in the midline posteriorly, and where there is circumferential extension the opening will usually be found at this site. Most tracts can be felt as indurated ridges.

An Eisenhammer anal retractor is then inserted into the anus and the internal opening sought in the indurated quadrant. A fine malleable probe can then be inserted into the internal and external openings. An internal opening will not be obvious in about 30% of cases.

Pathological examination

Granulation tissue from the tract and any skin tag or fibrous tissue removed must be submitted for microscopic examination to exclude any specific condition, particularly Crohn's disease.

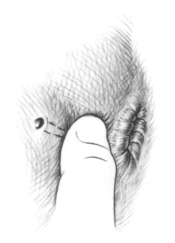

10a

Operations

SIMPLE LOW FISTULA

10a–c The external opening and induration around the tract are palpated. Digital examination of the anal canal is then carried out to feel for an internal opening. An Eisenhammer retractor is inserted and the internal opening sought at the dentate line. Anterior tracts are often radial; posterior tracts may be horseshoe-shaped. A probe is then gently inserted into the external opening, and in a radial fistula it may pass directly through the internal opening. Even in radial fistulae, however, the tract is not always straight, and the probe must never be forced or a false passage will result. If a probe director easily passes through the fistula to exit in the anus, the tract can simply be laid open with a knife or diathermy probe.

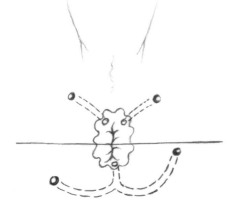

10b

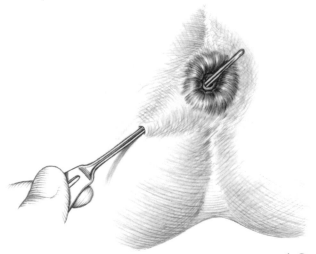

10c

11 The edges of the wound are held apart with a pair of Allis' forceps, and the granulation tissue curetted away. Careful search is made for any extensions of the fistula, particularly upwards in the intersphincteric plane, and the granulation tissue is carefully curetted away from such an extension.

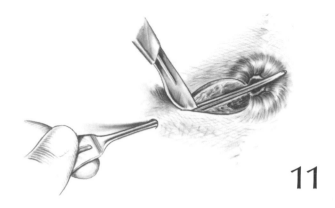

11

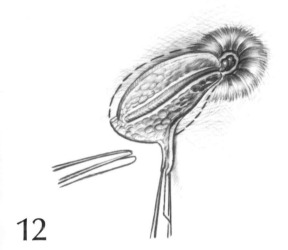

12

Extension of the wound

12 The wound is extended outwards for a short distance beyond the external opening, which is removed. The granulation tissue is sent for histology. When a probe cannot be passed through the fistula, or the internal opening not found, the tract is laid open from the external surface using a pair of Miltex scissors. The granulation tissue can be followed and the tract laid open until either it enters the anal canal or stops short in the intersphincteric plane. It is usually necessary in these circumstances to divide the internal sphincter to the level of the tract in order to produce a flat wound and stop pocketing.

High intersphincteric fistula

13 After the lower part of the tract has been opened, it may become apparent that a higher intersphincteric tract is present because of induration in the region of the anorectal ring. A probe is then passed upwards and the tract laid open to its upper limit by dividing the internal sphincter. There may be a secondary opening which usually depicts the upper extent of the tract. It should be remembered that the tract may not run straight upwards, but may curve around.

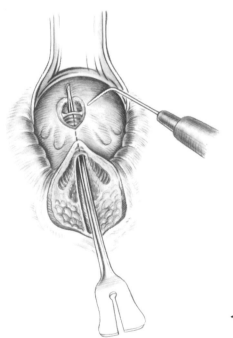

13

Trans-sphincteric fistula

Course of the main tract

14 The main tract of this type of fistula follows the roof of the ischiorectal fossa, i.e. it lies on the under-surface of the puborectalis and pubococcygeal muscles. The tract is horseshoe-shaped if both sides are involved, with the anterior extension on each side passing deep to the transverse perineal muscles. The communication with the anal canal is most commonly in the midline posteriorly, but not invariably so. The tract leading to the external opening on the skin is usually vertical and may descend from any part of the main circumferential tract, or multiple tracts may be present. The communication with the lumen is usually angled upwards and is often missed for this reason. If a probe is passed into the external opening, it will enter deeply parallel to the anal canal, and its tip may be palpated through the rectal wall at a level apparently above the anorectal ring. It must never be forced through at this level, or opened into the rectum, as this will result in a high fistula. The real internal opening is almost always below the anorectal ring, most commonly at the level of the dentate line.

In an extensive fistula, the internal opening may be quite small and only take a lachrymal probe angled upwards. By palpation over the fistula, the internal opening may be apparent by the appearance of a bead of pus. Injection of dyes via a small cannula placed in an external opening is not helpful in determining the extent of the tract.

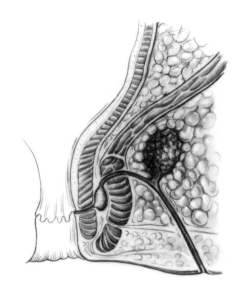

14

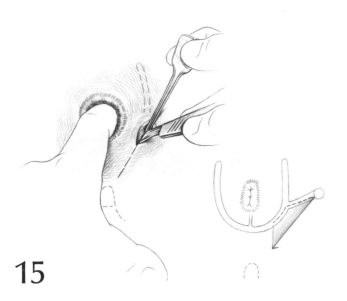

15

15 The external part of the tract is always opened first, either with a scalpel slid along a grooved director or with fistula scissors. The tract is followed by the pyogenic granulation tissue, which is curetted from the tract. It is followed backwards towards the midline and is usually extrasphincteric, but being essentially circumferential it does not cut muscle.

16 The edges of the wound are held open with a pair of Allis' forceps and the whole extent of the fistula is laid open, with any upward extensions curetted out. It is possible to leave part of the skin intact if the tract is curetted out beneath, but it is usually preferable to lay open the whole of the tract.

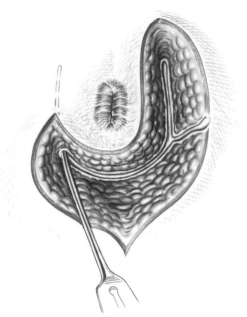

16

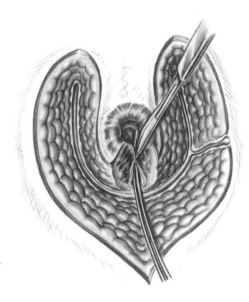

17

17 The tract may extend to the opposite ischiorectal fossa, but there is usually an abscess cavity full of chronic granulation tissue lying posteriorly, which may extend upwards in the precoccygeal space, occasionally extending through Waldeyer's fascia. When this posterior abscess has been laid open, the tract into the anal canal will become apparent and can be laid open if it is certain that the internal opening is below the anorectal ring. If there is any doubt, the superficial muscles only are divided, and a seton is placed around the deep part of the muscle. Muscles should always be divided at right angles to their fibres if possible, and not obliquely.

18 The wound is trimmed by bevelling the skin edges and removing part of the underlying fibrous tissue from the fistula to produce a saucer-shaped wound which will heal readily. All granulation tissue is meticulously curetted away, and a careful search should ensure that no section of the tract has been overlooked.

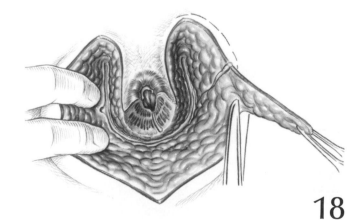

18

USE OF THE SETON

A seton or ligature around part of the sphincter may be used in three ways. The first is to mark the fistula if the surgeon is uncertain of the height of the tract in relation to the puborectalis muscle and does not wish to proceed with the operation. This will allow the tract to be evaluated when the patient is awake and allow definitive surgery to be carried out later.

19 The second use of the seton is to tie it loosely around the muscles after laying open the external part of the tract and draining any upward ischiorectal abscess. The internal opening is curetted out and as much granulation tissue removed as possible. The seton is then placed around the undivided muscle of the external and internal sphincter to allow drainage and healing. If this method is adopted, repeated examination under anaesthesia will be required, with further curetting of the tract, often over many months. About 50% of fistulae may heal by this method, but the other 50% will eventually require laying open before healing is obtained. It is difficult to achieve adequate drainage of high intersphincteric or trans-sphincteric extensions by this method. Its only certain place is in the treatment of fistulae associated with Crohn's disease, when a ligature of silk or Ethibond can be left in place for many months or indeed indefinitely.

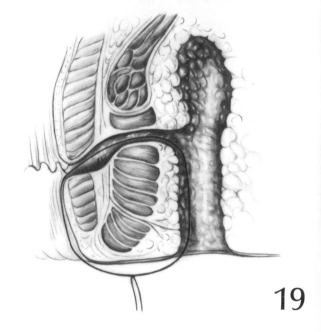

19

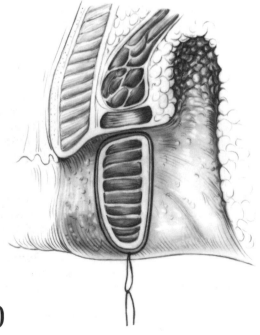

20

20 When the fistula involves the whole of the external sphincter or a substantial part of it, the surgeon may elect to use the seton as a cutting ligature. The external part of the fistula is laid open to drain it completely, and the internal sphincter laid open to the level of the primary tract, or above, until the level of the penetration of the external sphincter. The skin and mucosa are removed as if the fistula was to be laid open, but the external sphincter is preserved. A ligature of 1 silk or Ethibond is then placed around this muscle and tied tightly with a loop externally, and the ends left long.

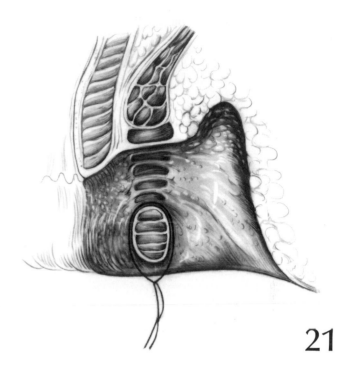

21, 22 After 2 weeks, the ligature will have cut through approximately half of the external sphincter and will be quite loose. The wound is curetted and a further seton inserted in the same tract by threading the end of the ligature through the loop tied in the previous suture and then cutting one end of the ligature and pulling the new suture through the remaining muscle. In this way, a false passage is not made. The ligature is again tied tightly, and this ligature or a successive one will cut through the muscle completely, but without allowing the ends to retract. The wound will heal and continence be achieved.

21

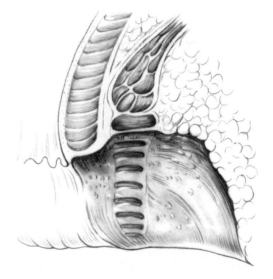

22

RECTAL ADVANCEMENT FLAP

The third method of treatment is the rectal advancement flap. This has a place in treating certain high trans-sphincteric fistulae, but is often used unnecessarily in low intersphincteric fistulae when the only piece of muscle to be divided is the internal sphincter to the dentate line, as is commonly done in any anal internal sphincterotomy.

23 With an Eisenhammer retractor in place, a rectal muscle flap of the whole rectal wall is fashioned with a broad base and elevated in the anal canal from the underlying internal sphincter muscle, exposing the perirectal fat above the anal canal.

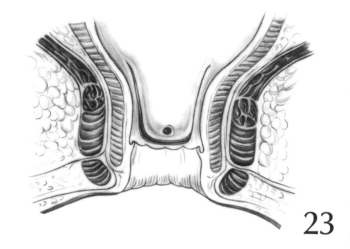

23

24–26 The internal opening is then excised with the base of the flap and the granulation tissue curetted out where the tract pierces the internal sphincter and the intersphincteric abscess. The external opening of the fistula is laid open and all the granulation tissue is curetted out. The defect in the internal sphincter is sutured with interrupted 2/0 polyglactin sutures or alternatively the internal sphincter can be double-breasted longitudinally and sutured. The flap is then sutured around its margins with interrupted 2/0 polyglactin sutures.

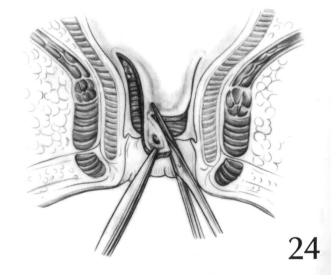

24

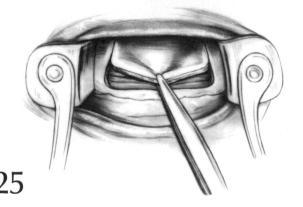

25

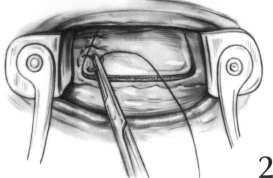

26

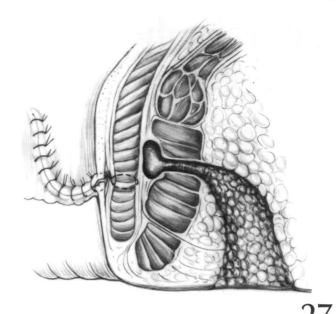

27

27, 28 The trans-sphincteric or intersphincteric part of the wound is left open to drain. It is not surprising that breakdown of these wounds commonly occurs, as they are akin to anastomoses made in an infected field. With a low intersphincteric fistula, a good result will be obtained even if the flap breaks down, but with a high trans-sphincteric or suprasphincteric fistula, breakdown of the flap will result in a further fistula, often larger than the original.

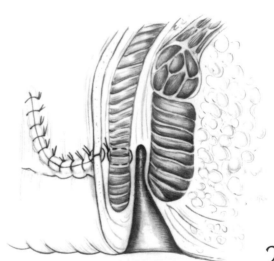

28

Postoperative care

Skin excision should be kept to a minimum, and scars should be fashioned circumferentially away from the ischial tuberosities. These are infected wounds, and cleansing and granulation tissue is stimulated with the use of 1:40 sodium hyperchlorite solution applied to flat gauze dressings. If there is significant bleeding, gauze wrung out in 1:1000 topical adrenaline solution should be inserted into the wound.

The wound heals slowly, the final scar being much smaller than the initial wound, and the anal appearance may not be grossly altered. Sphincter function is usually adequate, even when a considerable amount of the external sphincter has been divided. If necessary, the wound should be reviewed under anaesthesia, particularly if there is a persistent discharge of true pus.

Illustrations by Gillian Oliver

Lateral subcutaneous internal anal sphincterotomy for anal fissure

M. J. Notaras FRCS, FRCSEd, FACS
Consultant Surgeon, Barnet General Hospital and Honorary Senior Lecturer and Consultant Surgeon, University College Hospital, London, UK

Principles and justification

Examination of the lower half of the anal canal by separation of the buttocks to open up the perianal region will reveal the presence of any simple anal fissure, as they are located below the dentate line and are always confined to the anoderm in the mid-posterior position (90%) or the mid-anterior position (10%). The anoderm is that part of the anal skin that lies between the dentate line and the anal verge and is the squamous lining of the anal canal.

1 An acute fissure is a superficial splitting of the anoderm and may heal with conservative management. Once the fissure is recurrent or chronic, operation is required for a permanent cure. A chronic fissure is recognized by the presence of transverse fibres of the internal sphincter in its floor. A late stage in the development of a chronic fissure is the formation of a large fibrous polyp from the anal papilla on the dentate line at the upper end of the fissure. Infection of the sentinel pile that develops at the lower end of the fissure at the anal verge may lead to the formation of a superficial fistula.

Fissures that are multiple or extend above the dentate line should be viewed with suspicion as a simple anal fissure never extends above the dentate line. These complex fissures are usually signs of more serious diseases, such as ulcerative colitis, Crohn's disease, tuberculosis, or syphilis. When associated with large rubbery inguinal lymph nodes, they may indicate a primary syphilitic infection, and smears from the anal canal should be taken for dark-ground illumination before digital or endoscopic examination contaminates the field with lubricant.

It must be remembered that anal sexual intercourse is necessary for the transmission of anal syphilis, so this infection must be considered in patients suspected of, or known to engage in, this form of sexual activity. Serological tests must be performed, and the possibility of acquired immune deficiency syndrome considered.

Human immunodeficiency virus (HIV)-positive patients with anal conditions should be identified, as it is important to distinguish fissures from ulcers. Biopsies should be taken from any suspicious fissure or ulcer, and in HIV-positive patients viral culture of part of the biopsy specimen is essential. Sphincterotomy performed for an HIV-positive homosexual patient infected with cytomegalovirus or herpetic ulcer may result in faecal incontinence combined with slow healing of the wound.

An intersphincteric sinus or abscess may be mistaken for a chronic anal fissure unless excluded by careful examination. A subcutaneous fistula may also be present in a sentinel haemorrhoid (*see Illustration 1*).

Treatment of anal fissure

Lateral subcutaneous internal anal sphincterotomy has been shown to have many advantages over other forms of treatment, such as anal dilatation and mid-posterior internal sphincterotomy performed through the floor of the fissure. It has rapidly gained acceptance as it may be performed as an outpatient procedure under local or general anaesthesia. Its main advantages are that it avoids an open intra-anal wound, the divided internal sphincter is bridged by skin, there is minimal anal wound care, postoperative anal dilatation is unnecessary and relief from symptoms is almost immediate, with the fissure becoming painless and healing within 3 weeks.

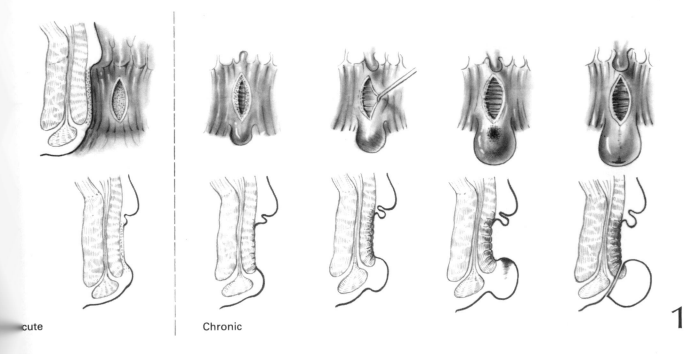

cute   Chronic   1

Preoperative

The author prefers no bowel preparation so that the urge to defaecate after the operation is not delayed. The patient may be placed in the lithotomy, lateral or jack-knife position according to the preference of the surgeon. Sigmoidoscopy should be performed on all patients.

Anaesthesia

The procedure may be performed under general or local anaesthesia or a combination of methods. The author supplements general anaesthesia with local anaesthesia, which permits a lighter general anaesthetic to be used. A local anaesthetic combined with dilute adrenaline solution helps to reduce bleeding and immediate postoperative pain.

Approximately 10 ml of local anaesthetic agent (0.5%

lignocaine hydrochloride with 1:200 000 adrenaline) is infiltrated subcutaneously into the perianal area on each side of the anus. The inferior haemorrhoidal nerves are blocked on each side by injection of 5–7 ml into each ischiorectal space along the medial aspect of each ischial tuberosity. A further 5 ml is injected directly into the external sphincter muscle on each side of the anus.

When local anaesthesia is used alone, it should be supplemented by diazepam, 10–20 mg intravenously (according to age and weight), and sometimes also pethidine hydrochloride, 50–100 mg intravenously. This technique sedates patients adequately, and although conscious throughout the procedure, they usually have no memory of the event. After the operation patients will need to rest for 1–2 h until the effects of local anaesthesia have subsided and the sphincters have recovered.

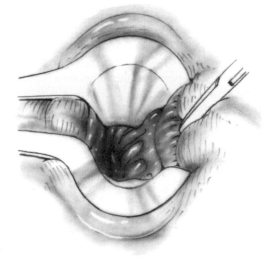

 2a

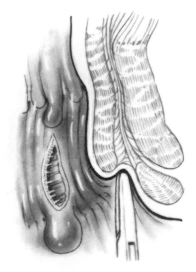

2b

Operations

CLOSED TECHNIQUE

The lithotomy position is used.

2a, b A bivalved anal speculum (Parks', Eisenhammer or Goligher) is introduced into the anal canal and opened sufficiently to stretch the anus slightly. The internal sphincter is then felt as a tight band around the blades of the speculum. Its lower border is easily palpated and can be demonstrated by gently pressing a pair of forceps into the intersphincteric groove. The floor of the fissure should be probed for a sinus or fistula.

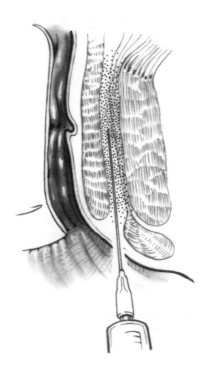

3a

3a, b Local anaesthetic agent, 2–3 ml, is introduced under the mucosa and anoderm. The anal lining is lifted away from the internal sphincter by the infiltration of local anaesthetic, thus reducing bleeding and the risk of perforation by the scalpel blade in the closed technique. It also facilitates dissection if the open technique is used.

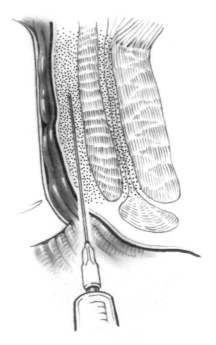

3b

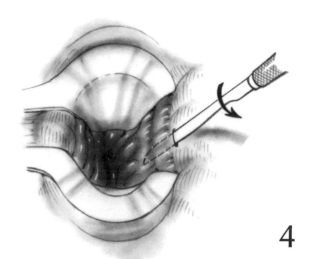

4

4,5 After the internal sphincter has been identified, a narrow-bladed scalpel (52L 'Beaver' cataract knife) is introduced through the perianal skin at the mid-lateral aspect of the anus (3 o'clock). It is pushed cephalad with the flat of the blade sandwiched between the internal sphincter and the anoderm until its point is just above the dentate line.

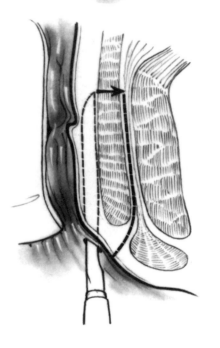

5

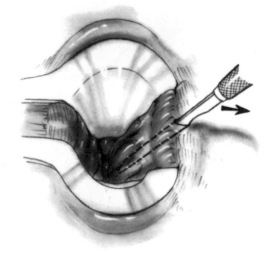

6

6 The sharp edge of the blade is then turned towards the internal sphincter, and by incising outwards and laterally the internal sphincterotomy is performed. As the scalpel blade cuts through the internal sphincter there is a characteristic 'gritty' sensation, and with completion of the division there is a sudden 'give', indicating that the blade has reached the outer surrounding ring of external sphincter muscles.

7 Another variation of the technique is to introduce the blade between the external and internal sphincter muscles via the intersphincteric groove, and then to perform the sphincterotomy by cutting inwards towards the mucocutaneous lining.

Whichever technique is used, the aim is to preserve the skin bridge over the divided internal sphincter.

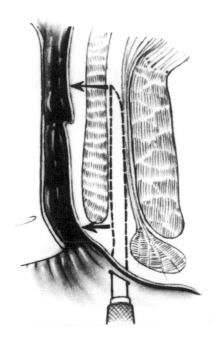

7

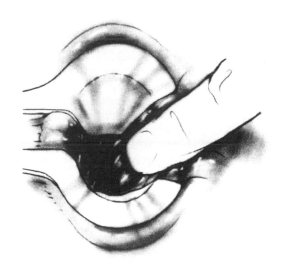

8

8 After division of the internal sphincter the completeness of the sphincterotomy may be assessed after withdrawal of the knife by pressure of the finger tip over the site. This will rupture any residual internal sphincter fibres.

Usually, there is a slight ooze of blood from the small external wound, but this is soon arrested by tamponade as the external sphincters recover and contract around the internal sphincter. The external wound is left open to allow drainage.

9 If there is a large sentinel tag, it is removed with sharp-pointed scissors without damaging the sphincters and with minimal excision of the perianal skin. All overhang is removed. Fibrous polyps are excised if present.

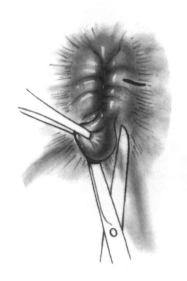

10a, b A fistula in a sentinel tag (when present) should be laid open. The tract passes through some of the superficial fibres of the lower border of the internal sphincter. It is tempting also to perform a complete internal anal sphincterotomy through the fissure and the rest of the sphincter above the sentinel tag, but results are better if the surgeon confines himself merely to laying open the fistula and then performing a lateral subcutaneous sphincterotomy. This avoids the development of a 'key-hole' deformity in the mid-posterior position, which may lead to perianal soiling.

A dressing is laid on the anal area. Intra-anal dressings are contraindicated as they cause postoperative pain. Once bleeding has ceased no dressings are required. The patient is encouraged to have a bowel action as soon as the inclination develops.

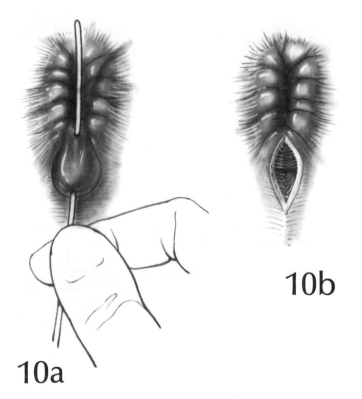

OPEN TECHNIQUE

If the surgeon is not happy with the closed technique because of fear of damage to the external sphincter muscle, the open method is equally applicable. The author originally practised this technique, but with experience found the closed technique simpler and more expeditious.

11a, b
A bivalved anal speculum is inserted into the anus to stretch the internal sphincter slightly to assist its identification, as described in the closed method.

A local anaesthetic with adrenaline is injected into the subcutaneous area selected for the procedure. A radial incision is made into the perianal skin just below the inferior border of the internal sphincter. This incision is preferred to the circumferential type, as the wound is left unsutured and open for drainage and the edges of the wound will approximate naturally.

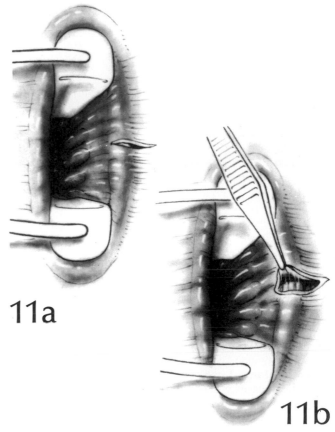

11a

11b

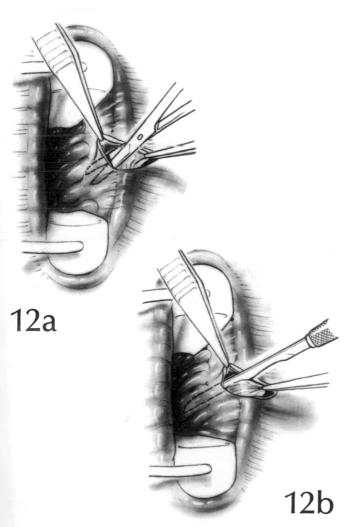

12a

12b

12a, b
The upper end of the incision is grasped with a pair of forceps and dissection with narrow-bladed scissors is carried out to separate the anoderm from the internal sphincter. The latter is recognized by its white fibres. To facilitate dissection and the sphincterotomy, its lower border may be grasped with forceps.

The exposed internal sphincter is then divided by a narrow scalpel blade or scissors.

13 The wound is left open to allow free drainage. A 'lay-on' dressing of gauze is placed over the anus. Intra-anal dressings should not be used, as they cause postoperative pain.

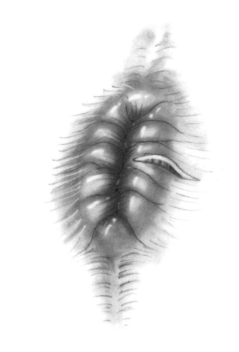

13

ANAL STENOSIS

14a–c Patients may have marked anal stenosis caused by chronic and repeated ulceration. It may also follow a previous haemorrhoidectomy or the prolonged use of mineral oils ('paraffin anus').

In those cases where there has been no previous anal surgery, bilateral subcutaneous lateral sphincterotomy may be of value. The sphincterotomy is performed on one lateral side, and if considerable tension remains in the internal sphincter on the opposite side, a second lateral subcutaneous sphincterotomy is indicated.

When there has been a previous haemorrhoidectomy, it is usual for scarring of the anoderm to extend beyond the dentate line to the rectal mucosa. There is usually fibrosis in the internal sphincter deep to these areas. In such cases, the author selects a site for the sphincterotomy in the healthiest tissue between the areas of scarring. It may also be necessary to make release incisions in the scarred mucosal areas but these are made superficially. Patients are advised to use an anal dilator for up to 2 months after the procedure.

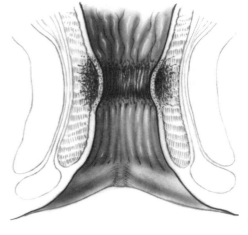

14a

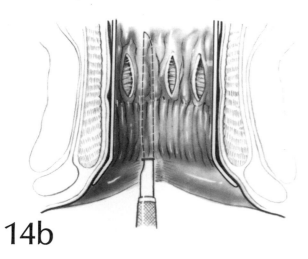

14b

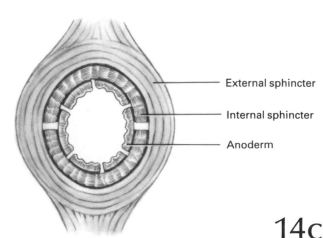

External sphincter

Internal sphincter

Anoderm

14c

Perianal and anal condylomata acuminata

James P. S. Thomson DM, MS, FRCS
Consultant Surgeon and Clinical Director, St Mark's Hospital for Diseases of the Rectum and Colon, London,
Honorary Consultant Surgeon, St Mary's Hospital, London, Honorary Lecturer in Surgery, The Medical
College of St Bartholomew's Hospital, London, Civil Consultant in Surgery, Royal Air Force and Civilian
Consultant in Colorectal Surgery, Royal Navy, UK

R. H. Grace FRCS
Consultant Surgeon, The Royal and New Cross Hospitals, Wolverhampton, UK

Principles and justification

Condylomata acuminata are caused by infection of stratified squamous epithelium with human papilloma virus (HPV); HPV types 6, 11, 16 and 18 are those usually recovered. A significant proportion of affected patients are homosexual.

This disease has an interesting natural history, because although most patients require treatment, spontaneous regression does occur. The presence of purple or black lesions among the more usual pink warts indicates that spontaneous regression might occur. Malignant change has been reported, but in the majority of patients the disease follows an entirely benign course with varying numbers of warts.

The condition known as 'giant condylomata', however, is a different and rare lesion. This is a very well differentiated squamous cell carcinoma, which usually extensively involves the anal canal and perianal skin and requires radical treatment.

Assessment

The diagnosis of perianal condylomata acuminata is usually obvious, but it is important to determine accurately the extent of the disease, because warts may also be present within the anal canal or lower rectum and on the external genitalia. In women (approximately one-fifth of affected patients), the vulva, vagina and cervix must be assessed. For all patients, recurrence is likely if not all the lesions are treated.

Differential diagnosis of perianal warts is condylomata lata, a secondary manifestation of syphilis. Condylomata acuminata are commonly transmitted by sexual contact, and other forms of sexually transmitted disease should be excluded. The cooperation of a physician who specializes in these diseases should be sought in the management of patients, not only to diagnose but also to screen for other sexually transmitted disorders, and contacts should be traced.

Principles of treatment

Small numbers of warts confined to the perianal skin may be treated by the repeated application of 25% podophyllum resin in compound benzoin tincture. Surgical treatment, however, will be required if: (1) there is no response to podophyllum, (2) there is extensive involvement of the perianal skin, and (3) if there is involvement of the anal canal and lower rectum.

The traditional method of removing condylomata acuminata used diathermy or electrocautery. Although this technique satisfactorily removed the lesions, it resulted in damage to the surrounding normal skin and to the base of the small wounds created after removal of the warts. Treatment of adjacent lesions resulted in a confluent area of tissue destruction with considerable discomfort in the postoperative period. Healing was slow, and scarring occasionally resulted in stenosis of the anal canal.

Scissor excision avoids the use of diathermy or cautery except in controlling the occasional persistent bleeding point. A solution of adrenaline 1:300 000 in physiological saline is injected subcutaneously and submucosally. This separates the warts from each other, because even large lesions have an area of normal skin between them. This allows the maximum amount of healthy skin and mucosa to be preserved when individual warts are removed by sharp-pointed scissors. The resulting small wounds heal rapidly with minimal discomfort to the patient. Usually, it is possible to remove all the warts on one occasion, but if there is a large number, removal may best be done in two stages with an interval of approximately 1 month.

Occasionally confluent lesions in the upper anal canal cannot be removed individually. Total circumferential submucosal excision is feasible, and as the extent is seldom more than 2 cm, the wound can be closed by inserting interrupted catgut sutures to approximate the lower rectal mucosa at the dentate line.

Laser equipment may be used, and an operating microscope may be of value, particularly for intra-anal lesions, which may be rendered white by applying acetic acid.

Preoperative

The rectum should be empty; a disposable enema the evening before operation usually provides adequate preparation.

Anaesthesia

This operation is best performed under general anaesthesia, but caudal anaesthesia provides adequate relaxation of the anal canal.

Small scattered lesions involving only the perianal skin can be excised after infiltration of local anaesthetic, but many patients find this difficult to endure.

Operation

1 Adrenaline 1:300 000 in physiological saline is injected subcutaneously. Approximately 50–75 ml solution is injected into each perianal area. This is best done in quadrants so that the solution is injected in a particular area immediately before excision is begun; if all the solution is injected initially, absorption occurs and the benefit of the 'ballooning' effect is lost. While the injection is being given, the needle of the syringe should be moving so that an intravenous injection is avoided.

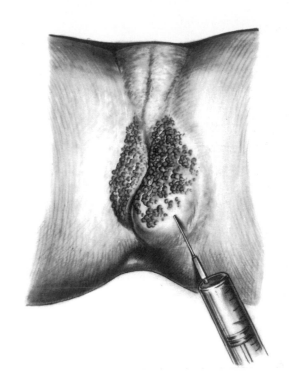

1

Excision of warts

2, 3 Warts are individually removed, preserving as much normal skin as possible using a pair of fine-toothed forceps and scissors. There is usually little haemorrhage, but a persistent bleeding point may be controlled by diathermy.

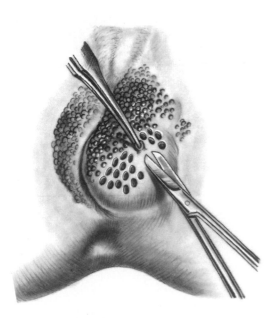

2

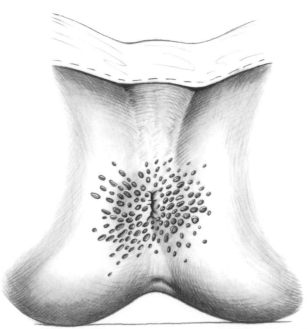

3

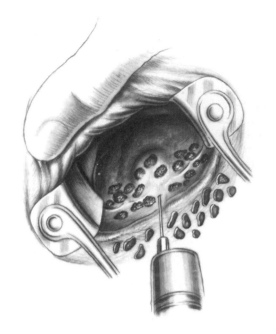

4

Removal of warts from within the anal canal

4, 5   With the aid of an anal retractor, such as the Parks' retractor, adrenaline is injected submucosally. The warts are again removed individually, preserving the mucosa between them. A large mucosal defect may be sutured with 3/0 chromic catgut to approximate the mucosa of the lower rectum to the dentate line.

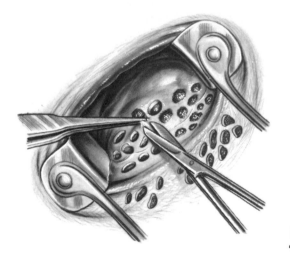

5

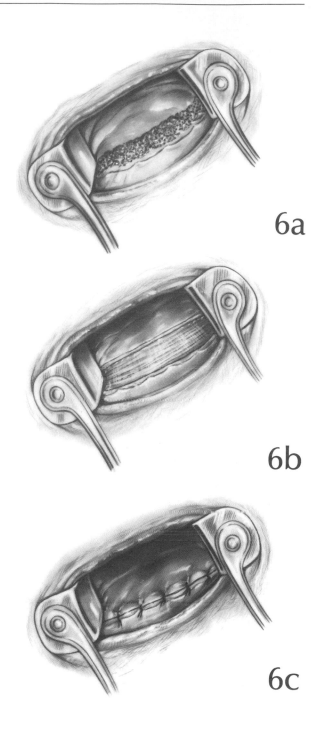

6a

6b

6c

Circumferential lesions

6a–c Circumferential lesions may be removed in the same way. The defect, which is seldom more than 2 cm in length, is closed by approximating the distal rectal mucosa to the line of the anal valves with about 12 fine catgut sutures.

Wound dressing

When all the warts have been removed, a gauze dressing soaked in physiological saline and enclosed within a sheet of Surgicel is inserted into the anal canal and used to cover the perianal area. A pressure dressing is then applied with the aid of a T bandage or with a pair of close-fitting elastic pants. The Surgicel acts as a haemostatic agent and also makes a very satisfactory non-stick dressing, because after 24 h it becomes very slippery, thus facilitating its removal.

Postoperative care

Little discomfort is experienced after this procedure, and the patient requires minimal analgesia. A normal diet should be started immediately after the operation, and the passage of a satisfactory stool is ensured by prescribing a bulk laxative. If extensive warts are removed from the anal canal, an anal dilator (No. 1 St Mark's dilator) should be passed twice a day with the aid of 1% lignocaine gel.

The warts can recur, and patients should be warned about this possiblity. If warts continue to recur after repeated operations, a chemotherapeutic ointment (5-fluorouracil) may be used. The role of this agent, however, in the treatment of condylomata acuminata requires further study.

Further reading

Prasad ML, Abcarian H. Malignant potential of perianal condyloma acuminatum. *Dis Colon Rectum* 1980; 23: 191–7.

Simmons P, Thomson JPS. Sexually transmitted diseases (and warts). In: Decosse JJ, Todd IP, eds. *Anorectal Surgery*. Edinburgh: Churchill Livingstone, 1988: 132–48.

Thomson JPS, Grace RH. The treatment of perianal and anal condylomata acuminata: a new operative technique. *J R Soc Med* 1978; 71: 180–5.

Procedures for pilonidal disease

John U. Bascom MD, PhD, FACS
Consulting and Attending Surgeon, Sacred Heart General Hospital, Eugene, Oregon, USA

History

Surgeons pursuing inappropriate goals may create pilonidal problems. The result can be great disability, long hospitalization and persistent open wounds, but the fault may not lie with the surgeon who only follows published but out-of-date recommendations. Both simple primary treatments that avoid complications and a curative operation for the complications of ill-advised surgery will be described.

Pilonidal disease was first described 150 years ago. It seemed a simple condition, but resulted in unexpected healing problems and unexplained recurrences. Some indolent wounds defied all treatment, although wide excision seemed to offer a solution. The use of wide excision increased during World War II until nearly 80 000 men had been hospitalized by 1945 for an average of 55 days each, in a vain attempt to cure the disease. Immobilization of these needed troops led the

Surgeon General in the USA to issue an edict prohibiting wide *en bloc* excision and mandating simple linear incision.

In the past, the surgical approach has been to treat the secondary abscess rather than the two aetiologic issues: the nearly invisible midline cutaneous 'pits', and the potent but invisible forces across the natal cleft.

In pilonidal disease, less treatment is better than more. The condition is often self-limiting and nonoperative methods can cure[1]. Most pilonidal lesions create only a mild nuisance, and they are rare in patients older than 40 years. By contrast, most substantial problems associated with pilonidal disease are iatrogenic and therefore the surgeon must understand and confront the factors that create the disease to prevent these complications.

Principles and justification

Pilonidal cysts are not embryonic in origin and the disease is not congenital but acquired. Occasionally, congenital dimples will appear over the distal sacrum, but they do not give rise to pilonidal disease. Dimples are easily distinguished from pilonidal pores and are seldom a source of symptoms. Unusual midline epidermal cysts may develop over the lower spinal cord and communicate with the skin, but they are easily distinguished from pilonidal disease.

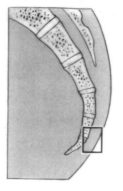
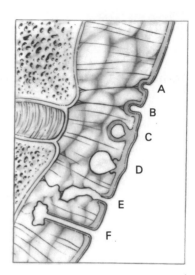

1

1 Pilonidal disease is a condition of the epidermis that begins with forces that stretch the normal hair follicle (A) in the natal cleft[2]. This results in a small hole in the skin called a 'pit' (B), which represents an enlarged hair follicle. Histological sections taken near a pilonidal pit show various sizes of enlarged hair follicles in otherwise normal skin. Each follicle holds a single hair surrounded by rings of keratin, and under these influences it becomes inflamed. When the mouth of the follicle becomes closed by inflammation (C), the combination of a 'vacuum' beneath the follicle and the pressure within the follicle drives keratin into the subcutaneous fat creating an acute abscess (D) with its associated pain caused by pus under pressure. A chronic abscess (E), the most common form of the disease, appears and persists after spontaneous or surgical drainage. Thus, by definition, this pilonidal lesion is an abscess and not a cyst because it has no epithelial lining.

In long-standing lesions, however, a tube of epithelium (F) may develop by slow growth down the wall of a chronic abscess. This lining develops no rete pegs and no skin structures or hair follicles. Tubes develop in approximately 10% of patients and are usually only 2–5 mm in length, but occasionally they may extend to 2 cm or more. Epithelial tubes must be removed or marsupialized to prevent the development of epithelial inclusion cysts.

The reduced subcutaneous pressure in the natal cleft, which is one of the factors that causes keratin to be drawn down through the thin base of the hair follicle, was identified and measured by Brearley[3]. The negative pressure develops because of the tension between the skin attachment to the midline skeleton and the weight of the hanging buttocks when a patient is in the erect position. Measurements show that most pilonidal pits develop precisely over the angle of the sacrum where the maximum negative pressure leads to follicle stretching and rupture.

Although hair shafts may play a role in the origin of the disease, hair appears in only half of these abscesses. Hair is often a secondary invader, however, gathered into the natal cleft and then sucked into the abscess cavity by the negative pressure already discussed and propelled by rubbing of tissue against the scales of shed hairs.

The natal cleft itself is of great aetiological importance. Pilonidal lesions occur only in skin clefts, most commonly the natal cleft, and never on convex surfaces. In severe disease, a surgeon's attempt to preserve the natal cleft may not only allow the condition to persist, but complex wounds sometimes develop because of the creation of a deep residual cleft, and the tension that pulls the skin away from the sacrum. Wounds under such tension do not heal, and the moist conditions in the cleft encourage the growth of anaerobic bacteria[4], which also interfere with healing. Thus, in severe disease, treatments to obliterate the cleft are always useful, while in primary disease, treatments to obliterate the cleft are only occasionally helpful.

Operations

ACUTE PILONIDAL ABSCESS

Indications and contraindications

All patients with acute pilonidal abscesses seek treatment for a hot, red, exquisitely tender bulge deep in the natal cleft; aspiration or open drainage provides relief of symptoms, with antibiotics being necessary after aspiration but not after open drainage.

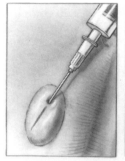
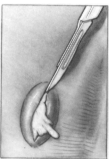

Anaesthesia

2 Patients appreciate the comfort of oral oxycodone before anaesthesia, but it is prompt drainage that relieves the pain. The effects of local anaesthesia are blunted in inflamed tissue, thus extensive infiltration is impractical and can be very painful. Slow superficial injection of the local anaesthetic mixture into the area of the incision is sufficient (bupivacaine hydrochloride, 0.5%, with adrenaline, 1:200 000, and buffered 1:10 with sodium bicarbonate solution, 50 mmol/l).

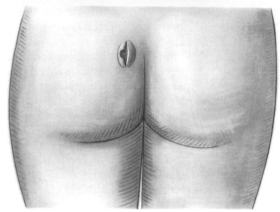

2

Incision

The abscess can be aspirated, but this author prefers to incise it laterally. If an incision is used, the surgery to be performed on the abscess in its chronic form 1 week later can be anticipated by incising 2.5 cm from the midline. The knife blade is advanced through the fat towards the midline. When pus appears, advancement of the knife is stopped. The pus does not need to be cultured and the abscess cavity should not be packed. A 1-cm button of skin is cut away from the lateral edge of the incision, which prevents premature resealing and is less painful than packing. Daily showers should be encouraged, and a mini-pad to protect clothing from drainage is useful.

Outcome

Patients with an acute pilonidal abscess treated in this fashion will obtain comfort within hours of aspiration or open drainage. Although this treatment is incomplete, the abscess seldom requires redrainage within 7 days, by which time the midline pits become visible and can be excised (see method for chronic pilonidal abscess described below).

CHRONIC PILONIDAL ABSCESS

Indications and contraindications

A chronic abscess is the most common form of pilonidal disease and is best treated by abscess drainage and pit excision, but other options are also discussed below. Patients with a midline pit who complain of a discharge or natal cleft pain and those with recent acute drainage (even if they are currently asymptomatic) should be treated surgically, because a pocket of granulations is usually present.

Midline wounds larger than 1 cm, congenital midline dimples, pilonidal pits without symptoms and the chronic abscess of many years' duration which has multiple deep tracts (such tracts may extend in several layers down toward the sacrum and are better laid open and allowed to heal by second intention) are not suitable for this treatment. Care must be taken to identify the patient who complains of pain on sitting and has no natal cleft pit, but has a sharp spur on the coccyx. Removal of the spur through a laterally placed incision gives relief.

Drainage and pit excision

This procedure attacks the source of the disease but does not create a large unhealing wound. It is simple enough for office or outpatient use and patients can return to work the following day.

Preoperative

Preoperative aspirin users are best deferred for 3 weeks without aspirin to allow for platelet recovery. One hour before surgery, oxycodone is given for comfort during injection of local anaesthetic agent. Oral cephalexin, 250 mg, and metronidazole, 400 mg, are given orally at the same time. Before taping the buttocks apart, the separated buttocks are pulled in all directions to help identify all the pits; magnification and good lighting are of value.

Anaesthesia
Bupivacaine hydrochloride, 0.5%, with adrenaline, 1:200 000 (for less bleeding), provides prolonged local anaesthesia. Patients appreciate warmed solutions being applied to the skin and slow infiltration through a fine (number 30) needle is advocated. The addition of 1 ml of sodium bicarbonate solution (50 mmol/l) to each 10 ml of anaesthetic solution neutralizes the irritating effect of the local anaesthetic. Except for exceedingly sensitive patients, general anaesthesia is unnecessary.

Incision

Incisions in the midline should be avoided whenever possible. The forces and conditions that created the pilonidal problem will tend to disrupt a suture line. Thus, when entering the abscess cavity, one or more incisions should be placed laterally away from the midline.

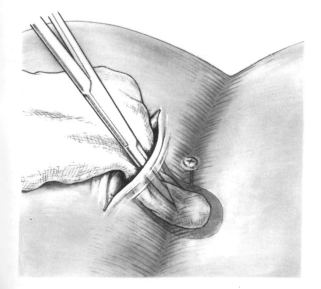

3 An incision is made 2.5 cm to one or both sides of the midline. The fat is left *in situ* on the overlying skin. The incision is made long enough to be able to see inside the entire cavity quite clearly. Incision length adds nothing to disability and does not delay healing. Scrubbing with gauze removes granulations, hair and debris. This scrubbing reveals a fibrous wall. Branch cavities must be carefully sought, and these need to be opened and scrubbed. In 10% of patients it is necessary to excise a small segment of fibrous abscess wall when infiltrated with hair.

3

4 The point of the haemostat is thrust into the cavity, directing it against the underside of the midline skin, and rubbed firmly. This identifies the follicle that started the trouble and other enlarged follicles that require removal.

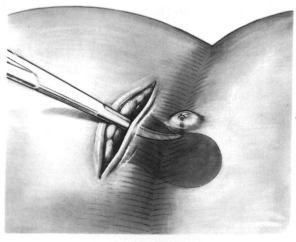

4

5 All enlarged pits are cut out, cleaned out and removed. The tip of a number 11 blade is used to excise the pit by taking a piece of tissue the size of a grain of rice. Multiple pits are excised individually as far as is feasible. The deep end of the removed specimen is inspected. A complete excision shows either soft, ill-defined, red-brown granulations or fibrous tissue. A tiny, clean, and 'macaroni-like' end, which is seen in about 5% of cases, indicates that a deeper part of an epithelial tube remains. This must be excised or inclusion cyst formation is likely.

Skin punches or curettes used vigorously is an alternative method of pit excision. The resulting small defects may be sutured with a subcuticular removable monofilament or allowed to heal secondarily.

The large lateral wound is left open to allow drainage. The lateral wound should not be packed because packing causes pain and serves no purpose.

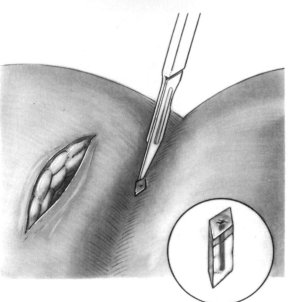

5

Postoperative care

Antibiotic coverage is continued for three doses. The patient should be encouraged to wash the wound with soap and water during a twice-daily shower. An immediate return to normal sitting and other activity should also be suggested. A dressing to protect clothing is useful. After 2 days a mini-pad inside the underwear suffices.

Sutures are removed on the seventh day. The patient is examined each week until certain of solid midline healing. Most patients need only one or two postoperative visits.

Complications
The most common complication is a slowly healing midline wound, which occurs in about 10% of patients. Most respond to careful local hygiene and shaving, but occasionally a wound will require a small pack, silver nitrate, or minimal marsupialization. The rare non-

healing wound will yield to a smaller repeat of pit excision or to a Karydakis procedure. On rare occasions, patients have increasing pain and watery drainage in the postoperative period and this indicates superficial cellulitis which should be vigorously treated with appropriate antibiotics.

Outcome

The technique described above for lateral drainage of the abscess and excision of pits has been used in over 430 patients. Follow-up of 92% of 200 patients showed no large unhealed wounds. Treatment approached the ideal of no disability because half the patients returned to school or work the day following treatment. Mean healing time was 3 weeks and recurrent abscess or epithelial inclusion cysts appeared in only 5% of patients, with all recurrences being smaller than the original presenting problem.

Other treatment options

Non-operative management

6 The picking out of invading hairs, a few weekly local hair shavings, and emphatic instruction on cleanliness have healed many lesions, but the approach requires diligence. Results are not as prompt as those associated with pit excision, but the freedom from complications is unequalled.

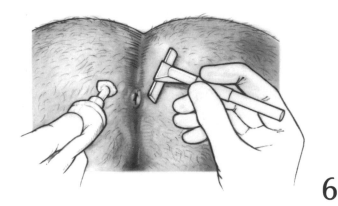

6

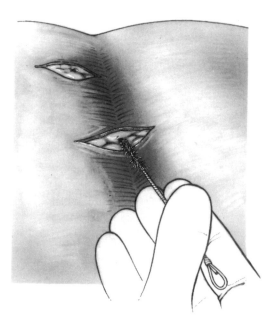

7

Pit excision and cavity brushing

7 This limited surgery is worth considering[5]. A transverse excision of the pit gives access to the cavity which can then be thoroughly cleaned. Unlike a vertical incision, the tissue tension associated with transverse incisions will tend to pull the wound closed rather than open.

Midline incision

8 A midline incision is acceptable if it lays open the cavity through all openings, but it is not recommended as initial treatment. Trimming back the skin edges prevents early closure. Deep tissues should not be removed. Marsupialization (suturing down the edges of the wound) may speed healing but may increase wound tension. The two disadvantages of midline vertical incision are the need for packing and the occasional resistant wound which does not heal. Such wounds, formerly disastrous, now fortunately respond to secondary repair described below. Primary closure should never be used after a midline incision because it is very often followed by recurrent sepsis and local skin breakdown.

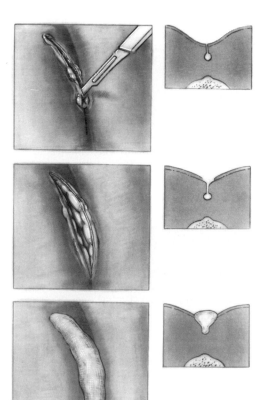

8

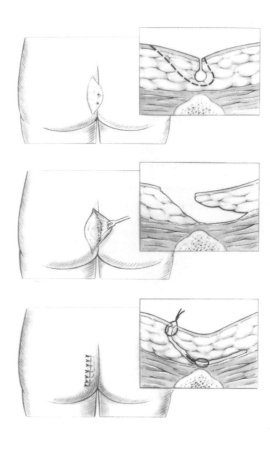

Karydakis operation[6]

9   An eccentrically placed skin excision is used followed by a limited excision of subcutaneous tissue. This method offers the advantages of incision closure, fresh skin is brought into the midline, and the natal cleft is flattened. The main disadvantages of the operation are the removal of substantial amounts of tissue and the mobilization of fat, which may risk postoperative abscess formation under the skin flap.

Procedures not recommended

There is no place in the treatment of chronic pilonidal abscess or any other pilonidal problem for wide midline excisional surgery. *En bloc* excisions down to the sacrum should never be used. This procedure attacks the wrong target. Such wounds suffer from slow healing or non-healing. Thus, the use of retention sutures or pressure packs have no place in current treatment of pilonidal disease.

9

COMPLEX PILONIDAL WOUNDS

Cleft closure

Indications and contraindications

Excessive and inappropriate pilonidal surgery may give rise to considerable patient morbidity with weeks in hospital, wounds packed open for years, or a succession of failed operative procedures. The cleft closure operation can resolve these problems and is indicated for any wound that remains unhealed at 3 months, for primary treatment of large or complex defects, and for any major secondary surgery. This operation should not be used, however, for most primary treatments nor for a small recurrent abscess with only a pinhole midline opening, which should be treated as a primary chronic abscess.

The four advantages of the operation are prompt and secure healing in even the largest wounds, stability in the presence of complications, suitability for outpatient surgery, and a low rate of recurrence. Furthermore, the operation moves the suture line away from the midline natal cleft. It heals without functional defect or significant cosmetic changes.

Preoperative

The patient should be assessed while he is standing, by marking the outer line of contact of the buttocks with a felt pen. A tentative repair is sketched on the patient's skin and then a gloved finger is used to explore the natal cleft with the patient sitting, bending and standing until the geometry of the closure is familiar.

Anaesthesia

General anaesthesia is required. Local anaesthetic suffices for smaller versions of this procedure. At the start of the operation, intravenous cefapirin sodium, 1 g, and metronidazole, 1 g, are given to protect against common pathogens including anaerobes.

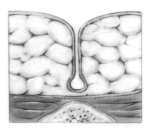

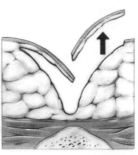

General principle

10 The general principle of the procedure is shown in the illustration. It accomplishes a skin transfer by lifting a flap of extra skin from the donor buttock and drawing it across the midline onto the recipient buttock.

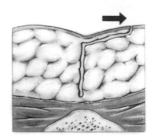

10

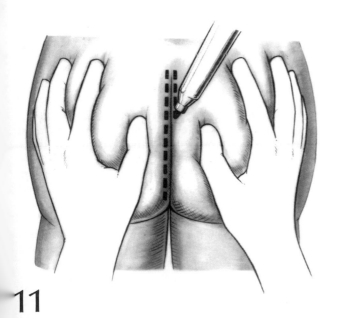

11

Incision

11 The patient is re-examined in the jack-knife position for rectal fistulae, a potent source of failure. The buttocks are pushed together and the outer line of their contact is marked with a felt pen.

12 The buttocks are taped apart and before skin preparation, bupivacaine hydrochloride and adrenaline are infiltrated to limit blood loss and give prolonged postoperative comfort. The incision for the donor flap should be sketched, with a view to raising the flap from the least damaged side of the natal cleft, full thickness and fat free.

The incision is commenced on the recipient side, off the midline and above the top of the natal cleft. The knife should slant down and across the midline at an acute angle just above the unhealed wound. Inferiorly, the incision turns sharply to cross the midline at right angles cephalad of the anus, and then it should turn again so that the lower end of the incision points towards the anus.

The skin from the midline incision is elevated to the surface of the donor buttock at the line of natural contact. Cephalad to the anus the perianal skin is weak. Therefore, the surgeon should leave some extra subcutaneous tissue attached. It may be necessary with low-lying wounds to extend undermining of the anal

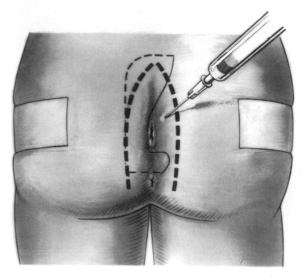

12

flap into the subcutaneous sphincter fibres. Rotation of this anal flap will relieve tension at the anal end of the closure and prevent skin necrosis. At the upper end of the incision, undermining continues above the top of the natal cleft, because leaving the upper cleft attached to the sacrum invites recurrence.

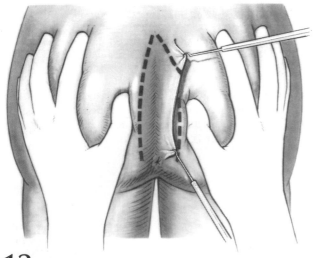

13 The recipient side is measured. The donor flap itself is used as a template. The tapes are released and the buttocks are pushed together. The donor flap is gently pulled across the midline. Any skin overlapped by the donor flap is marked for removal. A loose donor flap, which would fold down between the fat layers, should be avoided. Below the level of the end of the sacrum, the skin is marked for removal to the natural line of contact, but not beyond. The removal of more skin risks postoperative discomfort from skin tension while the patient is in the sitting position.

13

14 Skin to be discarded is elevated out to the marked limit of removal. This prepares a bed to receive the donor flap. It also unroofs the unhealed wound.

From the bed of the unhealed wound, granulations and debris are scrubbed away with gauze. The 2–3-mm sheet of scar that forms the base of the wound is excised. The scar will heal if left in place, but removal often relieves tissue tension to a surprising extent. To further free tissues, a knife is pulled across strands of scar in the fat between sacrum and buttock skin on each side. Fat or muscle should not be mobilized. As much fat as possible is saved to provide padding. Bleeders should be carefully cauterized.

Exposed fat over so vast an area gives alarm, but with release of the retracting tapes, the fat falls to the sacrum. Most of the raw surface disappears as fat from right meets fat from left. The donor flap covers the remainder. After a final check 'fit', skin from the recipient side is excised.

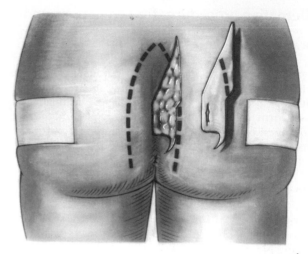

14

Wound closure

15 To finish cleft closure, a suction drain is pulled through a stab wound. The Blake drain gives the least pain on removal. The drain is sewn and taped securely because accidental removal delays healing. Fat is approximated with small bites of 4/0 polydioxanone suture to position the skin for closure. Closure is started by tacking the rotated anal flap roughly into position. The skin edges should now lie together without tension. Deep bites in fat for wound strength are unnecessary. The skin incision is closed with a subcuticular pull-out using 3/0 polypropylene and bringing a cross-stitch to the surface at intervals to simplify later removal. Sutures are reinforced with skin tapes. The wound is covered with a light dressing.

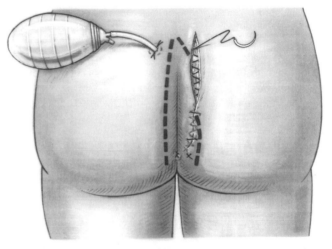

15

Postoperative care

The patient may be discharged after recovery from anaesthesia and may sit in the car on the way home. Written instructions should be given for daily showers, twice daily iodophore swabbing, changes of absorbent cotton near the anus four times daily, and 4 days of oral cephalexin and metronidazole at 250 mg each four times daily. The drain is removed at 4 days and the pull-out suture at 1 week. Examination should be performed weekly until healing is complete. Most patients resume activities on the fourth postoperative day.

Complications
Complications of cleft closure are uncommon. Infection responds quickly to opening the inferior 2 cm of the wound and administering antibiotics. Small patches of skin necrosis heal and do not affect the result.

Haematomas respond best to evacuation under anaesthesia and reclosure over a drain. Postoperative discomfort on sitting is rare and largely avoidable. Irritated areas quickly respond to careful cleansing. Small recurrences respond to local revision and flattening.

Outcome

Thirty-five referred patients underwent cleft closure. They had sought help for recurrent disease after one to five operations, or for surgical incisions unhealed after periods of 6 months to 20 years. Most patients left the outpatient facility the day of cleft closure. Most wounds healed primarily, a few with minor intermittent discomfort. All wounds were healed within 3 months, and at 6 months to 7 years all wounds remain healed. Three chronic unhealed perineal wounds after total colectomy for Crohn's disease responded similarly.

Alternative procedures for complex wounds

Local care

Repeated local shaving and meticulous hygiene may help some complex wounds. Holding the buttocks apart with tape to allow the cleft to dry may occasionally help. This form of treatment, however, should not be prolonged because the likelihood of a good outcome is small.

Skin grafts

Split-thickness skin grafts to a granulating surface are seldom successful, and if on occasion a preliminary healing is achieved, the skin surface remains vulnerable. Therefore, split-thickness skin grafts are not recommended.

Z-plasty

16 Full thickness Z-plasty requires mobilization of fat and carries a suture line across the risk-prone midline natal cleft. The distal end of the Z is placed beside the cleft and not within it. In the author's experience, the cleft closure procedure is to be preferred.

References

1. Allen-Mersh TG. Pilonidal sinus: finding the right track for treatment. *Br J Surg* 1990; 77: 123–32.

2. Bascom JU. Pilonidal disease: long-term results of follicle removal. *Dis Colon Rectum* 1983; 26: 800–7.

3. Brearley R. Pilonidal sinus: a new theory of origin. *Br J Surg* 1955; 43: 62–8.

4. Marks J, Harding KG, Hughes LE. Staphylococcal infection of open granulating wounds. *Br J Surg* 1987; 74: 95–7.

5. Lord PH, Millar DM. Pilonidal sinus: a simple treatment. *Br J Surg* 1965; 52: 298–300.

6. Karydakis GE. Easy and successful treatment of pilonidal sinus after explanation of its causative process. *Aust NZ J Surg* 1992; 62: 385–9.

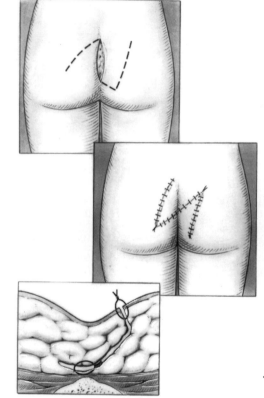

16

Surgical approaches to the kidney, upper third of the ureter and inferior vena cava

H. N. Whitfield MA, MChir, FRCS
Consultant Urologist, St Bartholomew's Hospital and St Mark's Hospital for Diseases of the Colon and Rectum, London, UK

Principles and justification

The correct choice of an incision is fundamental for successful surgery. A knowledge of the surface anatomy of organs will ensure that an incision is placed accurately. Where there is a choice of incision the pros and cons of each must be understood and the decision made in the light of the pathology to be dealt with and the patient's habitus and general health. Sometimes the decision will be a compromise between what is easiest for the surgeon and what will provide the most effective recovery for the patient: the smaller the incision, the less the morbidity for the patient. With increasing surgical experience it becomes possible to reduce the length of an incision and yet still provide adequate exposure. There should be no shame in enlarging an incision, however, if during the operation exposure is found to be inadequate. Correct positioning of the patient on the operating table, the use of sandbags and table tilt and the availability of a range of retractors are all vital adjuncts to ensuring that any incision affords adequate exposure. Inevitably, the choice of incision will sometimes be influenced by the surgeon's experience with one particular approach, which becomes the preferred option. Where there is a choice it is advantageous, after the learning phase, to take a view on the merits of different incisions and to become practised at one or two in any situation.

In this and the following two chapters, the details of the surgical approaches to the urinary tract will be accompanied by a critical appraisal of each. As postoperative recovery will be influenced by the incision made and by the pain produced, it is important to discuss with the anaesthetist the need for postoperative analgesia, so that pain relief can be planned carefully in advance.

Incisions

TRANSCOSTAL 12TH RIB INCISION

This incision provides good exposure, but a considerable bulk of muscle is cut, and there may be some weakness of the anterior abdominal wall as a result. The pleura is at risk and must be identified.

Position of patient

1 The patient should be positioned so that the gap between the 12th rib and the iliac crest occurs over the 'break' of the operating table. The patient's back should be at the edge of the table and vertical. The patient can be secured by strapping or table supports or a combination of both. In an elderly patient when the spine is osteoarthritic, the extent to which the table is broken must be reduced. In other cases the maximum amount of break possible (30–40° from the horizontal) should be used. A pillow is placed between the legs and the lower knee bent to 90°. The upper arm is supported in a cradle.

During the breaking of the operating table, major cardiovascular changes can occur, with diminished venous return because of partial occlusion of the inferior vena cava. It is essential that before this manoeuvre is undertaken, the patient must be being ventilated and cardiovascular monitoring instituted. The permission of the anaesthetist must be obtained before the position of the patient is altered.

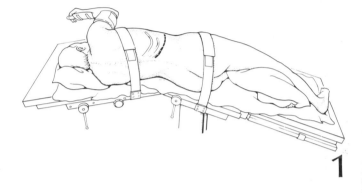

Incision

The incision extends from the angle of the 12th rib posteriorly to 8–15 cm beyond the tip of the 12th rib anteriorly. The length of the incision needs to be increased in obese patients. Exposure is not increased significantly by further anterior extension.

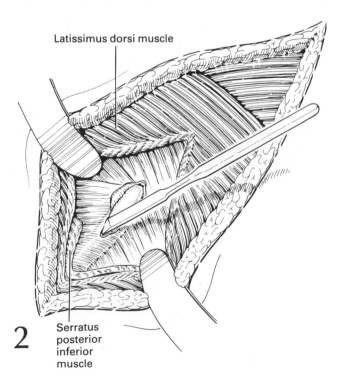

Latissimus dorsi muscle

Serratus posterior inferior muscle

2

2 The subcutaneous tissue and the external oblique and latissimus dorsi muscles are incised directly where they overlie the 12th rib, which is exposed.

3 The periosteum is elevated from the rib using a periosteal elevator and a raspatory. The mobilized rib is removed by cutting it across at its angle with rib shears, and then removing the fibrous attachments of the anterior cartilaginous end with a knife or scissors.

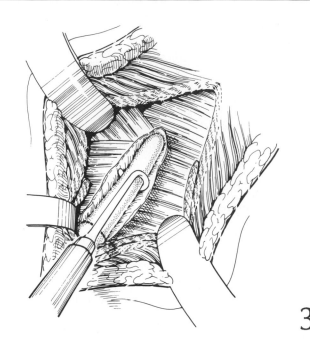

3

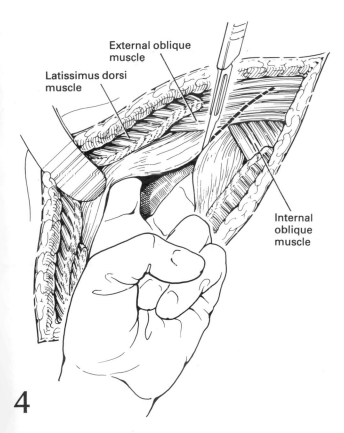

External oblique muscle

Latissimus dorsi muscle

Internal oblique muscle

4

4 The first and second fingers are inserted into the defect created by incising the lumbar fascia immediately anterior to the tip of the 12th rib. The peritoneum is stripped off from the undersurface of the abdominal wall musculature and pushed medially. The muscles of the anterolateral abdominal wall are then incised using a knife. Care should be taken to identifiy and avoid the subcostal vessels and nerve. Haemostasis of the cut muscles is secured by electrocoagulation.

5 The incision may be extended as far anteriorly as the lateral border of the rectus sheath. Posteriorly, access is improved by carefully incising the lowest diaphragmatic fibres as far posterolaterally as possible, and then gently pushing the pleura superiorly.

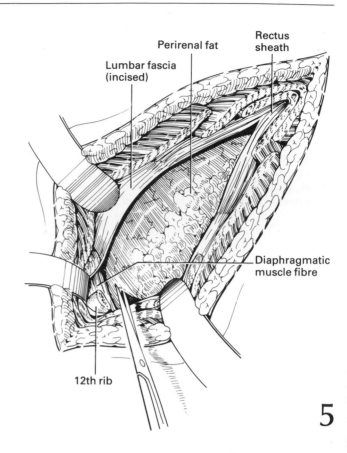

6 The muscles are closed in two layers, using interrupted 1 chromic catgut sutures for the first layer, and a continuous 1 chromic catgut suture to the perimysium of the latissimus dorsi muscle. All the sutures of the first layer are placed before tying. The operating table is then unbroken and the closure can be performed without tension. Care should be taken to avoid transfixing the pleura in the posterior angle of the wound. The subcostal nerve and vessels should also be preserved.

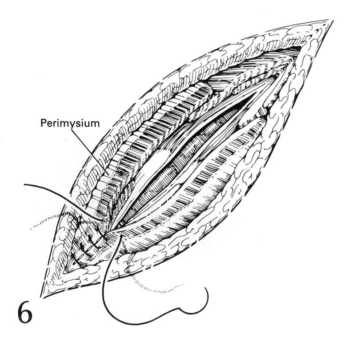

Wound closure

SUBCOSTAL INCISION

This incision provides good exposure to the upper ureter and pelviureteric junction, but restricted access to the renal pedicle and upper pole. Postoperative pain is less than in those incisions in which a rib is excised.

Position of patient and incision

7 The patient is positioned as for the 12th rib incision. The incision extends from the lateral border of the erector spinae 1 cm below the 12th rib, anteriorly as far as necessary, but not beyond the lateral border of the rectus sheath.

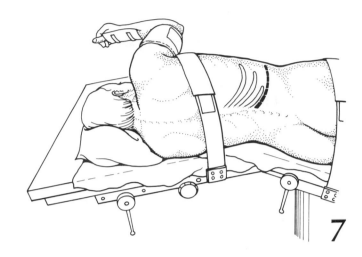

8 The latissimus dorsi and the serratus posterior inferior muscles are incised in the posterior half of the wound to expose the lumbar fascia. The lumbar fascia in turn is incised and two fingers are inserted to sweep the peritoneum medially.

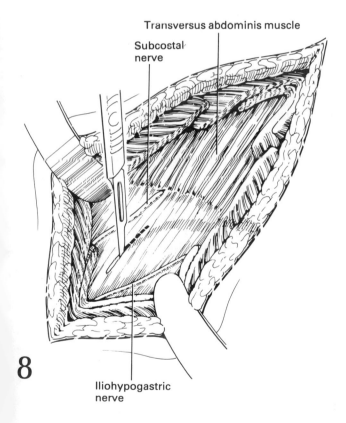

Transversus abdominis muscle

Subcostal nerve

Iliohypogastric nerve

9 The incision in the lumbar fascia is extended anteriorly through the transversus abdominis muscle. At the posterior end of the wound, the costovertebral ligament should be cut as far laterally as possible to allow the 12th rib to be retracted superiorly. The subcostal nerve should be mobilized superiorly and the iliohypogastric nerve inferiorly.

Wound closure

The deep layer of interrupted 1 chromic catgut sutures and the continuous 1 chromic catgut layer to the perimysium are inserted as for a 12th rib incision.

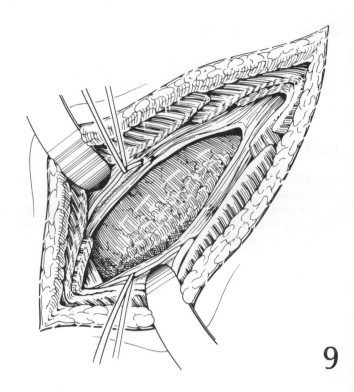

9

SUPRACOSTAL INCISION

This incision provides good exposure, but is technically more difficult than the transcostal incision. It is difficult to see the costovertebral ligament, which may have to be incised blind. The source of any bleeding from diaphragmatic vessels behind the 12th rib may be difficult to identify and control. The pleura is at risk. Closure is quick and easy.

Position of patient and incision

10 The patient is placed as for the 12th rib exposure, but the incision is usually placed between the 11th and 12th ribs. If the 12th rib is short, however, better exposure may be gained by making a supra-11 incision.

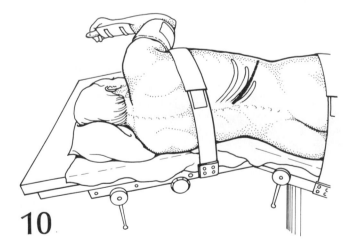

10

11 The latissimus dorsi, serratus posterior inferior and the internal and external oblique muscles are divided to expose the 12th rib and the intercostal muscle.

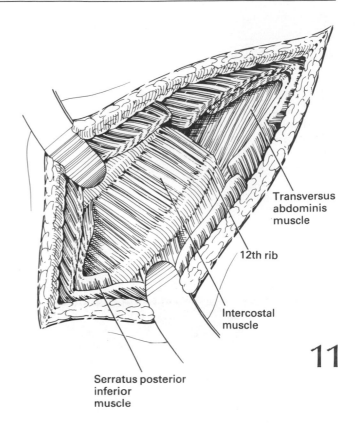

Transversus abdominis muscle

12th rib

Intercostal muscle

11

Serratus posterior inferior muscle

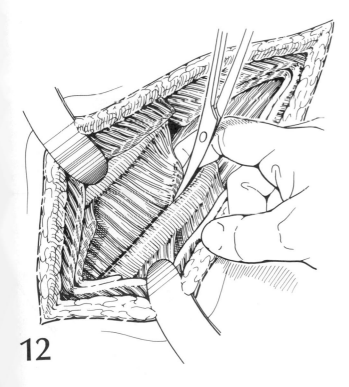

12

12 The intercostal muscle is incised at its insertion into the superior aspect of the 12th rib, starting at the tip of the 12th rib. A finger is inserted between the intercostal muscle and the pleura and the incision continued posteriorly.

Using the same finger, the costovertebral ligament is identified in the posterior angle of the incision. The ligament is divided at the upper border of the rib using scissors.

13 The pleural attachments to the undersurface of the rib can be palpated and divided to expose the diaphragm.

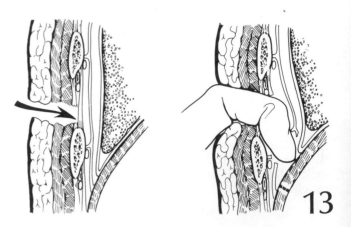

13

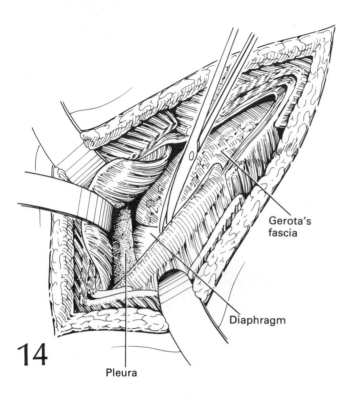

Gerota's fascia

Diaphragm

14

Pleura

14 The diaphragm should be incised as posteriorly as possible, and the pleura and diaphragm are swept superiorly with a finger. Gerota's fascia then lies in the floor of the incision and can be further exposed by mobilizing the peritoneum medially.

Wound closure

15 The amount of break on the operating table is reduced, and the tips of the 11th and 12th ribs approximated with 1 chromic catgut. Using interrupted 1 chromic catgut the diaphragm and the superior margin of the intercostal muscle are approximated to the upper cut border of the latissimus dorsi muscle anteriorly and the upper border of the serratus posterior inferior muscle posteriorly.

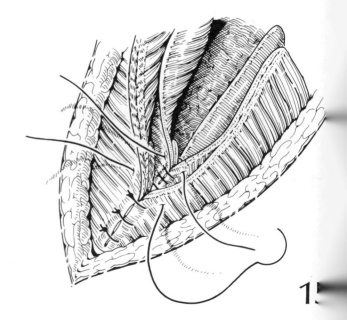

15

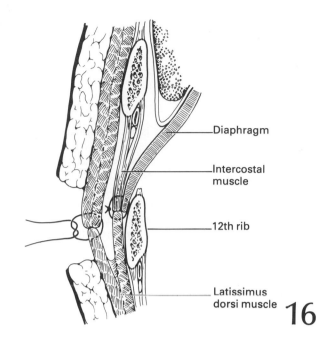

16 This is not a precise anatomical closure, but will have the advantage that the pleura will be closed if it has been accidentally opened. A small wound drain would then be needed to prevent surgical emphysema.

Diaphragm

Intercostal muscle

12th rib

Latissimus dorsi muscle

16

LUMBOTOMY INCISION

This incision produces significantly less postoperative pain than any other surgical approaches to the kidney, the pelviureteric junction and the upper ureter. Access is not easy, however, and the incision should not be used by inexperienced surgeons nor in overweight patients.

Position of patient and incision

17 The position is as for all other lateral approaches to the kidney, except that the patient should be tilted prone 20° from the vertical. The incision extends from the upper border of the 12th rib at the lateral side of the erector spinae downwards and forwards to the iliac crest for a distance of approximately 10 cm.

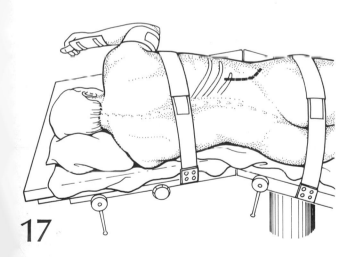

17

18 The latissimus dorsi is incised in the line of its fibres. An assistant holds the muscle bundles apart by repositioning Langenbeck retractors while the incision is progressively deepened. In the inferior aspect of the incision, the serratus posterior inferior muscle is incised across its fibres. The lumbar fascia is opened midway between the subcostal neurovascular bundle, which is mobilized inferiorly, and the 11th intercostal nerve.

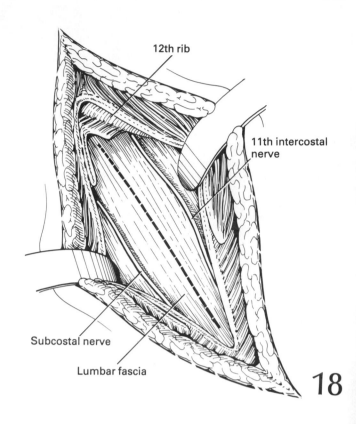

19 Gerota's fascia is then exposed. A ring retractor provides the most effective exposure. Additional exposure is gained by removing 1 cm of the 12th rib and, if necessary, dividing the 11th rib. Care must be taken to avoid damaging the pleura at the superior aspect of the incision.

Wound closure

Closure is quick, by approximating the edges of the lumbar fascia, using interrupted 1 chromic catgut. The subcostal and 11th intercostal neurovascular bundles are identified and preserved. The perimysium of the latissimus dorsi is sutured with a continuous 1 chromic catgut suture.

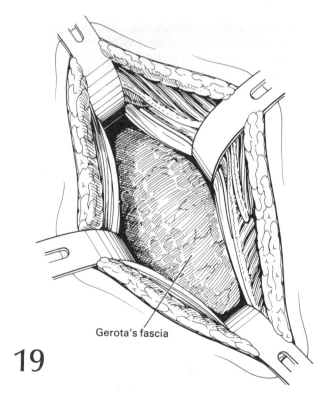

NAGAMATSU INCISION

This incision provides excellent exposure of the renal artery, and during tumour nephrectomy early arterial control can be established with minimum mobilization of the kidney or Gerota's fascia.

Position of patient and incision

20 The patient is placed in the lateral position. The incision extends from above the 11th rib at its angle inferiorly to the angle of the 12th rib and thence along the line of the 12th rib towards the umbilicus, as far as the lateral border of the recti.

The latissimus dorsi and serratus posterior inferior muscles are incised in the line of the incision. The periosteum is removed over a 2-cm length of the 11th and 12th ribs as described above, and these segments are removed. The anterior end of the incision is opened by incising the external and internal oblique muscles, as described for a transcostal incision.

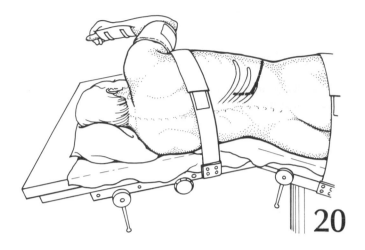

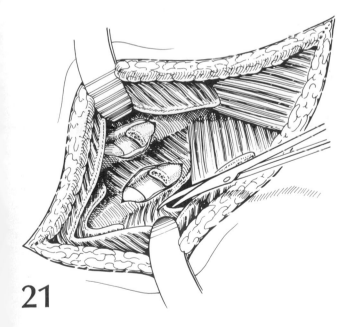

21 The lumbocostal ligaments, extending between the lowest two ribs and the transverse processes of L1 and L2 are identified and divided between marker sutures, enabling the myocostal flap of costal margin to be mobilized upwards with the diaphragm and pleura.

The kidney is retracted medially, and gentle dissection (to avoid any large perinephric veins) will allow the plane between Gerota's fascia and the quadratus lumborum and psoas major to be opened up to reveal the renal artery or arteries, which are controlled.

Wound closure

22 The lumbocostal ligament is approximated, and closure thereafter is the same as for a transcostal approach.

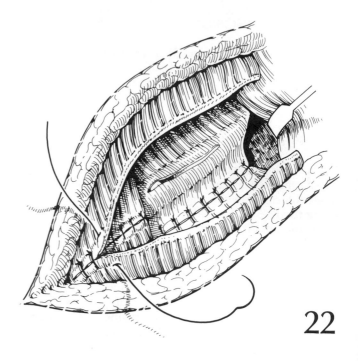

22

THORACOABDOMINAL INCISION

This incision provides good access for large renal tumours, particularly those arising from the upper pole and/or invading the inferior vena cava. Retroperitoneal lymphadenectomy may also be performed through this incision.

Position of patient and incision

23 The patient is positioned supine with a sandbag under the ipsilateral shoulder and buttock. The incision may be made over the eighth, ninth or tenth rib, extending from the posterior axillary line to the midline and continuing as a midline incision as far inferiorly as required. By breaking the table, hyperextension of the spine can provide further exposure.

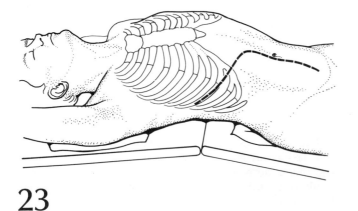

23

24 The latissimus dorsi, serratus posterior inferior and external oblique muscles are incised either with cutting diathermy, scissors, or a knife, and the chosen rib is exposed. The intercostal muscle above the rib is divided or the rib is resected. The incision is extended anteriorly and the internal oblique and rectus muscles are incised.

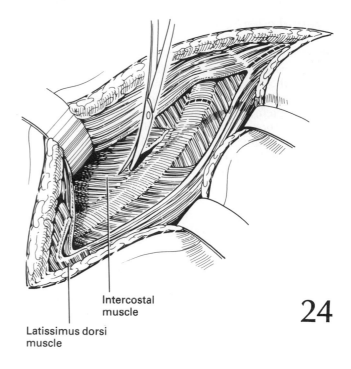

Intercostal muscle

Latissimus dorsi muscle

24

Transversalis muscle

Costal cartilage

Internal oblique muscle

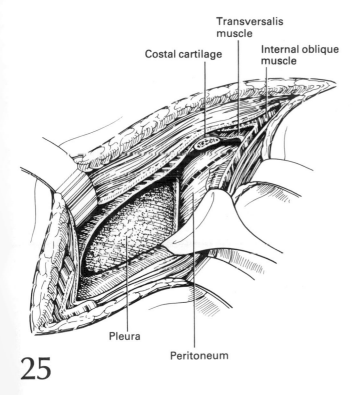

Pleura

Peritoneum

25

25 The costovertebral ligament is divided posteriorly and the costal cartilage anteriorly. The pleural cavity is opened where it comes into view on deep inspiration. The lung is retracted and the diaphragm and its attached pleura are incised. The peritoneum is opened and two large self-retaining retractors are inserted to reveal the liver, gallbladder, duodenum, colon and Gerota's fascia.

Wound closure

26 The peritoneum is closed first, using a chromic catgut suture. The diaphragm is approximated with 2/0 silk sutures. The costal cartilage is approximated with a 1 nylon suture, and the intercostal muscle and the pleura are brought together with an absorbable polydioxanone suture (PDS; Ethicon, Edinburgh, UK) or chromic catgut. The latissimus dorsi, serratus posterior inferior and the external oblique muscles are closed with an interrupted absorbable suture which may include the intercostal muscle.

An underwater drain is inserted separately, and the peritoneal cavity should also be drained.

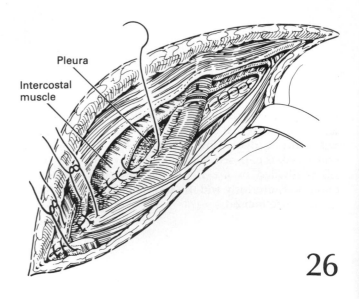

Pleura

Intercostal muscle

26

TRANSVERSE INCISION

This incision provides wide exposure of both sides of the retroperitoneum, which is particularly useful for left-sided renal tumours extending along the renal vein and into the inferior vena cava. Bilateral renal tumours and para-aortic lymphadenectomy may also be performed through this incision.

Position of patient and incision

27 The patient is positioned supine with the spine hyperextended. The incision extends from the tips of the 11th rib 3–4 cm below the costal margin.

27

28 The incision is deepened through the sub-cutaneous fat as far as the anterior rectus sheath, which is then incised. The recti are divided with cutting diathermy, and the superior epigastric arteries are identified and ligated. The posterior rectus sheath, the external and internal oblique muscles and the transversus abdominis muscle are divided. The peritoneum is then exposed and is opened to reveal the falciform ligament, which is ligated and divided.

Wound closure

The peritoneum, posterior rectus sheath and transversalis aponeurosis are closed as the posterior layer with interrupted absorbable sutures. The anterior rectus sheath and internal and external oblique muscles are closed with interrupted sutures as the anterior layer.

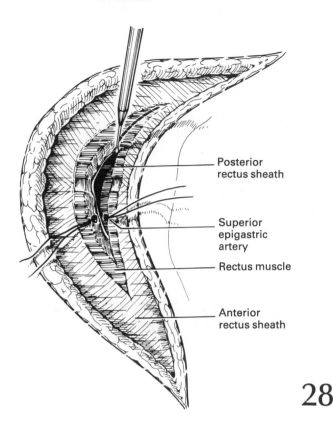

Posterior rectus sheath

Superior epigastric artery

Rectus muscle

Anterior rectus sheath

28

MIDLINE INCISION

This is a very useful incision for many urological procedures, including nephrectomy, nephroureterectomy, urinary diversion, bladder augmentation and replacement, and ureterolysis. Great care must be taken in closing to ensure that no hernia can occur.

Position of patient and incision

29 The patient is placed supine. Depending on the procedure to be performed, some Trendelenburg, anti-Trendelenburg, or lateral tilt may be advantageous. The incision extends from the xiphoid process inferiorly, skirting the umbilicus, and continuing inferiorly as far as is necessary.

29

30 The subcutaneous tissues are divided in the midline to expose the linea alba, which is incised to expose the peritoneum. Using two pairs of forceps the peritoneum is tented upwards, and after palpating the peritoneal fold to ensure that no intestine has been picked up, the peritoneum is incised. The incision in the peritoneum and the linea alba is then continued to the extent of the skin incision. A ring retractor allows good exposure.

Wound closure

Using a non-absorbable continuous monofilament nylon suture, the linea alba and peritoneum are closed together. The knot should be buried. An absorbable subcutaneous suture is needed in all but the thinnest patient.

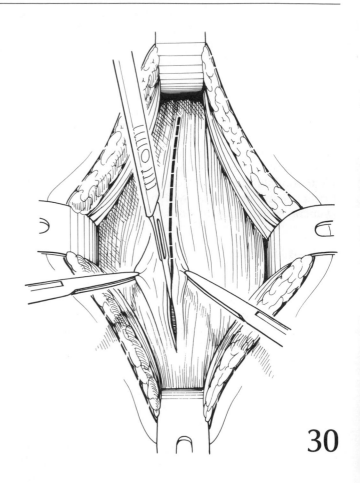

30

PARAMEDIAN INCISION

This incision has lost popularity. The wound, though closed in two layers, is no stronger than a midline incision. There is a risk of the rectus becoming devascularized. Tissue planes are opened up, which creates the potential for infection. The rectus muscle may be split instead of mobilized to try to avoid these problems.

Position of patient and incision

31 The patient is positioned supine. The length and position of the incision caudally and in a cephalad direction may be varied to suit the operation. The incision is made through subcutaneous tissues 3 cm lateral to the midline.

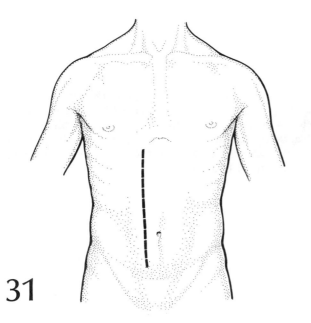

31

32 The anterior rectus sheath is incised and the more medial border grasped with holding forceps. The rectus muscle is freed medially and posteriorly and haemostasis secured, particularly at the tendinous intersections. The rectus muscle is then retracted laterally and the peritoneum is exposed and incised.

Wound closure

The incision is closed in two layers: the peritoneum and posterior rectus sheath together with an absorbable suture, and the anterior rectus sheath with a non-absorbable suture.

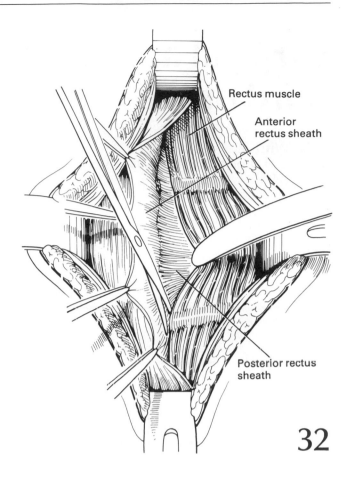

Rectus muscle

Anterior rectus sheath

Posterior rectus sheath

32

Illustrations by Gillian Oliver

Surgical approaches to the middle third of the ureter

H. N. Whitfield MA, MChir, FRCS
Consultant Urologist, St Bartholomew's Hospital and St Mark's Hospital for Diseases of the Colon and Rectum, London, UK

Incisions

EXTRAPERITONEAL MUSCLE SPLITTING

Exposure of the ureter as it crosses the bifurcation of the common iliac artery is very good. By extending the incision inferiorly the lowest end of the ureter may be exposed. The middle third of the ureter can be exposed by extending the incision superiorly. Extending the incision may necessitate some cutting of the internal oblique muscle.

1 The incision is made on the lateral side of the anterior abdominal wall at a site and for a length that will vary depending on the operation to be performed.

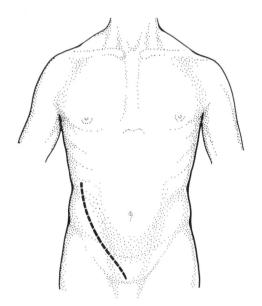

1

2 The external oblique muscle is exposed and the muscle bundles and the aponeurosis are split in the line of their fibres and retracted medially and laterally to expose the internal oblique muscle.

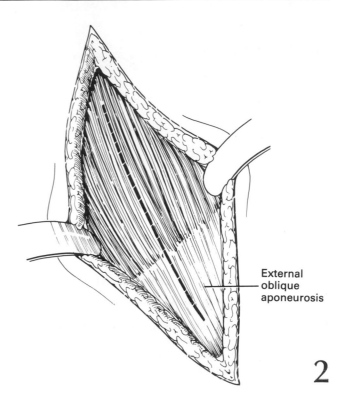

External oblique aponeurosis

2

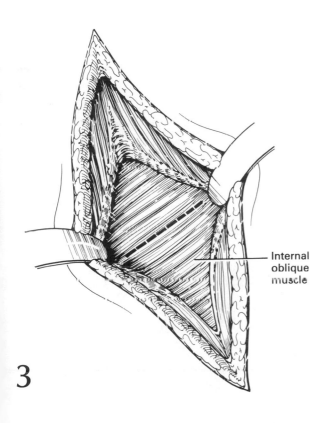

Internal oblique muscle

3

3 The internal oblique muscle is also split in the line of its fibres in the middle of the wound and retracted superiorly and inferiorly. The lateral edge of the transverse fascia to which the peritoneum is attached comes into view and is swept medially.

4 Mobilization of the peritoneum is aided by dividing the inferior epigastric artery and the round ligament of the uterus as it emerges from the internal inguinal ring. In the male, the vas deferens may be divided (with the patient's consent) or mobilized inferiorly.

Wound closure

The incision is closed using a layer of absorbable interrupted sutures to the internal oblique perimysium and a continuous layer of absorbable sutures to the external oblique muscle.

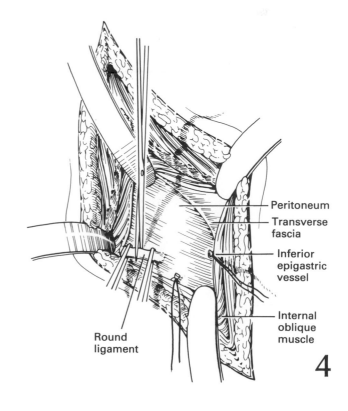

Peritoneum

Transverse fascia

Inferior epigastric vessel

Internal oblique muscle

Round ligament

4

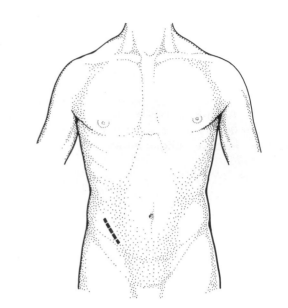

5

EXTRAPERITONEAL MUSCLE CUTTING

$5, 6$ Where greater exposure is needed than is easily provided by a muscle-splitting incision, the internal oblique muscle may be incised. This may be necessary in obese patients.

Wound closure

Closure is performed as for a muscle-splitting incision, taking particular care to close the internal oblique muscle to avoid hernia formation.

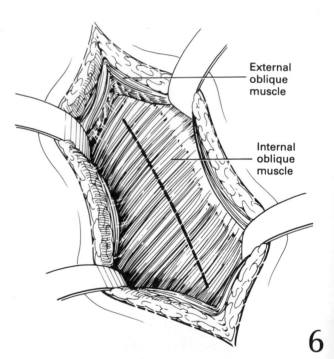

External oblique muscle

Internal oblique muscle

6

Surgical approaches to the lower third of the ureter, bladder and prostate

H. N. Whitfield MA, MChir, FRCS
Consultant Urologist, St Bartholomew's Hospital and St Mark's Hospital for Diseases of the Colon and Rectum, London, UK

Incisions

PFANNENSTIEL INCISION

This incision gives good extraperitoneal exposure to the bladder and to the prostate. The ureter may also be exposed transperitoneally by opening the peritoneal cavity at the level of its reflection from the bladder.

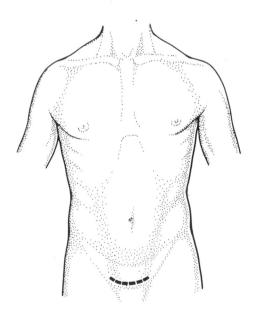

1 The length of the incision and its distance above the pubic symphysis may be varied by several centimetres.

1

2   On incising the subcutaneous tissues, the recti come into view and the pyramidalis muscles inferiorly.

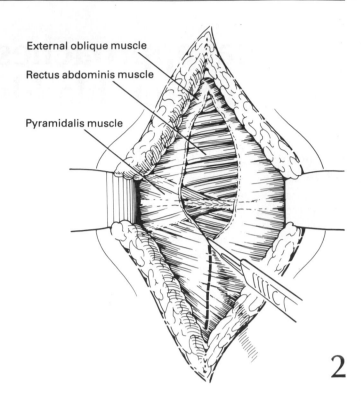

External oblique muscle

Rectus abdominis muscle

Pyramidalis muscle

2

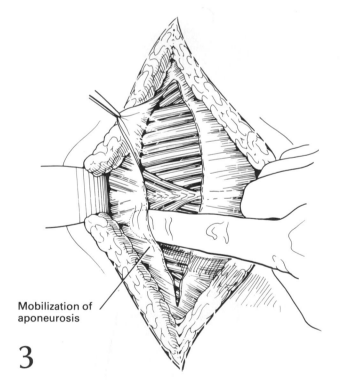

Mobilization of aponeurosis

3

3   The incised aponeurosis of the external oblique is grasped with holding forceps and inferiorly the plane between its undersurface and the underlying muscles is developed by sweeping the finger across. Superiorly the same mobilization is performed, coagulating a constant vessel on each side which runs between the rectus muscle and the anterior rectus sheath.

4 The midline raphe between the recti is divided to the level of the mobilized aponeurosis of the external oblique muscle. The peritoneum is swept superiorly and the bladder is exposed.

Additional exposure can be obtained by dividing the tendinous insertions of the recti muscles.

Wound closure

Closure is performed by approximating the medial borders of the recti with interrupted absorbable sutures, and closing the external oblique aponeurosis transversely with a continuous absorbable suture. The tendinous insertions of the recti should be sutured if they were divided.

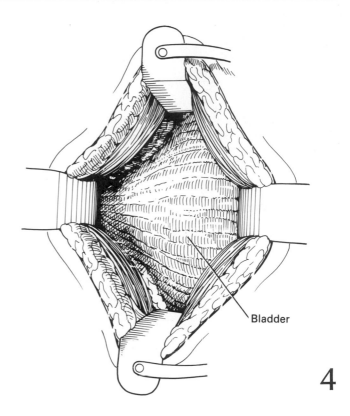

Bladder

4

LOWER MIDLINE EXTRAPERITONEAL INCISION

The exposure from this incision is better inferiorly than with a Pfannenstiel incision and it is a faster incision both to make and to close. The incidence of subsequent inguinal herniae may be less than following a Pfannenstiel incision which may cause weakness to the posterior wall of the inguinal canal.

5 The incision extends from below the umbilicus to the pubic symphysis.

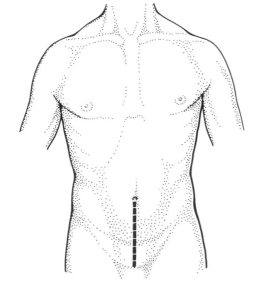

5

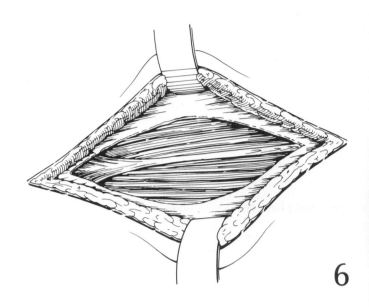

6 The anatomy is displayed as with a Pfannenstiel incision (pp. 893–895) and the subsequent steps are the same.

Wound closure

Closure is performed by using a continuous absorbable suture to the rectus sheath.

SUPRAPUBIC V INCISION (TURNER-WARWICK)

The skin incision is as for a Pfannenstiel incision (page 893).

7 A V-shaped incision is made in the rectus sheath, not extending out beyond the sheath laterally. The horizontal base of the V should be 4–5 cm long over the upper border of the pubic symphysis.

8 The rectus sheath flap is mobilized superiorly, coagulating vessels running between the recti and the underside of the rectus sheath. By undermining the inferior margin of the rectus sheath where it overlies the pubic symphysis and suturing the mobilized sheath to the skin edge, exposure inferiorly is improved. The recti are divided in their midline raphe, and exposure is completed using a Turner-Warwick ring retractor.

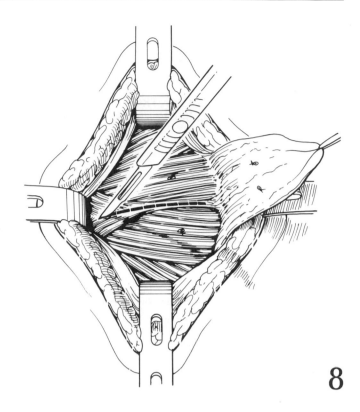

8

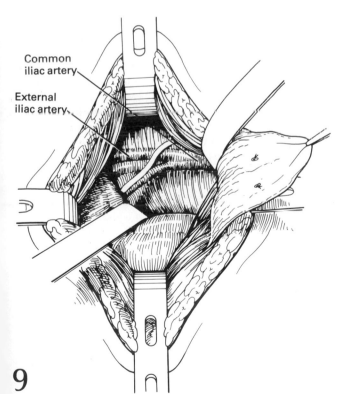

Common iliac artery

External iliac artery

9

9 Additional exposure, as far as the lower border of the kidney, can be obtained by extending the incision through the muscles of the anterior abdominal wall superiorly and laterally, but without dividing the rectus, the belly of which on the side of the extension is retracted medially.

Illustrations by Gillian Oliver

Surgery for renal stones

H. N. Whitfield MA, MChir, FRCS
Consultant Urologist, St Bartholomew's Hospital and St Mark's Hospital for Diseases of the Colon and Rectum, London, UK

History

The advent of percutaneous nephrolithotomy (PCNL) and extracorporeal shock wave lithotripsy (ESWL) during the 1980s has dramatically reduced the need for open renal surgery. Only 5% of patients with renal stones will require open surgery if both PCNL and ESWL are available. In those centres without ESWL, up to 10% of patients with renal stones may require open surgery.

The specialized techniques that were developed during the 1960s and 1970s depended on an appreciation of extrarenal anatomy and recognition of the need to perform intrarenal surgery under ischaemic conditions. Methods of preserving renal function during ischaemia were refined. Most patients requiring open surgery for renal stones today have complex stone disease, and the techniques that were developed remain of paramount importance.

Preoperative

Radiography

Availability of an up-to-date intravenous urogram is essential. Retrograde ureterography is very seldom required, as high-dose urography will define the pelvicaliceal anatomy accurately unless there is severe impairment of renal function. If the stones are of low density, plain tomography may be required as part of the intravenous urography.

Plain radiography of the urinary tract on the day of surgery is absolutely essential as stones can move unexpectedly.

Biochemistry

If intravenous urography shows no evidence of renal damage and the serum creatinine is normal, there is no need for a creatinine clearance measurement. This becomes important, however, when there is impairment of renal function, to identify those patients who must be monitored biochemically particularly carefully after operation and those who may require preoperative or postoperative dialysis.

Renography

If there is extensive stone disease or if there is impaired overall renal function, it is important to estimate differential renal function. If the stone-bearing kidney contributes less than 10% to overall renal function and the other kidney is normal, nephrectomy is usually indicated. When the percentage function is greater than this, a number of other factors will influence the decision, such as the age and symptoms of the patient, the overall renal function, and the chances of achieving complete stone clearance.

Urine culture

A sample for urine culture must be taken before operation. Although the result may not be available by the time of surgery, a decision must be taken whether or not to give prophylactic antibiotics. Cloudy urine is usually infected. Staghorn stones, even if primarily metabolic, have a significant infective element. Stones that are causing obstruction, either at the pelviureteric junction or in a caliceal neck, often provoke infection which may not be picked up by routine urine culture because the obstruction may prevent infected urine from reaching the bladder. In all these cases, prophylactic antibiotics should be given.

Blood cross-matching

For all open renal operations for stones except pyelolithotomy, two units of blood should be cross-matched.

Operations

PYELOLITHOTOMY

Indications

This operation is indicated when percutaneous renal surgical expertise or ESWL is not available. Very occasionally, patients with cystine or other very hard stones that cannot be distintegrated either by ESWL or endoscopically may require open surgery. If complications of percutaneous surgery have occurred previously, open surgery may occasionally be the best way to resolve the stone problem.

If a patient has a stone in the renal pelvis together with pelviureteric junction obstruction, open surgery is fully justified to combine stone removal and pyeloplasty. A percutaneous procedure to correct pelviureteric obstruction has been described, but there is less complete acceptance of this procedure than of other percutaneous renal surgery techniques for stones.

Preoperative

Results of a recent urine culture must be obtained and a parenteral antibiotic given before operation if any infection is demonstrated.

Intravenous urography should be performed to demonstrate urinary tract anatomy. Plain abdominal radiography immediately before surgery is mandatory. Peroperative radiographic screening facilities should be available in case difficulty is experienced in localizing the stone.

Renal function should be monitored. Measurement of serum creatinine in uncomplicated stone cases is all that is necessary. Where overall function is impaired, creatinine clearance should be measured and differential renal function estimated by isotope renography.

For a simple pyelolithotomy there is no need to cross-match blood.

In patients with impaired renal function, particularly those with infective stones, preoperative dehydration may exacerbate renal damage by a combination of renal underperfusion and infective interstitial nephritis. Intravenous fluids should be given to avoid such preoperative dehydration.

Incision

As full mobilization of the kidney is not necessary for a simple pyelolithotomy, a lumbotomy incision provides very satisfactory exposure in patients who are not overweight. In obese patients or in more complicated cases, one of the other standard incisions for exposing the kidney should be performed.

1 The perinephric fat in the region of the renal pelvis should be grasped with Duval forceps and retracted medially. Gentle dissection will expose the renal pelvis.

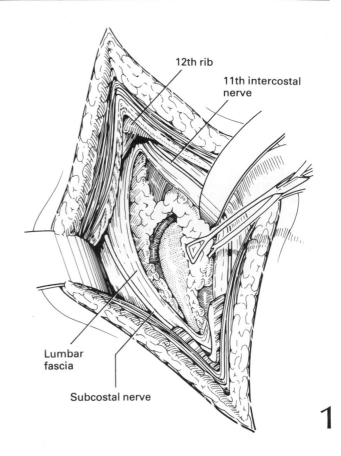

1

2 If the renal pelvis is small and intrarenal, a 'simple' pyelolithotomy may become very difficult. In such cases the kidney should be fully mobilized and the Gil-Vernet technique of extended pyelolithotomy becomes necessary[1].

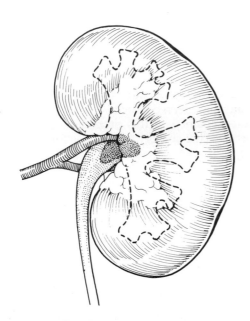

2

3 The renal pelvis is opened between stay sutures, usually on its posterior aspect. The course of the posterior branch of the renal artery is variable and care must be taken to avoid damaging it. The risk of devascularizing the renal pelvis and causing secondary pelviureteric junction stenosis is less if the incision in the renal pelvis is made longitudinally. The stone is grasped with stone forceps and removed.

Wound closure

The incision in the renal pelvis is closed with a continuous 3/0 or 4/0 absorbable suture. A drain is inserted down to the site of the pyelotomy.

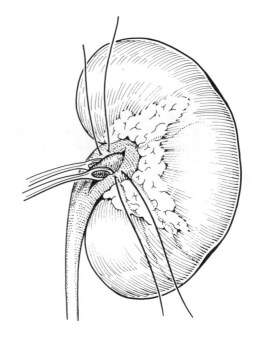

3

EXTENDED PYELOLITHOTOMY

This approach to complex renal stones has been popularized by Gil-Vernet[1]. By avoiding the need for a parenchymal incision, the risk of causing renal function to deteriorate postoperatively is reduced. It is possible to remove some complex stones by this technique; residual stones in calices that cannot be exposed may be removed through a radial nephrotomy (*see* page 907).

4a–c The anatomy of the renal sinus was first described by Henlé in 1966. The anatomical studies of Graves have shown the variations in the distribution of the posterior branch of the renal artery or arteries, which must be recognized to avoid infarcting the posterior segment of the kidney. The main trunk of the posterior branch may cross the superior or the inferior pelvicaliceal junction, and the extent to which the artery is hidden by parenchyma in the renal sinus varies.

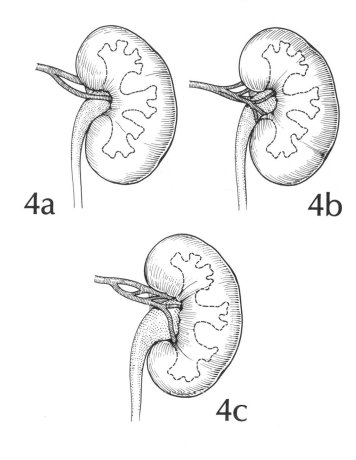

Indications

Exposure is easier when the renal pelvis is not small and intrarenal. Quite extensive branched calculi may be removed or a solitary caliceal fragment may be exposed.

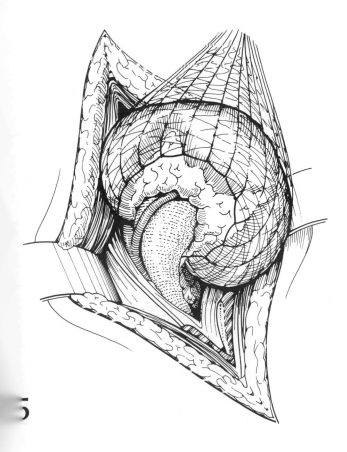

Incision

5 The kidney must be fully mobilized. A constant vein courses from the posterior aspect of Gerota's fascia to the posterior abdominal wall at the level of the middle of the kidney, and this vein should be identified and coagulated to avoid tiresome bleeding. A convenient method of supporting the kidney thereafter is within a netting sling. A ring retractor provides secure exposure.

6 The peripelvic fat from the posterior aspect of the renal pelvis is removed by scissor dissection, remaining close to the wall of the renal pelvis. If there has been renal infection, the fat may be very adherent. If possible, the fat should be allowed to remain attached towards the hilum, so that at the end of the operation it may be replaced over the pyelotomy.

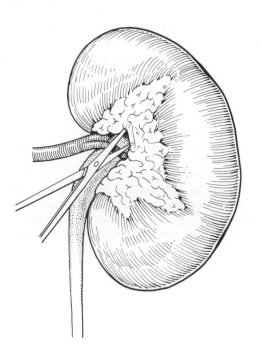

6

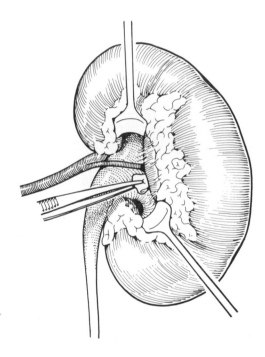

7

7 Small Gil-Vernet retractors are placed under the parenchyma, which is rolled back progressively off the renal pelvis; this can be achieved effectively with a pledget swab held in forceps. At this stage of the dissection, great care must be taken to avoid damaging the posterior branch of the renal artery.

8 The renal pelvis is opened transversely. The incision should be made as far away from the pelviureteric junction as possible, to reduce the risk of devascularizing the junction, which will result in stenosis. The length and direction of the incision can be varied to conform to the shape of the intrarenal anatomy and the contained stone.

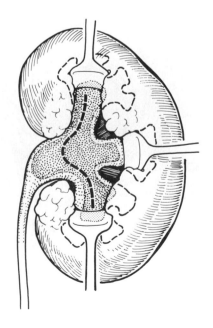

8

9 If a solitary caliceal stone is to be removed through this approach, the incision should be made vertically in the infundibulum.

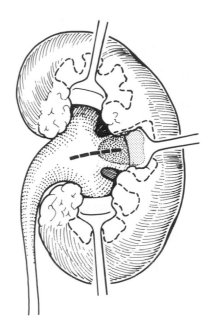

9

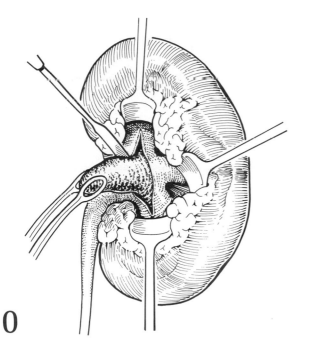

10

10 Stones are most readily removed by inserting a curved McDonnell's dissector behind them to assist the levering and twisting necessary to remove the stone.

Wound closure

The incision in the pelvis is closed using interrupted 3/0 or 4/0 chromic catgut. The peripelvic fat should be replaced over the incision and carefully kept in place by one or two absorbable sutures.

A tube drain is inserted down to the renal pelvis. The perinephric fat should also be replaced and the wound closed in layers.

COAGULUM PYELOLITHOTOMY

This procedure was first described by Dees in 1943 as being suitable for removing small mobile stones within the collecting system[2]. The prerequisite is that the renal pelvis should be extrarenal and the infundibula of the calices should be wide.

Indications

The advent of PCNL and ESWL has made the indications for this procedure very few.

Incision

The kidney is mobilized and held in a netting sling. The coagulum is prepared by mixing 12 ml of dried human fibrinogen solution with 1 ml of thrombin solution[3]. Methylene blue may be added to aid identification of any retained coagulum. The addition of calcium and/or cryoprecipitate weakens rather than strengthens the coagulum.

11 The ureter is occluded and the mixture is injected into the renal pelvis. The coagulum forms within 4 min, and the renal pelvis is opened between stay sutures. The coagulum and its contained stones are removed from the pelvis by gentle traction. Peroperative radiography may be required to check stone clearance (*see* page 908).

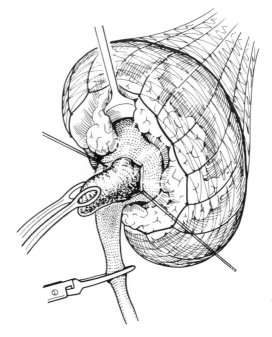

11

Wound closure

The renal pelvis is closed with 3/0 or 4/0 chromic catgut, and a tube drain is placed down to the pelvis. The wound is closed in layers.

Complications

If portions of coagulum are retained they will be dissolved by urokinase quite rapidly. The source of the blood products used must be free from contamination by human immunodeficiency virus. One report of a fatal complication due to pulmonary embolism with the coagulum[4] has highlighted the importance of avoiding overdistension of the collecting system with the mixture.

RADIAL NEPHROTOMY

The technique was first described by Wickham[5]. Anatomical studies by Graves had confirmed that there is a segmental arterial arrangement with no collateral circulation between segments, an observation first made by John Hunter in 1974. Venous tributaries are collected into large trunks around the anterior aspect of calices. Wickham showed that a nephrotomy causes minimum damage when placed as peripherally as possible on the posterior aspect of the kidney.

Indications

By combining the radial nephrotomy technique with a pyelotomy, even the most complex stones may be removed. There is still every justification for open surgery in patients with a staghorn calculus, particularly when there has been no previous surgery, when the bulk of the stone lies within the calices rather than within the renal pelvis.

Incision

12 The renal artery is exposed by exploring the posterior surface of the kidney. The pulsating artery is identified, often more towards the upper pole and more medially than would be expected. Small veins and a lymph node often overlie the artery, and these should be identified and exposed as far from the kidney as possible, before any of the arterial branches take off. On the right side the renal artery can be exposed as it emerges from under the inferior vena cava. Polar vessels exist in up to 20% of patients, and these should be identified and preserved. Adjustments to the netting sling may be required to achieve this.

13 It is useful to expose the renal vein by dissecting the anterior surface of the renal sinus. Soft rubber slings should be passed round the artery and vein, and round the upper ureter when it has been identified.

Before a nephrotomy is performed the renal artery must be clamped. If the period of ischaemia is confidently predicted to be less than 20 min no method of renal preservation is required. Longer ischaemia makes some form of renal preservation mandatory.

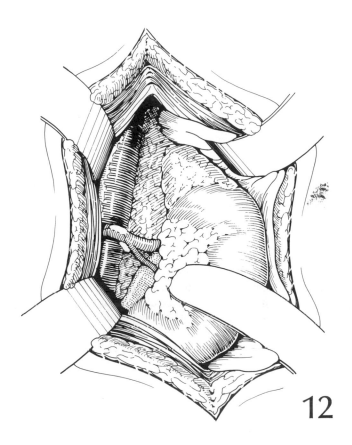

12

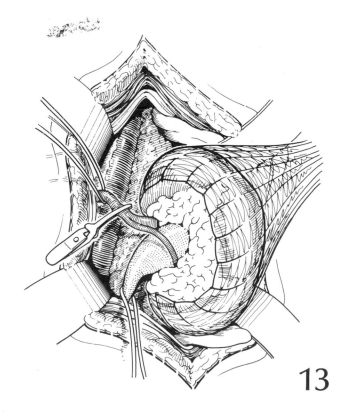

13

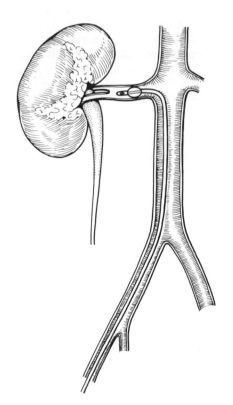

14, 15 The kidney will tolerate up to 3 h of ischaemia if cooled to 20°C. Cooling can be achieved either by applying plastic coils through which ice-cold fluid is circulated, by surrounding the kidney with sterile crushed ice, or by perfusing the kidney with cold saline intra-arterially through a Swan-Ganz catheter. After manipulating the catheter into the renal artery, a balloon is inflated through one channel of the catheter to occlude the artery while cold irrigant is injected through the other channel. At the end of the procedure the balloon is deflated. Close co-operation and co-ordination between urologist and radiologist are required.

If the period of ischaemia is not greater than 1 h, 2 g of inosine injected intravenously immediately prior to arterial clamping will provide protection of renal function.

An alternative to clamping the renal artery is to use B-mode ultrasonography to identify renal vessels. These are marked on the kidney, and the incision is made in a silent area in the same way as described for a radial nephrotomy performed under ischaemic conditions.

14

15

16 The renal pelvis is opened and as much as possible of the renal pelvic portion of the stone is removed. The stone-bearing calix is identified by using a fine needle as a transparenchymal probe. An incision is made, preferably on the posterior surface of the kidney as peripherally as possible, and the stone is extracted. Multiple nephrotomies will be necessary if a complex stone is to be removed completely. The nephrotomies can be held open by an assistant using stone forceps. The stones can best be removed by inserting a McDonnell's dissector behind them and levering them out.

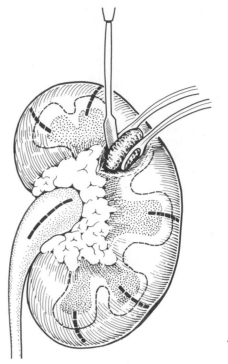

16

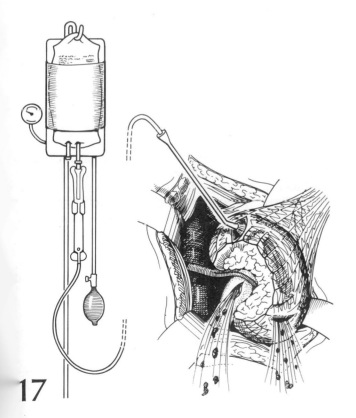

17 High-pressure irrigation with cooled normal saline will help to keep the kidney temperature at 20°C and to flush out residual fragments of stone.

17

18 Intraoperative radiography is essential to assess whether or not stone clearance is complete. Ligaclips (Ethicon, Edinburgh, UK) placed on the netting sling act as reference points for identifying any residual fragments of stones.

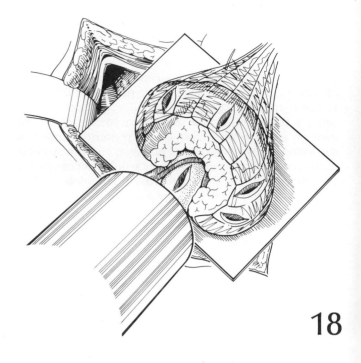

18

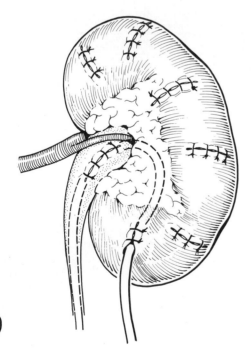

19

Wound closure

19 At the end of the procedure the nephrotomies should be closed with a continuous 3/0 or 4/0 chromic catgut suture. The suture closing the nephrotomy should pick up the capsule and 2–3 mm of underlying parenchyma. A 12-Fr nephrostomy tube should be brought through one of the nephrotomies.

A tube drain should be left down to the kidney, Gerota's fascia approximated over it, and the wound closed in layers.

ANATROPHIC NEPHROLITHOTOMY

Studies over a number of centuries have confirmed John Hunter's assertion that segmental renal arteries are end vessels. Hyrtl and Brodel both showed that an avascular plane exists on the posterior aspect of the kidney, marking the boundary of the territory between the posterior and anterior branches of the renal artery. The avascular line can be exploited as access to the collecting system.

Indications

Even since the advent of PCNL and ESWL, anatrophic nephrolithotomy remains of value in patients with staghorn calculi when the bulk of the stone is caliceal and infundibular rather than pelvic. If infundibular stenosis is present, the indications for this approach are particularly strong. If the decision is made to perform open surgery for a complex stone, the choice between an extended pyelotomy, radial nephrotomy or anatrophic nephrotomy will depend more upon the preference and experience of the surgeon than on any other consideration.

Incision

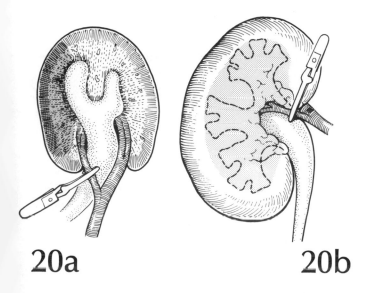

20a, b The kidney is fully mobilized as described for radial nephrotomy. The renal artery is dissected out to demonstrate the posterior branch. Intravenous mannitol is administered in a dose of 12.5–25 mg, and after 5 min the posterior branch of the renal artery is clamped. One or two ampoules of methylene blue are given intravenously, and the line of demarcation which results is marked on the renal capsule. The arterial clamp is removed for 5 min before the main trunk of the artery is clamped and ischaemia established, as described above.

20a   **20b**

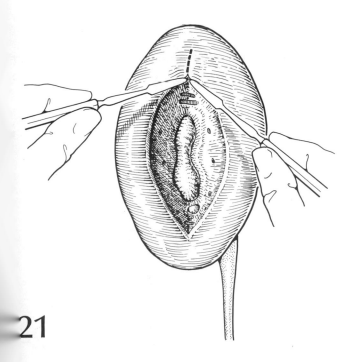

21 The incision into the renal capsule is deepened by blunt dissection to expose the infundibula and posterior aspects of the calices. As the posterior aspects of the upper and lower poles are supplied by the anterior branches of the renal artery, the incision should not be continued for the full length of the posterior surface.

21

22 The renal pelvis is opened and the posterior calices exposed by incising their infundibula, and all stones are removed. Access to anterior calices can be gained in a similar fashion.

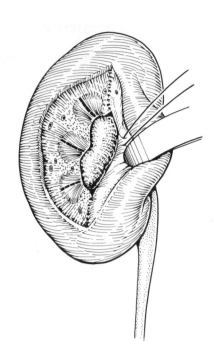

22

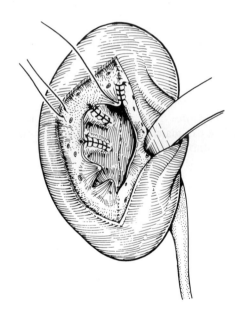

23

23 To correct the infundibular stenosis that is often present, the mucosal surfaces of longitudinal openings into adjacent infundibula are sutured together – a calicoplasty.

24 Alternatively, a calicorrhaphy is performed by suturing horizontally a vertical incision across a stenosed infundibulum.

Wound closure

A 12-Fr nephrostomy tube is inserted and the renal pelvis is closed with a continuous absorbable suture. The capsule is approximated similarly, Gerota's fascia is closed, and a drain is left down to the perinephric space.

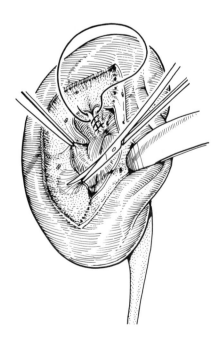

24

LOWER POLE PARTIAL NEPHRECTOMY

This technique was advocated by Hamilton Stewart as the treatment of choice for stones in the lower caliceal group. Renal stone disease, both primary and recurrent, occurs most commonly in the dependent calices of the lower pole, and by removing this region of urinary stasis the incidence of recurrent stones may be reduced.

Indications

Although PCNL and ESWL have reduced the indications for open surgery for stone disease, there are still some patients with a dilated lower caliceal group, often associated with a degree of infundibular narrowing, who form recurrent stones in the absence of infection or metabolic disorder. Such patients may benefit from lower pole partial nephrectomy.

Localized infection in the kidney may give rise to an abscess, and although this can be managed by minimally invasive surgical methods, there may be occasional indications for open surgery, particularly if there is an associated stone. Tuberculous infection may very occasionally result in infundibular stenosis and hydrocalicosis, which can only be managed by partial nephrectomy.

A tumour localized to one or other pole may also be amenable to partial nephrectomy.

Trauma may be localized and of sufficient severity to warrant partial nephrectomy if conservative management fails.

Incision

The kidney is fully mobilized, and the vascular pedicle is isolated so that slings can be placed around the artery and vein(s) to provide full control of any potential bleeding.

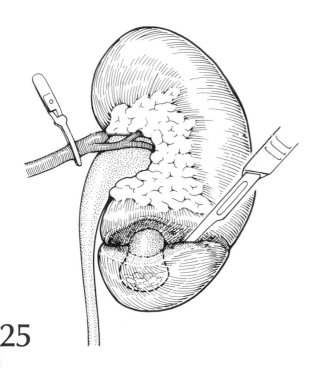

25 The incision into the parenchyma is made after the renal artery has been clamped. As the procedure can be completed within 20 min, hypothermic renal protection is not needed. Either a transverse or a wedge-shaped incision may be made, and in both cases the incision is deepened with a knife, ignoring parenchymal vascular anatomy.

Wound closure

26 The collecting system should be closed with fine absorbable sutures and the vessels ligated individually. Haemostasis is confirmed by removing the vascular clamp.

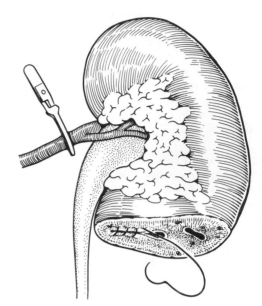

26

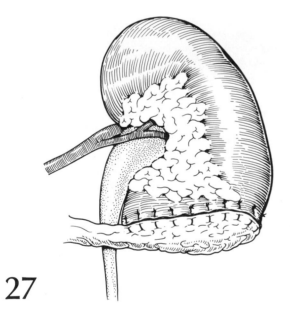

27

27 Adjacent perinephric fat should be sutured over the raw surface. After a wedge-shaped incision, it is a mistake to try to reconstitute the kidney with deep mattress sutures.

A drain should be left down to the kidney.

Postoperative care

Bleeding is the complication to be monitored carefully. Even after meticulous haemostasis, arterial or venous bleeding may occur in the first 12 h after operation that is sufficiently severe to require re-exploration. A urinary fistula can occur, but will usually settle spontaneously. The insertion of a JJ stent may hasten the resolution of such a fistula.

References

1. Gil-Vernet JM. New surgical concepts in removing renal calculi. *Urol Int* 1965: 20: 255–88.

2. Dees JE, Anderson EE. Coagulum pyelolithotomy. *Urol Clin North Am* 1981; 8: 313–17.

3. Norris RW, Colvin BT, Kenwright MG, Flynn JT, Blandy JP. *In vitro* studies on optimum preparation of coagulum for surgery of renal calculi. *Br J Urol* 1981; 53: 516–19.

4. Pence JR, Airhart RA, Novicki DE, Williams JL, Ehler WJ. Pulmonary emboli associated with coagulum pyelolithotomy. *J Urol* 1982; 127: 572–3.

5. Wickham JEA, Coe N, Ward JP. One hundred cases of nephrolithotomy under hypothermia. *J Urol* 1974; 112: 702–5.

Further reading

Alken P, Thüroff J, Reidmiller H, Hohenfellner R. Doppler sonography and B-mode ultrasound scanning in renal stone surgery. *Urology* 1984; 23: 455–60.

Assimos DG, Boyce WH. Operative surgery of renal stones by the anatrophic approach. In: Wickham JEA, Buck AC, eds. *Renal Tract Stone*. Edinburgh: Churchill Livingstone, 1990: 471–81.

Boyce WH. Surgery of urinary calculi in perspective. *Urol Clin North Am* 1983; 10: 585–94.

Brodel N. The intrinsic blood vessels of the kidney and their significance in nephrotomy. *Johns Hopkins Hosp Bull* 1901; 12: 10–22.

Fitzpatrick JM, Sleight MW, Braack A *et al*. Intrarenal access: effects on renal function and morphology. *Br J Urol* 1980; 52: 409–14.

Marberger M, Gunther R, Mayer EJ, Wiestler M. A simple method for *in situ* presentation of the ischaemic kidney during renal surgery. *Invest Urol* 1976; 14: 191–3.

Taylor WN, Boyce WH. An anatomical basis for surgery of the renal papillae. *J Urol* 1982; 128: 1052–4.

Illustrations by Philip Wilson

Operations for drainage: nephrostomy

H. N. Whitfield MA, MChir, FRCS
Consultant Urologist, St Bartholomew's Hospital and St Mark's Hospital for Diseases of the Colon and Rectum, London, UK

Principles and justification

Indications

Whenever renal failure is caused by an obstruction, relief of the obstruction must be established as early as possible. Percutaneous nephrostomy under local anaesthesia and the availability of JJ stents have combined to minimize the indications for open surgery. However, a nephrostomy tube may be required after open renal surgery for stones, trauma or pelviureteric junction obstruction, or any renal surgery where there is a risk of postoperative bleeding. In such circumstances a nephrostomy tube provides a very satisfactory method of drainage.

Tuberculosis, causing severe ureteric and bladder damage, used to be a not uncommon indication, but has declined with the enormous reduction in the incidence of genitourinary tuberculosis.

The only remaining indication for permanent nephrostomy tube drainage is if there is irrevocable ureteric obstruction and/or fistula following pelvic surgery with or without radiotherapy, which has also resulted in bowel damage precluding the use of intestine for ureteric and bladder replacement.

Preoperative

The patient should be made fit for general anaesthesia, with dialysis if necessary. Patients in renal failure always have a greater potential for bleeding than normal, which may be increased by the anticoagulation accompanying haemodialysis. Furthermore, patients with chronic renal failure are anaemic and it is therefore advisable to cross-match 2 units of blood.

Operation

There are two techniques: end nephrostomy and ring nephrostomy. In either case the patient is positioned on the operating table as for any renal operation and a suitable incision chosen on the basis of the position of the kidney, and depending on any other operation that is to be performed (*see* pp. 873–889).

1 The kidney is exposed and the lower pole cleared of fat but it is not necessary to fully mobilize the kidney. The renal pelvis is cleared of fat and a pyelotomy (1 cm) made transversely. A small malleable probe, through the head of which a hole has been drilled, is manoeuvred into a lower calix, pushed through the parenchyma and the capsule incised over it.

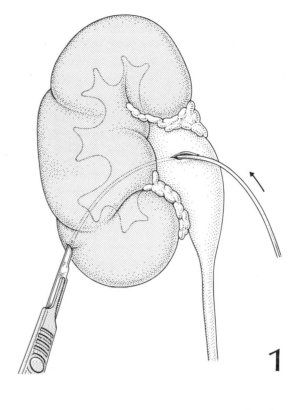

1

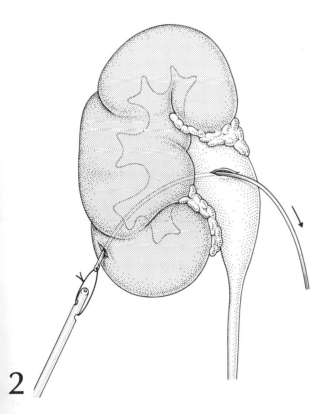

2

2 A nephrostomy tube is then attached to the probe with a suture and pulled back into the renal pelvis. It is not necessary to insert a nephrostomy tube larger than 18 Fr. The author prefers a straight tube or a Foley catheter to a Malecot or de Pezzer catheter since they are less traumatic to the kidney when removed.

3 The pyelotomy should be closed with continuous or interrupted absorbable sutures. The nephrostomy tube should be secured to the renal capsule with an absorbable suture, and should be brought out as anteriorly as possible on the abdominal wall (for patient comfort), with as straight a course as possible to facilitate changing the tube if necessary. There should be no need for a perirenal drain. Perirenal fat should be replaced.

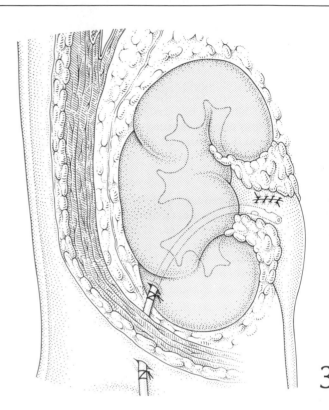

3

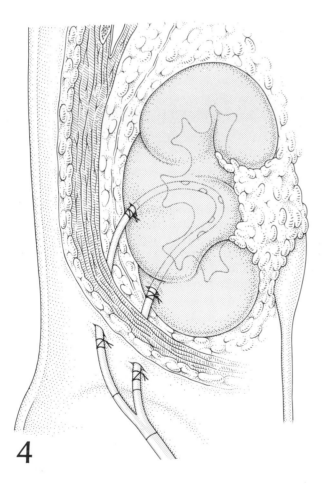

4

4 A ring nephrostomy has the advantage that it cannot be pulled out by accident. A second entry point to the collecting system is made through a middle or upper calix. A suture is attached to the malleable probe and drawn back into the renal pelvis and attached to the end of the nephrostomy tube before being drawn through the parenchyma and fixed to the capsule. The two ends of the nephrostomy tube are bought out as anteriorly as possible and attached to a Y piece and thence to a collecting device.

Postoperative care

The patient is likely to develop ileus for 24–48 h after surgery and will therefore require intravenous fluids and appropriate analgesia.

Complications

Bleeding may occur from the parenchyma; if this is persistent and severe selective arterial embolization should be performed.

If the side holes of the nephrostomy tube lie outside the parenchyma, because of initial misplacement or subsequent dislodgement, urinary extravasation will occur. Readjustment of the tube under radiographic control is necessary.

Illustrations by Joanna Cameron

Operations for renal ablation: tumour excision

M. Marberger MD
Professor and Chairman, Department of Urology, University of Vienna, Vienna, Austria

Principles and justification

With renal cell carcinoma presenting as a unilateral disease in over 97% of all cases, and surgical removal still being the only therapeutic approach offering a realistic chance of cure, radical nephrectomy is the standard treatment of choice. When renal cell carcinoma occurs in solitary kidneys or when bilateral renal cell carcinomas are found, this policy of radical surgery calls for chronic haemodialysis or renal allotransplantation, with significant morbidity and disappointing results. In the earlier stages of the disease, at least as long as the tumour is confined to the kidney, renal cell carcinoma tends to grow by direct expansion, compressing the surrounding renal parenchyma to form a pseudocapsule. The tumour is still localized at this stage and can be excised completely without sacrificing the kidney. Technically, this is most easily done by following the pseudocapsule as a preformed plane of cleavage, 'enucleating' the tumour from the bed of renal parenchyma. Dissection and microangiography studies, however, have clearly shown that the pseudocapsule is perforated by radial vessels nourishing the outer layer of the tumour at an early phase, and the tumour tends to spread through the layers of the pseudocapsule in a finger-like fashion. Although enucleation has proved successful with small tumours, the principles of oncological surgery clearly dictate that a good margin of healthy tissue must be excised around the specimen.

Organ-sparing removal of renal tumours should therefore be performed as tumour excision in a plane of healthy tissue well outside the pseudocapsule of the tumour. With the advantages offered by a bloodless field by virtue of renal ischaemia and regional hypothermia,

almost all tumours that are still confined to the kidney can be managed *in situ*, even if major segmental veins are involved. Complete removal of the kidney, tumour excision on a workbench and allotransplantation theoretically offer less risk of tumour cell spillage, but the considerably higher complication rate of the approach *ex situ* limits tumour excision *ex situ* to the rare exception.

Indications

The decision for parenchyma-sparing tumour excision is mainly influenced by the amount of renal parenchyma remaining after tumour nephrectomy as opposed to tumour excision, and the size, type and position of the tumour. This results in a spectrum ranging from mandatory organ-preserving surgery to relative indications where the benefit of the procedure has to be evaluated individually.

Tumours in solitary kidneys

This is an absolute indication where as much parenchyma as possible has to be saved without leaving tumour behind. Although renal function may gradually deteriorate at a later stage, one-third of a solitary kidney can sustain a quality of life unsurpassed by chronic haemodialysis and the possibility of later allotransplantation.

917

Bilateral tumours

The presence of bilateral tumours is an absolute indication for parenchyma-sparing operations, but the surgeon has more flexibility as the overall amount of healthy renal parenchyma is usually higher. The side with the tumour that is technically simpler to excise is managed first. If the procedure goes well and a tumour-free kidney of adequate quality is obtained, the decision to remove the contralateral kidney with the tumour that is more difficult to excise is facilitated. Simultaneous management of both sides should be avoided as transient postoperative renal insufficiency is balanced by the contralateral kidney, even when tumour-bearing. The second side is treated after the function of the first kidney has stabilized and this is documented by split radioisotope renography, usually after about 14 days.

Up to 80% of patients with von Hippel–Lindau disease develop renal mass lesions, which are usually multiple and frequently bilateral. Although at imaging masses often appear as cysts, at least half of these patients develop renal cell carcinoma. Neurological symptoms predominate and usually lead to routine imaging of the kidneys, so that the renal lesions are detected at an early stage. All renal masses in conjunction with von Hippel–Lindau disease should be excised with a parenchyma-sparing technique, even if only a unilateral lesion is diagnosed at first.

About 4% of patients with Wilms' tumour have synchronous bilateral tumours, and in about one-third of the patients this is only detected at routine surgical exploration of an apparently normal contralateral kidney. Here the situation differs from renal cell carcinoma as highly effective adjunctive chemotherapy and radiotherapy are available. Additional surgery is therefore limited to obtaining histological proof by biopsy. This is followed by conservative treatment as long as there is objective response in terms of tumour shrinkage. Only if there is no response, or less than a 50% reduction of tumour size, are kidneys re-explored, and the tumours are excised with maximum conservation of renal parenchyma.

Unilateral tumour in the presence of a poorly functioning contralateral kidney

This is an extension of the situation of a tumour in a solitary kidney, with more functional renal reserve. Particularly if tumours are smaller and easily excised, partial nephrectomy is the treatment of choice.

Small peripheral tumours in the presence of a normal contralateral kidney

With the free availability of ultrasonography and computed tomography (CT), asymptomatic solid renal masses represent up to one-third of all kidney tumours diagnosed at present. If solitary and smaller than 4 cm in diameter, approximately two-thirds of them are benign and the remainder are renal cell carcinomas of low grade and stage. With the exception of angiomyolipoma, imaging techniques and fine needle biopsies are unreliable in establishing a valid diagnosis. Even frozen sections often fail to distinguish adenomas from low-grade renal cell carcinoma. Rather than sacrificing the entire kidney, it appears justified to excise only the tumour. This is a relative indication at most, and burdens the surgeon with heavy responsibility. His technique must be absolutely reliable regarding complete tumour removal and obtaining a good margin of healthy tissue around the specimen. If there is even the least doubt in achieving this, organ-sparing excision has to be abandoned.

Benign renal tumours

With the exception of renal angiomyolipoma (hamartoma), the standard imaging techniques and fine-needle biopsy cannot distinguish benign tumours reliably enough from renal cell carcinoma to render surgical exploration unnecessary. The fat-containing areas within angiomyolipoma are diagnostic on CT, rendering further evaluation unnecessary. Although they are always benign, some angiomyolipomas may grow to a considerable size and may rupture spontaneously, resulting in haemorrhagic shock. Larger angiomyolipomas should therefore be excised with an organ-sparing technique. Renal hamartoma may be detected in as many as 80% of patients with tuberous sclerosis, often with bilateral and multiple lesions. Most can be managed conservatively, but if excision is required, this should be performed in an organ-sparing fashion.

Preoperative

Detailed knowledge of the position and extent of the tumour within the kidney, and its bearing on the vascular and collecting system, are the key to the procedure. Renal ultrasonography and axial CT with and without contrast dye usually establish the diagnosis and delineate the extent and location of the tumour. It is essential that CT is performed with 4-mm cuts to identify any smaller satellite tumours. A good-quality intravenous urogram is helpful in establishing any tumour involvement of the collecting system, but this information can also be obtained by coronal reconstruction of the CT scan or simple nephrotomography immediately after the investigation.

With every tumour to be excised, except peripheral T_1 lesions, selective renal arteriography should routinely be performed; commonly, the border between tumour and healthy parenchyma can clearly be seen from the vascular pattern. Tumour involvement of larger hilar veins requires meticulous dissection of the hilar structures at an early stage of the operation. In general, only involvement of the main stem and major branches of the renal vein is identified by CT. If tumours extend to the hilar region, evaluation of more peripheral tributaries by pharmacophlebography is recommended.

In the presence of non-resectable metastases, renal cell carcinoma cannot be cured. Evidence for systemic spread of the tumour therefore renders organ-preserving surgery even less justified than palliative nephrectomy in cases with a normal contralateral kidney. The retroperitoneal lymph nodes, liver, chest and mediastinum should therefore be scanned routinely by axial CT, and a bone scan should be obtained to rule out osseous metastases.

With the exception of very small peripheral tumours, renal ischaemia and regional hypothermia are routinely employed to provide a bloodless field during dissection of the tumour. Ischaemic tolerance is better if the kidney is well hydrated; 1500 ml of Ringer's lactate are therefore administered intravenously during the preoperative fasting period, and the patient is well hydrated throughout the procedure, aiming at a urine output of 5 ml/min at the time of clamping the renal artery. Nephrotoxic agents, in particular nephrotoxic antibiotics, should be avoided in the perioperative period.

Operation

The procedure is always performed under general anaesthesia with endotracheal intubation. A Foley urethral catheter is routinely inserted. If a long period of renal hypothermia is expected, body temperature should be monitored and maintained with the help of a warming system.

Position of patient and incision

Usually the kidney is approached through a generous 12th rib supracostal incision with the patient in a lateral jack-knife position (see pp. 878–881). This permits good retroperitoneal exposure of the entire kidney and pedicle and is easy to extend anteriorly if the aorta or vena cava has to be dissected. In cases of large tumours at the upper pole, it may be preferable to use an extrapleural 11th rib supracostal approach. Dissection should be carried backwards to the angle of the rib, incising the intercostal ligaments, so that the lower rib can swing downwards away from the one above.

With large perihilar tumours, a transverse upper abdominal incision from the umbilicus into the 11th intercostal space may be preferable, with the patient placed in a 45° oblique lateral decubitus position and the table flexed. This facilitates an anterior approach to the pedicle, but in contrast to transperitoneal tumour nephrectomy, the pedicle is approached extraperitoneally by reflecting the peritoneal fold and colon medially. Urinary extravasation may complicate this type of surgery and is easier to manage when confined to the retroperitoneal space.

Gerota's fascia is incised sharply in the line of the skin incision. Starting at the point most distant from the tumour, the fatty capsule is carefully dissected off the kidney, leaving it attached only in the area immediately adjacent to the tumour. Carefully avoiding compression of the tumour, dissection is now carried anteriorly and posteriorly around the kidney to the hilar structures. In doing so, the fatty capsule is preserved as an anterior and posterior leaf to be reused for covering the kidney at the end of the procedure.

1 A rib retractor or Wickham angulated ring retractor with malleable blades is inserted, exposing the entire kidney. The renal vein is identified anteriorly, dissected over a distance of at least 3 cm and snared. The renal artery is identified by palpation, dissected, usually from the posterior side of the kidney, and snared. The ureter is identified at the level of the lower pole, likewise snared, and followed upward to the pelvis. Having identified all important perihilar structures, they are stripped of the loose fat attached to them with forceps or a swabstick, carefully coagulating the many smaller veins in this area. This leaves the kidney completely mobilized, with only the tumour covered by perirenal fat, so that it can be suspended with umbilical tapes.

Attention is now focused on the perihilar lymph nodes, mainly the left para-aortic nodes for a left-sided tumour and the right paracaval nodes for a tumour on the right. A formal lymph node dissection is usually not performed, but very obvious nodes are removed and sent for frozen sectioning. If nodal involvement is significant, the procedure is terminated. In the presence of no more than one or two small positive nodes, the incision is extended anteriorly, and a formal lymph node dissection is carred out. As with radical nephrectomy, the prognosis is poor when nodes are involved, but in the absence of other metastases an occasional patient may be saved. With tumours in a solitary kidney or bilateral tumours, the indication for parenchyma-sparing surgery remains unchanged. In the unlikely event that nodal involvement occurs with a small peripheral tumour in the presence of a normal contralateral kidney, the kidney is removed, together with all fatty tissue and the ipsilateral adrenal gland.

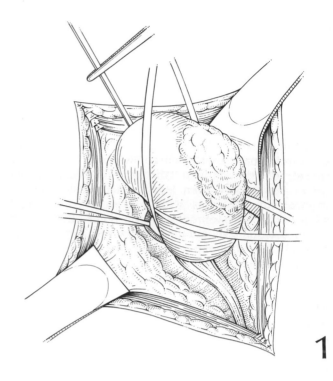

1

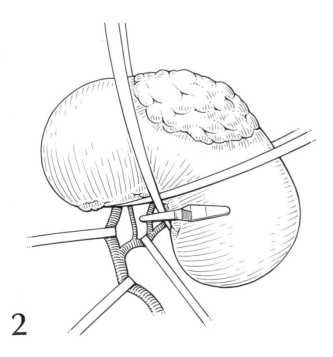

2

2 The renal artery is dissected until all its segmental subdivisions are identified. Branches that seem to supply the tumour are followed distally as far as possible. If they disappear within the tumour-bearing part of the kidney, they are clamped with a soft bulldog clamp. If healthy parenchyma does not blanch, they can be ligated, but this should be done with extreme caution as the arterial anatomy is highly variable and a non-perfused segment might be overlapped by parenchyma perfused from another artery, so that valuable parenchyma may be lost. Any accessory renal artery must also be dissected and snared, in order to control all of the arterial blood supply of the kidney.

With the exception of only the smallest peripheral tumours, excision should always be performed in a bloodless field. This requires regional hypothermia to avoid ischaemic damage to the kidney. Surface cooling with slush ice is the simplest and most universally applicable technique. Sterile slush is prepared by freezing standard saline packed in double-wrapped sterile vinyl bags. Vigorous shaking during the freezing process assures a soft consistency of the ice, but usually it is easier to simply crush bigger chunks on a side table under a sterile cloth with an orthopaedic hammer. In the mean time, 125 ml of 20% mannitol are rapidly administered intravenously.

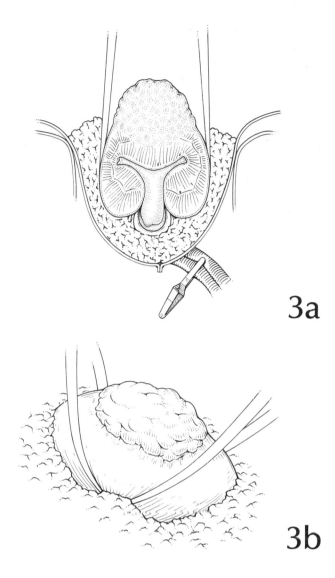

3a, b As soon as sufficient sterile ice is available, the renal artery is clamped as far proximally as possible with an atraumatic bulldog clamp; accessory arteries are treated in the same way. The renal vein is not occluded. Suspending the kidney with the tapes, a watertight dam is formed around it with a standard intestinal bag, such as that used for intestinal surgery. The blind end is cut open, and the bag is placed over the kidney, so that the original open end with its integrated string lace can be closed around the pedicle, distal to the clamp on the renal artery. The dam is filled with ice, so that only the immediate operative field remains exposed, the rest of the kidney being entirely covered. For optimum protection, renal core temperature should be maintained between 10°C and 20°C throughout the entire ischaemic period. This is usually achieved without the need for temperature monitoring, if the soft slush is continuously removed with suction and ice replaced as needed throughout the procedure.

3a

3b

4 Even with the fatty capsule preserved over the tumour, its extension into the parenchyma is usually well delineated. The fibrous capsule is incised sharply approximately 1 cm outside this margin all around the tumour.

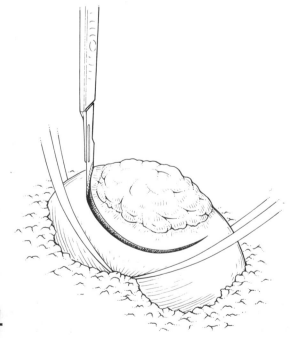

4

5 Using brain dissectors and malleable metal strips as retractors, the plane of cleavage is now developed by blunt dissection within the normal tissue, well outside the pseudocapsule of the tumour.

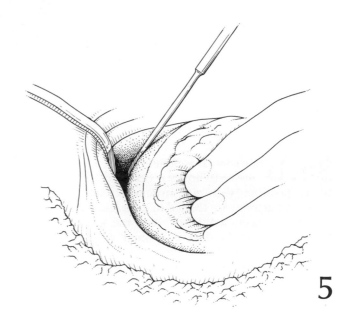

5

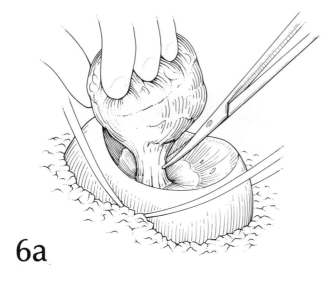

6a

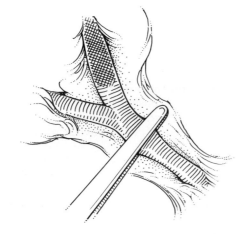

6b

6a, b This is seldom a problem in the periphery, but may become difficult with larger tumours as hilar structures are approached. With the kidney ischaemic, the extent of the tumour is usually easily palpable, so that dissection can be continued bluntly, skeletonizing the larger vessels and collecting system. To avoid tearing these structures, they are severed sharply with dissecting scissors. A tumour thrombus extending into a larger vein is usually clearly visible before the vessel is opened. In this event the vein is followed in the central direction until it can be ligated with 5/0 polyglycolic acid sutures beyond the tumour thrombus.

Larger tumours may displace major segments of the collecting system without invading them. It is preferable to preserve these drainage parts of the kidney and they can often be dissected and preserved to an extent that permits simpler closure or reconstruction.

7 Finally, the tumour remains attached only at its base, where it receives its major blood supply and where tumour extension into the collecting system, veins, or normal parenchyma is most likely to occur, but where neighbouring hilar vessels, important for the remaining kidney, are very close. Holding the tumour and the attached parenchymal layer gently in one hand, the remaining bridge is severed step by step by sharp dissection. With any evidence for tumour extension into the plane of dissection, and in the author's experience this is easily discernible with optical loops, dissection is continued several millimetres more centrally until healthy tissue is reached.

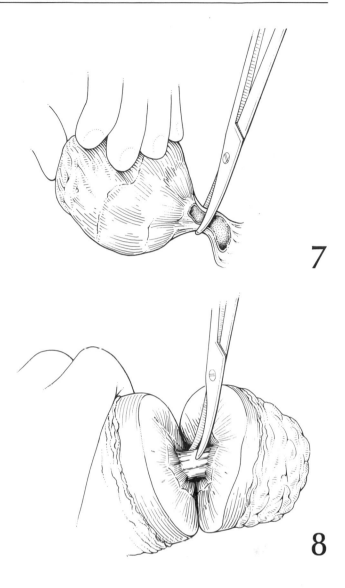

8 The same basic technique is used regardless of the location of the tumour. If the tumour involves most of the upper or lower pole, it is preferable to remove the entire pole rather than to leave a tongue of poorly perfused and drained parenchyma. After incising the fibrous capsule 1 cm proximal to the tumour's edge, the parenchyma is divided bluntly with the same technique down to the hilar structures. These are then dissected and transected step by step, leaving a guillotine-type nephrotomy plane.

The entire specimen is sent off for frozen sectioning after marking the tumour base. It is more reliable if the pathologist selects the biopsies for assessing the completeness of excision, rather than the surgeon taking random biopsies in the cleavage plane. With the kidney protected by hypothermia against ischaemic damage, there is adequate time to certify reliably the completeness of excision. If histology reveals residual tumour and the procedure is being performed for a small peripheral tumour in the presence of a normal contralateral kidney, excisional surgery becomes too risky and the kidney should be removed. If the tumour was excised from a solitary kidney or there are bilateral tumours, the conservative approach has to be continued by taking another 5-mm slice of tissue from the area involved, which is again assessed by frozen sectioning. When the perihilar fat is reached the vessels should be dissected to avoid damage to segmental arteries needed for the remaining kidney. With central tumours, this may result in almost complete separation of the upper and lower poles, which are only connected by the skeletonized vessels and the remaining parts of the collecting system.

Tumour involvement of the major renal vein indicates a poor prognosis. This situation should already have been identified at the preoperative diagnostic examination. In the rare event that there is no evidence of lymphatic or distant metastases, this situation is the exception where workbench excision is simpler. The kidney is approached as for standard radical nephrectomy, ligating the renal artery as close to its origin from the aorta as possible and severing the renal vein flush to, or even with a cuff of, vena cava. Tumour excision can be performed *ex situ* on the abdomen of the patient, without severing the ureter, but the delicate reconstruction is simpler if the kidney is completely removed and the procedure performed on a separate side-table under ideal conditions.

If tumour involvement of the main renal vein is detected unexpectedly at surgery, complete tumour removal may still be possible *in situ* by tumour thrombectomy and repair of the renal vein. Nephrectomy, rendering a patient anephric, with subsequent chronic haemodialysis and allotransplantation, has a considerably higher morbidity rate than excisional surgery and should always be absolutely the last resort if radical excision cannot be achieved with the other techniques.

Wound closure

9 While waiting for the results of the frozen sections, a watertight closure of the collecting system is performed with running 5/0 chromic catgut sutures.

Care must be taken not to deprive segments of renal parenchyma of appropriate drainage by inadvertently occluding a caliceal infundibulum. If the collecting system cannot be reconstructed with a flap of mucosa that remains, the parenchyma drained by this calix has to be removed. With larger defects, an internal 7 Fr indwelling ureteric stent should be inserted in an antegrade direction to secure unimpeded drainage; it is a wise precaution in the case of very elaborate reconstruction also to insert a soft 10 Fr nephrostomy tube which is led out through the nephrotomy.

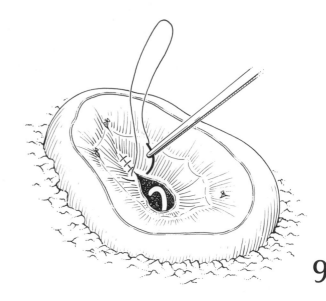

9

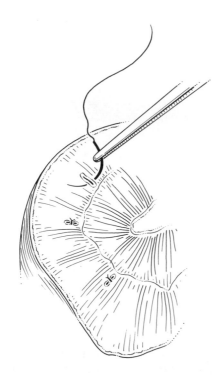

10

10 All transected arteries and veins are carefully suture-ligated with 5/0 polyglycolic acid sutures. Coagulation should not be used. Haemostasis should be performed meticulously and with optical magnification. This usually takes up all the time the pathologist needs for the frozen sections to confirm tumour-free margins.

11 The ischaemic kidney is supple and can usually be folded over the defect from which the tumour was taken, so that nephrotomy planes can be approximated against each other. The two-component fibrin adhesive Tissucol (Immuno, Vienna, Austria) facilitates closure, although it is not essential. The two components are mixed and prewarmed separately as specified, and applied simultaneously to the nephrotomy planes.

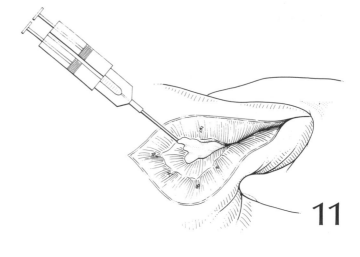

12 An assistant then approximates the two opposite nephrotomy planes with swabsticks, so that they are in contact, and holds them in this position for 3–5 min. During this time, the defect in the capsule is closed with a running 4/0 chromic catgut suture, which grasps the fibrous capsule and only the most superficial layers of the renal parenchyma.

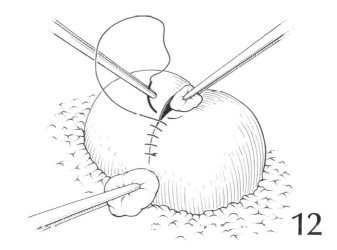

In the rare event that the planes of the nephrotomy cannot be brought into contact, the defect is covered with a free graft of peritoneum or absorbable collagen (Helistat, US Surgical, Norwalk, Connecticut, USA), which is secured using the same technique.

After rapid intravenous infusion of 125 mg of 20% mannitol, the renal circulation is restored. The kidney rapidly regains a uniform pink colour and firm consistency. Oozing from the nephrotomy can usually be controlled by manual compression for several minutes and occasionally a reinforcing superficial running suture over the suture line, closing the capsular defect. If this fails to stop the bleeding, an arterial lesion has to be suspected. With only a small nephrotomy for a peripheral small tumour, this may be controlled by one deeper figure-of-eight parenchymal suture of 3/0 chromic catgut. If the nephrotomy is large, deep parenchymal sutures are unreliable, and only result in

damage to the remaining parenchyma. The renal artery has to be occluded again and the kidney recooled. The nephrotomy is opened, and the entire plane of dissection is scrutinized for the source of bleeding, which is carefully cross-sutured. The nephrotomy is closed again using the same technique. Under no circumstances should renal circulation be re-established with the nephrotomy still open in an effort to identify the source of bleeding, as the blood-filled parenchyma can only be closed with deep parenchymal sutures resulting in significant renal damage and an unnecessary loss of blood.

The kidney is repositioned in the renal fossa. A 24 Fr tube drain is inserted through a separate stab incision and positioned so that its tip lies in the most dependent position within Gerota's fascia. The fatty capsule and Gerota's fascia are closed with a running suture, and the wound is closed as usual.

Postoperative care

In the immediate postoperative period, particular attention is paid to renal function and the possibility of haemorrhage. The patient is well hydrated, preferably with central venous pressure monitoring, aiming at a urine output of at least 100 ml/h. Extended surgery in a lateral jack-knife position may cause atelectasis of the contralateral lung, particularly in combination with regional hypothermia, so that attention is directed at adequate ventilation. If the pleura was opened inadvertently on the ipsilateral side, chest radiography is routinely performed to confirm correct expansion of the lung. Antibiotics need not be administered routinely.

If the recovery proceeds normally, the Foley catheter is removed after 24 h, and the patient is fully mobilized. Fluids are replaced intravenously until bowel function normalizes, which usually happens after an enema on the second postoperative day. The wound drain is removed as soon as it dries up, and any indwelling ureteric stent around the sixth or seventh day after operation.

Complications

Haemorrhage

If bleeding is significant the drain rapidly clogs up, so that a dry drain does not rule out a perirenal haematoma. If the clinical condition, circulatory parameters and dropping serum haemoglobin levels indicate this possibility, renal ultrasonography should be performed immediately. With an enlarging perirenal haematoma, early surgical revision with evacuation of the haematoma and haemostasis with the techniques described is recommended. Even if bleeding stops spontaneously due to tamponade, large retroperitoneal haematomas cause a prolonged ileus, so that they should be evacuated. When the collecting system has been opened, transient haematuria is common. In more severe cases, the Foley catheter should be exchanged for a three-way catheter and the bladder should be irrigated to avoid clot retention. In cases of persisting haematuria in the absence of a perirenal haematoma, selective renal arteriography will identify any intrarenal arterial lesion. At open surgical revision, these lesions are difficult to identify and can usually be managed only with deep parenchymal sutures. The treatment of choice is therefore superselective angioinfarction at the time of diagnostic angiography.

Impairment of renal function

Using a proper cooling technique, the kidney tolerates ischaemia without significant loss of function for at least 3 h; the kidney should produce urine within minutes of removing the bulldog clamp from the renal artery. For a solitary kidney, precise monitoring of urine output in the first hours after the procedure is essential. If the patient becomes oliguric despite a further 125 ml of 20% mannitol, acute thrombosis of the renal artery or tubular necrosis has to be suspected. As the former condition requires immediate surgical revision if the kidney is to be saved, technetium-99m pertechnate perfusion renography or Doppler ultrasonography of the renal artery should be performed at once; where this is not possible, venous digital subtraction angiography is indicated. If the major arterial branches are unequivocally perfused, the condition is caused by acute tubular necrosis. Renal function in general recovers after conservative treatment, although temporary haemodialysis may be needed.

Urinary extravasation

With more elaborate excision and reconstruction of the collecting system, urine may temporarily be discharged from the wound drain. If this continues beyond the third day after operation despite retracting the drain for 1–2 cm, a self-retaining ureteric stent is inserted endoscopically, which will usually dry up the wound at once. If a nephrostomy was placed at the time of surgery, it is only removed after nephrostomography has ruled out extravasation. If fever occurs, renal ultrasonography should routinely be performed to detect any urinoma. Percutaneous puncture and drainage as well as insertion of an indwelling ureteric stent effectively control the situation.

Ultrasonography of the kidney is routinely performed before the patient is discharged and will also reliably detect any abnormal fluid collection within the nephrotomy area, which may result from parenchyma still perfused but not properly drained. If the patient is asymptomatic, such formations are left for the routine follow-up examinations to see whether they grow. If this happens, or the patient has fever, they are drained percutaneously. Usually these small urinomas gradually disappear or remain constant in size, giving them the appearance of a 'normal' renal cyst.

Follow-up

The most obvious risk of organ-sparing tumour excision lies in the possibility of tumour recurrence. Large clinical series give an approximately 10% tumour recurrence rate within a mean follow-up of 3–5 years for patients with tumour excised from solitary or both kidneys. In the highly selected group where small peripheral tumours are excised in the presence of a normal contralateral kidney, the author has never observed a recurrent tumour, but the possibility of course exists. As recurrent tumours may again be excised or the kidney removed, scrupulous follow-up surveillance is therefore essential.

The renal anatomy differs significantly from the preoperative situation, particularly when very large tumours were excised. A careful ultrasonographic study and axial CT of the kidney with 4-mm cuts should therefore be routinely undertaken as a baseline examination within the first month after operation. This is followed by renal ultrasonography every 3 months over the following 2 years, supplemented by axial CT 6 months after surgery. The routine examinations after standard tumour nephrectomy must also be performed: chest radiography and ultrasonography of the liver and retroperitoneum every 3 months in the first year and every 6 months thereafter.

With the appearance of suspicious lesions that were not apparent at the baseline examinations, further examination is warranted. Despite the limitations of needle biopsies of renal tumours, this is usually the most direct approach; rather than fine-needle aspiration biopsies with thin needles, which bend easily and therefore tend to be misguided, core-needle biopsies with biopsy needles working on a vacuum basis, provide the most accurate approach. The biopsy should always be performed under CT guidance, with an image documenting the position of the tip of the needle in the suspicious area at the time of biopsy. If the biopsy is negative, further CT with 4-mm cuts is performed 3 months later. If evidence of a recurrent tumour is found, the kidney must be re-explored. Selective arteriography helps in planning the procedure and may be helpful in delineating the size of the recurrent tumour. The tumour can again be excised as described above, although perirenal scarring after the first operation renders the procedure more demanding.

Although hypertension has not been a significant problem, focal malperfusion after extensive surgery on the renal parenchyma can result in hypertension, so that blood pressure should be monitored at regular intervals. If serum creatinine levels are only slightly above the upper normal range, renal function can be expected to remain stable. If renal function is more severely impaired, i.e. endogenous creatinine clearance being below 30 ml/min, a gradual decline in renal function has been reported with long-term follow-up. It remains unclear whether this results from hyperperfusion or only from an age-related decline of renal function in cases where the amount of remaining renal parenchyma was already borderline. Conservative treatment, in particular of hypertension, slows the pace of deterioration, but ultimately the patient will need chronic haemodialysis and allotransplantation.

Outcome

The survival rates reported after organ-conserving excision are excellent if the tumour is confined to the kidney. In patients with a tumour in a solitary kidney, 5-year survival rates of well over 80% have been reported for T_1 and T_2 lesions, and these rates come close to 100% tumour-free survival for peripheral lesions smaller than 4 cm in diameter. Although all published series are retrospective analyses of highly selected patient groups treated at centres specializing in this field, and no statistically correct study is available randomizing the same tumours either to excisional surgery or radical nephrectomy, data are rapidly accumulating to show that excisional surgery is as successful as radical nephrectomy for T_1 and selected T_2 renal cell carcinoma. These results also provide the rationale for this approach in the presence of a normal contralateral kidney. The surgeon must, however, always be aware of the fact that surgical removal is the patient's only chance of cure. Excisional surgery therefore requires strict adherence to the criteria of patient selection, meticulous surgical technique and regular patient follow-up as outlined above.

Bilateral renal cancer has a poorer prognosis than unilateral cancer, patients with asynchronous renal cancer probably facing a more unfavourable outcome than those with synchronous disease. This is hardly surprising, as multiplicity of a malignant disease probably signifies a higher malignant potential, and it remains undecided whether the tumour on one side is a metastasis of the tumour on the other. Nevertheless, 5-year survival rates of about 50% have been reported, documenting excisional surgery as the treatment of choice.

Operations for ureterolithotomy

H. N. Whitfield MA, MChir, FRCS
Consultant Urologist, St Bartholomew's Hospital and St Mark's Hospital for Diseases of the Colon and Rectum, London, UK

Principles and justification

Indications

Most ureteric stones will pass spontaneously, a fact which is often forgotten or ignored in this era of extracorporeal shockwave lithotripsy (ESWL) and endoscopic ureteric surgery. There are sound reasons for pursuing a conservative policy of management in patients with a ureteric stone of 5 mm or less in size. Indications for intervention include persistent colic, deteriorating renal function (which should be monitored isotopically) and infection above the obstruction. Non-progress of a stone may also be an indication for intervention but the length of time for which a conservative policy can be pursued will depend on the site of the stone, the preference or prejudice of the surgeon and the wishes of the patient.

Since most ureteric stones can be dealt with endoscopically or with ESWL it has become increasingly difficult to identify indications for open ureterolithotomy. Not infrequently, the procedure is performed after the other methods have failed. In cases where technology or expertise is not available open surgery will still be necessary. However, since ureteric stones are frequently recurrent the new methods of treatment have obvious and enormous advantages.

Open ureteric surgery is still indicated as the primary intervention if there is an associated ureteric stricture below the stone. It can be difficult to identify such a stricture without direct endoscopic assessment, since the ureter below a stone often appears narrow because of spasm. If a large stone is impacted in the mid-ureter primary open surgery may be the best option, but to prove impaction usually involves a previous attempt to dislodge the stone from below, and the usual practice is to proceed to an attempt at some form of *in situ* disintegration with ultrasonic, electrohydraulic or laser disintegration.

Preoperative

A urine culture result should be available or the culture should be in progress. Plain abdominal radiography immediately before surgery is mandatory. Prophylactic antibiotics are not required in the absence of urinary infection.

Operations

General techniques

A stone may be difficult to palpate within the ureter, particularly if there has been previous open or recent failed endoscopic surgery, resulting in periureteric oedema and fibrosis. Surface anatomy markings in conjunction with radiographs should help to identify that part of the ureter which should be mobilized.

1 Rubber slings are passed around the ureter above and below the stone whenever possible.

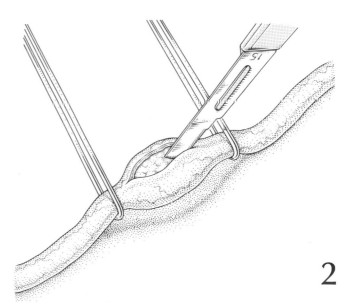

2 A longitudinal incision is made directly over the stone. No attempt should be made to 'milk' a stone up or down the ureter. If there is any suspicion of infection above the stone urine can be sent for culture.

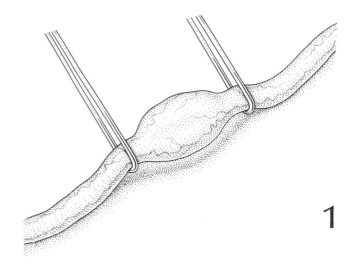

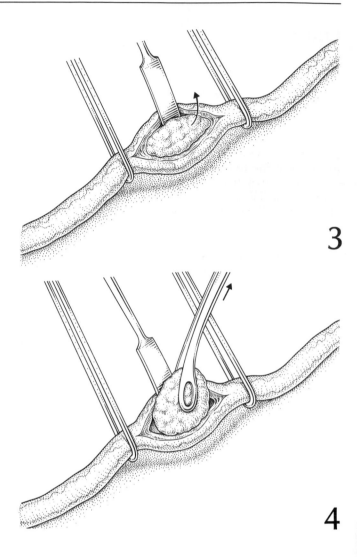

3

4

$3, 4$ The stone should be removed by inserting a blunt McDonald's dissector behind the stone, which can then be partially levered out, and grasped with stone forceps.

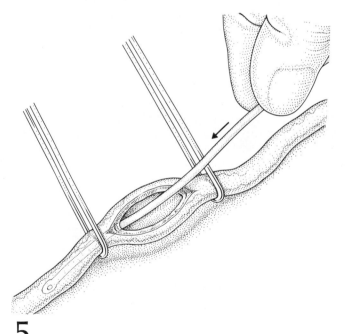

5

5 The patency of the ureter above and below the site of the stone should be confirmed by passing a 6–8-Fr gum elastic bougie.

6 The ureter should be closed using a single layer of fine interrupted absorbable sutures, which pass through the submucosa, muscle and serosa of the ureteric wall. The author does not recommend leaving the ureter to close spontaneously.

A drain should be placed down to the site of the ureterotomy, and can be shortened when urinary leakage begins to lessen and removed when leakage ceases.

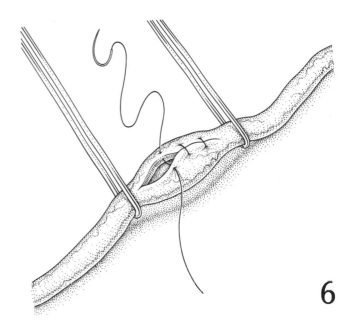

6

Upper third

7 The upper third of the ureter is best exposed through one of the approaches described for the kidney (*see* chapter on pp. 873–889). To minimize postoperative morbidity a subcostal or a lumbotomy incision is preferred to any of the incisions requiring rib resection. The ureter is identified by dissecting medially on the posterior abdominal wall at the level of the lower margin of the kidney. It is not necessary to mobilize the kidney but by retracting it upwards the ureter may be identified more easily. Sometimes palpation is the easiest way to find the ureter, as it feels like a whipcord. Slings should be placed above and below the stone at an early stage to prevent it from migrating.

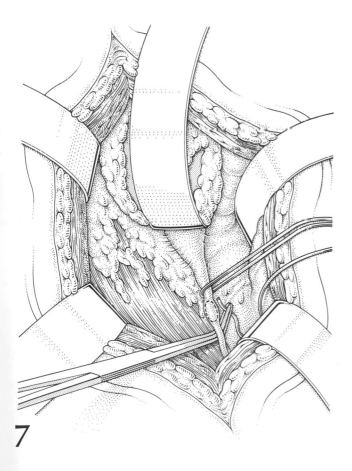

7

Middle third

8 A muscle-splitting or muscle-cutting incision will allow exposure of the middle third of the ureter (*see* chapter on pp. 890–892). If the line of the skin incision tends towards the vertical rather than the horizontal the incision may be extended in either direction if there is difficulty in locating the stone.

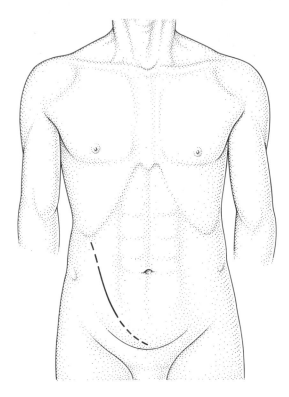

8

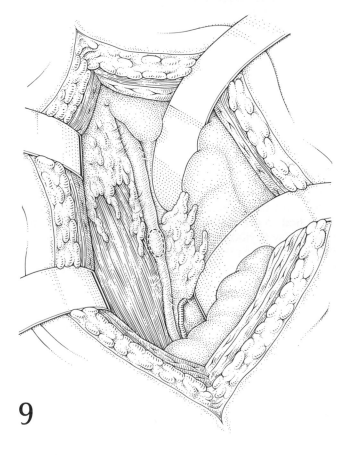

9

9 The ureter may be difficult to identify since it may be more medial than anticipated. Tilting the operating table away from the surgeon or placing a sandbag under the patient's buttock may help. Good retraction of the peritoneum is essential. Care must be taken that the ureter is not mobilized on the under surface of the peritoneum. There are relatively few landmarks at this level, except the gonadal vessels, which will help in the identification of the ureter.

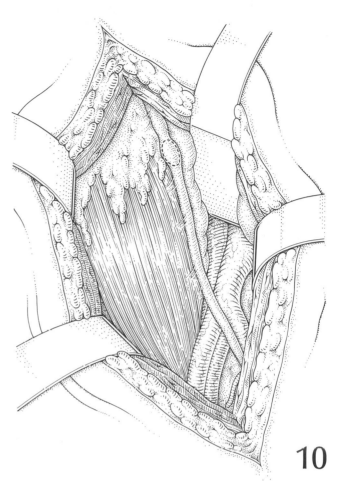

10 If difficulty persists, the ureter should be located where it passes over the bifurcation of the common iliac artery. It can then be traced superiorly.

Lower third

The lower third of the ureter can be exposed through a Pfannenstiel incision, but the author's preference is to use an oblique muscle-cutting incision, which must extend inferiorly over the public symphysis (*see* chapter on pp. 893–897).

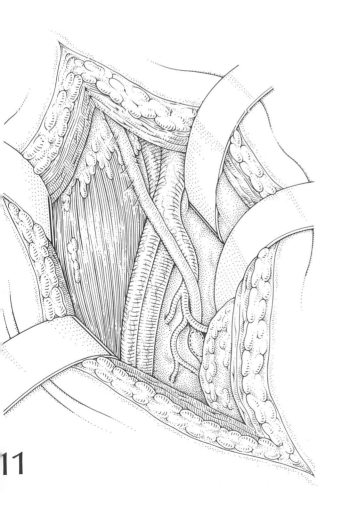

11 The ureter is identified as it crosses the bifurcation of the common iliac artery and can then be traced inferiorly. Ureteric branches of the superior vesical pedicle must be coagulated as the dissection proceeds.

12 The umbilical ligament will be encountered running medially some 3 cm below the bifurcation of the common iliac artery and must be ligated and divided, since it is seldom obliterated. The superior vesical pedicle is next identified, ligated and divided to enable the lowest part of the ureter to be exposed. If the dissection is kept close to the wall of the ureter the stone can usually be palpated.

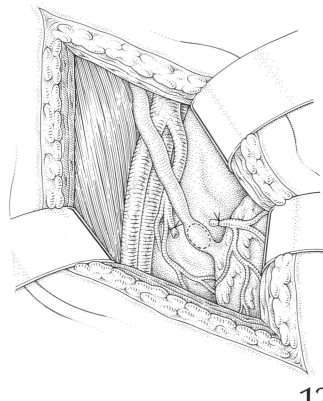

12

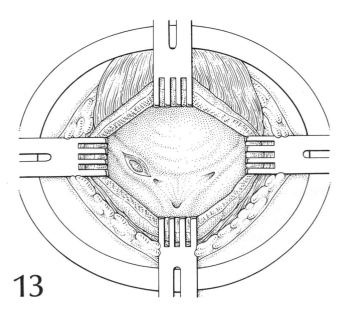

13

TRANSVESICAL URETEROLITHOTOMY

The only indication for a transvesical ureterolithotomy is if the stone is in the intramural ureter and the surgeon is unable to remove it endoscopically.

13 The bladder is exposed through a Pfannenstiel or lower midline extraperitoneal incision. A vertical vesicotomy is made and the stone is identified above the ureteric orifice. An incision is made on to the stone above the ureteric meatus and the stone removed. The ureterotomy does not need to be closed. The bladder is closed in two layers with absorbable sutures.

A drain should be left down to the site of the vesicotomy and the bladder should be drained with a urethral catheter for 1 week.

TRANSVAGINAL URETEROLITHOTOMY

In multiparous women in whom there is anterior vaginal wall descent the lowest 5 cm of the ureter can be exposed transvaginally. The operation is not suitable for stones in the intramural ureter. The stone must be palpable through the vagina.

14 With the patient in the lithotomy position the vagina is cleaned with an antiseptic solution. A weighted vaginal speculum is inserted to retract the posterior vaginal wall and the labia are sutured laterally. The cervix is held in a toothed forceps and pulled inferiorly. The full thickness of anterior vaginal wall is incised transversely, lateral to the cervix over the stone. The ureter is secured with a Babcock forceps and an incision made into it over the stone. The ureter and vaginal wall should be closed separately with interrupted absorbable sutures, and a small drain brought out through the vaginal incision.

This approach is used rarely. There is a risk of bleeding if the uterine vessels are damaged. It is impossible to remove the stone if it migrates proximally during ureteric mobilization. There is a risk of ureterovaginal fistula formation.

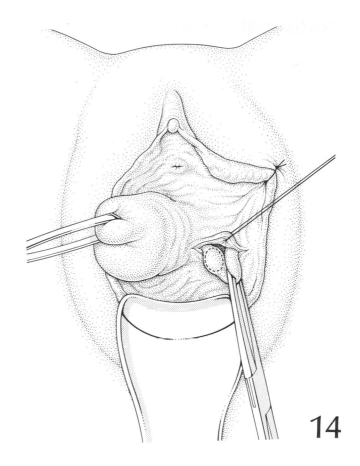

14

TRANSURETHRAL URETEROLITHOTOMY

A common site for a ureteric stone to become lodged is in the intramural ureter. If this occurs it can be difficult to pass a ureteroscope, a guidewire or a stone basket. An attempt should always be made to remove the stone endoscopically. If this fails it is reasonable to resect the anterior wall of the intramural ureter.

15 The stone can be identified cystoscopically as it bulges the intramural ureter. The resectoscope cutting loop is used to expose the stone. A ureteric catheter should be passed to check the patency of the upper ureter. If any difficulty is encountered during the operation a JJ stent should be left *in situ* for a few days.

Vesicoureteric reflux is a likely sequel to this procedure, but there is no evidence that in adults this has a harmful effect.

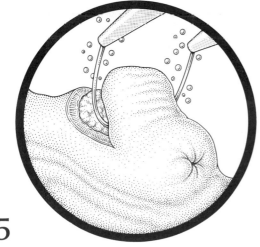

15

Postoperative care

After any open ureterolithotomy the patient usually has an intestinal ileus for 24–48 h, and intravenous fluids are required. Oral intake should be restricted until bowel sounds have returned and the patient has passed flatus.

Wound drains are shortened when any urinary leak has begun to settle, and can usually be removed on about the third day. A suction drain may provoke or perpetuate urinary leakage and should not be used.

Complications

A urinary fistula can occur and although a wound drain will keep the patient dry and comfortable there is some evidence that it may encourage a leak to continue. A drain should be shortened at the first sign of urinary leakage lessening, and removed as early as possible. Nevertheless, a fistula may arise. An expectant policy may be pursued, since fistulae will close spontaneously, providing there is no distal obstruction. Prolonged leakage can be managed by inserting a JJ stent. If it proves impossible to negotiate the site of the fistula from a cystoscopic approach then an attempt to insert a JJ stent antegradely may be made. If this is unsuccessful a percutaneous nephrostomy tube may encourage the fistula to close.

Severe bleeding may occur following removal of a stone from the lower ureter, resulting from a failure to secure the superior vesical pedicle. Such bleeding becomes obvious within the first few hours after operation: the patient must be returned to theatre and the vessel ligated.

A urinoma can arise if urinary leakage occurs once the drain is removed. Small urinomas may reabsorb spontaneously with no ill effects. Larger ones, or when there is evidence of infection, will require percutaneous drainage.

Urinary infection, particularly with *Staphylococcus*, can be associated with prolonged urinary leakage. Any urine infection must be treated early and vigorously with an appropriate antibiotic.

Ureteric stricture formation is a potential hazard after open ureterolithotomy and may be associated with poor surgical technique. Ureteric closure should not include the mucosa. If the ureter is oedematous and closure is difficult serosal sutures only should be inserted, or the ureter left to close spontaneously.

Illustrations by Philip Wilson

Retropubic prostatectomy

John P. Pryor MS, FRCS
Consultant Uroandrologist, King's College and St Peter's Hospital at The Middlesex Hospital, London, UK

History

Retropubic prostatectomy is the method of choice for removing the larger benign prostate that is causing bladder outflow obstruction. Each surgeon will have his own criteria for carrying out an open operation and this will depend upon the general condition of the patient, the experience of the surgeon and the equipment that is available to him.

The operation was first described in 1908 by Van Stockum, but its present popularity stems from the influence of Terence Millin, an Irishman who worked in London. He first exploited the retropubic route in 1945[1] and published his monograph, *Retropubic Urinary Surgery*, in 1947[2]. Retropubic prostatectomy rapidly became the method of choice for removing the benign prostate, and it 'undoubtedly yielded the most impressive results in larger subcervical adenomas where the ease of enucleation, good access to the prostatic bed and preservation of an intact bladder combined to make the mortality low and convalescence rapid'[3]. The recent development of fibre-optics, surgical diathermy and the rod lens have led to a resurgence in the use of transurethral resection and have led to a decline in the use of retropubic prostatectomy. The suggestion that late mortality is lower after retropubic prostatectomy[4] has led to renewed debate as to the merits of the two operations[5].

Principles and justification

All patients undergoing prostatectomy require preliminary cystourethroscopy, and the decision to perform a retropubic operation is made at that time in conjunction with the operative findings, the condition of the patient and the bimanual examination of the prostate when the bladder has been emptied. Urologists perform approximately 5% of prostatectomies by the retropubic route and reserve the open operation for a larger benign prostate or when it is also desirable to remove a large vesical calculus or diverticulum or to repair an inguinal hernia. A retropubic prostatectomy should not be performed if there is a concomitant bladder tumour or for a prostatic carcinoma. The size of the prostate influences the decision to perform an open operation, but other considerations, such as general fitness of the patient and the experience and equipment of the surgeon, are also important. In general, the decision not to proceed with a transurethral resection is made when the prostate is estimated to be between 40 and 100 g in size. Occasionally heavy bleeding occurs at the commencement of transurethral resection – usually in the hypertensive patient – and in these circumstances it may be wiser to proceed with an open operation.

It is rare for a patient to be too unfit for operation, but the operation is contraindicated if there is mental impairment.

Preoperative

Prophylactic antibiotics are unnecessary but any urinary tract infection should be treated with the appropriate antibiotics. A period of catheter drainage is necessary if there is evidence of an obstructive uropathy and the operation should be delayed until the blood urea level approaches normal.

Routine haematological tests should include haemoglobin estimation, blood grouping, the detection of sickle cell disease and the Australian antigen status of the patient. It is safer to have 2 units of blood available for transfusion, but there is a trend to conserve blood and only cross-match when blood is required. This necessitates the immediate availability of a full blood transfusion service within the hospital.

Active prophylaxis against pulmonary embolism is advisable when performing a retropubic prostatectomy. Intermittent calf vein compression is effective and can be applied once the decision to proceed by open operation has been made. Low-dose heparin prophylaxis is safe but requires planning before the patient is anaesthetized.

Anaesthesia

The services of a skilled anaesthetist are essential and a general or regional anaesthetic technique may be chosen. Spinal or epidural anaesthetics are particularly useful if the patient suffers with a respiratory tract disorder. Controlled hypotension is unnecessary and is best avoided as it carries a greater risk in the elderly. It is important that the abdominal musculature is relaxed and that there should be no impediment to the venous drainage such as occurs with coughing. It is essential to commence the administration of the intravenous fluids at the start of the operation, as some degree of blood loss is inevitable.

Operation

A preliminary cystoscopy should always be performed to ensure that there is no intravesical pathology and the bladder is left empty. Small papillary carcinomas of the bladder may be resected and the base fulgurated since the operation should not be performed in the presence of a tumour.

Position of patient

The patient is placed supine on the operating table with a 10° head-down tilt. The legs may also be flexed at the knee. Such a position facilitates abdominal access and also encourages venous drainage from the prostatic bed, thereby reducing haemorrhage.

Incision

The skin is thoroughly cleansed with a 10% povidone-iodine solution and the patient draped in such a way as to allow access to the penis once the prostate has been removed. The operation is performed through a transverse lower abdominal incision situated in the skin crease approximately 3 cm above the symphysis pubis. The incision is 10–15 cm long and depends upon the thickness of the abdominal wall fat. A right-handed surgeon stands on the patient's left, and performs most of the operation facing the patient's feet.

Separation of rectus muscles

1 The anterior rectus sheath is incised in the line of the skin incision and is mobilized from the underlying rectus muscles down to the pubic symphysis and upwards towards the umbilicus. It is necessary to coagulate small arteries entering the rectus sheath from the muscles. The rectus and the pyramidalis muscles are widely separated in the lower part of the incision, and it may be necessary to incise the lower part of the linea alba vertically in the upper part of the wound.

It is useful at this stage to insert a tube drain through a small incision in the midline of the lower flap of the anterior rectus sheath midway between the line of incision and the pubic symphysis. The ends of the drainage tube are clamped together with Kocher's forceps and secured to the drapes towards the patient's feet in such a way as to exert traction and obviate any subsequent need for a retractor in the inferior part of the wound.

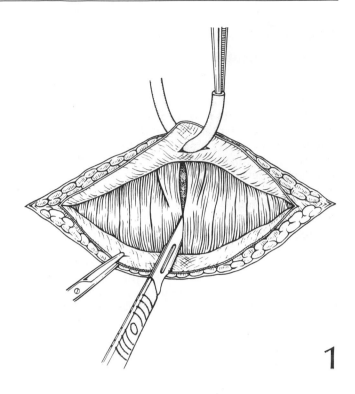

1

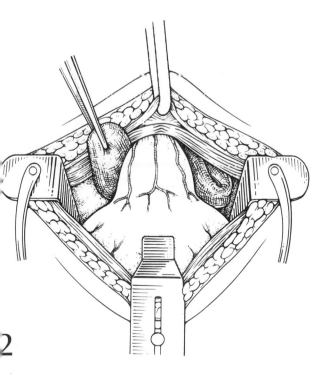

2

Exposure of anterior surface of prostate

2 The retropubic fat is gently separated to expose the bladder and prostate and the blades of a Millin self-retaining retractor are inserted. Further separation of the retropubic fat exposes the anterior surface of the prostatic capsule and any haemorrhage is controlled with diathermy. At this stage it is convenient to tuck two 10-cm gauze swabs into the retropubic space just lateral to the prostate. The third blade of the Millin retractor is introduced to retract the bladder, clearly displaying the anterior surface of the prostate and adjacent bladder wall.

Incision of prostatic capsule

3 Two stay sutures (0 chromic catgut on a curved needle) are then placed through the prostatic capsule in such a way as to occlude the vein(s) running longitudinally (a branch of the dorsal vein of the penis). The more proximal of these sutures is placed at the junction of the prostate and bladder neck. The correct situation is recognized by the longitudinal direction of the veins turning to run more laterally. These sutures are left long to facilitate identification of the incision into the prostatic capsule. A 3-cm incision is made in the prostatic capsule between the stay sutures and about 1 cm distal to the bladder neck. The incision is made through the full thickness of the capsule and stops when the white appearance of the prostate is identified. Any bleeding from the prostatic capsule should be controlled at this stage.

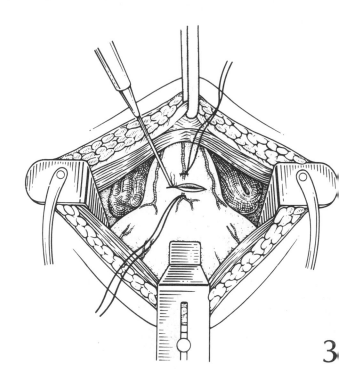

3

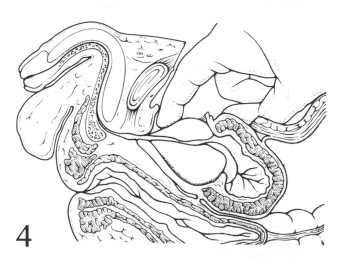

4

Plane of enucleation

4 A pair of scissors is used to commence the dista separation of the anterior surface of the prostatic adenoma from the prostatic capsule. This plane is developed by blind dissection with the pulp of the right index finger. The right lobe is freed first by separating the anterior surface, followed by the lateral and posterior surfaces from the prostatic capsule. The same procedure is repeated for the left lobe but the continuity of the urethra at the apex of the prostate is maintained. The finger dissection may be facilitated by removing the Millin retractor but this is not always necessary and the retractor should be reinserted once the dissection is complete.

Division of the urethra

5 It is possible to insert the index and middle fingers inside the prostatic capsule in such a manner as to straddle the urethra once the lateral lobes of the prostate have been freed. A pair of curved scissors is inserted inside the prostatic capsule and, guided by the position of the fingers, is used to divide the urethra cleanly in order to avoid avulsing any of the distal urethra, thereby damaging the sphincter mechanism. The scissors should be kept as vertical as possible to prevent damage to the distal part of the intrinsic urethral mechanism. It is often difficult to divide the urethra under direct vision but great care is essential at this stage of the operation if postoperative urinary incontinence is to be avoided. The lateral lobes now lie freely within the prostatic capsule.

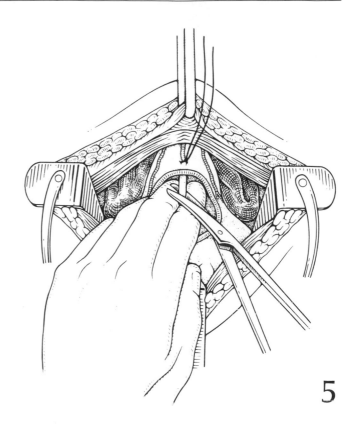

5

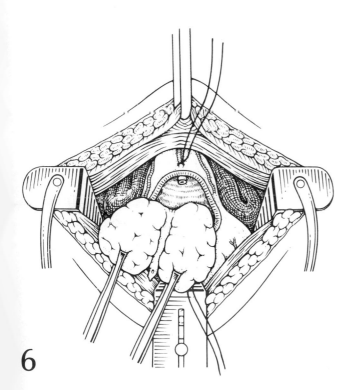

6

Dislocation of the adenoma

6 Each lateral lobe is securely gripped with a pair of vulsellum forceps and dislocated anteriorly out of the prostatic cavity. The proximal end of the divided urethra is identified and a pair of scissors placed inside the urethra, which is then divided anteriorly, together with the overlying prostatic tissue, as far as the bladder neck.

Removal of the adenoma and control of haemostasis

7 A pair of bladder neck spreaders is placed inside the bladder to define the bladder neck. The attachment of the prostate to the bladder neck is then divided by sharp dissection with a diathermy point and the prostate removed. Removal of the prostate is always accompanied by bleeding, and on rare occasions this may be profuse. Immediately the adenoma has been removed it is wise to pack the prostatic capsule with gauze swabs and control any bleeding by direct pressure.

The general status of the patient is then assessed and rapid fluid replacement given if required. The packs may then be removed and the prostatic cavity carefully inspected, remnants of prostatic adenoma excised and any bleeding vessels diathermized. It is sometimes difficult to control profuse bleeding from large veins in the prostatic capsule and in these circumstances the cavity is packed and external pressure applied with a swab in a holder for 5–10 min (timed to avoid impatience). It is neither necessary nor possible to arrest the capillary oozing from the prostatic bed; this will diminish by repacking the prostatic cavity with swabs.

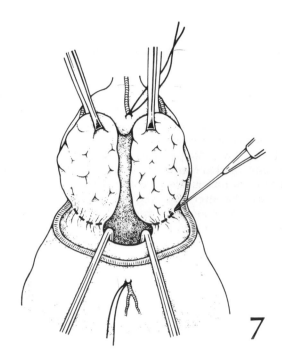

7

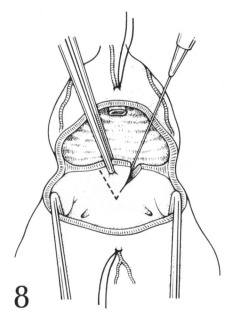

8

Excision of a wedge of bladder neck

8 Attention is next given to the bladder neck, which should be sufficiently large to admit two fingers easily. If this is not possible, a wedge is excised from the bladder neck. The ureteric orifices are first identified and the middle of the bladder neck is grasped by a pair of forceps. A V-shaped wedge is then excised as shown.

Anchoring the bladder mucosa

9 It is unnecessary to suture the bladder mucosa to the prostatic bed except in those patients where the prostate extended beneath the trigone. In these circumstances it is useful to anchor the mucosa to the floor of the prostatic cavity with two or three 2/0 chromic catgut sutures. This technique facilitates catheterization and is of particular benefit should the urethral catheter fall out or require replacement. Persistent haemorrhage from the bladder neck may be controlled by suturing, and in these circumstances the bladder mucosa may be anchored with the same suture.

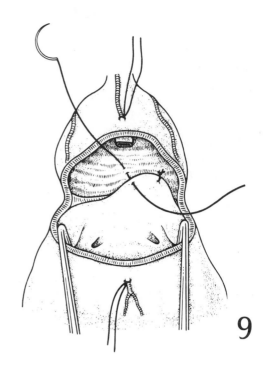

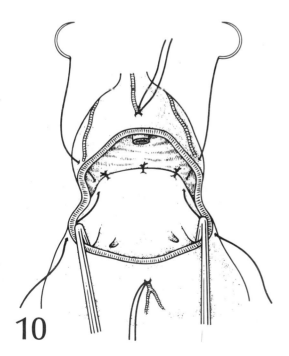

Insertion of catheter

10 Any swabs remaining within the prostatic capsule are removed and a marker suture (0 chromic catgut) is placed at each lateral corner of the capsular incision. These sutures act as a guide for the ends of the incision but are also haemostatic. The needle is inserted from without into the cavity of the bladder, then through the bladder mucosa and bladder neck into the prostatic cavity and finally through the prostatic capsule. Each of these sutures is tied and left long and a 20-Fr three-way Foley-type catheter is passed into the bladder. It is preferable that the catheter should be fairly rigid and have large eyes. It is seldom necessary to insert a suprapubic catheter into the bladder.

Closure of prostatic capsule

11 The prostatic capsule is closed with a continuous 0 chromic catgut suture which arrests any bleeding from the prostatic capsule and also ensures a watertight closure. It is easier to insert this suture by taking each edge of the capsule with separate bites of the needle. There may be some leakage through the prostatic capsule but it is seldom worthwhile attempting to insert any further sutures.

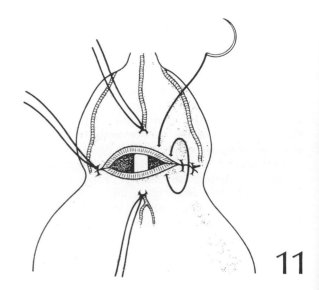

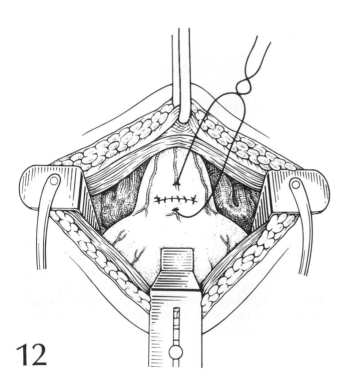

Final stages

12 At this stage it is useful to tie together the two initial stay sutures which were placed into the prostatic capsule. The bladder is then washed out to ensure that there is free catheter drainage. The two swabs which were placed on either side of the prostate at the start of the operation are removed and a final check is made for any bleeding from the vessels in the retropubic fat.

Wound closure

13a, b The tubular wound drain, which, inserted at the commencement of the procedure, has acted as a retractor throughout, is then unclipped and placed down to the suture line in the prostatic capsule. The rectus muscles are approximated with interrupted 0 chromic catgut sutures and the anterior rectus sheath is closed with a similar suture material. This may conveniently be a continuous suture line. The subcutaneous tissues are loosely approximated with plain catgut sutures and the skin closed with well-spaced interrupted sutures. At the conclusion of the operation the catheter is once again checked to make sure that it is draining freely and is then connected to a closed urine collection apparatus. The retropubic drain is also connected to a closed collection bag.

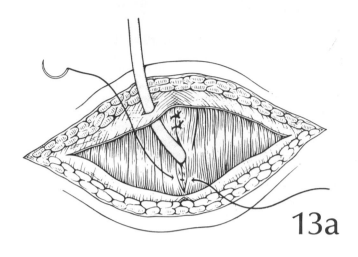

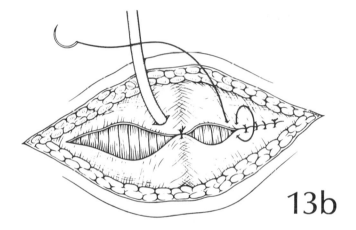

Additional procedures

It is often convenient to repair an inguinal hernia at the time of a retropubic prostatectomy, but this should be deferred until the prostatectomy has been completed safely. Vasectomy is no longer performed in order to reduce the risk of epididymitis

Postoperative care

Blood transfusion is unnecessary, except in the very large gland (greater than 250 g). Any fluid loss during the course of the operation should have been replaced by intravenous fluids and these are usually given to ensure a high urine output. In elderly patients, or in those with cardiac abnormalities, it is often wise to give frusemide, 40 mg, by intramuscular injection every 12 h to minimize the risk of cardiac failure and to prevent the occurrence of clot retention. This technique is particularly useful when there has been profuse bleeding at the time of operation. The use of a three-way catheter will also help obviate the need for a bladder washout. The urine should always be collected in a closed drainage system as this is helpful in lessening the risk of urinary infection. Careful attention should be given to cleansing the penis around the catheter in the postoperative period.

The patient is encouraged to drink at an early stage and intravenous fluids are unnecessary after the first 24 h. Early mobilization and physiotherapy are important in the prevention of pulmonary embolism and the retropubic drain is usually removed 48 h after the operation. The urethral catheter is removed when there is no longer any risk of clot retention – usually between the third and fifth day.

Complications

The general risks of myocardial ischaemia, chest infection and pulmonary embolism are ever present with an elderly group of patients undergoing surgery. These risks may be minimized by the skills of the supporting team of anaesthetists, nurses and physiotherapists. The risk of a urinary tract infection may be lessened if preoperative catheterization is avoided, and by the judicious use of antibiotics.

Prostatorectal fistulae have been reported following retropubic prostatectomy but tend to occur when the operation has been performed for an unsuspected carcinoma of the prostate. Urethral strictures are relatively uncommon after a retropubic prostatectomy but bladder neck stenosis occurs in 1% of patients. Regrowth of the prostate may occur but patients rarely present less than 10 years after the retropubic operation. The regrowth may be due to the occurrence of a prostatic cancer even though the histology of the original gland showed benign prostatic hyperplasia.

Urinary incontinence is common immediately after the removal of the urethral catheter but fortunately this only persists in approximately 1% of patients.

References

1. Millin T. Retropubic prostatectomy: a new extravesical technique, report on 20 cases. *Lancet* 1945; ii: 693–6.

2. Millin T. *Retropubic Urinary Surgery*. Edinburgh: E & S Livingstone, 1947.

3. Sandrey JG. Retropubic prostatectomy. In: Innes Williams, D, ed. *Operative Surgery: Urology*. 3rd edn. London: Butterworths, 1977: 253–61.

4. Roos NP, Wennberg JE, Malenka DJ *et al*. Mortality and reoperation after open and transurethral resection of the prostrate for benign prostatic hyperplasia. *N Engl J Med* 1989; 320: 1120–4.

5. Neal DE. Prostatectomy – an open or closed case. *Br J Urol* 1990; 66: 449–54.

Illustrations by Marc Donon

Testicular torsion

Su-Anna M. Boddy BSc, FRCS
Senior Registrar in Paediatric Surgery, St George's Hospital, London, UK

N. P. Madden MA, FRCS
Consultant Paediatric Surgeon, Westminster Children's Hospital, London, UK

Torsion of the testis must be the first consideration in any child or young adult with acute scrotal pain. There are two peaks in the incidence: in the perinatal period and between the ages of 10 and 25 years.

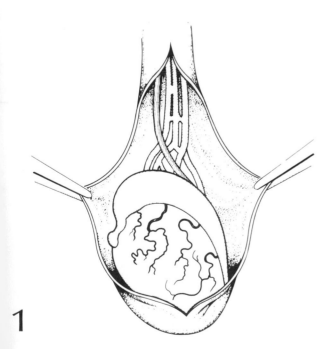

1

Diagnosis

Neonatal torsion

In the neonate the torsion is extravaginal. An intra-uterine or neonatal torsion may first present as an impalpable testis. If a baby is born with a non-tender unilateral scrotal lump, surgical exploration is unnecessary. Exploration is indicated if the diagnosis is uncertain or the testis painful. There is controversy as to whether the contralateral testis needs to be fixed, since it is unlikely that the contralateral testis is at risk of torsion and there is a real risk of damaging the testis by operation.

Intravaginal torsion of the testis

1 If the tunica vaginalis invests the whole of the epididymis and the distal part of the spermatic cord, the testis is in effect suspended in the scrotal cavity like a bell clapper and is free to rotate within the tunica vaginalis. This situation may be indicated by an abnormal horizontal lie of the testis. Testicular maldescent may also predispose to torsion. The torsion is usually towards the midline septum, that is, the right testis rotates in a clockwise direction and the left in an anticlockwise direction from the examiner's point of view.

Recurrent torsion

There is a history of episodic testicular pain, with or without swelling of the testis. On examination the testis may lie more transversely in the scrotum, but may otherwise appear completely normal. However, the history alone indicates that both testes should be fixed by early surgery.

Differential diagnosis

Torsion of a testicular appendage

Torsion of a testicular appendage presents at 4–10 years of age. Careful palpation will reveal a tender nodule associated with the upper pole of the testis; the lower part of the testis is not tender. On transillumination this nodule may appear as a dark spot. If the diagnosis of torsion of a testicular appendage can be made, neither hospital observation nor operation are mandatory.

Acute epididymo-orchitis

Unilateral epididymo-orchitis is common in adults but rare in children, in whom it is likely to be associated with infection or anomaly of the urinary tract.

Mumps orchitis

This rarely, if ever, occurs before puberty and appears within 3 days to 1 week after the onset of parotitis. It is usually bilateral.

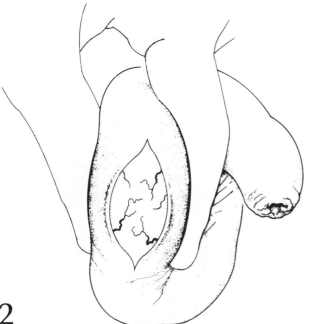

2

Idiopathic scrotal oedema

In this condition the erythema and swelling of the scrotal skin spread into the groin, perineum or base of the penis. Pain is not a major feature. The skin may be tender but the underlying testis and cord are normal. The peak incidence is at 4–6 years of age and the only treatment necessary is reassurance.

Incarcerated inguinal hernia

The symptoms and signs of torsion of an undescended testis closely resemble those of an incarcerated inguinal hernia – a painful tender swelling in the groin – but are associated with an empty scrotum. Since early surgical exploration is mandatory for both conditions differentiation is, perhaps, unnecessary.

Operation

Timing

In most cases the diagnosis of acute torsion of the testis must be made clinically unless techniques such as Doppler ultrasonography or radioisotope scanning are immediately available. Any delay in operation, once the diagnosis is suspected, will prejudice the survival of the testis.

2 The testis is delivered from the scrotum through a vertical incision over its longitudinal axis. The skin, dartos fascia and tunica vaginalis are all incised. As the tunica vaginalis is incised the haemoserous fluid of the secondary hydrocoele is released.

3 The testis is delivered from the tunica vaginalis and the cord untwisted.

The tunica albuginea is incised in order to release the pressure on the underlying tubules and to assess viability.

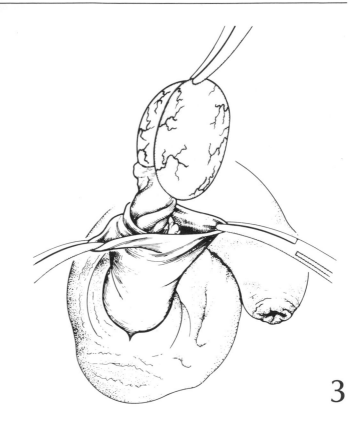

3

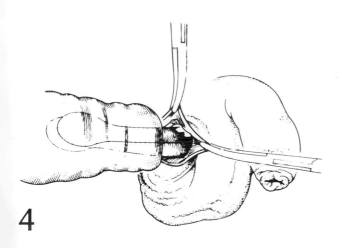

4

4 The untwisted testis is wrapped in moist, warm swabs and its colour carefully observed. While waiting to confirm whether perfusion has been re-established, the contralateral testis may be fixed.

Conservation or removal of the testis

If the testis is completely black and necrotic and is deemed non-viable then it should be removed. The spermatic cord is ligated within the scrotum with a strong absorbable suture and the testis removed. However, if there is any question that some perfusion might be re-established then the testis should be conserved. It is imperative to fix the contralateral viable testis.

Fixation of the testis

5 Testes should be fixed by three fine non-absorbable monofilament sutures such as 6/0 polypropylene. These should be placed between the tunica albuginea and the lateral wall of the scrotal cavity, at the upper and lower poles of the testis and at the equator.

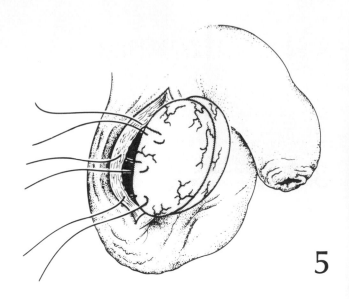

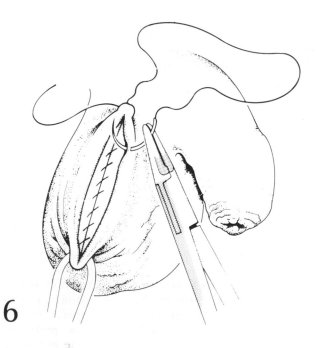

6 The wound is closed in layers using continuous 5/0–3/0 chromic catgut sutures, depending on the age of the patient. A scrotal support should be applied at the end of the operation.

Illustrations by Marc Donon

Orchidopexy

N. P. Madden MA, FRCS
Consultant Paediatric Surgeon, Westminster Children's Hospital, London, UK

Su-Anna M. Boddy BSc, FRCS
Senior Registrar in Paediatric Surgery, St George's Hospital, London, UK

Undescended testes occur in 21% of premature and 2.7% of full-term infants. The testes often spontaneously descend during the first year of life and by 1 year of age all but 0.2% of testes will have descended into the scrotum.

Three types of abnormal testicular position are recognized.

A *retractile testis* is pulled up into the inguinal canal by the cremasteric muscle. The testis is normal, will lie spontaneously in the scrotum when the cremaster relaxes, and can be coaxed well down into the scrotum by gentle manipulation from the groin. A retractile testis does not need orchidopexy, but should be kept under annual review until the hormonal drive at puberty ensures that it stays in the scrotum.

An *ectopic testis* has descended beyond the external ring but lies outside the scrotum, commonly in the superficial inguinal pouch but also in the perineum or prepubically. An ectopic testis requires a formal orchidopexy.

An *undescended testis* may be located anywhere along the line of descent from the kidney to the scrotum. If, on examination, the testis is palpable but incompletely descended, then it requires a formal orchidopexy. If, however, the testis is impalpable a laparoscopy should be performed to determine whether the testis has undergone intra-abdominal torsion, or whether it is intra-abdominal[1]. There is a 10–25% risk of malignancy in an intra-abdominal testis and it is probably best treated by orchidectomy, if the contralateral testis is normal. In the case of bilateral intra-abdominal testes specialized procedures such as Fowler–Stephens or microvascular transfer of the testis are required[2].

Age at orchidopexy

Degenerative changes commence in the undescended testis during the second or third year of life, so the optimal age for orchidopexy is about 2 years.

Preoperative

Anaesthesia

The operation is performed under general anaesthetic. This is usefully supplemented by local anaesthetic with bupivacaine which can be infiltrated into the wound at the time of operation. A caudal anaesthetic may be preferred, particularly in bilateral cases.

Skin preparation

The patient is laid supine with the legs slightly separated. The skin is prepared with povidone-iodine from the level of the umbilicus down to mid-thigh, being sure to include the scrotum and perineum.

Operation

A transverse incision is made in the skin crease overlying the appropriate inguinal canal.

1 The subcutaneous tissues are divided, taking care to control the superficial epigastric vessels with diathermy. The testis may be encountered superficial to the inguinal canal or at the external ring, in which case the gubernaculum should be divided with diathermy and the testis brought into the wound in order to expose the external ring. The external oblique is incised in the line of its fibres. Fine artery forceps are placed on either side of the incision, which is extended to the external inguinal ring, taking care not to divide the ilioinguinal nerve.

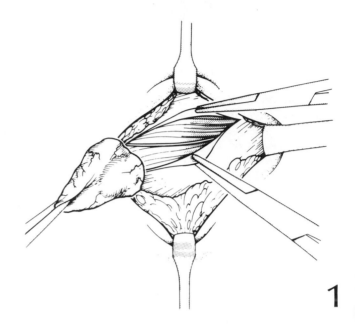

1

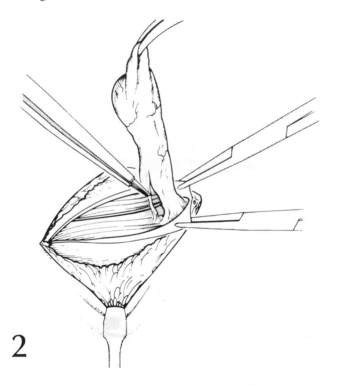

2

2 After division of the gubernaculum a fine artery forceps is placed on the lower pole of the testis on either the tunica vaginalis or the tunica albuginea. The testis and spermatic cord are mobilized, taking care to control the cremasteric vessels with bipolar diathermy as these frequently cause irritating bleeding.

3 A retractor is placed under the fibres of the internal oblique as they arch over the internal inguinal ring and a fine artery forceps is placed near the proximal end of the processus vaginalis, which lies superficial to the vas and vessels. The processus vaginalis may be completely patent or simply represented by the slight tenting of the peritoneum when the spermatic cord is put under tension. If a fully patent processus vaginalis is present it may be very fine and effectively surround the vas and vessels, making dissection difficult.

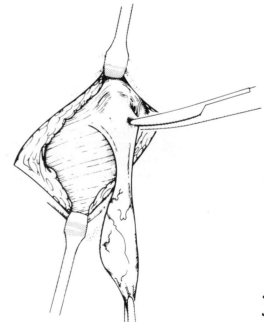

3

4 Initially an attempt should be made to dissect the vas and vessels from the processus vaginalis without opening it. This dissection should be carried out as distally as possible to prevent the processus from being accidentally torn deep to the internal ring. Great gentleness is required when dissecting adjacent to the vas and vessels, which must not be compressed.

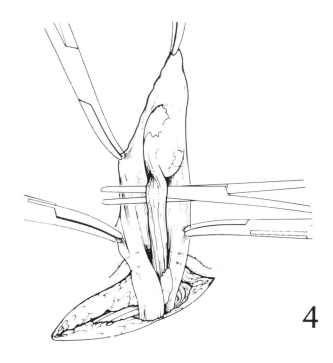

4

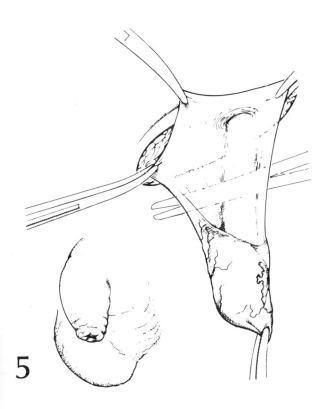

5

5 If the processus vaginalis is inadvertently opened placing fine artery forceps on its margins and putting tension on these forceps facilitates dissection of the vas and vessels from the deep layer of the processus, by blunt dissection with a fine artery forceps.

6 Once the processus vaginalis is secured in a single artery forceps it is divided and separated from the vas and vessels by blunt dissection as far as the internal ring. It is transfixed with fine monofilament absorbable suture such as 4/0 polydioxanone (PDS; Ethicon, Edinburgh, UK).

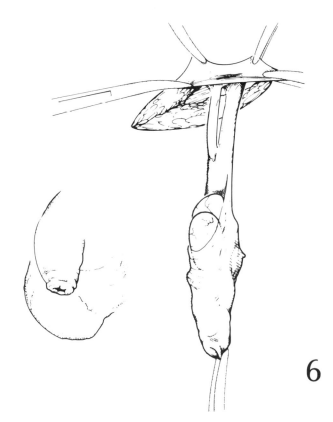

6

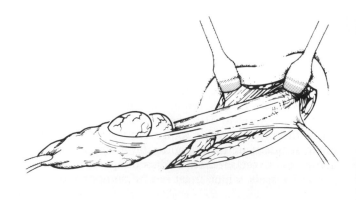

7 A retractor is then placed into the internal ring, retracting the neck of the sac and the arching fibres of internal oblique superiorly and laterally. The testicular vessels and vas are then put under tension by drawing the testis inferiorly and medially. Fibrous adhesions will thus be identified, and these need to be divided carefully, avoiding damage to the testicular vessels and vas. (If there is inadequate length of vas and vessels, the Jones preperitoneal approach should be considered[3].)

7

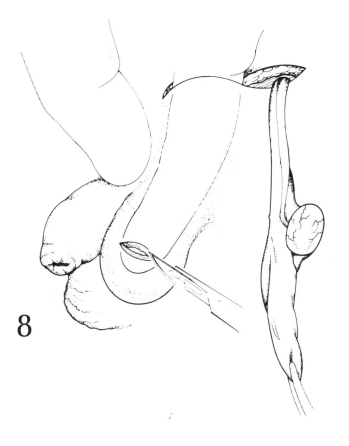

8

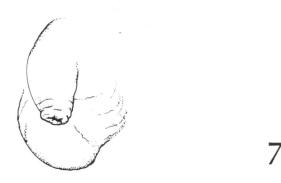

8 If the distal tunica vaginalis is still intact around the testis it should be incised and the testis everted from it. Once sufficient length of vas and vessels has been gained to allow the testis to be brought into the scrotum, a finger is passed along the line of the inguinal canal and into the scrotum. An incision is made in the upper half of the scrotum onto this finger, enough to allow adequate separation of the skin but leaving intact a significant thickness of the underlying fascia.

9 A fine artery forceps is then passed retrogradely up via the scrotal incision into the inguinal wound as the finger is withdrawn from this track. This forceps is used to draw the testis down into the scrotum, ensuring that the vas and vessels are not twisted. The scrotal fascia is gently teased open to allow the testis to emerge through the scrotal wound and this fascia will have the effect of 'buttonholing' the testis in the scrotum.

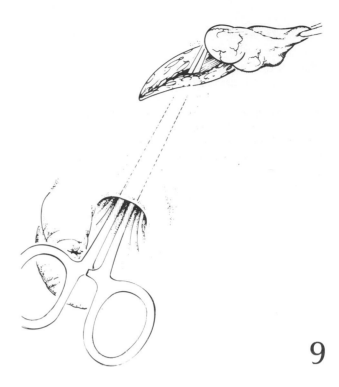

9

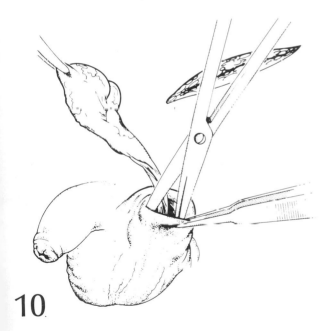

10

10 The testis is drawn superiorly onto the abdominal wall and a fine-toothed forceps placed on the inferior margin of the scrotal skin wound. By lifting the edge of the scrotal skin up an adequate scrotal pouch can be made by blunt dissection. If the testis has been brought down under some tension it may be desirable to pull some fascia from the base of this pouch into the wound so that a single fine absorbable suture can fix the lower pole of the testis to this fascia. The testis is then placed in the scrotal pouch with the remnants of the tunica vaginalis.

The scrotal skin is closed with continuous or interrupted 4/0 chromic catgut. The inguinal incision is closed with a fine absorbable monofilament suture to the external oblique aponeurosis, starting medially to avoid trapping the nerve. At this stage both wounds may be infiltrated with 0.25% bupivacaine. Scarpa's fascia may be closed with continuous or interrupted fine absorbable sutures. The skin is closed with fine absorbable subcuticular sutures such as 5/0 Vicryl (Ethicon, Edinburgh, UK).

Postoperative care

The operation can usually be performed as a day case, and the child discharged home with paracetamol elixir for analgesia, but older children may require an overnight stay. Contact sports and bicycle riding should be avoided for 3 weeks.

The position and viability of the testis should be assessed 3 weeks and 6 months after operation.

References

1. Boddy S-AM, Corkery JJ, Gornall P. The place of laparoscopy in the management of the impalpable testis. *Br J Surg* 1985; 72: 981–19.

2. Boddy S-AM, Gordon AC, Thomas DFM, Browning FSC. Experience with Fowler Stephens and microvascular procedures in the management of intra-abdominal testes. *Br J Urol* 1991; 68: 199–202.

3. Jones PF, Bayley FH. An abdominal extraperitoneal approach for the difficult orchidopexy. *Br J Surg* 1979; 66: 14–18.

Further reading

de Muinck Keizer-Schrama SMPF, Hazebroek FWJ. *The Treatment of Cryptorchidism: Why How When; Clinical Studies in Prepubertal Boys.* Alblasserdam: Decor Davids, 1986.

Hydrocoele and spermatocoele

Peter H. Lord *OBE*, MChir, FRCS
Formerly Consultant Surgeon, Wycombe General Hospital, High Wycombe, UK

Principles and justification

A hydrocoele may be primary and idiopathic or it may be secondary to an underlying condition affecting the testicle or epididymis. Primary hydrocoele can be treated by repeated aspiration, by aspiration and instillation of a sclerosant, or by surgery.

Repeated aspiration was accepted practice 50 years ago, but is now normally reserved for the very elderly and infirm patient with limited expectation of life. Apart from the inconvenience of repeated aspiration, there is a recurrent risk of infection or haematoma, and the tunica vaginalis tends to become thickened and is eventually unsuitable for the other forms of treatment.

Aspiration and injection of sclerosant is widely practised. The sclerosants used include phenol[1,2], ethanolamine oleate[3], sodium tetradecyl sulphate[4] and tetracycline[5,6]. Some authors report a high degree of success with a 95% cure rate[4], while others report a higher failure rate[6,7].

The problems that may be encountered are failure to cure, the need for more than one treatment, inflammation with or without infection, the appearance of multilocular cysts[8], and pain lasting several days, occasionally severe. The obvious advantage, particularly with a successful case, is that the patient is entirely ambulatory, and the treatment is rapid and inexpensive.

The plication operation to be described is a simple procedure. Cure of the hydrocoele is achieved in all cases. There is no haematoma if the procedure is carried out correctly. Complications, such as infection, are extremely rare. The patients are reasonably comfortable postoperatively and the procedure is normally carried out as a day-case under general or local anaesthesia[9].

There are few disadvantages to the plication operation, and they are outweighed by the fact that during the procedure the surgeon holds the testicle in his hand, and he can be entirely confident that the hydrocoele is idiopathic, and that there is no underlying pathology.

Usually the differentiation between a hydrocoele and a spermatocoele is not difficult in that in the spermatocoele the cyst lies above the testis and clinically it can be felt to be separate from the testis, whereas in hydrocoele the testis lies within the fluid. If the spermatocoele is large, the differential diagnosis may be difficult, but can be helped by transillumination in a blacked out room. Fortunately, even when an incorrect diagnosis is made, the appropriate procedure of the two to be described can be selected without difficulty once the operation has begun.

Operations

PLICATION OPERATION FOR HYDROCOELE

It is important to stress that the complete hydrocoele is not delivered out of the scrotum. The incision is made into the hydrocoele and the testis is delivered by turning the hydrocoele inside out. If any attempt is made to deliver the intact hydrocoele out of the scrotum some degree of haematoma is almost inevitable. Often the haematoma is large and causes considerable morbidity. In the plication operation there should be virtually no bleeding, and there should never be a postoperative haematoma.

Incision

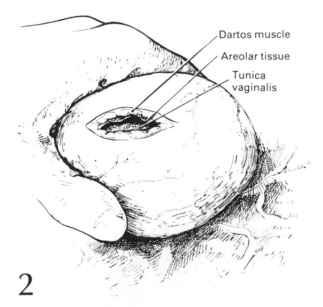

1 After the usual skin preparation and towelling, the hydrocoele should be grasped in such a way as to put the scrotum on the stretch at the point of incision. This skin tension compresses the scrotal skin vessels and the incision is virtually bloodless. In order to achieve this skin tension the surgeon, if right-handed, stands on the patient's right and grasps the hydrocoele with the left hand in such a way as to stretch the skin on the surface. The grip is maintained until stage three of the procedure when haemostatic control is taken over by the Allis' forceps. The left-handed surgeon would stand on the patient's left and grasp the scrotum with the right hand.

The direction of the incision should be determined by the position of the small vessels which can be seen through the skin, and orientated to avoid them. The position of the incision is determined by the position of the testis in the hydrocoele. The aim should be to incise the tunica vaginalis at the point furthest from the testis.

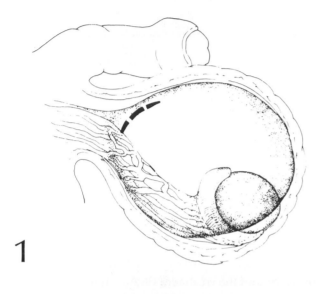

Dartos muscle
Areolar tissue
Tunica vaginalis

2 The tension on the skin is maintained while an incision is made large enough for the delivery of the testis, about 5 cm. The incision is deepened cautiously to go through skin, dartos muscle and areolar tissue, first with the knife and then with the small curved scissors, avoiding damage to the tunica vaginalis itself, as this should not be opened until the next stage of the operation has been achieved.

3a–c

Six Allis' forceps are applied, three to each side of the incision; in each case one blade of the Allis' forceps is slipped under the incised tissues, closed, and then turned over. When all six are in position, the divided vessels are controlled, and there should be no further bleeding during the procedure.

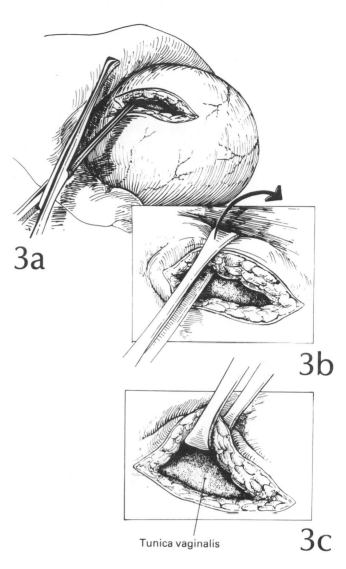

3a

3b

Tunica vaginalis

3c

4a

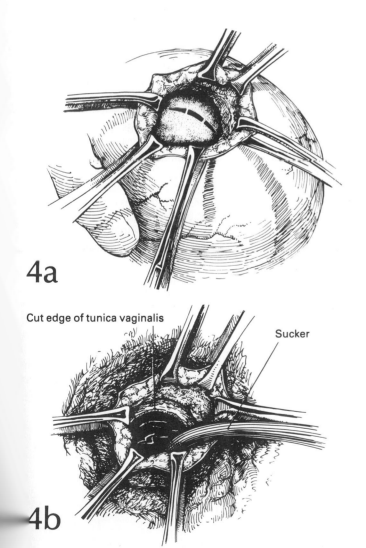

Cut edge of tunica vaginalis

Sucker

4a, b

An incision is made in the tunica vaginalis with the aspiration sucker ready to remove the fluid and keep the operation site dry.

4b

5 The incision in the tunica vaginalis is also enlarged to 5 cm. The testis is pushed up from below, exteriorized and held in the air. If the incision was made in the correct position, the testis will have a symmetrical curtain of tunica vaginalis hanging below it.

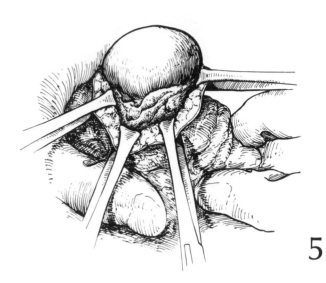

5

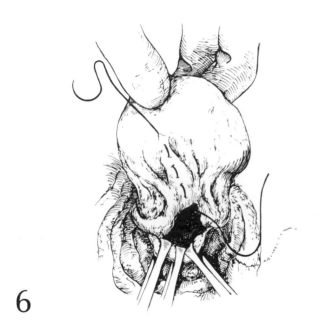

6

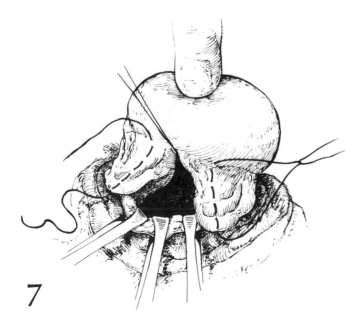

7

6 The curtain of tunica vaginalis must now be plicated to gather it up into a little ruff, which will lie along the mediastinum testis. This results in the testis being returned to the scrotum no longer covered by tunica vaginalis, so that no further hydrocoele can form. The plication sutures run from the cut edge of the tunica upwards to the mediastinum testis.

The suture material used for this plication is 3/0 polyglycolic acid suture (Dexon; Davis and Geck, Gosport, UK) or Vicryl (Ethicon, Edinburgh, UK). This material is much preferred to catgut. Catgut is a foreign protein which is removed by an inflammatory response. Polyglycolic acid is a polymer that hydrolyses at body temperature when moist, to form glycolic acid, a normal constituent of the body. There is almost no reaction by the tissues to this suture material which quietly fades away.

7 Eight or ten sutures are normally required. They lie parallel to each other. They may be inserted and left untied, secured by artery forceps until all are in place, and then finally all tied in succession, but it is equally satisfactory to tie each plication suture as it is inserted. This means that the tunica has to be picked up from within the folds caused by the previous stitch using fine-toothed forceps.

8 When all the plication sutures have been tied, the testis can be returned to the scrotum. This is the most difficult part of the operation, as there is no space within the scrotum to receive the testis now that the tunica sac has been obliterated. The areolar tissue in the scrotum has to stretch to accommodate the testis, and this is achieved if the six Allis' forceps are held apart and the testis is gently squeezed back into the scrotum. Once it is inside, the edges of the incision come together easily.

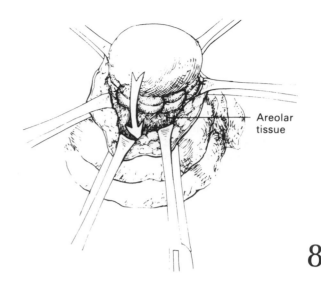

Areolar tissue

8

Wound closure

9 The incision is closed in two layers. First a Lane's forceps is applied to each end of the incision, and these are held apart to stretch the incision line. The first pair of Allis' forceps can now be removed and using the fine-toothed forceps the dartos is retrieved on each side and brought together with an interrupted 3/0 Dexon suture. A row of interrupted sutures is needed. They should be quite close together as they are taking over the haemostatic function previously performed by the Allis' forceps. As the row of sutures is put in, the Allis' forceps are progressively removed. It is tempting to close this layer with a continuous suture. This is inadvisable, as if the suture is too tight it will cause necrosis of the muscle and delay healing.

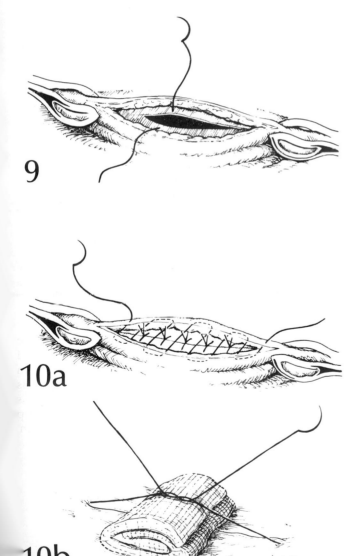

9

10a

10b

10a, b Finally the skin edges are brought together by a continuous subcuticular Dexon suture. The two ends of this suture are tied across a gauze or sponge pad which acts as a dressing.

OPERATION FOR SPERMATOCOELE (EPIDIDYMAL CYST)

When a spermatocoele forms, it arises as a tiny cyst in the head of the epididymis which gradually increases in size. As it does so, it carries its own blood supply with it and pushes aside the areolar tissue of the scrotum. It therefore follows that there is a plane of separation between the wall of the cyst and the surrounding scrotal tissue. To remove this cyst successfully that plane of cleavage must be found and exploited, as it is entirely bloodless. This bloodless plane may no longer exist if there have been attempts at treatment by aspiration or injection of sclerosants.

11a, b As with a hydrocoele, the scrotum is grasped with the left hand for a right-handed operator, and a small incision of 2 cm is made through the skin of the scrotum avoiding the vessels that can be seen there, and Allis' forceps are applied as before, one each side of the incision.

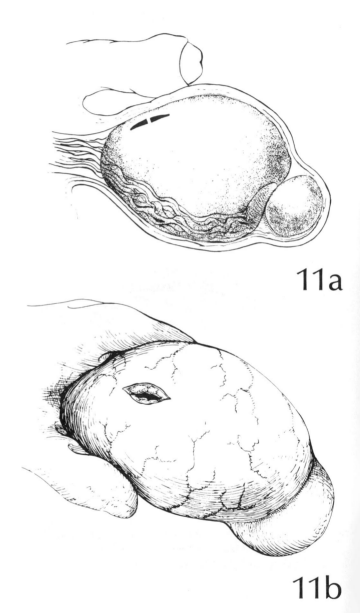

11a

11b

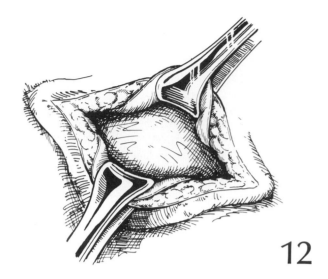

12 Using blunt dissection, the areolar tissue is pushed aside until the blue-looking shiny surface of the spermatocoele presents in the floor of the wound. This part of the operation is not easy and has to be done carefully, as it is important to avoid opening the cyst unintentionally.

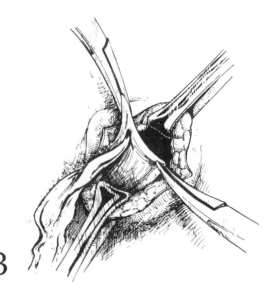

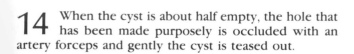

13 Once the shiny bluish surface of the cyst has been found, the areolar tissue should be pushed aside over a small area. Finally, the cyst is grasped in artery forceps and at the same time a small incision is made to let out some of the fluid.

14 When the cyst is about half empty, the hole that has been made purposely is occluded with an artery forceps and gently the cyst is teased out.

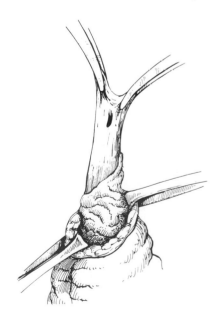

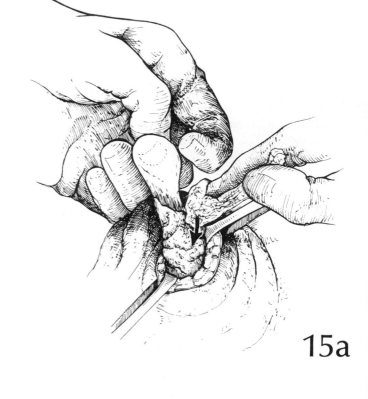

15a

15a, b To do this, the areolar tissue has to be pushed away from the cyst wall either using a swab or by lifting it away with fine-toothed forceps. As the cyst begins to leave the scrotum so does some of the fluid that has been left within the cyst. The presence of this fluid greatly aids the dissection, so care should be taken not to breach the wall of the cyst, and if it is inadvertently opened a further artery forceps should be clamped across the hole. The cyst is lax because half of the fluid has been removed and thus it can be completely delivered from the scrotum without provoking any bleeding.

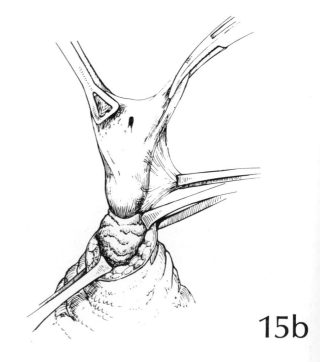

15b

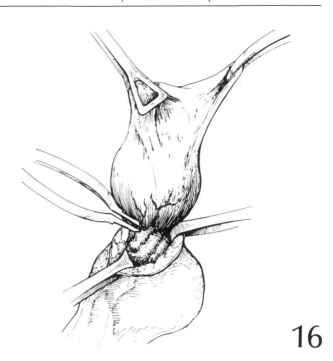

16 The cyst is then held up and the vessels that originate in the head of the epididymis and supply the wall of the cyst can be clearly seen and dealt with either by diathermy or by clamping with artery forceps and tying with Dexon.

16

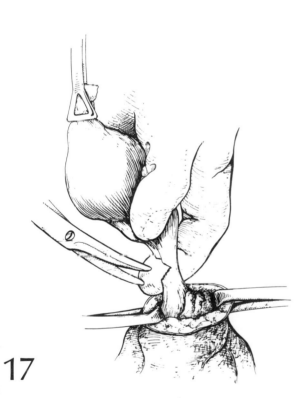

17

17 Once this blood supply has been controlled the cyst can be removed.

18 Lane's forceps are applied at each end of the wound and closure can be in two layers as described for hydrocoele, or more simply by three interrupted Dexon sutures taking skin and dartos muscle. These can be removed on the fifth or sixth postoperative day or left to fall away as the suture hydrolyses.

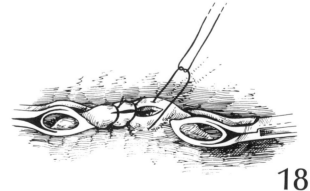

18

Postoperative care

The patient should wear a suspensory bandage for comfort. He can bathe the following day, but should be instructed to dry the wound by gently pressing with a clean towel, or by using a hair dryer. The sponge dressing used after operation for hydrocoele can be removed on the fifth, sixth or seventh postoperative day, and the Dexon subcuticular stitch can be cut flush with the skin and left to hydrolyse.

References

1. Maloney GE. Comparison of results of treatment of hydrocoele and epididymal cysts by surgery and injection. *BMJ* 1975; iii: 478–9.

2. Nash JR. Sclerotherapy for hydrocoele and epididymal cysts. *Br J Surg* 1979; 66: 289–90.

3. Hellström P, Tammela T, Kontturi M, Lukkarinen O. Ethanolamine oleate as a sclerosant for testicular hydrocoeles and epididymal cysts. *Br J Urol* 1988; 62: 445–8.

4. Macfarlane JR. Sclerosant therapy for hydrocoeles and epididymal cysts. *Br J Urol* 1983; 55: 81–2.

5. Kaye KW, Lange PH, Fraley EE. Spermatic cord block in urologic surgery. *J Urol* 1982; 128: 720–1.

6. Badenoch DF, Fowler CG, Jenkins BJ, Roberts JV, Tiptaft RC. Aspiration and instillation of tetracycline in the treatment of testicular hydrocoele. *Br J Urol* 1987; 59: 172–3.

7. Thomson H, Odell M. Sclerosant treatment for hydrocoeles and epididymal cysts. *BMJ* 1979; ii: 704.

8. Rencken RK, Bornman MS, Reif S. Multilocular hydrocoele after sclerotherapy. *Br J Urol* 1988; 62: 92–3.

9. Kaye KW, Clayman RV, Lange PH. Outpatient hydrocoele and spermatocoele repair under local anaesthesia. *J Urol* 1983; 130: 269–71.

Further reading

Blandy J. Surgery of the testicle. In: *Operative Urology*. Oxford: Blackwell Scientific, 1978: 226–42.

Hellström P, Malinen L, Kontturi M. Sclerotherapy for hydroceles and epididymal cysts with ethanolamine oleate. *Ann Chir Gynaecol Col* 1986; 75: 51–4.

Lord PH. A bloodless operation for the radical cure of idiopathic hydrocoele. *Br J Surg* 1964; 51: 914–16.

Lord PH. A bloodless operation for spermatocoele or cyst of the epididymis. *Br J Surg* 1970; 57: 641–4.

Rencken RK, Bornman MS, Reif S, Olivier I. Comparative trial of sclerotherapy for hydrocoeles. *Br J Urol* 1990; 65: 382–4.

Sharlip ID. Surgery of scrotal contents. *Urol Clin North Am* 1987; 14: 145–8.

Circumcision

J. P. Blandy MA, DM, MCh, FRCS, FACS
Professor of Urology, The Royal London Hospital, London, UK

History

The records of circumcision antedate history[1-4], and this ancient ritual mutilation is a subject of intense anthropological interest. The majority of circumcisions are today still done for ritual reasons rather than for any medical indication.

Principles and justification

Indications

There are a number of important surgical indications for circumcision. If a male cannot retract the prepuce to keep the glans clean and free from smegma, infection is liable to lead to recurrent balanitis. From time to time the prepuce is affected by balanitis xerotica obliterans – a thickening of the skin accompanied by contracture, which leads to slowly worsening phimosis. Not only may this be complicated by secondary balanitis, but it may also cause pain on intercourse. Occasionally, a very tight prepuce becomes trapped behind the glans leading to paraphimosis, which becomes increasingly difficult to reduce the longer it is neglected.

Certain diseases are more likely to affect the uncircumcised penis, notably herpes virus infection, chancroid and primary syphilis, and there is plausible evidence that the human immunodeficiency virus finds an easier entry through the delicate moist skin of the uncircumcised penis than through the dry keratinized skin of the circumcised one[5-7]. A case can be made for offering circumcision to every male homosexual practising buggery.

Preoperative

In the presence of severe suppurative balanitis, it is wise to perform a dorsal slit to permit drainage, give antibiotics and allow the inflammation to subside for a few days. In most cases this is unnecessary; most cases of balanitis of this type do better with an immediate circumcision.

Anaesthesia

Local anaesthesia may be provided by 1% lignocaine without adrenaline in a ring around the base of the penis. Most adults and children prefer a general anaesthetic.

Operation

Incision

A clean cut with the knife leaves a clean skin edge without the ragged outline left by scissors.

1 The incision through the outer surface of the prepuce is made to overlie the corona glandis; this avoids removing too much skin.

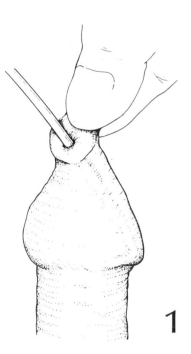

1

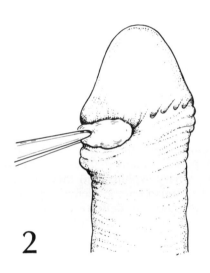

2

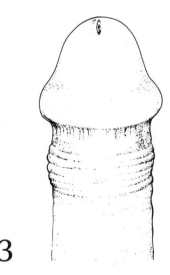

3

2, 3 The prepuce must be fully retracted and cleaned again with water-soluble antiseptic. A second incision is made 3 mm proximal to the coronal sulcus.

4 The two incisions are held up with forceps and a straight incision made between them to join the circular incisions.

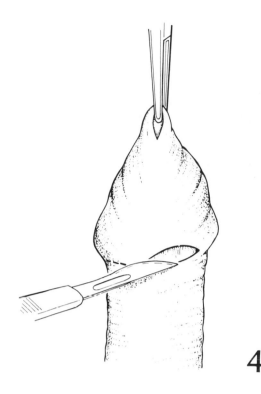

4

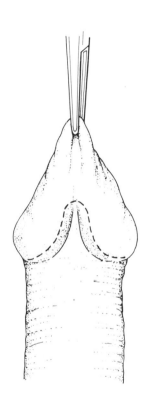

5

5, 6 The plane of cleavage under the sleeve of skin that has thus been outlined is developed with scissors and the prepuce removed.

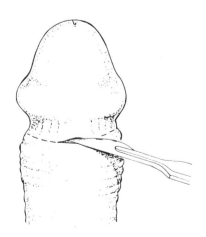

6

7a–e Haemostasis must be exact and complete. Very small vessels may be closed by diathermy with bipolar diathermy forceps; larger ones should be tied with 5/0 chromic catgut.

It is safe to use monopolar diathermy only if great care is taken to surround the penis with a swab soaked in saline, giving a large pedicle for the return of the current to earth. If monopolar diathermy is used in the penis of the tiny baby, there is a high risk that the main arteries of the penis will be coagulated, and there have been many cases where the penis has sloughed, with disastrous consequences for patient and surgeon.

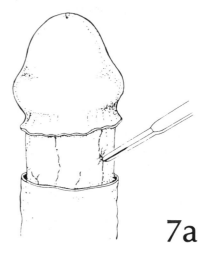

7a

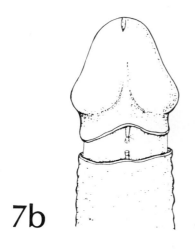

7b

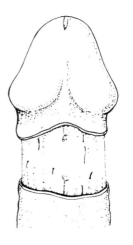

7c

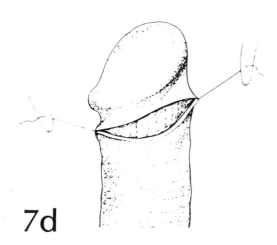

7d

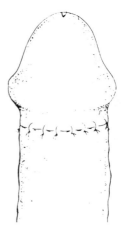

7e

Postoperative care

The best dressing for circumcision is fresh air. The wound may be covered with a thin layer of vaseline gauze and a dry dressing for the rest of the day. Haemostasis should be so perfect that there is no need for any pressure dressings, particularly none that encircle the penis and can give rise to 'garotting' of the glans. As long as the wound is kept clean and dry, no further attention should be necessary.

Outcome

In adults the foreskin should always be sent for histological section; balanitis xerotica obliterans is a common indication for cirumcision, and in view of the suspicion that this is a premalignant condition, the findings of this diagnosis should indicate lifelong follow-up.

References

1. Remondino PC. *History of Circumcision*. London: Davis, 1891.

2. Ghalioungui P. *Magic and Medical Science in Ancient Egypt*. London: Hodder and Stoughton, 1963.

3. Frazer, JG. *The Golden Bough*. London: Macmillan, 1922.

4. Blandy JP. Circumcision. *Hosp Med* 1968; 3: 550–3.

5. Fink AJ. A possible explanation for heterosexual male infection with AIDS. *N Engl J Med* 1986; 315: 1167; 1987; 316: 1546–7.

6. Cameron DW, D'Costa LJ, Maitha GM *et al*. Female to male transmission of human immunodeficiency virus type I: risk factors for seroconversion in men. *Lancet* 1989; ii: 403–7.

7. Oates JK. Genital herpes. *Br J Hosp Med* 1983; 29: 13–22.

Further reading

Snowman LV. *The Surgery of Ritual Circumcision*, 3rd edn. London: The Initiation Society, Weinberg, 1962.

Vasectomy

H. N. Whitfield MA, MChir, FRCS
Consultant Urologist, St Bartholomew's Hospital and St Mark's Hospital for Diseases of the Colon and Rectum, London, UK

Principles and justification

Indications

Some urological surgeons advocate that a bilateral vasectomy should be performed at the time of transurethral prostatectomy to reduce the incidence of epididymo-orchitis. The incidence of this complication following prostatectomy is in the region of 6% and a vasectomy may reduce it by half[1]. Other surgeons believe that a vasectomy is unnecessary, even if prophylactic antibiotics are not administered[2].

Vasectomy is very commonly performed as a method of contraception. A patient who requests a vasectomy for this purpose must be counselled carefully. No hard and fast rules can be laid down about the criteria to be expected of those wishing to undergo a vasectomy. The influence of age, marital status and previous children is best left for the patient and his surgeon to discuss. Psychological screening is difficult if not impossible in a relatively short consultation and the recommendation of the patient's general practitioner is important.

The medicolegal cases which arise following vasectomy serve to illustrate the vital importance of covering the following points during counselling:

1. The operation should be regarded as irreversible. Sperm banks may offer the chance to retain 'fertility'. Successful vasectomy reversal in terms of the presence of spermatozoa will occur in 90% of cases, but the pregnancy rate is approximately 50%.
2. Bleeding and infection are both recognized as short-term complications. No long-term sequelae have been confirmed, although a number have been suggested, e.g. atheroma, testicular cancer.
3. Other methods of contraception must be employed until two consecutive samples of semen have been demonstrated to be completely azoospermic.
4. The decrease in ejaculatory volume will be of the order of 10%.
5. A vasectomy does not improve or impair libido and erections.
6. A recanalization risk exists which is of the order of 3–5 per 1000 cases[3, 4].

Preoperative

The patient should always be examined at the preoperative visit so that anatomical or pathological problems such as varicocoele or absent vas deferens can be identified. A consent form for the operation must be signed by the patient and surgeon. There is no legal necessity for the patient's partner to sign too.

The scrotum, the base of the penis and adjacent pubic hair should be shaved.

The operation can be performed under local or general anaesthesia, and the choice may be left to the patient. However, those of a nervous disposition may benefit from having a general anaesthetic. In either case it is essential for the surgeon (and the anaesthetist) to recognize that, although this appears to be a minor procedure, potentially catastrophic cardiovascular problems can arise. When there is a traction on the vas deferens the patient may become bradycardic because of a vasovagal reflex and cardiovascular collapse can ensue. For this reason, whenever and wherever the operation is performed, a resuscitation trolley must be available and atropine, 0.6 or 1.2 mg, must be given intravenously if there are any signs of a vasovagal episode.

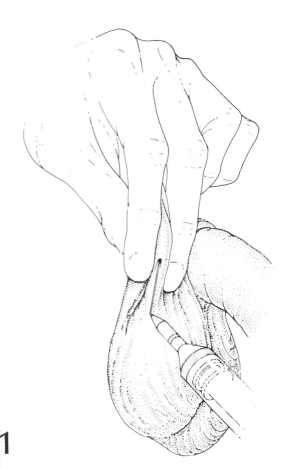

1

Operation

1 The key to the technique is that the vas deferens must be located and then held firmly. If local anaesthetic is being used it becomes more difficult to identify the vas deferens and to hold it and surgeons in training benefit from the opportunity to learn the operation when a patient is under general anaesthesia. The vas deferens lies posteriorly in the scrotum and the right-handed surgeon should stand on the right of the patient and use the left hand to fix the vas between the first and second fingers on the front of the scrotum on each side, with the thumb posteriorly pushing it between the two fingers. The vas deferens, once located, should be gently rolled round towards the anterior scrotal wall, allowing other cord sutures to slip posteriorly. When it is immediately beneath the anterior scrotal wall 5 ml of local anaesthetic (1% lignocaine) can be infiltrated into the skin and around the vas deferens, concentrating on the proximal vas, keeping as close to it as possible.

2 A 0.5-cm incision is made at right angles over the vas deferens where it is still held by the two fingers and thumb of the left hand and deepened until it is exposed, when it is grasped with a pair of Allis' forceps.

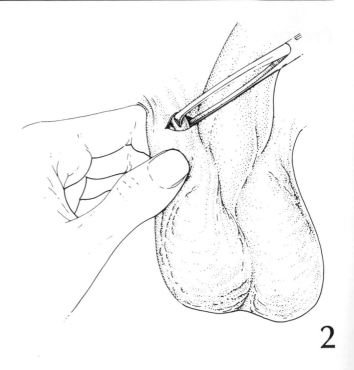

2

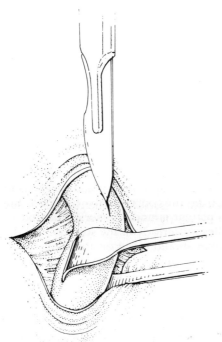

3a

3a, b The fascial coverings of the cord are incised and the vas deferens regrasped with a pair of toothed dissecting forceps and drawn out of the wound. Clips are applied proximally and distally 2–3 cm apart and the intervening vas is excised, leaving 0.5–0.75 cm proximally.

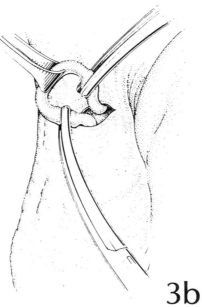

3b

4 The distal end is tied off with an absorbable suture, and the proximal end is tied off similarly after it has been looped back on itself.

The cremasteric muscle layer is closed separately from the skin with an absorbable suture.

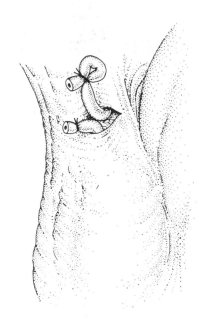

4

Postoperative care

The patient should wear tight underpants for a week to support the scrotum and should avoid baths, showers and strenuous physical activity for 48–72 h. Semen analyses should be performed, starting 6 weeks after the operation, until two consecutive specimens have shown a complete absence of spermatozoa in a centrifuged aliquot.

Complications

Bleeding occurs occasionally, but is rarely severe enough to cause a scrotal haematoma which requires evacuation. Such bleeding is usually due to a failure to secure the artery to the vas deferens.

Infection can arise, but will usually respond to antibiotics; spermatozoa granulomas are found in about 25% of patients but very few provoke symptoms. The incidence of recanalization of the vas deferens is in the order of 1 in 3000–4000 cases, but whether this is due to a technical failure on the part of the surgeon or to true recanalization is never possible to ascertain for certain.

References

1. Mebust WK, Foret JD, Valk WL. Transurethral surgery. In: Harrison JH, Gittes RF, Perlmutter AD, Stamey TA, Walsh PC, eds. *Campbell's Urology* Volume 3. Philadelphia: Saunders, 1979: 2361–81.

2. Chilton CP, Morgan RJ, England HR, Paris AMI, Blandy JP. A critical evaluation of the results of transurethral resection of the prostate. *Br J Urol* 1978; 50: 542–6.

3. Sherlock DJ, Holl-Allen RTJ. Delayed spontaneous recanalisation of the vas deferens. *Br J Surg* 1984; 71: 532–3.

4. Schmidt SS. Prevention of failure in vasectomy. *J Urol* 1973; 109: 296–7.

Exposure of major blood vessels

P. R. F. Bell MD, FRCS
Professor of Surgery, Leicester Royal Infirmary, Leicester, UK

The work of the peripheral vascular surgeon ranges widely through the anatomy of the whole body and he is required to command a wide range of anatomical knowledge. This chapter outlines the standard technique for exposure of the major arteries.

Both diseased and healthy arteries may be surprisingly friable, and rough dissection may cause severe damage and be sufficient to jeopardize the result of the vascular reconstruction. Gentleness must be observed at all times and, in general, it is desirable to dissect a little way from the exterior surface of the vessel so that the inadvertent division of a branch can be treated by ligation rather than requiring a suture flush with the vessel wall. Good angiography is essential to forewarn the surgeon of the presence of anatomical variations and to minimize the need for fruitless exposure of vessels which are not appropriate for the proposed operation. In some cases the role of angiography has now been replaced by duplex ultrasonography and shortly, possibly, by magnetic resonance imaging.

Exposure of the carotid artery

The patient is placed on the back with the head extended and placed on a rubber ring. The head is then turned away from the side to be operated on. The incision is placed along the anterior part of the sternocleidomastoid muscle as far as the angle of the jaw and passes slightly backwards.

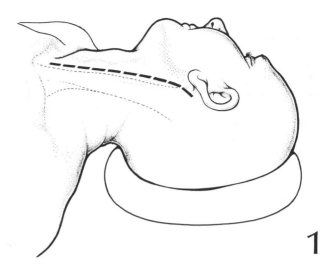

1

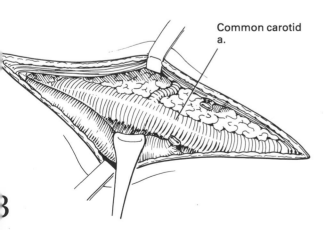

Anterior facial v.

Sternocleidomastoid m.

2

2 After incising the skin and platysma, the sterno-cleidomastoid muscle is displaced posteriorly and the internal jugular vein comes into view. The anterior facial vein can be seen passing forwards.

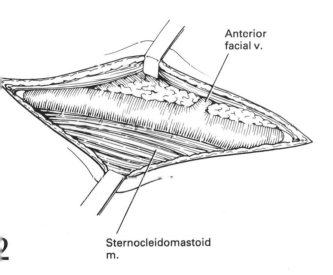

Common carotid a.

3

3 The anterior facial vein is divided and the internal jugular vein is retracted posteriorly exposing the internal carotid artery covered with a layer of areolar tissue.

4 By dissecting along the medial border of the common carotid artery the superior thyroid artery will be seen and can be encircled with a sling. The external carotid artery can also be controlled in the same way, care being taken to locate the hypoglossal nerve as it crosses the vessels high up in the wound. The internal jugular vein is retracted backwards and the vagus nerve will be seen between these two vessels. The descending hypoglossal nerve runs down the front of the common carotid artery. The slings around the superior thyroid and external carotid arteries can be used for retraction to expose the internal carotid artery more fully.

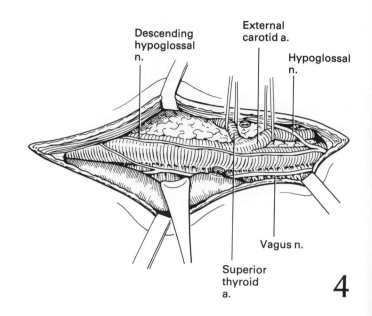

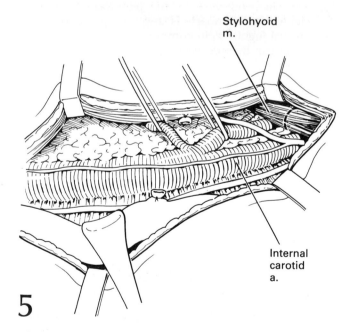

5 If it proves necessary for more of the internal carotid artery to be exposed then the stylohyoid muscle should be divided as shown. More of the internal carotid artery can be exposed by division of the digastric tendon or subluxation of the jaw in a forward direction.

Exposure of the vertebral artery

6 For exposure of the vertebral artery an incision is made obliquely just lateral to the sternocleido-mastoid muscle.

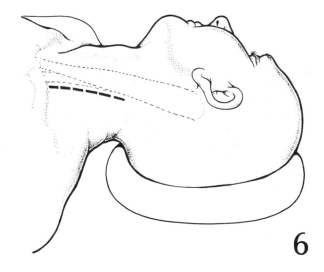

6

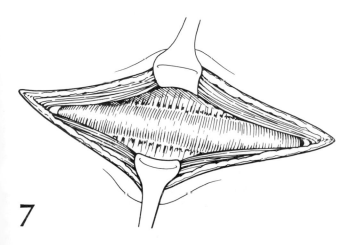

7

7 The internal jugular vein is exposed after dividing the lateral part of the muscle.

8 The internal jugular vein is retracted laterally to expose the vagus nerve which is also retracted laterally. The carotid artery will be seen medially and this should be dissected sufficiently to allow medial retraction. Dissection in the angle between the artery and the vein reveals the vertebral vein and behind it the vertebral artery crisscrossed by branches of the cervical sympathetic chain.

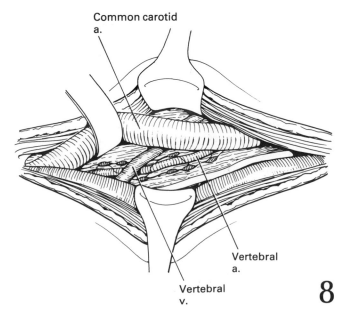

Common carotid a.

Vertebral a.

Vertebral v.

8

9 The vertebral vein and some elements of the sympathetic trunk are divided with downward extension of the incision to expose the whole of the lower part of the vertebral artery before it passes towards the vertebral bodies and also to expose the subclavian artery from which it arises.

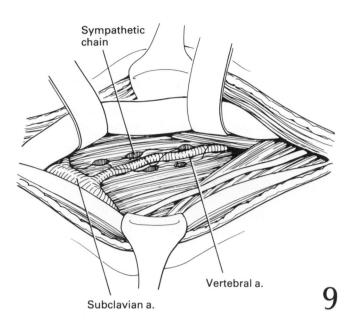

10 For exposure of the distal vertebral artery an incision should also be made along the line of the sternocleidomastoid muscle which, after exposure, is retracted medially. The dissection should proceed posteriorly, the carotid artery and vein being retracted medially if necessary. The accessory nerve will be found crossing the levator scapulae muscle and should be protected. The upper end of the levator scapulae should be divided with a scalpel passing an appropriate instrument behind it to protect the structures lying there.

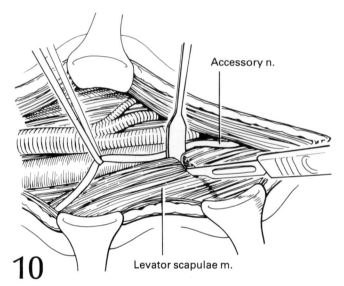

11 When the levator scapulae muscle has been divided the anterior primary ramus of C2 will be seen crossing the cervical part of the artery. Further access to the artery can be obtained by dividing C2.

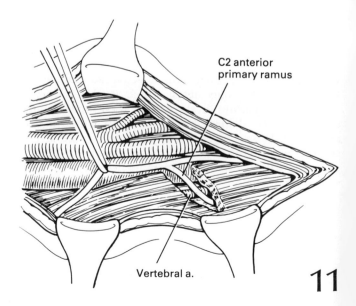

Exposure of the subclavian artery

12 An incision is made above the scapula, lateral to the insertion of the sternocleidomastoid muscle.

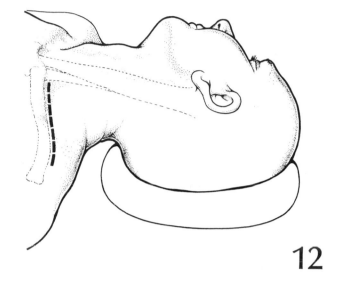

12

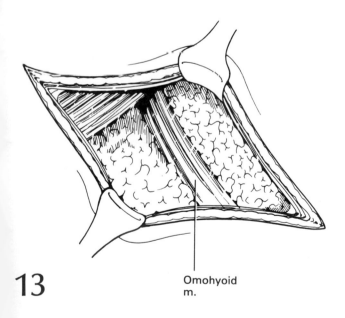

13

Omohyoid
m.

13 The platysma and fascia are dissected to reveal the omohyoid muscle, lymph nodes and fat. The lymph nodes and fat should be displaced upwards.

14 The phrenic nerve will be seen beneath the deep fascia overlying the anterior scalene muscle which can be felt as a band passing downwards and medially. The brachial plexus will easily be seen or felt laterally. A curved blunt instrument is passed behind the anterior scalene muscle.

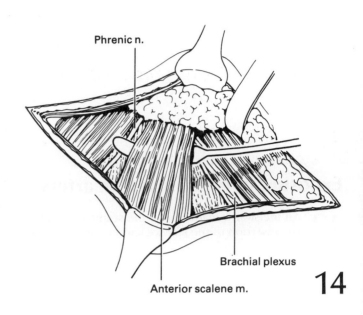

Phrenic n.

Brachial plexus

Anterior scalene m.

14

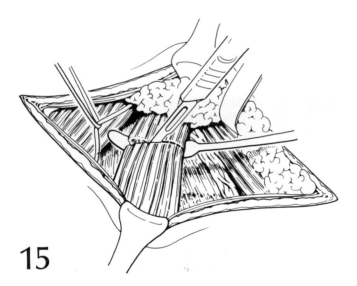

15

15 The anterior scalene muscle is divided carefully, protecting the phrenic nerve which is best performed by passing a sling around it.

16 Division of the anterior scalene muscle reveals the subclavian artery and its suprascapular and internal mammary branches. The vertebral artery can also be seen medially.

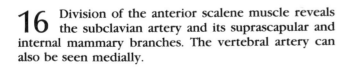

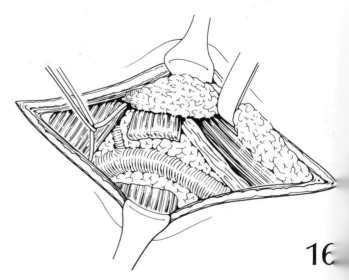

16

Exposure of the distal subclavian and proximal axillary artery

17 The subclavian artery should be exposed as already described, the incision being taken across the clavicle. This can be divided as shown.

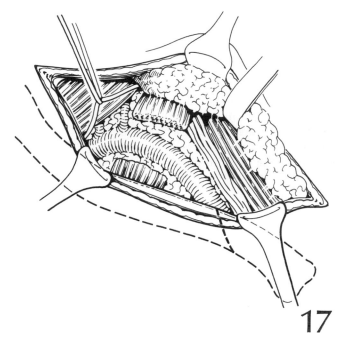

17

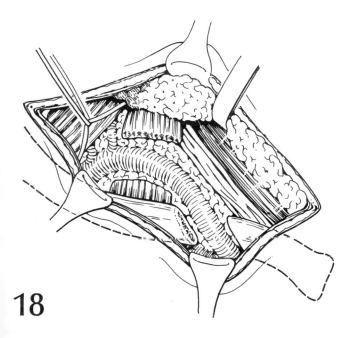

18

18 After division of the clavicle downward retraction reveals the distal part of the subclavian artery as it crosses the first rib and the upper part of the axillary artery beyond this.

19 The middle part of the axillary artery is exposed by making an incision below the middle third of the clavicle.

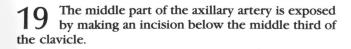

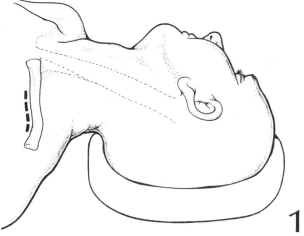

19

20 The skin and deep fascia are incised and branches of the acromioclavicular artery can be seen coming through the clavipectoral fascia. The pectoralis major muscle lies above and below these branches.

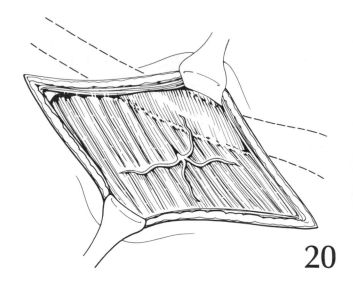

20

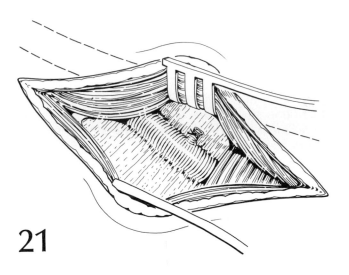

21

21 The muscle fibres of the pectoralis major are divided after tying off the branches of the acromioclavicular artery. The axillary artery can be felt in the depths of the wound and exposed by sharp dissection. One or two branches need to be tied to expose it fully.

22 For more distal exposure the pectoralis minor muscle in the lateral part of the wound needs to be divided completely. Retraction is required to access the artery.

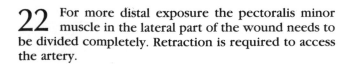

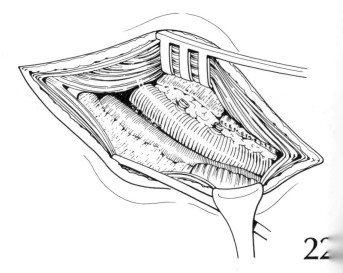

22

Exposure of the brachial artery

23 This can be exposed throughout the upper arm by an incision placed along its medial border just behind the biceps muscle.

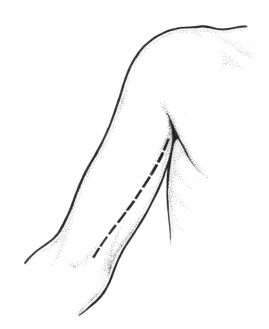

23

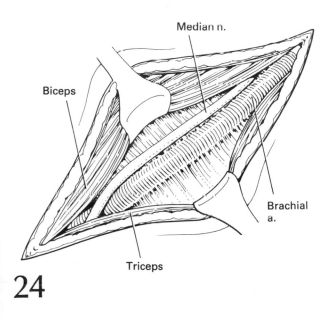

24

24 After incising the skin and deep fascia the biceps muscle is retracted anteriorly and the triceps posteriorly. The median nerve can be seen lying superior to the brachial artery.

25 Further dissection will reveal the brachial vein which can be retracted posteriorly to expose the ulnar nerve.

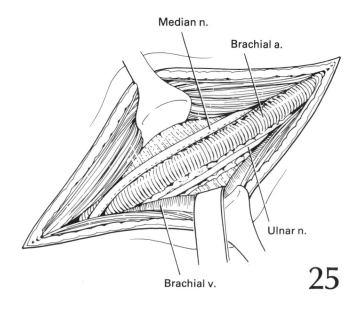

25

26 For exposure of the bifurcation of the brachial artery an S-shaped incision should be made in the antecubital fossa.

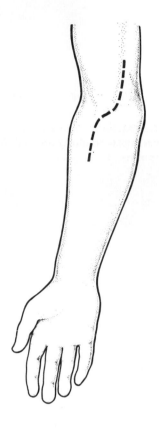

26

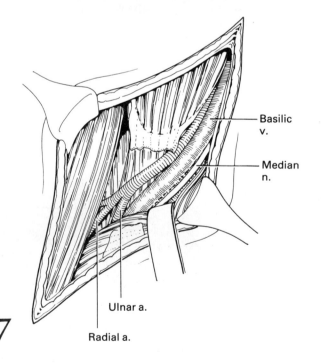

Basilic v.

Median n.

Ulnar a.

Radial a.

27

27 After division of the bicipital aponeurosis the brachial artery and its bifurcation into the radial and ulnar arteries will be seen where they pass between the brachioradialis and flexor muscles. The median nerve and basilic vein can be seen posteriomedial to the artery.

28 The ulnar and the radial arteries are exposed through incisions on the anterior surface of the forearm.

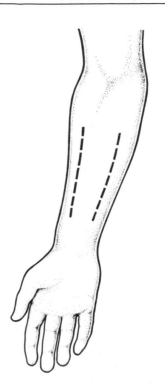

28

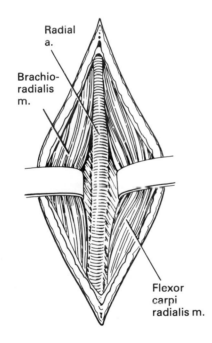

Radial
a.

Brachio-
radialis
m.

Flexor
carpi
radialis m.

29

29 By dissection between the brachioradialis muscle medially and the flexor carpi radialis muscle laterally the radial artery will be exposed along with its associated veins.

30 By dissection of the pronator teres and brachioradialis muscles laterally and the flexor digitorum sublimus muscle medially the ulnar artery will be seen.

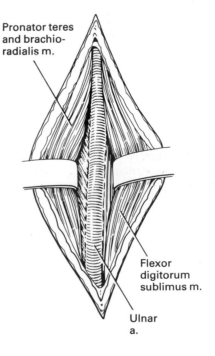

Pronator teres
and brachio-
radialis m.

Flexor
digitorum
sublimus m.

Ulnar
a.

30

31 For exposure of the ulnar and radial artery at the wrist the incisions should be made as indicated.

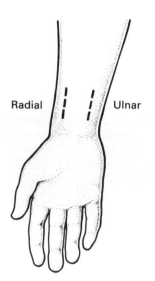

Radial   Ulnar

31

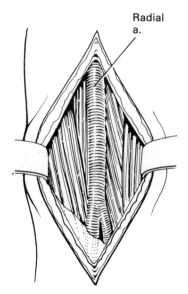

Radial
a.

32

32 The radial artery is very superficial and may be palpated and exposed easily.

33 The ulnar artery is a little deeper but again is relatively superficial and can be exposed before it enters the deep aspect of the hypothenar eminence.

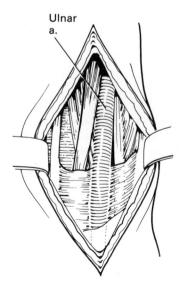

Ulnar
a.

33

Exposure of the ascending aorta and arch branches

34 Various incisions are made to expose the ascending aorta and its branches in the neck. The most commonly used is a vertical incision.

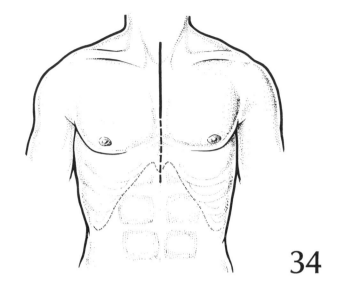

34

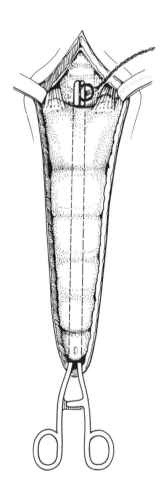

35

35 The incision is deepened to the sternum from the manubrium sternum to the xiphisternum. An appropriate clamp such as a Roberts is passed behind the sternum and a Gigli saw pulled through the tunnel. This is then used to divide the sternum. An electric saw can, as an alternative, be used to divide the sternum from the front.

36 After the sternum has been divided it is held apart by self-retaining retractors.

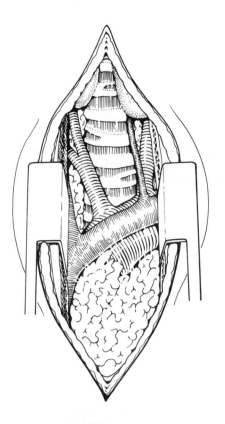

36

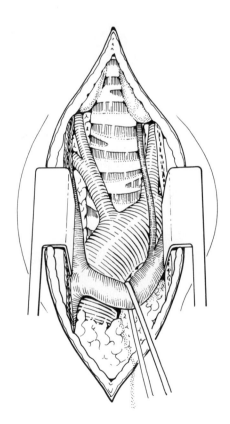

37

37 The brachiocephalic vein will be seen and should be retracted downwards to expose the aortic arch and the roots of the brachiocephalic, left carotid and subclavian arteries.

38 In order to expose the branches of the aortic arch in the neck a transverse limb is added to the vertical incision.

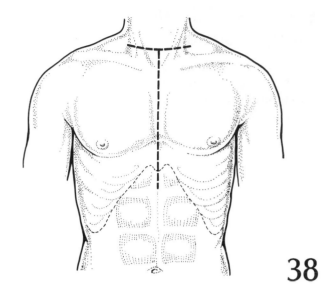

38

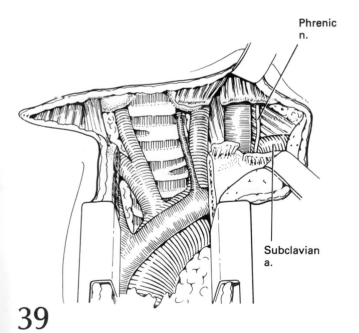

Phrenic n.

Subclavian a.

39

39 By division of the sternocleidomastoid and anterior scalene muscles, the subclavian artery can be seen and the phrenic nerve protected. This allows various types of graft to be inserted between the ascending aorta and its branches in the neck.

Exposure of the descending thoracic aorta

40 This is exposed through an incision in the fifth or eighth intercostal space, depending upon which level is to be exposed.

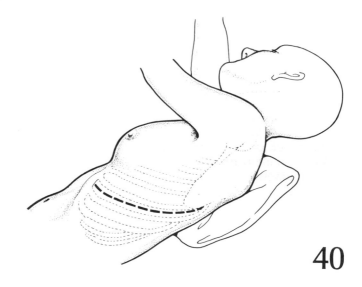

40

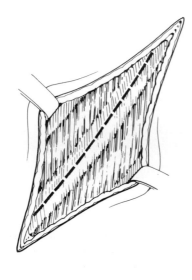

41a

41a, b The thoracic cavity is entered by removing the rib and the lung is displaced forwards. The descending aorta will be seen posteriorly.

Lung displaced forward

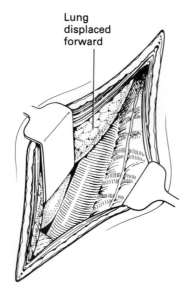

41b

Exposure of the lower thoracic and upper abdominal aorta

42 For exposure of the descending thoracic and upper abdominal aorta a midline incision is made in the abdomen with an extension through the costal margin along the seventh rib for exposure of the lower thoracic aorta and the fifth for exposure of the upper thoracic aorta.

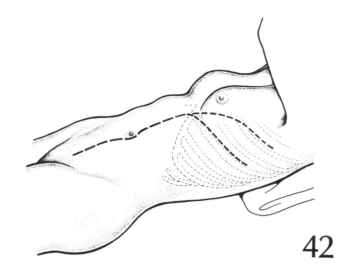

42

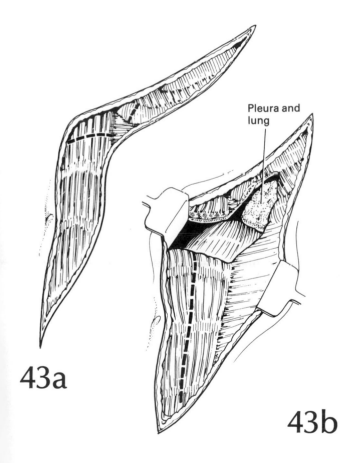

Pleura and lung

43a

43b

43a, b The rectus muscle and costal margin are divided to allow exposure of the pleura which is then opened.

44 The diaphragm can be divided either transversely close to the costal margin which avoids damage to the phrenic nerve, or vertically which damages the phrenic nerve but gives much better exposure.

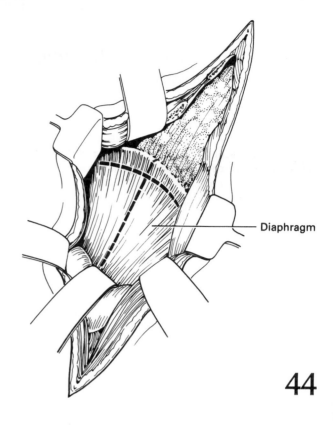

Diaphragm

44

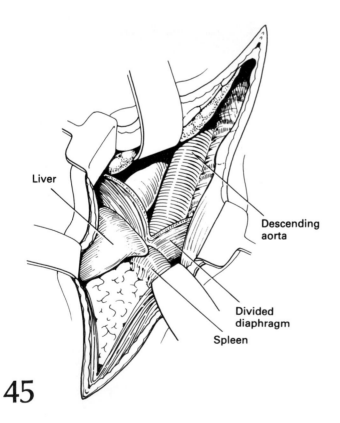

Liver

Descending aorta

Divided diaphragm

Spleen

45

45 After division of the diaphragm the thoracic aorta, liver, abdominal contents and spleen can be seen.

46 An incision is made in the peritoneum along the lateral border of the spleen and colon.

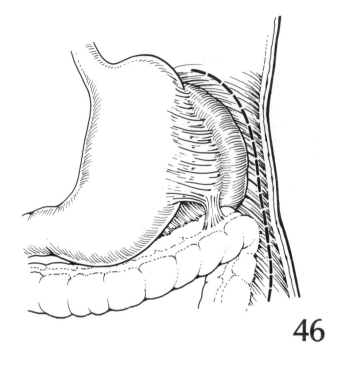

46

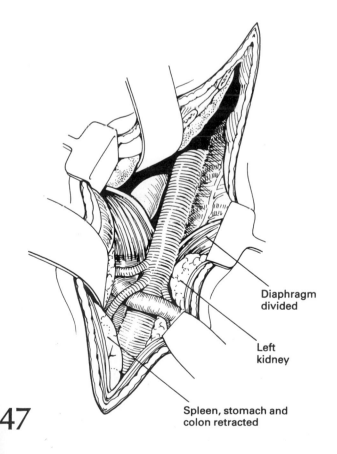

47 The colon, spleen and pancreas are mobilized to the right which exposes the abdominal aorta and its main branches, the coeliac axis, the superior mesenteric artery and the renal vessels. The left renal vein can be seen crossing the abdominal aorta.

Diaphragm divided

Left kidney

Spleen, stomach and colon retracted

47

Exposure of the abdominal aorta and its branches

48 This is accomplished through a number of transverse incisions (A), a midline incision (B), or an oblique incision (C).

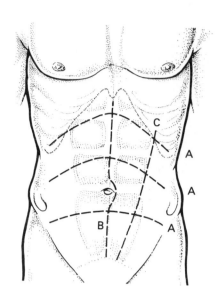

48

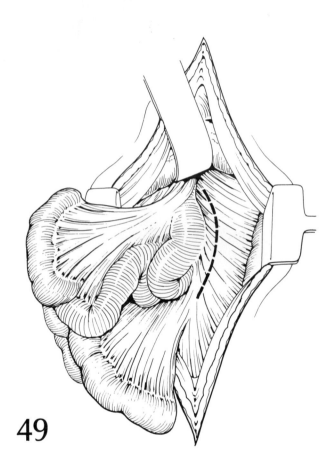

49

Superior mesenteric artery

49 The peritoneum on the left side of the duodeno-jejunal flexure is incised carefully and the bowel pushed to the right. This will expose the aorta.

50 Alternatively a transverse abdominal incision can be used with the same incision in the peritoneum close to the duodenojejunal flexure in order to expose the aorta.

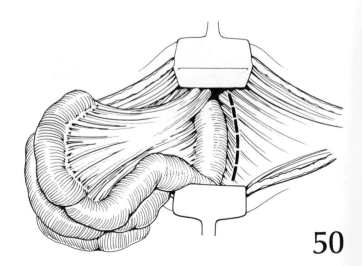

50

51 For a retroperitoneal exposure the abdominal muscles are divided as shown in *Illustration 48* (line C) and the peritoneum displaced to the right. This will expose the aorta and the kidney.

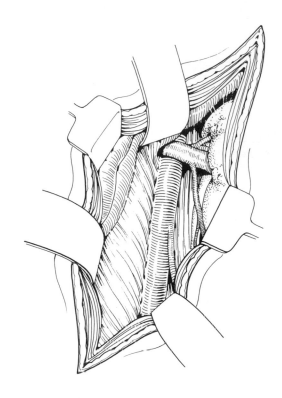

51

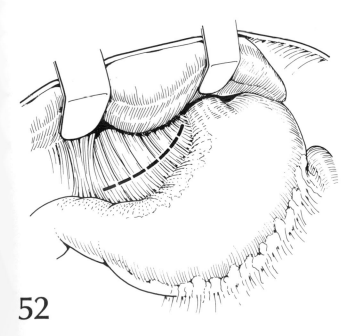

52

Coeliac axis

52 The coeliac axis is exposed after opening the abdomen through a transverse or vertical incision and opening the lesser omentum.

53 After ligating the vessels in the greater omentum the pancreas can be seen at the back of the lesser sac and the aorta felt just above the level where the crura cross it.

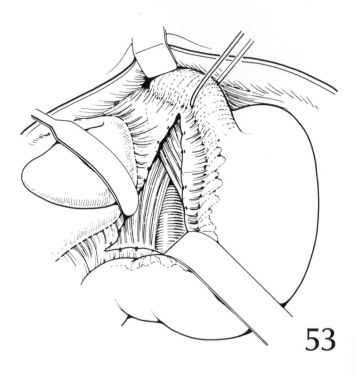

53

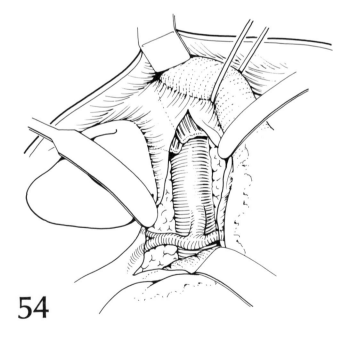

54

54 The crura are divided to expose the aorta and just above the stomach the origin of the coeliac axis will be seen.

Splenic artery

55 The splenic artery is exposed by dividing the greater omentum along the lower border of the stomach and displacing that organ proximally.

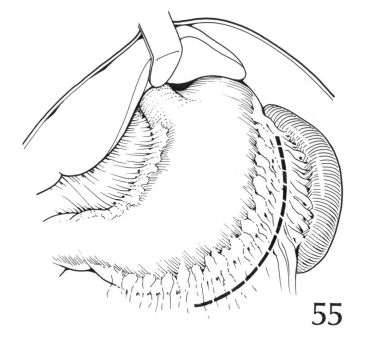

55

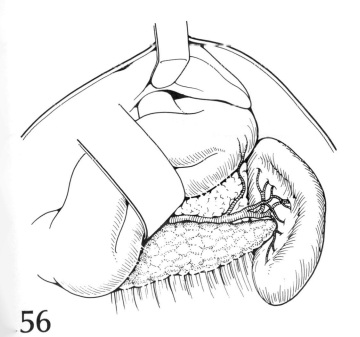

56

56 The artery will be seen running along the upper part of the pancreas.

Superior mesenteric artery origin

57 The origin of the superior mesenteric artery can be exposed through a transverse or vertical incision in the peritoneum lateral to the spleen and colon.

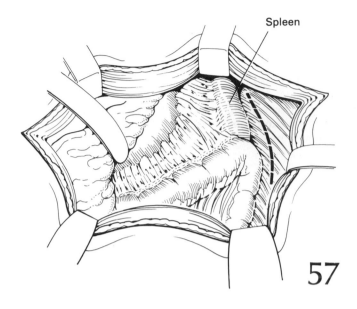

57

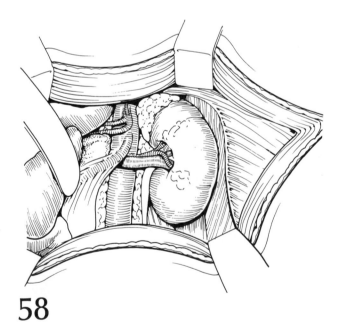

58

58 The spleen, pancreas and stomach are mobilized to the right exposing the kidney, the aorta, its major branches and the renal veins. The origins of the coeliac and superior mesenteric artery and other branches can be accessed in this way.

59 For exposure of the superior mesenteric artery lower down the intestine is mobilized to the right and the artery, along with the superior mesenteric vein, palpated in the free edge of the mesentery above the jejunum. Incising the peritoneum will expose the artery here.

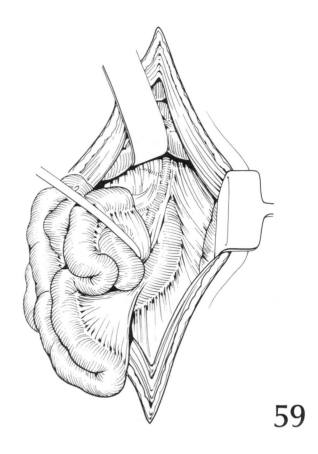

59

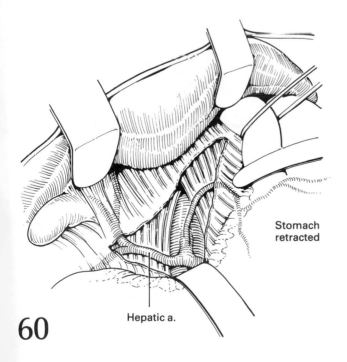

60

Stomach retracted

Hepatic a.

Hepatic artery

60 Division of the lesser omentum allows exposure of the hepatic artery as it crosses from the coeliac artery.

Renal arteries

61 The renal arteries are exposed using a transverse or vertical incision after passing a sling around the left renal vein which is pulled downwards.

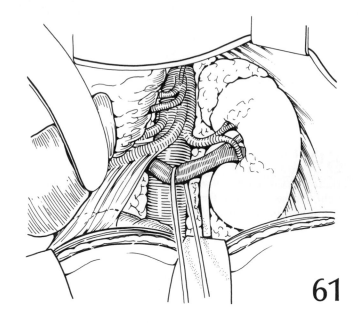

61

62, 63 The right renal artery is exposed by incising the peritoneum lateral to the duodenal loop and displacing it medially.

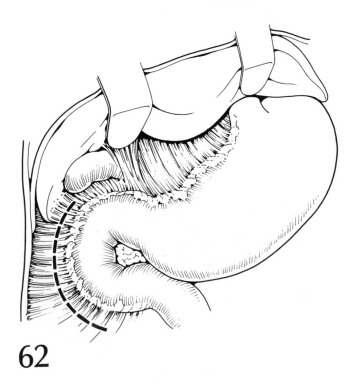

62

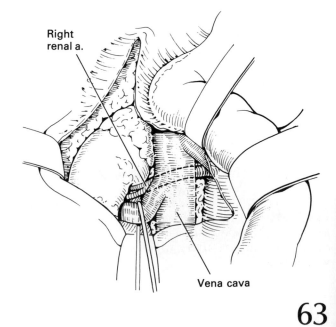

Right
renal a.

Vena cava

63

Exposure of the iliac artery

64 An oblique incision is made in the left iliac fossa.

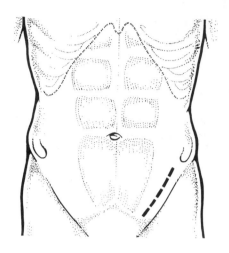

64

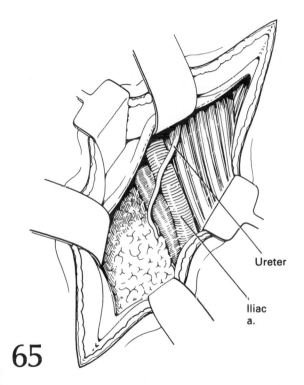

Ureter

Iliac
a.

65

65 To expose the iliac artery and vein the muscles are divided and the peritoneum mobilized medially, taking care to avoid the ureter which crosses the bifurcation of the common iliac artery.

Exposure of the internal iliac artery

66 In order to expose this vessel, the common and external iliac arteries are encircled with slings and pulled laterally. This allows exposure of the origin of the internal iliac artery which can be dissected free with scissors.

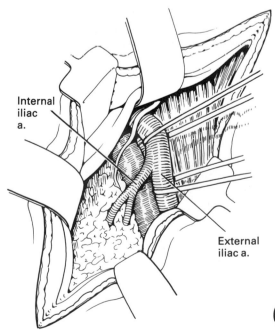

Internal
iliac
a.

External
iliac a.

66

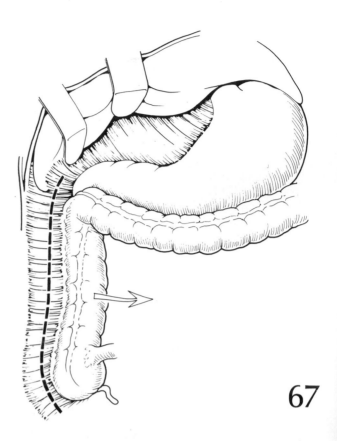

67

Exposure of the inferior vena cava

67, 68 The vena cava is exposed by opening the patient's abdomen through a transverse or vertical incision, incising the peritoneum lateral to the duodenal loop and ascending colon, and displacing these structures medially to expose the entire vena cava retroperitoneally.

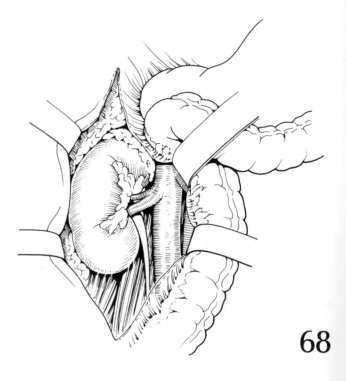

68

Exposure of the portal vein

69 This is exposed in the free edge of the porta hepatis. The hepatic artery is mobilized medially and the bile duct likewise. The portal vein lies behind these vessels.

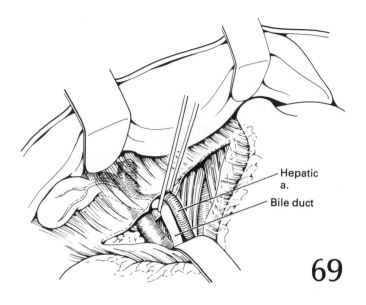

Hepatic a.

Bile duct

69

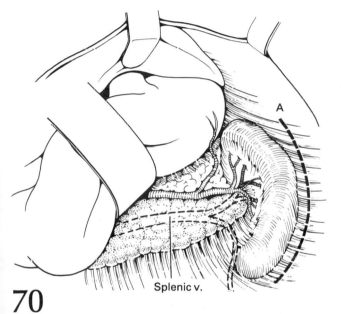

A

Splenic v.

70

Exposure of the splenic vein

70 As this structure lies behind the pancreas it is best exposed by incising the peritoneum lateral to the spleen as shown at A.

71 The spleen is then mobilized medially and the vein will be seen running along the back of the pancreas where it can be isolated if necessary.

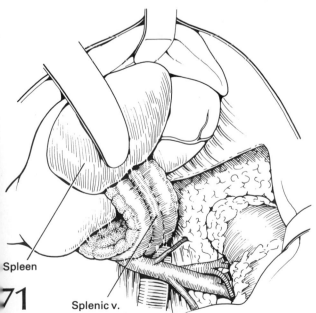

Spleen

71

Splenic v.

Exposure of the superficial and deep femoral arteries

72 A vertical or oblique incision is made in the groin.

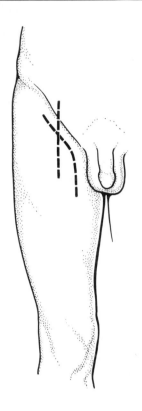

72

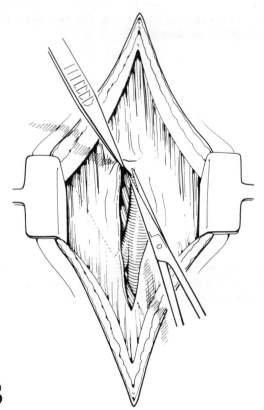

73

73 The fascia overlying the vessels is cut with a pair of scissors.

74 A pair of Lahey forceps is passed behind the artery and a sling passed around it.

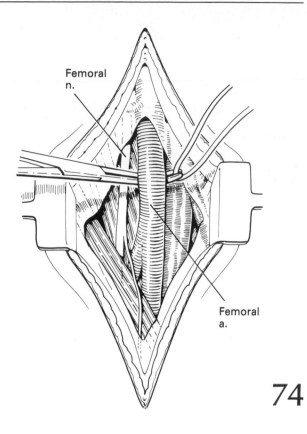

Femoral n.

Femoral a.

74

75 Slings are similarly passed around the common and superficial femoral arteries and the upper branches of the deep femoral artery.

Deep femoral v.

75

76 For extensive exposure of the deep femoral artery the small veins which often cross its origin and lower down the circumflex femoral vein are divided and the vessel fully exposed.

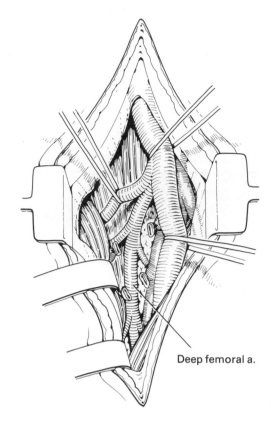

Deep femoral a.

76

Exposure of the femoral artery

77 For exposure of the femoral artery in the mid thigh a vertical incision is made.

78 The vastus medialis and adductor longus muscles are separated and the artery exposed.

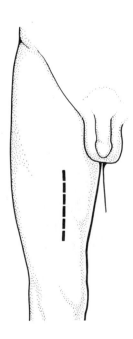

77

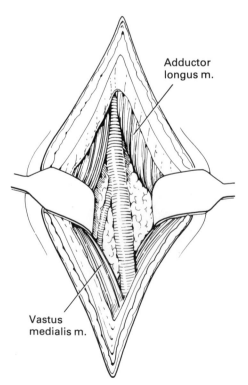

Adductor
longus m.

Vastus
medialis m.

78

Exposure of the popliteal artery

79 Using a posterior approach an S-shaped incision is made.

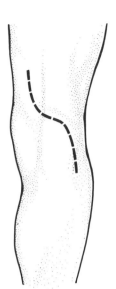

79

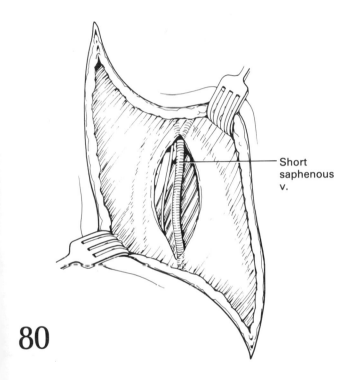

Short
saphenous
v.

80

80 When the fascia and fat have been divided the short saphenous vein will be seen. This has to be divided to gain access to the popliteal fossa.

81 The medial popliteal nerve and vessels will be seen passing between the two heads of the gastrocnemius muscle and are suprisingly superficial.

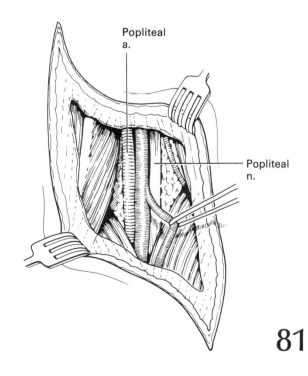

Popliteal
a.

Popliteal
n.

81

82 For exposure of the above knee popliteal artery an incision is made in the lower medial part of the thigh along the anterior border of the sartorius muscle.

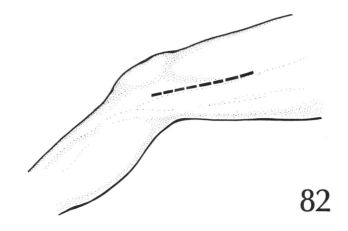

82

Long saphenous n.

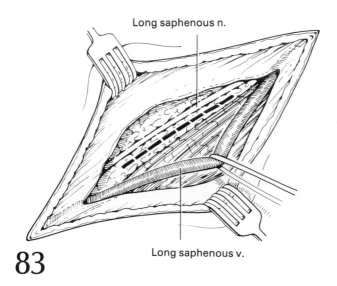

Long saphenous v.

83

83 The incision is deepened until the long saphenous vein can be seen and should be protected. An incision is made in the deep fascia behind the nerve and the sartorius muscle retracted posteriorly.

84 Using finger dissection the popliteal artery is felt in the popliteal fossa lying anteriorly medial to the vein.

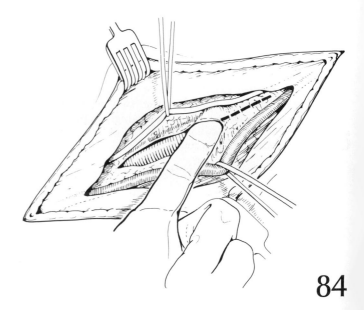

84

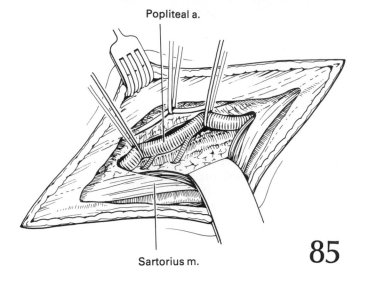

85 Appropriate retraction allows a sling to be passed around it to provide access.

86 The below knee popliteal artery is exposed by using an incision just behind the tibia, passing backwards slightly near to the knee joint.

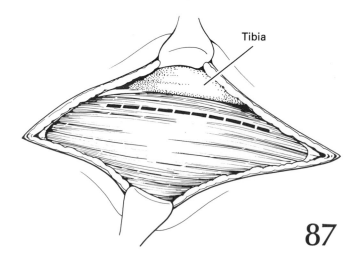

87 An incision is made in the deep fascia anterior to the gastrocnemius muscle.

88 The gastrocnemius muscle is retracted posteriorly and the soleus muscle can be seen attached to the tibia. The vessels passing behind it can be felt above in the popliteal fossa.

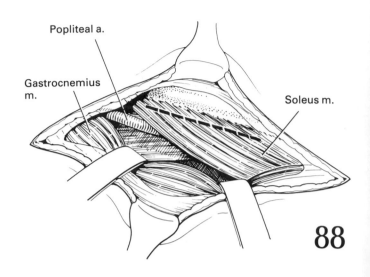

89 By dividing the tendon of the soleus muscle where it is attached to the tibia, the artery and vein can be followed downwards. The artery in particular is crossed by many small venous branches which require careful ligation.

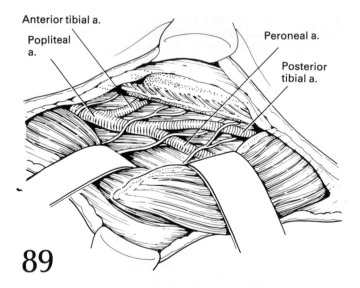

Exposure of the long saphenous vein

90 In order to remove the long saphenous vein multiple incisions are made along it and the vein exposed.

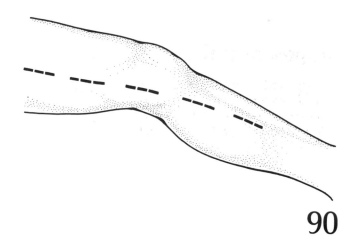

90

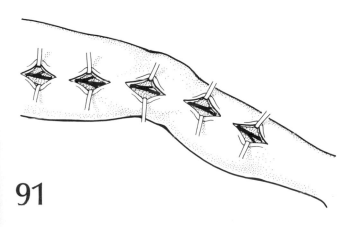

91

91 It is then removed by undermining the skin bridges. The upper end of the vein can be found first where it joins the saphenofemoral junction from where it can be traced by duplex ultrasonography and marked before surgery.

92 The vein is then removed through a continuous incision. This is probably better as it does less damage to the vein.

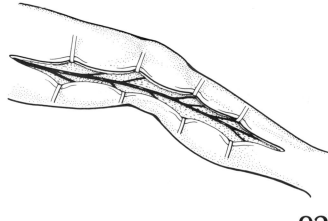

92

Exposure of the crural vessels

93 The posterior tibial and peroneal arteries are exposed by further detachment of the soleus muscle from the tibia until the peroneal artery disappears through the interosseous membrane half way down the leg.

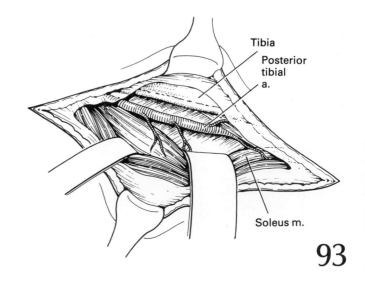

93

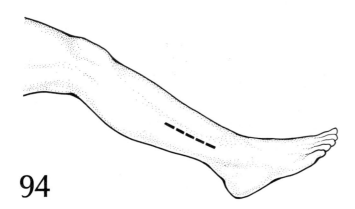

94

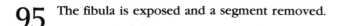

94 The peroneal artery is exposed in the lower half of the leg by an incision on the lateral side.

95 The fibula is exposed and a segment removed.

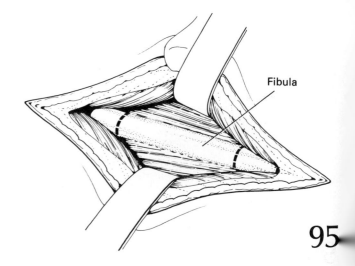

95

96 Once the fibula is removed the artery can be seen behind it.

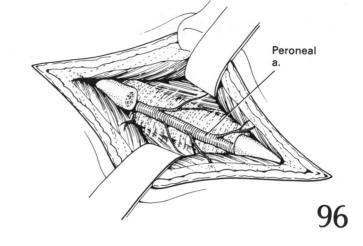

Peroneal a.

96

97 The anterior tibial artery is exposed by an incision over the anterior tibial muscles.

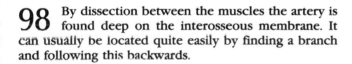

97

98 By dissection between the muscles the artery is found deep on the interosseous membrane. It can usually be located quite easily by finding a branch and following this backwards.

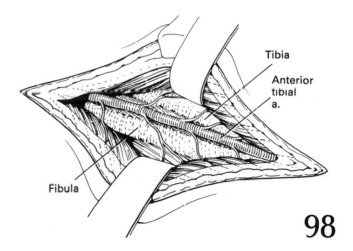

Tibia

Anterior tibial a.

Fibula

98

99 The anterior tibial and posterior tibial arteries are exposed at the foot or ankle by incisions over the posterior tibial artery behind the medial malleolus or anterior tibial artery on the dorsum of the foot.

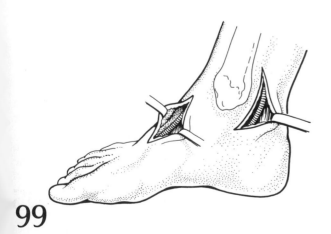

99

Illustrations by Mark Iley

Arterial suture and anastomosis

P. L. Harris MD, FRCS
Consultant Vascular Surgeon, Royal Liverpool University Hospital, Liverpool, UK

History

The principles of vascular repair with sutures were established in the first decade of the 20th century by Alexis Carrel, who in 1912 was awarded the Nobel Prize for Medicine for this work. Since then, technical refinements of suture materials have made possible surgical reconstruction of most arteries, from the root of the aorta to microvascular anastomosis or repair of the smallest vessels, e.g. digital arteries or those on the surface of the brain. Fine sutures on atraumatic needles are best for arterial anastomosis. Silk was used for many years, but it has now been replaced by synthetic fibres, which are less traumatic to the vessel walls.

Principles and justification

Indications

There are three principal indications for operating on an artery: injury, aneurysmal dilatation and occlusion. Injury may result from sharp or blunt trauma and may be associated with damage to other structures, e.g. fractures of long bones. Iatrogenic injuries are increasingly common, arising from arterial access either for investigation or treatment. Another growing prob-

lem is that of self-induced arterial injury in main-line drug abusers. Occasionally, radical surgery for malignant disease may necessitate arterial repair. In most circumstances reconstruction of a damaged major artery is preferable to tying its ends, and this is particularly true in the lower limb.

Although elective and emergency treatment of aneurysmal and occlusive arterial lesions is mostly within the province of vascular specialists, the need for vascular repair may be encountered in all branches of surgery and it is therefore essential that all surgeons are familiar with the principles of arterial suture and anastomosis.

Contraindications

Total ischaemia of a limb for several hours resulting in massive muscle death is an absolute contraindication to vascular repair, because not only will the limb not be salvaged but fatal metabolic disturbance may ensue. Severe compound or crushing injury with gross tissue loss may also be an indication for amputation rather than vascular repair.

Arterial repair is superfluous where there is an adequate collateral circulation, as for example in the case of an injury to the radial artery at the wrist with an intact palmar arch.

Wherever possible, arterial suture should be avoided in the presence of infection.

Instruments

Clamps, needle holders and suture clamps

A wide selection of vascular clamps is essential. For large intra-abdominal and thoracic vessels the DeBakey Atraugrip range is effective, while for smaller arteries, for example femoral, popliteal, subclavian, brachial and carotid arteries, paediatric clamps of the Castaneda type are suitable. A range of small bulldog clamps is useful for controlling back bleeding from side branches, and for delicate vessels the Schofield–Lewis type is safe and effective.

Small peripheral arteries, including those distal to the popliteal and brachial arteries, should never be clamped as they are very sensitive to clamp damage. These vessels should be controlled with fine atraumatic plastic loops and by smooth round-ended atraumatic intraluminal catheters. Plastic loops may be colour-coded for easy identification.

Arteries must be handled gently and only with atraumatic non-toothed forceps.

Needle holders for vascular work must have fine points in order to facilitate accurate placement of sutures, and the jaws should be constructed from high-quality materials such as tungsten in order to ensure a firm grip of the needle. The range of sizes available should take account of the fact that arteries may be close to the surface or at considerable depth.

Rubber-shod clamps fashioned from small haemostats with the jaws cushioned by fine rubber or plastic tubing should be attached to the loose end of the suture in order to keep it out of the way. Unprotected metal instruments must never be applied to monofilamental sutures, which are relatively brittle and easily damaged.

Suture materials

Non-absorbable sutures on atraumatic needles are essential for arteries and there are three types in common usage.

1. Monofilamental material, such as polypropylene (Prolene), is very smooth and slips easily through the tissues. This property allows the anastomosis to be tightened easily by applying longitudinal tension on the suture. Its main disadvantage is a tendency to brittleness, and sutures of this type also tend to have a 'memory' causing twist (kink). It is essential to use several throws in each knot to ensure security.
2. The second type of suture is braided material coated with an outer layer of polyester to make it smooth. These sutures are less brittle and have no 'memory', but do not slide so easily through tissues.
3. Polytetrafluoroethylene (PTFE) sutures are available specifically for use with PTFE grafts. They are swaged onto very fine needles in order to overcome the problem of needle-hole bleeding from these grafts. The suture material itself is very strong and has excellent handling properties, but the needles are comparatively fragile and are unsuitable for suturing tough or calcified vessels and knots slip easily.

Arterial sutures may be single-ended with one needle or double-ended with two. They are available in varying sizes from 2/0 to 10/0. In general, the finest suture that is strong enough for the job should be used. As a rough guide, the following sizes are appropriate: 3/0 for the aorta; 4/0 for the iliac arteries; 5/0 for the femoral artery; 6/0 for the popliteal and brachial arteries; and 7/0 for tibial arteries.

For very fine work, a monofilament stitch is always necessary, and magnifying loops should be used.

Preoperative

Heparin

In non-traumatic situations, it is usual to give systemic heparin before application of the clamps. A standard dose of 5000 IU may be given. Alternatively, the dose may be related to the weight of the patient, for example 1000 IU/kg body weight. It is not always necessary to reverse the heparin, but one common practice is to reverse half of the dose of heparin originally used with the appropriate amount of protamine sulphate. (Protamine sulphate, 2 mg, neutralizes heparin, 1000 IU.)

For all arterial operations, a solution of heparinized saline should be prepared for irrigation of open vessels and instillation into vessels distal to a clamp. This is made up from heparin, 5000 IU in 500 ml normal saline.

Operation

SIMPLE SUTURE

Arteries are best opened longitudinally rather than transversely for three reasons. First, a longitudinal arteriotomy is easier to close; secondly, any thrombus that accumulates on the suture has less tendency to narrow the lumen; thirdly, it can easily be extended. A transverse arteriotomy is difficult to close because the intima retracts away from the outer layers and there is a greater risk of intimal dissection and flap formation.

1 Longitudinal arteriotomies in large or medium-sized arteries can usually be closed by simple lateral suture. The needle must pass through all layers of the arterial wall with every stitch, and care should be taken to ensure that the intima turns outwards. It is important to maintain a firm, even, tension on the suture line and optimal spacing and size of each bite, which can only be learned by experience. Even, regular spacing is usually best, but occasionally irregular stitches may be required to take account of calcified atheromatous plaques.

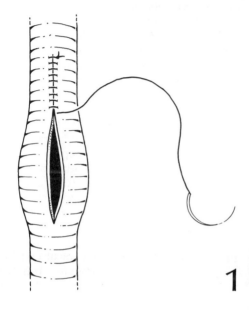

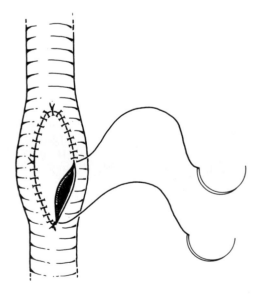

CLOSURE WITH A PATCH

2 For vessels of less than 4 mm in diameter (which usually includes the brachial artery) and where there is loss of substance of the arterial wall that would cause linear closure to narrow the lumen too greatly, it is preferable to close the artery with a patch. This technique can also be used to widen the lumen of a vessel that has become stenosed by disease, for example the deep femoral artery. For small vessels, a patch of autologous vein should be used (the long saphenous vein should not be sacrificed for this purpose). In larger vessels, prosthetic material (either Dacron or PTFE) may be used. An oval or rectangular patch is better than an elliptical one with sharp points which tends to narrow the vessel at each end.

END-TO-END ANASTOMOSIS

This is most easily accomplished by the triangulation technique, as described originally by Carrel.

Stay sutures

3 The transected ends of the vessels are first carefully cleared of excess adventitia, because if this should intrude on the lumen it will promote thrombosis. Three stay sutures are inserted, the first being placed in the centre of the back or deepest aspect of the anastomosis, with the other two positioned so as to divide the circumference of the vessels equally into three. Any disparity in calibre can be compensated for at this stage. Everting horizontal mattress or simple sutures may be used. Sometimes it may be simpler to use just two stay sutures placed either at the anterior and posterior points or at each side, but this is not recommended as a routine.

Interrupted sutures

4 Interrupted sutures should always be used for small or medium-sized vessels. By applying gentle traction to the stay sutures, each of the three segments of the anastomosis is completed in turn commencing with the two at the deepest aspects.

Continuous sutures

5 For larger vessels a continuous suture may be used, commencing on each side of the deepest part of the anastomosis. Care must be taken not to pull the suture too tight and cause a purse-string effect.

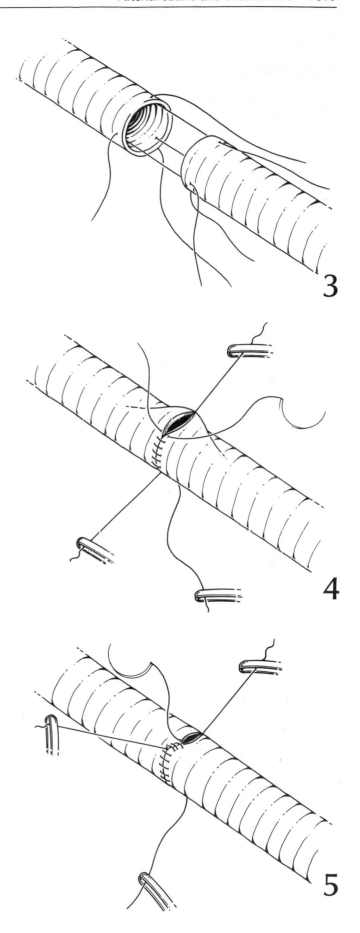

Single-stitch method

6 If there is difficulty in rotating the vessels, for example at a large bifurcation, a single stitch may be used. Commencing on the side nearest the operator, the sutures are inserted from within the lumen to complete the deep or posterior aspect and then continued across the anterior aspect to the starting point. Alternatively, a double-ended suture may be commenced at the midpoint posteriorly and each side completed in turn.

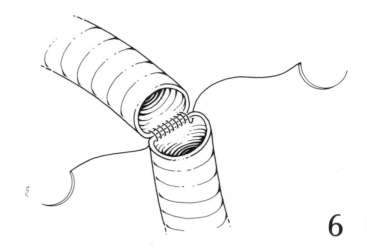

Inlay technique

7 This is the method used for abdominal aortic aneurysms. A horizontal mattress stitch using a double-ended suture is started in the middle of the back of the graft, picking up a double layer of the aortic wall at the neck of the aneurysm and inserting the needles from inside the lumen.

The suture may then be tied and each side of the anastomosis completed in turn. The needle should pass from graft to aorta, and it is essential to take large bites of the aorta to include all layers.

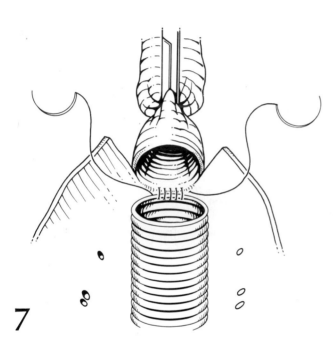

Parachute technique

8 Alternatively, the double-ended suture may be left untied in order to allow a number of stitches to be placed on each side before the graft is pulled down onto the artery.

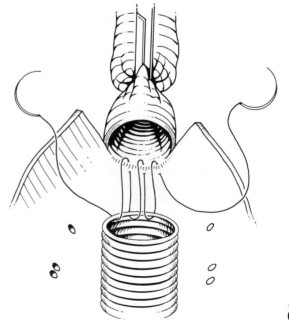

END-TO-SIDE ANASTOMOSIS

This is the usual method of anastomosis for bypass operations. The anastomosis should be oblique, and its length should be approximately twice the diameter of the lumen of the graft. The end of the graft should be fashioned into a spatulate shape, so that on completion of the anastomosis it adopts a 'cobra head' appearance.

Four-quadrant technique

9 A double-ended suture is placed at the 'heel' of the anastomosis and stitching is completed along each side of the anastomosis to the mid-point. If the 'toe' is left free at this stage, the inside of the anastomosis can be inspected to ensure apposition of the intima.

The 'toe' of the graft is then trimmed accurately to size and secured with a double-ended suture to the apex of the anastomosis. The procedure is completed by closing the two remaining quadrants. The 'toe' and 'heel' are the most crucial points of an end-to-side anastomosis, where there is the greatest risk of vessels becoming narrowed. To avoid this risk at the toe, the starting point should be offset to one side or other of the apex. Alternatively, a number of interrupted sutures can be placed around the toe.

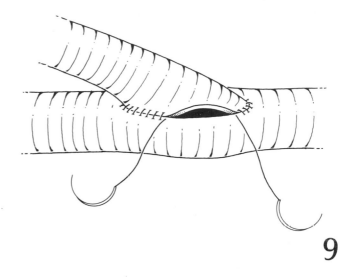

Parachute technique

10 Where access is difficult or good visualization of the anastomosis is impaired, this technique may be advantageous. Using a double-ended monofilament suture, a series of running stitches is placed at what will become the 'heel' of the anastomosis, with the graft and artery separated. These sutures are then pulled tight as the vessels are approximated.

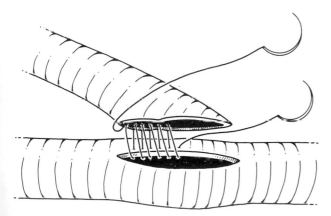

SUTURING THE DISEASED ARTERY

Stronger material may be used for suturing densely sclerotic or calcified vessels. Wherever possible the needle should be passed from within the lumen to the outside of the arterial wall in order to 'pin back' loose plaques, and this requires the suture to pass from graft to artery rather than vice versa. In the presence of calcification it may be necessary to insert a large suture around the whole plaque, in which case additional fine adventitial stitches may be required for complete haemostasis. Care must be taken that sutures are not cut or frayed by calcified plaques. Caution must be exercised in removing plaques or performing local endarterectomy when suturing arteries.

Kunlin suture

11 If an endarterectomy has been performed, there is a risk of intimal flap dissection at the downstream edge. To eliminate this risk, sutures are inserted to secure the intima. The needle passes from outside to inside through an endarterectomized part of the wall and back from inside to outside through the atheroma to be finally tied on the outside.

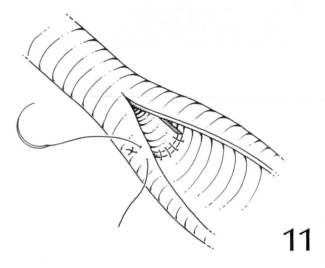

11

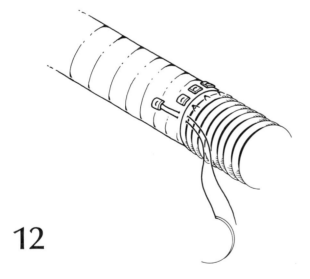

12

Buttressing sutures

12 Disease may sometimes cause the arterial wall to be friable so that it will not hold sutures, which then cut out. This can be a cause of serious haemorrhage. In these circumstances, the sutures should be buttressed with pads of Dacron for large arteries or small pieces of muscle for small arteries.

NON-SUTURED ANASTOMOSIS

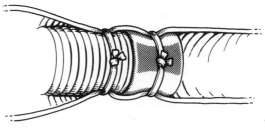

13 This technique has a limited application for the treatment of dissecting aneurysms and some atherosclerotic aneurysms involving the thoracic aorta, where it may confer some advantages over conventional suturing[1]. A rigid, Dacron-covered polypropylene ring attached to the end of the graft is inserted on an applicator within the lumen and held in place by tapes ligated around the outside of the aorta.

13

References

1. Harris PL, Moody AP, Edwards PR, Cave-Bigley DJ. Technical advantages of a ringed intraluminal graft in the management of difficult aortic aneurysms. *Eur J Vasc Surg* 1990; 4: 355–9.

Technique of endarterectomy

C. W. Jamieson MS, FRCS
Consultant Surgeon, St Thomas' Hospital, London, UK

Principles and justification

Indications

Endarterectomy of an artery is indicated in the presence of a short stenotic lesion (open endarterectomy) or, less frequently, in longer occlusions, particularly when the insertion of a synthetic bypass is contraindicated because of the risk of infection.

Preoperative

Good quality angiograms are more important in patients selected for endarterectomy than in those selected for bypass because the exact nature of the stenotic process must be evaluated with great care to make sure the correct segment is treated surgically. In bypass it is only really necessary for surgeons to know that the area selected for the origin of the bypass and that selected for the outflow tract are adequate.

Operations

OPEN ENDARTERECTOMY

Incision

1 The diseased segment is isolated between arterial clamps after full systemic heparinization of the patient. A small incision is made longitudinally in the artery, using a size 15 blade. The incision is deepened very carefully and the knife is withdrawn as soon as fresh blood is encountered, indicating that the arterial lumen has been opened.

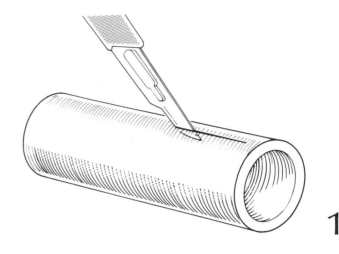

1

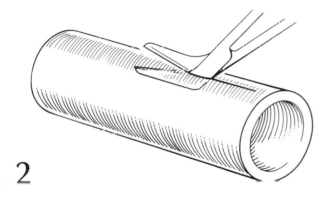

2

2 The incision is extended proximally and distally with a pair of Pott's scissors to cover the extent of the stenotic lesion.

3 One side of the arteriotomy is lifted by the surgeon and the other by the assistant. The surgeon seeks to enter a plane of endarterectomy in the arterial wall using a Watson–Cheyne dissector.

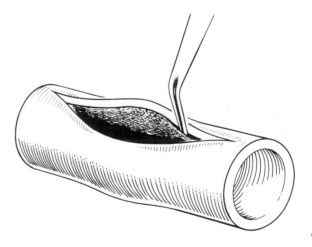

3

4 When a good plane is located the dissector is passed around the apex of the arteriotomy to ensure that the plane remains constant on both sides of the artery. The dissector is only passed around the proximal extremity of the arteriotomy. The inner layers of the vessel distal to the site of endarterectomy are carefully left adherent to their attachments to the remainder of the arterial wall.

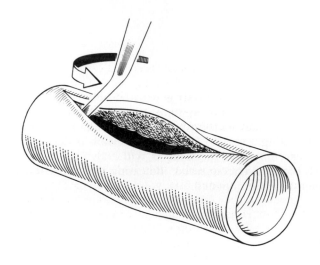

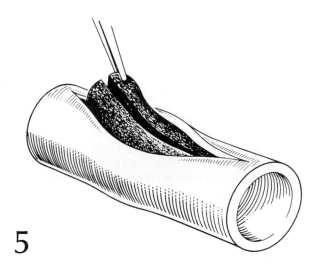

Removal of plaque

5 Using the dissector, the plane of endarterectomy is extended around the whole circumference of the vessel in the proximal part of the arteriotomy, totally freeing the plaque, which is then divided at the proximal end of the arteriotomy and lifted out of the vessel.

6 The distal extremity of the stenosing plaque is then carefully divided with Pott's scissors, exactly at the point at which it remains attached to the arterial wall, so that no loose free flap remains which might lift in the restored blood flow and cause occlusion of the artery.

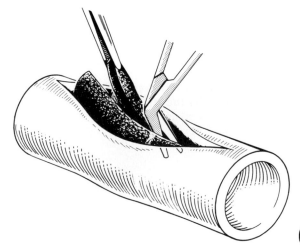

7 If there is any suggestion that this distal extremity of the endarterectomized segment may be loose, two anchoring sutures are passed through the arterial wall, through the endarterectomized segment and out through the unendarterectomized intima, to anchor it in place.

It is sometimes possible to divide the most distal extremity of the plaque first, with sharp dissection, and then to extend the plane of endarterectomy proximally, dividing the endarterectomized core at the proximal extremity of the arteriotomy; this is particularly useful in carotid endarterectomy, where the plaque tails off distally into thin, healthy artery.

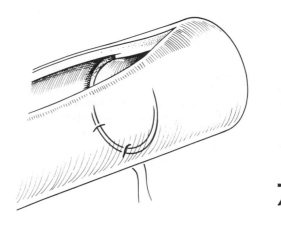

7

Closure

Downflow and backflow are tested by momentary release of each clamp. The arteriotomy is closed with appropriate calibre polypropylene sutures, using 3/0 polypropylene for large vessels such as the aorta and 4/0 or 5/0 for smaller arteries. It is best not to close arteries smaller than 5 mm in diameter directly but to use a patch to avoid the inevitable slight stenosis associated with direct closure.

8 An interrupted suture is placed in the proximal extremity of the arteriotomy and tied. A continuous suture then starts at the distal extremity of the arteriotomy and is advanced to meet the proximal suture. After completion of the suture line the proximal clamp is removed to drive air from the isolated arterial segment before the distal clamp is removed.

After removal of the clamps the vessel is palpated distal to the reconstruction to ensure that a palpable pulse has returned, and the vessel distal to the arteriotomy is observed closely for a few minutes to ensure that dissection has not taken place in the newly endarterectomized segment; this is immediately visible as a blue discoloration of the arterial wall, as blood is forced into it as the flap of intima lifts, and is associated with a loss of the distal pulse, though a strong pulse may persist in the dissection itself.

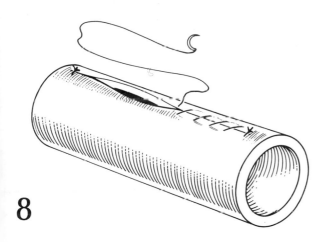

8

SEMI-CLOSED ENDARTERECTOMY

Incision

This technique is suitable for longer occlusions and may be performed through one or two arteriotomies. After systemic heparinization the occluded segment of vessel is exposed and clamps are applied above and below the occluded area.

9 An arteriotomy is made distal to the area of occlusion, extending into the occluded segment to permit exposure of the distal extremity of the stenosing plaque.

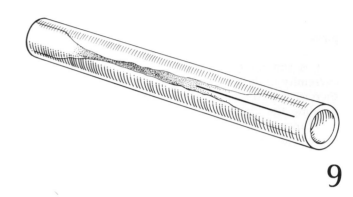

9

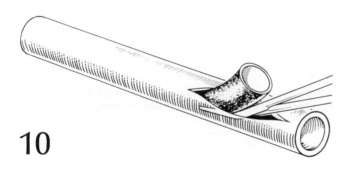

10

Removal of plaque

10 Using the same technique as for open endarterectomy, the arteriotomy is opened and the distal extremity of the plaque is dissected free using a Watson–Cheyne dissector, with a combination of sharp dissection and Pott's scissors.

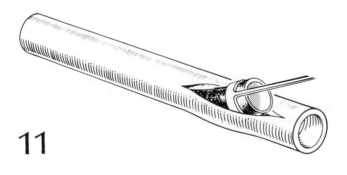

11

11 A loop or arc stripper is then passed up in the plane of endarterectomy to the proximal extremity of the occluding lesion. A loop stripper is relatively safe but, unfortunately, will not easily traverse an artery of varying lumen. An arc stripper will traverse such a vessel, but there is a danger that it may be caught in the wall if it is twisted as it is passed up and down the vessel.

12 After passage of the stripper proximally, arterial forceps are gently closed on the arterial wall with sufficient force to break the inner plaque but not the outer layer of the wall. The artery is held in the finger and thumb of the other hand while the clamp is applied and the plaque can be felt to break, with adequate pressure. The plaque is then milked distally from the vessel by a combination of traction with a pair of forceps and pressure of the finger and thumb of the other hand.

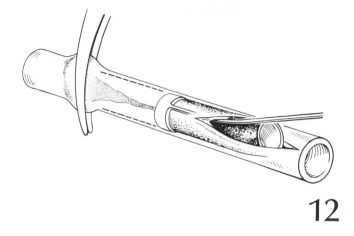

12

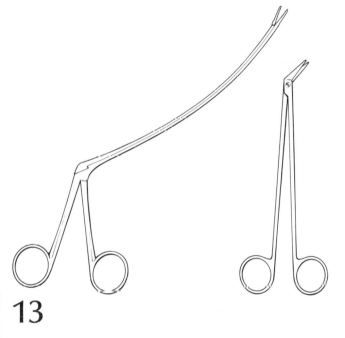

13

13 The plaque may not rupture satisfactorily, or fragments of atheroma may be left in the vessel lumen; these may be removed using a pair of Martin's thrombectomy forceps.

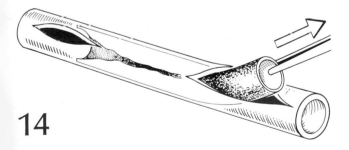

14

14 If the plaque will not rupture it is important that excessive pressure is not applied as this may destroy the arterial wall. A second arteriotomy is then made at the proximal extremity of the occlusion and the plaque is divided under direct vision, to be withdrawn distally.

Closure

The proximal arteriotomy is sutured first, as downflow may then be tested to assess the adequacy of clearance of the obstructed segment. The distal arteriotomy is then closed, again ensuring that there is no evidence of a dissection of the distal end of the intima which may have to be anchored.

EVERSION ENDARTERECTOMY

This elegant variation on the closed endarterectomy technique was described by Wiley.

15 After systemic heparinization the occluded segment of the vessel is clamped proximally and distally and divided transversely at the distal extremity of the occlusion.

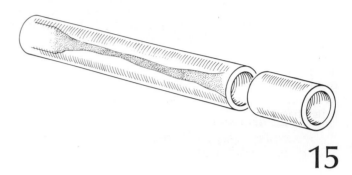

15

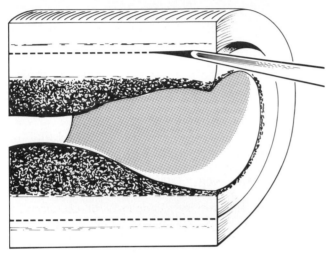

16

16 A Watson–Cheyne dissector is inserted into the plane of endarterectomy in the arterial wall and the adventitia and outer layer of the media are everted, allowing precise division of the adherent bands between the core and the outer wall. After division of the core the eversion is reduced.

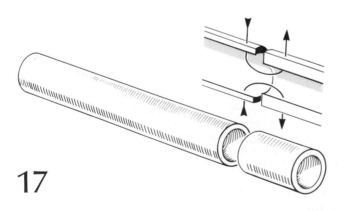

17

17 The divided artery is then resutured, using interrupted sutures to avoid stenosis. This effectively anchors the distal, undivided intima. The sutures should pass from the outer wall of the endarterectomized vessel into the lumen of the unendarterectomized vessel and out again, thereby anchoring the distal intima.

Outcome

Endarterectomy is technically more demanding than a bypass procedure and for this reason it has been practised less frequently in recent years, but it does have the advantage that sepsis is not so disastrous as is infection of a synthetic graft, and the long-term results of endarterectomy in most sites are comparable with those of bypass.

Aortoiliac reconstruction: thromboendarterectomy and bypass grafting

John J. Ricotta MD
Professor of Surgery and Director, Division of Vascular Surgery, State University of New York at Buffalo, Buffalo, New York, USA

James A. DeWeese MD
Professor of Surgery and Chief Emeritus of Cardiothoracic and Vascular Surgery, University of Rochester Medical Center, Rochester, New York, USA

History

Aortoiliac reconstruction began with thromboendarterectomy of the aortoiliac and femoral segments. Open endarterectomy was developed first by Dos Santos, followed by the semiclosed technique and, finally, eversion endarterectomy, still used by some. Concerns about the technical challenge of thromboendarterectomy and the better long-term patency of aortofemoral bypass have caused many surgeons to abandon this procedure. In recent years, attention has turned to extending the bypass more proximally to adequately address disease in the perirenal and visceral aorta, most commonly through an extended retroperitoneal approach. At the same time there has been a resurgence of interest in iliofemoral bypass for patients with unilateral iliac occlusion. Stenotic iliac lesions are now often treated by percutaneous balloon angioplasty, sometimes accompanied by distal cross-femoral reconstruction. An axillobifemoral bypass is occasionally used. Thus, there are now many alternatives in aortoiliac reconstruction, and the approach is currently tailored to each clinical situation[1,2].

Principles and justification

Reconstruction of the aortoiliac segment is usually justified in patients with symptomatic arterial insufficiency of one or both lower extremities. The relatively low morbidity and mortality rates associated with aortofemoral bypass (2–5%) and excellent long-term patency rates (about 90%) justify this approach in patients with symptoms of claudication who are otherwise fit for surgery[3]. Patients with claudication who are at increased risk for aortofemoral bypass can often be treated by lower risk procedures, e.g. iliofemoral bypass, cross-femoral bypass, axillobifemoral bypass, or percutaneous angioplasty with or without cross-femoral bypass. If there is an indication from the physical assessment that one of these approaches is possible, then angiography is appropriate to evaluate higher risk patients with claudication for such intervention.

Impending tissue loss with severe aortoiliac disease is a firm indication for arterial reconstruction. Because amputation is often the alternative in these patients, a higher degree of operative risk is acceptable. As in patients with claudication, however, the treatment selected must be matched to the patient's arterial anatomy and clinical condition.

As a general guideline, patients with diffuse aortoiliac involvement are best treated by aortofemoral bypass. Unilateral iliofemoral reconstruction is reserved by the authors for those patients with significant disease restricted to a single iliac system and a relatively normal aortic bifurcation. Percutaneous angioplasty has been helpful in patients with discrete (usually less than 5 cm) stenosis or occlusions of the iliac vessels. While some clinicians advocate angioplasty in lesions up to 10 cm in length, iliofemoral bypass is preferable if possible in these cases. In poor-risk patients with bilateral iliac disease, i.e. occlusion with contralateral discrete stenosis, the authors have not hesitated to employ unilateral angioplasty with cross-femoral bypass. In these cases, a Palmaz stent is currently employed in conjunction with angioplasty to protect the downstream reconstruction.

Preoperative

Assessment

In addition to a thorough history and physical examination non-invasive vascular evaluation is important. This should include segmental limb pressures and Doppler waveform recording from the common femoral arteries. Duplex ultrasonography may be helpful in some patients to identify discrete iliac lesions amenable to angioplasty, but it cannot currently replace biplane angiography[4]. Angiography should include anteroposterior views of the entire abdominal aorta including the visceral vessels. Lateral aortic views are important when perirenal disease is suggested on the anteroposterior aortogram or when a meandering mesenteric artery is identified. Lateral aortography is the only way to identify posterior aortic plaque and to visualize the orifices of the coeliac and superior mesenteric arteries. If stenoses of the iliac arteries are suggested, oblique films may be necessary to delineate the extent of disease further. Finally, when questions still remain as to the significance of aortoiliac disease, pullback pressure measurements may be necessary, often with the use of a vasodilator such as papaverine. A pressure gradient of more than 10 mmHg following injection of a vasodilator is diagnostic of a haemodynamically significant lesion. Distal films should include tibial run-off.

From the foregoing it is obvious that transfemoral aortography is preferred whenever possible. This provides the best information on distal run-off and permits pressure measurement. In some cases of severe iliac disease or aortic occlusion, transfemoral aortography is not possible. Transaxillary or translumbar aortography is an acceptable alternative. Use of small catheters and the digital subtraction technique has reduced complications from the transaxillary approach. Lateral aortography is often needed in these cases and may be cumbersome if a translumbar approach is used. Intravenous digital subtraction techniques are seldom detailed enough to provide information not available after a thorough physical examination and non-invasive study.

General evaluation focuses on the heart, lungs and abdominal viscera. A history of angina, exertional dyspnoea, postprandial abdominal pain, or hypertension is sought. Laboratory evaluation includes chest radiography, electrocardiography, clotting profile and serum creatinine concentrations. A history of untreated angina, unstable angina, or unexplained cardiographic abnormalities requires further evaluation, currently by stress nuclear cardiography or 24-h electrocardiographic monitoring. Patients with ischaemic myocardium at risk may require coronary angiography, particularly before elective surgery for claudication. Significant dyspnoea or abnormal chest radiographic findings should prompt preoperative pulmonary function tests. Patients with hypertension and abnormal or borderline serum creatinine concentrations should have a creatinine clearance performed before surgery, particularly if angiography suggests renovascular disease.

Patient preparation

Patients should be admitted on the evening before surgery for hydration. Intravenous hydration is particularly important if angiography is performed on the day before operation. Intensive preoperative monitoring (including peripheral arterial and pulmonary artery catheters) is indicated in patients with visceral vessel involvement as well as in those at increased cardiac risk. Optimal preoperative control of intravascular volume, cardiac performance and vascular resistance is essential in these patients to reduce perioperative morbidity.

Prophylactic antibiotics are administered within 1 h before skin incision and continued until all invasive monitoring is removed. General anaesthesia is preferred for these procedures. Supplemental epidural anaesthesia may be useful in some patients, and this can be continued for 24–48 h after surgery in selected cases.

Operations

Aortoiliac endarterectomy is still indicated in some patients whose disease is limited to the distal aorta and common iliac arteries. Although it may be technically more challenging than bypass procedures, it avoids the use of a prosthetic material. The more extensive dissection of the aortic bifurcation required with this procedure may increase the frequency of ejaculatory dysfunction in men and is used sparingly in men for this reason. Cases of aortic hypoplasia are best treated by aortofemoral bypass. Endarterectomy is occasionally useful when re-establishing flow in a contaminated field or treating a graft infection. Thromboendarterectomy can be performed through a standard retroperitoneal or transabdominal approach.

STANDARD RETROPERITONEAL APPROACH

Position of patient and incision

1 For the standard retroperitoneal approach, the patient is positioned with the left side elevated to 30–45°. This is readily achieved by a rolled towel or bean bag. Reverse flexion of the table (jack-knife position) is helpful for additional exposure. The incision is begun just below the umbilicus just medial to the lateral border of the rectus muscle and extends laterally to the tip of the 12th rib.

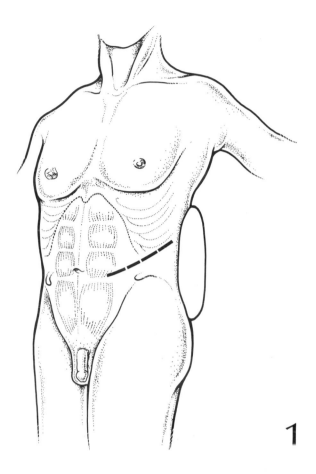

1

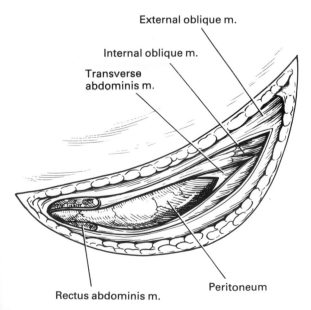

External oblique m.

Internal oblique m.

Transverse abdominis m.

Rectus abdominis m.

Peritoneum

2 The anterior rectus sheath is incised and the rectus muscle is retracted (or occasionally transected) for adequate medial exposure. The medial portion of the incision is the most usual point at which the peritoneal cavity is entered, and care should be taken to avoid this. If the peritoneum is incised, it is immediately closed with a running absorbable suture (3/0 or 4/0). The external oblique, internal oblique and transverse abdominis muscles are transected along the line of the skin incision.

2

Exposure of the aorta and iliac vessels

3 The retroperitoneal space is entered laterally and the peritoneum and its contents are swept medially using a gauze laparotomy pad. Mobilization proceeds above the retroperitoneal fat and psoas muscle and the genitofemoral nerve. In this approach, dissection is anterior to the left kidney. The inferior mesenteric artery is identified and divided for additional exposure. From this point on the operation is identical to the transperitoneal approach. At the conclusion of the endarterectomy the rectus sheath, transverse abdominis and oblique muscles are closed individually with 0 or 2/0 absorbable sutures.

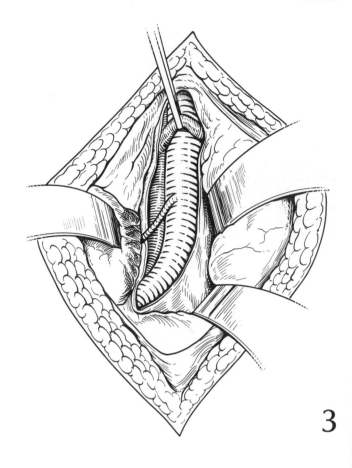

3

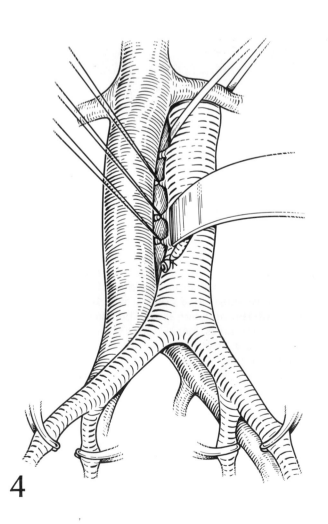

4

Mobilization of the aorta and iliac vessels

4 Completion of the thromboendarterectomy requires extensive mobilization of the aorta and iliac arteries including their tributaries. Mobilization should extend 2–3 cm proximal and distal to the known area of disease and may include the distal abdominal aorta, common external and internal iliac arteries, middle sacral and lumbar arteries. The smaller arteries can be controlled by Pott's ties or small bulldog clamps.

Arterial incision

5 Incisions are made to encompass the proximal and distal aspects of the proposed thromboendarterectomy. This can be accomplished by using two incisions: one placed to the right of the inferior mesenteric artery and extending down the right common iliac vessel and a separate longitudinal incision on the left common iliac artery. This technique minimizes disruption of the preaortic autonomic plexus, which is located to the left side of the aortic bifurcation.

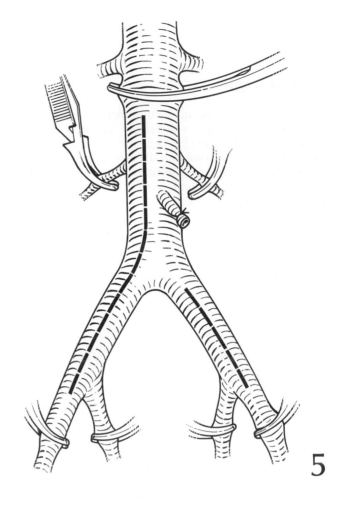

5

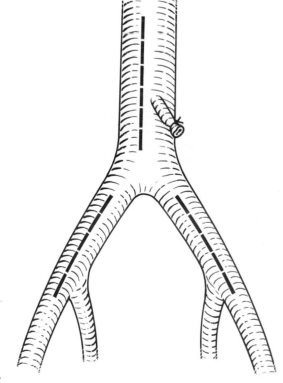

6

6 Alternatively, three incisions can be made, separating the aortic and right iliac arteriotomies. In either event the iliac arteriotomies must extend distally past the end of the endarterectomy (usually at the iliac bifurcation).

Endarterectomy

7 The plane of cleavage is identified just deep to the intima. This plane is developed using a clamp or endarterectomy spatula. The dissection is carried circumferentially throughout the diseased segment. The inner core is divided proximally and distally with scissors and the plaque is removed. Endarterectomy may be facilitated by dividing the plaque proximally early in the procedure to aid in developing the cleavage plane. The endarterectomy is completed in a semiclosed fashion using an intraluminal dissector between the incisions. The endarterectomy is ended where the plaque becomes attenuated, most often at the common iliac bifurcation. The intima is cut flush at this point with Pott's scissors to avoid loose flaps.

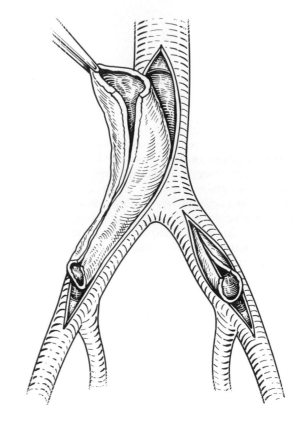

7

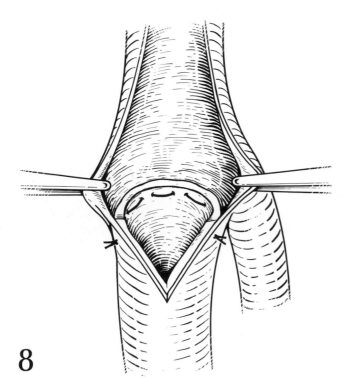

8

Securing the intima

8 Following transection of the intima, it is inspected closely and the area irrigated with heparinized saline solution. If the intima is loose at its distal cut margin, it should be anchored to the vessel with a series of interrupted mattress sutures tied outside the vessel. After inspection of the distal operative site, the entire endarterectomy is flushed with heparinized saline to remove any loose debris and thrombus.

Closure of arteriotomies

9 The arteriotomies are closed with running 4/0 or 5/0 monofilament sutures. Before completion of the closure, clamps are momentarily released first distally and then proximally to flush out residual debris or thrombus.

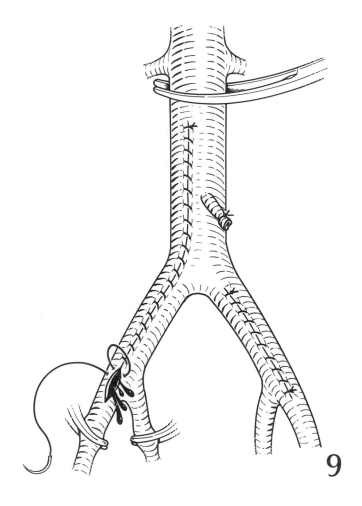

9

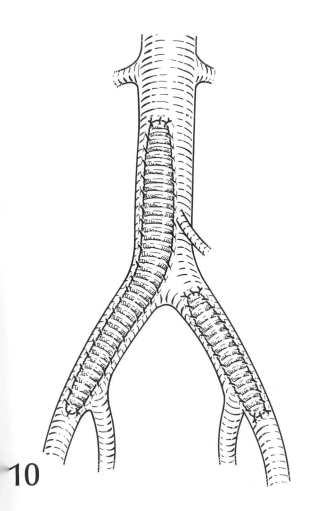

10

10 If necessary, the arteriotomies may be closed with a patch of Dacron or polytetrafluorethylene (PTFE). This is particularly helpful when the aorta is small. The ends of the patch are rounded or squared off to widen the distal ends of the arteriotomy. After release of the clamps, bleeding is controlled by packs with light pressure. Liquid thrombin or microcrystalline collagen may occasionally be required. Significant suture line leaks are repaired with interrupted 6/0 sutures.

Alternative methods of endarterectomy

11 Eversion endarterectomy and semiclosed endarterectomy have been used as alternatives to the method described here. Eversion endarterectomy involves complete mobilization and transection of the vessel involved, which is then turned back on itself.

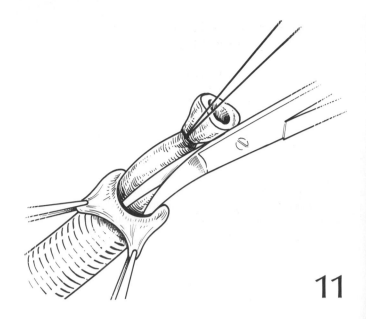

11

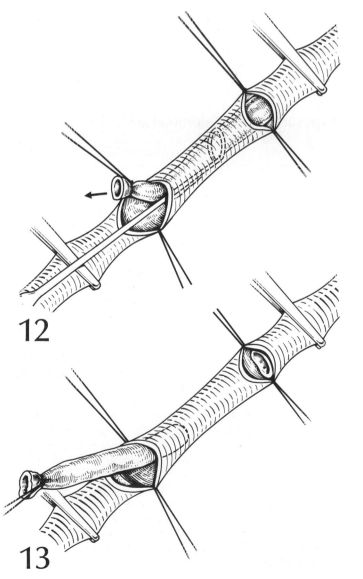

12

13

12, 13 The semiclosed technique usually involves multiple transverse arteriotomies and the use of a looped endarterectomy stripper. These techniques are difficult for long segments unless the operator is very familiar with them. They offer no advantages over the approach described above.

TRANSPERITONEAL AORTOILIAC AND AORTOFEMORAL BYPASS GRAFT

This remains the most common procedure performed for aortoiliac occlusive disease. A variety of prosthetic materials is used. Currently, the authors' preference is collagen-impregnated Dacron or PTFE because of the impermeable nature of the material. If standard knitted or woven Dacron is used, it must be preclotted before implantation. Using this approach, the proximal anastomosis is infrarenal; while the distal anastomosis can be to the common iliac, external iliac, or femoral arteries, the authors believe that common femoral anastomosis is indicated in the overwhelming majority of operations performed for occlusive disease and is associated with better long-term patency.

Incision

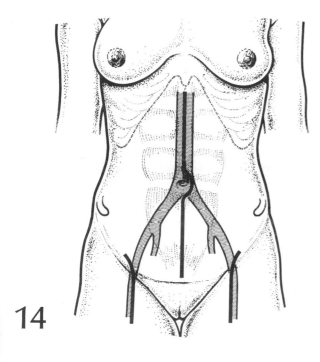

14   The preferred incision is a long midline one extending from the xiphoid process to the pubic symphysis, although a left paramedian or even a transverse incision is employed by some surgeons. When the graft is to be carried to the femoral arteries, these are exposed by longitudinal incisions beginning above the level of the inguinal ligament and extending down over the femoral arteries low enough to expose the common femoral bifurcation. Additional proximal exposure of the distal external iliac artery can be gained by curving the incision laterally parallel to the inguinal ligament. The ligament can be retracted superiorly and the artery exposed, often without transecting the ligament.

Exposure of the abdominal aorta

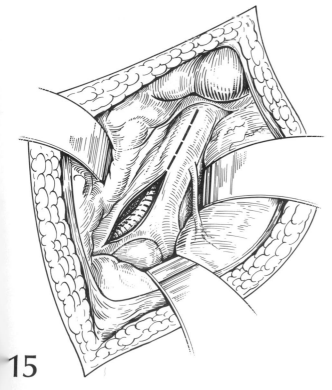

15   The retroperitoneum is entered by incising the retroperitoneal attachments of the duodenum and mobilizing the ligament of Treitz. This incision is begun as close to the duodenum as possible and continued down the right side of the aorta. A flap of posterior peritoneum is developed based to the left of the aorta. This flap is used after completion of the bypass to separate the graft from the visceral organs. The lymphatic vessels overlying the aorta are divided between ligatures or clips. Dissection proceeds proximally until the renal vein is identified. Failure to encounter this structure must alert the operator to the possibility of a retroaortic renal vein. During dissection the inferior mesenteric vein is mobilized and retracted. Although the inferior mesenteric vein may be ligated if necessary, this has not occurred in operations for occlusive disease in the authors' experience.

Infrarenal aortic dissection begins just below the renal vein and continues for 2–3 cm distally. The importance of placing the proximal (aortic) anastomosis high on the infrarenal aorta cannot be overemphasized. This area is most often free of disease and most amenable to precise anastomosis. One or more pairs of lumbar arteries may be sacrificed to obtain adequate mobilization of the aorta. The aorta is encircled using finger dissection if possible, although a curved vascular clamp may be required. During these manoeuvres care must be taken to avoid damage to the vena cava or lumbar veins.

Mobilization of the renal vein

16, 17 In especially high lesions, additional exposure can be gained by mobilizing or dividing the renal vein. The authors prefer mobilization to division and ligature. Mobilization may require division of the gonadal vein to allow the renal vein to be retracted superiorly. If the renal vein must be divided this should be done close to its junction with the vena cava and the ends oversewn with a double layer of 5/0 monofilament suture. When dividing the renal vein it is important to preserve both the gonadal and adrenal veins to provide venous outflow for the left kidney. Whenever possible the decision to transect the renal vein should be made before the gonadal vein is sacrificed during mobilization of that structure.

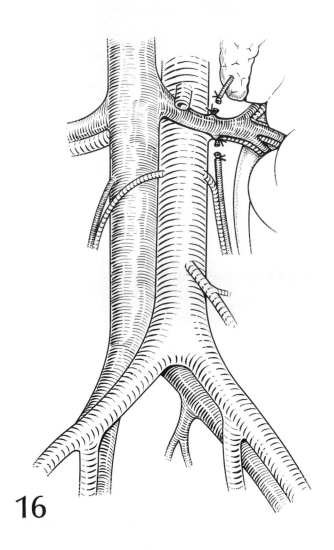

16

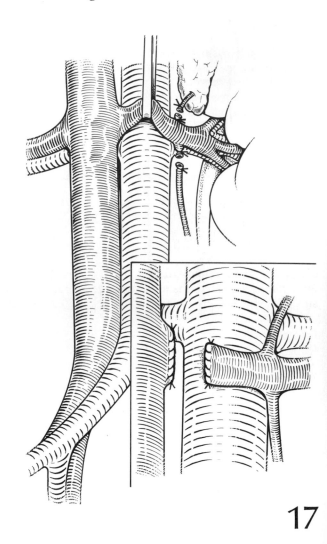

17

Clotting the graft

This step is always necessary when a non-coated knitted Dacron graft is used, although it is not as important when the less porous woven grafts are employed. Preclotting serves two purposes: to seal the graft effectively against leakage and to provide a smooth fibrin lining at the blood–graft interface. When newer impervious prosthetics are used, this step is not required.

18, 19 Before systemic heparinization, fresh blood, 100 ml, is withdrawn from the aorta or vena cava and placed in a basin. An appropriately sized graft is selected for use. The graft should be isodiametric or slightly smaller than the artery for aortic reconstruction. In the authors' experience the graft selected is more often too large than too small for the vessels. One end of the graft is clamped, and fresh blood is forced through the graft using a catheter-tipped or bulb syringe. This procedure is continued until leakage through the prosthesis is minimal. The prosthesis is then flushed with heparinized saline to remove any loose debris.

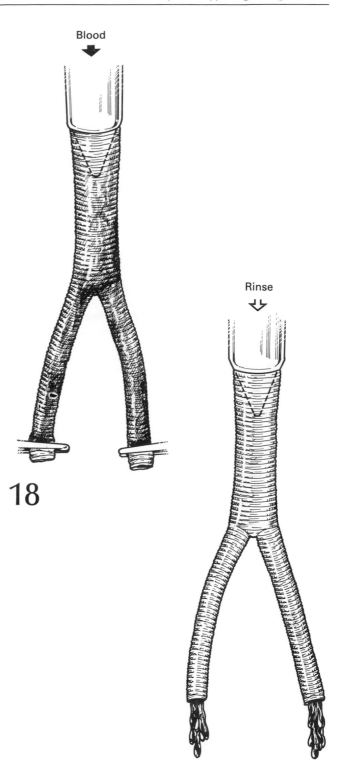

Making the tunnel

20 Following removal of blood for clotting, the retroperitoneal tunnel is made using blunt dissection. Tunnelling is accomplished using finger dissection from the abdominal and femoral incisions. The tunnel begins in the abdomen behind the ureter and directly over the iliac artery. Failure to remain behind the ureter can result in postoperative ureteric obstruction. In the groin, the plane is found immediately over the femoral artery. Tunnelling is completed bluntly and a long vascular clamp is guided through the tunnel from below upwards. Dacron tape is left in the tunnel.

The patient is anticoagulated with intravenous heparin, 100–150 units/kg. The arteries are clamped distally first to avoid embolism, and the prosthesis is inserted. At this point the inside of the prosthesis is inspected, and any loose fibrin or clot is removed using forceps or flushing techniques. After completion of the proximal anastomosis, the graft will be filled with blood to test for leakage and then flushed with blood to remove debris before performing the distal anastomosis.

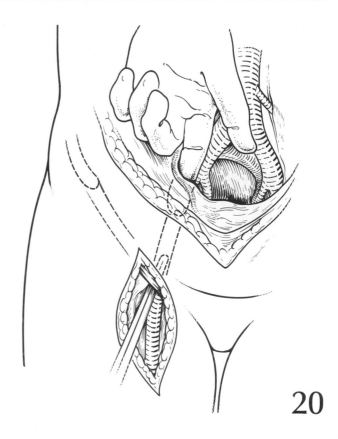

20

End-to-end proximal anastomosis

The proximal anastomosis may be end-to-end or end-to-side. The former is preferable because of less turbulent flow and more accurate suture placement. End-to-end anastomoses have a particular advantage when there is extensive juxtarenal aortic disease, as they permit inspection of the proximal aorta, limited thromboendarterectomy, and accurate placement of sutures in the proximal anastomotic line. Every effort is made to locate the proximal anastomosis high on the infrarenal aorta.

21 The aorta is clamped proximal and distal to the area proposed for anastomosis, and the aorta is transected. The distal end of the aorta is oversewn with a double layer of 3/0 or 4/0 polypropylene (Prolene).

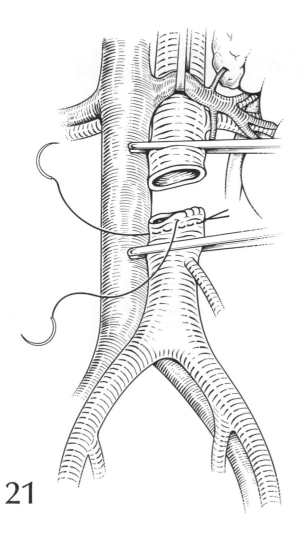

21

22 A preclotted graft of appropriate size is then anastomosed to the cut end of the aorta using a running 3/0 or 4/0 polypropylene suture. The anastomosis is begun on the posterior wall of the aorta. This suture may be tied or a running parachute technique may be used. The two ends of the suture are then continued posteriorly and anteriorly to complete the suture line. Whenever possible, the sutures proceed from intima to adventitia on the aorta.

Alternative techniques include placing two equidistant sutures to bisect the anastomosis or using interrupted mattress sutures for the posterior wall or the entire circumference of the anastomosis. While these methods have their advocates, the authors have not found them to be particularly advantageous in the usual aortic reconstruction. It is most important that the aortic sutures are placed in relatively good aorta with a single motion whenever possible. Excessive torque on the artery can result in needle hole bleeding or even disruption of the proximal suture line.

End-to-side proximal anastomosis

End-to-side grafts are indicated in specific circumstances where it is important to preserve prograde flow to the pelvis through the hypogastric vessels[5]. This is most common when there are bilateral external iliac occlusions with less disease in the aorta and common iliac vessels. If inferior mesenteric flow is to be preserved, proximal end-to-side anastomosis may be used, although an end-to-end anastomosis with reimplantation of the inferior mesenteric artery may be preferable. End-to-side anastomosis is also preferred in patients with a small aorta. It may be used in patients where the aortic segment to be used is soft and disease-free. The exposure of the aorta is identical to that already described.

23 A side-biting partial occlusion clamp may be used; however, two aortic occlusion clamps are preferred because this allows better exposure of the arteriotomy. The upper clamp is applied in the standard fashion above the level of anastomosis. The lower clamp is applied from below in the axis of the aorta to occlude the lumbar vessels as well as the distal aorta. End-to-side anastomosis does not require mobilization of the posterior aortic wall. An elliptical incision is cut in the graft and the suture is begun at the distal aorta and the 'heel' of the graft as a mattress suture, which is tied and then carried up each side. One suture is carried around the apex of the graft so that this critical area can be completed under direct vision. Suturing should always proceed from inside to outside on the artery to avoid raising a flap of intima. When the anastomosis is complete, it is tested as described below.

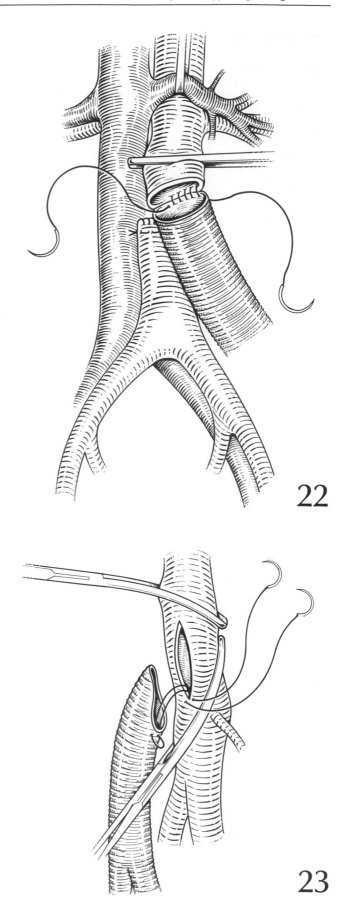

22

23

Testing the proximal suture line

24 The limbs of the aortic graft are clamped and the aortic clamp briefly removed to allow the graft to fill with blood. The graft is reclamped close to the suture line and the aortic clamp again released to test anastomotic integrity. Bleeding from needle holes is usually controlled with pressure. Any large leaks, however, are best repaired with interrupted sutures at this point. Once the suture line is secure, the proximal aorta is reclamped.

Prolonged clamping of the graft should be avoided unless the character of the aorta precludes reclamping the vessel safely. A cuff of graft may be placed over the limbs of the bifurcation graft and brought proximally to cover the anastomosis. This is particularly helpful when the aortic cuff is friable and has been used routinely by some surgeons with the hope of decreasing aortoenteric fistulae.

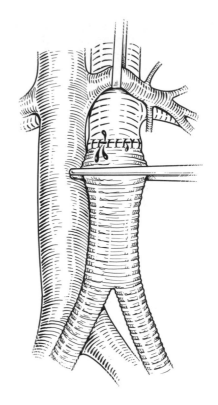

24

End-to-side distal anastomosis

The distal anastomosis may be performed to the common iliac, external iliac or common femoral artery. While there are some advantages to avoiding an anastomosis in the groin (lower incidence of wound problems and avoiding an area of flexion), the long-term patency of aortofemoral grafts may be superior to that of aortoiliac grafts when performed for occlusive disease. For this reason the distal anastomosis is usually carried to the common femoral artery. As progressive disease is frequent in the superficial and common femoral arteries, it is important to site the femoral anastomosis low on the common femoral artery over the orifice of the deep femoral artery. A long vascular clamp is pulled through the tunnel with the umbilical tape previously placed. Each limb of the graft is grasped and pulled down into the groin, care being taken not to twist it.

25 The distal end of the graft is carefully bevelled for the distal anastomosis. The graft should be cut in an S shape with heavy scissors. The distal end should be tailored to accommodate the distal arteriotomy. The distal anastomosis can then be performed.

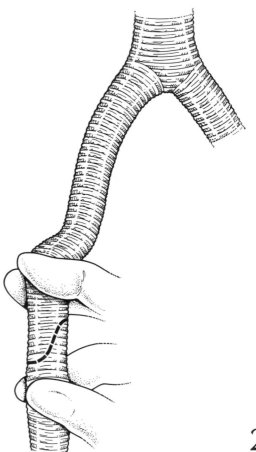

25

26 The technique of distal anastomosis is the same in the iliac and femoral arteries. A segment of artery is isolated between clamps and a longitudinal arteriotomy made. In the femoral artery the origins of the superficial and deep femoral arteries are dissected free, and these arteries are clamped. As stated above, the incision should extend down to the common femoral bifurcation so that the orifice of the deep femoral artery is visualized. If the superficial femoral artery is occluded or there is disease at the orifice of the deep femoral artery, the arteriotomy can be extended down the deep femoral artery, and the distal anastomosis can be extended as a tongue over the deep femoral artery as a deep femoral reconstruction. The anastomosis is begun by placing double-ended 5/0 or 6/0 polypropylene sutures at each corner of the graft. These are carried from the inside to the outside of the artery.

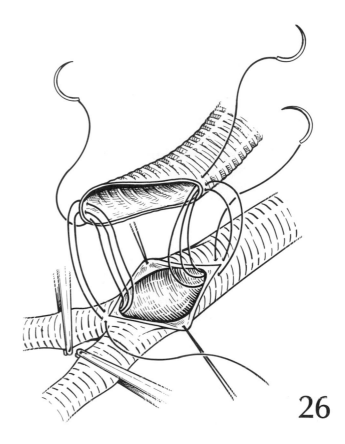

26

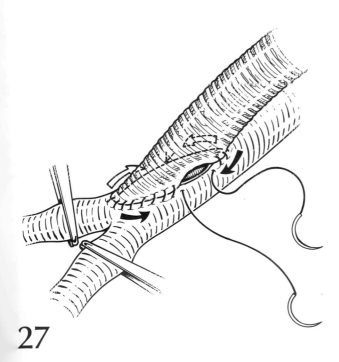

27

27 With the graft suspended, three or four sutures are placed at each corner under direct vision. The sutures are then drawn taut, the graft brought down to the artery, and the anastomosis completed by running sutures placed towards the middle of the suture line from each apex. This technique permits optimal visualization of the corner stitches, which is important to avoid compromising both inflow and outflow.

In an alternative technique, a mattress suture is placed at the 'heel' of the graft and then run around the top of the graft under direct vision. Following completion of one anastomosis the distal clamp is removed, allowing retrograde flow to flush out clot and debris through the opposite limb of the graft. This contralateral limb is then clamped near the bifurcation, and the proximal clamp is slowly released to prevent a drop in systolic blood pressure of more than 20 mmHg. The same procedure is carried out after completion of the second anastomosis.

Reimplantation of inferior mesenteric artery

In most patients the inferior mesenteric artery can be sacrificed with impunity, but in a small number the collateral circulation is inadequate. A large meandering artery seen on preoperative arteriography may help to identify these patients. Larger arteries (5 mm diameter or more), particularly those without back-bleeding, are more likely to require reimplantation.

28 If reimplantation is necessary, a button of aortic wall with the inferior mesenteric artery at its centre is excised and sewn onto the side of the graft. At operation the inferior mesenteric artery may be tested by temporary occlusion. During this time the colour of the intestine is observed and Doppler flow can be studied in the inferior mesenteric artery and along the antimesenteric border of the intestine.

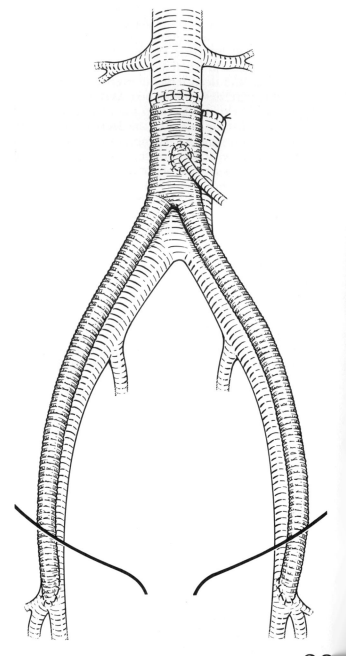

28

Closure of retroperitoneum

29 Following insertion of the graft, the retroperitoneum is closed. The purpose is to prevent contact of the intestine, particularly the duodenum, with the aortic prosthesis. The retroperitoneal incision is approximated with a running absorbable suture. A double-layer closure has been suggested to separate the aorta more effectively from the abdominal viscera. Every attempt is made to leave the mobilized duodenum free rather than to reattach it to its retroperitoneal position. If necessary, an omental pedicle may be placed between the aorta and the intestine to provide further coverage.

The groin wounds are closed meticulously in layers. At least two subcutaneous layers are employed. Haemostasis and avoidance of lymphatic leaks are of utmost importance in prevention of wound complications. Subcuticular closure of the skin avoids transcutaneous sutures in the groin.

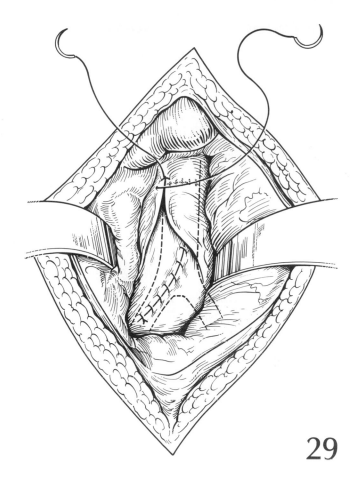

29

TREATMENT OF JUXTARENAL AORTIC OCCLUSIONS

Following aortic occlusion, thrombus may extend to the level of the renal vessels. In these instances the atherosclerotic plaque ends below the renal arteries, but the perirenal artery is occluded by organized thrombus. A standard aortofemoral bypass can be accomplished using minor modifications of the techniques just described. The goal of these modifications is to establish a segment of infrarenal aorta suitable for anastomosis.

30 Exposure is identical to that described for transperitoneal aortic procedures. In this case, however, the renal vein is mobilized and both renal arteries, as well as the suprarenal aorta, are exposed. After heparinization, the renal arteries are controlled by bulldog clamps or soft loops, and the aorta is transected 3–4 cm below the renal vein. The occluded proximal aortic segment is then transposed anterior to the left renal vein to facilitate exposure and a thrombectomy is begun. The dissection plane is between the organized plug of thrombus and the intima. This proceeds circumferentially until the thrombus is extruded from the aorta by the combined forces of dissection and prograde aortic flow. It should be noted that the aorta is *not* clamped during this portion of the dissection, but rather controlled by the operator's fingers or an open clamp.

When prograde flow is established, the aorta is occluded by digital pressure followed by application of a vascular clamp. The thrombectomized portion of the aorta is inspected and flushed to remove debris and the aortic clamp is reapplied below the renal vessels. The aorta is then repositioned behind the renal vein and a standard end-to-end bypass is performed as previously described.

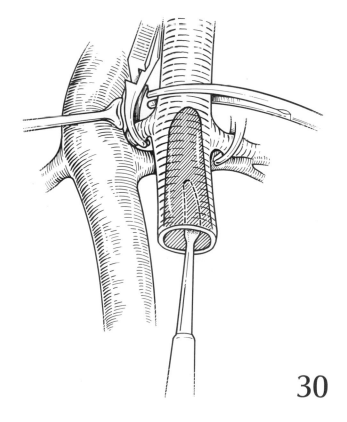

30

SUPRACOELIAC CONTROL OF AORTA

Not uncommonly, the aorta is significantly diseased at the level of the renal vessels or in the portion involving the origins of the mesenteric arteries. This is often not appreciated on standard anteroposterior angiography. While infrarenal aortofemoral bypass is often performed in these cases, clamping a diseased infrarenal aorta may result in embolism, bleeding from the proximal suture line, or late false aneurysm. If significant perirenal disease exists, it is better to clamp the aorta above the renal vessels. When this is done the proximal anastomosis can often be placed just distal to the origins of the renal arteries, avoiding visceral revascularization. The authors prefer to obtain aortic control above the coeliac axis at the level of the diaphragm. This can be done either transperitoneally or by an extended retroperitoneal exposure.

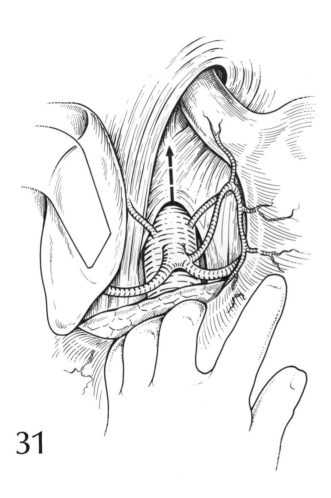

31

Transperitoneal exposure of supracoeliac aorta

31 The supracoeliac aorta is approached through the gastrohepatic ligament[6]. The triangular ligament is incised and the left lobe of the liver is mobilized and retracted to the right. The aorta is located by palpation, and the muscular fibres of the aortic hiatus are divided by ligature or cautery. It is not necessary to isolate the oesophagus at this point, as the aorta is easily distinguished from this structure. After the crural fibres are dissected away from the aorta, the vessel can be encircled by finger dissection. A tape is not placed around the aorta; when the clamp is to be applied, the vessel is encircled by the thumb and index finger of the left hand, lifted off the spinal column and occluded with a straight vascular clamp.

Treatment of perirenal aortic disease

32 With the aorta clamped above the coeliac artery, the aorta is transected below the renal vessels. In most instances an anastomosis can be performed at the level of the renal vessels without further manipulation. If necessary, an endarterectomy of this segment can be performed, although the plane is somewhat more superficial than is usually taken in peripheral vessels. Back-bleeding encountered from the mesenteric vessels is usually modest and can be controlled by pressure, or the field can be kept clear with suction. Use of autotransfusion is suggested in these cases. After the aorta is deemed satisfactory, anastomosis is performed.

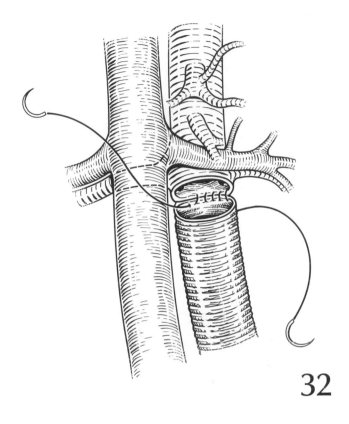

32

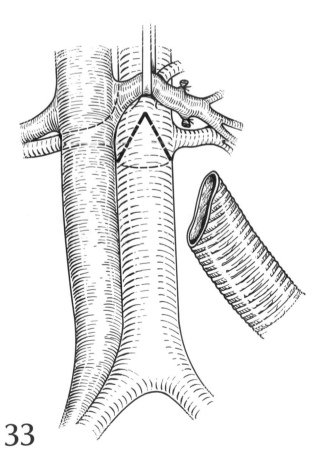

33

33 Very occasionally, endarterectomy must be continued just above the orifices of the renal vessels. If this can be anticipated the retroperitoneal approach is preferred. Additional exposure, however, can be gained by incising the anterior aspect of the aorta to just below the superior mesenteric artery. After endarterectomy, the proximal portion of the graft is bevelled to facilitate closure of this defect.

EXTENDED RETROPERITONEAL APPROACH TO THE AORTA

When the aorta at the origins of the mesenteric and renal vessels is involved in the atherosclerotic process, the extended retroperitoneal approach is preferred[7]. In this exposure, the supracoeliac aorta is approached on its posterolateral aspect and the viscera are reflected anteriorly. By dividing the diaphragm at the aortic hiatus, the aorta can be exposed to the level of the 10th thoracic vertebra. A thoracoabdominal incision is avoided, along with its attendant morbidity. The major drawback of this approach is limited access to the visceral and right renal vessels. Therefore, it should only be used when disease is confined to the origin of these arteries and can be treated by endarterectomy.

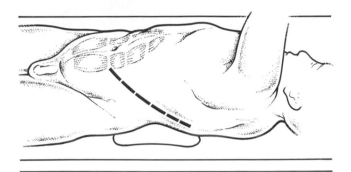

34

Patient position and incision

34 The patient is placed in a modified left thoracotomy position with shoulders almost perpendicular to the operating table but hips rotated as much as possible parallel to the plane of the table. A bean bag is used to stabilize this position. Exposure is facilitated by placing the table in a jack-knife position. The operating surgeon is positioned at the patient's back.

The incision begins 3–5 cm below the umbilicus at the lateral border of the rectus muscle and extends laterally between the 10th and 11th or 11th and 12th ribs, depending on the level of aortic control desired. The authors initially carried this incision to the border of the paraspinous muscles, but in recent years have shortened its posterior extent considerably. This appears to have decreased the incidence of intercostal neuralgia and 'pseudohernia' from denervation of the lateral abdominal musculature. It is important to try to spare the intercostal bundles as much as possible. When the superior incision is used, the chest is commonly entered at the lateral border of the incision. This is of no great consequence and the fibres of the diaphragm are reapproximated over a temporary tube at the conclusion of the operation while the lungs are expanded.

35 The oblique and transverse abdominis muscles are divided in the line of the skin incision, and the retroperitoneal space is entered. Mobilization begins laterally and extends medially as described for the standard retroperitoneal approach. In this case, however, dissection is carried behind the left kidney, which is displaced anteriorly with the other viscera. In the unusual circumstance of a retroaortic renal vein, the kidney is left posteriorly.

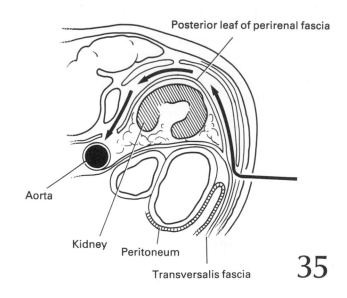

Dissection of the aorta

36 A large lumbar vein is usually encountered, which helps identify the origin of the left renal artery. Dissection of the aorta begins along the vertebral column and continues posteriorly. The most important landmark is the left renal artery, which should be identified early. The aortic dissection should proceed posterior to this vessel. Lymphatic and lumbar vessels are ligated in continuity as necessary with 3/0 silk ligatures. Dissection is carried through the diaphragm, diaphragmatic crura and, if necessary, to the lower thoracic aorta. This allows the aorta to be clamped in a disease-free area. No attempt should be made to dissect the aorta circumferentially from this approach, as this could result in troublesome venous bleeding. The vessel is mobilized enough to allow placement of a larger vascular clamp above the level of disease and below the renal arteries.

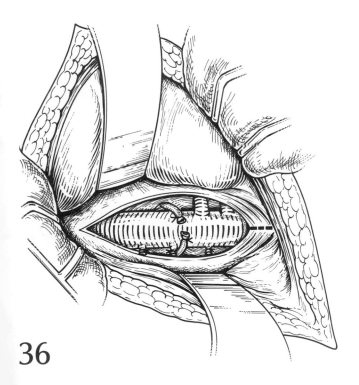

Endarterectomy of suprarenal abdominal aorta

37a, b The aorta is incised posterior to the left renal artery. An endarterectomy plane is established at this point. This plane is more superficial than would be taken in the femoral or carotid systems. Back-bleeding from the renal and superior mesenteric and coeliac arteries is controlled with Fogarty balloon catheters. If necessary, endarterectomy of one or more of the renal and visceral arteries may be carried out at this point. After the aortic segment has been endarterectomized, the repair proceeds in one of two ways.

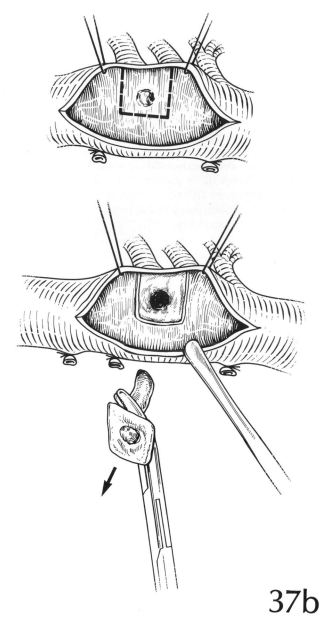

37b

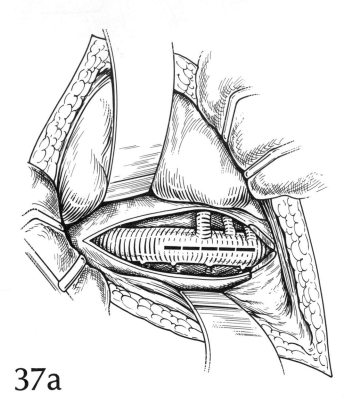

37a

38 If the distal aorta is normal, the arteriotomy may be closed with 4/0 or 5/0 monofilament after the distal intima has been secured to avoid dissection. This approach is only applicable in a small minority of patients.

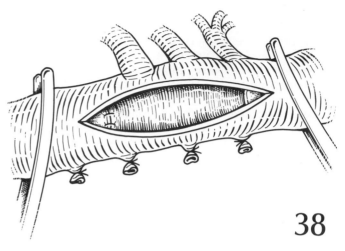

38

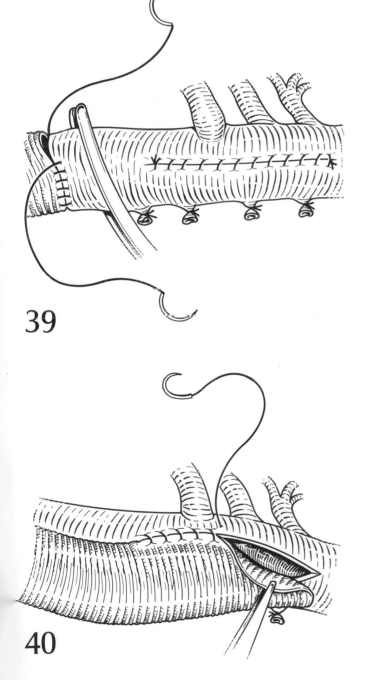

39

Endarterectomy with aortofemoral bypass

39 When there is extensive aortoiliac disease, this procedure may be combined with standard aortofemoral bypass. The endarterectomy is extended into the proximal cuff of the infrarenal aorta (without extending the arteriotomy), which is then transected 2–3 cm below the renal arteries. The aortotomy is closed with a running 5/0 polypropylene suture, and the transected endarterectomized aorta is reclamped below the renal arteries. Following this, a standard end-to-end aortofemoral graft is placed. Once again, however, 4/0 or 5/0 polypropylene on a fine needle is used for the proximal suture line. Fine sutures and use of felt pledgets to buttress the aortic closure diminish bleeding problems.

40 Alternatively, the aortic anastomosis can be made directly to the visceral aorta by bevelling the graft. Although this extends the suprarenal clamp time minimally, it avoids two suture lines and in recent years has become the authors' preferred approach. The aorta is usually clamped above the renal arteries for no more than 30–45 min, and this is tolerated without ill effects in most patients.

Wound closure

Following completion of the reconstruction, the wound is closed in layers. If the pleura has been entered, it is closed around a 20-Fr red rubber catheter which is then removed. The muscle layers are then closed individually using running 0 or 1 absorbable sutures. Scarpa's fascia is closed with a 3/0 running suture, and the skin is approximated in the usual fashion.

40

ILIOFEMORAL BYPASS

This procedure is reserved for patients with significant disease limited to one iliac artery. Ideally, a portion of common iliac artery should be available for the proximal anastomosis. This procedure can still be performed, however, if the origin of the involved iliac vessel is occluded, provided that the aortic bifurcation is free of disease. The authors prefer this procedure to cross-femoral bypass in appropriate cases, because it avoids operation on an asymptomatic limb and involves a single groin incision. Long-term patency of this type of reconstruction is comparable with or superior to that reported with cross-femoral bypass.

Exposure of iliac artery

41 The involved iliac artery is exposed retroperitoneally as previously described on page 38. On the right side the vena cava does not interfere with exposure.

When the origin of the common iliac vessel is patent, the artery is clamped at this point after heparinization. If the ipsilateral hypogastric artery is perfused in a prograde fashion, an end-to-side anastomosis to the common iliac artery is performed as previously described.

If the common iliac artery is occluded, the iliac artery is transected and an end-to-end anastomosis is constructed. This is done with a 4/0 monofilament suture using an 8-mm or 10-mm prosthesis. Tunnelling and distal anastomosis are as described on page 202.

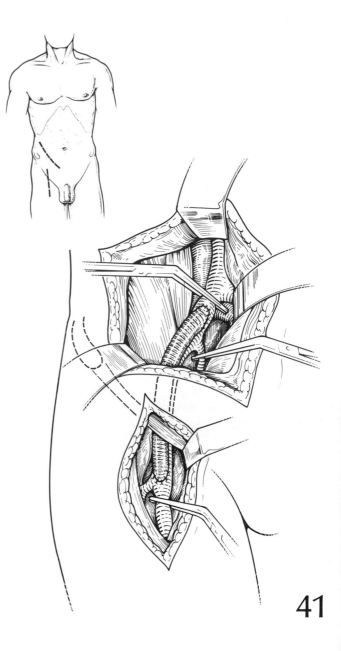

41

42 If the common iliac artery is completely occluded but the aortic bifurcation is not severely diseased, control is obtained by clamping the distal aorta and contralateral iliac vessel. In these cases, the common iliac artery is transected and its origin thrombectomized. An end-to-end anastomosis can be performed to the disobliterated proximal common iliac vessel. Tunnelling and distal anastomosis are performed and wounds closed.

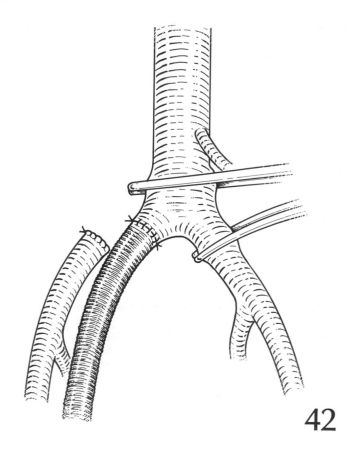

42

Postoperative care

Patients who undergo aortic reconstruction are monitored for 24–48 h in an intensive care unit. The authors routinely use indwelling urinary catheters, radial arterial lines and measurements of central venous pressure. In patients with cardiac dysfunction, pulmonary artery catheters are employed, and this is routine in patients in whom supracoeliac manipulation has been performed.

Complications

Major postoperative problems are hypovolaemia, bleeding and distal ischaemia. These are best anticipated by aggressive monitoring and treated early. The authors routinely reverse anticoagulation with protamine sulphate and assume that continued blood loss is due to a technical error. While this is a rare event, prompt re-exploration is required. Alteration in distal perfusion can be diagnosed by physical examination and confirmed by Doppler blood pressure measurement. When it occurs, prompt re-exploration is required, which can usually be performed transfemorally. Operative angiography may be required to identify the cause of

graft failure. Prophylactic fasciotomy may be required if the ischaemic interval exceeds 4–6 h. Patients with evidence of atheroembolism and intact pulses are treated expectantly.

Colonic ischaemia may occur, often heralded by bloody diarrhoea, and is best documented by flexible sigmoidoscopy[8]. Ischaemia limited to the mucosa may be treated non-operatively with nasogastric suction, intravenous antibiotics and repeated endoscopic evaluation. Transmural ischaemia requires prompt resection and colonic diversion.

43 Impotence, or more commonly retrograde ejaculation, can occur as a result of disruption of the parasympathetic nerves around the aortic bifurcation. This can be prevented by careful dissection in this area.

Pelvic ischaemia can occur after revascularization of the infrarenal aorta and can be associated with ischaemia of the distal spinal cord. It is often due to pelvic devascularization caused by a proximal end-to-end aortic anastomosis in the face of bilateral external iliac occlusions, which prevent retrograde perfusion of the hypogastric arteries and distal aorta. This can be prevented by attention to the preoperative arteriogram and use of an end-to-side aortic anastomosis in these cases. If an end-to-side anastomosis is technically difficult, some attempt to revascularize at least one hypogastric artery is warranted.

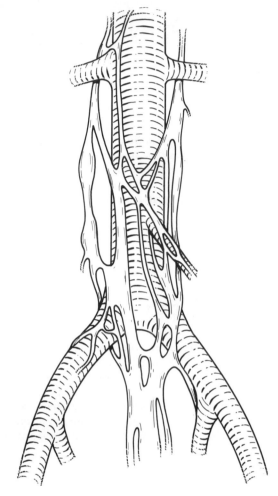

43

References

1. Davies AH, Ramarkha P, Collin J, Morris PJ. Recent changes in the treatment of aortoiliac occlusive disease by the Oxford Regional Vascular Service. *Br J Surg* 1990; 77: 1129–31.

2. Brewster DC. Clinical and anatomical considerations for surgery in aortoiliac disease and results of surgical treatment. *Circulation* 1991; 83(Suppl): 142–52.

3. Szilagyi DE, Elliott JP Jr, Smith RF, Reddy DJ, McPharlin M. A thirty year survey of the reconstructive treatment of aortoiliac occlusive disease. *J Vasc Surg* 1986; 3: 421–36.

4. Langsfeld M, Nepute J, Hershey FB, Thorpe L, Auer AI, Binnington HB *et al.* The use of deep duplex scanning to predict hemodynamically significant aortoiliac stenoses. *J Vasc Surg* 1988; 7: 395–99.

5. Picone AJ, Green RM, Ricotta JJ, May AG, DeWeese JA. Spinal cord ischemia following operations on the abdominal aorta. *J Vasc Surg* 1986; 3: 94–103.

6. Green RM, Ricotta JJ, Ouriel K, DeWeese JA. Results of supraceliac aortic clamping in the difficult elective resection of infrarenal abdominal aortic aneurysm. *J Vasc Surg* 1989; 9: 124–34.

7. Shepard AD, Tollefson DF, Reddy DJ, Evans JR, Elliott JP, Smith RF *et al.* Left flank retroperitoneal exposure: a technical aid to complex aortic reconstruction. *J Vasc Surg* 1991; 14: 283–91.

8. Zelenock GB, Strodel WE, Knol JA, Messina LM, Wakefield TW, Lindenauer SM *et al.* A prospective study of clinically and endoscopically documented colonic ischemia in 100 patients undergoing aortic reconstructive surgery with aggressive colonic and direct pelvic revascularization, compared with historic controls. *Surgery* 1989; 106: 771–80.

Illustrations by Raymond Evans

Abdominal aortic aneurysm resection

Averil O. Mansfield ChM, FRCS
Consultant Vascular Surgeon, St Mary's Hospital, London, UK

Principles and justification

The decision to operate on an abdominal aortic aneurysm is made on consideration of two factors: the size of the aneurysm and the fitness of the patient. If an aneurysm ruptures, the community mortality rate is in the region of 90%. If the patient reaches hospital and has an operation, the mortality rate is around 50%. If, however, the operation is elective and the aneurysm is intact, the operative mortality rate should be under 5%.

It is generally accepted that the risk of rupture becomes significant when the transverse diameter of the aneurysm reaches about 5 cm, hence a patient with an aneurysm of this size or greater should be offered an operation unless general fitness for major surgery precludes this.

Preoperative

General assessment

Ischaemic heart disease is a commonly associated problem and is the most common cause of postoperative mortality. The author prefers patients to have an exercise test and, if this reveals a problem, guidance about further tests is sought from the cardiologist. When necessary the operation is delayed in order to improve the patient's fitness; an aortocoronary bypass may be performed if indicated.

Renal function is routinely assessed and if the creatinine is elevated further investigation of the cause is undertaken with the assistance, where necessary, of the nephrologist. This may involve renal scans, arteriography and sometimes biopsy.

Pulmonary function tests are performed when indicated and, when necessary, treatment including drugs and physiotherapy is given.

Specific investigations

Clinical examination will be comprehensive but particular attention must be paid to other common sites of aneurysm, e.g. the popliteal arteries. Occlusive disease in the legs is sometimes associated, in which case ankle pressure indices should be recorded. The abdomen should be auscultated in order to detect bruits and particularly to detect an aortocaval fistula by the mechanical murmur which is sometimes audible. Rectal examination will be routine but may occasionally demonstrate a pelvic aneurysm.

Ultrasonography is a useful screening test and in some centres is the only specific preoperative test carried out routinely. It is operator dependent and a skilled ultrasonographer not only can measure the aneurysm but can demonstrate the renal arteries and their relationship to the aneurysm.

Computed tomography is the author's preferred routine preoperative investigation and will demonstrate the size, relationships, characteristics and extent of the aneurysm as well as other intra-abdominal problems. Particularly useful features to note are: the wall thickness (if greatly thickened anteriorly it will give warning of an inflammatory aneurysm); the course of the ureters; the site of the left renal vein (whether anterior or posterior to the neck of the aneurysm); the origin of the visceral arteries and their relationship to the sac; and the presence of iliac aneurysms.

Magnetic resonance imaging may in time replace other investigations as, in addition to providing transverse sections, it supplies some information equivalent to that of arteriography, while avoiding irradiation and administration of contrast media.

The specific indications for arteriography in the author's work-up are involvement of the visceral arteries and intermittent claudication.

Prophylactic antibiotics, usually flucloxacillin or a cephalosporin, are administered.

Anaesthesia

The operation is performed under general anaesthesia. The patient is monitored by means of an arterial line, a central venous line and, in the author's unit, a Swan–Ganz catheter.

An epidural catheter is inserted at the end of the operation for the delivery of epidural opiates for pain control. A bladder catheter is essential for the close monitoring of urinary output.

Operation

Incision

1a–c Normally the incision is made in the midline from the xiphisternum to the pubic symphysis (*Illustration 1a*).

Occasionally, when preoperative investigations indicate that a straight graft is definitely all that will be needed and there have been no previous abdominal operations, a transverse incision sited just above the umbilicus can be used (*Illustration 1b*).

If there is doubt about the upper limits of the aneurysm provision should be made to extend the incision across the costal margin if necessary (*Illustration 1c*).

Occasionally the external iliac arteries are aneurysmal and in this case the graft will have to be taken down to the groins. These should always be prepared but will seldom be incised.

Laparotomy

The peritoneal cavity is carefully examined for any additional pathology. In the author's experience the most common additional findings are gallstones, diverticular disease and colonic cancer.

Throughout the laparotomy care must be taken to avoid manipulation of the aneurysm because of the danger of macroemboli and microemboli, the latter being commonly referred to as 'trash'. Individual decisions will need to be taken if additional unexpected problems are revealed but no procedure that might spill organisms can be carried out at the same operation as the insertion of a prosthesis into the aorta.

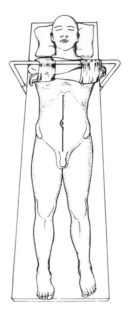

1a

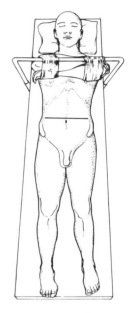

1b

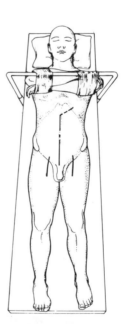

1c

Exposure of the aorta

The author stands on the patient's right but other surgeons find it easier to stand on the left.

2 The whole of the small bowel has to be mobilized to the right of the abdomen. The base of the mesentery runs across the posterior abdominal wall and overlies the aorta. This process of moving the gut to the right may be visualized as turning the pages of a book with the spine of the book being the base of the mesentery. This must be done completely in order to avoid danger to the vessels in the small bowel mesentery.

When adhesions are encountered these must be dealt with very carefully as invasion of the gut lumen will result in the need to abandon the operation in an unruptured case.

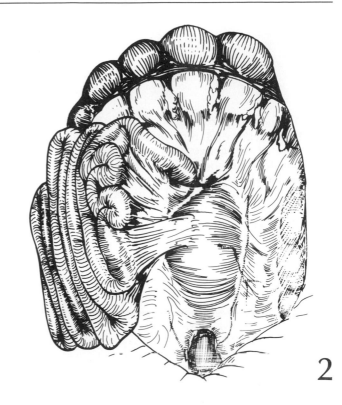

2

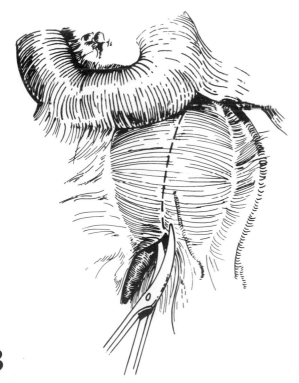

3 The posterior peritoneum is divided along the line of divide between the small bowel mesentery to the right and the large bowel mesentery to the left, avoiding the blood supply of both. Division is continued upwards to the duodenojejunal junction, easily identified by the inferior mesenteric vein. Great care is needed to avoid damage to the serosa of the duodenum.

3

4 The most important landmark in the exposure of the aorta is the left renal vein. This normally crosses the aorta at or above the neck of the aneurysm. Occasionally it runs behind the aorta and may have been identified there by computed tomography. Failure to recognize a retroaortic renal vein can result in severe haemorrhage.

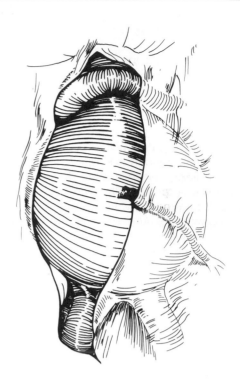

4

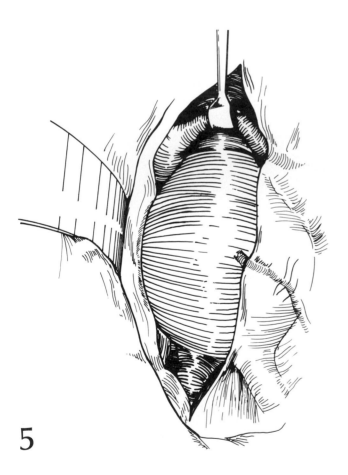

5

5 The lower edge of the left renal vein and its junction with the inferior vena cava is displayed. It can be gently freed from the underlying aorta so that it can be displaced upwards if necessary before clamping. Tributaries should be left intact at this stage because it is occasionally necessary to divide the left renal vein and the tributaries are then important collaterals.

Preparation of the neck of the aneurysm

The area of the aorta where normal aorta suddenly expands to become aneurysmal is first identified. If possible 1 cm of normal aorta is needed in order to place the clamp. The dissection is entirely limited to the sides of the normal aorta. The dissection never needs to extend to the posterior surface of the aorta, and to trespass there with finger, instrument or sling is to invite disaster from bleeding lumbar arteries or veins.

During the preparation of the sides of the aorta the aim is to clear an area big enough to place the clamp and to be able to reach the lumbar spine on either side. The renal arteries are nearby and may even be arising in whole or in part from the neck of the aneurysm, and the possibility of a lower pole renal artery arising here or even from the aneurysmal segment should be recognized. The renal arteries must be carefully preserved.

Once it is clear that the clamp can be placed when required, the other end of the aorta is approached.

Tilting the table towards the surgeon, if standing on the patient's right, is a considerable advantage.

Exposure of the iliac arteries

The lower end of the aorta is uncovered, care being taken to avoid the inferior mesenteric artery which arises from the anterior surface of the aorta towards its left side.

6 At this stage the gut may be wrapped in a towel and placed in a gut bag. Some surgeons are able to cope with the gut packed into the right iliac fossa but the author prefers to wrap it and lift it outside the abdomen.

It is difficult to identify the nerves which run over the aortic bifurcation but in males this area should be avoided for fear of subsequent abnormal sexual function. Male patients should be warned of the possibility during preoperative counselling.

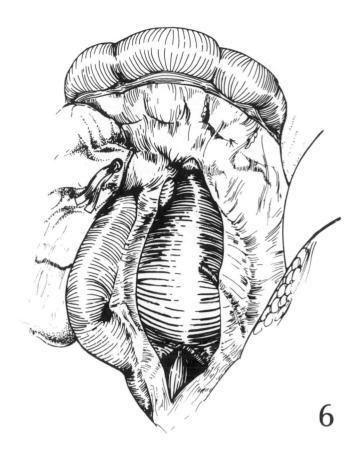

6

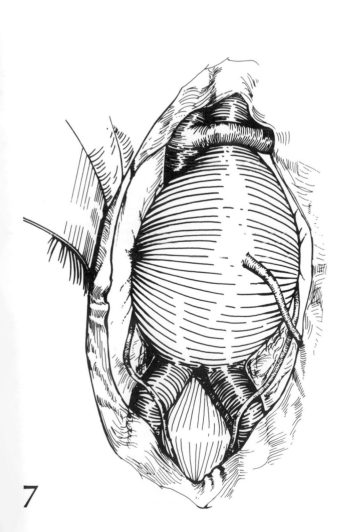

7

Right iliac artery

7 The ureter is the only structure of importance lying anterior to the iliac artery apart from the gut. The ureter obviously should not be damaged but perhaps less obviously nor should its blood supply. Hence it should be identified but not moved and the dissection should take place on each side of it. This is particularly important when it is stretched out over a large iliac aneurysm and there is a great temptation to mobilize it off the aneurysm. The ureter must, however, be left undisturbed in the certain knowledge that when the aneurysm is deflated by the operation the ureter will no longer be stretched and its blood supply will be intact.

Left iliac artery

8 This is more difficult as the sigmoid colon and its mesentery is a barrier to extensive dissection from above. The iliac artery can easily be clamped above the sigmoid colon but, if it is aneurysmal and the whole artery needs to be explored, it is easier to divide the peritoneal reflection lateral to the sigmoid colon and reflect the sigmoid colon towards the aorta. This enables the whole of the left iliac artery and the ureter to be displayed.

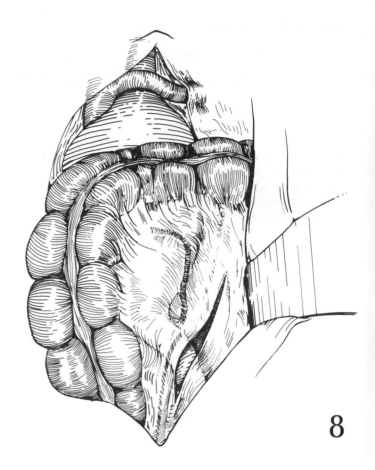

8

Site of distal clamping

This site will depend on the presence and extent of iliac aneurysms and will be beyond them. If the common iliac artery is aneurysmal but there are no aneurysms beyond the bifurcation, then both internal and external iliac arteries need to be displayed. Care must be taken to avoid dissection around these arteries because of the risk of bleeding from the closely applied vein. Venous injury in the depths of the pelvis from the internal iliac vein can cause haemorrhage which is difficult to control. It is better to accept the possibility that both the vein and the artery may be clamped than to risk tearing the vein by separating the two.

An alternative to iliac clamping is intraluminal balloon tamponade introduced from the aorta.

Iliac aneurysms

When these are present the first essential is to exclude them from the circulation so that they do not pose a future threat. The second aim is to leave one internal iliac artery in circulation. It this is impossible because of bilateral internal iliac aneurysms then the deep femoral arteries assume great importance and must be preserved. Consideration will also need to be given to the reanastomosis of the inferior mesenteric artery.

Insertion of the graft

If a woven graft is used there is no need to preclot the graft before heparin is given. If a knitted graft is preferred then preclotting is very important and in these cases a graft would be selected and 20 ml of blood from the aorta placed in the graft at this stage. If the patient has a coagulopathy then a sealed graft which is impervious to blood may be employed. Grafts can be sealed with gelatin, collagen or albumin.

When everything is prepared for clamping the anaesthetist gives heparin intravenously. The author uses a standard but rather unscientific dose of 5000 units.

9 After allowing time for circulation the iliac arteries are clamped with Dardik clamps.

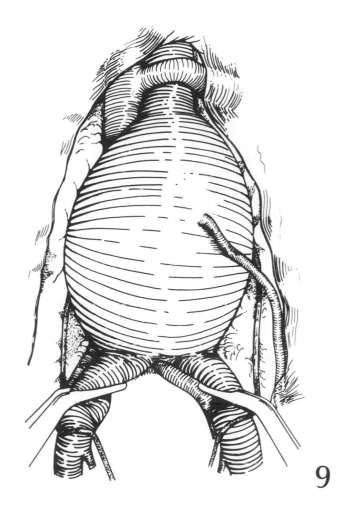

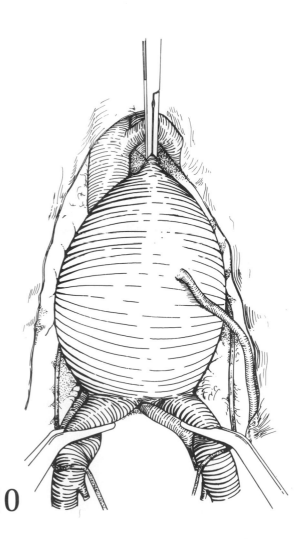

10 A clamp is placed on the aorta in the normal segment just above the neck. A Glover's coarctation clamp may be used and placed from front to back and not from side to side. It should be closed only as tightly as is necessary to stop the aortic pulsation below it. It can be steadied by the use of a tape or sling.

11 The aorta is opened towards its right side in order to avoid the origin of the inferior mesenteric artery. The incision passes upwards to the midline at the neck and the edge of the neck is transected with scissors in its anterior half. A Dardik clamp is placed across the free edge of the aortic wall to control the inferior mesenteric artery.

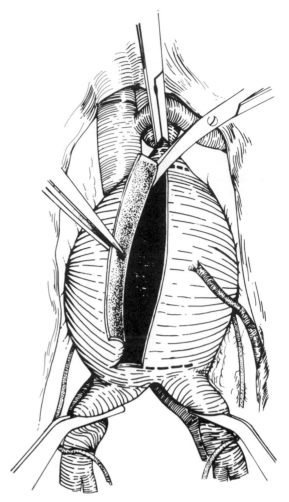

11

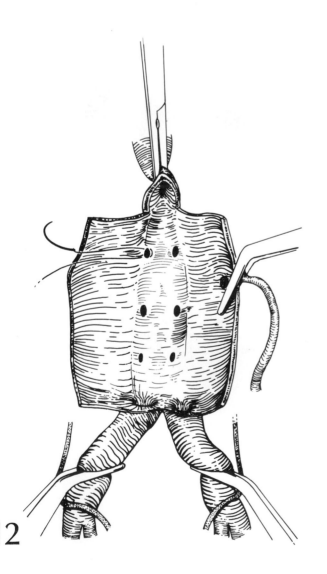

12

12 The incision is extended down to the bifurcation. The thrombus is scooped out and a specimen sent for culture. There may be quite profuse haemorrhage at this time from the lumbar arteries. These need to be oversewn but if they are surrounded by atheroma it may be more efficient to remove some of this in order to be able to place an accurate and effective suture. A silk suture may be used. All bleeding from lumbar arteries must be completely controlled because they will not be in continuity with the circulation hereafter and bleeding can be an avoidable cause for a return to theatre.

If a graft has not yet been prepared, one is now selected to match as far as possible the size of the arteries.

Straight graft

13 The proximal anastomosis is between the neck of the aneurysm and the edge of the Dacron graft. Using 3/0 polypropylene (Prolene) the suture line is begun in the middle of the back. Each bite goes through the artery and graft separately and the bites are about 1 mm apart. The depth from the edge should vary so as not to produce a neat and fragile row of perforations, but each bite needs to be at least 1 mm and often 2 or 3 mm deep. Any tendency to slip onto the aneurysmal section must be resisted as this will result in a future weakness of the wall.

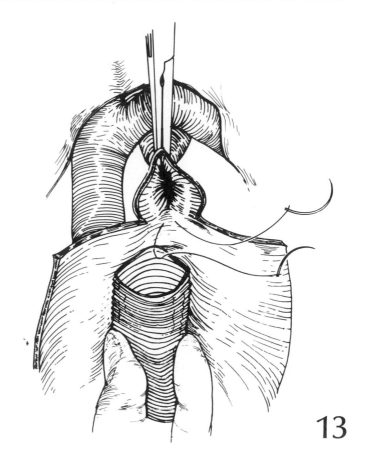

13

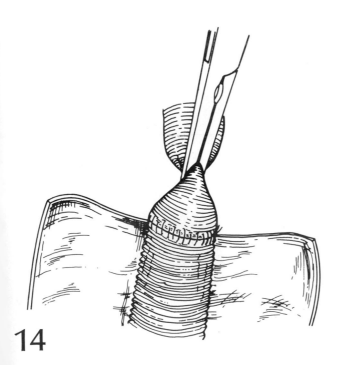

14

14 The knot should be placed towards the left lateral wall so that it is away from the duodenum.

15a–e When the proximal anastomosis is complete it can be tested by clamping the graft and releasing the aortic clamp. The advantage of this test is that any leak at the back becomes impossible to get to once the lower anastomosis is completed. The clamp may be left on the graft until the completion of the second anastomosis.

The graft is stretched and cut to fit. It should not be left so long that it bulges forwards when flow is restored, nor should it be so tight that there is tension. The distal anastomosis on the aortic bifurcation is similar to the proximal anastomosis and can be started either in the middle of the back or at a lateral corner. The bites need to be substantial, as at the proximal anastomosis, but one should bear in mind the fact that the left common iliac vein may be a close posterior relation.

The parachute technique may be used for both anastomoses when polypropylene or similar suture material is being used. In this method a number of sutures are placed before being tightened, giving the benefit of clear vision in a difficult corner.

Before completion of the distal anastomosis all the components are allowed briefly to flush back to remove thrombus or debris and air. It is usual to allow flow into only one iliac artery initially and to remove the second iliac clamp when the anaesthetist is ready. Back-bleeding from the inferior mesenteric artery is checked and, if satisfactory, the artery is oversewn from within. This avoids damage to its first branch which might be responsible for the continuity of the vascular supply to the colon from the superior mesenteric artery.

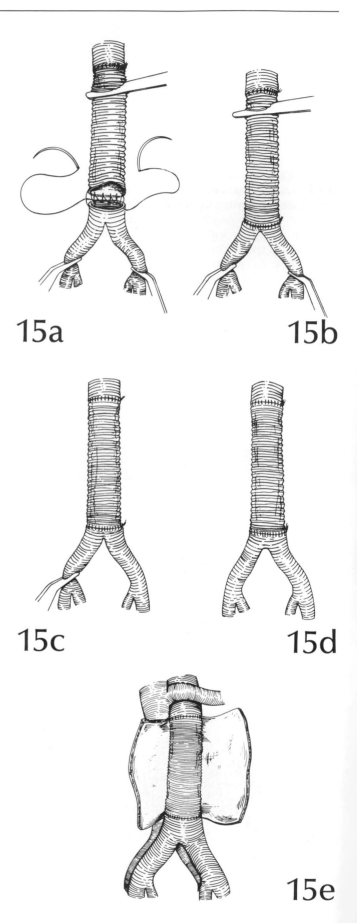

15a

15b

15c

15d

15e

16 The sac is closed around the graft thus avoiding direct contact between graft and gut.

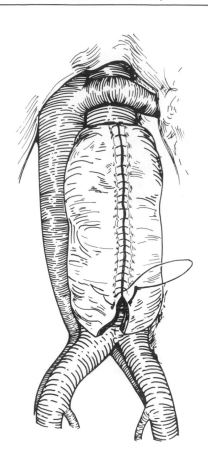

16

Bifurcation graft

The trunk of the bifurcation graft is cut short but should be long enough to enable a branch to be joined onto it should the need arise.

The top anastomosis is identical to that of the straight graft.

17 Each distal anastomosis is placed at the most proximal point consistent with excluding all the aneurysms. Ideally, if there are no aneurysms beyond the iliac bifurcation, the anastomosis is onto the conjoined orifices of the external and internal iliac arteries. The graft then lies inside the opened iliac aneurysm or is tunnelled through it and always lies behind the ureter.

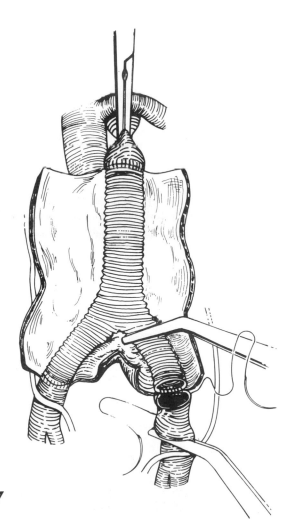

17

18 If the internal iliac artery is not aneurysmal but the bifurcation is diseased it is sometimes possible to join the proximal external iliac artery to the proximal internal iliac artery and then to join the graft end-to-side onto the external iliac artery, thus preserving internal iliac flow.

If the internal iliac artery is aneurysmal then it must be ligated or oversewn and the distal anastomosis is end-to-end to the external iliac artery.

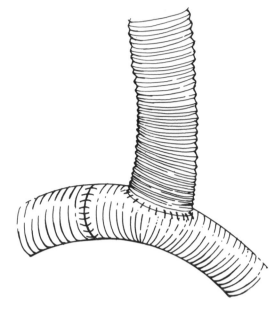

18

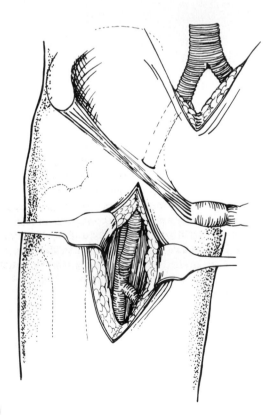

19

19 Very occasionally even this level proves to be unsatisfactory and the distal anastomosis is in the groin onto the common femoral artery.

In aneurysmal disease it is important to avoid longer grafts than necessary so that the intervening structures are still supplied with blood. Dacron, unlike arteries, does not have branches.

Aortocaval fistula

20, 21 Operative management, especially if the condition is unexpected, may prove difficult because of profuse haemorrhage. The communication between aorta and inferior vena cava should be closed with a running 3/0 polypropylene suture from within the aorta.

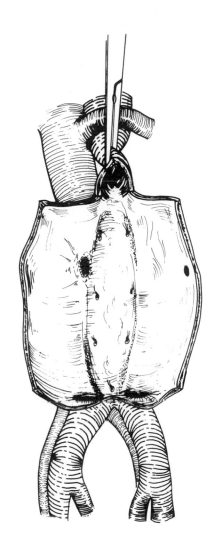

20

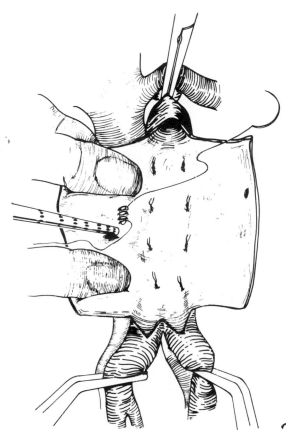

21

22 Digital pressure as in *Illustration 21* is usually enough to control the venous bleeding but when in difficulty a useful technique is to use balloon tamponade, either introduced directly through the fistula or remotely inserted. The latter is a most useful adjunct to the control of venous bleeding and a caval occlusion catheter is passed up from the saphenous vein while packs control the bleeding. When correctly positioned they are inflated and the bleeding is usually easily controlled. Sometimes there is more than one fistulous opening.

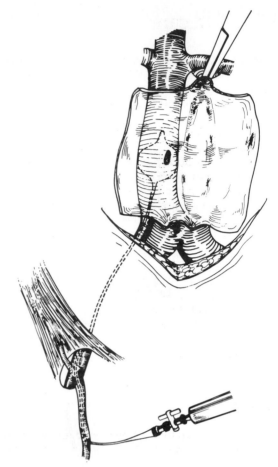

22

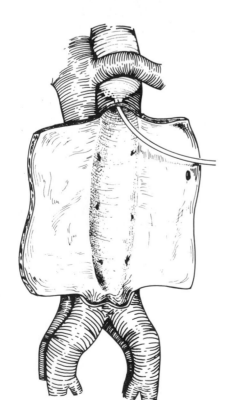

23

Variation when aneurysm is ruptured

The patient is not paralysed until the drapes are in place and the operation can begin. Heparin is omitted in most cases.

The proximal clamp is placed first.

23 Occasionally a balloon catheter is used for proximal control on a temporary basis.

Very rarely the aorta is controlled by a clamp at the hiatus. Although regarded by some as a useful emergency measure the author has not found it to be required in the great majority of operations. It is not as easy as it sounds, it results in considerable haemodynamic disturbance, and because it is above the renal arteries it probably increases the risk of renal failure.

When the graft is inserted some time should be spent looking for vessels such as lumbar arteries which may not have bled when the patient was hypotensive initially but which can cause postoperative problems with bleeding.

Postoperative care

All patients require close postoperative monitoring, ideally in an intensive care unit. The latter is essential in the emergency case. It is unusual in the author's unit for a patient to be ventilated after surgery for an unruptured infrarenal aneurysm but it would be routine to ventilate the patient for a period after an emergency operation.

Urinary output is closely monitored and appropriate support such as renal dopamine given as necessary.

Clotting parameters need to be measured and when necessary corrected. After emergency operations it is often necessary to give platelets and fresh frozen plasma.

Cardiac and respiratory monitoring and treatment are given as required and as the patient warms up every effort is made to maintain a stable blood pressure and cardiac function.

Adequate pain control is essential and is usually satisfactorily taken care of by epidural opiates. The method of choice will depend on local preference but reliable relief from pain must be provided.

Antibiotics are continued until the lines are removed. Heparin is used for prophylaxis against thromboembolism unless there is a contraindication.

Complications

Early problems are usually technical and most often concerned with bleeding. Occasionally patients will have to return to theatre for this problem but every effort must be made at the original operation to avoid this.

Renal dysfunction is one of the more frequent problems, especially in cases of rupture, and occasionally patients will require dialysis.

Prolonged ventilation, usually following massive transfusion, can be a problem and some patients may eventually need a tracheostomy.

Myocardial infarctions may occur after the repair of an aneurysm, hence the desire to improve cardiac function before operation when this is possible.

'Trash' embolization should be prevented as far as possible by avoiding manipulation of the aneurysm, by using heparin, by clamping distally before proximally, and by flushing the vessels before flow is restored. If, in spite of this, problems occur embolectomy will sometimes help, but when this is not appropriate an infusion of prostacyclin may be given.

Infection is a major concern and graft infections are usually later problems which can be life threatening and generally require the removal of the graft.

False aneurysms can sometimes occur at the anastomoses and again these are usually late complications.

Aortoenteric fistula, when it occurs, is usually a very late complication and when a patient with an aortic graft presents with gastrointestinal haemorrhage it should be the major component of the differential diagnosis.

Outcome

The majority of patients can expect to have a normal life span after repair of the aneurysm.

Future work on abdominal aneurysm resection should address the following key issues: (1) what size of aneurysm requires operation; (2) should patients be screened for abdominal aortic aneurysm; (3) which graft should be used; (4) is there a familial genetic disposition; and (5) will endoluminal methods become the treatment of choice?

Carotid endarterectomy

Michael D. Colburn MD
Resident, Department of General Surgery, University of California at Los Angeles School of Medicine, Los Angeles, California, USA

Wesley S. Moore MD
Professor of Surgery, Chief, Section of Vascular Surgery, University of California at Los Angeles School of Medicine, Los Angeles, California, USA

History

Most cerebrovascular accidents (approximately 60%) are related to atheromatous disease of the extracranial carotid arteries[1]. The first carotid reconstruction was reported in 1954[2]. In 1988, the Rand Corporation published a report which reviewed the indications for carotid endarterectomy and concluded that the operation was being overused[3], and the role of carotid endarterectomy has been questioned. Recently, the efforts of a number of experts in the field have resulted in the initiation of several randomized prospective clinical trials designed to determine precisely the natural history and associated stroke risk of carotid artery atheromatous lesions[4-6]. The preliminary results of these trials are now available, and some 40 years after Eastcott's initial report describing operative repair of a carotid artery lesion, the proper role of carotid surgery is finally being clearly defined.

Pathology of carotid bifurcation occlusive disease

Atherosclerosis

Atherosclerosis is the most common pathological process affecting the cerebral circulation. The manifestations of atheromatous change in this area, however, can vary, and both occlusive and degenerative aneurysmal lesions are well known. Occlusive stenoses, however, are by far the most common. Clinically important histological characteristics include: the relative proportions of fatty, fibrous and calcified material; the presence of surface clot or ulceration; and the degree of intraplaque haemorrhage. Soft irregular fatty plaques which are not calcified represent high-risk lesions. On the other hand, smooth fibrous and calcified lesions are more stable and represent a lower embolic risk.

Fibromuscular dysplasia

The precise incidence of fibromuscular dysplasia is not known, but it is not common. Many different histological subtypes have been described, including intimal fibroplasia, medial fibroplasia, medial hyperplasia and perimedial dysplasia[7]. The most common subtype found in the extracranial carotid arteries is medial fibroplasia. Mural dilatations forming microaneurysms are common and form the basis of the classic 'string of beads' appearance observed angiographically. Intracranial aneurysms are commonly associated with carotid artery fibromuscular dysplasia and have been reported in approximately 30% of patients. In addition, a significant percentage of patients who present with a spontaneous carotid artery dissection are found to have evidence of fibromuscular dysplasia in the contralateral artery.

Intimal hyperplasia

Intimal hyperplasia is the abnormal sustained proliferation of cells and extracellular connective tissue matrix that occurs as the result of injury to the arterial wall. In the carotid bifurcation this injury typically occurs following an endarterectomy. Grossly, these lesions appear firm, pale and homogeneous. The involved area is smooth and uniformly located beneath the endothelium. Several mechanisms by which injury to the vascular endothelium may lead to activation of the medial smooth muscle cell have been suggested. Postulated theories include haemodynamic factors, alterations in lipid metabolism and complex interactions between the arterial wall and circulating factors such as platelets and components of the inflammatory system.

Radiation injury

Radiation therapy has become a common form of treatment for a variety of neoplasms, including those affecting the head and neck. Damage to the vascular wall alters its permeability to circulating lipids and impairs its ability to repair structural tissue. Over the course of the next few weeks endothelial regeneration and medial fibrosis begin to appear. Finally, within several months, the luminal surfaces become thickened and irregular. These changes are characterized by fatty infiltration, fibrosis and intimal regeneration. The medial fibrosis and intimal thickening are responsible for the eventual luminal narrowing seen following radiation injury.

Clinical patterns of cerebral ischaemia

Neurological events resulting from cerebrovascular pathology can conveniently be divided into three general categories based on the duration of symptoms. The first group of patients are those who experience a transient ischaemic attack (TIA), defined as an ischaemic event that lasts no longer than 24 h. Typically, the patient will report a focal neurological deficit, such as weakness in a limb or slurred speech. It is implied in this definition that neurological recovery is complete and no residual deficit is present. If the neurological deficit persists beyond 24 h, but completely resolves within 7 days, it is termed a resolving ischaemic neurological deficit (RIND). Lastly, if the ischaemic symptoms last longer than 7 days, the event is labelled a stroke. The clinical significance of a RIND is unclear, and it is considered by some to simply represent a stroke with rapid and full recovery. The term stroke implies irreversible brain tissue damage, even when clinically some patients appear to recover full function following a deficit which lasted longer than 7 days. It remains unclear whether a RIND represents permanent or reversible brain tissue damage.

Principles and justification

Indications

Atherosclerotic plaques

The role of carotid surgery in patients with asymptomatic carotid occlusive disease remains controversial. The case for endarterectomy in asymptomatic patients is based primarily on retrospective reviews studying patients with appropriate lesions who were followed but not operated on. To summarize the available data, the mean stroke rate/year in asymptomatic patients not treated by operations is about 5.0%, which could be expected to lead to a 5-year stroke rate of about 25%

(*Table 1*). In surgical patients, the mean operative mortality in patients with asymptomatic lesions is 1–2%, with a 30-day perioperative stroke rate of about 1.5%. The long-term stroke rate in operated patients is 1.3% in the first year and 0.5% each year thereafter (*Table 1*)[8]. This would predict a 5-year incidence of stroke of 4.8% (including perioperative strokes), which represents an absolute reduction in the expected stroke risk of 20.2% in favour of surgically treated patients.

Unlike asymptomatic lesions, the indication for surgery in patients with symptomatic carotid lesions is no longer controversial. Three prospective randomized studies have now analysed the results of carotid surgery in patients with a symptomatic ipsilateral lesion (*Table 2*).

Fibromuscular dysplasia

The mechanism by which fibromuscular dysplasia of the extracranial carotid arteries causes symptoms is controversial. Platelet clots or cholesterol emboli may arise from the irregular luminal surface. Alternatively, decreased flow through a single critical stenosis, or through a number of non-critical stenoses aligned in series, may be the operative mechanism. It is likely that the true aetiology in any given patient varies, and combinations of these processes may also occur. Unfortunately, the natural history of fibromuscular dysplasia of the extracranial carotid artery in an otherwise asymptomatic patient is not known. Most authors agree, however, that currently asymptomatic lesions should be carefully followed and that surgical intervention should be reserved for those patients who later develop symptoms[1].

Recurrent carotid stenosis

The mean incidence of asymptomatic carotid restenoses ranges between 7% and 15%, and between 1% and 5% of developed restenoses are associated with recurrent

Table 1 Natural and modified history of atherosclerotic carotid bifurcation lesions

Symptoms at presentation	Stroke risk in first year (%)	Stroke risk yearly thereafter (%)	Stroke risk after 5 years (%)
Natural history			
Asymptomatic	5.0	5.0	25.0
Transient ischaemic attack	10.0	6.0	34.0
Completed stroke	9.0	9.0	45.0
Best medical therapy			
Asymptomatic	5.0	5.0	25.0
Transient ischaemic attack	8.5	5.0	28.5
Completed stroke	9.0	9.0	45.0
Surgical management			
Asymptomatic	1.3	0.5	3.3
Transient ischaemic attack	3.0	1.5	9.0
Completed stroke	7.0	2.2	15.8

Table 2 Prospective randomized trials comparing carotid endarterectomy with the best available medical treatment

Study	Number of patients	30-day operative mortality (%)	Percentage reaching endpoint (surgery group)	Percentage reaching endpoint (medical group)	Mean follow-up (months)
Asymptomatic*					
Veterans Administration Cooperative[4]	444	1.9			
Symptomatic					
Veterans Administration Cooperative[4]	189		7.7	19.4	11.9
>70% stenosis			7.9	25.6	
<70% stenosis			7.1	6.7	
North American Symptomatic Carotid Endarterectomy Trial[5]					
Stenosis (30–69%)*					
Stenosis (70–99%)	659	0.6	8.0	18.1	24
European Carotid Surgery Trial[6]					
Stenosis (0–30%)	374	1.4	11.8	6.2	36
Stenosis (30–69%)*					
Stenosis (70–99%)	778	0.9	12.3	21.9	36

*Results not yet available

symptoms[9, 10]. It has long been recognized that the natural history of recurrent carotid stenoses is not the same as that of the original lesion in a given patient. The risk of subsequent stroke or ischaemic events in these patients is clearly different from that of primary atherosclerotic lesions. This is probably related to the pathology of the recurrent lesion. Smooth, fibrous, intimal hyperplastic recurrent lesions, even of the same or greater degree of stenosis than the original atherosclerotic plaque, are well tolerated by most patients. This is probably due to the low risk of embolic events related to these lesions relative to the soft necrotic atherosclerotic plaques originally found in these patients.

Preoperative

Evaluation

Atherosclerosis is a systemic disease, and involvement in other vascular beds must be identified. The association between carotid and coronary involvement with atherosclerotic changes is well known and must be looked for. Any patient with a history of coronary artery disease, suggestive symptoms, or silent abnormalities on routine electrocardiography (ECG), should undergo a comprehensive cardiac assessment prior to any cerebrovascular reconstruction.

Traditionally, most surgeons have held to the belief that the complete evaluation of patients with cerebrovascular symptoms must include an accurate anatomical delineation of the aortic arch, carotid bifurcation and intracranial vasculature. Recently, however, the role of diagnostic arteriography has diminished and duplex scanning is emerging as an acceptable preoperative evaluation technique. The duplex scan is an accurate non-invasive imaging technique, and this, combined with increased knowledge of the natural history of these lesions, has caused the need for routine arteriography in all patients with cerebrovascular disease to be questioned. The arguments for carotid endarterectomy with or without preoperative arteriography have been outlined recently by Gelabert and Moore[11]. To summarize, there is no question that arteriography exposes patients to an increased risk which must be added to the operative morbidity when calculating the overall risk of surgical therapy; however, the need to image the entire cerebrovascular tree from the arch to the intracranial vessels is debatable. Clinically important proximal disease is uncommon and is usually apparent on physical examination. Furthermore, in the presence of a critical bifurcation lesion, identification of additional intracranial disease does not ordinarily alter the patient's management. Thus, the combination of a careful history and physical examination, combined with a reliable evaluation of the carotid bifurcation, should safely identify candidates for operative intervention.

Anaesthesia

Both local and general anaesthesia are accepted procedures for carotid surgery. Local techniques usually include a regional cervical block in combination with direct skin infiltration of anaesthetic agents. Initial sedation is normally achieved by gentle administration of parenteral diazepam or a related agent. Mental confusion, respiratory depression and hypoxia must be avoided. Regional cervical block is easily accomplished by infiltrating the cervical plexus with a mixture of 1% lignocaine hydrochloride and 0.5% bupivacaine hydrochloride. Rapid skin anaesthesia with a prolonged duration can also be obtained by this combination. Subcutaneous injections, as well as deep injections along the posterior border of the sternocleidomastoid muscle to anaesthetize the superficial nerves of the cervical plexus, complete the local block. Occasionally, additional injections within the carotid sheath may be required.

The advantages of local anaesthesia during carotid endarterectomy are related to avoidance of the cerebral and myocardial depressant effects of general anaesthesia. First, neurological assessment during carotid surgery is critical, and an awake patient is a very sensitive cerebral monitor. Secondly, neurological status in the immediate postoperative interval, a period during which patients who undergo general anaesthesia are not well monitored, is easily assessed. Finally, the improved tolerance of the elderly or cardiac-impaired patient to local anaesthesia allows a safer operation in these high-risk groups of patients.

Despite these advantages, most surgeons prefer general anaesthesia for patients undergoing carotid surgery. General anaesthesia provides the most controlled operative setting, including excellent airway control and less movement in the operative field. Physiological advantages include improved oxygenation, reduced cerebral metabolic demand and increased cerebral blood flow, particularly when halogenated anaesthetic agents are utilized.

Regardless of the method of anaesthesia, accurate blood pressure monitoring during carotid surgery is essential. Therefore, all patients should have a radial arterial catheter inserted prior to the induction of anaesthesia. This line can also be used to measure arterial blood gases and should be left in place to monitor blood pressure during the immediate postoperative period.

Operations

CAROTID ENDARTERECTOMY

Position of patient

The patient should be positioned supine on the operating table with the head rotated away from the operative side. The head of the table is raised 10–15° which reduces venous pressure and minimizes incisional blood loss. Depending on individual differences in body habitus, the neck can be extended by the placement of a small towel roll beneath the shoulders.

Incision

1 A longitudinal incision is made which follows the ventral border of the sternocleidomastoid muscle. The approximate position of the carotid bifurcation can often be determined from the preoperative diagnostic studies. Ideally, the incision should be centred longitudinally so that the bifurcation is below the midpoint. When necessary for additional exposure, this incision can be continued caudad to the sternal notch, and cephalad to the mastoid process[2].

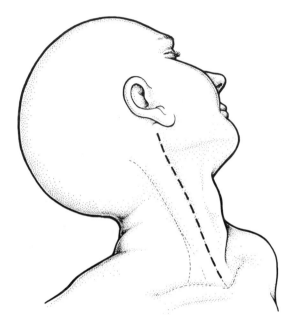

1

Dissection

2 The plane of dissection remains along the anterior border of the sternocleidomastoid until the belly of this muscle can be reflected off the carotid sheath. Often the posterior tail of the parotid gland is encountered at this level, and when this occurs further dissection is required. The gland should be mobilized and reflected anteriorly rather than divided, which can cause excessive bleeding and occasionally lead to a salivary fistula. Once the carotid sheath is visualized, it should be opened along the anterior border of the jugular vein, which can easily be identified through the sheath. The jugular vein is mobilized completely and any large branches identified. The common facial vein is a broad-based tributary, which commonly joins the jugular vein just above the carotid bifurcation. This vein provides a useful marker for the location of the carotid bifurcation and, once identified, it should be divided between ligatures. Particularly in high bifurcations, the hypoglossal nerve can also be located deep to the facial vein, and care must be taken to avoid inadvertent injury to this structure.

After dividing the facial vein, the jugular vein can be reflected laterally, providing exposure of the carotid vessels. The vagus nerve which is ordinarily posterior, can be located anywhere within the carotid sheath. Therefore, in each case, its course must be identified and protected to avoid injury. The laryngeal nerve, which is usually recurrent, can arise directly off the vagus and cross anterior to the carotid artery at this level where it enters the vocal musculature. When not recognized, division of this nerve will lead to vocal paralysis. It should also be mentioned that, although this anomaly is more common on the left side, its presence has also been described on the right.

Once the sheath has been entered and all pertinent structures identified and protected, the common carotid artery is sufficiently mobilized proximally to allow complete delineation of the extent of disease, and to provide sufficient length in case a bypass shunt is required. The bifurcation, external and internal carotid arteries are then mobilized in a similar fashion. Reflex bradycardia can occur during manipulation of the carotid bulb due to stimulation of the carotid body. This can be prevented, or reversed when necessary, by local injection of an anaesthetic agent to block the nerves arising from the carotid body. The external and internal carotid arteries must be mobilized for a sufficient length to clearly identify the distal extent of the disease. The hypoglossal nerve must be carefully identified, particularly when mobilizing the internal carotid artery.

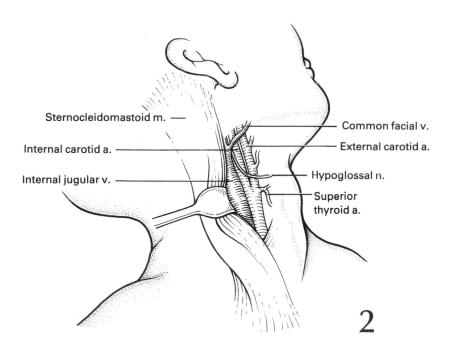

Sternocleidomastoid m. —

Internal carotid a. —

Internal jugular v. —

Common facial v.

External carotid a.

Hypoglossal n.

Superior thyroid a.

2

Carotid artery back-pressure measurement

3 Selective cerebral protection based on the measurement of distal internal carotid artery back-pressure was originally described by Moore *et al*. Using this method, the adequacy of the collateral blood flow to the ipsilateral hemisphere during proximal artery occlusion is determined by measurement of the back-pressure. A 22-Fr needle is bent 2 cm from the tip at an angle of 45° and connected to an arterial pressure transducer. The needle is inserted into the common carotid artery with the angulated tip lying longitudinally in the lumen and directed toward the bifurcation. First, an open carotid artery pressure is measured, and this should be compared with the radial artery line to ensure that the pressure transducer is functioning correctly. Then, with the external and proximal common carotid arteries temporarily occluded, the internal carotid artery back-pressure is recorded.

Although no precise consensus has been reached, most reviews define the range of 30–50 mmHg as the pressure below which cerebral protection is mandatory, If this is the case, the clamps on the external and proximal common carotid arteries are removed, and preparations are made for the use of an internal bypass shunt. Commonly cited objections to this method include the inaccuracy of extracranial pressures in the presence of an undiagnosed intracranial lesion and variations in the values obtained with different levels of anaesthesia, ventilation and other metabolic parameters.

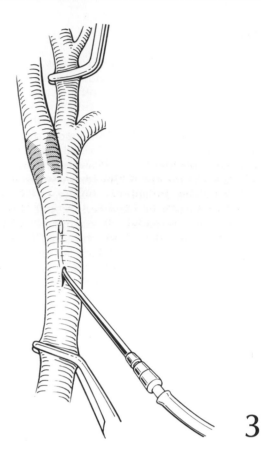

3

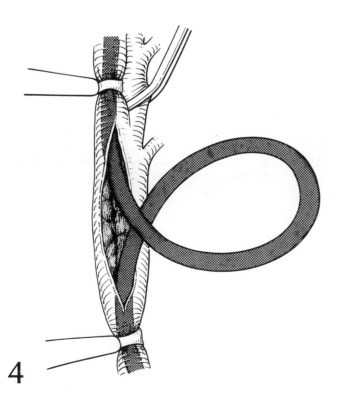

4

Insertion of shunt

4 When an internal carotid shunt is required, several principles should be appreciated. Most importantly, full exposure of all three major carotid vessels is mandatory. This allows for complete proximal common carotid control and full appreciation of the distal extent of disease in both the internal and external carotid arteries. With the internal and external carotid arteries controlled, the common carotid is occluded proximally with a soft clamp. The arteriotomy should extend comfortably beyond the distal extent of the luminal disease. The distal internal carotid is allowed to back-bleed, and an internal shunt with an appropriate diameter is gently inserted. The authors prefer to use the Javid shunt; however, other types are available. The shunt is flushed, clamped and subsequently inserted into the common carotid artery proximally. Snares (Rumel tourniquets) are used to secure the shunt at its insertion points, and the occluding clamp on the common carotid is removed. Thus in the final configuration, the shunt is in place with only a single occluding clamp in its mid portion. This clamp is removed slowly, watching carefully for air or debris which may be visible through the proximal portion of the shunt. Once the shunt is in place and cerebral protection accomplished, attention can be directed to the performance of a technically excellent operation.

Clamping of carotid arteries

5 Performance of a technically perfect carotid endarterectomy requires appreciation of several time-honoured principles. Once adequate exposure is achieved and cerebral protection (if necessary) assured, the internal, external and finally common carotid arteries are clamped, in that order. The clamps should be placed in such a way that the bifurcation can be rotated exposing the lateral surface directly opposite the orifice of the external carotid artery.

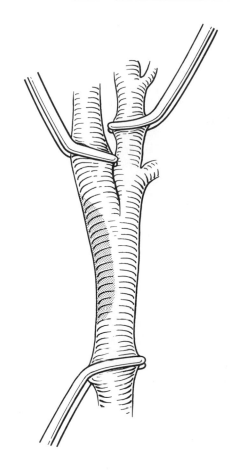

5

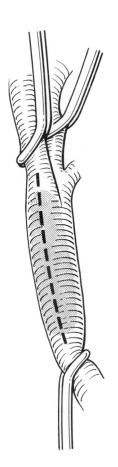

6

Arteriotomy

6 The arteriotomy is placed longitudinally along this surface. This minimizes the risk of damaging the bifurcation flow divider. Furthermore, by placing the arteriotomy here, there is less chance of narrowing the endarterectomized lumen during closure.

Endarterectomy

7a–c Once the arteriotomy is complete, a thorough inspection of the luminal surface is made, and any ulceration or mural thrombosis is noted. The precise depth of the endarterectomy plane is critical. Care should be taken to select the plane between the diseased intima and the circular fibres of the media. This allows complete removal of the atheromatous process without compromising the endpoint. More superficial planes risk incomplete removal of complex plaques, and deeper dissections inevitably lead to an abrupt step-up at the endpoint of the endarterectomy.

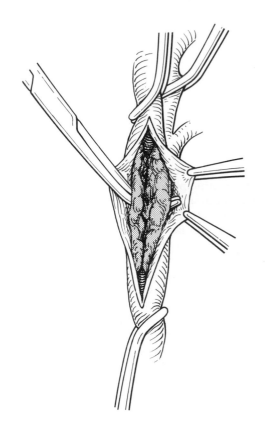

7a

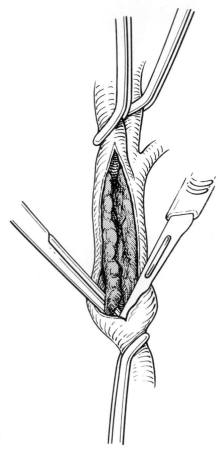

7b

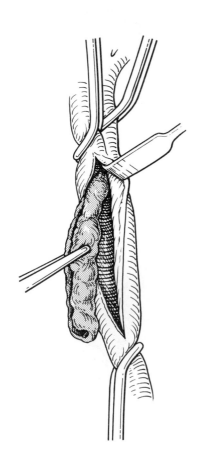

7c

Completion of endarterectomy

8 Once the endarterectomy is completed, including clearing of the external carotid artery and direct visualization of both the proximal and distal endpoints, the endarterectomy surface should be mechanically irrigated with liberal amounts of heparinized saline solution. This serves to remove small bits of atheromatous or medial debris and can help to identify occult intimal flaps. Any debris or small flaps that are identified should always be removed by gentle downward or lateral traction. Removing a fragment in the cephalad direction can lead to inadvertent extension of the dissection distally. It is of utmost importance to carefully examine the external carotid artery, as it is well known that technical failures in the orifice of this vessel can lead to serious postoperative complications.

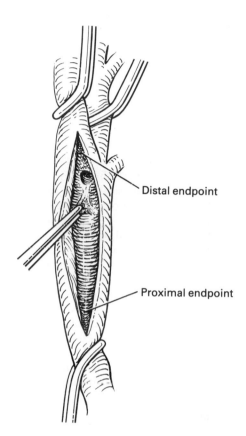

Distal endpoint

Proximal endpoint

8

Closure of endarterectomy

9a, b Closure of the endarterectomy site is critical, and the tendency to hurry this step of the procedure is perhaps the most common cause of postoperative complications. If an adequate evaluation of the collateral circulation has been made, and if appropriate cerebral protection (if necessary) has been instituted, there is absolutely no need to rush this portion of the procedure. Primary closure with 6/0 polypropylene suture is preferable and well tolerated. If a shunt has been placed, the arteriotomy is closed with the exception of an approximately 1-cm segment in the middle of the defect. The common carotid is again controlled, the shunt is clamped and removed, and the carotid vessels are again flushed, beginning distally as always. The arteriotomy closure is then completed, with the vessels temporarily occluded. Alternatively, a Satinsky partially occluding clamp can be used to maintain flow while the arteriotomy is repaired.

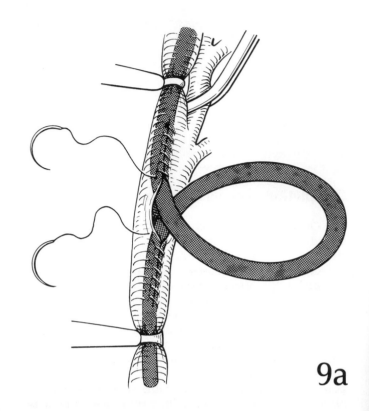

9a

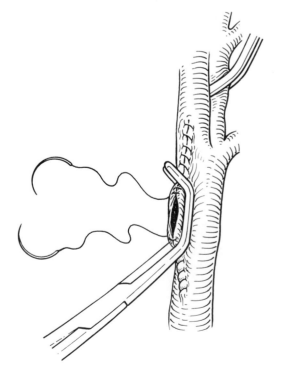

9b

PATCH ANGIOPLASTY

Patch angioplasty is appropriate for small vessels, particularly in women, and in reoperative cases. Prosthetic material is chosen in most situations (Dacron or expanded polytetrafluoroethylene (PTFE)), except in cases of recurrent carotid stenosis where autologous vein is preferable. An important principle when patching a bifurcation arteriotomy is not to attempt to construct the largest luminal diameter possible. Rather, the original size of the vessel should simply be approximated, and any unnatural luminal narrowing avoided. This prevents large patulous arteries which can become culs-de-sac for the later development of mural thrombi.

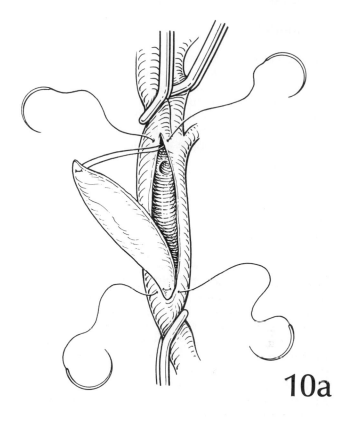

10a, b Whichever method is chosen, the closure begins distally, and closely placed sutures incorporating small bites of artery are inserted until the carotid bulb and common carotid artery are reached. Proximally, a second suture is begun which proceeds distally. Before the suture line is completed, the internal, external and common carotid arteries are flushed. After the sutures are tied, the internal carotid artery is allowed to back-bleed and completely fill the carotid bulb. The proximal internal carotid artery is again gently occluded and flow is restored through the external system by removing the clamps on the external and common carotid arteries respectively. Finally, after several seconds the occluding clamp is removed from the internal carotid artery. When sutures are placed carefully and in an unhurried manner, suture line bleeding is seldom a problem. On occasion, pledgets of thrombin-soaked Gelfoam or fibrin glue may be necessary, particularly when prosthetic material is used.

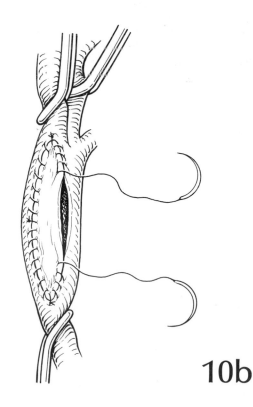

EXTERNAL CAROTID ENDARTERECTOMY

Technique

Endarterectomy of lesions of the external carotid artery is indicated when flow reduction or ulceration in this vessel has been determined to be the cause of significant cerebrovascular symptoms. Most commonly this circumstance occurs following chronic occlusion of the internal carotid artery. In this setting, the external carotid artery can supply a significant portion of the intracranial circulation via well-developed collaterals. Therefore, embolization or the development of a flow-limiting lesion in the origin of the external cerebral circulation can cause significant symptoms in the distribution of the previously occluded internal carotid artery. This procedure is also very occasionally performed to repair a proximal lesion before an extracranial-to-intracranial bypass.

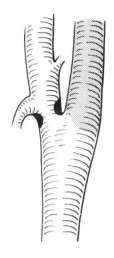

11 Dissection of the carotid bifurcation is carried out in a fashion similar to a standard carotid endarterectomy. After mobilizing the bifurcation and all its major branches, a moment should be taken to confirm that the internal carotid artery is totally occluded. Occasionally, this vessel will be found to be still patent, permitting a conventional carotid endarterectomy to be performed with restoration of antegrade flow through the internal cerebral circulation. If internal carotid occlusion is confirmed by direct inspection, the proximal carotid artery is clamped and the origin of the internal carotid artery is divided flush with the carotid bifurcation.

The arteriotomy through the orifice of the internal carotid artery is positioned on the posterior lateral aspect of the carotid bulb and continued distally onto the external carotid artery beyond the distal extent of the atherosclerotic lesion in that vessel. Under direct vision, an endarterectomy of the external carotid artery is performed. The plane of the dissection and the handling of the endpoints is managed in the same manner as a carotid bifurcation endarterectomy.

The arteriotomy is closed primarily. Great care should be taken to contour the repair to provide a smooth, tapered transition from the common carotid artery to the endarterectomized external carotid artery. Any residual luminal irregularities, such as a retained stump at the site of the divided internal carotid, may provide a cul-de-sac for the development of thrombotic or platelet aggregates, leading to emboli and recurrent cerebrovascular symptoms. If the external carotid artery is small, it may be necessary to close the arteriotomy with a patch. Either a prosthetic or autologous tissue patch may be used. Both vein and a segment of the chronically occluded internal carotid artery have been used successfully for this purpose.

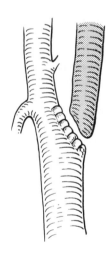

11

INTERNAL CAROTID ARTERY DILATATION

Technique

Early in the experience with the surgical management of fibromuscular dysplasia, most patients underwent resection of the diseased arterial segment and reconstruction by either primary anastomosis or construction of an autologous interposition graft. In 1968, Morris *et al.* described the technique of internal carotid artery dilatation, which has greatly simplified the surgical correction of these lesions.

This procedure is best performed while the patient is under general anaesthesia. The positioning, exposure and initial dissection of the carotid bifurcation are the same as for carotid endarterectomy. For this procedure, however, it is particularly important to mobilize the entire extracranial portion of the internal carotid artery. In this way, the dilatation can be carried out under direct visual and palpable control. Thorough mobilization of the carotid bifurcation will also aid in the cephalad passage of the carotid dilators by allowing caudal countertraction during the procedure.

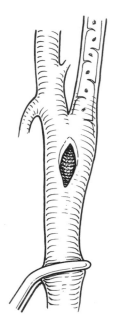

12 Once the arteries are all identified and mobilized, the patient is systematically heparinized and the common carotid artery is clamped proximally. A 1-cm longitudinal arteriotomy is made in the carotid bulb adjacent to the origin of the internal carotid artery. A 2-mm coronary dilator is then introduced into the orifice of the internal carotid artery proximally and carefully advanced. As mentioned, gentle caudal countertraction on the carotid bulb while advancing the dilator can be very helpful. The intraluminal position of the dilator should be assessed continually by a combination of visual inspection and external palpation. The dilator is passed to the base of the skull and then carefully removed. During the dilation, the surgeon will often feel the disruption of each intraluminal septum as the dilator is advanced.

Progressively larger diameter dilators of 0.5-mm increments up to a maximum of 4.0 mm are passed through the diseased arterial segment in a similar fashion. After each passage, the artery is allowed to back-bleed though the arteriotomy to remove any debris dislodged by the dilatation.

An alternative technique to progressive intraluminal dilatation is the use of intraoperative balloon angioplasty. One theoretical advantage of this method is avoidance of the potential arterial traction injury caused by the repetitive longitudinal motion of the intraluminal dilators. The results of this technique, however, though favourable, have not been shown to be superior to the standard dilatation procedure.

At the completion of the dilatation, the arteriotomy is closed and antegrade blood flow is restored. As always, completion arteriography is highly recommended to confirm an adequate technical result.

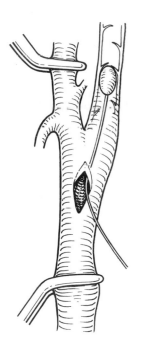

12

EXTENDED EXPOSURE TECHNIQUES

When a carotid artery bifurcates high in the neck, or when there is extensive distal disease involving the internal carotid artery, it may be necessary to obtain additional exposure in the superior aspect of the incision. Several techniques have been described to increase the length of internal carotid artery that can be approached. Surgeons performing carotid surgery should be familiar with these manoeuvres.

The simplest and most important technique is to extend the skin incision completely across the mastoid process behind the ear. This allows additional mobilization of the sternocleidomastoid muscle up to its tendinous insertion. The spinal accessory nerve enters the muscle at this level and must be preserved.

When additional exposure is necessary, the posterior belly of the digastric muscle can be detached from its insertion onto the mastoid process. The digastric muscle consists of two muscle bellies united by a rounded tendon. The posterior belly arises from the mastoid process and the anterior portion inserts on the mandibular symphysis. It is useful to appreciate the superficial anatomical position of the posterior digastric muscle when dissecting in this area. All important neurovascular structures lie deep to the digastric muscle at this level. Only the external jugular vein and branches of the facial and great auricular nerves pass superficial to the posterior belly of the digastric muscle. Below the muscle, particular care must be taken to avoid injury to the hypoglossal and spinal accessory nerves, as well as the facial branch of the external carotid artery. The stylohyoid muscle can also be divided. This muscle stretches between the styloid process and hyoid bone and its removal, along with the styloid process, can provide additional exposure of the distal internal carotid artery at the base of the skull.

When the disease extends very distally, it is possible to gain additional exposure by anteriorly subluxating the condylar process of the mandible. The displaced mandible can be secured in place with wires. This manoeuvre alters the geometry at the base of the skull by turning a triangular space into a rectangle and thereby enlarging the operative field.

Lastly, techniques by which the ramus of the mandible is divided have also been described. This is an involved procedure that greatly complicates the postoperative course, and the authors have never found this manoeuvre to be necessary.

RECURRENT STENOSIS

The incision and principles of exposure when approaching a recurrent carotid lesion are the same as described for a standard endarterectomy (page 1076). The dissection is invariably more difficult due to scarring from the previous procedure, and extra care must be taken to avoid injury to the cranial nerves. The hypoglossal nerve is particularly vulnerable as it can be draped over the bifurcation by the scar tissue. Once completely dissected, the common, external and internal carotid vessels are clamped, and the bifurcation opened using a longitudinal arteriotomy.

The histological property of carotid bifurcation atherosclerotic lesions, which allows for the performance of a standard endarterectomy, is the ability to easily develop a plane of dissection between the plaque and the circular medial fibres of the arterial wall. Unfortunately, recurrent carotid lesions composed of hyperplastic intimal tissue do not share this property. These lesions are formed by intrinsic medial cells which migrate across the internal elastic lamina and replicate within the neointima. Thus, it is not possible to form a precise plane of dissection that allows the removal of the luminal narrowing disease without dangerously thinning the remaining arterial wall. The surgical approach to recurrent carotid lesions therefore, is patch angioplasty rather than endarterectomy. On the other hand, when the recurrent lesion is found to be composed of ordinary atheroma, a standard endarterectomy can be performed.

The choice of patch material includes prosthetic material and autologous vein. There is a theoretical argument that prosthetic material may contribute to the hyperplastic intimal process, but this has not been proved experimentally. In fact, it has been suggested that autologous vein, with its intact endothelium elaborating humoral growth factors, may be a greater stimulus to a continued hyperplastic reaction in the patched arterial segment. When vein is chosen, saphenous vein is most commonly used, as experience has shown that vein segments taken from the neck are ordinarily too thin and should be avoided. Regardless of the material chosen, the patch should always be constructed in such a way as to approximate the original size of the carotid bulb. Large patulous repairs may lead to the accumulation of laminar thrombus and result in distal embolism.

Occasionally, the recurrent disease is so advanced that patch angioplasty is not feasible. In these rare cases, reconstruction can be accomplished by the use of an interposition graft.

Wound closure

Closure of the incision following a carotid operation should be meticulous and adhere to all the basic principles of surgery. The wound should be irrigated generously with warm saline solution and perfect haemostasis confirmed. The platysma is reapproximated with a running suture, and the skin is closed with stainless steel staples. Some surgeons prefer to place a closed suction drain beneath the platysmal layer and bring it out through a separate stab wound. A sterile dressing is applied, and the patient is observed carefully while awakening from anaesthesia.

Postoperative care

Immediately after awakening from anaesthesia, a preliminary neurological assessment should be made. The patient is subsequently transferred to the recovery room followed by the intensive care unit for careful monitoring during the first 24 h following surgery. Particular attention should be made to assess systemic blood pressure and neurological function frequently during this period. In addition, careful wound observation is essential to detect the formation of a haematoma, which may compromise the reconstruction or threaten the airway. After 24 h, the intra-arterial line and the closed suction drain, if placed, can be removed, and the patient is returned to the general ward. Most patients undergoing carotid surgery are admitted to hospital the morning of surgery and are discharged home on the second or third day after operation. Before discharge, the skin staples are replaced with adhesive Steri-Strips and an appointment is made for the patient to return within 2–3 weeks for the first follow-up after the operation.

Complications

An uncomplicated carotid endarterectomy is a well-tolerated operation. Tissue trauma and operative blood loss are normally minimal, and patients are routinely discharged from hospital on the second or third day after surgery. For this reason, perioperative complications are particularly discouraging and must be avoided at all costs. Operative intervention, particularly in asymptomatic patients, will only continue to be justified by keeping operative morbidity and mortality to a minimum.

Technical errors

By definition, technical errors occurring during the operation are preventable by adherence to good surgical principles. One major cause of a technical complication is incomplete or inadequate removal of plaque from the endarterectomized segment. Distal intimal flaps are common if care is not taken to directly assess this endpoint. This complication can be minimized by extending the arteriotomy beyond the distal extent of the visible luminal disease. When a shunt has been inserted, this manoeuvre becomes critically important, otherwise it is not possible to adequately visualize the distal endpoint. Very occasionally, tacking sutures may be required to ensure a smooth transition to normal intima. Regardless of the visual appearance of the endarterectomized surface, a completion angiogram should always be obtained to document the absence of defects or narrowing following the arteriotomy closure.

Embolism occurring during or after carotid endarterectomy is probably the most common cause of postoperative neurological deficits. These events can occur while the carotid artery is being mobilized. Alternatively, embolism occurs during cross-clamping, following the insertion of the internal carotid artery shunt, or after restoration of flow. Placing the distal end of a shunt first allows back-bleeding and removal of any residual air or debris. Inserting the proximal portion while the shunt is clamped at its midsection, allows visualization of air or debris from the proximal common carotid artery while the shunt is slowly opened. Following completion of the endarterectomy, any residual plaque should be carefully removed. Irrigating the lumen with heparinized saline can be very helpful in identifying and completely removing small fragments. After closure of the arteriotomy, flow should first be restored into the external carotid system to capture any remaining intraluminal debris. Antegrade flow can then be safely re-established into the internal system by slowly removing the clamp on this vessel.

Cranial nerve injury

As described above, several peripheral nerves must be identified and protected during the exposure of the carotid bifurcation. Injury to these structures is another source of postoperative morbidity following carotid endarterectomy. In 1980, Hertzer reviewed the postoperative complications in a series of patients undergoing carotid endarterectomy and found a 16% incidence of cranial nerve injuries[12]. All cranial nerve injuries occurring during carotid surgery can be prevented by becoming familiar with the normal and possible abnormal anatomical neurovascular relationships and carefully protecting these structures during the procedure.

Hypertension/hypotension

Blood pressure changes, both during and immediately following carotid endarterectomy, are common and potentially serious if not treated appropriately. The aetiology of blood pressure fluctuations following carotid surgery is multifactorial. One proposed mechanism is damage to the baroreceptor mechanism located in the carotid sinus. Devascularization or interruption of the afferent nerves emerging from this structure potentially reduce the sensitivity of this receptor to changes in blood pressure. Conversely, endarterectomy of the carotid bifurcation may lead to overdistension of the thin-walled bulb and increased stimulation of the carotid sinus.

Intraoperative hypotension associated with bradycardia due to stimulation of the carotid body should respond promptly to the local injection of 0.5% lignocaine hydrochloride into the tissues adjacent to the carotid sinus. If this manoeuvre fails to restore normal haemodynamics, an immediate cardiac evaluation should be performed. Hypertension during or following carotid endarterectomy can usually be easily treated with intravenous sodium nitroprusside. The requirement for intravenous antihypertensive therapy seldom lasts beyond the first 24 h after operation, and patients with long-standing essential hypertension can be started on their oral medications following this interval.

References

1. Gelabert HA, Moore WS. Carotid endarterectomy: current status: *Curr Probl Surg* 1991; 28: 181–262.

2. Eastcott HHG, Pickering GW, Robb C. Reconstruction of internal carotid artery in a patient with intermittent attacks of hemiplegia. *Lancet* 1954; ii: 994–6.

3. Winslow CM, Solomon DH, Chassin MR, Kosecoff, J. Merrick NJ, Brook RH. The appropriateness of carotid endarterectomy. *N Engl J Med* 1988; 318: 721–7.

4. Towne JB, Weiss DG, Hobson RW. First phase report of cooperative Veterans Administration asymptomatic carotid stenosis study – operative morbidity and mortality. *J Vasc Surg* 1990; 11: 252–9.

5. North American Symptomatic Carotid Endarterectomy Trial Collaborators. Beneficial effect of carotid endarterectomy in symptomatic patients with high-grade carotid stenosis. *N Engl J Med* 1991; 325; 445–53.

6. European Carotid Surgery Trialists' Collaborative Group. MRC European Carotid Surgery Trial: interim results for symptomatic patients with severe (70–99%) or with mild (0–29%) carotid stenosis. *Lancet* 1991; 337: 1235–43.

7. Stanley JC, Gewertz BL, Bove EL, Sottiurai V, Fry WJ. Arterial fibrodysplasia: histopathologic character and current etiologic concepts. *Arch Surg* 1975; 110: 561–6.

8. Thompson JE. Carotid endarterectomy for asymptomatic carotid stenosis: an update. *J Vasc Surg* 1991; 13: 669–76.

9. Hertzer NR, Martinez BD, Benjamin SP, Beven EG. Recurrent stenosis after carotid endarterectomy. *Surg Gynecol Obstet* 1979; 149: 360–4.

10. Zierler RE, Bandyk DF, Thiele BL, Strandness DE. Carotid artery stenosis following endarterectomy. *Arch Surg* 1982; 117: 1408–15.

11. Gelabert HA, Moore WS. Carotid endarterectomy without angiography. *Surg Clin North Am* 1990; 70: 213–23.

12. Hertzer NR, Feldman BJ, Beven EG, Tucker HM. A prospective study of the incidence of injury to the cranial nerves during carotid endarterectomy. *Surg Gynecol Obstet* 1980; 151: 781–4.

Femorodistal reversed vein bypass

D. Bergqvist MD, PhD
Professor, Department of Surgery, University Hospital, Uppsala, Sweden

T. Mätzsch MD, PhD
Associate Professor, Department of Surgery, Lund University, Malmö General Hospital, Malmö, Sweden

History

Reconstructive surgery for femoropopliteal occlusive disease, most commonly caused by arteriosclerosis, is the most commonly performed procedure in peripheral vascular surgery. A great step forward was taken by Kunlin[1], who used autologous vein as a bypass graft for superficial femoral artery occlusions, although reversed vein grafts had already been used after trauma during World War I. For many years the use of reversed vein dominated, but since the mid 1970s the *in situ* technique has increasingly been performed. Both techniques have pros and cons, and discussion of them can be vivid and aggressive. Few randomized studies have compared *in situ* and reversed vein bypass, and with the use of optimal techniques for both there seems to be little difference in outcome in terms of long-term patency. This discussion will not be further addressed here, and for analysis of results the reader is referred to Taylor and Porter[2] and Calligaro *et al*[3]. In addition to being used by some surgeons as first choice of treatment, knowledge of the reversed technique is needed when it is impossible to perform an *in situ* bypass.

Principles and justification

Whenever possible, the authors' preference is the *in situ* technique. The choice of whether to use the *in situ* technique or a reversed autologous vein grafting procedure depends on several factors. If the ipsilateral vein is missing because of previous variceal or other surgery, is unsuitable due to extensive varicosities, or is too small in calibre, the need for alternative conduits arises.

If the procedure aims at reconstruction on a crural level, i.e. below the popliteal artery, the reversed vein bypass is less suitable because of difficulties in harvesting a sufficiently long conduit and of discrepancies in luminal size between the proximal reversed vein segment and the small calibre arterial vessels in the lower leg.

Indications

The main clinical indications are intermittent claudication, chronic critical leg ischaemia, acute chronic ischaemia and popliteal aneurysm.

Intermittent claudication is a somewhat controversial indication. Some surgeons are fairly liberal, while others are very conservative and perform femorodistal bypass surgery only occasionally when the claudication is disabling. An argument supporting the more conservative approach is the often benign natural course, with increasing walking distance after training and stopping smoking.

Chronic critical leg ischaemia is defined on the basis provided by the Ad Hoc Committee[4] or the Second European Consensus document on chronic critical leg ischaemia[5]. Clinically, this means patients with rest pain, ischaemic ulcers, or frank gangrene.

Acute on chronic ischaemia must be differentiated from embolic disease, where embolectomy often is sufficient. On the other hand, an attempt with a Fogarty catheter in patients with acute on chronic ischaemia will often fail or aggravate the condition. In many cases, thrombolysis and balloon angioplasty will solve the problem; in others a bypass procedure is necessary.

Preoperative

Assessment and preparation

In addition to measurements of ankle–brachial index and toe pressure, preoperative assessment should always include angiography. Attention is directed towards acceptable run-in and run-off conditions. A poor run-in with significant atherosclerotic lesions in the suprainguinal segment will jeopardize the patency of the bypass, as will an inadequate run-off. Assessment of the run-off must be made with caution, as at times the arteries distal to an occlusion and the continuity of the pedal arch may not be visualized on the arteriogram due to poor contrast filling of the vessels if proper care is not taken during arteriography. A 'blind' popliteal segment, however, is not a contraindication to this type of operation.

Assessment of the vein is also important. Gross varicosities constitute a contraindication, but limited variceal sacculae can be accepted and corrected during operation. A vein less than 4 mm in diameter is less suitable for use as a bypass. If doubts concerning the quality of the vein arise, mapping with duplex ultrasonography can be helpful. Preoperative investigation of the vein should always be performed with the patient standing in order to achieve sufficient filling of the vein.

The patient should be prepared with a whole body scrub using a chlorhexidine-containing soap in order to minimize the risk of infection that is increased whenever performing a groin incision. For this reason, antibiotic cover is also provided. The antibiotic chosen should be active against *Staphylococcus epidermidis*, as this is the most commonly encountered organism in graft infections. If the extremity has overt gangrene, it has been recommended that antibiotics should be chosen according to the organisms identified in cultures of the gangrenous area.

Anaesthesia

General, spinal or epidural anaesthesia can be used.

Operation

Position of patient

The lower abdomen, groin and both legs are prepared and draped. The foot is placed in a sterile plastic bag in order to make inspection possible during the operation. A small cushion under the knee allows easier access to the popliteal artery. Special attention is directed towards the heel of the foot; during the operation and for as long as epidural or spinal analgesia is provided, a pad should be in place to prevent pressure necrosis.

Skin incision

1a, b For exposure of the proximal saphenous vein and common femoral artery, a laterally convex incision lateral to the vessels is preferred in order to minimize damage to the lymphatic vessels. For exposure of the popliteal artery proximal to the knee, the incision is placed just above the femoral epicondyle and two fingerbreadths behind the femur along the anterior border of the sartorius muscle. For exposure of the distal popliteal artery, the 10–15-cm incision is placed just behind the tibial margin.

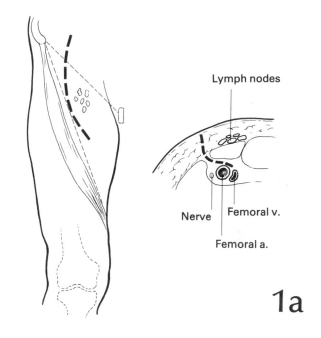

1a

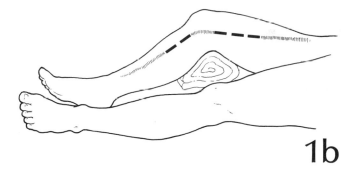

1b

Groin dissection

2 A slightly arched incision just lateral of the femoral artery is preferred to a vertical one above the artery in order to avoid damage to the lymph nodes or vessels, which could lead to prolonged lymphorrhoea or infection. A separate fascial incision over the saphenous vein at the foramen ovale about one fingerbreadth below and lateral to the pubic tubercle also helps to maintain the lymphatics intact. Utmost care must be taken not to create undue skin flaps in order to minimize risk of skin edge necrosis and infection, which may be disastrous for the reconstruction, the leg and the patient.

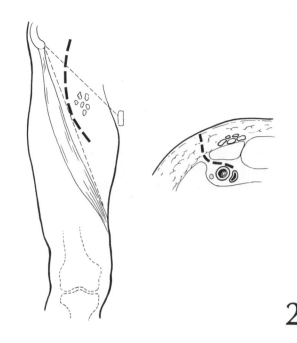

2

3a, b The femoral artery and its branches are exposed, controlled and taped.

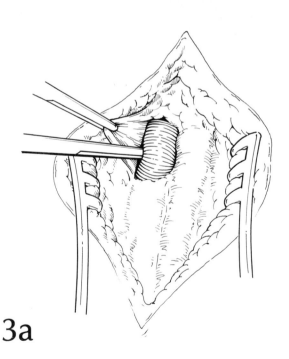

3a

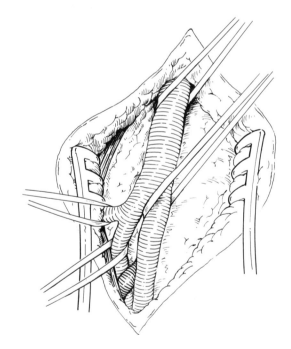

3b

Preparing the site of distal anastomosis

4a–d Before the vein is freed and prepared, the recipient artery should be dissected and checked for patency and suitability for anastomosis. If the distal anastomosis is to be placed at the proximal popliteal artery, an incision just above the femoral epicondyle and behind the medial edge of the femur is chosen. This is usually also the location of the saphenous vein, so care must be taken not to injure it during dissection. The incision is extended through the adductor fascia, and the artery is gently mobilized and held with soft rubber tapes. Major branches are preserved.

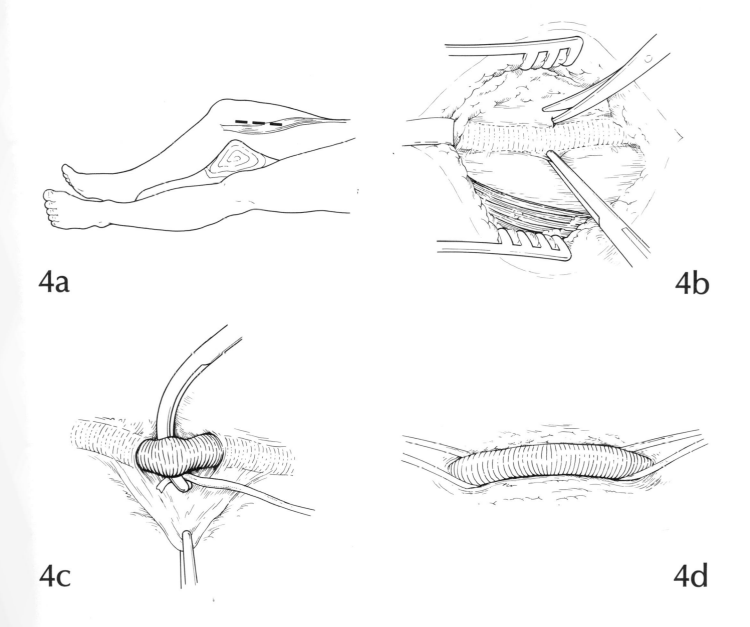

4a

4b

4c

4d

5a, b If the distal anastomosis is to be at the distal popliteal artery, an incision behind the tibial margin is chosen. The saphenous vein runs in close proximity to this incision and is easily injured if care is not taken. The fascia is divided 1–2 cm behind the tibial edge and the gastrocnemius muscle is retracted backwards. The tendons of the hamstring muscles must sometimes be divided, which can be done without risk. The popliteal artery, vein and nerve are found in the fatty tissue of the popliteal fossa. Usually there are two veins with the artery in between, which makes careful dissection necessary in order to avoid troublesome bleeding. The approach is made easier if a cushion is placed under the distal thigh. The artery should be mobilized to the point where it enters the soleus muscle and branches off into the tibiofibular trunk, and the anterior tibial artery. It is secured with rubber tapes and checked for suitability as a recipient artery.

Access to the crural vessels is described in detail on page 1014.

6a, b The saphenous vein is divided and the proximal stump suture ligated at its junction with the femoral vein. All small tributaries are ligated with 4/0 non-resorbable material near the vein and with resorbable material on the peripheral side.

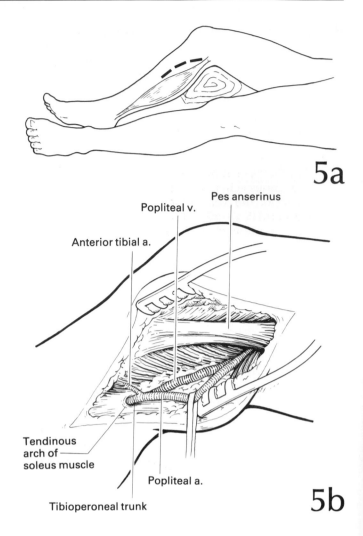

5a

Pes anserinus

Popliteal v.

Anterior tibial a.

Tendinous arch of soleus muscle

Popliteal a.

Tibioperoneal trunk

5b

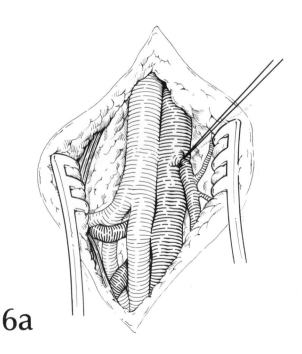

6a

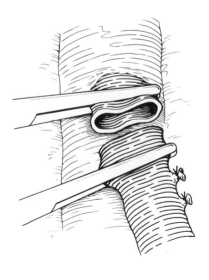

6b

7 The ligatures should be placed neither too near the saphenous vein nor too peripheral in order to avoid narrowing of the vein lumen or blind stumps where thrombosis will occur, which can ultimately progress and cause acute graft occlusion or distal embolization.

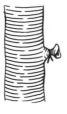 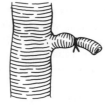 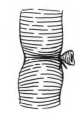

Correct   Wrong – too long   Wrong – too close

7

Freeing the vein

8 Using either multiple short incisions or one continuous incision along the vein, it is dissected free with all branches tied off and divided as described. Creating flaps or superficially undermined areas must be avoided at all times and hence a continuous incision that is sequentially extended distally with respect to the course of the vein is preferred. This method also minimizes the risk of undue tension on the vein, which must be avoided. The vein should be handled with utmost care at all times and desiccation prevented by frequent irrigation.

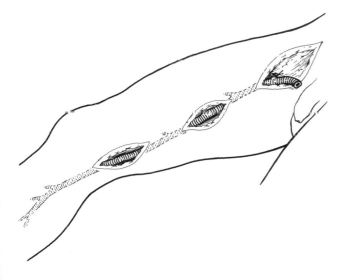

8

Use of short saphenous vein or arm veins

In cases where the long saphenous vein is absent due to earlier surgery or unsuitable as a conduit, the short saphenous vein or arm veins can be used as alternatives.

Harvesting the short saphenous vein

Ideally, the patient is placed in the prone position while the vein is dissected. This necessitates repositioning of the patient during operation, which can be cumbersome. With adequate assistance it is not very difficult to make the dissection with the patient supine. By flexion and inward rotation of the hip joint with the knee joint flexed it is also possible to gain access to the vein.

9 The vein is located just behind the lateral malleolus. When freeing the vein, care must be taken not to injure the sural nerve which runs in very close proximity to it.

After locating the vein and the nerve, the incision is extended along the vein up the calf. About halfway between knee and ankle, the vein penetrates the muscular fascia and runs underneath it. All branches are carefully ligated and divided.

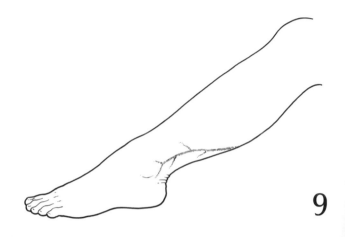

9

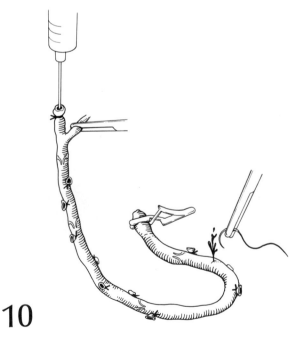

10

10 The short saphenous vein is particularly prone to spasm, which may be counteracted by irrigation with a solution of papaverine.

When harvesting the short saphenous vein, it is particularly important not to create any undermined skin flaps, in order to avoid skin edge necrosis. After having freed the vein for a sufficient length it is ligated, divided and handled as described for the long saphenous vein on page 1094. The skin incision should be closed immediately.

Harvesting arm veins

11a–d If no other options for obtaining an autologous vein are available, the veins of the arm can be utilized. For this purpose, the patient's arm must be prepared and draped so that it can be moved freely. A separate table supporting the arm is preferable.

The cephalic vein can be harvested from the radial side of the wrist to the confluence with the subclavian vein in the deltoid–pectoral triangle. The basilic vein is less suitable for harvesting as it disappears underneath the fascia shortly above the elbow. Techniques have been described for using both the cephalic and the basilic vein as one conduit[6].

The main drawbacks of using arm veins as conduits are the great anatomical variations in size and conformation and the abundant branches. The arm veins are also very adherent to the skin, making dissection more difficult. The use of arm veins however, should always be considered if no other possibilities exist for obtaining an autologous vein graft.

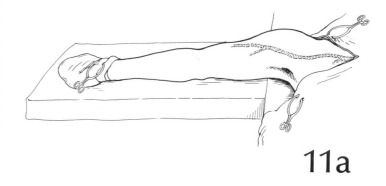

11a

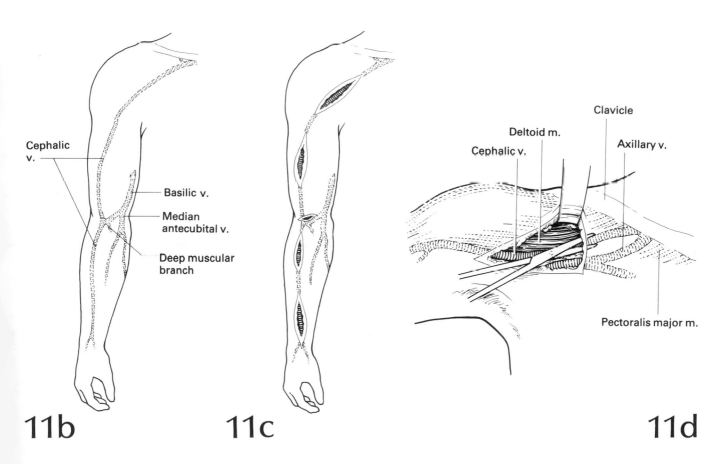

11b   **11c**   **11d**

Distension of vein and checking for leakage

12a, b After the vein has been dissected free it is curved through 180° and flushed (preferably) with cold heparinized blood. Pure saline solution is not optimal, but balanced salt and albumin solutions containing heparin and papaverine may be used as an alternative. In order to avoid damage to the endothelium the vein should never be distended above a pressure of about 200 mmHg – a pressure that is very easily achieved with a syringe if care is not taken. If papaverine has been used for relaxation of a contracted vein, it is particularly vulnerable to increased pressure.

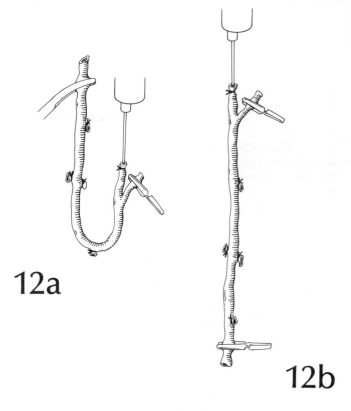

12a

12b

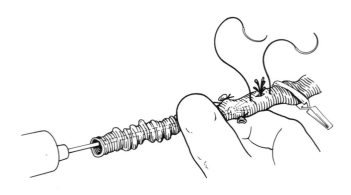

13

13 The vein is checked for points of leakage from divided and missed branches which, if present, are carefully sutured with a fine (8/0) monofilament. Luminal narrowing must be avoided. Magnification glasses (2.5 ×) are very useful for this step.

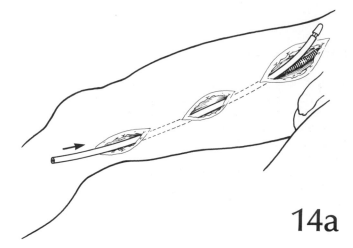

14a

Tunnelling

14a–c The vein is placed in a tunnel, preferably along the superficial femoral artery or subcutaneously. The tunnel is created with a tunneller, a curved steel tube containing a rod with has a coned end. The tunneller is passed from the point of the distal anastomosis subfascially to the groin incision. If the distal anastomosis is below the knee, care is taken to ensure that the tunneller is passed laterally to the medial tendons of the gastrocnemius. The end of the vein is attached to a pair of long grasping forceps after the rod has been removed, and pulled through the steel tube. Utmost care must be taken in order not to twist the vein as it is passed through the tube. The tunneller is then removed.

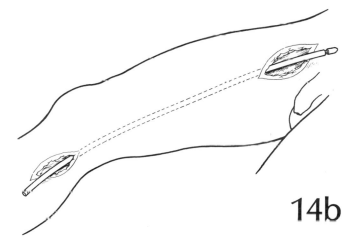

14b

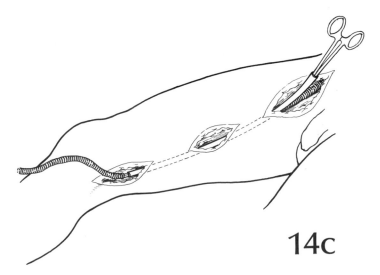

14c

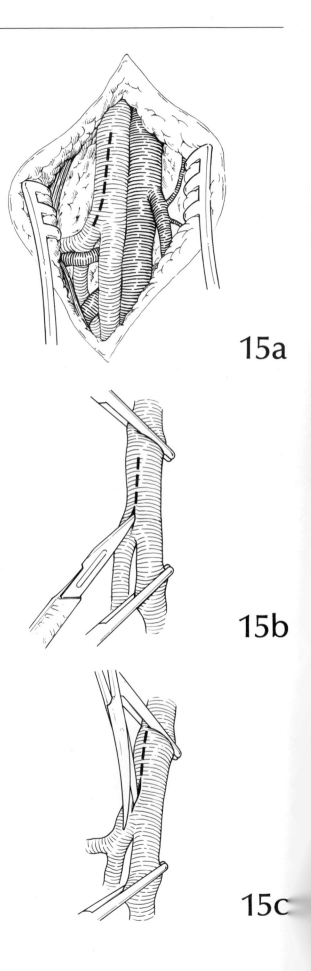

15a

15b

15c

Preparing the artery for anastomosis

15a–c Following systemic heparinization, the exposed common, superficial and deep femoral artery in the groin are clamped with vascular, atraumatic clamps. An arteriotomy is made as a stab incision in the common femoral artery with a number 11 scalpel blade. The intima of the posterior wall must be carefully avoided so as to eliminate the risks of intimal dissection and occlusion. The incision is extended with angled Pott's scissors. The distal end of the arteriotomy is placed so that it can be easily extended down into the deep femoral artery if there is a stenosis of the orifice.

Anastomosing the vein to the common femoral artery

16a–e The end of the vein is cut obliquely to fit the arteriotomy without tension. The suture always begins at the heel with double-ended monofilament sutures. The authors prefer polytetra-fluoroethylene (PTFE), which appears to be superior to the stiffer polypropylene sutures in handling. The sutures are always placed from the inside of the artery outwards in order to avoid separation of the thickened intimal layer. The first suture is tied down and the next is placed from the outside of the vein to the inside of the artery to form a continuous suture. Great attention is paid to avoid causing narrowing of the heel. This is avoided if the first two stitches are placed along the axis of the artery. A continuous suture is inserted for about half the length of the arteriotomy, and the same procedure is repeated on the other side. A second suture is then passed from the inside through the vein and artery at the toe of the arteriotomy, tied down and completed continuously to join the other two sutures where it is tied.

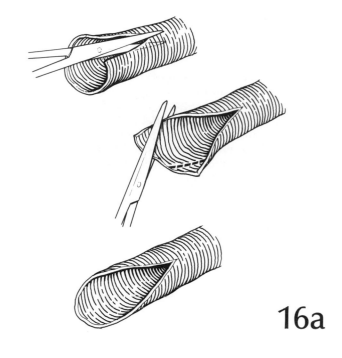

16a

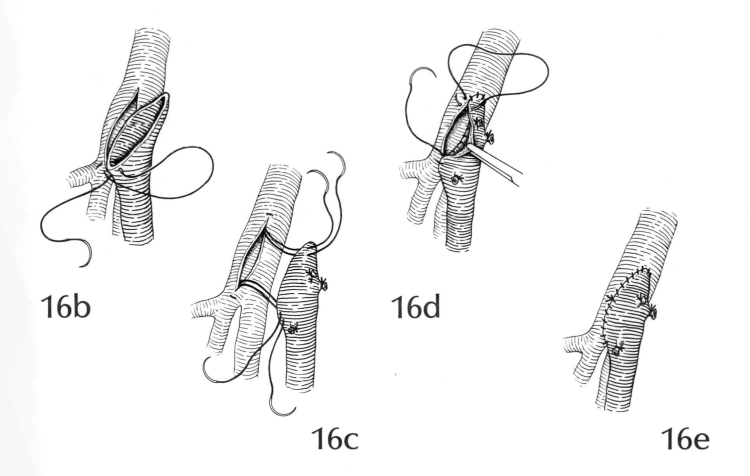

16b

16c

16d

16e

Completion of the anastomosis

17 Before the anastomosis is completed and the last two or three sutures are placed, adequate back-flow and down-flow are checked by briefly opening the clamps. The anastomosis is then irrigated with heparinized saline (5000 units in 0.51 sodium chloride). The anastomosis is completed and the flow in the artery re-established while the vein is clamped just distal to the anastomosis. Minor bleeding from the anastomosis will mostly stop after applying a dry swab for a few minutes.

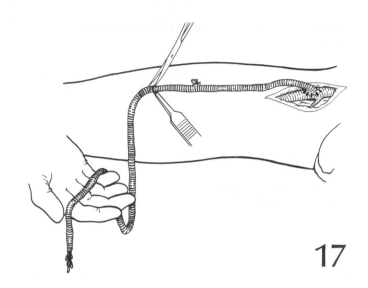

17

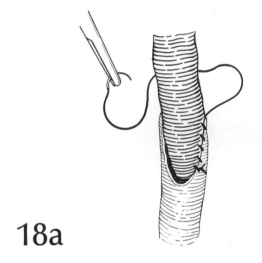

18a

Distal anastomosis

18a, b After an arteriotomy in either the above-knee or below-knee popliteal artery, the vein is trimmed and cut to fit the length of the arteriotomy having extended the knee fully to measure the required length. The anastomosis is performed using the same method as for the proximal anastomosis. Here, care must be taken to avoid narrowing of the distal end of the recipient vessel. If the vessel is of small calibre, three separate sutures should be placed at the toe and tied separately.

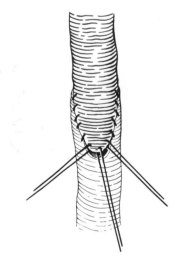

18b

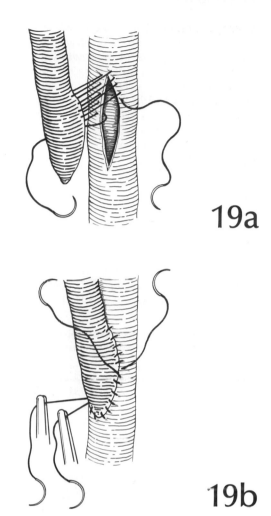

19a, b Alternatively, and if the vessel is located deep with a difficult approach, a parachute or sliding technique may be used for the distal anastomosis at the heel. The first stitch is made slightly below the corner of the proximal edge of the arteriotomy. Without tying, the next suture is placed proximal to the first and then the next around the corner of the heel, whereafter it is gently pulled down. Polypropylene monofilament sutures are better suited for this kind of technique than PTFE sutures, as they allow more sutures to be placed before approximation. The sutures may have to be tightened one by one using a nerve hook. In this way every suture can be placed exactly under visual control, even under difficult conditions.

Just before completion of the anastomosis, back-flow and on-flow are tested and the anastomosis is rinsed and irrigated as previously described.

Completion angiography

If there is any question about the function of a distal anastomosis, angiography is performed. This can often be done using a branch that has been saved for this purpose. Contrast medium, 20 ml, is injected and films are taken over the distal anastomosis and distal to it to ensure adequate filling of the recipient vessel.

Wound closure

After haemostasis has been ensured, the skin wounds are closed. The skin edges must be handled gently in order to avoid necrosis and infectious complications.

Errors and complications

Several technical errors are possible during dissection, harvesting and preparation of an autologous vein as a bypass conduit. Most of them will lead to acute or early graft occlusion and must thus be avoided at all times. Some of the most commonly encountered faults and complications and how to avoid them will be summarized.

Pitfalls during dissection and harvesting

20a, b Incorrectly tied branches will lead to either narrowing of the lumen or creation of blind stumps that can act as the origin of progressing thrombosis. The branches should be tied 1–2 mm away from the vein wall or oversewn if too short. One branch near the proximal anastomosis should be kept longer for use when performing completion angiography and tied correctly afterwards.

Rotation of the vein in excess of 90° will cause flow impairment, thrombosis and acute graft failure. This can be prevented by, for example, marking the vein with dye before the tunnelling procedure. Gentle filling of the vein with heparinized blood will also help to reveal any twists.

Undue traction and distension of the vein will cause damage to the endothelium, thus causing denuded and thrombogenic areas.

If the vein is too short it can be lengthened by using either the short saphenous vein or arm veins. If no other alternatives exist, a composite graft can be created by anastomosing a thin-walled 6-mm PTFE graft for the proximal part to the autologous vein graft that is used to make the critical distal anastomosis and to bridge the knee joint. The synthetic graft should be as short as possible. If only a short distance has to be gained, a thromboendarterectomy of the most proximal part of the superficial femoral artery may be enough, making it possible to anastomose the vein more distally than to the common femoral artery.

Numerous errors are possible when performing the anastomosis and in order to avoid these, the reader is referred to the chapter on pp. 1016–1023. At all times it must be remembered that the key to successful bypass surgery is meticulous technique.

Intraoperative prophylaxis against clot formation

When cross-clamping it is important to avoid blind segments as far as possible and, if such segments occur, to rinse them with heparinized saline and to check that they are free from clots before unclamping. Intravascu-

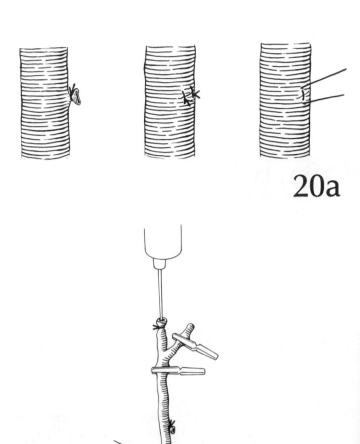

20a

20b

lar clots can be prevented with either dextran or heparin. Dextran, 500 ml, is given as an intravenous infusion during surgery, and this is repeated daily for 2–4 days after operation[7]. In addition to influencing platelet adhesion and clot formation, dextran also has beneficial rheological properties. Most vascular surgeons use heparin given by one of several regimens. Either 5 000 units or a total of 100 units/kg body weight is given at cross-clamping. Some surgeons recommend reversal with protamine sulphate after restoration of flow, using 1–2 mg/100 units heparin.

Postoperative care

Adjuvant therapy

Postoperative graft occlusion is a multifactorial process, and therefore it has proved difficult to study the pharmacological prevention of graft occlusion. The scientific background for practical recommendations is thus rather weak. There seems to be no doubt, however, that continuing smoking increases the risk of graft occlusion. Although difficult, it is important to motivate patients to stop smoking. Various antiplatelet drugs have been tried which appear to be beneficial when started preoperatively, at least in technically difficult femorodistal bypasses. Increasing patency with oral anticoagulants has not been proved. Both oral anticoagulant and antiplatelet drugs seem to increase patient survival.

Follow-up

During the hospital stay, the circulation is frequently checked with pulse palpation and/or Doppler ultrasonography. Routine surveillance after departure from hospital is still a matter of debate, but most vascular surgeons have some form of surveillance programme. Since the introduction of duplex scanning it has become clear that postoperative development of asymptomatic stenotic lesions occurs in both the inflow and outflow tracts and also within the graft, often at the site of the valve cusps. Simple measurement of the ankle–brachial index is not sensitive enough to detect these stenoses at an asymptomatic stage, and the presence of stenoses indicates an increased risk of graft occlusion. The majority of graft stenoses develop during the first year, and there are data indicating that it is possible to increase the overall patency of infrainguinal vein grafts by a systematic surveillance programme with reintervention at the stenotic sections of the graft[8]. Duplex scanning (or digital subtraction angiography) is recommended at least every 3 months during the first year with the first examination performed 3–6 weeks after the operation.

Complications

Early occlusion

Besides poor run-in and run-off, early occlusion of reversed vein grafts (within 30 days) is most often due to technical problems. If some form of measurement of flow or resistance has been made intraoperatively and there is an indication of a high-resistance, low-flow outflow tract, amputation is a reasonable choice following occlusion. If not, a revision procedure is indicated, thereby increasing secondary patency. If occlusion occurs during hospitalization, a technical failure should be suspected. The patient should immediately undergo catheter thrombectomy, followed by mandatory angiography or angioscopy to identify the cause of occlusion and then correct it. If occlusion occurs after 14 days or more, local thrombolysis is probably the most gentle technique that avoids destroying the vein. Thrombolysis is followed angiographically and again revision with either percutaneous angioplasty or a surgical procedure (patch or short-jump bypass) is directed to the cause of the graft occlusion. The longer the time lapse after the primary bypass the more likely it is that balloon angioplasty will succeed. Early in the postoperative course a graft stenosis will be too elastic and recur immediately. Simple Fogarty catheter thrombectomy is not often very successful in vein graft occlusions, which is one reason for instituting an aggressive surveillance programme to detect stenoses before occlusion occur.

References

1. Kunlin J. Le traiment de l'artérite oblitérante par la greffe veineuse. *Arch Mal Coeur* 1949; 42: 371–2.

2. Taylor LM, Porter JM. Reversed *vs in situ*: is either the technique of choice for lower extremity vein bypass? *Perspect Vasc Surg* 1988; 1: 35–55.

3. Calligaro KD, Friedell ML, Rollins DL, Semrow CM, Buchbinder D. A comparative review of *in situ* versus reversed vein grafts in the 1980s *Surg Gynecol Obstet* 1991; 172: 247–52.

4. The Ad Hoc Committee on Reporting Standards, Society for Vascular Surgery. Suggested standards for reports dealing with lower extremity ischemia. *J Vasc Surg* 1986; 4: 80–94.

5. Second European Consensus Document on Chronic Critical Leg Ischemia. European Workshop Group on critical leg ischemia. *Circulation* 1991; 84(Suppl 4): 1–26.

6. LoGerfo FW, Paniszyn CW, Menzoian Y. A new arm vein graft for distal bypass. *J Vasc Surg* 1987; 5: 889–91.

7. Rutherford R, Jones DN, Bergentz S-E *et al*. The efficacy of dextran 40 in preventing early postoperative thrombosis following difficult lower extremity bypass. *J Vasc Surg* 1984; 1: 765–73.

8. Harris P. Follow-up after reconstruction arterial surgery. *Eur J Vasc Surg* 1991; 5: 369–73.

Illustrations by Peter Cox

Operations for varicose veins

C. V. Ruckley MB, ChM, FRCS(Ed), FRCPE
Professor of Vascular Surgery, University of Edinburgh, and Consultant Surgeon, Vascular Surgery Unit, Royal Infirmary, Edinburgh, UK

Principles and justification

Pathology of venous disease

1a, b Approximately 20% of the adult population have chronic venous disease. Primary varicose veins constitute the great majority and these are mainly of the 'stem' type, the principal incompetent channel being the long or short saphenous vein, or both. In the face of proximal valvular incompetence the thin-walled tributaries draining into these stems form typical variceal patterns. They have a familial tendency and usually become conspicuous in early adult life or even earlier. The valvular dysfunction is believed to be secondary to structural deficiencies in the vein walls.

A variety of pathological processes may either damage valves or obstruct venous outflow and thereby promote the development of secondary varicose veins. Most are due to deep vein thrombosis, but other conditions include pelvic masses, enlarged lymph nodes, bony displacements and tricuspid incompetence.

The pattern of post-thrombotic secondary varicose veins is determined by the site and extent of the original thrombosis and the relative predominance of obstruction or valve imcompetence. Secondary varicose veins, however, tend to be associated with deep vein reflux, incompetent perforators and the skin changes of chronic venous insufficiency, whereas only a minority of patients with primary varicose veins progresses to chronic venous insufficiency.

Chronic venous insufficiency is the syndrome resulting from continuous venous hypertension in the erect posture, whether stationary or exercising, in contrast to the normal individual in whom the superficial venous pressure falls with contraction of the calf muscles. Chronic venous insufficiency consists of postural discomfort, swelling, varicose veins and the changes in skin and subcutaneous tissues collectively known as lipodermatosclerosis: pigmentation, inflammation, induration, eczema and ulceration.

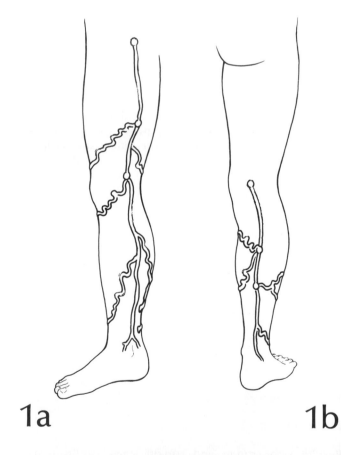

1a   **1b**

About one-third of patients with chronic venous insufficiency have incompetence of the superficial veins with or without perforator incompetence, a further one-third have added incompetence of the deep system, and one-third have evidence of previous deep vein thombosis rendering the deep veins obliterated, or incompetent, or both. The term post-thrombotic syndrome should be reserved for the last group.

2 Varices of atypical distribution may be a feature of congenital venous anomalies, the best known of which are the Klippel–Trenaunay syndrome (varicose veins, cutaneous naevus, soft tissue and bone hypertrophy) and the Parkes–Weber syndrome, in which the varices and overgrowth are due to multiple, diffuse arteriovenous fistulae.

Venous flares or spider naevi are common, particularly in women, but are not a suitable subject for surgery. The same applies to the unusually conspicuous but non-varicose veins, the so-called athlete's veins, which sometimes worry young, lean, well-muscled men who have very little subcutaneous fat.

3 Vulval and perineal varices occur in women associated with pregnancy and pelvic inflammatory disease. They may cause discomfort before menstruation or during coitus. They commonly diminish after pregnancy. These varices, which drain into the internal iliac or gonadal systems, extend as multiple channels down the medial aspect of the thigh from the perineum.

Management of varicose veins

Varicose veins are a condition of progressive deterioration. Nevertheless, the high proportions of patients with recurrent or residual varicose veins after operation and of patients who, despite treatment, progress to chronic venous insufficiency and recurrent ulcers, testify to the deficiencies in management of chronic venous disease in general and of varicose veins in particular. This is partly a reflection of poor-quality care and partly due to the fact that the condition is too common and the workload too great for effective care to be provided for all who need it under a state-funded health care system.

Varicose veins should be treated by experienced surgeons who are fully conversant with the anatomical variations so common in the venous system, and who are willing and able to allocate the time and care necessary to achieve satisfactory, long-lasting results.

The first essential is careful preoperative assessment, employing vascular laboratory techniques and radiology in the more complex cases. The surgery must be thorough and must deal with all sites of major reflux from deep to superficial systems in the groin, thigh and calf. Treatment does not end with the operation. Despite careful surgery a proportion of patients will have residual varices or will develop new sites of incompetence. They should therefore be followed up, and any persisting or recurring veins dealt with by sclerotherapy.

Follow-up sclerotherapy should be regarded as an intrinsic part of the surgical treatment of varices, and patients should be clearly informed of this before operation.

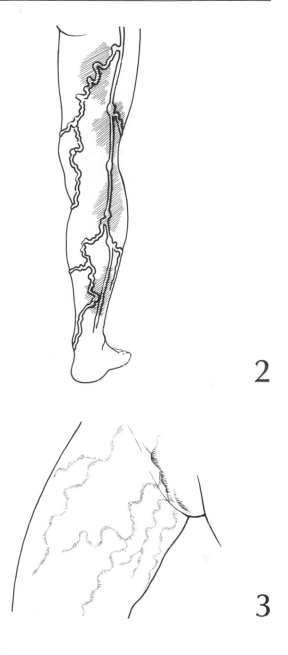

Indications

Varicose surgery is performed: (1) to relieve symptoms; (2) for cosmetic reasons; (3) for prophylaxis; and (4) to reverse skin changes and effect ulcer healing.

Many varicose vein operations are quite justifiably performed on cosmetic grounds. It is unusual for varices to give rise to distinct pain, although tiredness, heaviness and swelling in the leg are common, as is an aching discomfort in distended veins. An important factor in the minds of many surgeons is prevention, as the natural history is one of progressive deterioration, progressing in a minority of cases to the skin manifestations of chronic venous insufficiency. Varicose veins also predispose to phlebitis, deep vein thrombosis and bleeding in the event of trauma.

Preoperative

Assessment

Preoperative assessment is crucial to the success of varicose vein surgery, and so should be done by the surgeon who is to perform the operation. Some patients with uncomplicated primary varices who are lean and in whom the variceal pattern is easily traced do not require any special investigations, other than those required to assess general fitness for surgery and suitability for day care. Recurrent or residual varicose veins, however, are often the result of saphenofemoral and/or saphenopopliteal incompetence being missed at the original preoperative assessment. Logically, the more frequent deployment of additional investigations should promote more effective surgery and fewer recurrences.

Examination

4   The limb is examined in a good light, with the patient standing on a cloth-covered elevated platform in a warm room, a few minutes being allowed for the veins to distend fully. The leg being examined should be slightly flexed at hip and knee to allow superficial venous filling. Common sites of superficial valvular incompetence give rise to typical distributions of varices. Knowledge of these, verified by palpation and percussion along the line of the vein, allows the varicose venous tree to be fully marked without any further tests in the great majority of cases.

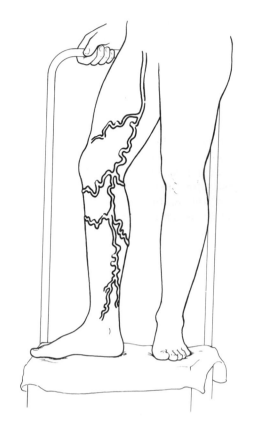

4

Testing for reflux

5a–c   Levels of deep-to-superficial reflux can also be verified by the application of venous tourniquets, applied with the patient supine and the leg elevated. On standing it becomes evident whether the tourniquet is controlling reflux or not, and by repeating the test with the tourniquet moved up or down the levels can be precisely identified. In a simpler form of this test, preferred by the author, suspected points of incompetence are controlled by the finger tips.

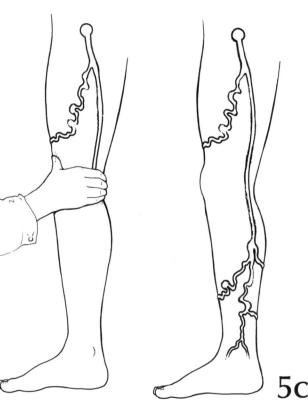

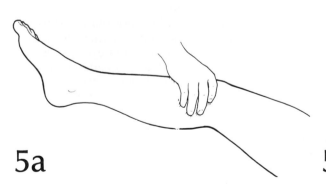

5a

5b

5c

Short saphenous incompetence

6   In patients with short saphenous incompetence it is important, in view of the high frequency of anatomical variations in the area, to detect accurately the point at which the saphenous vein turns inwards to join the deep vein. In thin individuals this may be relatively obvious, and the use of Doppler ultrasonography may assist, but in many patients it is advisable to define the junction preoperatively with either duplex scanning or varicography.

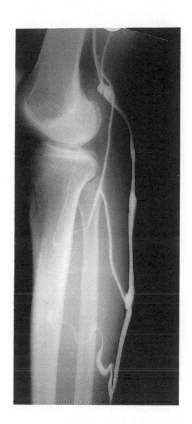

6

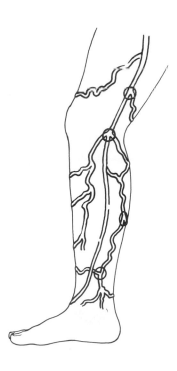

7

7   All varices in the thigh and calf are mapped out as parallel lines with an indelible marker, with specific marks for the sites of incompetent perforators and blow-outs. It is a useful precaution to ask the patient, before completing the marking, whether he or she is aware of any varices that have been missed.

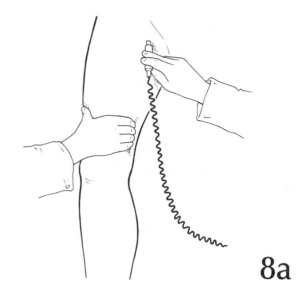

8a

8a, b The continuous wave hand-held Doppler ultrasonographic device will give useful information as to whether reflux is occurring in the region of the saphenofemoral or saphenopopliteal junctions and at suspected sites of perforators.

It is important to be aware, however, that although continuous wave Doppler ultrasonography will demonstrate the presence of reflux, it may not always be clear whether this is occurring in the deep or the superficial veins. Where there is remaining doubt as to the existence of saphenofemoral or saphenopopliteal incompetence, or where it is difficult to distinguish between varices feeding from thigh perforators and incompetence in the groin or perineum, duplex colour-coded scanning and/or varicography become essential.

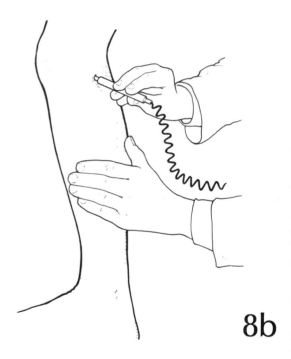

8b

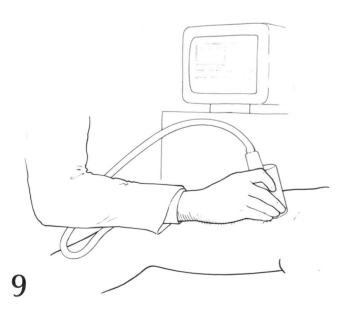

9

9 Colour-coded duplex scanning may be taken as the reference standard for delineating venous anatomy and function at the present time and should be frequently deployed as a guide to accurate varicose vein surgery.

The particular place of varicography is in the investigation of recurrent varices, where it has the advantage of displaying the anatomy as a guide to dissection in the operating theatre.

Operations

SAPHENOFEMORAL LIGATION

This is not an operation for the inexperienced, unsupervised surgeon, for two principal reasons. First, the recurrence of varices due to inadequately performed saphenofemoral ligation is very common. Secondly, the risk of damage to the femoral artery or vein in the groin, with serious consequences for the patient and medicolegal consequences for the surgeon, is considerable.

Anaesthesia and position of patient

10 The operation is performed under epidural anaesthesia, and unless only the short saphenous system requires attention, it begins with the patient supine and in the Trendelenburg position.

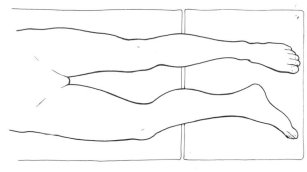

10

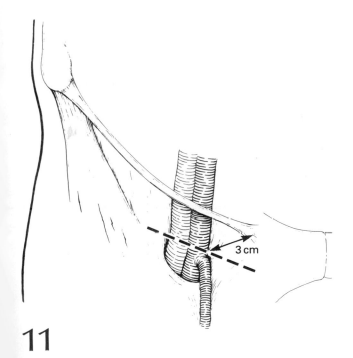

11

Incision

11 The knee is slightly flexed and rotated externally. The surface marking of the saphenofemoral junction is 3–4 cm below and lateral to the pubic tubercle. The incision is centred on this point and is made about 6–8 cm in length, in the skin crease below the inguinal ligament. As these incisions usually heal with a virtually invisible scar, a small incision is no advantage, and indeed is positively conducive to an unsatisfactory operation for reasons made clear below.

The incision is deepened through the membranous layer of the superficial fascia, until the long saphenous vein is encountered. A Travers self-retaining retractor is inserted.

Identification of the long saphenous vein

12 As anatomical variants are common and as in thin or heavily muscled individuals the femoral vein and artery may be close to the surface, the long saphenous vein is not divided until it has been unequivocally identified by sufficient dissection to ascertain the locations of the femoral artery and vein and to identify the saphenofemoral junction.

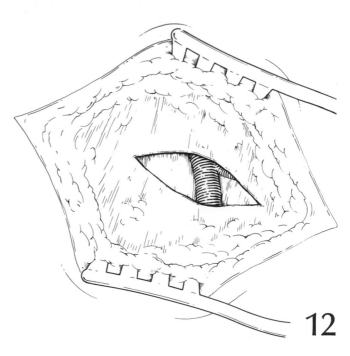

12

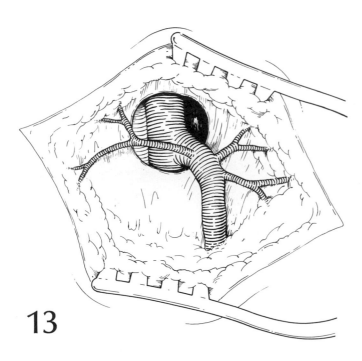

13

Saphenous tributaries

13 Expected tributaries are the superficial external pudenal, the superficial external iliac and superficial inferior epigastric veins, although variations are common. Each of these, when dissected out 2–3 cm from the point of junction with the saphenous vein, will be found to divide into two or more tributaries.

14 These subdivisions are individually ligated with 3/0 absorbable polyglactin (Vicryl) ligature or sealed by diathermy distally. If this dissection is not done and the tributaries are simply ligated where they join the long saphenous vein, there remains a network of superficial veins connecting the veins of the thigh with those of the perineum, the lower abdominal wall and the iliac region, thus promoting recurrence of varices.

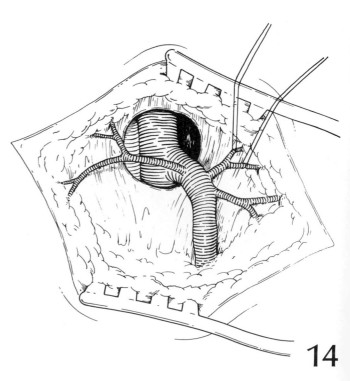

14

Dissection of the saphenofemoral junction

15a–c The long saphenous vein is divided and the upper end lifted up on Mayo's artery forceps, this manoeuvre greatly facilitating mobilization of tributaries and definition of the saphenofemoral junction. The upper end of the vein is mobilized with a pledget mounted on a haemostat, and the investing fascia is cleared from the vein with a DeBakey arterial dissecting forceps, great care being taken not to traumatize tributaries such as the deep external pudendal vein, which joins the femoral vein or the long saphenous vein itself on the medial side of the junction. The deep external pudendal vein is tied by passing a ligature round it. This must be done with care, as avulsion of this vessel followed by efforts to control the bleeding is a potential cause of femoral vein damage.

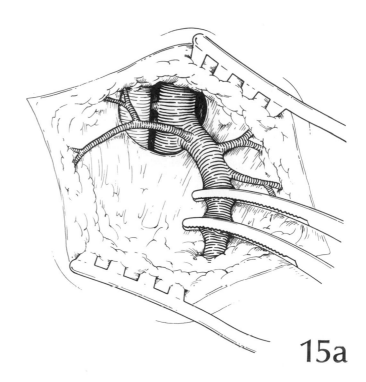

15a

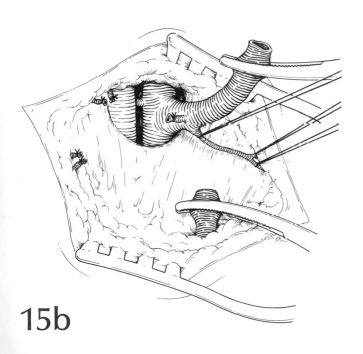

15b

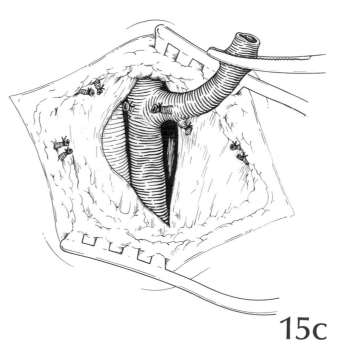

15c

16 To visualize the femoral vein below the junction it is usually necessary to divide the superficial external pudendal artery which crosses below the junction in the lower rim of the foramen ovale. At the end of this manoeuvre the junction plus 2–3 cm of the proximal and distal femoral vein should be clearly seen.

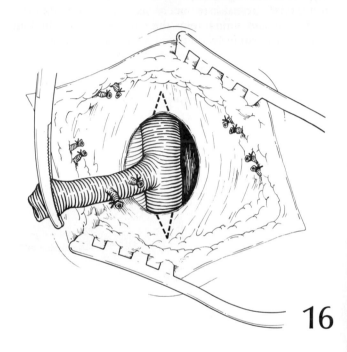

16

Anatomical variants

17a–c Common anatomical variants include: (*a*) double saphenous veins; (*b*) major thigh tributaries joining near the saphenofemoral junction and therefore readily mistaken for the main veins; and (*c*) major tributaries which, instead of joining the long saphenous vein, join the superficial external iliac or the superficial external pudendal veins.

These are all common causes of surgical error and must be sought. They are some of the reasons why a small incision is inappropriate for this part of the operation.

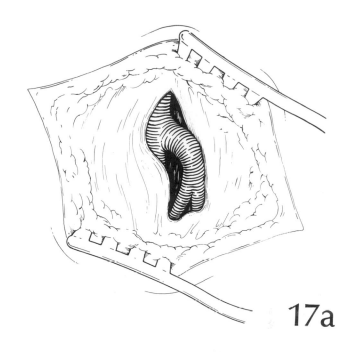

17a

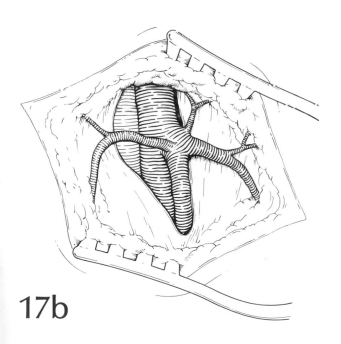

17b

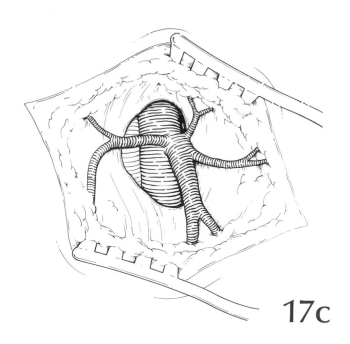

17c

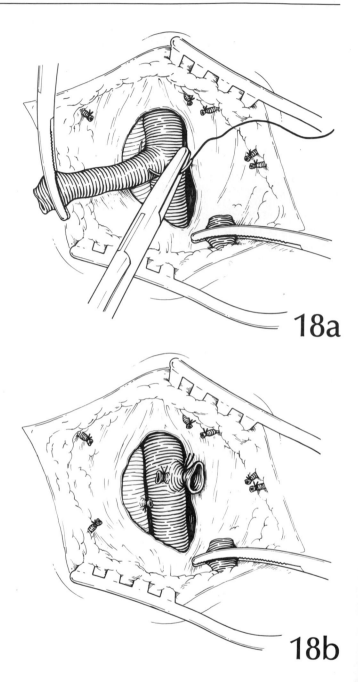

Flush ligation

18a, b The long saphenous vein is transfixed with a 3/0 polyglactin suture almost flush with the femoral vein, care being taken neither to tent up the latter nor to leave a blind sac. It is divided, the lower end being held in a haemostat.

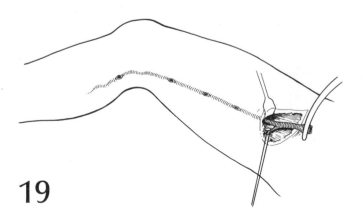

Upper thigh tributaries

19 The next step is to ligate the upper thigh tributaries. The self-retaining retractor is removed, the lower edge of the wound elevated by the assistant and the knee flexed. Traction is put on the saphenous vein, which is then mobilized down the thigh by finger dissection. By this means the posteromedial tributary and occasionally other tributaries can be reached through the groin incision. They are ligated with 2/0 polyglactin.

Removal of the thigh portion of long saphenous vein

In order to minimize the likelihood of recurrence, extirpation of the thigh portion of the long saphenous vein is advocated. It may be advisable to conserve the saphenous vein if the patient has risk factors for arterial disease, such as a strong family history of arterial disease, hypercholesterolaemia, diabetes, or smoking. As a generalization, however, the population of patients with varicose veins and the population prone to obliterative arterial disease tend to be two different groups.

Full-length stripping of the long saphenous vein has been abandoned in favour of thigh stripping, as no benefit is derived from stripping the calf portion and saphenous nerve damage in the calf has often been reported.

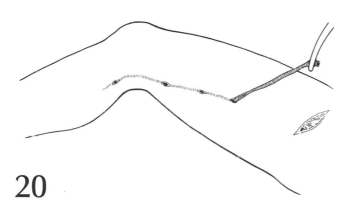

20

20 The author's practice is to remove the long saphenous vein from the groin to the main trifurcation, about 3–4 cm below the knee joint. This may be done without a stripper, through a series of small incisions about 10 cm apart through which the saphenous vein is extracted and the tributaries individually ligated. This method minimizes haematoma formation, allows the groin wound to be closed early and facilitates the performance of the remainder of the operation under tourniquet. It also avoids the not uncommon difficulty encountered in passing the stripper.

Traction on the saphenous vein from above allows it to be readily palpable through the skin. A 5–10-mm incision is made 10 cm below the groin and the vein hooked out. With care any local tributaries can be pulled to the surface and ligated. Serial incisions are made at intervals down to the upper calf and the steps repeated. At the 'goose's foot' trifurcation below the knee, the long saphenous vein is ligated and divided.

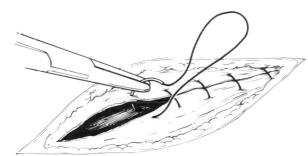

21a

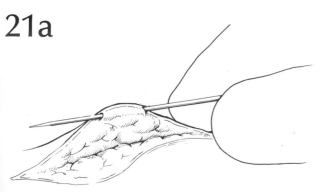

21b

Closure of thigh wounds

21a, b At this stage all thigh wounds are closed. The groin wound is closed with subcutaneous and subcuticular synthetic absorbable sutures and the lower wounds can usually be closed simply with wound tapes. If any sutures are needed, 4/0 subcuticular polyglactin is employed. The remainder of the operation is conducted under tourniquet.

Phlebectomy

22 The removal of varices through multiple incisions (phlebectomy) is performed under tourniquet. The leg is elevated and exsanguinated by means of a pneumatic exsanguinator or a sterile Esmarch bandage, and a tourniquet is applied around the mid-thigh. This remains in place for the remainder of the operation and is only removed after the final bandage has been applied. The illustration shows a Lofqvist pneumatic tourniquet which is held in position by means of a small rubber wedge.

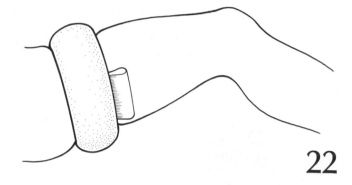

22

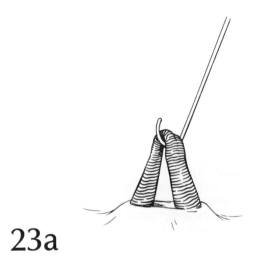

23a

23a, b Varices are removed through 5-mm incisions. These are placed at intervals of 5–10 cm along the lines of the veins, the aim being total removal of the underlying varices. As they are very tiny they can be either longitudinal or transverse. At each incision the vein is mobilized with a combination of fine instruments including a small phlebectomy hook and mosquito forceps and brought to the surface, freed from subcutaneous tissues and avulsed.

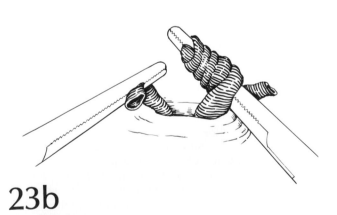

23b

Perforators

A medial ankle venous flare or lipodermatosclerosis in the classical gaiter distribution are two signs that incompetent perforators are present and should be intercepted.

24a, b
Perforators are approached through slightly larger incisions, sufficient to admit the tip of the little finger to palpate the point of passage of the perforator through the deep fascia where it is ligated flush.

Perforators embedded in areas of indurated lipodermatosclerosis cannot be dissected out and are dealt with by a subfascial approach as described below.

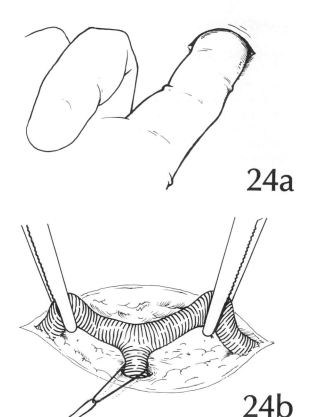

24a

24b

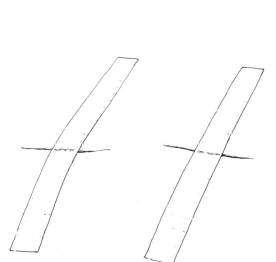

25

Wound closure

25
The majority of the wounds do not require any formal closure other than wound tapes. Larger ones are closed with subcuticular 4/0 synthetic absorbable sutures.

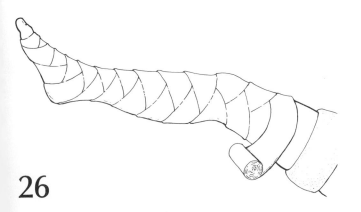

26

Bandaging

26
The leg is bandaged with a cohesive elastic bandage using a figure-of-eight technique over a layer of orthopaedic wool, before the tourniquet is released. The bandage begins at the base of the toes and is continued to the upper thigh. The foot is positioned at a right angle and the turns of the bandage are fashioned so as to allow flexion at the knee and ankle.

SHORT SAPHENOUS LIGATION

Position of patient

If no surgery to the long saphenous system is required, the patient is positioned prone after a tourniquet has been applied to the thigh. If it is part of a more extensive vein operation which is begun with the patient in the supine position, then it is the author's policy to close the thigh wounds, leave the tourniquet in position and turn and redrape the patient for the posterior approach. Some surgeons prefer to position the patient on one side, with the leg to be operated on uppermost and the other knee flexed. This, however, limits access if varices need to be followed onto the medial aspect.

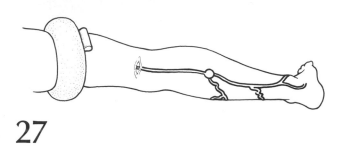

27

Incision

27 It is vital that the saphenopopliteal junction should have been accurately mapped out beforehand and incisions placed appropriately. If the junction is in its normal location 2–3 cm above the transverse skin crease, a transverse 3-cm incision placed in the crease is satisfactory. In about one-third of cases the junction is several centimetres higher, and in 15% of cases the short saphenous vein does not end in the popliteal vein at all but passes medially to join the long saphenous vein.

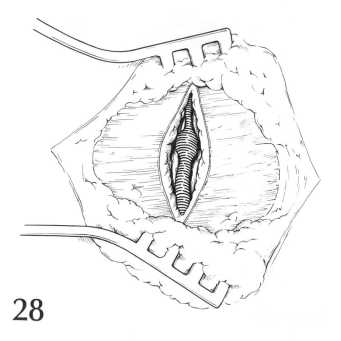

28

Exposure of the junction

28 The deep fascia is opened vertically, which allows the veins to be followed some distance in either direction should it become necessary. The short saphenous vein is identified and carefully mobilized. It usually only has one significant superficial tributary, a median vein running down the back of the thigh. This may connect above with the posteromedial thigh vein or sometimes it is large and connects via perforating veins to the deep femoral vein. It is divided and ligated.

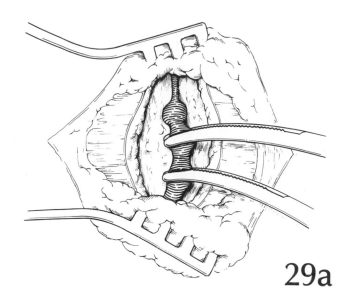

29a

29a, b
The short saphenous vein is freed by blunt dissection from the sural nerve and popliteal fat. Once it has been identified with certainty, it is divided between haemostats and the proximal end mobilized.

Mobilization must be done with care. Nerve damage is not uncommon in short saphenous vein surgery. The common peroneal nerve runs down the lateral side of the popliteal fossa adjacent to the medial edge of the biceps femoris, becoming quite superficial as it crosses the back of the biceps tendon and winds around the head and neck of the fibula. The tibial nerve is less likely to be damaged being deep to the popliteal vessels.

The saphenopopliteal junction is less distinct than the saphenofemoral junction, and the popliteal vein may be quite mobile. Care must therefore be taken not to tent up and damage the popliteal vein.

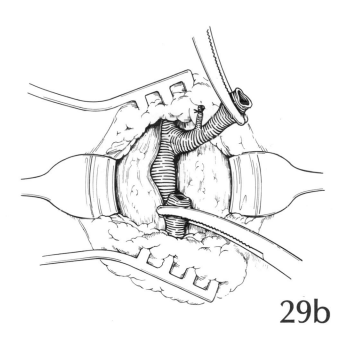

29b

Flush ligation

30 The short saphenous vein is transfixed and flush ligated with 3/0 polyglactin. Gastrocnemius veins sometimes join the short saphenous vein rather than the popliteal vein direct. They should not be ligated, as this can give rise to troublesome discomfort on standing and even venous claudication in the gastrocnemius muscles. When these veins join the short saphenous vein the latter is ligated peripheral to the junction.

It is seldom necessary to strip the short saphenous vein down to the ankle, particularly as this is liable to cause sural nerve damage. A stripper may, however, be useful as a guide, as it is much more difficult to feel the short saphenous through the skin than the long saphenous vein. The downward passage of a stripper can be helpful in identifying the short saphenous vein distally where incisions are placed to intercept tributaries.

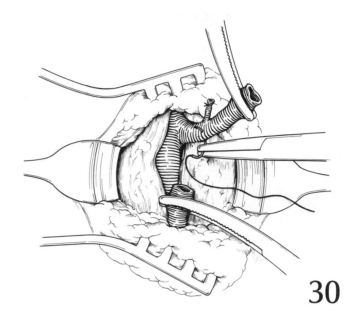

30

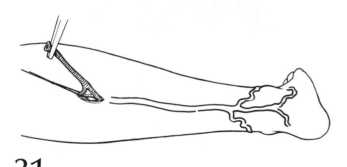

31

31 Tributaries are dealt with through small incisions. In particular there is often a large blow-out at mid-calf, which may connect with the long saphenous system. In dealing with the short saphenous system at all levels great care must be taken not to damage the sural nerve.

Wound closure

Wound closure and bandaging are the same as described above, except that the bandaging is only taken to the level of the tibial tuberosity.

RECURRENT VARICOSE VEINS

It may be difficult to decipher the sources of deep-to-superficial reflux in patients with recurrent veins by clinical examination alone. Hand-held Doppler ultrasonographic probes can be useful, but this technique has limitations in distinguishing between deep and superficial reflux and also between reflux arising at the saphenofemoral junction and thigh varices that are filled from perforators.

Colour-coded duplex scanning is very helpful in examining the venous anatomy and carries the advantage of allowing the reflux to be visualized, but it is not a substitute for the 'road map' guide to surgery provided by varicography.

Approach to the saphenofemoral junction

Assuming that a groin scar indicates a previous attempt at saphenofemoral ligation, the aim of the approach is to avoid the mass of vascular scar tissue that usually overlies the junction.

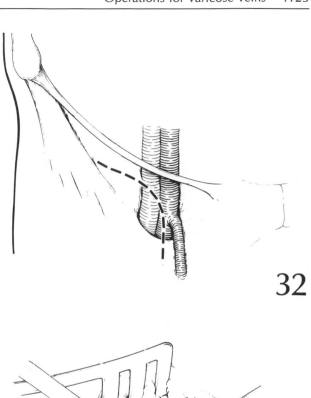

32

32 A 'hockey-stick' incision is centred over the saphenofemoral junction, beginning in the groin skin crease laterally and turning down along the line of the saphenous vein medially.

Exposure of the femoral artery

33a, b The incision is deepened to expose the femoral artery. Dissection is then carried medially to expose the saphenofemoral junction. This will usually be found to be patent. The long saphenous vein at the junction is mobilized and divided between clamps. The stump is transfixed and flush ligated with a 3/0 polyglactin suture.

The more difficult part is to eradicate the tributaries converging on the scar tissue overlying the saphenofemoral junction. It can most easily be achieved by a block removal of the scar tissue, but this carries the possibility of lymphatic damage with subsequent leg swelling or even lymph fistula. Therefore, the alternative course adopted by the author is to dissect around the perimeter, intercepting with ligation or diathermy all converging veins.

The remainder of the operation is conducted as described for primary varicose veins.

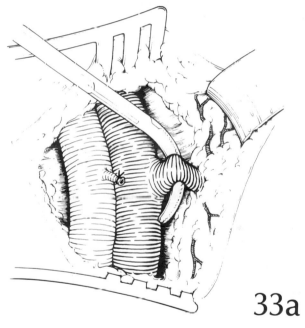

33a

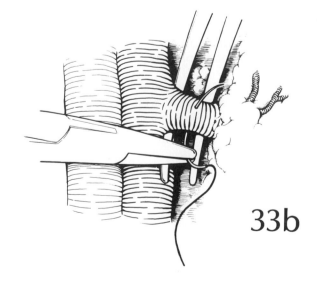

33b

SUBFASCIAL LIGATION

The dense scar tissue of chronic lipodermatosclerosis may render the dissection of perforators outside the deep fascia almost impossible, so that a more radical approach is required. Patients should receive prophylaxis such as subcutaneous heparin against deep vein thrombosis, as slow healing may necessitate several days of bed rest and these patients often constitute a high-risk group.

Subfascial ligation is not usually a 'stand-alone' operation, but requires all proximal sites of deep-to-superficial incompetence also to be dealt with.

Incision

34 The positioning of the skin incision depends on the location of the incompetent perforators and the extent of the skin changes. In the vast majority of patients the important perforators are in the gaiter area on the medial side of the calf at the anterior border of the soleus muscle.

35 If the skin changes are not extensive, the perforators can be approached through a short (4–8-cm) longitudinal incision placed medially.

36 The author's preference, however, particularly if there are also lateral perforators requiring attention, is a posterior 'stocking seam' incision. The operation is performed under tourniquet.

37 The incision is carried straight down through the deep fascia, resisting all temptation to undermine the skin by dissecting out any superficial veins encountered. The deep fascia is elevated with skin hooks, and the subfascial plane is easily developed to expose all perforators. These are ligated with polyglactin and divided.

The deep fascia is not closed. The skin is closed with fine subcuticular absorbable monofilament sutures and bandaged as described on page 565 before tourniquet release.

Several days of rest and elevation of the leg are essential, because these wounds are prone to delayed healing and early ambulation can be damaging.

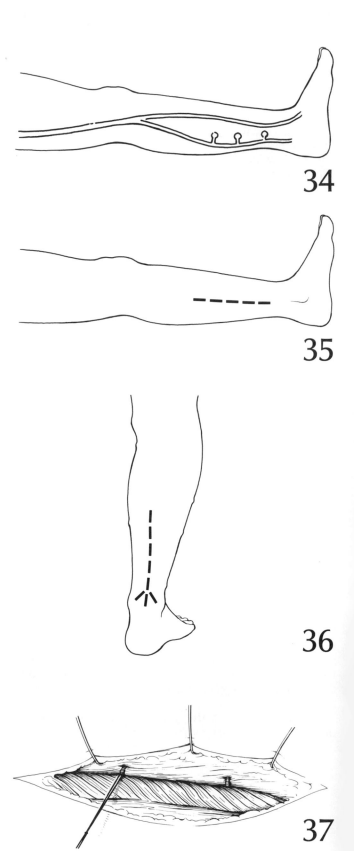

SUBFASCIAL ENDOSCOPY

38 An attractive alternative to subfascial ligation is the use of a subfascial endoscope to visualize and intercept the perforators.

The procedure is performed under tourniquet. Proximal sites of incompetence are ligated and varices avulsed.

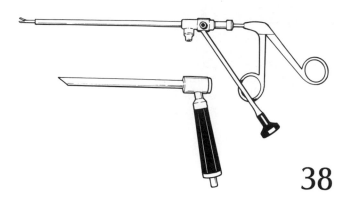

38

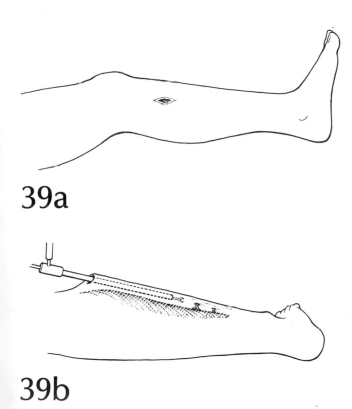

39a

39b

39a, b The endoscope is introduced through a small incision in the upper medial calf. The incision is carried through the deep fascia. The endoscope is then introduced and advanced down the medial border of the tibia.

Dissection can be performed through the endoscope to bring into view the perforators, which can then be clipped, avulsed, or sealed by diathermy.

This procedure allows rapid postoperative recovery and can be incorporated into day surgery practice.

Acknowledgment

Illustration 6 is reproduced from *A Colour Atlas of Surgical Management of Venous Disease*, 1988 with permission of Wolfe Medical Publications.

Ligation of ankle perforating veins

J. H. Scurr BSc, FRCS
Senior Lecturer and Honorary Consultant Surgeon, Department of Surgical Studies, University College and Middlesex School of Medicine, London, UK

Principles and justification

Perforating veins communicate between the deep venous system and the superficial venous system, the two systems being separated by an encircling layer of deep fascia. The presence of these veins has been recognized for a long time, the first description being attributed to von Loder in 1803. Incompetence of the valves in these veins has been implicated in the development of venous ulceration, and this led to the development of operations specifically to ligate them. The original operation for dealing with these veins was described by Linton in 1938, and was modified by Dodd and Cockett[1] in 1956. The operations described involved an extrafascial or subfascial approach, with a long incision extending almost the whole length of the calf, either medially or posteriorly, with a recommendation that any pre-existing ulcer should also be excised. These procedures allowed the fascia to be reflected and the perforating veins to be identified and ligated using absorbable suture material. The operations have been associated with poor wound healing, extensive scarring and reduced ankle mobility.

If the purpose of these operations was to improve venous function and to aid ulcer healing, then recent advances in our understanding of venous physiology and studies looking at ulcer recurrence rates[2] have suggested that there is no improvement in venous function and that ulcer recurrence rates are as high as 55%.

Studies show that between 40% and 60% of venous ulcers are due to superficial venous insufficiency alone[3]. Operations to correct superficial venous insufficiency will therefore result in ulcer healing rates of between 40% and 60%. In those patients in whom the ulcer is due to deep venous insufficiency, the presence or absence of incompetent perforating veins may be irrelevant to long-term ulcer healing.

Anatomical, radiological and more recent duplex ultrasound studies of the perforating veins show that they are present in the normal limb. They range from less than 1 mm in diameter to 10 mm or more. Only the larger veins seem to have valves, but not all valves direct flow from the superficial to the deep system. In 25 studies on fresh post-mortem specimens, Hadfield[4] found no valves in smaller perforating veins and only rudimentary ones in the larger veins. Nicolaides[5] has suggested that outward flow in medial calf perforating veins can only occur if there is axial deep vein incompetence. The importance of incompetent medial calf perforating veins in venous ulceration has not been established and makes the extensive surgical procedures of Linton, Dodd and Cockett unacceptable.

Indications

The indications for surgery are by no means precise and await further clarification. Large perforating veins, contributing significantly to superficial venous insufficiency, should be managed surgically. The common perforating veins include the saphenofemoral junction, the saphenopopliteal junction, a mid-thigh Hunterian perforator, and medial and lateral calf perforating veins. Ligation of the saphenofemoral junction and removal of the long saphenous vein will interrupt most perforating veins in the distribution of the long saphenous system. The presence of duplex long saphenous veins and anatomical variations can result in missed communications between the deep and superficial system. With persisting superficial venous insufficiency, progressive skin changes – lipodermatosclerosis – leading to frank ulceration, may occur. The best results from surgery are obtained when intervention takes place before these changes occur.

Preoperative

Assessment

1 All patients should undergo a formal non-invasive venous assessment. The use of Doppler ultrasound, photoplethysmography and strain gauge plethysmography provides a useful screening mechanism to separate out those patients with superficial venous insufficiency, those with deep venous insufficiency, and those with a combination. A further assessment with B-mode duplex ultrasound will allow direct visualization of the veins, a demonstration of reflux and an opportunity to visualize perforating veins and to determine whether the flow is inward or outward. In most patients with significant superficial venous insufficiency, surgery should be undertaken.

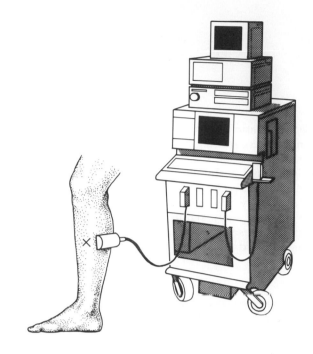

1

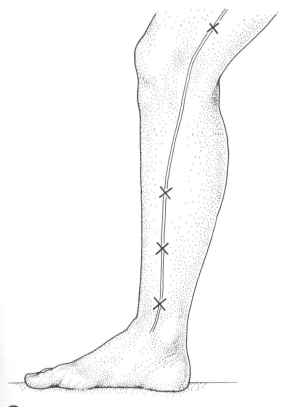

2

Marking

2 All patients with skin changes, a history of venous ulceration or recurrent varicose veins should be accurately assessed and marked before surgery using either venography or ultrasonographic imaging. With the patient's leg dependent but non-weightbearing, the veins of the superficial system are marked. By applying calf and then foot compression, the presence of perforating veins can be identified and the direction of flow noted. In those patients with large perforating veins with outward flow, a small mark can be placed on the skin to identify the site.

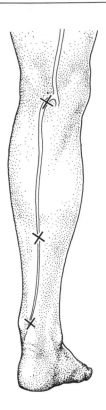

3 A systematic check of the whole leg should be undertaken, starting at the groin and moving down the medial side of the leg, returning then to the posterior aspect of the leg to identify the origin of the short saphenous vein, moving down the short saphenous vein before returning to the lateral border of the leg. In practice, only significant perforating veins are marked and these tend to be in excess of 4 mm, with obvious outward flow.

3

Operation

Position of patient

The patient is placed supine on the operating table under general anaesthesia (local anaesthesia can be used for a small number of perforating veins). The legs are elevated, the skin is prepared, and the patient is draped.

If there are significant posterior perforating veins, including the short saphenous vein, the operation is best started in the prone position, the patient being turned during the course of the procedure.

Incisions

4a, b Small incisions ranging from 1.5 to 3 mm are used over the site of the perforating vein. Even with the leg elevated, bleeding can be quite profuse. The perforating vein is then brought to the surface with a micro-Halstead or an Oesch hook. Gentle traction is applied and a very significant portion of superficial vein, with its connection to the perforating vein, is then removed. Digital pressure is applied to control bleeding.

This operation is repeated until all the perforating veins have been interrupted. The wounds are dressed with small plasters; no sutures are required. Once the skin has been cleaned, a high compression (35–45 mmHg) stocking is applied to the limb.

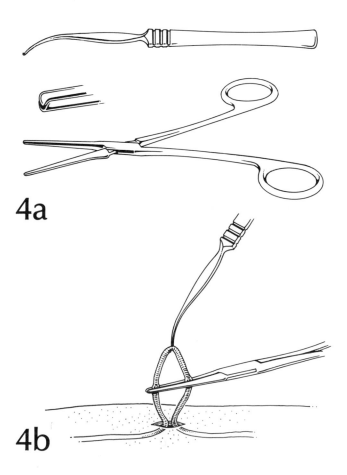

4a

4b

Postoperative care

The patient is returned to the ward with 15° of foot elevation. This is maintained for 12 h, after which the patient is encouraged to walk maximally and told to rest on the bed or a settee with the feet up if not walking, and to avoid standing still. The stockings can be removed for washing and the patient can shower.

Complications

There are relatively few postoperative complications, but all patients should be warned that they will have considerable bruising, they may have small areas of numbness, and that these areas of numbness may be associated with quite intense tingling pain. Cutaneous nerve damage occurs in an unpredictable manner and may cause the patient considerable distress unless prior warning is given.

Postoperative venous thrombosis is a rare event. Deep vein thrombosis prophylaxis should be administered to those patients with a past history of venous thrombosis, those patients who are relatively elderly, or who are likely to remain immobile.

Superficial thrombophlebitis and cellulitis can occur after these procedures. With adequate compression this is an unusual occurrence, but when it does occur it is associated with considerable pain. This can be managed with non-steroidal anti-inflammatory drugs, rest and compression.

Editors' note

The editors would agree that there is little formal haemodynamic evidence to justify extensive perforator vein ligation and that identification with duplex scanning has proved very valuable, as has varicography. Many surgeons would prefer to ligate all significant perforating veins formally via a slightly longer incision rather than rely upon avulsion with Oesch hooks. The varices are traced deeply through a 2–3 cm longitudinal incision to the site at which the perforating vein penetrates the deep fascia. The vein is divided between ligatures at this point and thereby formally ligated.

References

1. Dodd H, Cockett FB. *Pathology and Surgery of the Veins of the Lower Limb*. 2nd edn, Edinburgh: Churchill Livingstone, 1976.

2. Burnand K, Lea Thomas M, O'Donnell T, Browse NL. Relation between postphlebitic changes in the deep veins and the results of surgical treatment of venous ulcers. *Lancet* 1976; i: 936–8.

3. Coleridge-Smith P. Noninvasive venous investigations. *Vasc Med Rev* 1991; 1: 139–66.

4. Hadfield JII. *The Anatomy of the Perforating Vein of the Leg in the Treatment of Varicose Veins by Injection and Compression*. Stoke: Manubus and Bergen, 1991: 4–11.

5. Zukowski AJ, Nicolaides AN, Szendro G, Irvine A, Lewis R, Malouf GM *et al*. Haemodynamic significance of incompetent calf perforating veins. *Br J Surg* 1991; 78: 625–9.

Illustrations by Marc Donon

Treatment of venous ulcers

C. W. Jamieson MS, FRCS
Consultant Surgeon, St Thomas' Hospital, London, UK

Principles and justification

Venous ulcers represent a common and debilitating condition. Many are associated with pure superficial venous incompetence and varicose veins[1], but a large number, varying from 49%[2] to 87%[3], are due to either deep venous obstruction or deep venous valvular incompetence[2]. In the assessment of any apparent venous ulcer, it is most important that the state of the arterial circulation should be investigated with Doppler ultrasound and, if necessary, angiography if a diminished ankle systolic blood pressure is found[3]. The possibility of squamous neoplastic change in a venous ulcer must also be borne in mind (Marjolin's ulcer), and a biopsy of the ulcer rim should be taken if there is any evidence to suggest that it might be neoplastic. A squamous carcinoma developing in an ulcer usually causes piling up and prominence of an otherwise shelving rim and multiple biopsies of the suspicious areas make the diagnosis, although the disorganized epithelium at the healing edge of an ulcer can confuse the histologist in making a categorical diagnosis of squamous carcinoma and the biopsy must, therefore, be generous. If evidence of squamous carcinoma is found, the prognosis is poor and treatment must involve wide radical excision of the ulcer and a search for associated metastatic nodes in the groin. If present, these should be treated by formal block dissection. Involvement of bone is not uncommon, in which case the only definitive treatment is amputation.

Evidence of associated arterial insufficiency should indicate the need for arterial reconstruction, which may in itself heal the ulcer although there is a venous component in its aetiology and occult arterial disease is common. Routine ankle blood pressure recording should be included in the assessment of all 'venous' ulcers[4].

The basic treatment of venous ulcers consists of local measures to improve the venous circulation and control the oedema, together with treatment of the primary venous cause.

Local treatment of venous ulcers

Local antibiotics and complex antiseptics should be avoided as these patients have a strong risk of allergy to any complex molecule. Indeed, a superimposed hypersensitivity reaction should be considered in every case of venous ulceration; the patient may be sensitive to the rubber in elastic bandages, to their stockings, to detergents or any lotion, and exposure to such immune stimulants must be avoided. Obvious necrotic tissue should be treated by debridement under general anaesthesia. The ulcer should be cleaned regularly with normal saline, swabs taken and specific pathogens treated with the appropriate antibiotics if culture is positive. Some form of firm supporting bandage or stocking should be applied from the forefoot to the knee or to the upper thigh if there is oedema of the whole lower limb. The types of support available are legion, but excellent results have been claimed for the double-bandaging technique advocated by Charing Cross Hospital[5]. Their technique comprises an inner layer of orthopaedic wool (Velband) to absorb exudate and equilibrate compression pressure. Over this is applied a standard crepe bandage, followed by a compression bandage and finally a lightweight elasticated Cohesive bandage. All the layers of bandage are applied at mid-stretch, so that compression is achieved by elasticity rather than tension.

Care must be observed in the use of stockings and bandages on the legs of patients with arterial disease in whom further arterial thrombosis or skin necrosis may be precipitated[6, 7]. Failure to diagnose arterial disease is indefensible and emphasizes the need for routine ankle blood pressure recording in patients with ulcers.

Patients with severe deep venous obstruction may find firm bandages intolerable as they increase the pressure that accompanies exercise in the deep compartments of the limb. Indeed, this symptom is a good indicator of deep venous obstruction. Tight bandages must also be avoided in patients with associated arterial insufficiency as they may cause cutaneous necrosis and even loss of the limb.

After the ulcer has healed, the patient should continue to wear a graded compression stocking exerting a force of between 40 and 60 mmHg. The foot of the bed should be elevated by approximately 10 cm to encourage reduction of oedema at night, and the patient may benefit from the use of a rhythmic compression pneumatic boot such as the Flotron pump which helps to control the oedema and is particularly useful in patients living in a hot climate where a supporting stocking is intolerable.

Surgical treatment of venous ulcers

Venous ulcers develop in areas of dermatoliposclerosis in which there is increased fibrosis and vascularity[8, 9], with a diffusion barrier in the capillary walls because of leakage of fibrin through the capillaries. It is thought that this diffusion barrier is the main factor in their aetiology. Appropriate treatment of the cause of venous hypertension may help to reverse this vicious circle, but in many instances the damage has progressed to such an extent locally that the area of skin is unstable.

Preoperative

Any pathogens cultured from the ulcer are treated with appropriate antibiotics for at least 2 days before operation and the antibiotics are continued for 5 days afterwards. The whole limb is prepared using an aqueous antiseptic and towelled.

Operation

Excision of venous ulcer

1 The limb is elevated through 45° by reverse breaking the operating table to reduce venous pressure.

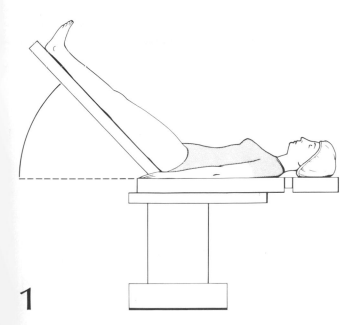

1

2 The whole area of liposclerosis, including the ulcer, is excised down to the deep fascia.

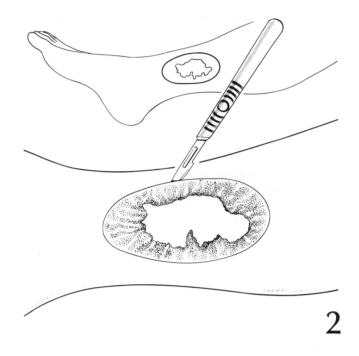

2

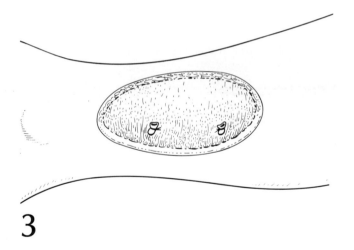

3

3 Large perforating veins are usually found penetrating the fascia and these are oversewn with fine absorbable sutures.

4 A thin split skin graft is taken from the ipsilateral thigh, meshed and applied to the defect after immaculate haemostasis. This graft is held in position by circumferential interrupted sutures. The graft is covered with paraffin gauze and then with a pad of proflavine wool and a gentle crepe bandage over cotton wool. Great care must be taken when applying the crepe bandage not to twist the dressing and dislodge the graft from its correct position.

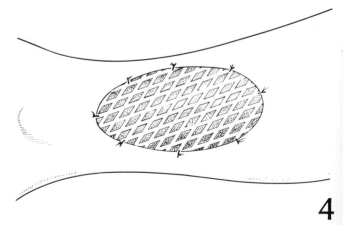

4

Postoperative care

Excess split skin taken at the time of grafting is retained in normal saline in a refrigerator. The dressing is removed after 5 days and areas of graft which have not taken are regrafted using this skin. The wound is then exposed whenever possible, but covered at night to prevent damage. The graft should mature within 9 days.

This operation does not deal with the primary cause of venous hypertension and the patient must still be diligent in protecting the limb with elevation and the use of an elastic stocking or pneumatic compression to prevent recurrence of ulceration.

References

1. Sethia KK, Darke SG. Long saphenous incompetence as a cause of venous ulceration. *Br J Surg* 1984; 71: 754–5.

2. Cornwall JV, Doré CJ, Lewis JD. Leg ulcers: epidemiology and aetiology. *Br J Surg* 1986; 73: 693–6.

3. McEnroe CS, O'Donnel TF, Mackey WC. Correlation of clinical findings with venous hemodynamics in 368 patients with chronic venous insufficiency. *Am J Surg* 1988; 156: 148–52.

4. Callam MJ, Harper DR, Dale JJ, Ruckley CV. Arterial disease in chronic leg ulceration: an underestimated hazard. Lothian and Forth Valley leg ulcer study. *BMJ* 1987; 294: 929–31.

5. Blair SD, Wright DDI, Blackhouse CM, Riddle E, McCollum CM. Sustained compression and healing of chronic venous ulcers. *BMJ* 1988; 297: 1159–61.

6. Heath DI, Kent SJS, Johns DJ, Young TW. Arterial thrombosis associated with graduated pressure antiembolic stockings. *BMJ* 1987; 295: 580.

7. Callam MJ, Ruckley CV, Dale JJ, Harper DR. Hazards of compression treatment of the leg: an estimate from Scottish surgeons. *BMJ* 1987; 295: 1382.

8. Burnand KG, Whimster I, Naidoo A, Browse NL. Pericapillary fibrin in the ulcer bearing skin of the leg: the cause of lipodermatosclerosis and venous ulceration. *BMJ* 1982; 285: 1071.

9. Hopkins NFG, Spinks TJ, Rhodes CG, Ranicar ASO, Jamieson CW. Positron emission tomography in venous ulceration: a study of regional tissue perfusion. *BMJ* 1983; 286: 333.

Injection treatment of varicose veins

J. T. Hobbs MD, FRCS
Formerly Consultant Surgeon, St Mary's Hospital and St George's Hospital, London and Honorary Senior Lecturer in Surgery, University of London, UK

History

During the past century the treatment of varicose veins by injection became established and was in widespread use. There were many complications and the results were not consistently good. Surgery evolved rapidly and injection treatment fell into disrepute. Outspoken and influential surgeons failed in their dogmatism to differentiate between good and bad methods of sclerotherapy.

Principles and justification

In the past, ineffective sclerosants have been injected with the patient standing and minimal application of pressure. This has resulted in large painful thrombi with surrounding inflammation; the vein often reopened, sometimes with additional valve damage, and pigmentation was frequent. However, sclerotherapy has continued to be practised in Europe during the past 60 years, often to the exclusion of surgery. Fegan established a large clinic in Dublin 30 years ago and the success of his enthusiastic but careful approach resulted in a revival of sclerotherapy. The importance of adequate compression for a sufficient period of time is now well established. Having demonstrated that varicose veins can be eliminated by effective sclerotherapy, several clinical trials have been undertaken to compare surgery and sclerotherapy in the treatment of varicose veins. The late results of these trials have produced three clear conclusions:

1. In the presence of proximal incompetence of the long and/or short saphenous veins surgery is indicated; sclerotherapy is effective for eliminating dilated superficial veins and incompetent lower leg perforating veins.
2. When proximal incompetence is present, it should be eliminated first by surgery as subsequent injection treatment is simpler and often confined to the lower leg.
3. Trials have shown that stripping the incompetent long saphenous vein to the knee is preferable to a combination of proximal ligation plus injection or proximal ligation plus phlebectomies because a rapid and gross recurrence may occur if a large vein is left *in situ*.

Treatment of varicose veins

No treatment

Patients with minor vein problems and symptoms from other causes can be reassured that the veins may not become worse or cause complications.

Elastic stockings

Patients with minor problems for which curative treatment is not indicated or desired can be made symptom-free by wearing elastic stockings.

Surgery

This is described in the chapter on pp. 1106–1125.

Sclerotherapy

If the veins are to be eliminated, either sclerotherapy or surgery must be used. There is a place for both methods and good results will be consistently obtained only when there is proper assessment, careful planning of treatment and precise execution. This requires the surgeon to be competent and equally enthusiastic for both methods of treatment.

Principles of sclerotherapy

The aim of treatment is to inject a small volume of an effective sclerosant into the vein lumen, which is then compressed to avoid thrombus formation. Compression must be maintained until permanent fibrosis has obliterated the lumen. Good results depend on careful technique. Important aspects of treatment include consideration of where to inject, how to inject and how to bandage.

1 Treatment can be planned according to the flow diagram illustrated.

Sclerosants

It has been established that the most effective sclerosant for eliminating large veins is 3% sodium tetradecyl sulphate (Sotradecol in USA, STD in UK, and Trombovar in France), which is effective in small volumes but must be placed in the vein lumen. If accidentally placed in the skin or subcutaneous tissue necrosis will occur. Allergic reactions are rare but increase if STD is used repeatedly. For smaller veins, such as reticular or dilated superficial veins, it has been recommended that the sodium tetradecyl sulphate solution is diluted, but there is still a risk of skin necrosis. Polidocanol (Aethoxysklerol in Germany, Sclerovein in Switzerland) is preferable for the smaller veins but less effective for large veins. It is painless and available in a range of concentrations from 0.5% to 5%. A 2% preparation is normally effective for small veins, with 3% for larger veins, but this is less effective than 3% STD for the largest veins. The weaker concentrations (0.5% and 1%) have been recommended for the smallest veins and dilated venules, but may cause necrosis with ulceration. Here Scleremo (1.1% sodium chromate in glycerine) is preferable, being the most effective and safest.

Plan of treatment

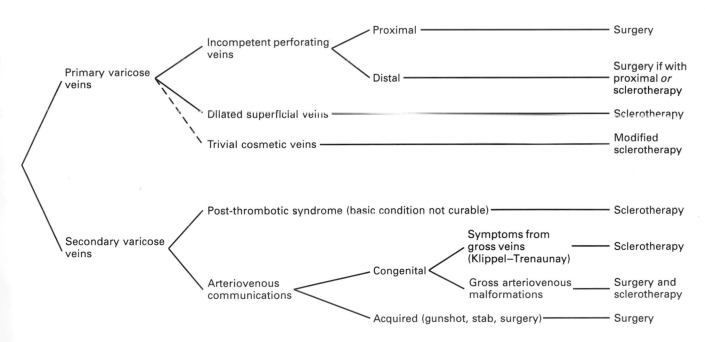

1

Preoperative or pretreatment assessment

Varicose veins are common; it has recently been estimated that 27% of the adult population of the USA have lower extremity venous abnormalities, with 2–3% having clinical manifestations of deep or superficial insufficiency. Veins and their associated problems are usually seen in general surgical or vascular clinics where the potentially serious conditions rightly deserve most attention. Less severe vein problems are often seen and treated by an unsupervised junior team member. A dedicated clinic which is properly equipped and staffed by competent doctors and nurses with adequate secretarial support, so allowing large numbers of patients to be effectively treated, is important.

Record card

$2a, b$ The patient's details are recorded on a specially designed record card for easy reference.

Once the history is complete, the patient is examined after standing on an appropriate stool with hand support for several minutes. Dilatation of the veins will be seen to extend progressively up the leg over a 5-min period and cannot be properly assessed by a cursory inspection. The pattern of veins is drawn on the reverse side of the record card and other relevant notes added.

It is essential that all significant incompetent perforating veins are located. Involvement of the long and short saphenous veins is usually obvious, but proximal incompetence may not be apparent when the patient first stands, particularly in obese legs. The proximal short saphenous vein is obscured when the leg is fully extended. Veins on the lateral aspect of the thighs suggest the possibility of an incompetent lateral thigh perforator, or may arise from the saphenofemoral junction via the anterolateral or posterolateral tributary. Veins on the upper medial aspect of the thigh may not arise from the saphenofemoral junction but pass behind the adductor tendon to communicate with the pelvis via the posterior vulval area (internal pudendal and obturator veins). Significant incompetent perforating veins on the medial aspect of the leg include the mid- and low-thigh perforators above the knee, and below the knee the Boyd's perforator as it joins the medial gastrocnemius vein. On the lower leg the posterior arch vein joins the important ankle perforating veins. Other significant perforating veins are the mid-calf joining the gastrocnemius vein, and a perforator on the lower lateral calf joining the soleal vein.

The points of control are located by sliding the fingers along the vein to empty them and noting the sites of refilling. These points are presumed to include the sites of incompetent perforating veins. Hand-held Doppler instruments will confirm the presence of reflux but cannot always locate the source. At the back of the knee it is not possible to differentiate between the deep veins, gastrocnemius veins, short saphenous vein and vein of the popliteal fossa (sometimes referred to as an accessory short saphenous vein).

When the exact site of incompetence is in doubt and when the state of the deep veins requires assessment, the patient should be referred to a vascular laboratory for further studies. Non-invasive investigations include duplex ultrasonography with or without colour imaging. Invasive studies include measurement of venous pressure and venography (ascending or descending varicography). When proximal incompetence is demonstrated, surgical treatment is preferred and on-table venography can be used if there is doubt about the level and pattern of the proximal incompetence.

If surgical treatment is not indicated the veins can be eliminated by injection compression although, in the presence of proximal incompetence, recurrence will occur progressively after several years. However, the treatment can easily be repeated.

When there is no proximal incompetence and adequate compression can be maintained, injection compression is effective. This is particularly so below the knee where the bandages are less likely to move.

A burst bleeding vein is easily controlled by injecting the adjacent feeding vein and sometimes ulcers which are healing slowly can be rapidly improved by injecting the adjacent veins.

Materials

A suitable stool is required for the patient to stand on, so allowing the doctor to sit comfortably to examine and mark the legs, and a hand rail must be available to support the patient (this may be fixed to the wall). A couch is required for the patient to lie horizontally during treatment (the head may be elevated for comfort so that the patient can sit comfortably while being bandaged). A trolley provides the required materials for treatment. These include: 2-ml plastic disposable syringes fitted with 16-mm, 25-gauge or 27-gauge needles having a transparent hub and each loaded with 1 ml of 3% sodium tetradecyl sulphate; cotton wool balls; 1-inch (2.5-cm) hypoallergenic tape (Micropore or Dermicel); Tubipad (large), inverted, cut in 1-foot (30-cm) lengths; 3-inch (7.5-cm) limited stretch bandages (elastocrepe or STD export); 4-inch (10-cm) limited stretch bandages (elastocrepe or STD export); Tubigrip, flesh coloured, size D; applicators for Tubigrip; plastic tape for fixing bandages; and scissors. Resuscitation equipment must be immediately available.

Clinic No.	**St. Mary's Hospital** London, W.2.	Vein Clinic Mr John T. Hobbs						Hospital No.	

Surname	Christian name	M S W D	DOB	SEX M F	First seen Age Date		Referred by	Cosmetic Primary Recurrent

Address	Occupation	G.P.
Telephone:	Posture	

Symptoms		R	L	Past treatment	R	L	Family history	
Pain				Support				
				Other				
Prominent veins	Thigh			Injection				
	Calf						Pregnancies	
Dilated venules								
Pigmentation				Surgery				
Eczema				Groin tie			Thrombophlebitis	
Ulceration				LSV strip			Superficial L R	
Oedema				Local ties			DVT { Calf Proximal	
Night cramps				Subfascial				
Restless legs				SSV tie			Pulm. embolus	
Liposclerosis				SSV strip			Allergy Skin	
Bleeding				Skin graft			Other	

General health	Past illness	Photos
		Venogram
		Isotope venogram
Smoking No/Yes		Ultrasound
Weight range		
Skeletal	Haemorrhoids	Venous pressure
Back	Constipation	Impedance plethy.
Hip/Knee	Menopause	Photoplethysmography
Feet	Hormones	
Medication BP	Weight	Height	

2a

Physical examination

Right   Left

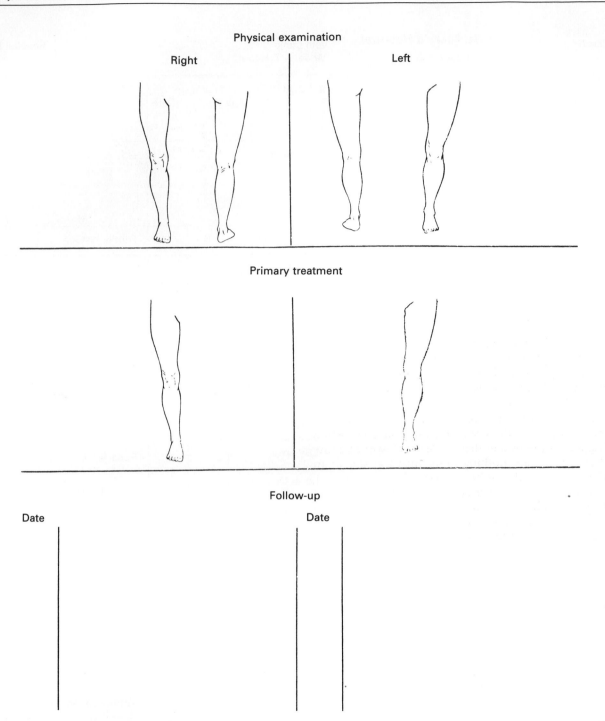

Primary treatment

Follow-up

Date   Date

2b

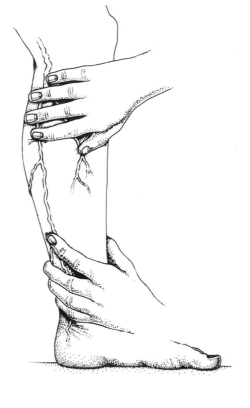

Marking the leg

3a, b With the patient standing, the vein pattern is drawn on the record card and the leg is then carefully assessed by palpation and the sliding finger method to determine points of control. These are intended to include all sites of incompetent perforating veins. Fascial defects are sometimes easily palpable on the medial aspect of the lower leg and pain is felt when the fingertip is pressed in these defects. However, some so-called defects are nothing more than the site of an emptied varix in the subcutaneous tissue. The sites where sections of the vein can be controlled and kept empty are circled with an indelible marker (Pentel N-50, bullet tip). The convention is to use red circles for injection sites and blue outlines for the veins before surgery.

3a

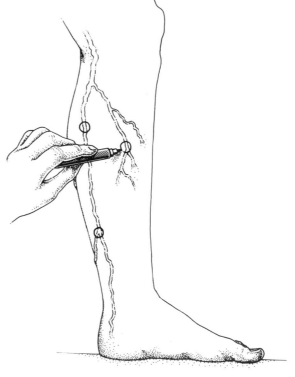

3b

Placement of needle in vein

4 The patient then lies on the couch, either face down or on the back as appropriate. Using a 2-ml syringe containing 1 ml of 3% sodium tetradecyl sulphate, a 25-G needle is placed obliquely into the vein at the marked site, having previously checked easy movement of the plunger and patency of the needle.

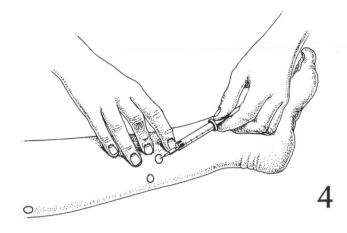

4

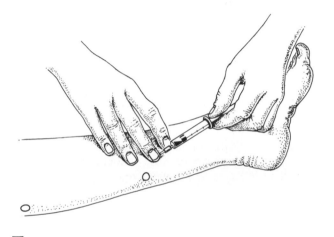

5

Monitoring injection

5 The segment of vein being injected is isolated between the index and ring fingers of the other hand. These fingers are then moved apart to empty the vein being injected. The middle finger is placed over the needle to monitor the injection. Blood is then drawn into the hub of the needle to check its correct placement. If the needle is in an artery, pulsation will be seen on careful observation and the needle must be withdrawn immediately.

Injection of sclerosant

When it is certain that the needle is in the vein lumen, a small volume of sclerosant, 0.25 or 0.5 ml (rarely, 0.75 ml in very large veins) is injected smoothly and rapidly (slow injection allows dilution) into the vein lumen. The feel of the plunger and palpation over the needle are monitored with both hands. Any perivenous leak must be prevented and if there is doubt the injection must be stopped.

Local pressure

6 As the needle is removed a pad of cotton wool is placed over the injection site and held in place with a suitable length of non-allergic adhesive tape. Cotton wool balls are ideal, being conveniently and economically supplied in bags of 250 or 500. When grossly dilated veins are injected, the leg should be elevated onto the operator's arm or shoulder to empty the veins and so ensure an adequate concentration of sclerosant at the injection site.

Sorbo rubber pads are unnecessary and less practical but are useful when bandaging superficial thrombophlebitis. Shaped rubber pads are helpful over ulcers.

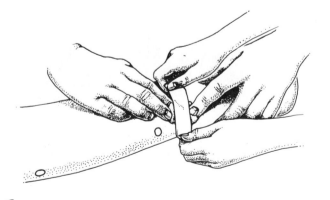

6

Bandaging

Once all the injections are complete (up to ten sites with a maximum of 6 ml of 3% sodium tetradecyl sulphate), the legs are firmly bandaged from the foot to well above the highest injection.

7 A 3-inch (7.5-cm) limited stretch, strong cotton bandage is applied from the head of the metatarsals up to the mid-calf with the leg elevated. The application of the bandage is most important and must be smooth, with steadily reducing pressure on the leg and no constricting turns. This is achieved by using one hand to feel the tension; the active hand is moved to maintain the correct tension at each edge of the bandage. The operator's wrist is abducted or adducted to adjust the tension at the bandage edges.

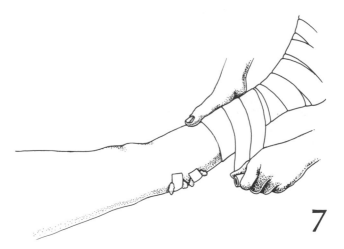

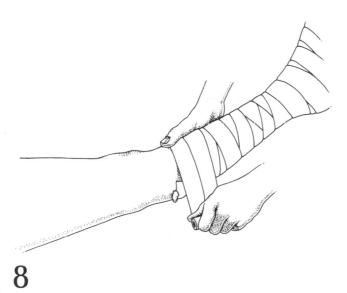

8 After the first bandage has been fixed in place, a 4-inch (10-cm) bandage is then placed over it and continued up to just below the knee, taking the same care with its application. The bandage is cut when sufficient has been applied. The bandages must be firm and remain in place to be effective.

Application of Tubigrip

9a, b Finally, the bandages are covered by a length of flesh-coloured elasticized tubular bandage (Tubigrip size D). The Tubigrip is easily applied by means of an applicator and is finished by folding the ends inside which leaves a smooth and neat appearance, holding the bandage in place.

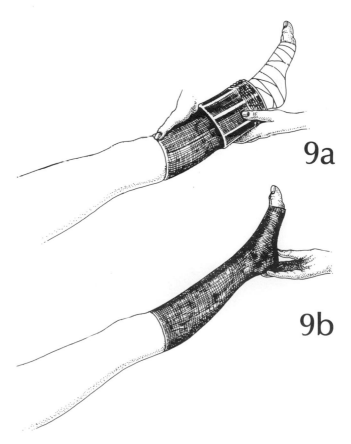

Bandaging above knee

When the veins which have been injected continue across the knee and when injections are made above the knee, then the whole leg must be bandaged to prevent thrombophlebitis developing in the thigh.

10 A length of tubular elastic bandage with a wide foam strip (Tubipad, large size) is first placed over the knee joint to prevent the bandages cutting into the back of the knee. It should be inverted before application so that the foam is not in direct contact with the skin.

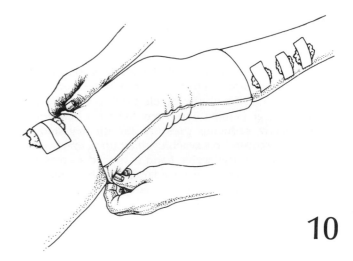

10

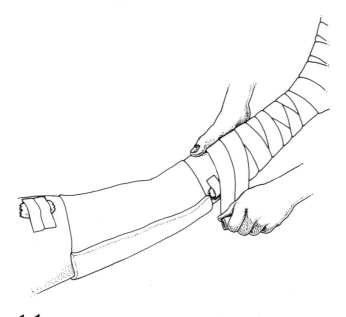

11

11 The 3- and 4-inch bandages are then applied as before, continuing the 4-inch bandage up the thigh to above the highest injection site.

Sometimes, when there are no veins crossing the knee and there are no injections at this level, it is advantageous to apply the 3-inch bandage up to the knee and the 4-inch bandage above the knee, so avoiding bandages over the knee joints.

In obese legs, when it is apparent that the bandages will move, a self-adherent (Cohepress) bandage can be placed over the upper part of the bandage.

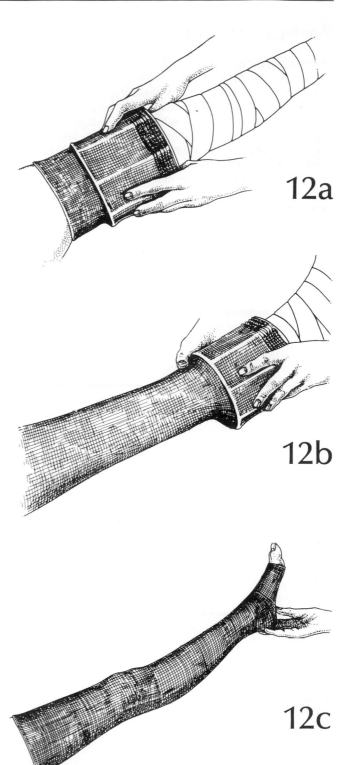

12a

12b

12c

12a–c Flesh-coloured tubular elastic bandage is then applied over the bandages.

Post-treatment management

Immediate care

The patient will have been resting quietly for up to 30 min during treatment and it has been shown that there is no movement of sclerosant from the injected superficial veins until walking is resumed. This allows sufficient time for the sclerosant to have permanently damaged the intima at the injection site. When treatment is complete the patient should walk to the waiting room and rest there for half an hour, taking gentle strolls. This observation period is important to ensure that no allergic or anaphylactic reaction will occur after leaving the clinic. During this time the nurses and secretary should be watching the treated patient to detect the first signs of reaction since prompt treatment is essential.

On sitting or lying, when the bandages feel tight, the patient is instructed to plantarflex and dorsiflex the ankle joint alternately.

The patient is then told to walk whenever there is any discomfort and to include two half-hour walks in each day's routine. If the legs are inactive, swelling will cause the bandages to be uncomfortable.

Bandages below the knee remain in place because of the shape of the leg, but if the upper calf is obese, the bandages should be continued over the knee to avoid a sharp edge. Bandages continued over the knee and on the thigh will roll down unless supported. Suspenders must therefore be worn and fixed to the outer tubular bandage. For patients with overweight legs, a panty girdle is preferable as support.

Some people find the bandages very uncomfortable when worn in bed and this discomfort and subsequent difficulty in sleeping can be relieved by taking promethazine hydrochloride (Phenergan) 25 mg in the evening (available over the counter).

Long-term care

After injection of large veins, the patient returns for review after 3 weeks. The bandages and all dressings are removed and the leg is inspected.

Intravascular haematoma

Occasionally a clot is found in the vein at the injection site. This collection forms because of inadequate compression resulting from bandage movement after a large vein has been injected. If left it will cause local pain, may result in skin staining, and eventually may allow the vein to recanalize by preventing obliteration of the lumen. However, if the clot is promptly evacuated there is no disadvantage, pain is immediately relieved and complications averted. The haematoma is pricked with a 19-G 50-mm disposable hypodermic needle and manually evacuated.

Further bandaging

When large veins are injected in the lower leg, the bandages are reapplied for a further period of 2–3 weeks. Often it is only necessary to rebandage the lower leg. When dealing with the prevention of recurrent leg ulcers in post-thrombotic limbs, it may be necessary to wear the bandages for more than 6 weeks. If the compression is removed too early, the leg is more painful, and bandaging for too long a period is preferable to too short a period.

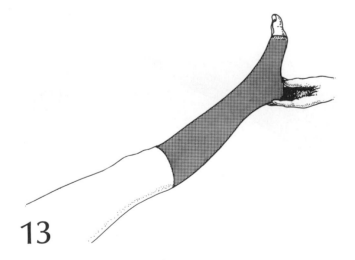

13 After discarding the bandages, class III elastic stockings (thigh or below-knee length as indicated) are then provided and worn during the day for a further 4 weeks. For the first 2 weeks this is all day, every day, and for the second period the stockings may be removed in the evening and for social occasions.

When smaller dilated superficial veins are treated the bandages can be removed at 2 weeks and elastic stockings then worn for 2–4 weeks depending on the degree of resolution of the treated veins.

Providing injection therapy is carefully applied, consistently good results can be obtained and during treatment patients can continue their normal occupation with minimal discomfort.

Complications

Complications rarely occur when the method is correctly performed. However, there are occasional problems, particularly during the initial period of learning while the technique is being perfected. The complications range from trivial skin staining to unexpected sudden death. In general the complications are less serious and less common than those associated with surgical treatment, much of which is unsupervised.

Immediate complications

Vasovagal collapse
This is the most common complication and may be dramatic and without warning. Recovery is rapid on elevation of the legs.

Allergic reaction
Patients with a history of asthma and other allergic phenomena must be treated with extra care. Early signs are urticarial blisters and red blotches spreading from the area surrounding the injection sites. When these signs are recognized injection should be stopped. Chlorpheniramine maleate (Piriton, 10 mg) should be given intravenously and followed by 4 mg orally. The oral dose of 4 mg three times a day can be continued for 24–48 h as necessary.

Anaphylaxis
This is rare, but is dramatic and immediately life-threatening. When treating veins by injection, the operator must always be aware of this so that it is immediately recognized and promptly treated. The early warning signs are the sudden onset of a persistent dry cough and the patient will complain of tightness in the chest and increasing breathing difficulties. Once recognized, treatment should be stopped immediately and 10 mg of antihistamine administered intravenously. If there is a marked reaction with urticaria, wheezing, coughing and anxiety, adrenaline should be given subcutaneously as 0.2–0.5 ml of 1:1000 solution. If the patient collapses without detectable pulse and blood pressure, adrenaline should be given intravenously, 1 ml of 1:10 000. Corticosteroids have no place in the emergency situation but will prevent recurrence several hours later. An intravenous infusion of 0.9% saline should be set up and the patient admitted to hospital. Resuscitation equipment must be immediately available in the treatment room, including airways, ventilation bags and oxygen.

Incorrect placement
If any sclerosant is injected into the subcutaneous tissue, there will be immediate pain and later an area of inflammation will persist and will often resemble an area of lipodermatosclerosis. If near or in the skin, ulceration will occur.

Intra-arterial injection
Accidental injection into an artery is a serious complication which must always be guarded against. The possibility of intra-arterial injection is minimized by using a careful injection technique. If there is the slightest doubt then the injection must be stopped. Most cases of this complication have involved the posterior tibial artery which is close to the skin in an area where significant incompetent perforating veins are found, and injection into this artery will result in some tissue loss in the foot. In thin legs, when attempting injection of the long saphenous vein, the superficial femoral artery has been accidentally injected, resulting in amputation.

Intra-arterial injections cause immediate and persistent severe pain. A sludge forms in the vessels and occludes the microcirculation. There is intense vasospasm. This always results in acute ischaemia, proceeding to gangrene and tissue loss.

Treatment is immediate administration of heparin, vasodilators and analgesics. The limb should be cooled and procaine injected around the artery at the site of injection.

Ocular disturbances
Rarely, patients have described flashing lights, blurred vision or partial visual field loss within 30 min of starting sclerotherapy. This has always recovered spontaneously within hours. In migraine sufferers, an acute episode may be precipitated by the stress of the treatment and should be treated in the usual way.

Early complications

Toxic overdose
This is preventable because excessive volumes of sclerosant should not be administered. There is a wide safety margin because large volumes have been administered without any adverse long-term effects.

Intravenous haematoma
If a large vein is not emptied by leg elevation when the injection is performed, and if the bandages fail to maintain adequate compression, a clot may develop. This should be evacuated and pressure maintained to avoid pain, skin staining and recurrence.

Ascending thrombophlebitis
If the vein is not fully compressed throughout its length, the reaction at an injection site may spread above the bandages. This is most often seen above the bandage in a fat thigh or in the long saphenous vein above the knee when bandaging is only applied below the knee. It responds to adequate compression helped by aspirin or non-steroidal anti-inflammatory drugs.

Thromboembolic phenomena

These are extremely rare when the legs are adequately bandaged and the patient fully mobilized. Occasionally they can happen without obvious reason but usually follows injection into a large vein, such as the proximal part of the long or short saphenous vein.

Problems of bandaging

The most common complication of injection treatment is trouble with the necessary bandaging. This is frequently seen during the learning period of the first year until the method has been mastered. It is also seen when poor quality bandages are used. Most problems relate to bandaging above the knee because of the shape of the leg. Self-adherent bandages (Cohepress) are helpful in this situation, as is the use of a panty girdle. Fat thighs are not suitable for this form of treatment.

Late complications

Injection ulcer

This results from extravenous injection of sclerosant, causing necrosis of subcutaneous tissue and skin. It is slow to heal and only painful during the initial period when there is inflammation. The final result is similar to a vaccination mark without excessive scarring.

Persisting local pain

This is caused by extravenous injection or leakage resulting in inflammatory necrosis of the subcutaneous tissue deep to an intact skin. It is slow to recover and resembles lipodermatosclerosis. It may respond to non-steroidal anti-inflammatory drugs.

Skin staining

If there is longstanding intravenous haematoma or perivenous blood, the skin may be discoloured and this disfigurement can be permanent, because of the deposition of haemosiderin and some melanin. Treatment is not effective and so skin staining must be avoided by careful injection of small volumes of sclerosant followed by adequate compression.

Telangiectatic matting

The appearance of new very fine red vessels is occasionally seen after sclerotherapy, as after surgery. It may be associated with the injection of excessive volumes of sclerosant under pressure in small superficial vessels and the lack of adequate compression. It is seen more often after injection with hypertonic saline. Its appearance cannot always be explained but it is difficult to treat, though it does usually show some resolution with time. Presumably small vertical feeding veins persist.

Thyroidectomy

Robert Udelsman MD, FACS
Associate Professor and Director of Endocrine and Oncologic Surgery, The Johns Hopkins Hospital, Baltimore, Maryland, USA

History

Although enlargement of the thyroid gland (goitre) had been appreciated as early as 2700 BC, it has only been in the past 100 years that thyroid surgery has become safe and efficacious. In the mid 1800s, Theodor Bilroth of Vienna and Theodor Kocher of Berne began to improve the technique of thyroidectomy. They appreciated the importance of recurrent laryngeal nerve protection and contributed to the understanding of iatrogenic hypothyroidism (cachexia strumipriva) and postoperative tetany. Shortly thereafter, William Halsted of Baltimore, Charles Mayo of Rochester, and George Crile of Cleveland refined the operative techniques. It is noteworthy that each of these American surgeons had visited the famous European clinics and were no doubt influenced by their colleagues. In 1909, Kocher received the Nobel Prize for Medicine for his contributions to thyroid physiology, pathology and surgery.

Principles and justification

Routine thyroidectomy is performed for thyroid nodules, well differentiated thyroid cancers, multinodular goitre and Graves' disease and includes unilateral subtotal thyroid lobectomy, unilateral total thyroid lobectomy with or without isthmus resection, and total thyroidectomy. The extent of surgery is dependent upon the operative indications and, to some extent, the experience of the surgeon.

The most common indication for thyroid surgery is the diagnosis or treatment of thyroid nodules. Routine use of fine needle aspiration for thyroid nodules has resulted in a net decrease in thyroid surgery due to the ability to select patients for surgery who have either indeterminate aspirates or aspirates suggestive or diagnostic of malignancy. Additional indications for surgery include a multinodular goitre with obstructive symptoms, a unilateral toxic adenoma, or selected patients with Graves' disease.

The routine operative procedure for indeterminate thyroid nodules is a thyroid lobectomy which may include the isthmus. There is an increasing trend, especially among experienced endocrine surgeons, to perform total thyroidectomies for well differentiated thyroid cancers, as well as in patients with nodular thyroid disease with a history of prior childhood exposure to radiation of the head and neck. A total thyroidectomy can be performed safely, but risks to the recurrent laryngeal nerves, the parathyroid glands and the external branch of the superior laryngeal nerves are ever present. A bilateral subtotal thyroidectomy has historically been performed for Graves' disease. However, in many institutions Graves' disease is treated with radioactive iodine, and subtotal resection is reserved for those patients who either fail to respond to radioactive iodine treatment or refuse its administration. In addition, the concept of leaving the appropriate amount of thyroid gland behind is frequently unsuccessful, and many advocate total or near-total thyroidectomy for Graves' disease since it is easier to place the patient on life-long thyroid hormone replacement than to risk recurrent Graves' disease from the thyroid remnant.

Subtotal resection is a commonly performed operation for a multinodule goitre which often extends inferiorly into the anterior superior mediastinum. These multinodular glands, which can be massive, can almost always be resected through the cervical approach and a median sternotomy is rarely required.

Preoperative

All patients are evaluated with a detailed history and physical examination focused on the head and neck. A history of radiation therapy in childhood or familial history of thyroid cancer, especially medullary carcinoma, is exceedingly important. The physical examination includes a general assessment for the risk of anaesthesia and the potential for airway compromise, as well as examination for signs of the toxic thyroid. The neck is carefully examined for the presence of thyroid nodules and for cervical adenopathy. Either indirect or direct laryngoscopy should be performed routinely in all patients to rule out vocal cord paresis. Imaging studies, including sonography and radioactive scans, are only used in selected cases. Fine needle aspiration is the diagnostic procedure of choice for patients with dominant thyroid nodules. However, an experienced aspirator and an experienced cytopathologist are essential. Assessment of tracheal compression can be obtained by radiography of the chest including the neck. Patients with thyroid function disorders including both hyperthyroidism and hypothyroidism require preoperative treatment before undergoing general anaesthesia.

Anaesthesia

General endotracheal anaesthesia is routinely employed. Deep muscle relaxation aids the surgeon and simplifies the anaesthetic management. Neuromuscular blockade is avoided when neck dissections are to be included with the procedure, since intraoperative assessment of nerve function is critical during a neck dissection. Patients are routinely admitted the morning of surgery.

Operation

1 The position of the patient in the operating room is critical in order to gain adequate exposure and to minimize injury to the patient. After satisfactory general endotracheal anaesthesia has been obtained, an oesophageal stethoscope is inserted which aids the anaesthetist and can also be of benefit for palpating the oesophagus when dealing with retro-oesophgeal goitres. An inflatable thyroid pillow is placed behind the patient's shoulders (an inflatable intravenous fluid cuff is an acceptable and inexpensive substitute). This inflatable device allows the anaesthetist to assist by inflating or deflating the cuff as needed. The operation is performed in the reverse Trendelenburg position with the patient in the flexed position and the head extended on the head ring. Both arms are tucked at the patient's sides after padding, especially of the elbow region to prevent injury to the ulnar nerves. Intravenous access is obtained by a peripheral intravenous line in one or both arms. Urinary bladder catheterization is not routinely employed. The neck and chest from the level of the mandible to the nipples are included in the operative field.

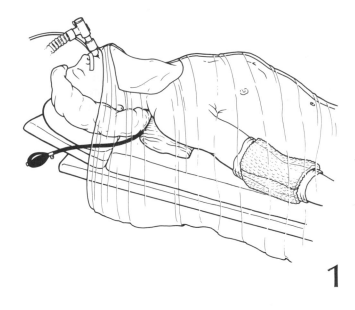

1

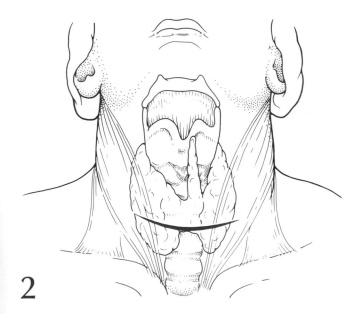

2

2 The incision is made approximately 1–1.5 finger breadths above the sternal notch. Often, a skin crease can be identified which is ideally suited for a cosmetic result. If no skin crease is available, a stretched silk suture is pressed against the skin, which results in a symmetrical and gentle curve. The excision extends just beyond the medial borders of the sternocleidomastoid muscles. For large goitres the incision can be extended.

3 Skin retractors are pulled superiorly, and subplatysmal flaps are raised, preserving the anterior jugular veins. The plane of dissection is directly superficial to these veins.

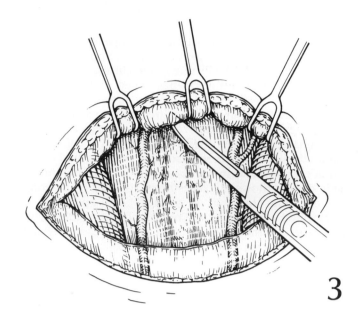

3

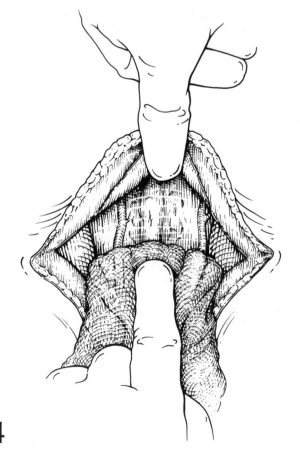

4 Countertraction is applied with the left hand on a gauze pad and, using the right thumb, the superior flap is raised utilizing blunt dissection in the subplatysmal plane.

4

5 The superior extent of the dissection extends to the notch on the thyroid cartilage and bilaterally beyond the medial borders of the sternocleidomastoid muscles. The inferior dissection is performed in a similar manner. This flap, although short, allows access to the anterior mediastinum.

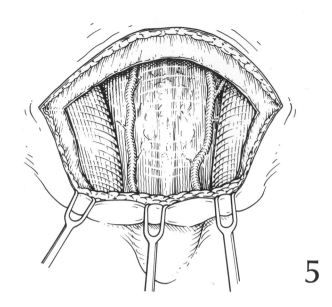

5

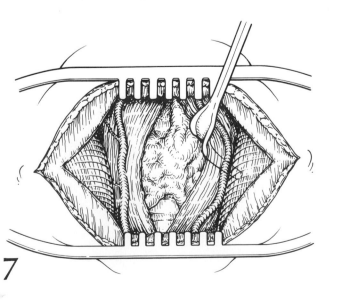

6

6 The median raphe is divided between the strap muscles which are retracted bilaterally. Transection of the strap muscles is rarely required, but can be performed for an unusually large gland. Furthermore, the surgeon should not hesitate to resect strap muscles, particularly the sternothyroid muscle, when there is evidence of direct tumour invasion. A self-retaining retractor (Hamburger–Brennan–Mahorner) is inserted to hold the skin, subcutaneous tissue and platysma muscle. This self-retaining retractor is extremely useful as it allows the assistant to participate actively.

7 Both the sternohyoid and sternothyroid muscles are retracted bilaterally, preserving the anterior jugular veins. The extent of contralateral dissection is dependent upon the operative indication, but in all cases the contralateral thyroid lobe is palpated to rule out nodular disease. In cases of bilateral resection mobilization of the strap muscles is performed bilaterally.

7

8 The self-retaining retractor has a side arm that allows self-retaining lateral traction of the strap muscle which results in exposure of the thyroid gland.

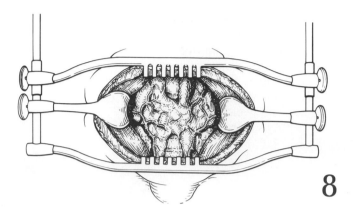

9 A unilateral thyroid lobectomy is shown. The surgeon utilizes a gauze sponge to retract the thyroid gland medially which brings the middle thyroid vein into view. The thyroid lobe is rotated by applying traction on a gauze pad and pulling the gland in a medial direction. A fine-tipped right angled clamp is used to pass 3/0 silk ties around the middle thyroid vein.

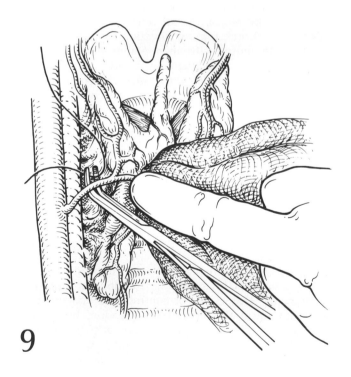

10 After the middle thyroid vein has been ligated, additional medial rotation is achieved exposing the inferior thyroid artery which usually runs anterior to the recurrent laryngeal nerve. The parathyroid glands are supplied by end arteries which usually arise from the inferior thyroid artery.

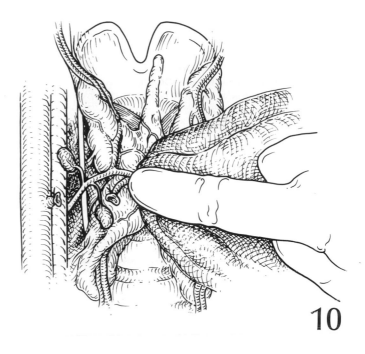

10

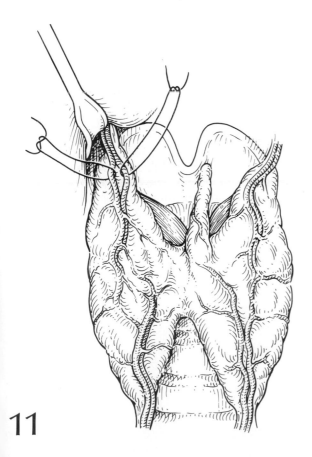

11

11 Once the recurrent laryngeal nerve has been identified in its normal anatomical position, attention is focused on the upper pole. The superior pole vessels branch before entering the thyroid parenchyma and can be ligated directly on the thyroid capsule. Additional exposure of the upper pole can be facilitated by the use of an additional retractor held by the assistant. The external branch of the superior laryngeal nerve often runs close to the superior pole vessel. It can be preserved by ligating the superior pole vessels individually directly on the thyroid capsule. Additional exposure to the upper pole can be obtained by mobilizing the space between the cricopharyngeus muscle and the medial position of the upper pole, which allows medial access to the superior pole vessels. In addition, a superior parathyroid gland is occasionally noted in this location.

12 In the case of a unilateral thyroid lobectomy for a small nodule in the right lobe, a pair of fine-tipped clamps is passed behind the thyroid gland and anterior to the trachea and clamped. The extent of resection can include the isthmus and/or the pyramidal lobe.

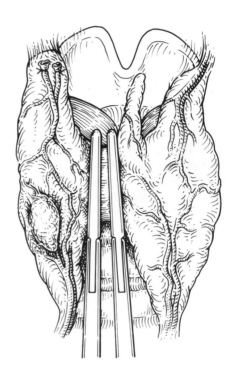

12

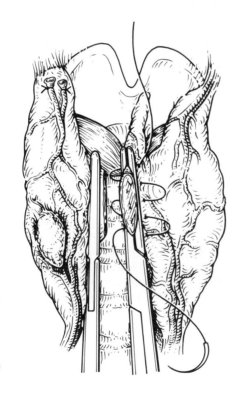

13

13 The tissue between the clamps is then cut and the residual portion left *in situ* is undersewn with a 2/0 cardiovascular silk suture. The suture begins at the superior end of the clamp and is sewn behind the clamp without removing it. The clamp is then removed and the suture continued from inferior to superior, so the final knot is tied in the superior aspect. This manoeuvre allows the tissue to be compressed to ensure haemostasis. For the resected lobe a similar suture technique can be used, although this step can be expedited due to its temporary nature.

14 An Allis-type clamp is used to grasp the medial portion of the resected lobe, and a no. 15 scalpel blade is used to transect the pretracheal fascia sharply. Removing the pretracheal fascia in this fashion allows for a clean resection and minimizes the uptake on a postoperative radioactive thyroid scan. This dissection continues laterally to the mid lateral portion of the trachea. Additional dissection is not advised due to the proximity of the recurrent laryngeal nerve.

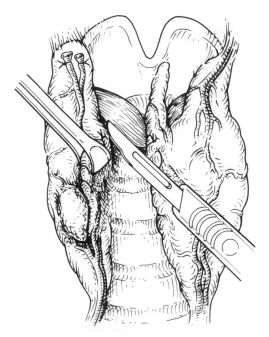

14

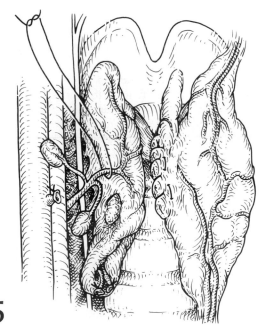

15

15 At this point, the gland is once again rotated medially and the recurrent laryngeal nerve and the anatomy of the inferior thyroid artery are again defined. If necessary, the parathyroid glands are peeled off the thyroid gland and the inferior thyroid artery is ligated on the thyroid capsule, preserving the blood supply to the parathyroid glands. If a total thyroidectomy is performed, an identical resection is completed for the contralateral lobe.

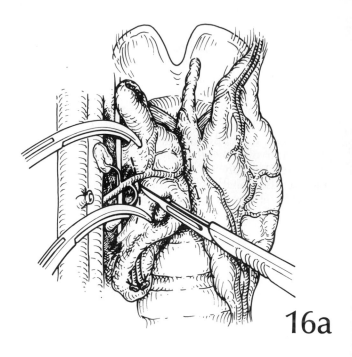

16a

16a,b For a subtotal resection, a series of fine-tipped Crile clamps are placed across the thyroid in an attempt to leave approximately 3–5 g of thyroid tissue. The thyroid gland is then transected sharply and these clamps are undersewn with silk sutures. It is extremely important to remember that the recurrent nerve is still at risk during the placement of these clamps, and especially during the placement of sutures behind the clamps. The lateral view (*Illustration 16b*) shows that the patient's right side has already been sutured to the trachea, and a similar procedure is being performed on the left side. This pexing procedure allows for additional haemostasis as the thyroid capsule is placed directly onto the pretracheal fascia. Again, the importance of preserving the recurrent laryngeal nerve cannot be over emphasized.

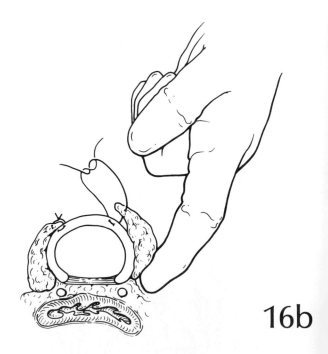

16b

17 Drains of both closed and open types have been employed by many surgeons but are not necessary in most patients as a dry operative field is the expectation and not the exception. However, if a drain is used, it can be placed through a separate stab incision or brought out through the lateral aspect of the wound. Closure of the strap muscles is performed in the midline using a continuous suture of 3/0 polyglactin (Vicryl). It is very important to avoid injury to the anterior jugular veins which are in close proximity.

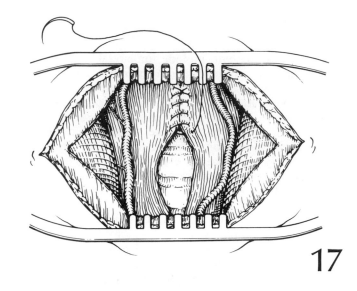

17

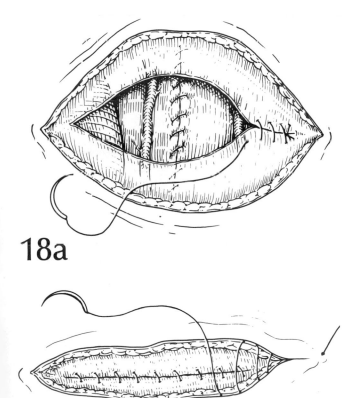

18a

18b

18a,b The platysma is also closed in a running, continuous fashion with a 3/0 polyglactin suture. It is important for cosmetic reasons not to include the subcutaneous tissue in this closure as this will result in tethering and dimpling of the skin.

A subcuticular closure of 5/0 polypropylene (Prolene) on a cutting needle is used. Many other options exist, including the use of a stapler and polyglactin sutures, but the author prefers the use of the polypropylene suture as it is essentially non-reactive and is easily removed 4–7 days after surgery.

Postoperative care

Patients are routinely extubated in the operating room and transported with their heads elevated at approximately 1 h they are transported to a routine floor where the head of the bed is kept elevated at approximately 30°. They are offered clear liquids the evening of surgery and a regular diet the next morning. Patients are routinely discharged on the first postoperative day.

Outcome

Risks to the patient include unilateral or bilateral recurrent and/or superior laryngeal nerve injury, neck haematoma with subsequent airway compression, iatrogenic hypoparathyroidism, and the rare occurrence of thyroid storm. Wound infections are exceedingly rare. Meticulous operative technique is the mainstay for injury prevention. Complication rates of less than 1% are routinely reported by experienced surgeons. The surgeon and the surgical team must be aware, however, that neck haematoma and recurrent nerve injury are potential life-threatening problems in the immediate postoperative day. The serum calcium level is measured in the postoperative period. Asymptomatic hypocalcaemia will almost always normalize without calcium supplementation. Symptomatic postoperative hypoparathyroidism requires treatment with calcium and occasionally vitamin D. In emergency situations, calcium can be administered intravenously.

Further reading

Chen H, Nicol TL, Udelsman R. Follicular neoplasms of the thyroid: does frozen section evaluation alter operative management? *Ann Surg* 1995; 222: 101–6.

Clark OH. Total thyroidectomy: the treatment of choice for patients with differentiated thyroid cancer. *Ann Surg* 1982; 196: 361–70.

Mazzaferri EL, Jhiang SM. Long-term impact of initial surgical and medical therapy on papillary and follicular cancer. *Am J Med* 1994; 97: 418–28.

Patwardhan NA, Moront M, Rao S, Rossi S, Braverman LE. Surgery still has a role in Grave's hyperthyroidism. *Surgery* 1993; 114: 1108–13.

Thompson NW, Olsen WR, Hoffman GL. The continuing development of the technique of thyroidectomy. *Surgery* 1973; 73: 913–27.

Udelsman R. Thyroid carcinoma. In: Cameron JL, ed. *Current Surgical Therapy*. 4th edn. St Louis: Mosby, 1992: 568–72.

Welbourn RB. *The History of Endocrine Surgery*. New York: Praeger Publishers, 1990.

Parathyroidectomy

A. G. A. Cowie MA, FRCS, FICS
Consultant Surgeon, University College Hospital and St Peter's Hospital at The Middlesex Hospital, London, UK

History

The first good record of a deliberate parathyroidectomy described an operation in Vienna in 1925 by Mandl. It was not until 1948, however, when Fuller Albright in America recognized that osteitis fibrosa cystica (Von Recklinghausen's disease of bone) was due to hyperparathyroidism, that proper criteria for diagnosis and principles of treatment were established. Only minor changes in principle have been made since then, though there have been many refinements in diagnostic biochemistry and in preoperative localization techniques. While parathyroid exploration is usually straightforward and does not take long, unfortunately the operation can unexpectedly be extremely difficult, and so it should only be undertaken by a surgeon who is familiar with possible anatomical variations and pathological pitfalls, and who is accustomed to evaluating the tactical considerations raised by the different forms of hyperparathyroidism.

Principles and justification

As mild forms of hyperparathyroidism exist and patients with either adenomatous or hyperplastic disease have been followed up for many years without coming to harm, it is clearly not enough simply to make the diagnosis and to act on it. During long-term follow-up, however, about 20% of previous asymptomatic patients develop symptoms or complications requiring surgery in the course of the first 5 years. The symptoms and complications of the disease can be disabling or painful, and indeed may be life-threatening. For patients in need of treatment, there is no satisfactory long-term solution other than surgery. The ideal situation for the surgeon is to be presented with a patient in whom the diagnosis is secure and all that is required is the finding and removal of the abnormal parathyroid tissue.

At the time of presentation, patients may be suffering the major complication of bone disease, the effects of stones in the urinary or biliary tracts, or peptic disorders (e.g. ulceration) or pancreatitis. Other complaints, such as psychiatric disturbances, hypertension or myopathy, are common. Many patients complain only of malaise, lethargy, depression, thirst or constipation, and a large proportion are asymptomatic, having been picked up during routine biochemical screening. Because the early symptoms are vague and easily misinterpreted, and because many conditions interfere with calcium metabolism, it is essential that the parathyroid team should have special endocrine and metabolic expertise. In many ways the surgery is the easier part of the treatment.

The diagnosis of primary (or tertiary) hyperparathyroidism depends upon the finding of persistent sustained hypercalcaemia, after making due allowance for variable levels of calcium binding and ionization. If there is diagnostic uncertainty after the myriad alternative causes for hypercalcaemia have been considered, confirmation may be sought by estimating the level of parathyroid hormone in peripheral blood. Parathyroid hormone estimation can be misleading, however, depending on which assay is employed and to which part of the 83 amino acid chain the specific antibody is raised; in addition, the level of parathyroid hormone is not necessarily persistently high. Tests such as hydrocortisone suppression or discriminant analysis are still useful, and in doubtful cases provocation tests may be employed, in which calcium levels are deliberately raised or lowered temporarily and the effect on parathyroid hormone levels determined.

Secondary hyperparathyroidism should be suspected in patients with calcium-losing disorders, such as enteropathy or chronic renal failure, and in such cases parathyroid hormone estimation is again very helpful.

Parathyroid carcinoma should be considered in patients with aggressive disease and rapid onset of exaggerated symptoms, particularly if there is a palpable nodule in the neck (normally even large parathyroids are impalpable because they are so soft).

Indications

All patients with proven hyperparathyroidism should be considered for surgery, even if symptoms are mild and a decision to operate is deferred. Patients selected for observation will need regular long-term supervision. All parathyroid surgeons will recognize that patients often declare after operation that they feel so much better and that they only now appreciate how chronically unwell the disease made them feel.

Symptomatic patients and those who have already suffered complications should be offered surgery without delay, and patients with the familial form of the disease or who suffer a multiple endocrine neoplastic disorder merit special consideration. The principal indications for operation in secondary hyperparathyroidism are the development of painful osteodystrophy or deterioration in renal function thought to be calcium-related.

Patients who have stones and obstruction should have the obstruction relieved, but the stones may be better removed after the parathyroid abnormality has been corrected, because new stones may form while awaiting the parathyroid operation. This principle applies to both the renal and the biliary tracts.

Contraindications

Parathyroid disease in pregnancy has special risks to mother and baby and should be managed with advice from a specialist centre.

Preoperative

In experienced hands, parathyroid exploration has a low mortality and morbidity, and patients may safely be managed at both extremes of life. Preparation is the same as for other routine operations, with a few additions. Vocal cord function should be checked and recorded, as unilateral paresis can be virtually asymptomatic. If paresis is discovered, surgery will still continue exactly as before, but the record may well be found to be of medicolegal importance.

Prophylactic use of heparin is not contraindicated and seldom causes problems of additional blood loss. Some patients present with dangerously high calcium levels, and almost all of these will benefit from treatment to lower the level. Rehydration and the establishment of a diuresis is often enough. Other measures include the use of steroids (prednisolone, 10–20 mg three times daily for 4–5 days), phosphate infusion (100 mmol in 6 h), calcitonin (100–200 units subcutaneously twice daily for 4–5 days), diphosphonates (etidronate disodium, 7.5 mg/kg daily by slow intravenous infusion for 3 days), or mithramycin (25 µg/kg single dose). Very occasionally, in a patient with long-standing and severe bone disease in whom profound postoperative hypocalcaemia may be anticipated, it may be wise to create a pseudohyperparathyroid state by pretreatment with vitamin D.

Many attempts have been made to localize parathyroid glands before operation. Ultrasonography is the most simple and useful technique, and it can detect a gland of 5 mm or more in size; small glands may be missed, and the retrosternal space cannot be reached by this scanning method. Radionuclide scanning using subtraction techniques to locate both thyroid and parathyroid parenchyma with ^{75}Se-methionine and the thyroid alone with ^{125}I can be helpful with the bigger glands. Venous samples for parathyroid assay, particu- larly from small veins near the thyroid, obtained by catheterization using a Seldinger technique and access from the groin under radiographic control, are particularly useful in patients after a failed first operation. Computed tomography has been disappointing, but magnetic resonance imaging shows promise. In difficult cases selective arteriography has been effective, but only in the most skilful hands. Despite these multiple modalities, however, no localization technique can surpass careful exploration by an experienced and skilled surgeon.

At operation some surgeons like to use vital staining with methylene blue, 5–7.5 mg/kg intravenously 1 h before operation, to differentiate tissues. The author prefers to rely on his appreciation of shades of red, brown and yellow, which do not change in the course of an operation, however long the procedure may last. Shades of blue due to methylene blue infusion tend to intensify with time and to spread from the selected tissue to all other tissues, leading to the greatest confusion in the most difficult cases, particularly if the operation is prolonged.

Anaesthesia

A well-secured endotracheal tube and special protection for the cornea with a suitable eyepad and possibly a conjunctival ointment are important. It is helpful if monitoring wires and tubes are routed away from the operative field. Some surgeons like hypotensive anaesthesia with the blood pressure maintained at about 70–80 mmHg, but this is not essential. Meticulous attention to haemostasis throughout the procedure is perhaps the most important aspect of the whole operation.

Operation

Position of patient

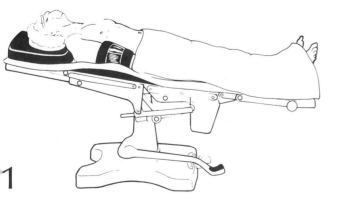

1   The patient is placed supine, with a 30° head up inclination of the upper body, the shoulders resting on a small sandbag and the head steadied on a head ring. The neck is gently extended for best access, but care must be taken with elderly patients with cervical vertebral pathology, as it is easy to overstrain the neck.

1

Incision

2 Draping is as for thyroidectomy. If the head towel is firmly fixed, it can be used to anchor a traction suture at a later stage, making it possible to avoid using cumbersome retractors.

The incision is planned to lie 1 cm above the heads of the clavicles and to be 4–5 cm in length. It lies in or parallel to the skin creases of the neck, following Langer's lines and just crossing the medial edge of the sternomastoid muscle. In patients with a long neck, a rather higher incision will be necessary to reach the upper margins of the dissection. Infiltration of the line of the planned incision with adrenaline solutions may make the earliest part of the operation a little less haemorrhagic, but it is unnecessary and may well distort tissue planes, making the dissection unnecessarily untidy. The author prefers an incision just through the skin with the scalpel, deepened through other layers (including the platysma) with a diathermy needle.

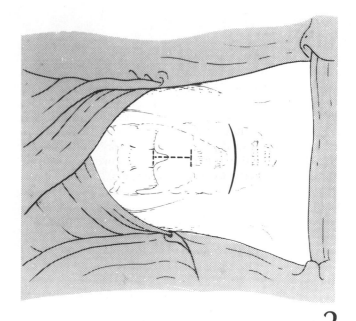

2

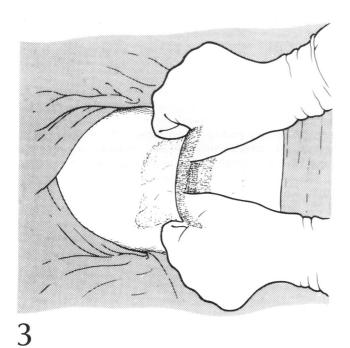

3

3 The plane between the platysma and the anterior jugular veins is opened and developed by gauze dissection using thumb pressure. Exposure is taken up above the thyroid cartilage, laterally to the surface of the sternomastoid muscle and down to the manubrium sterni.

4 The skin edges are retracted by traction sutures anchored to the head towel. Sutures work well for this and avoid the encumbrance of fixed metal retractors.

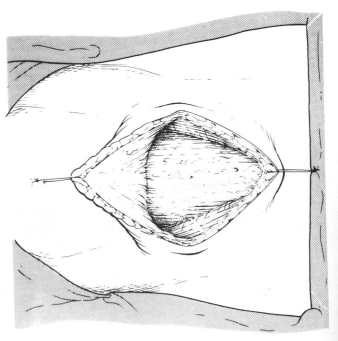

4

Mobilization of muscles

5 On each side, the medial edge of the sternomastoid muscle is lifted and dissection taken beneath it to expose the carotid sheath, the jugular vein and the hyoid part of the omohyoid muscle. This dissection allows free retraction and so much improves the exposure later.

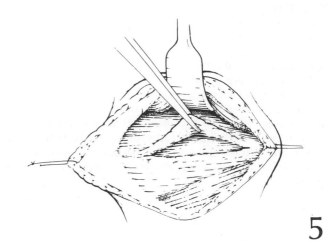

6 The medial edge of the sternohyoid muscle is lifted and separated from the sternothyroid muscle beneath. The upper end of the sternothyroid muscle is clearly defined, and it is lifted off the thyroid gland, opening a plane that is crossed by many small blood vessels which bleed easily and tend to obscure the view unless special care is taken with haemostasis.

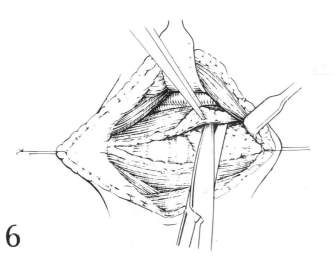

7 The sternothyroid muscle may be cut from its attachment to the thyroid cartilage and reflected downwards. Division of the sternothyroid muscle in this way improves the exposure for difficult cases, but it is not always necessary.

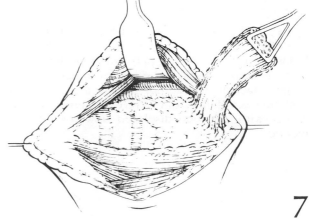

8 A stay suture is placed in the lobe of the thyroid and used to lift it out of its bed, drawing it to the opposite side. Filmy adhesions between thyroid and muscle are divided close to the muscle itself, leaving as much tissue as possible attached and related to the thyroid lobe. A lower parathyroid may lie within this tissue and can be missed if this precaution is not taken. The middle thyroid vein or veins are tied and divided if present.

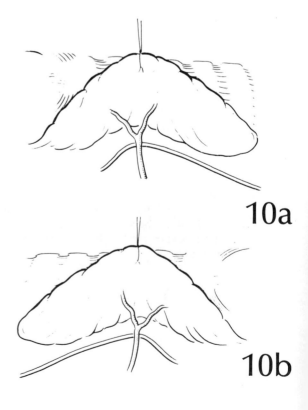

8

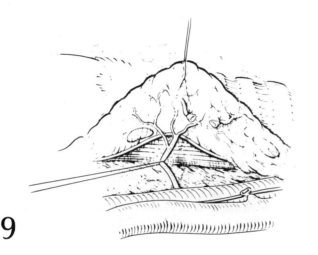

9

9 When the lobe of the thyroid is lifted out of its bed and is pulled to the opposite side, the inferior thyroid artery can be identified as it passes deep to the carotid artery. The recurrent laryngeal nerve may be identified and any anatomical variation can be recognized.

10a, b Recording the operative findings, and particularly the site and number of each biopsy, is very important, particularly in difficult cases or reoperations, and may be crucial in decisions about surgical tactics. The author prefers a pictorial representation as if the thyroid were viewed from the lateral aspect with the lobe displaced upwards out of the wound.

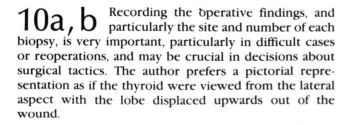

10a

10b

11,12 The surgeon must be prepared for anatomical variations of the inferior thyroid artery and the recurrent laryngeal nerve.

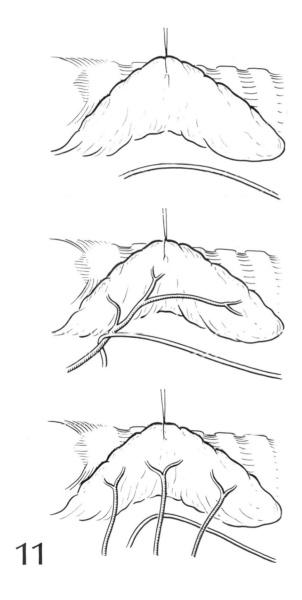

11

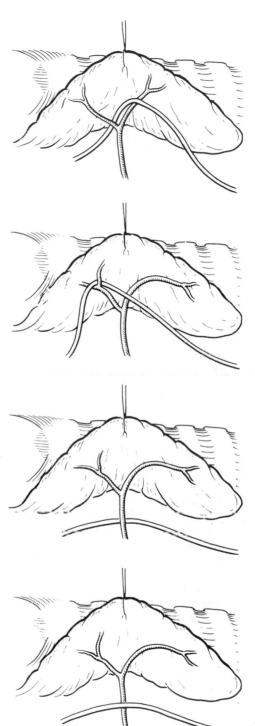

12

13, 14 Meticulous haemostasis and careful exposure has prepared the field for a search for the parathyroid glands. A surgeon must be aware of the expected site to find each gland. The operative locations in 1000 cases in the author's series are summarized by the shaded areas in *Illustrations 13* and *14* for the right superior parathyroid and right inferior parathyroid respectively.

The thyroid and parathyroid glands are covered by a thin fascia which obscures the anatomical outlines. This fascia is gently peeled away with quick attention to any bleeding that occurs to avoid suffusing the tissues with blood. Parathyroid glands are identified by their colour, shape and mobility, and their soft texture. When bruised, they 'blush' from intracapsular haemorrhage and when cut (as for biopsy) they bleed profusely. Most parathyroid surgeons quickly learn the characteristic 'brown' colour of the gland and the soft texture is striking – if it can be felt, it is probably a lymph node. Positive identification is by frozen section histopathology of very small biopsies.

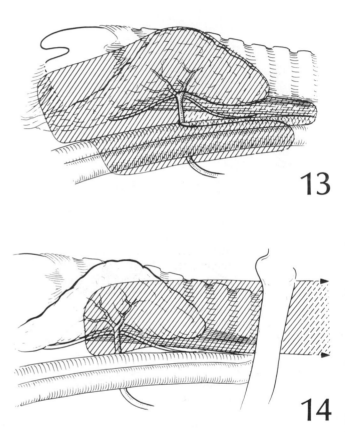

13

14

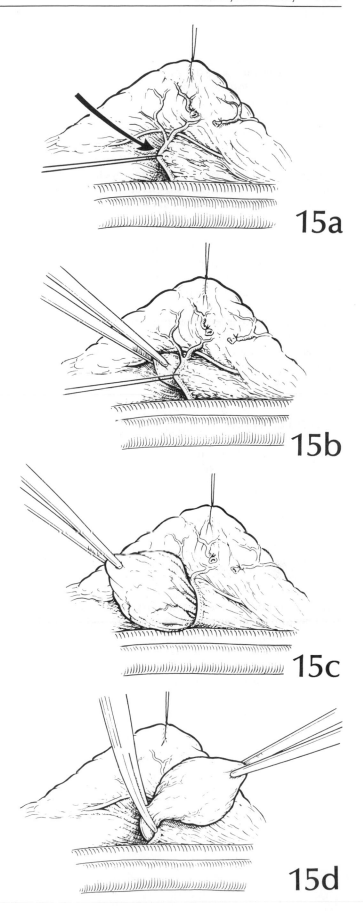

15a–d

If not easily visible, inferior glands are most likely to be found in the cervical tongue of the thymus which is accessible from the neck. Superior glands often migrate deep to the inferior artery to lie alongside the pharynx. Ideally, all four glands are identified and confirmed by frozen section. The adenoma is then removed.

A single adenoma and three normal glands are found in 83% of patients with simple parathyroid disease. Removing the adenoma is curative. Multiple adenomas are found in 6% of patients with adenomatous disease. Three adenomas may safely be removed; one normal parathyroid gland is more than enough for normal calcium haemostasis. In patients with hyperplastic glands at a first operation, three and a half glands will normally be removed. The most normal looking half gland should be chosen and marked with a non-absorbable suture with long tails, removing all the rest. In the long term, it may be necessary to go back and remove the remaining half gland. At one time, there was a vogue for transplantation of parathyroid tissue in these cases to a more accessible site such as the forearm. Unfortunately, such transplants tend to migrate and are often impossible to locate at a future operation. Along with most other parathyroid surgeons, the author has given up the practice of transplantation.

16 In carcinoma of the parathyroid, if the diagnosis is a histological surprise and a whole tumour has been excised intact, nothing more should be done at the first operation, and the patient should be followed up. If the tumour was adherent to muscle or thyroid, the tumour should be excised *en bloc* with the muscle and/or the relevant hemithyroid. If the tumour is multiple, total clearance of the neck should be undertaken, including all the parathyroid glands, the whole of the thymus and any accessible anterior lymph nodes.

If a tumour is not found and the neck exploration has been thorough, the operation should be concluded and the diagnosis and localization reappraised. Even when four normal parathyroids are found, it should be remembered that there may be five, six or seven glands. Only when the diagnosis has been reconfirmed and the patient judged suitable for a thoracic operation should mediastinal exploration be considered. A mediastinal adenoma requiring a sternal split to remove it occurs in about 3% of patients with hyperparathyroidism.

Wound closure

The wound is closed in layers, usually with a small vacuum drain. The skin is closed with clips or with subcuticular sutures. Povidone-iodine irrigation of the wound has reduced the small but significant risk of wound sepsis.

Postoperative care

Patients should be mobilized early, and in most cases the drip and drain are removed after one night. The clips in the skin may be removed in 2–3 days.

Temporary hypocalcaemia is common, and observations for Chvostek's and Trousseau's signs are useful. Calcium measurements on blood samples taken from an

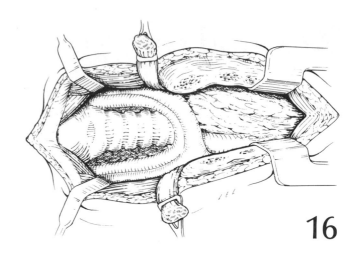

16

uncuffed vein are made regularly – in simple cases on days 1, 3 and 5 and in complex cases daily. If tetany threatens, 10 ml of 10% calcium gluconate is given intravenously after a blood sample has been taken. Usually, however, it is sufficient to give oral calcium as milk or effervescent calcium tablets. Occasionally, it may be necessary to give some form of vitamin D as a parathyroid substitute. It is necessary to watch for problems due to oedema or haemorrhage, as in thyroid surgery.

In most cases parathyroid exploration is a quick, satisfying and safe procedure, and the patient will often be able to go home within a week.

Further reading

Cowie AGA. Morbidity in adult parathyroid surgery. *J R Soc Med* 1982; 75: 942–5.

Dent CE, Watson L. The hydrocortisone test in primary and tertiary hyperparathyroidism. *Lancet* 1968; ii: 662–4.

Tomlinson S, O'Riordan JLH. The parathyroids. *Br J Hosp Med* 1978; 19: 40–53.

Illustrations by Paul Richardson

Adrenal surgery

J. S. P. Lumley MS, FRCS
Professor in Vascular Surgery, St Bartholomew's Hospital, London, UK

P. Hornick FRCS
Department of Cardiothoracic Surgery, Harefield Hospital, Middlesex, UK

Principles and justification

Indications

The indications for adrenalectomy are as follows:

1. Hyperplasia (primary nodular adrenocortical hyperplasia; adrenal medullary hyperplasia; pituitary-dependent bilateral adrenocortical hyperplasia; ectopic ACTH production).
2. Neoplasia (adrenocortical adenoma; adrenocortical carcinoma; phaeochromocytoma; ganglioneuroma; neuroblastoma).
3. Removal of adrenal glands as part of the management of an endocrine-dependent disease process.

Preoperative

In the preparation of the patient with complex endocrine manifestations of adrenal disease, a co-ordinated team approach is vital. The optimal timing of surgery is decided between surgeon, endocrinologist and anaesthetist. Specific preparations include rendering the patient normotensive (or there should be a significant reduction in blood pressure and postural hypotension), normalizing blood biochemistry and correction of metabolic alkalosis, and the correction of severe tachycardia and arrhythmias.

The use of steroids at the induction of anaesthesia is usually reserved for bilateral adrenalectomy. Steroid replacement therapy is occasionally needed in cases of unilateral adrenalectomy for primary adrenal tumours to compensate for suppression of the opposite adrenal gland by low ACTH levels. For such cases, hydrocortisone hemisuccinate infusion (400 mg/24 h) is started with the premedication. Alternatively, hydrocortisone hemisuccinate (100 mg) is given intravenously with the premedication and 6-hourly thereafter for the first day after surgery.

All patients should receive a three-dose regimen of a third-generation cephalosporin antibiotic as prophylaxis. Similarly, all patients should wear thromboembolic-deterrent stockings and receive subcutaneous heparin, 5000 units twice daily, until mobile.

Operation

Anterior (transperitoneal) approach

This is a transabdominal approach. Inspection of both adrenal glands is facilitated by this approach and it is thus suitable for patients with bilateral adrenal disease, large tumours and, if concomitant oophorectomy is planned, with advanced breast cancer.

The patient is placed in the supine position and the abdomen is opened by a transverse, or rooftop, abdominal incision (*see* pp. 886–887). The surgeon stands on the side of the table opposite the adrenal gland to be removed.

Access to the right adrenal gland

1 The second part of the duodenum is mobilized to the left and the right kidney and the hepatic flexure of the transverse colon are mobilized downwards. This exposes the right kidney and the inferior vena cava.

The liver is retracted superiorly, and the duodenum inferiorly and to the left. The adrenal vein may now be observed entering the vena cava superior to the right kidney.

The kidney is stabilized with the surgeon's non-dominant hand, and the posterior parietal peritoneum is incised above its upper pole, directly over the adrenal gland.

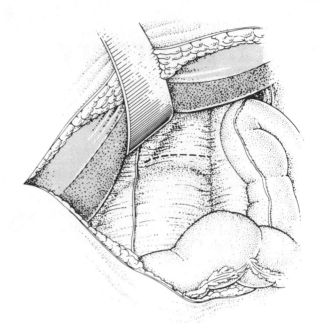

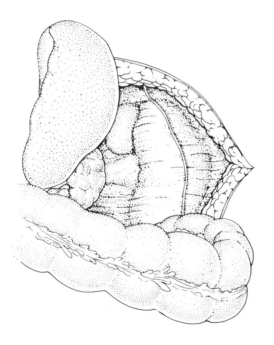

Access to the left adrenal gland

2 The spleen and pancreas are mobilized by division of the left or posterior leaf of the lienorenal ligament. The spleen and tail of the pancreas are now mobilized and displaced downwards to reach the upper pole of the kidney and the adrenal gland situated on its anteromedial aspect.

Posterior approaches

The adrenals may be approached through any of the standard incisions described in the chapter on pp. 873–889 for the exposure of a kidney. The lumbotomy incision is suitable only for tumours less than 5 cm in diameter. A thoracoabdominal incision may be required for very large tumours.

ADRENALECTOMY

Whatever the approach selected, the subsequent dissection follows the same technique.

Identification

Each adrenal gland lies on the respective diaphragmatic crus. It has a yellow-ochre colour and a firm consistency on palpation. It is separated from the kidney by perinephric fat and fascia. The right adrenal caps the upper pole of the kidney and the left adrenal is related to the upper medial border of the kidney

Right adrenalectomy

3 A short adrenal vein runs to the right side of the inferior vena cava. The vein is exposed by blunt dissection of the fat between the inferior vena cava and the adrenal gland, using cotton pledgets; the dissection is facilitated by stabilizing the kidney using the non-dominant hand.

The vein is ligated and divided. If this vein is avulsed from the inferior vena cava, brisk haemorrhage will ensue. The wound should be packed for at least 5 min, after which the pack is removed and a sucker is used to identify the tear. This should be controlled with a vascular clamp and the defect repaired with 5/0 Prolene (Ethicon, Edinburgh, UK).

The arteries supplying the adrenal are small and variable and may be coagulated by diathermy or controlled with metal clips.

The fascial connections between the gland and the kidney are divided last to prevent the gland from retracting upwards to a more inaccessible level.

Left adrenalectomy

4 The left adrenal vein is longer than the right and enters the left renal vein. The vein is ligated and divided at its point of entry to the left renal vein. The arterial supply is dealt with by diathermy or clip. The fascial connections are divided and the gland removed.

Having ensured that haemostasis is complete, suction drains are placed to each adrenal bed and brought out to the exterior through separate stab incisions. If the pleura has been entered and the defect not repaired, a chest drain should be inserted.

The wound is closed in layers.

Postoperative care

All patients receive intravenous fluids until gastrointestinal function is sufficient to maintain fluid balance. Antibiotic cover may be discontinued following the second and third doses at 8 and 16 h after surgery.

A check chest radiograph is taken of all patients who have undergone rib bed exploration. A significant pneumothorax will require the insertion of a chest drain.

Chest physiotherapy is important, especially after rib resection. Prophylaxis against deep venous thrombosis should be continued until the patient is fully mobile.

Steroid requirements

Steriod replacement is indicated for all cases of bilateral adrenalectomy and in cases of unilateral adrenalectomy where the remaining gland is hypoplastic as a result of low ACTH levels. In the latter, the supplements can

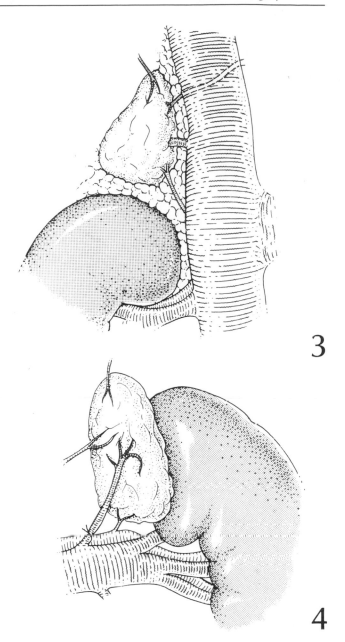

3

4

usually be withdrawn gradually over a period of 2–3 months.

Hydrocortisone hemisuccinate (100 mg) is given intravenously until swallowing is reinstituted, and is then substituted by oral hydrocortisone (20 mg four times daily) and reduced to a maintenance dose of 10 mg three times daily. Then the dose of hydrocortisone is reduced to below 50 mg in 24 h, 0.1 mg fludrocortisone is introduced. The dose of steroids is increased if postoperative complications develop, or if there are manifestations of adrenocortical insufficiency, vomiting, hypotension or skin desquamation.

Upon discharge from hospital, the patient must be advised on the importance of taking medication, and issued with a steroid user's card with the instruction to carry it at all times.

Index